Medical-surgical nursing for Australian students

A systems approach

FIRST EDITION

Anne-Marie Brady

Catherine McCabe

Margaret McCann

Jacqueline Brewer

Zachary Byfield

Ellen Dyke

Sara Geale

Renjith T Hari

Sarah Mills

Penelope Sweeting

Josephine Tighe

WILEY

First edition published 2022 by
John Wiley & Sons Australia, Ltd
42 McDougall Street, Milton Qld 4064

Typeset in 10/12pt Times LT Std

A catalogue record for this book is available from the National Library of Australia.

Wiley acknowledges the Traditional Custodians of the land on which we operate, live and gather as employees, and recognise their continuing connection to land, water and community. We pay respect to Elders past, present and emerging.

Creators/contributors
Anne-Marie Brady (author), Catherine McCabe (author), Margaret McCann (author), Jacqueline Brewer (author), Zachary Byfield (author), Ellen Dyke (author), Sara Geale (author), Renjith T Hari (author), Sarah Mills (author), Penelope Sweeting (author), Josephine Tighe (author)

Wiley
Chris Gray (Vice-President, APAC Education), Mark Levings (Publishing Manager, Tertiary and Professional), David Hobson (Product Manager), Kylie Challenor (Senior Manager, Education Content Management), Jess Carr (Senior Production Editor), Tara Seeto (Publishing Coordinator), Liam Gallagher (Production Assistant), Renee Bryon (Copyright & Image Research), Delia Sala (Cover Design)

Cover image: © rubberball / Getty Images

Typeset in India by diacriTech

Printed in Singapore
M115693_070921

BRIEF CONTENTS

CONTENTS

CHAPTER 15

Nursing care of conditions related to the digestive system 353

CHAPTER 16

Nursing care of conditions related to the urinary system 381

CHAPTER 17

Nursing care of conditions related to the endocrine system 423

CHAPTER 23

Nursing care of conditions related to reproductive health 609

CHAPTER 24

Principles of emergency and high dependency nursing 643

CHAPTER 25

Antipodean considerations 663

PREFACE

This book is designed to provide a broad overview and a practical understanding of the principles related to adult and paediatric medical-surgical nursing. It examines the principles underpinning medical and surgical nursing and includes contemporary developments in clinical care and places a focus on the national health priority areas. Using a systems approach, the book is designed to provide a comprehensive application of the relevant anatomy and physiology, which will inform medical and surgical nursing practice.

The book comprises 25 chapters and is presented in two sections designed to guide readers to reach an understanding of the context and the key aspects of medical and surgical nursing practice.

The text is not an unwieldy encyclopedia of medical-surgical nursing. Instead, it is a practical tool for students to learn the 'need to know' skills in order to become a safe provider of care.

- Part 1: The Australian healthcare system and common principles underlying medical and surgical nursing practice.
- Part 2: Nursing care of conditions by system.

In Part 1, the text introduces the reader to the structure, funding and access to the Australian healthcare system. Chapter 2 discusses healthcare in relation to Indigenous health and challenges in rural and remote settings. Chapters 3 to 9 address common principles that underpin medical and surgical nursing practice and the principles underlying comprehensive nursing assessment of patient care needs. The management of medications is a major component of the everyday work of the nurse in a medical-surgical environment, and a comprehensive overview of the principles underlying care and the nurses' responsibilities in relation to drug administration, both oral and parenteral are discussed. Nutritional assessment, the prevention and control of infection, caring for the older person, provision of appropriate and individualised care to families at the final stage of life, the principles of perioperative, high dependency care and a detailed review of paediatric-specific care are included.

In Part 2, a systems approach is taken to afford an overview of adult nursing in medical and surgical acute care environments. The nursing care related to all the systems is discussed in chapters 12–23 and covers topics related to the integumentary, respiratory, circulatory, digestive, urinary, endocrine, neurological, immune, haematological, musculoskeletal, eye/ear/nose/throat and reproductive systems. Each chapter presents an overview of the related anatomy and physiology to enhance students' understanding. All of the main conditions are considered, with a focus on relating the main concerns and priorities of medical and surgical nursing. Each chapter is associated with *additional sources of information* such as further reading, professional organisations and online resources.

Chapter 24 discusses special nursing care and gives the reader an overview of emergency department nursing and an understanding of the diverse nature of presenting medical/surgical emergencies, trauma and shock. Chapter 25 discusses antipodean considerations, such as snake and spider bites and jellyfish stings and their treatment.

In addition, *case studies* that follow the clinical reasoning cycle are employed throughout the chapters to enable the reader to consolidate their learning based around realistic patient scenarios. Case studies on the normal as well as the deteriorating patient prompt students to think, take cues and make decisions that encourage them to think like a nurse. *Multiple-choice questions* are also provided to enable self-evaluation.

ABOUT THE EDITORS

Anne-Marie Brady

Anne-Marie Brady is Chair of Nursing & Chronic Illness in the School of Nursing & Midwifery at Trinity College Dublin and has been involved in undergraduate and postgraduate education since 2000. She has completed a PhD, PG Diploma in Clinical Health Sciences Education and in Statistics at Trinity College Dublin, and a MSc and BSN at Northeastern University Boston, Massachusetts, USA. Her particular areas of research and teaching interest are general nursing and healthcare management. She has considerable international nursing experience, having worked in the UK, USA and the Irish Republic.

Catherine McCabe

Catherine McCabe is Associate Professor and Dean of Students Illness in the School of Nursing & Midwifery at Trinity College Dublin. Her particular area of interest in teaching is general nursing and advanced nursing practice. Her research primarily explores the effect of technology and multimedia systems on enhancing communications systems and quality of life for patients with chronic and life-threatening illnesses both in acute care settings and in the home. She has written a great deal on communication in nursing and published a number of papers on her research on communication and technology in healthcare.

Margaret McCann

Margaret McCann has been an Assistant Professor in the School of Nursing and Midwifery, Trinity College Dublin since 2005 and was previously employed as a lecturer in the Faculty of Nursing and Midwifery, Royal College of Surgeons in Ireland. She obtained an MSc in Nursing from the University of Manchester and Royal College of Nursing in 2001. She has been involved in nurse education since 1996. Margaret's primary teaching and research interests lie in the area of urology and renal care. Her research focuses on the prevention and control of vascular access infection in haemodialysis, and she has published a number of papers on issues relating to renal care and vascular access.

ABOUT THE ADAPTING AUTHORS

Jacqueline Brewer

Jacqueline Brewer is an adjunct academic at The University of Newcastle. She has been involved in undergraduate and postgraduate education of nurses and medical education since 2004. She has completed a Diploma of Herbal Medicine, Graduate Certificate in ICU and has a Masters of Medical Education. Her main area of interest is critical care, and she has been a clinical nurse specialist in operating theatres, has worked in ICU, CCU, NICU and ED and currently coordinates two postgraduate programs in acute care and emergency nursing.

Zachary Byfield

Zach Byfield is a Lecturer in Nursing. Clinically, Zach worked predominantly in acute clinical areas, specifically paediatric and emergency nursing. Zach has held a number of roles with nursing professional bodies and has been predominantly employed in education-focused roles for the majority of his professional practice. Zach holds a number of qualifications, including Bachelor of Philosophy, Bachelor of Nursing, Graduate Diploma in Paediatric Nursing, Master of Nursing, Master of Philosophy and is a Fellow of the Higher Education Academy.

Ellen Dyke

Ellen Dyke is a Lecturer at the University of Queensland and has been teaching in pre-registration nursing courses since 2014. Ellen has more than 20 years of clinical nursing experience covering medical, surgical and rehabilitation nursing, with a major part of her career spent in spinal cord injuries nursing. She has completed a Bachelor of Nursing, Bachelor of Nursing Informatics and a Master of Philosophy. She is passionate about nursing education and research and is currently undertaking a PhD with a focus on e-learning for registered nurses.

Sara Geale

Dr Sara Kathleen Geale is a Senior Lecturer at the Australian Catholic University. Sara has completed a PhD in Healthcare, Emergency and Disaster Management, a Masters in Healthcare, Postgraduate Applied Science Nursing and BA in Library and Information Science. Sara has considerable experience in nursing, working in Australia and Saudi Arabia. Sara continues to research and publish in nursing education and review for nursing and healthcare journals globally.

Renjith T Hari

Renjith Hari started academic nursing as a lecturer at Charles Darwin University and currently works at the University of New England. He has been involved in undergraduate and post graduate education since 2013. He has completed a Master of Clinical Education, Master of Nursing and Graduate Diploma in Nursing with critical care specialisation from Flinders University. His areas of research and teaching interest are digital health, clinical education, simulation, online education and clinical supervision. He has considerable clinical nursing experience in critical care, having worked in India, the United Arab Emirates and Australia.

Sarah Mills

Sarah Mills is an Associate Lecturer in Nursing at Charles Darwin University Australia and has been involved in undergraduate education since 2015. She holds a Masters of Advanced practice in critical care nursing, a Bachelor of Nursing (honours) and a Graduate Certificate of tertiary and adult education. She is a PhD candidate with Charles Darwin University Australia. Her particular areas of research and teaching interest are medical-surgical and critical care nursing and missed nursing care. She has international nursing experience, having trained and worked in the UK.

Penelope Sweeting

Penelope Sweeting is a Lecturer in nursing at Charles Darwin University and is heavily involved in undergraduate nursing education. Penelope also has extensive clinical experience in emergency nursing and is a PhD candidate studying human factors and suicide prevention. Her qualifications include a Bachelor of Nursing from the University of Technology Sydney, Graduate Certificate in Acute Care Nursing from the University of New England, and a Master of Advanced Nursing from the University of Technology Sydney.

Josephine Tighe

Josephine Tighe works as a Lecturer in the Bachelor of Nursing program at Swinburne University of Technology in Melbourne. After a gratifying career as a critical care nurse in a number of states and territories across Australia, Josephine has worked in undergraduate and postgraduate nursing education since 2015. She has completed a Master of Clinical Education (Research), Graduate Diploma of Clinical Education, Critical Care Certificate (ICU), and a Bachelor of Science (Nursing). Josephine's research interests are in innovative learning and assessment and preparation for clinical practice.

CHAPTER 1

The Australian healthcare system and nursing in Australia

LEARNING OBJECTIVES

After studying this chapter, you should be able to:

1.1 discuss the Australian healthcare system and how it seeks to provide universal care

1.2 identify the authorities that regulate healthcare in Australia and how they support safety and health in the community

1.3 review the systems in place to support equality and health literacy in Australian healthcare

1.4 distinguish between the roles of healthcare practitioners in Australia

1.5 reflect on the role of nursing and midwifery within the Australian healthcare system.

Introduction

The World Health Organization (WHO) states that health is 'the state of complete physical, mental and social wellbeing and not merely the absence of disease or infirmity' (WHO 2020). The WHO goes on to say that health is a fundamental right 'of every human being without distinction of race, religion, political belief, economic or social condition' (WHO 2020).

This chapter will discuss the Australian healthcare system, including both the public and private systems and the primary health network. We also look at the Australian government departments' responsibilities, the challenges facing the healthcare system, as well as healthcare providers in Australia and the standards of practice and codes of conduct that support them.

1.1 The Australian healthcare system

LEARNING OBJECTIVE 1.1 Discuss the Australian healthcare system and how it seeks to provide universal care.

The Australian healthcare system is arguably one of the best in the world, providing affordable healthcare for all Australians. The Australian healthcare system provides access to key health and family services through:

- family and children's services
- aged and community care services
- disability programs
- public health initiatives
- pharmaceutical benefits
- hospital and healthcare funding
- health services for Indigenous Australians
- emergency services for people in crisis.

Primary healthcare

Primary healthcare is usually the first contact the Australian population has with the healthcare system. Primary healthcare is provided by a general practitioner (GP) and allied healthcare professionals, including physiotherapists, occupational therapists, registered Chinese medicine practitioners, community health workers, midwives, nurse practitioners, pharmacists, dentists and Indigenous health practitioners. To learn more about allied health services in Australia, search the Allied Health Services Australia website.

The primary healthcare system allows people to receive treatment for the management of acute and chronic health conditions (Healthdirect n.d.). Primary Health Networks (PHNs) support primary healthcare providers and hospitals to coordinate the health services a person may need as part of this treatment. More information about PHNs can be accessed from PHN's website (Healthdirect n.d.).

Australian Primary Healthcare Nurses Association (APNA) is an example of a primary health network. More information on APNA can be accessed from their website: www.apna.asn.au/about.

Secondary healthcare

Specialist healthcare — also called secondary health services — requires a referral from a primary health service physician such as a GP. During a health assessment, a GP may conclude that the patient requires a more specialist review for a specific health condition. For example, they may refer a patient to a psychiatrist to treat a mental health condition, a diabetic patient to an endocrinologist or a pregnant woman to an obstetrician for ongoing management of her pregnancy. Other referrals include those to an imaging service for X-rays or scans (Australian Institute of Health and Welfare [AIHW] 2018).

The Australian Charter of Healthcare Rights

The Australian Commission on Safety and Quality in Health Care (ACSQHC), together with consumers (patients and their families/carers), health professionals, clinicians and policymakers, have worked together to create a charter of the care the Australian public has a right to expect when seeking treatment (see figure 1.1). The Charter applies wherever healthcare is provided, in both public and private facilities (ACSQHC 2019a).

FIGURE 1.1 The Australian Charter of Healthcare Rights

My healthcare rights

This is the second edition of the **Australian Charter of Healthcare Rights.**

These rights apply to all people in all places where health care is provided in Australia.

The Charter describes what you, or someone you care for, can expect when receiving health care.

I have a right to:

Access

- Healthcare services and treatment that meets my needs

Safety

- Receive safe and high quality health care that meets national standards
- Be cared for in an environment that makes me feel safe

Respect

- Be treated as an individual, and with dignity and respect
- Have my culture, identity, beliefs and choices recognised and respected

Partnership

- Ask questions and be involved in open and honest communication
- Make decisions with my healthcare provider, to the extent that I choose and am able to
- Include the people that I want in planning and decision-making

Information

- Clear information about my condition, the possible benefits and risks of different tests and treatments, so I can give my informed consent
- Receive information about services, waiting times and costs
- Be given assistance, when I need it, to help me to understand and use health information
- Request access to my health information
- Be told if something has gone wrong during my health care, how it happened, how it may affect me and what is being done to make care safe

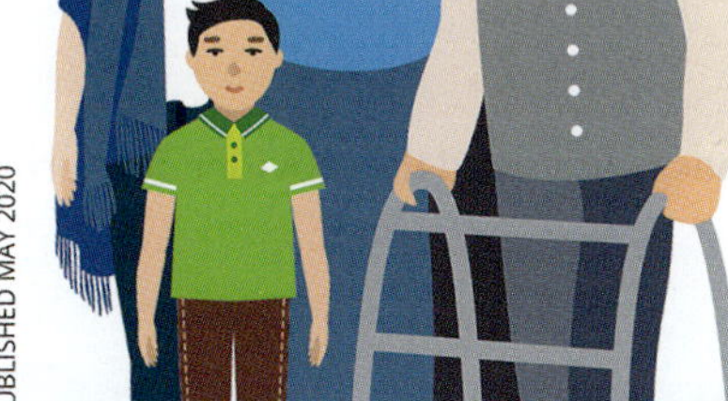

Privacy

- Have my personal privacy respected
- Have information about me and my health kept secure and confidential

Give feedback

- Provide feedback or make a complaint without it affecting the way that I am treated
- Have my concerns addressed in a transparent and timely way
- Share my experience and participate to improve the quality of care and health services

PUBLISHED MAY 2020

AUSTRALIAN COMMISSION ON SAFETY AND QUALITY IN HEALTH CARE

For more information, ask a member of staff or visit **safetyandquality.gov.au/your-rights**

Source: ACSQHC (2020).

1.2 Authorities responsible for healthcare in Australia

LEARNING OBJECTIVE 1.2 Identify the authorities that regulate healthcare in Australia and how they support safety and health in the community.

The Australian healthcare system uses the network of federal, state and territory, and local Australian government departments, all of which have distinct roles, to support fair and equitable healthcare. Figure 1.2 shows the distinct and shared responsibilities of each government department.

FIGURE 1.2 Main roles of the government in Australia's health system

Australian Government
- Sets national policies
- Is responsible for Medicare (including subsidising medical services and joint funding, with states and territories, of public hospital services)
- Funds Pharmaceutical through the Pharmaceutical Benefit Scheme
- Funds community-controlled Aboriginal and Torres Strait Islander primary healthcare
- Supports access to private health insurance
- Regulates private health insurance
- Organises health services for veterans
- Is a major funder of health and medical research, including through the National Health and Medical Research Council
- Regulates medicines, devices and blood

State and territory Governments
- Manage public hospitals
- License private hospitals
- Are responsible for public community-based and primary health services (including mental health, dental health, alcohol and drug services)
- Deliver preventive services such as cancer screening and immunisation programs
- Are responsible for ambulance services
- Are responsible for handling health complaints

Local Governments
- Provide environmental health-related services (for example, waste disposal, water fluoridation, water supply, food safety monitoring)
- Deliver some community- and home-based health and support services
- Deliver some public health and health promotion activities

Shared
- Regulation of health workforce
- Education and training of health professionals
- Regulation of Pharmaceuticals and pharmacies
- Support improvements in safety and quality of healthcare
- Funding of public health programs and services
- Funding of Aboriginal and Torres Strait Islander health services

Source: AIHW (2016).

Figure 1.3 provides a picture of the primary services, funding responsibilities and the provider delivering the services.

My Health Record

My Health Record is a secure, national digital health record system that provides healthcare providers with a summary of a patient's health information (Healthdirect n.d.b). Every Australian has a choice to use the My Health Record system — or they can 'opt-out'. Using My Health Record, healthcare providers can access up-to-date information, including health summaries, discharge summaries, prescription and dispense records, and pathology and diagnostic imaging reports.

FIGURE 1.3 Health services funding and responsibility 2013–14

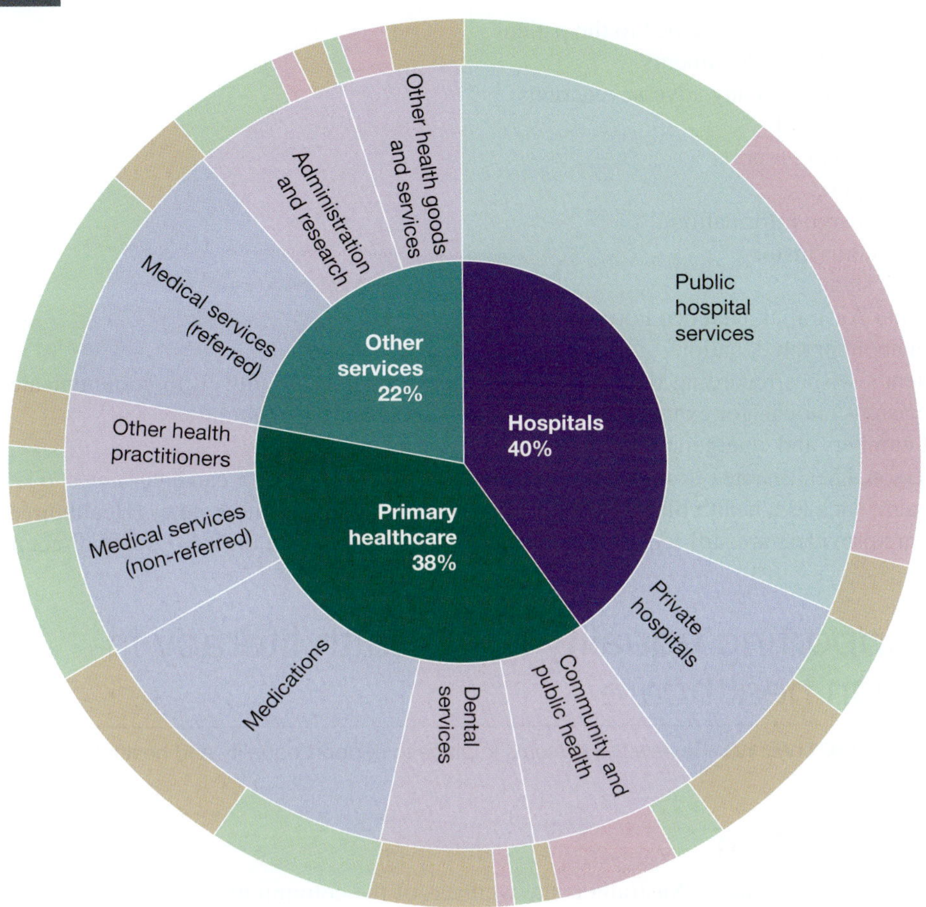

Share of recurrent expenditure

- Hospitals
- Primary healthcare
- Other services

Responsibility for services

- Combined public and private sector
- State and territory governments
- Private providers

Source of funding

- Australian Government
- State and territory governments
- Private

Note: The inner segments indicate the relative size of expenditure in each of the three main sectorsof the health system ('Hospitals', 'Primary healthcare' and 'Other services'). The middle ring indicates both the relative expenditure on each service in the sector (shown by the size of each segment) and who is responsible for delivering the service (shown by the colour code). The outer ring indicates both the relative size of the funding (shown by the size of each segment) and the funding source for the different services (shown by the colour code).

Source: AIHW (2016).

Primary healthcare providers have access to a patient's My Health Record by default. This supports a holistic approach to healthcare as providers involved in patient care can see what other treatments and/or medications the patient has received. This ensures that in a medical emergency, information about allergies, previous adverse reactions, drug interactions and medical conditions are available to the healthcare **provider**. The patient has control over who sees the information and can change access controls if and when they wish to — there are strict regulations about who can see or use My Health Records to protect an individual's digital health information records (Healthdirect n.d.b).

My Health Records can include:

- a written record by a doctor
- details of medications prescribed to the patient
- specialist and referral documents
- details of allergies and any adverse reactions
- immunisation record
- diagnostic imaging reports
- pathology reports
- hospital discharge information
- Medicare claims history
- Indigenous status
- veteran and Australian Defence Force status
- decision about organ donation
- the patient's wishes regarding their healthcare if they become too unwell to communicate and make their decisions known (for example, a living will or advance care planning)
- contact numbers and emergency contact details
- other personal health notes — the patient or a nominated representative can enter notes to keep track of their health, such as a health diary. Healthcare providers cannot see these notes (Healthdirect n.d.b). Healthcare providers are still required to keep their own patient care records (Healthdirect n.d.b).

1.3 Supporting equality and health literacy in Australian healthcare

LEARNING OBJECTIVE 1.3 Review the systems in place to support equality and health literacy in Australian healthcare.

Health promotion

A major focus of healthcare in Australia is the wellness of the community. The role of health promotion is to provide education to the public on health issues, prevent avoidable health conditions and improve Australians' overall health. Health promotion or **health literacy** provides the public with access to health information, allowing them to make informed healthcare decisions. Two examples of successful wellness campaigns are reducing deaths due to unsafe driving, with road fatalities falling from 30 to 5.4 per 100 000 people between 1970 and 2016. The second noteworthy campaign was alerting the public to the dangers of tobacco smoking. The National Drug Strategy Household Survey (NDSHS) estimated that 11.6 per cent of adults smoked daily in 2019. This rate has halved since 1991 and since declined an estimated 12.8 per cent in 2016 (AIHW 2020).

The Australian education system takes an active role in the promotion of healthy behaviours. School policies can be used to regulate the food available for purchase at canteens, and programs can be implemented to encourage students to take part in physical activity.

Immunisation and population-based cancer screening programs are major areas of health promotion in Australia. Routine immunisation begins at birth and incorporates vaccines against 17 diseases, including measles, mumps and whooping cough. The national program has achieved an immunisation rate of more than 90 per cent for all children at the ages of one, two and five. Participation in Australia's three national cancer screening programs ranges from 41 per cent of the target population for bowel cancer screening, 55 per cent for breast cancer screening and 55 per cent for cervical cancer screening.

Medicare: Australia's universal healthcare

Australia's public health system is based on the principle of universal access for Australian citizens and permanent residents. Universal access is a goal set by the WHO and means that people can obtain required health services without the risk of financial hardship from out-of-pocket payments. Universal coverage includes health promotion, preventative care, treatment, rehabilitation and palliation (WHO 2020).

Medicare is the publicly-funded Australian universal healthcare insurance scheme operated by Services Australia. It gives all Australians a wide range of health and hospital services at no or low cost (Healthdirect 2020).

If you live in Australia, have enrolled and are eligible for Medicare, you are entitled to receive:

- free healthcare in public hospitals
- bulk-billed (free) or subsidised treatment in facilities such as GP clinics, allied health services and specialist service rooms
  - The cost of the service is a standard amount agreed by the government to be paid to the provider. The service is bulk billed if there is no 'gap' between these amounts. A gap is a difference between the fee the provider charges for the service or investigation and the standard amount. The gap payment is the responsibility of the individual and is either covered by out-of-pocket expenses, by private health cover or a mix of both (Krassnitzer & Willis 2016).
- diagnostic investigations such as X-rays, ultrasounds, CT and MRI scans — there may be a gap fee for these services/investigations
- some surgeries and procedures
- free eye tests
- subsidised medications on the PBS.

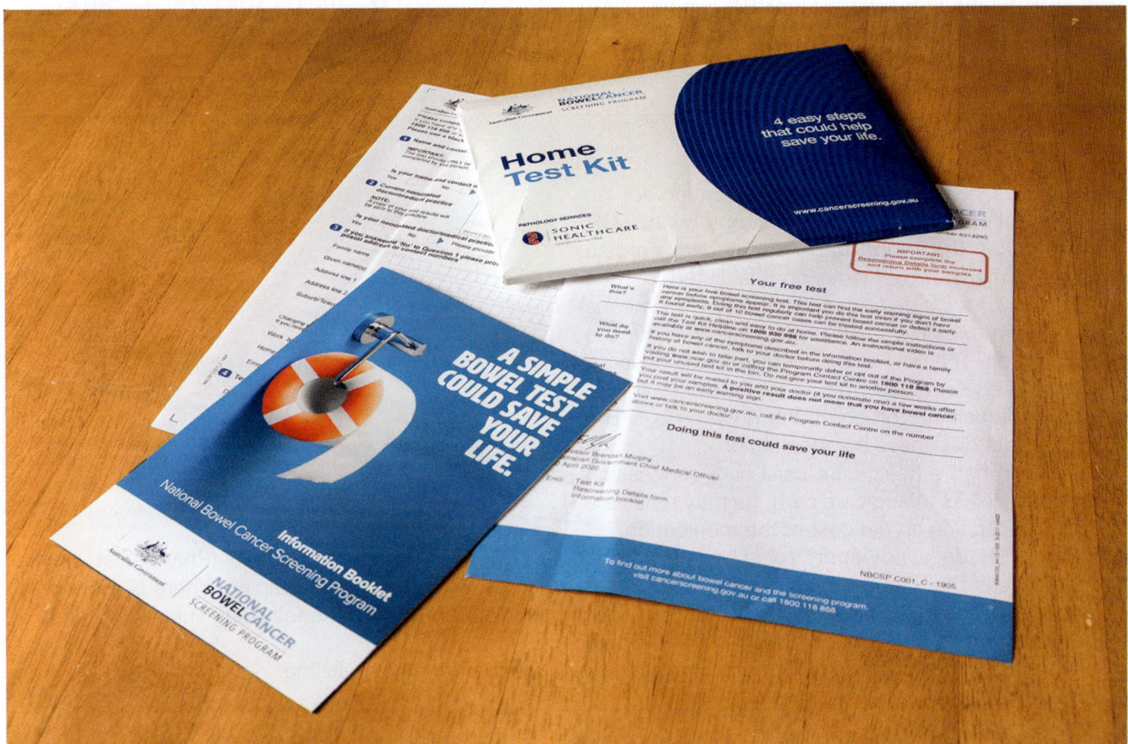

The Medicare Benefits Schedule is a list that identifies the medical services that are subsided by the Government (Krassnitzer & Willis 2016).

Emergency and non-emergency ambulance transport are not covered by Medicare. People pay for ambulance cover directly with the ambulance service within their state and or with their private health insurance (PrivateHealth.gov.au n.d.). See table 1.1 for a summary of what is covered by individual states for patient transport in an ambulance.

TABLE 1.1 **State ambulance services**

States	Ambulance service
Queensland and Tasmania	Emergency ambulance services are provided to residents for free by the State Government.
NSW and ACT	Provide free emergency ambulance services for Pensioners and Concession Card Holders.
Northern Territory	NT Centrelink Pensioner Concession Card or Health Care Card holders are exempt from ambulance fees.

(continued)

TABLE 1.1 *(continued)*

States	Ambulance service
Victoria	Victorian Pension Concession/Healthcare Card holders are covered for clinically necessary ambulance transport but Commonwealth Seniors Health Card holders are not covered.

Individuals that do not fall into any of the above categories above can arrange ambulance cover from the ambulance authority in their state or territory, or from a health insurer.

Source: Adapted from PrivateHealth.gov.au (n.d.).

Pharmaceutical benefits scheme (PBS)

The PBS was created as part of the Australian National Medicines Policy. Some of the policy's major goals were to ensure all Australians have access to affordable medications, and that they meet specific standards of quality, health and safety. The PBS is part of *Australia's National Health Act* 1953 (Clarke 2016).

BOX 1.1

How Australia's PBS works

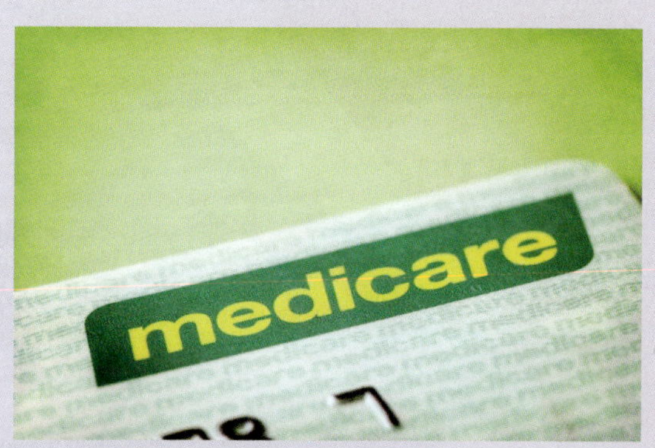

Kevin has been prescribed a medication for an illness and has been given a script by his GP. Kevin takes the script and his Medicare card to the pharmacy. The medication is listed on the PBS list of subsided medications, which means that Kevin does not have to pay full price for the medication. The cost of the medication is covered by the predetermined portion that Kevin will pay, and the subsided portion by the government. The pharmacist dispenses the medication.

If Kevin had a healthcare card or a concession card, as well as a Medicare card, he may receive a further reduction on the cost of the medication.

The PBS does not apply to schedule 2 (Pharmacy Medicine) and schedule 3 (Pharmacist only) medications that can be bought 'over the counter', such as paracetamol and aspirin. There is more on medication scheduling in the chapter on medication administration and at the following link: www.findapharmacy.com.au/advice/scheduling-of-medicines.

The PBS list can be accessed here: www.pbs.gov.au/browse/medicine-listing.

The Medicare safety net

To help ensure all Australians access affordable healthcare, low-income earners who have large out-of-pocket expenses are eligible for the Medicare Safety Net. This means they are entitled to higher Medicare benefits — they will get more money back for certain medical services (Services Australia n.d.).

Funding Medicare

Australians help pay for Medicare through two income taxes: the Medicare levy and the Medicare levy surcharge. The Medicare levy is a federal tax that that is based on a person's taxable income and currently starts at two per cent, providing some of the funding to support Medicare (Krassnitzer & Willis 2016). For individuals who do not have the appropriate level of private health insurance, the Medicare levy surcharge is also deducted from earnings in addition to the Medicare levy. The Medicare levy surcharge is used to further support Medicare by encouraging high-income wage earners to provide their own (private) health insurance.

Private health insurance and Medicare

The Australian government incentivises Australians to take out private health insurance through the Medicare levy surcharge (myDr.com 2019). People who earn over a predetermined level and do not have private hospital cover will be required to pay an additional surcharge of between 1 and 1.5 per cent of their taxable income in addition to the two per cent Medicare levy.

Private health insurance covers those services not covered by Medicare (depending on the level of cover chosen), for example:

- private hospital care
- dentistry
- physiotherapy
- chiropractic services
- optometry
- remedial massage
- natural therapies, i.e. aromatherapy, homeopathy, kinesiology, herbal medicine, yoga, pilates and naturopathy.

Those who opt for private health insurance are entitled to a government-funded rebate of 30 per cent on their insurance premiums. It increases to 35 per cent for those older than 65 and 40 per cent for those older than 70. Private health insurance covers over 50 per cent of the Australian population, with some level of health insurance (Flynn 2016).

In addition to Medicare, private health insurance is available for:

- private and sometimes public hospital charges (patients who elect to be private patients to be treated by the doctor of their choice)
- a portion of medical fees for inpatient services
- allied health/paramedical services (physiotherapist and podiatry services)
- some aids and appliances such as hearing aids, prosthetic or artificial limbs, TENS machines, orthotics, blood pressure and blood glucose monitors, etc.

Private hospital

People with private health insurance are encouraged to seek services through the private system, thereby reducing the demand on the public hospital system. Private healthcare means that patients and their families or carers can choose whom they would like to provide their specialists' service and the private hospital they would like to receive the treatment in. Other choices include where they go for dental treatments and allied health services (Krassnitzer & Willis 2016).

If you have private health insurance and are treated in a private hospital, waiting times for elective or non-emergency surgeries are usually shorter than in the public hospital system (Healthdirect n.d.c). Individuals have the opportunity to choose their own physician and may be entitled to a private room. Private hospitals also provide inpatient and outpatient services, depending on the specialty (Healthdirect n.d.c).

Private patient in a public hospital

Private patients can choose to be treated in a public hospital (Healthdirect n.d.c). That means they will be treated by their choice of doctor and be given a single room if available. Should they need follow-up care, they may be transferred to a private hospital.

Public hospital

Public hospitals in Australia are free of charge to Australian citizens and permanent residents and provide high-quality medical care (Healthdirect n.d.c). Public hospitals tend to be more widely accessible, offer more services and are usually better equipped to handle more complex cases than private hospitals. Public hospitals are usually the first choice for emergent or emergency healthcare issues. However, the waiting periods for elective surgery are usually longer in public hospitals. Public hospitals provide treatment for inpatients (a person admitted to hospital) and outpatients (non-admitted patients). An example of an outpatient is a who person attends the emergency department for treatment but is not admitted to a ward in the hospital, they go home instead. After some inpatients have been discharged, they may attend a specialist outpatient clinic for ongoing treatment, health checks and/or management of new health issues (Krassnitzer & Willis 2016).

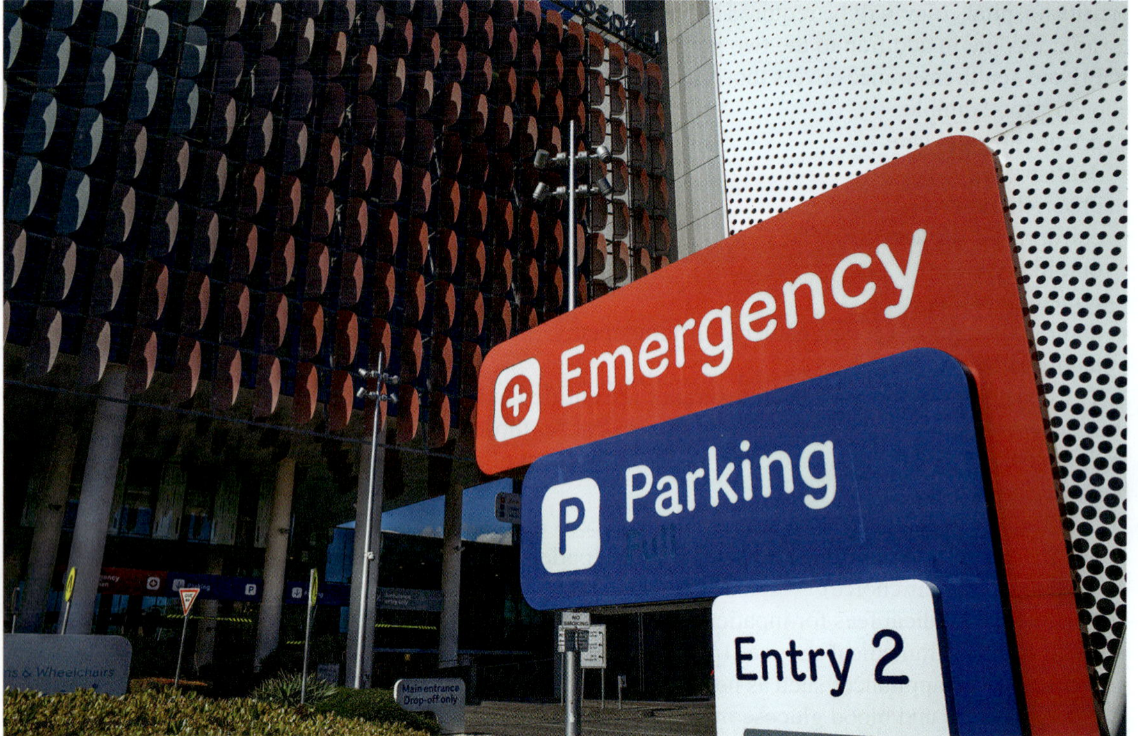

National Disability Insurance Scheme

One in five Australians lives with a disability that has, in some way, impacted their mental health, sensory function or mobility (Disability 2020). People who live with disability are more likely to have poorer health, develop mental health conditions, experience physical challenges associated with ageing at a younger age and are less likely to access the support they need than those living with disability (Ellison & Lante 2016).

Australians living with a disability have the same rights as other Australians and are entitled to the necessary support to help them reach their physical, emotional, social and intellectual potential. In 2014, Medicare was expanded to financially support the National Disability Insurance Scheme (NDIS), to provide individualised support and funding to assist those with disabilities (Ellison & Lante 2016). The NDIS is Australia's first national scheme for people with disability.

Veterans

The Department of Veterans Affairs (DVA) assist eligible Australian veterans and their families in accessing a range of healthcare and support services. Veterans can receive reduced costs for healthcare, medications, rehabilitation, transportation and some utilities. They also provide free mental healthcare for all veterans and resources to help manage their overall wellbeing. Other support services are provided to assist veterans in managing any service injuries or diseases (DVA 2019).

Aged care

Australia's aged care system is designed to help people who need extra support in their daily life. The aged care system is funded by the Australian government and is available to Indigenous Australian's over 50 years of age and to all other Australians over 65 years of age (Parliament of Australia 2019). There are several programs in place to help support the healthcare needs of older Australians and their families, including the following.

- The Commonwealth Home Support Programme: which offers a range of supports to assist a person living in their own home who may need domestic help, home maintenance, nursing care, personal care, meals, allied health services and respite care (a temporary break for carers) (Warburton & Mahoney 2016).
- Residential care: permanent care that is provided in an aged care facility when a person can no longer remain living in their own home, funded by government subsidies and the person needing care. The care needs and means of the resident determine how much funding they will receive to help pay for their care (Parliament of Australia 2019).

- Flexible care: which includes a range of care models to help people transition from care back into their homes after discharge from hospital. This covers those who may need extra short-term support at home while they recover from a setback or coordination of healthcare and services for people who live in rural and remote communities (Parliament of Australia 2019).

Rural and remote health

People who live in rural and remote areas of Australia have reduced access to healthcare because of geographical distances, reduced availability of services and reduced use of available primary health services (AIHW 2019). Consequently, people who live in rural and remote areas have poorer overall health, decreased life expectancy and higher death rates than people who live in cities (Tham & Ward 2016) and higher rates of injury and hospital admissions (AIHW 2019). Other factors that may impact the health of people in rural and remote areas include higher rates of engagement with activities that risk health — smoking and alcohol use — higher risk of physical injury from work or transport-related incidents, as well as reduced health literacy due to lower levels of education and reduced employment opportunities (AIHW 2019).

Indigenous healthcare

On 1 July 2014, the Australian Government established the Indigenous Australians' Health Programme (IAHP). The IAHP supports the delivery of comprehensive, high-quality and culturally sensitive primary healthcare, child and maternal healthcare and support for people with chronic diseases, as well as other specific health activities to improve the health of Aboriginal and Torres Strait Islander peoples. The aim is to improve health, life expectancy and to reduce child mortality.

'Closing the Gap' between Aboriginal and Torres Strait Islander peoples' health is a high priority in the Australian healthcare system (Healthdirect n.d.d). The ACSQHC (2019) has implemented a user guide that has been developed to support health service organisations implement the six Aboriginal and Torres Strait Islander health-related actions (see figure 1.4).

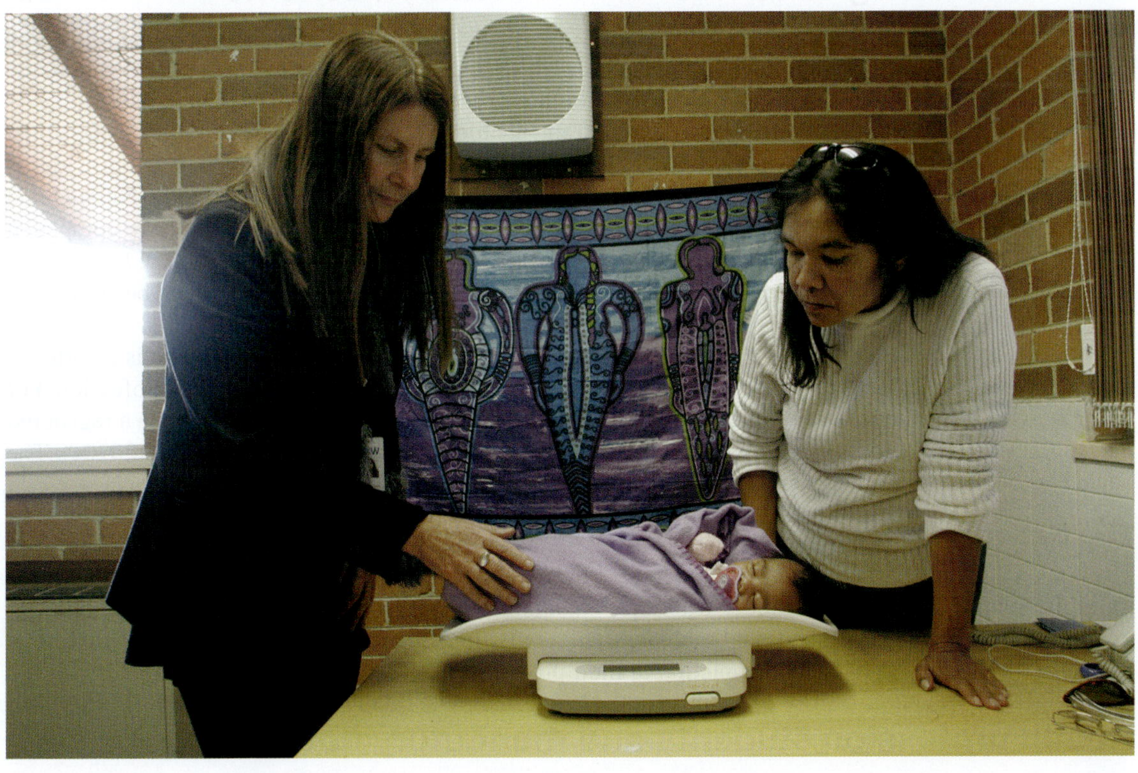

FIGURE 1.4 Six actions to meet the needs of Aboriginal and Torres Strait Islander people

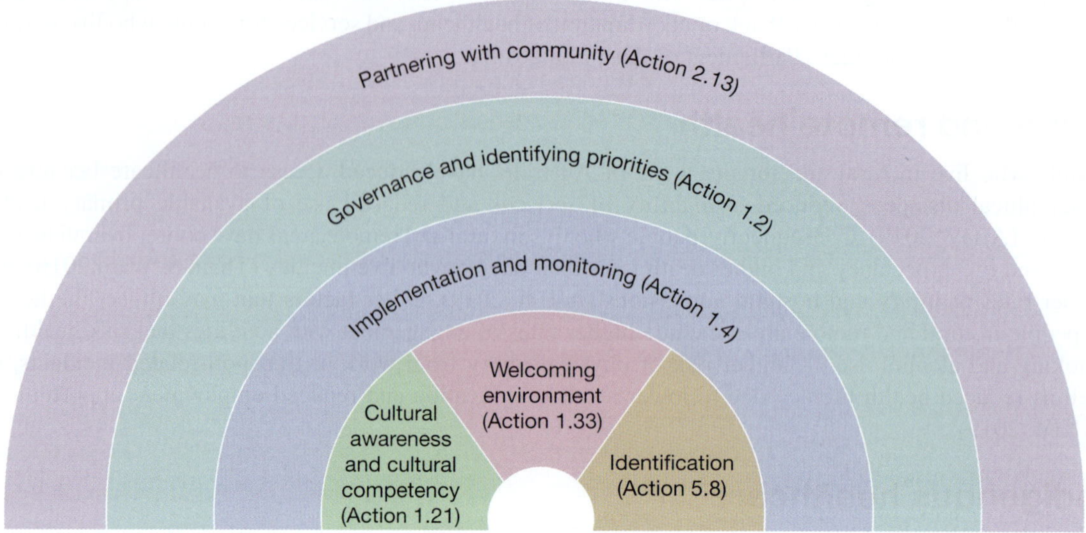

Source: ACSQHC (2017).

1.4 The role of healthcare providers in the Australian health system

LEARNING OBJECTIVE 1.4 Distinguish between the roles of healthcare practitioners in Australia.

The national registration and accreditation scheme

The National Scheme is designed to keep Australia's public safe from harm by ensuring that registered health practitioners have appropriate training and qualifications, provide competent and ethical care to the public, and foster the public's trust and confidence in those providing their care (AHPRA 2020c).

The National Scheme sets the standards and requirements for a person to register with their professional body. Yearly registration is required to continue working under the protected title for which a provider is registered. Nurses, registered nurses, nurse practitioners and midwives must register with the Nursing and Midwifery Board of Australia. For nurses and midwives, providing yearly evidence they have completed 20 hours of continuing professional development (CPD) is a requirement for registration. CPD demonstrates that nurses and midwives have maintained or further developed their skills in order to be competent in their work (AHPRA 2020c).

The National Scheme protects the titles of the registered health professions. This means it is an offence for a person to use a protected title if they are not registered with the National Board for that profession. For example, A person cannot use the title of registered nurse or give the impression that they are a registered nurse if they are not registered with the Nursing and Midwifery Board of Australia (AHPRA 2020c). The objectives of The National Scheme are shown in figure 1.5.

The National Scheme and health profession students

The National Scheme ensures that students have achieved the educational and skill requirements to apply for registration as a health practitioner with their National Board upon completing a study program. For example, student registered nurses and midwives will apply to register with the **Nursing and Midwifery Board of Australia (NMBA)** on completion of their program (AHPRA 2020c).

Health profession students and mandatory notifications

Mandatory notifications about a registered student can be made when there are concerns the student has an impairment (physical or mental, disability, condition or disorder) that affects their ability to participate in their training. If there are concerns the student has an impairment, the concerned registered health professional must decide if there is a risk of harm to patients or the broader community (AHPRA 2020b).

More information on mandatory reporting for registered health professionals and students can be found at www.ahpra.gov.au/Notifications/mandatorynotifications/Mandatory-notifications.aspx

FIGURE 1.5 The National Registration and Accreditation Scheme

Protecting the public
Setting national standards
Auditing compliance
Managing complaints (notifications) about health practitioners*
Publishing the online register
Accrediting training and education
Facilitating a mobile health workforce
Registering 700 000+ health practitioners
15 National boards
National registration and accreditation scheme
AHPRA

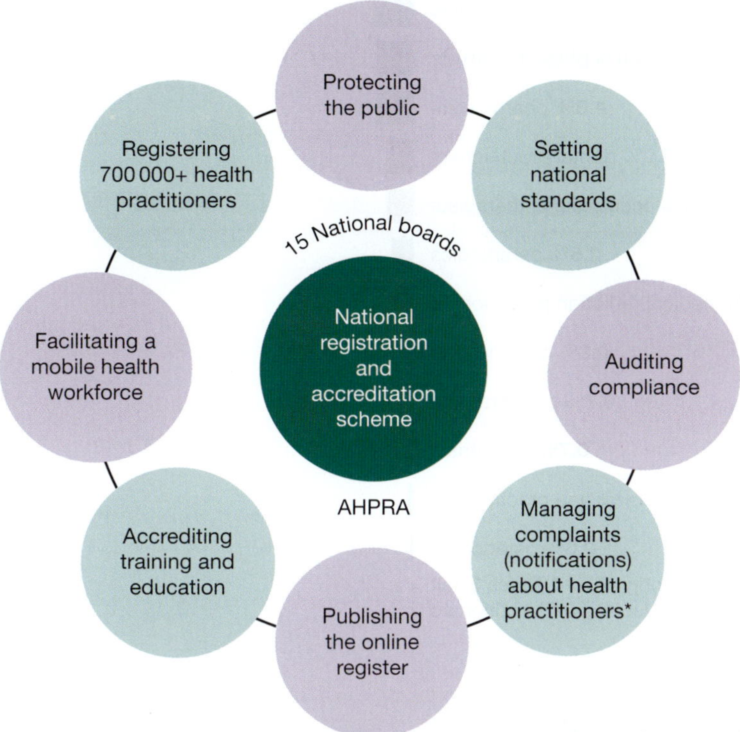

*Nationally, except in NSW and QLD where this is managed by the health professional councils authority and the 15 health professional councils, and the office of the ombudsman, respectively.

Source: AHPRA 2020c.

The Australian Health Practitioner Regulation Agency (AHPRA)

The Australian Health Practitioner Regulation Agency (AHPRA) oversees the National Registration and Accreditation Scheme for the 15 National Boards of the different health professions. The boards include:

- Aboriginal and Torres Strait Islander Health Practice Board of Australia
- Chinese Medicine Board of Australia
- Chiropractic Board of Australia
- Dental Board of Australia
- Medical Board of Australia
- Medical Radiation Practice Board of Australia
- Nursing and Midwifery Board of Australia
- Occupational Therapy Board of Australia
- Optometry Board of Australia
- Osteopathy Board of Australia
- Paramedicine Board of Australia
- Pharmacy Board of Australia
- Physiotherapy Board of Australia
- Podiatry Board of Australia
- Psychology Board of Australia.

Figure 1.6 provides a comparison of Australia's registered health professions by size and gender. Nursing and midwifery is the largest health workforce and in 2020, had a total of 415 433 members. The most recent profession to join registered health professionals is paramedicine, who became regulated in December 2018, and has almost 20 000 members (AHPRA 2020).

FIGURE 1.6 Relative size of registered health professionals

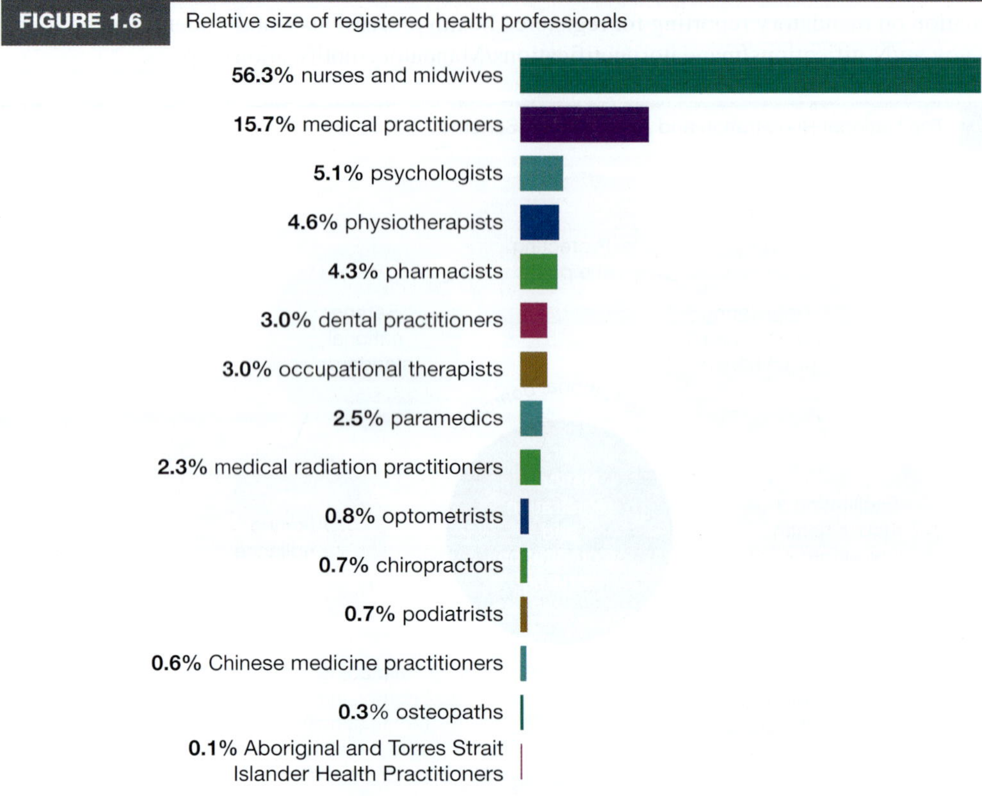

Source: AHPRA (2020).

Medical professionals

The Medical Board of Australia is supported by the **Australian Health Practitioner Regulation Agency (AHPRA)**. The Medical Board of Australia is responsible for the registration of medical practitioners and students (AHPRA 2018). The Medical Board of Australia develops standards, codes and guidelines that support Australia's medical professions and ensure high-quality medical care. They are responsible for investigating any notifications or complaints about a medical professional. Where needed, they conduct hearings and have the authority to transfer serious concerns to tribunal hearings. The Medical Board of Australia is also responsible for assessing international medical graduates who wish to practise in Australia to support a high standard of care and ensure that these individuals can provide that care. In addition, the Medical Board of Australia approves accreditation standards and accredited courses of study.

AHPRA has a national office based in Melbourne and offices in other states and territories to support local boards and committees (AHPRA 2018). The Medical Board of Australia National Board is supported by boards in each state and territory. These boards have been delegated powers to determine individual registration and notification decisions based on the national policies and standards established by the National Board. Each state and territory board has a registration committee, health committee, immediate action committee and notifications committee to deal with decisions at the local level.

Figure 1.7 identifies how many registered health practitioners as a whole work in each state and territory across Australia. New South Wales and Victoria have the biggest populations, which correlates to where most health practitioners work (AHPRA 2020).

Australia's National Standards in Healthcare (NSQHS)

The **Australian Commission on Safety and Quality in Health Care (ACSQHC)** oversees and coordinates improvements to the delivery of healthcare in Australia. Strategies and improvements to healthcare are made to:

- optimise patient safety
- encourage partnering with patients, consumers and communities
- ensure quality, cost and value
- support health professionals to provide care that is informed, supported and organised to deliver safe and high quality.

The ACSQHC developed **the National Safety and Quality Health Service (NSQHS)** Standards in collaboration with patients and their families, clinical experts, public and private healthcare providers and federal, state and territory governments. The standards are designed to help protect the public from harm and improve the healthcare provided to patients, their families and the communities in which they live (ACSQHC 2019b).

The Standards are applied in all Australian states and territories to provide consistent standards of care. The goal is that healthcare provided to patients is high quality, equal and consistent across Australia. (ACSQHC 2019b).

FIGURE 1.7 Number and percentage of registered health practitioners by state and territory

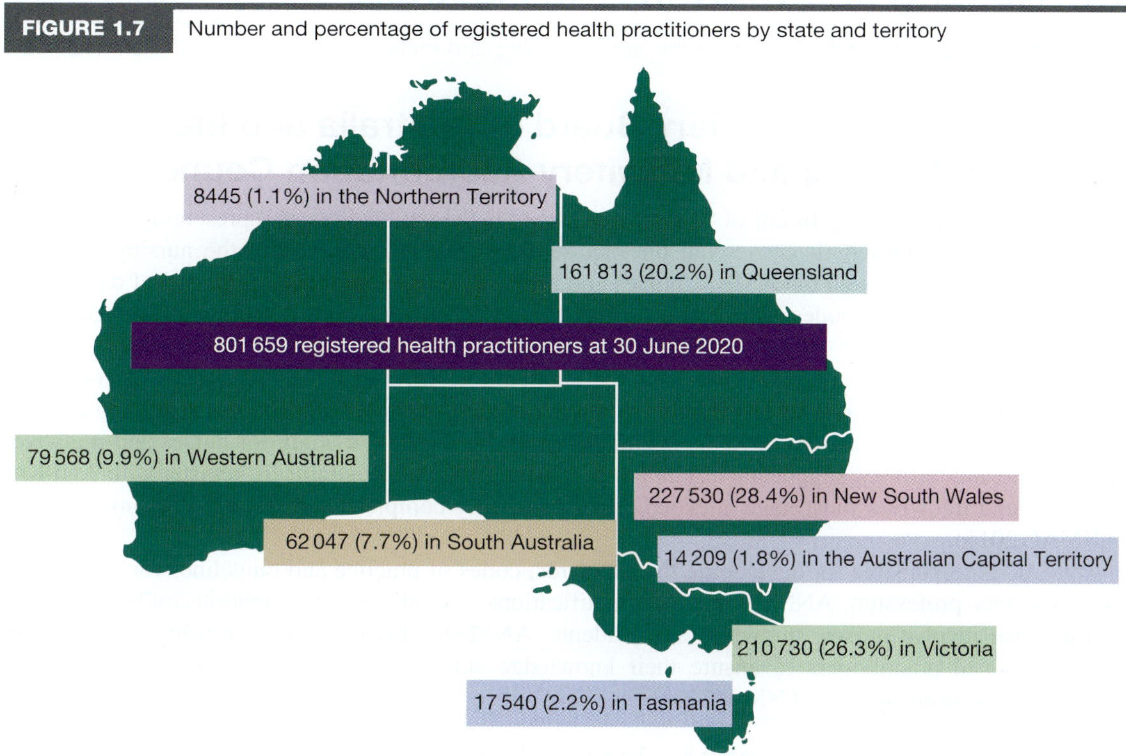

19 777 (2.5%) registered health practitioners have no principal place of practice (includes overseas-based registrants).

Source: AHPRA (2020).

The National Law

The Health Practitioner Regulation National Law (the National Law) was enacted in each Australian state and territory in 2009–10. The goal of the National Law was to create a national registration and accreditation scheme for registered health practitioners (National Health Practitioner Ombudsman 2020). **The National Law** protects **the National Registration and Accreditation Scheme (NRAS)**. The benefit is that once a healthcare provider registers with AHPRA, they are then allowed to practice within their scope of registration across Australia. Under the National Law, nurses and midwives are required to make a mandatory report to AHPRA of 'notifiable conduct by another health professional'. The law is consistent across Australia; however, each state and territory also has its own specific state law and reporting requirements (AHPRA 2020a).

The four national criteria for mandatory reporting to AHPRA are:

1. practised while intoxicated by alcohol or drugs
2. sexual misconduct in the practice of the profession
3. placing the public at risk of substantial harm because of an impairment (health issue)
4. placing the public at risk because of a significant departure from accepted professional standards.

The National Law and students

The National Law requires students to notify AHPRA within 7 days if they have:

- been charged with an offence punishable by 12-months imprisonment or more
- been convicted, or are the subject of, a finding of guilt for an offence punishable by imprisonment or registration under another country's law that provides for students' registration that has been suspended or cancelled (NMBA 2019).

1.5 Nursing and midwifery in Australia

LEARNING OBJECTIVE 1.5 Reflect on the role of nursing and midwifery within the Australian healthcare system.

The Nursing and Midwifery Board of Australia and the Australian Nursing and Midwifery Accreditation Council

The Nursing and Midwifery Board of Australia (NMBA) is the national board representing nursing and midwifery within AHPRA. It carries out the requirements for the regulation of the nursing and midwifery professions. Through the NMBA, nurses and midwives pay their annual professional registration fees, access professional codes, standards and guidelines for practice, and position statements for the professions.

The NMBA is also the national board for the **Australian Nursing and Midwifery Accreditation Council (ANMAC)**. The role of ANMAC is to register nurses, midwives and students studying in those fields, as well as review and approve the accreditation of the courses of study for nurses and midwives in each state and territory, supporting a standard of education across Australia. To register with AHPRA, all nurses and midwives must have attended and successfully completed accredited programs of study (ANMAC 2016).

ANMAC is responsible for developing the standards, codes of practice and guidelines for the nursing and midwifery profession. ANMAC manages notifications, complaints, investigations and disciplinary hearings that involve nurses, midwives and students. ANMAC also takes responsibility for assessing overseas trained practitioners to ensure their knowledge skills and attitudes are consistent with the Australian healthcare system (ANMAC 2016).

Nursing and midwifery students standards for practice and registration

Nurses and midwives use both the NSQHS and the NMBA standards for practice to help guide, plan and deliver nursing care for patients. The NSQHS standards can be found under the National Safety and Quality Health Service Standards website (www.safetyandquality.gov.au).

Nursing and midwifery students are required by the National Law to be registered as students with the NMBA. Education providers will complete this for students when study commences on an NMBA-approved program.

The purpose of student registration is to manage any notifications that may be received about a student. For example:

- if the student has a health impairment that poses a real risk of them causing harm to a patient
- if the student has committed an offence that is punishable by 12-months imprisonment or more
- if the student has a conviction of, or are the subject of, a finding of guilt for an offence punishable by imprisonment
- if the student has contravened an existing condition or undertaking.

The Australian nursing workforce

The development of new models of care is changing healthcare in Australia and means that nurses now provide care in such diverse settings as:

- nurse-led clinics
- day-surgery clinics
- community care facilities
- hospital in the home
- healthcare homes.

The nursing workforce must reflect the multicultural population it cares for. There are four categories for nursing roles in Australia.

1. Assistant in nursing (AIN) or patient care assistant (PCA)
   - Unregulated by a body — they are not registered with AHPRA and there are no standardised national training courses.
   - Acute care AINs require training from a registered education provider body.
   - Residential aged care organisations often provide on-the-job training for these roles.
   - Provide nursing care under the direction and supervision of a registered nurse.
   - Supervision may be direct or indirect according to the nature of the work.
2. Enrolled nurse (EN)
   - Registered under AHPRA and regulated under ANMAC.
   - Undertake an 18-month or 2-year course at TAFE or related health facilities to achieve a Diploma in Enrolled Nursing
   - Provide nursing care under the direction and supervision of a registered nurse.
   - Supervision may be direct or indirect according to the nature of the work.
3. Registered nurse (RN)
   - Registered under AHPRA and regulated under ANMAC.
   - Involves 3 years of accredited study at university to achieve a bachelor's degree with 800 clinical experience hours (minimum) in various healthcare settings.
   - High level of responsibility and accountability.
4. Nurse practitioner (NP)
   - Registered under AHPRA and regulated under ANMAC.
   - Authorised to function autonomously.
   - Works collaboratively in an advanced and extended clinical role.
   - Requires three years of study/training at university to achieve a Bachelor Degree in Nursing plus 1.5–2 years of additional study.
   - Minimum 3 years of post-registration practice in a speciality area.
   - Demonstrates commitment to and capacity to innovation and leadership in their speciality area.

The NMBA standards for practice across all nursing levels can be found under the NMBA website — Regulating Australia's nurses and midwives.

The codes, guidelines and standards for nursing and midwifery practice can be accessed from the NMBA website: www.nursingmidwiferyboard.gov.au/Codes-Guidelines-Statements.aspx.

Resources for nurses

The Australian College of Nursing (ACN) is Australia's leader of the nursing profession that provides a range of resources to help nurses deliver high standards of healthcare to Australians (ACN n.d.).

JBI (formally the Joanna Briggs Institute) is an Australian-based international research organisation based in the Faculty of Health and Medical Sciences at the University of Adelaide, South Australia. 'JBI develops and delivers unique evidence-based information, software, education and training designed to improve healthcare practice and health outcomes provides information that is used by healthcare practitioners' (JBI n.d).

SUMMARY

This chapter described how the Australian healthcare system is a network of federal, state and territory, and local government departments that have distinct roles in supporting each other to ensure all Australians have access to high-quality healthcare. We discussed the public and private healthcare systems, the primary health network, the Australian government departments' responsibilities, challenges to the healthcare system, and the healthcare providers in Australia, their standards of practice and codes of conduct.

KEY TERMS

Australian Commission on Safety and Quality in Health Care (ACSQHC) The ACSQHC oversees and coordinates improvements to the delivery of healthcare in Australia.

Australian Health Practitioner Regulation Authority (AHPRA) The national organisation responsible for implementing the National Registration and Accreditation Scheme across Australia.

Australian Nursing and Midwifery Accreditation Council (ANMAC) The role of ANMAC is to register nurses, midwives and students who are studying in those fields and to review and approve the accreditation of courses of study for nurses and midwives.

health The overall condition of the body or mind, free from disease or disorder.

health literacy The ability to understand and using information about a person's health to access care and make informed decisions about healthcare and treatment options.

healthcare Maintaining or improving physical and mental health through prevention, diagnosis, treatment, recovery, or cure of disease, illness, injury, and other physical and mental impairments in people.

Medicare Australia's universal health insurance scheme.

My Health Record A digital summary of a patient's medical conditions,medications and allergies, shared across a health system.

NMBA (Nursing and Midwifery Board of Australia) The National Board for nursing and midwifery. Carries out the functions for AHPRA and the nursing and midwifery professions.

provider Healthcare professionals or organisations that offer specialised healthcare.

The National Law An Act to make provision for a national legislative scheme for the regulation of health practitioners (the National Registration and Accreditation Scheme).

The National Safety and Quality Health Service (NSQHS) Healthcare standards developed by the ACSQHC to guide the delivery of safe healthcare anywhere in Australia.

The National Registration and Accreditation Scheme (NRAS) Ensures all regulated health professionals are registered against consistent, high-quality, national professional standards and can practise across state and territory borders.

REFERENCES

ACN. (n.d.) About us — Australian College of Nursing. www.acn.edu.au/about-us

ACSQHC. (2019a) Australian Charter of Healthcare Rights (second edition). www.safetyandquality.gov.au/publications-and-resources/resource-library/australian-charter-healthcare-rights-second-edition-a4-accessible

ACSQHC. (2019b) The NSQHS Standards. www.safetyandquality.gov.au/standards/nsqhs-standardsAHPRA

ACSQHC. (2017) User guide for Aboriginal and Torres Strait Islander health. www.safetyandquality.gov.au/topic/user-guide-aboriginal-and-torres-strait-islander-health

AHPRA. (2020) The regulated health workforce in 2019/20. www.ahpra.gov.au/Publications/Annual-reports/Annual-Report-2019/Overview.aspx

AHPRA. (2020a) Legislation. www.ahpra.gov.au/About-AHPRA/What-We-Do/Legislation.aspx

AHPRA. (2020b) Mandatory notifications. www.ahpra.gov.au/Notifications/Raise-a-concern/Mandatory-notifications.aspx

AHPRA. (2020c) The National Registration and Accreditation Scheme. www.ahpra.gov.au/About-AHPRA/What-We-Do.aspx

AHPRA. (2018) Medical Board. Role of the Board. www.medicalboard.gov.au/About.aspx

ANMAC. (2016) About ANMAC. www.anmac.org.au/about-anmac

Australian Institute of Health and Welfare (AIHW). (2019) *Rural and remote health. Summary.* www.aihw.gov.au/reports/rural-remote-australians/rural-remote-health/contents/summary

Australian Institute of Health and Welfare (AIHW). (2018) *Australia's health 2018. Australia's health series 16. How does Australia's health system work?* Canberra. www.aihw.gov.au/getmedia/63fe0895-b306-4375-95ff-162149ffc34b/aihw-aus-221-chapter-2-1.pdf.aspx.

Australian Institute of Health and Welfare (AIHW). (2016) *Australia's health 2016. Australia's health series no. 15. Cat. no. AUS 199.* Canberra. www.aihw.gov.au/getmedia/9844cefb-7745-4dd8-9ee2-f4d1c3d6a727/19787-AH16.pdf.aspx

Clarke, P. (2016) 'The Pharmaceutical Benefits Scheme: recent trends and options for reform'. In L. Reynolds & H. Keleher (Eds.). *Understanding the Australian Healthcare System* (pp. 106–120). Chatswood, Australia: Elsevier.

Commonwealth of Australia Department of Health. (2020) The Australian health system. www.health.gov.au/about-us/the-australian-health-system

Disability, A. N. O. (2020) What is a disability? www.and.org.au/pages/disability-statistics.html

DVA. (2019) Who we are. www.dva.gov.au/health-and-treatment/veteran-healthcare-cards/veteran-card

Ellison, C. & Lante, K. (2016) 'People living with a disability; navigating support and health systems'. In L. Reynolds & H. Keleher (Eds.). *Understanding the Australian Healthcare System* (pp. 181–193). Chatswood, Australia: Elsevier.

Flynn, K. V. N. (2016) Financial fraud in the private health insurance sector in Australia. Perspectives from the industry. *Journal of Financial Crime*. 23(1): 143–158. doi: DOI10.1108/JFC-06-2014-0032

Healthdirect. (2020) What is Medicare? Australian Government, Department of Health. www.healthdirect.gov.au/what-is-medicare

Healthdirect. (n.d.a) Primary Healthcare Networks (PHNs). Australian Government, Department of Health. www.healthdirect.gov.au/primary-health-networks-phns

Healthdirect. (n.d.b) About My Health Record. Australian Government, Department of Health. www.healthdirect.gov.au/my-health-record

Healthdirect. (n.d.c) The public and private hospital systems. Australian Government, Department of Health. www.healthdirect.gov.au/understanding-the-public-and-private-hospital-systems

Healthdirect. (n.d.d) Indigenous health. Australian Government, Department of Health. www.healthdirect.gov.au/indigenous-health

JBI. (n.d.) About JBI. https://joannabriggs.org/jbi-approach-to-EBHC

Krassnitzer, L. & Willis, E. (2016) 'The public health sector and Medicare'. In L. Reynolds & H. Keleher (Eds.). *Understanding the Australian Healthcare System* (pp. 18–34). Chatswood, Australia: Elsevier.

myDr.com. (2019) Australian health system: how it works. www.mydr.com.au/first-aid-self-care/australian-health-system-how-it-works

National Health Practitioner Ombudsman. (2020) The National Scheme. www.nhpo.gov.au/the-national-scheme

NMBA. (2020) Professional codes and guidelines. www.nursingmidwiferyboard.gov.au/Codes-Guidelines-Statements.aspx

NMBA. (2019) Fact sheet: Student registration. www.nursingmidwiferyboard.gov.au/Registration-and-Endorsement/Student-Registration/Fact-sheet-FAQ-student-registration.aspx

Parliament of Australia. (2019) Aged care. A quick services guide. www.aph.gov.au/About_Parliament/Parliamentary_Departments/Parliamentary_Library/pubs/rp/rp1617/Quick_Guides/Aged_Care_a_quick_guide

PrivateHealth.gov.au. (n.d.) How health insurance works. Overview of health system. www.privatehealth.gov.au/health_insurance/what_is_covered/index.htm#ambulance

Services Australia. (n.d.) Medicare safety nets. www.servicesaustralia.gov.au/individuals/services/medicare/medicare-safety-nets

Tham, R. & Ward, B. (2016) 'Rural health systems: spotlight on equity and access'. In L. Reynolds & H. Keleher (Eds.). *Understanding the Australian Healthcare System*, 3rd ed. (pp. 139–152). Chatswood, Australia: Elsevier.

Warburton, J. & Mahoney, A. M. (2016) 'The aged care sector: residential and community care'. In L. Reynolds & H. Keleher (Eds.). *Understanding the Australian Healthcare System*, 3rd ed. (pp. 122–137). Chatswood, Australia: Elsevier.

WHO. (2020) WHO remains firmly committed to the principles set out in the preamble to the Constitution. www.who.int/topics/health_systems/en

ACKNOWLEDGEMENTS

Figure 1.1: © Australian Charter of Healthcare Rights (second edition) — A4 Accessible. © ACSQHC. Reproduced with permission of Australian Commission on Safety and Quality in Health Care.

Figure 1.2: © Australian Institute of Health and Welfare.

Figure 1.3: © Health services — funding and responsibility, 2013–14, Australia's Health 2016; p. 28. Australian Institute of Health and Welfare. Licensed under CC BY 3.0 AU.

Figure 1.4: © User Guide for Aboriginal and Torres Strait Islander Health, Australian Commission on Safety and Quality in Health Care. © ACSQHC. Reproduced with permission of Australian Commission on Safety and Quality in Health Care.

Figure 1.5: © The National Registration and Accreditation Scheme. © Ahpra. Reproduced with permission of Ahpra.

Figure 1.6: © The regulated health workforce in 2018/19, Overview, © Ahpra. Reproduced with permission of Ahpra.

Figure 1.7: © The regulated health workforce in 2018/19, Overview, © Ahpra. Reproduced with permission of Ahpra.

Table 1.2: © Overview of Health System, Australian Government. Licensed under CC BY 3.0 AU.

Photo 1A: © Chris de Blank / Alamy Stock Photo

Photo 1B: © Robyn Mackenzie / Shutterstock.com

Photo 1C: © Shuang Li / Shutterstock.com

Photo 1D: © david hancock / Alamy Stock Photo

CHAPTER 2

Indigenous health and remote area nursing

LEARNING OBJECTIVES

After studying this chapter, you should be able to:

2.1 understand the social determinants of health faced by Indigenous Australians
2.2 explain the impact of the 'Closing the Gap' initiative in Australia
2.3 discuss the role of the remote area nurse in Australia
2.4 discuss the common conditions experienced by Indigenous Australians.

Introduction

Access to healthcare in Australia can be challenging for people living and working in remote areas due to the vast geographical spread of the population across Australia; a landmass of 7 617 930 square kilometres with a population of 26 million people. The majority of Australia's population reside in urban areas (Australian Bureau of Statistics [ABS] 2021). People who live in remote areas may have limited access to health services and transport and feel isolated. The majority of people living in remote areas are **Indigenous Australians** who already face more health challenges than non-Indigenous Australians due to several issues, including socioeconomic disadvantage.

Across Australia, the Northern Territory has the highest proportion of Indigenous residents among its population — an estimated 31 per cent in 2020 (ABS 2018). In 2020, an estimated 33 per cent of Indigenous Australians (286 600 people) lived in New South Wales and 28 per cent (241 100) in Queensland (Health & Welfare 2020a). This chapter will address the social determinants of health for Indigenous Australians and outline the role of the remote area nurse in Australia. It will also discuss the nursing care of patients with common conditions seen in remote areas.

2.1 The social determinants of health for Indigenous Australians

LEARNING OBJECTIVE 2.1 Understand the social determinants of health faced by Indigenous Australians.

For human beings to have a healthy body and a healthy mind depends on many different factors related to an individual or group, including access to health services, an individual's knowledge of health and capabilities, environmental factors, education and income. These are referred to as the **social determinants of health** and have a powerful connection to individual health outcomes. The social determinants of health can adversely affect a persons' physical or mental health in a number of ways, such as increasing their risk of infectious disease or injury, smoking or alcohol use, the diet they consume, or by causing psychological stress or lack of control over life's circumstances due to financial constraints. Early childhood development is another social determinant affecting health outcomes over the whole life course. Access to healthcare is a significant determinant of health in its own right, which is a major concern in rural and remote Australia, particularly for Indigenous Australians.

A number of reviews published by the United Nations in recent years have documented the common factors underlying the continuation of health and social inequalities experienced by Indigenous populations across the globe, including loss of culture and language, economic and social marginalisation and disposition from traditional territories (Economic et al. 2009; King et al. 2009). For Indigenous Australians, cultural identity, family and connection to their traditional land are essential for Indigenous community functioning and their health and wellbeing outcomes (Health & Welfare 2020c).

2.2 Closing the Gap

LEARNING OBJECTIVE 2.2 Explain the impact of the 'Closing the Gap' initiative in Australia.

Closing the Gap is a strategy that has been developed to improve the life and health outcomes of Aboriginal and Torres Strait Islander peoples. It is a commitment made by the Australian governments to achieve health equality for Indigenous Australians. The Closing the Gap campaign was initially established in 2008. The Council of Australian Governments (COAG) set six ambitious targets across the areas of health, education and employment to drive progress. Some of the targets, such as halving the gap in child mortality by 2018, for 95 per cent of all Indigenous four-year-olds to be enrolled in early childhood education by 2025, and halving the gap in Year 12 attainment by 2020, have either been met or are on track. However, some targets, such as closing the gap in life expectancy by 2031, and halving the gap in employment by 2018, have not been achieved or are not on track (Commonwealth of Australia 2018). This led has to the development of the National Agreement on Closing the Gap, known as the National Agreement, in 2020.

The National Agreement aims to improve Indigenous Australians' life outcomes. The National Agreement, has been developed in partnership between the National Federation Reform Council (NFRC) (representing the Australian Commonwealth Government, state and territory governments, and the Australian Local Government Association) and the Coalition of Peaks, which is a representative body of around 50 Aboriginal and Torres Strait Islander community-controlled peak organisations and members.

The National Agreement adopts a different approach to the Closing the Gap strategy, with Aboriginal and Torres Strait Islander people using a strengths-based approach to determine what is important to them. It outlines 16 socioeconomic targets and four priority reforms. The four priority reform targets aim to change the way governments at the national, state and community levels work to improve the life outcomes of Aboriginal and Torres Strait Islander people (Commonwealth of Australia 2018; Department of Health 2020). These are as follows.

1. *Formal partnerships and shared decision making.* Building and strengthening structures to empower Aboriginal and Torres Strait Islander people to share decision making with governments.
2. *Building the community-controlled sector.* Building formal Aboriginal and Torres Strait Islander community-controlled sectors to deliver services to support Closing the Gap.
3. *Transforming government organisations.* Systemic and structural transformation of mainstream government organisations to improve accountability and better respond to the needs of Aboriginal and Torres Strait Islander people.
4. *Shared access to data and information at a regional level.* Enable shared access to location specific data and information to support Aboriginal and Torres Strait Islander communities and organisations achieve the first three priority reforms.

The 16 socioeconomic targets aim to improve the following outcome areas: health and wellbeing, education, employment, justice, safety, housing, land and water, and languages (Australian Indigenous Health Info Net n.d.).

2.3 Nursing in a remote area

LEARNING OBJECTIVE 2.3 Discuss the role of the remote area nurse in Australia.

Nursing in a **remote area** can present many challenges but also be very rewarding. **Remote area nurses (RANs)** work in various settings from isolated Indigenous Australian communities and mining and refugee communities. Working in a remote area can leave some nurses feeling isolated with limited access to resources. RANs need to have advanced clinical competencies as they often work alone and have to deal with emergencies 24 hours a day (Dunbar et al. 2019). This can be extremely challenging due to the lack of resources and limited medications held in remote clinics. Nurses can also be rewarded by developing new skills and working in an autonomous role in some incredible geographic locations. Working as a RAN offers some unique travel opportunities and a chance to explore the more remote areas of Australia.

Remote nursing scope of practice

RANs have an advanced scope of practice compared to their metropolitan counterparts. RANs need to have exceptional assessment and critical thinking skills as they can be dealing with a great variety of medical conditions, from maternal emergencies to chronic disease checks, mental health and trauma or medical emergencies that may arise. Most Australian states and territories have procedures to allow RANs to supply and administer medications according to local protocols or standing orders. One such protocol is the CARPA Standard Treatment Manual, which directs nurses and Aboriginal health practitioners on caring for people presenting with various conditions, from medical emergencies to chronic disease checks. The CARPA Manual also includes a step-by-step approach to managing acute and chronic conditions using simple language. The Nursing and Midwifery Board of Australia (NMBA) also offers an endorsement for scheduled medicines for rural and remote nurses. This is a mandatory requirement for nurses working in rural and remote settings in Queensland and Victoria (NMBA 2019).

Air retrieval services

Due to the remote nature of many Indigenous communities, acutely unwell patients will need to be transported to their closest major hospital. It is the role of the RANs to communicate effectively with the air retrieval service, so they are best prepared to manage the patient's condition and send the right team of health professionals. A midwifery emergency will require a qualified midwife to attend. A critical care emergency will require a team equipped to intubate and ventilate a patient on arrival to the community. The RAN will need to stabilise the unwell patient and continue providing care while waiting for the air retrieval service to arrive. The nurse should also complete a transfer checklist to ensure that their patient is ready to be transported via plane or helicopter. They will need to provide ongoing care and transport the patient to the airport to meet the retrieval aircraft and hand over their patient's care (see figure 2.1), then the patient will be transferred to their local hospital.

FIGURE 2.1 A patient transfer with CareFlight

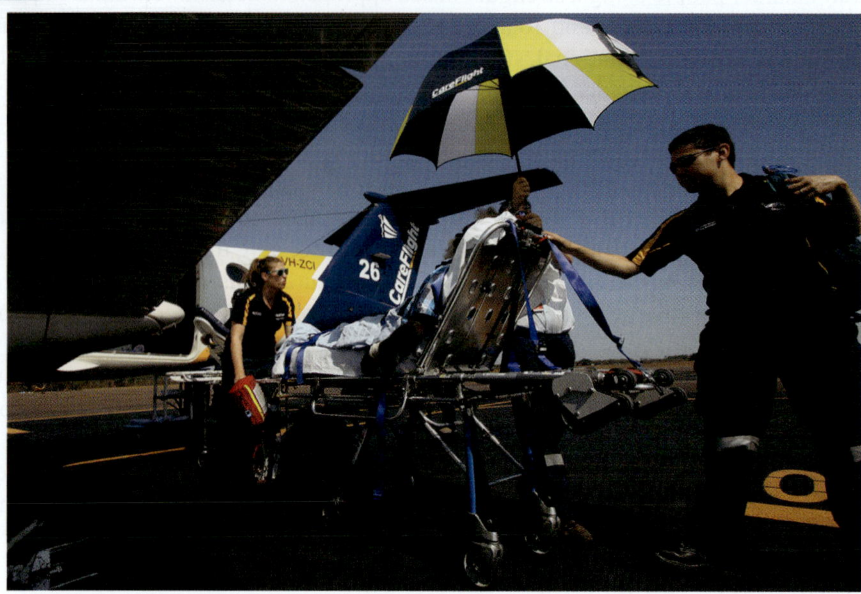

Source: CareFlight (2021).

Digital health records

My Health Record is an initiative from the Australian Department of Health to simplify access to medical records and expedite patient information access. Many Indigenous Australians move between communities regularly and may seek medical support from an alternate clinic. The ability for doctors and nurses to easily access this information could prove to be lifesaving, as they can easily access a summary of the patient's medical conditions, medications and allergies (Australian Digital Health Agency n.d.).

Telehealth

Video conferencing software has improved access to health services for many patients living in rural or remote areas. This advancement in technology has removed the need for many patients to travel long distances to a specialist appointment. Instead, they have a virtual consult in collaboration with their local health service provider (Department of Health 2015). **Telehealth** services have recently been expanded to include mental health to improve access to psychological services for patients living in rural and remote locations (Department of Health 2019).

2.4 Common conditions experienced by Indigenous Australians

LEARNING OBJECTIVE 2.4 Discuss the common conditions experienced by Indigenous Australians.

Many Aboriginal and Torres Strait Islander people suffer from poorer health and experience higher mortality rates than other Australians (Department of Health 2020). They suffer from higher rates of **diabetes**, **chronic kidney disease**, heart disease and **acute rheumatic fever**. While some of these conditions are discussed in greater detail throughout the relevant chapters in this text, key considerations for Indigenous Australians will be highlighted here.

Acute rheumatic fever and rheumatic heart disease

Australia has one of the highest incidences of acute rheumatic fever globally, with the highest rates found in Indigenous Australians, particularly in the Northern Territory (Australian Institute of Health and Welfare 2019; Menzies School of Health Research n.d.). It is a preventable condition connected to low socioeconomic disadvantage, particularly overcrowding due to the higher exposure of group A Strep in the environment, which can be easily transmitted from person to person (RHDAustralia 2020). Acute rheumatic fever is a condition cause by an abnormal immune response following an untreated bacterial infection with group A Streptococcus. It can affect a patient's heart, skin, blood vessels and joints (see figure 2.2). Acute rheumatic fever is caused by Strep throat, infected scabies and school sores (impetigo) and is more common in children aged 5–14 years old (Australian Institute of Health and Welfare 2019).

FIGURE 2.2 Clinical manifestations of acute rheumatic fever

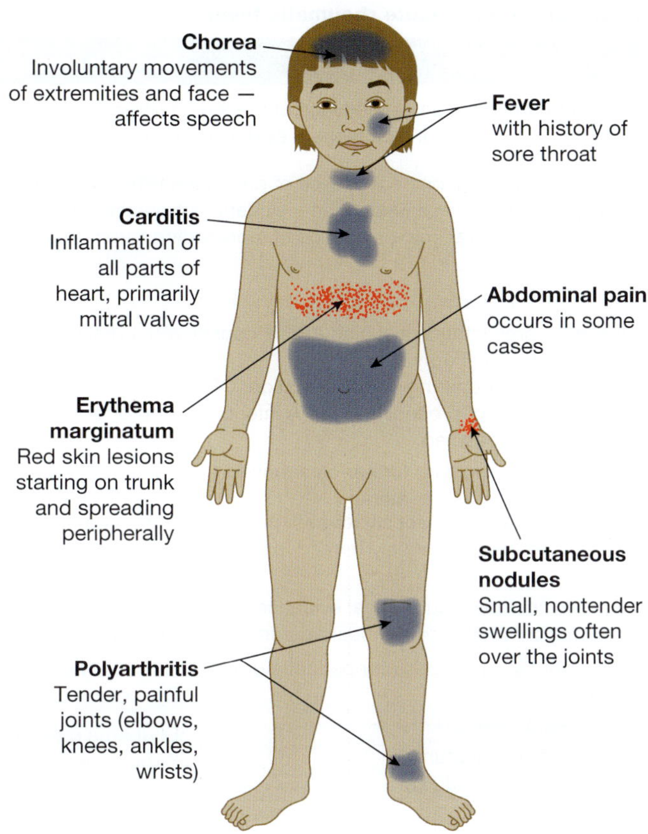

Rheumatic heart disease (RHD) occurs when the heart valves have been damaged by a single or repeated episode of acute rheumatic fever. It is related to overcrowded living conditions and remains a rare condition in established economies. Despite this, there continues to be a high prevalence of the condition in Aboriginal and Torres Strait Islander population of Australia. RHD can cause heart failure, so it is important to know the condition, particularly if you wish to work in the Northern Territory or a remote area. RHD can lead to complications such as mitral valve stenosis, atrial fibrillation and heart failure (Australian Institute of Health and Welfare 2019; RHDAustralia, 2020). Mitral valve stenosis (as shown in figure 2.3) needs to be repaired surgically in some cases. This operation would need to be conducted in a large metropolitan facility and means that patients are away from their family for extended periods. Surgical repair of a mitral valve can leave the patient on long-term anticoagulants to prevent the development of blood clots.

FIGURE 2.3 Mitral valve stenosis

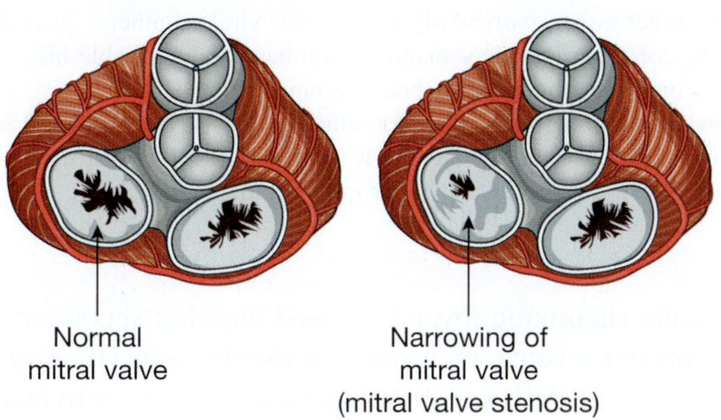

Nursing considerations

Nurses working with Indigenous Australians need to be aware of the diagnostic criteria for acute rheumatic fever to prevent a missed opportunity for secondary prevention treatment. These diagnostic criteria have been summarised in table 2.1.

TABLE 2.1 The diagnostic criteria for acute rheumatic fever

	High-risk groups†	Low-risk groups
Definite initial episode of ARF	2 major manifestations + evidence of preceding Strep A infection, OR 1 major + 2 minor manifestations + evidence of preceding Strep A infection[‡]	
Definite recurrent episode of ARF in a patient with a documented history of ARF or RHD	2 major manifestations + evidence of preceding Strep A infection, OR 1 major + 2 minor manifestations + evidence of preceding Strep A infection[‡], OR 3 minor manifestations + evidence of a preceding Strep A infection[‡]	
Probable or possible ARF (first episode or recurrence)	A clinical presentation in which ARF is considered a likely diagnosis but falls short in meeting the criteria by either: • one major or one minor manifestation, OR • no evidence of preceding Strep A infection (streptococcal titres within normal limits or titres not measured). Such cases should be further categorised according to the level of confidence with which the diagnosis is made: • probable ARF (previously termed 'probable: highly suspected') • possible ARF (previously termed 'probable: uncertain').	
Major manifestations	Carditis (including subclinical evidence of rheumatic valvulitis on echocardiogram) Polyarthritis[¶] or aseptic monoarthritis or polyarthralgia Sydenham chorea[††] Erythema marginatum[‡‡] Subcutaneous nodules	Carditis (including subclinical evidence of rheumatic valvulitis on echocardiogram) Polyarthritis[¶] Sydenham chorea[††] Erythema marginatum[‡‡] Subcutaneous nodules
Minor manifestations	Fever§§ ≥38°C Monoarthralgia[¶¶] ESR ≥30 mm/h or CRP ≥30 mg/L Prolonged P-R interval on ECG[†††]	Fever ≥38.5°C Polyarthralgia or aseptic monoarthritis[¶¶] ESR ≥60 mm/h or CRP ≥30 mg/L Prolonged P-R interval on ECG[†††]

† High-risk groups are those living in communities with high rates of ARF (incidence >30/100 000 per year in 5–14-year-olds) or RHD (all-age prevalence >2/1000). Aboriginal and Torres Strait Islander peoples living in rural or remote settings are known to be at high risk. Data are not available for other populations but Aboriginal and Torres Strait Islander peoples living in urban settings, Māori and Pacific Islanders, and potentially immigrants from developing countries, may also be at high risk.

‡ Elevated or rising antistreptolysin O or other streptococcal antibody, or a positive throat culture or rapid antigen or nucleic acid test for Strep A infection.

§ Recurrent definite, probable or possible ARF requires a time period of more than 90 days after the onset of symptoms from the previous episode of definite, probable or possible ARF.

¶ A definite history of arthritis is sufficient to satisfy this manifestation. Note that if polyarthritis is present as a major manifestation, polyarthralgia or aseptic monoarthritis cannot be considered an additional minor manifestation in the same person.

†† Chorea does not require other manifestations or evidence of preceding Strep A infection, provided other causes of chorea are excluded.

‡‡ Care should be taken not to label other rashes, particularly non-specific viral exanthems, as erythema marginatum.

§§ In high-risk groups, fever can be considered a minor manifestation based on a reliable history (in the absence of documented temperature) if anti-inflammatory medication has already been administered.

¶¶ If polyarthritis is present as a major criterion, monoarthritis or arthralgia cannot be considered an additional minor manifestation.

††† If carditis is present as a major manifestation, a prolonged P-R interval cannot be considered an additional minor manifestation.

CRP, C-reactive protein; ECG, electrocardiogram; ESR, erythrocyte sedimentation rate.

Source: RHDAustralia (2020).

Patients diagnosed with acute rheumatic fever will need ongoing secondary prophylaxis with monthly benzathine penicillin injections to prevent a recurrence of the disease. This can reduce the level of damage to the heart. Patients diagnosed with RHD will still need ongoing prophylactic treatment with monthly benzathine penicillin injections and may need ongoing treatment with anticoagulants if they develop atrial fibrillation or undergo heart valve surgery. Recall registers are commonplace in rural and remote health centres to enable nurses to be aware of which patients are due for their monthly injections.

Diabetes

Aboriginal and Torres Strait Islander people are almost four times more likely to suffer from type 2 diabetes. Diabetes can lead to a cascade of events that leads to the development of other chronic diseases. Ultimately, patients with uncontrolled diabetes can develop microvascular disease, leading to chronic kidney disease, cardiovascular disease, diabetic retinopathy, and diabetic foot ulcers. Many of these complications can be prevented, delayed and type 2 diabetes can even be reversed in its early stages if patients make positive lifestyle changes and maintain a normal blood glucose level. Effective diabetes management should be a priority for patients.

The management of diabetes is complex and requires the patient to have a sound understanding of their condition, including how to self-manage it. The local health team's role is to help educate and empower patients to manage their condition within the community. The local health clinic provides blood glucose monitors and supplies with support from the National Diabetes Services Scheme (NDSS). RANs and Aboriginal health practitioners are pivotal to providing sound education to patients that are newly diagnosed with diabetes. There are often diabetes educators that visit remote communities and consult with patients via telehealth.

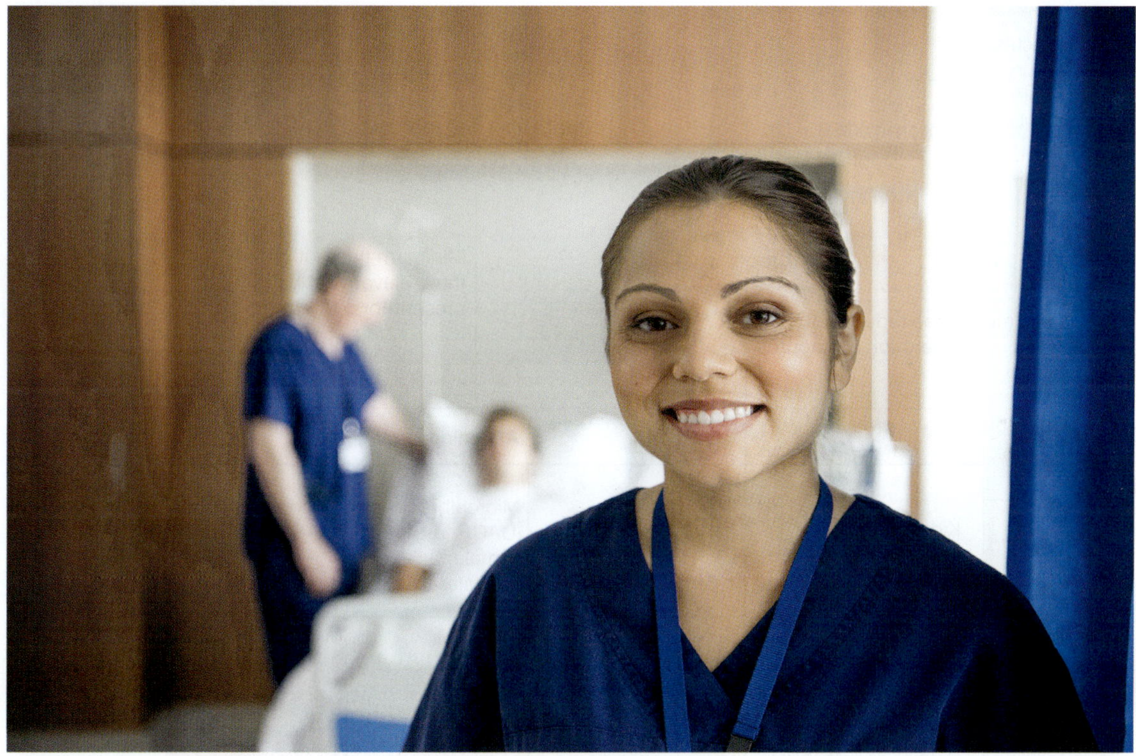

Chronic kidney disease

Almost one in five Indigenous Australian adults show signs of chronic kidney disease (CKD). The likelihood of having CKD increases with age and is higher among people with high blood pressure or diabetes and those living in remote areas. Hospitalisation rates for kidney disease or treatment for end-stage kidney disease among Indigenous Australians tend to be highest in remote areas, particularly in Central Australia (Health & Welfare 2020b).

CKD refers to all kidney conditions that last for more than three months, affecting the filtration and removal of waste from the blood by the kidneys or leakage of protein or albumin in the urine (see figure 2.4 for the algorithm used to detect CKD). CKD is a preventable condition related to lifestyle factors such as smoking and obesity, and other chronic diseases, including type 2 diabetes and hypertension. As many Aboriginal and Torres Strait Islander people live in remote locations, this can affect their access to specialists and be more costly to manage in its end stage.

FIGURE 2.4 Algorithm for initial detection of CKD

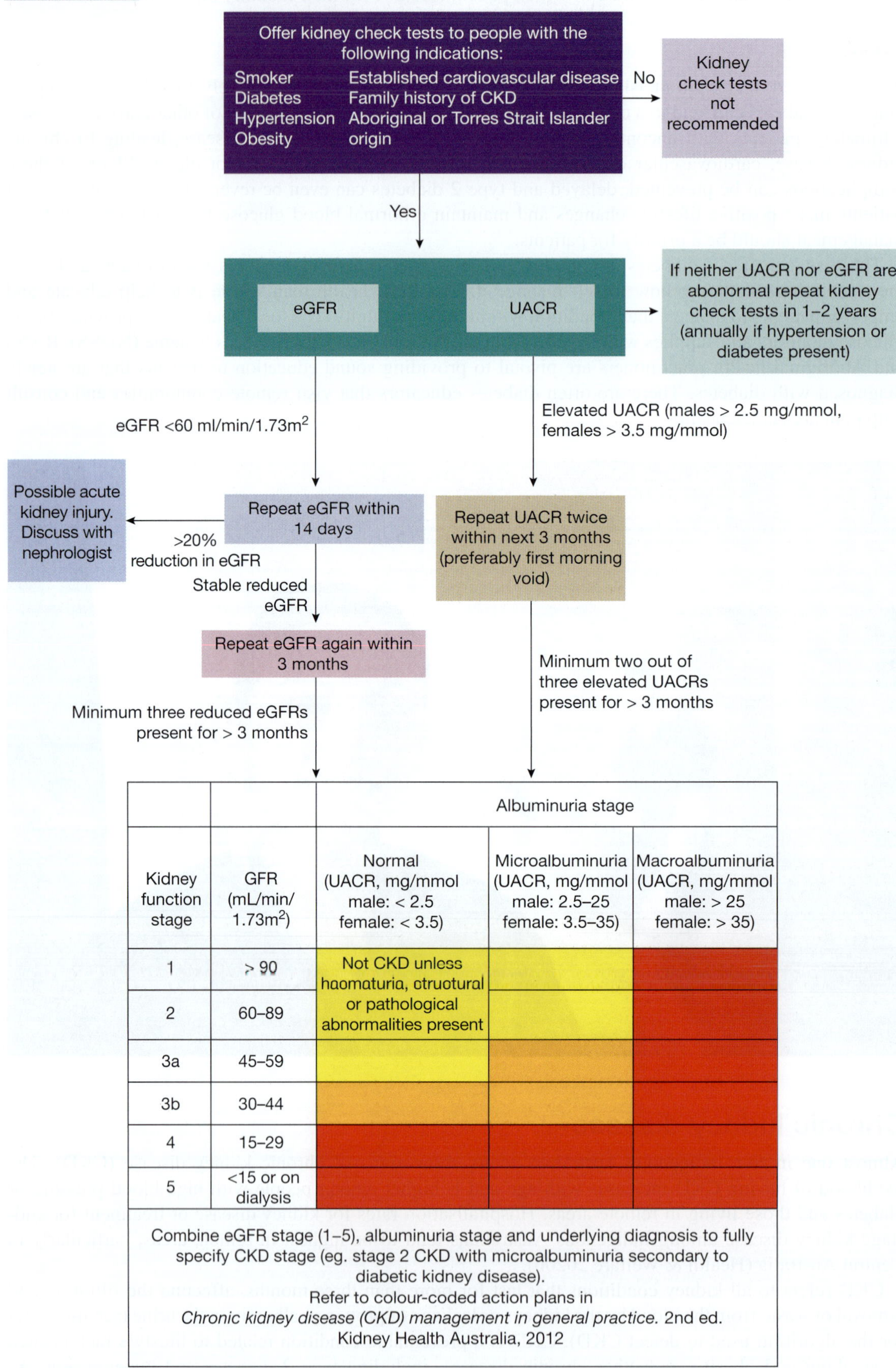

		Albuminuria stage		
Kidney function stage	GFR (mL/min/1.73m²)	Normal (UACR, mg/mmol male: < 2.5 female: < 3.5)	Microalbuminuria (UACR, mg/mmol male: 2.5–25 female: 3.5–35)	Macroalbuminuria (UACR, mg/mmol male: > 25 female: > 35)
1	> 90	Not CKD unless haematuria, structural or pathological abnormalities present		
2	60–89			
3a	45–59			
3b	30–44			
4	15–29			
5	<15 or on dialysis			

Combine eGFR stage (1–5), albuminuria stage and underlying diagnosis to fully specify CKD stage (eg. stage 2 CKD with microalbuminuria secondary to diabetic kidney disease).
Refer to colour-coded action plans in *Chronic kidney disease (CKD) management in general practice.* 2nd ed. Kidney Health Australia, 2012

Source: Johnson et al. (2012).

The impact of CKD on Aboriginal and Torres Strait Islander people is profound, particularly in the latter stages of the disease. To ensure ongoing, effective treatment, some patients may need to be away from their family and community for lengthy periods to attend specialist appointments, undergo surgical procedures, such as the formation of a fistula to facilitate dialysis, or learn to self-dialyse in the community, if that is an option. The increasing use of telehealth and remote dialysis services are allowing more Aboriginal and Torres Strait Islander patients to remain in their community while receiving care for CKD.

Stages of CKD are categorised into six stages according to the level of remaining kidney function. Two tests can be conducted to measure the level of kidney function/damage, including a serum estimated glomerular filtration rate (eGFR) and a urine sample to determine a patient's albumin to creatinine ratio (ACR). The normal range for eGFR is between 90 and 130 ml/min/1.73m^2, depending on a person's gender, although it naturally decreases as a person ages. The normal range for ACR is 1.0 – <2.5 mg/mmol for males and 1.0 – <3.5 mg/mmol for females. Figure 2.4 identifies the stages of CKD.

CASE STUDY 2.1

Working as a remote area nurse: a true story

As an English migrant to Australia, I was very interested in learning more about the Indigenous culture and seeing more of Australia. This led to me working as a RAN in a remote community in the Northern Territory. When I first arrived, I felt completely out of my comfort zone. My ICU scrubs were replaced by more casual attire, and my work hours had changed from 12-hour shifts to Monday to Friday clinic hours, plus a number of on-call shifts over the week. I worked in a large clinic compared to smaller communities — four RANs, two Aboriginal health practitioners and one doctor serviced the community with about 1200 people.

We started the day with a handover of the overnight patient presentations and determined which one needed follow up in the clinic. One nurse and Aboriginal health worker would then drive around the community to collect the patients and bring them to the clinic to be followed up. Patients would present to the clinic with a vast array of problems or concerns in addition to regular health checks. I realised how varied this role was and just how multi-skilled RANs and Aboriginal health practitioners were.

As I started to learn more about the role and consult with patients, I realised the anxieties I had about communicating with Indigenous Australians. I felt like I was walking on eggshells initially, scared to say or do anything wrong, but my confidence grew the more I engage with them. I realised that they had so much to teach me, and I loved working collaboratively with families, learning about their culture, and teaching them a little about mine. Some days and weeks were harder than others. The on-call shifts could be very busy and leave us short staffed in the clinic the following day if the nurse needed a sleep break. Nevertheless, this was the most clinically diverse, autonomous, enriching role I had worked in and I would encourage any nursing student to consider the option of remote area nursing in the future.

Question

Imagine working as a RAN for the day. What common conditions do you think you may come across?

Answer

The role of a RAN is incredibly varied. You could be consulting with patients presenting with infections such as pneumonia, skin sores (impetigo) or mental health problems, and those coming for their monthly Bicillin injections, chronic disease checks, maternity check-ups or emergencies.

CASE STUDY 2.2

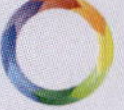

Nursing care of a stable patient

Mr Jaragba is a 46-year-old Indigenous man who presented to the local clinic for his chronic disease check. His blood test revealed that his eGFR has reduced from 34 to 29. The patient has a medical history of being hypertensive and was a smoker. He states that he has been feeling tired and not passing urine often. He noticed that his ankles are more swollen than what they were a few days ago.

A physical examination and observations revealed the following:

- temperature: 37.1°C
- heart rate: 90 beats per minute
- blood pressure: 150/90 mmHg
- respiratory rate: 20 breaths per minute
- oxygen saturation: 96% on room air.

Question

Using the information above, describe what action you would take as the nurse caring for this patient. Use the clinical reasoning cycle to guide you through the process and devise a care plan for your patient.

Answer

- *Step 1: Consider the patient.* Mr Jaragba, a 46-year-old Indigenous man.
- *Step 2: Collect cues/information.* Include subjective and objective data here, include the appearance of the patient, and their past medical history. He states that he is feeling tired and has a reduced urine output. His eGFR has reduced from 34 to 29. Objective data will include measurable information such as his vital signs.
- *Step 3: Process information.* Separate the relevant and irrelevant data — cluster the clues together to formulate an inference about the patient. Mr Jaragba's recent blood tests revealed that he has worsening kidney function, which could explain the excess fluid in his ankles. He is now considered a stage 4 CKD patient.
- *Step 4: Identify problems/issues.* Nursing problems or diagnosis should be listed here. Mr Jaragba's priority nursing problems are renal perfusion, risk of infection, and risk of fluid volume and electrolyte imbalance.
- *Step 5: Establish goals.* Goals of care for Mr Jaragba should focus on preserving his kidney function and planning for renal dialysis.
- *Step 6: Take action.* The nurse should weigh the patient to determine if he has any excess fluid on board (his dry weight will be documented on file). The nurse should discuss their findings with the patient and arrange for a review by the renal physician. This may be done via telehealth if the patient would like to stay in his community. The nurse may also ask the doctor to consider prescribing a diuretic, such as furosemide, to remove the excess fluid. A full medication review will need to be completed by the doctor to ensure the patient is not taking any medications that are toxic to the kidneys.
- *Step 7: Evaluate outcomes.* The patient will return to the clinic for a review in 24 hours and be weighed by the nurse to determine whether the excess fluid has been removed.
- *Step 8: Reflect on the process and new learning.* Reflect on any aspects of care that could have been done better.

CASE STUDY 2.3

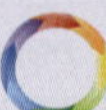 Nursing care of an unstable patient

David is an 11-year-old Indigenous male. He presents with a fever of 39 degrees, joint pain and swelling, along with subcutaneous nodules. The symptoms have been present now for 4 days. Two days ago, his right knee was painful and swollen, but today it has improved. The joints involved today include the right ankle and left knee. They are quite tender, painful and swollen. He is now unable to walk because of the pain.

David's observations are:

- temperature: 39°C
- heart rate: 120 beats per minute
- respiratory rate: 22 breaths per minute
- blood pressure: 100/60 mmHg
- oxygen saturation: 95% on room air
- he has a history of a sore throat 2 weeks ago.

Question

Using the information above, describe what action you would take as the nurse caring for this patient. Use the clinical reasoning cycle to guide you through the process and devise a care plan for your patient.

Answer

- *Step 1: Consider the patient.* David, an 11-year-old Indigenous male.
- *Step 2: Collect cues/information.* Include subjective and objective data here, including the patient's appearance and their past medical history.
  - Temperature of 39 degrees.
  - Joint pain and swelling.
  - Subcutaneous nodules.
  - History of a sore throat 2 weeks ago.

  The symptoms have been present now for 4 days. Two days ago, his right knee was painful and swollen, but today it has improved. The joints involved today include the right ankle and left knee. He is now unable to walk because of the pain.

- *Step 3: Process information:* Separate the relevant and irrelevant data — cluster the clues together to formulate an inference about the patient. David has a history of a sore throat 2 weeks ago, and has since developed polyarthritis, a fever and subcutaneous nodules. These symptoms are characteristic of acute rheumatic fever.
- *Step 4: Identify problems/issues.* Nursing problems or diagnosis should be listed here. David's priority nursing problems are risk of infection, impaired physical mobility and acute pain.
- *Step 5: Establish goals.* Goals of care for David should focus on treating his pain.
- *Step 6: Take action.* The nurse should focus on administering analgesia to relieve the patient's pain. A doctor will also consider prescribing an anti-inflammatory to reduce the swelling and penicillin to treat the infection. Blood tests will need to be taken, and the nurse should always follow the clinical guidelines for treating acute rheumatic fever.
- *Step 7: Evaluate outcomes.* The patient will continue to have their observations reassessed for signs of improvement.
- *Step 8: Reflect on the process and new learning.* Reflect on any aspects of care that could have been done better.

SUMMARY

The social determinants of health undermine the health of the population. For Indigenous Australians, cultural identity, family and connection to their traditional lands are essential for their health and wellbeing outcomes. This chapter discussed the Closing the Gap strategy and the National Agreement, which employs Aboriginal and Torres Strait Islander people in a strengths-based approach to determine what is important to them.

The role of the RAN is varied and complex. It encompasses a family-centred approach to care and the ability to care for patients with a great variety of conditions. This chapter discussed the much higher risk of chronic disease that face Indigenous Australians with poorer access to healthcare for those living in rural or remote communities.

KEY TERMS

acute rheumatic fever A condition caused by an abnormal immune response following an untreated bacterial infection with group A streptococcus.

chronic kidney disease (CKD) A progressive disease of the kidneys which leads to worsening kidney function.

diabetes A medical condition affecting the release of insulin from the pancreas. There are two types: type 1 is an autoimmune disease where the patient is wholly dependent upon insulin. Type 2 is caused by a poor lifestyle, and patients may or may not be dependent upon insulin.

Indigenous Australians People with familial heritage to groups that lived in Australia before British colonisation. They include the Aboriginal and Torres Strait Islander peoples.

remote area An area that is distant from a metropolitan or rural area and has limited access to services.

remote area nurses (RANs) Nurses working in a remote area of Australia with an advanced scope of practice.

social determinants of health A number of factors that can affect health outcomes for individuals, including access to health services, an individual's knowledge of health and capabilities, environmental factors, education and income.

telehealth A consultation with a healthcare provider by phone or video call.

REFERENCES

Australian Bureau of Statistics (ABS). (2018) Estimates of Aboriginal and Torres Strait Islander Australians. www.abs.gov.au/statistics/people/aboriginal-and-torres-strait-islander-peoples/estimates-aboriginal-and-torres-strait-islander-australians/latest-release

Australian Bureau of Statistics (ABS). (2021) *Population clock.* www.abs.gov.au/ausstats/abs%40.nsf/94713ad445ff1425ca25682000192af2/1647509ef7e25faaca2568a900154b63?OpenDocument

Australian Digital Health Agency. (n.d.) *What is in a My Health Record?* www.myhealthrecord.gov.au/for-healthcare-professionals/what-is-in-my-health-record

Australian Indigenous Health Info Net. (n.d.) *Closing the Gap.* https://healthinfonet.ecu.edu.au/learn/health-system/closing-the-gap/

Australian Institute of Health and Welfare (AIHW). (2019) *Acute rheumatic fever and rheumatic heart disease in Australia.* www.aihw.gov.au/getmedia/59ea3d1b-dc00-42df-8831-d40f7bdf2bad/Acute-rheumatic-fever-and-rheumatic-heart-disease-in-Australia.pdf.aspx?inline=true

Commonwealth of Australia, D. o. t. P. M. a. C. (2018) *Closing the Gap Prime Minister's report 2018.* www.pmc.gov.au/sites/default/files/reports/closing-the-gap-2018/sites/default/files/ctg-report-20183872.pdf?a=1

Department of Health. (2015) *Telehealth.* www1.health.gov.au/internet/main/publishing.nsf/Content/e-health-telehealth

Department of Health. (2019) *Better access telehealth initiative for rural and remote patients guidelines.* https://tinyurl.com/y3zcabt5

Department of Health. (2020) *Aboriginal and Torres Strait Islander health.* www.health.gov.au/health-topics/aboriginal-and-torres-strait-islander-health

Economic, U. N. D. o., Issues, P. F. o. I. & Division, U. N. S. (2009) *State of the world's indigenous peoples* (Vol. 9). United Nations Publications.

Health, A. I. o. & Welfare. (2020a) *Profile of Indigenous Australians.* www.aihw.gov.au/reports/australias-health/profile-of-indigenous-australians

Health, A. I. o. & Welfare. (2020b) *Profiles of Aboriginal and Torres Strait Islander people with kidney disease.* www.aihw.gov.au/reports/indigenous-australians/profiles-of-aboriginal-and-tsi-people-with-kidney

Health, A. I. o. & Welfare. (2020c) *Social determinants and Indigenous health.* www.aihw.gov.au/reports/australias-health/social-determinants-and-indigenous-health

Johnson, D. W. et al. (2016) Chronic kidney disease and measurement of albuminuria or proteinuria: a position statement. *Medical Journal of Australia.* 197: 224– 225.

King, M., Smith, A. & Gracey, M. (2009) Indigenous health part 2: the underlying causes of the health gap. *The Lancet.* 374(9683): 76–85.

Menzies School of Health Research. (n.d.) *Rheumatic heart disease.* www.menzies.edu.au/page/Research/Global_and_Tropical_Health/Rheumatic_Heart_Disease/#:~:text=Australia%20has%20one%20of%20the,people%20die%20from%20the%20disease

Nursing and Midwifery Board of Australia. (2019) *Endorsement for scheduled medicines for registered nurses (rural and isolated practice).* www.nursingmidwiferyboard.gov.au/Codes-Guidelines-Statements/FAQ/Fact-sheet-RN-endorsement-for-scheduled-medicines-rural-and-isolated-practice.aspx

RHDAustralia. (2020) *What is acute rheumatic fever?* www.rhdaustralia.org.au/what-acute-rheumatic-fever

RHDAustralia. (2020) *The 2020 Australian guideline for prevention, diagnosis and management of acute rheumatic fever and rheumatic heart disease*, 3rd ed. (pp 74–75). www.rhdaustralia.org.au/arf-rhd-guideline

ACKNOWLEDGEMENTS

Figure 2.1: © CareFlight.

Figure 2.4: © Johnson, D. W. et al. (2012) Chronic kidney disease and measurement of albuminuria or proteinuria: a position statement. *Medical Journal of Australia.* 197: 224–225. Reproduced with permission of John Wiley & Sons.

Table 2.1: © RHDAustralia (ARF/RHD writing group). *The 2020 Australian guideline for prevention, diagnosis and management of acute rheumatic fever and rheumatic heart disease* (3rd edition); 2020 pp. 74–75. Reproduced with permission of Menzies School of Health Research.

Photo 2A: © Johnny Greig / Getty Images

Extract 2.1: © Productivity Commission, 'Priority Reform 1, Formal partnerships and shared decision-making'. Licensed under CC BY 3.0 AU.

CHAPTER 3

Principles of infection prevention and control

LEARNING OBJECTIVES

After studying this chapter, you should be able to:

3.1 discuss the pathology of infection to support infection prevention and control in the clinical setting

3.2 explain the relevance of infection prevention and control in healthcare-associated infections (HAIs)

3.3 identify the role of the nurse in reducing and preventing antimicrobial resistance

3.4 apply the established clinical protocols that protect patients and staff in healthcare settings

3.5 reflect on the clinical reasoning cycle and its application to infection prevention and control

3.6 discuss the importance of patient-centred care in infection prevention and control.

Introduction

Healthcare-associated infections (HAI) and antimicrobial resistance are a significant threat to public health (Burnett 2018). The World Health Organization (WHO) defines HAI as 'an infection occurring in a patient during the process of care in a hospital or other healthcare facility which was not present or incubating at the time of admission' (WHO 2020b). All healthcare providers must understand the importance of **infection** prevention and control (National Health and Medical Research Council [NHMRC] 2019). According to the WHO, HAI can affect patients in any care setting and can present after discharge. HAI include occupational infections among healthcare providers and other persons who work in healthcare settings. Global data indicates that millions of patients contact HAI (WHO 2020b).

As new and resistant organisms continue to emerge and evolve, and antimicrobial agents become less effective, infection prevention and control are vital in maintaining public health, particularly among vulnerable patient groups such as the elderly, people with chronic diseases, people on immune suppressant therapy, people undergoing cancer treatment and young children (Caresearch 2020). As members of the healthcare team, nurses are leaders in practising infection prevention and controlling the spread of infection (Benson & Powers 2011). This is a fundamental element of nursing practice, and all healthcare professionals have the responsibility to adhere to evidence-based guidelines to control infection in the clinical setting. This chapter will discuss the pathology of infection, HAI and infection prevention and control, such as hand hygiene, personal protective equipment (PPE).

3.1 The pathology of infection

LEARNING OBJECTIVE 3.1 Discuss the pathology of infection to support infection prevention and control in the clinical setting.

Most infectious agents are **microorganisms**. Microorganisms live in continuous interaction with their environment — the human body is part of that environment. Dependent on the host's susceptibility, parasites, prions and some classes of microorganism such as bacteria, viruses, fungi and protozoa can be involved in either colonisation or infection. **Colonisation** occurs when bacteria grow on the body but do not cause infection. This is a natural process. An infection occurs when microorganisms enter the body, increase in number and then cause the body to react to the microorganism (Centers for Disease Control [CDC] 2016). The main gateway for microbes to enter the human body is the skin and mucosal surfaces of the gastrointestinal, respiratory and urogenital tracts. Interaction with bacteria leads to colonisation of these mucous membranes.

For an infection to occur, there must be a:

- causative agent: i.e. a **pathogen**
- a source: places where microorganisms live, including, but not limited to, other patients, visitors, healthcare workers, patient care equipment and dust or debris
- a susceptible person: a person who is not vaccinated or has a weak immune system
- a **locus**: a way for the microorganisms to enter the body, such as the mouth, or a wound
- a means of transmission: a way for the microorganisms to move to the susceptible person via other people, the environment and/or medical equipment.

A patient is more vulnerable to infection due to:

- invasive procedures such as insertion of a central or peripheral line or surgery
- pharmaceutical agents, such as immunosuppressants
- increased exposure to pathogens in the care setting
- compromised circulation
- chronic disease
- rupture of amniotic membrane
- lack of immunisation
- trauma, such as tissue damage and broken skin
- decreased haemoglobin and suppressed immune system
- an inflammatory response
- lack of knowledge or performance of infection control measures by the patient or the healthcare provider (Doenges et al. 2019).

Microorganisms that cause healthcare-acquired infection (HAI) can be acquired in various ways. **Endogenous microbes** are infections caused by an overgrowth of the bacteria present in a person's normal gut flora. This may be triggered by tissue damage and the transmission of bacteria to sites outside their natural habitat. For example, gram-negative bacteria in the digestive tract can cause surgical site infections after abdominal surgery, or urinary tract infections can occur if a urinary catheter was used and appropriate infection control and prevention procedures were not followed. Inappropriate use of antibiotic therapy can also allow for the overgrowth of organisms, such as *Clostridioides difficile* or a pathogenic yeast species such as *Candida albicans*.

Exogenous microbes or cross-infections are caused by the transmission of microorganisms from another patient or member of staff.

Microorganisms are transmitted to patients:

- through direct contact between patients via hands, saliva droplets or other body fluids
- via contaminated droplets or dust in the air
- via staff engaged in direct patient care who become transient or permanent **carriers**, subsequently transmitting microorganisms to other patients by direct contact during care via hands, clothes or nose and throat
- via objects contaminated by the patient, including equipment, the staff's hands, visitors, or other environmental sources such as food and water.

Endemic or epidemic exogenous environmental infections are caused by the transmission of microorganisms from the healthcare environment. In a healthcare setting, the modes of transmission of infectious agents are direct and indirect contact, including bloodborne pathogens, droplet transmission and airborne transmission. Figure 3.1 shows the chain of infection transmission. Several microorganisms survive well in the hospital environment. Examples of these are pseudomonas, acinetobacter and mycobacterium.

They can be found in:

- water, damp areas and occasionally in **sterile** products or disinfectants
- linen, equipment and supplies used in care provision. Good hygiene typically limits the risk of bacteria surviving since most microorganisms require humid or hot conditions as well as nutrients to survive
- food
- fine dust and droplet nuclei generated by coughing or speaking.
  Microorganisms smaller than 10 microns in diameter remain in the air for several hours and can be inhaled in the same way as fine dust.

FIGURE 3.1 The chain of infection transmission

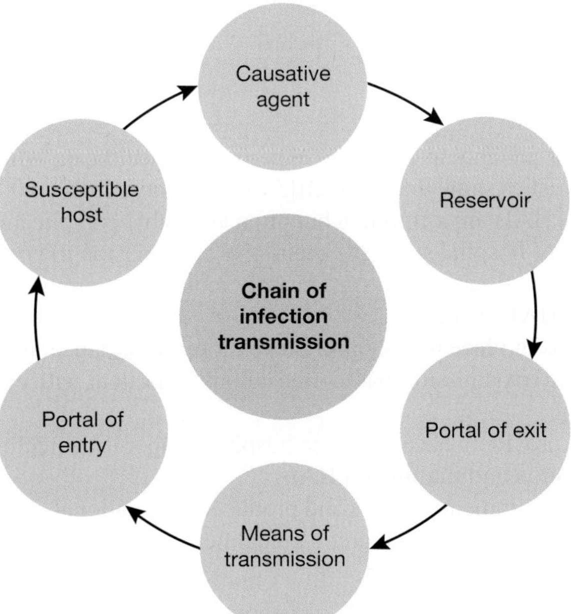

Source: National Health and Medical Research Council (NHMRC), *Australian Guidelines for the Prevention and Control of Infection in Healthcare* p. 15.

3.2 Healthcare-associated infections (HAIs)

LEARNING OBJECTIVE 3.2 Explain the relevance of infection prevention and control in healthcare-associated infections (HAIs).

Healthcare-associated infections (HAIs), in most cases, come from other patients, healthcare providers, healthcare workers and visitors to a healthcare setting. Infection is a complex interrelationship between a **host** and the infectious agent. People respond to a pathogen in different ways. Some people are colonised but never develop symptoms; some exhibit minor symptoms and recover quickly, while others become acutely ill, which may result in death. The outcome of exposure to a pathogen depends on the pathogen's virulence, the individual's immunity, their age and **comorbidities** such as diabetes or COPD (see figure 3.2).

FIGURE 3.2 Factors affecting susceptibility to HAIs

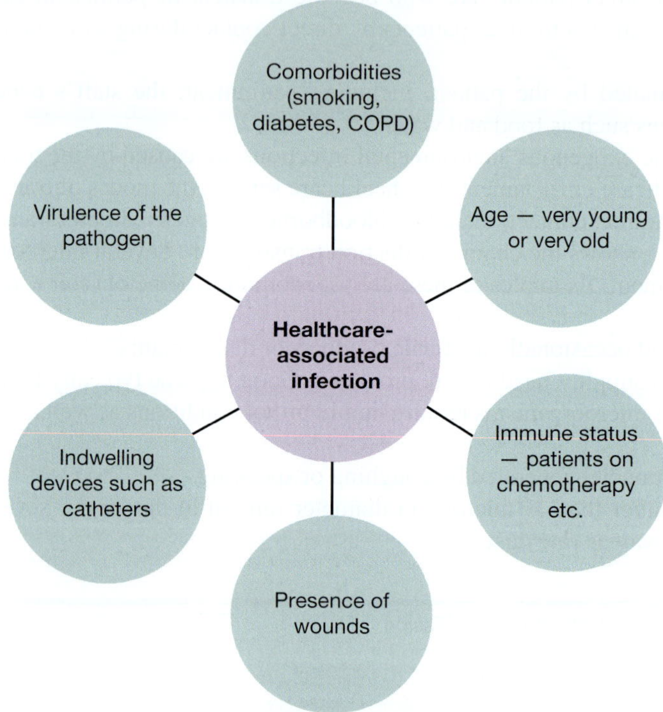

Source: Adapted from ACSQHC (2018).

Each year, many hospital patients in Australia experience a healthcare complication in the form of a HAI (ACSQHC 2018). Statistics show that from 2015 to 2016, more than 60 000 HAIs were diagnosed in Australian public hospitals. HAIs are a common but often avoidable complication of hospitalisation. They increase morbidity, lengths of hospital stays and the risk of readmission to hospital within 12 months.

All HAIs and their complications can be significantly reduced by providing patient care that reduces risks. Risk management of HAIs includes:

- safety and quality systems in place that support prevention, surveillance, management of care
- processes for standard and transmission-based precautions consistent with evidence-based best-practice guideline
- ensuring that healthcare providers have access to hospital-supported guidelines
- providing ongoing education and training on HAIs
- ensuring that all medical equipment, devices and products meet national and international standards are available for use consistent with manufacturer's guidelines
- ensuring a clean and hygienic environment.

Standard precautions

Standard precautions are work practices that apply to everyone (see figure 3.3). Standard precautions act as a first-line approach to infection prevention and control. Healthcare providers employ standard precautions to reduce the potential for HAIs and to reduce the risk of transmitting pathogens to public areas or taking them home. Standard precautions include:

- hand hygiene following the '5 Moments for Hand Hygiene'
- practising respiratory hygiene and cough etiquette
- appropriate use of and appropriate putting on and taking off of PPE, which include gloves, gowns, plastic aprons, masks, eye protection and face shields
- aseptic technique, which aims to prevent microorganisms on hands, surfaces or equipment from being introduced into a susceptible site, such as an open wound or broken skin
- safe handling and disposal of sharps
- appropriate handling of waste and linen
- Routine environmental cleaning
- appropriate reprocessing of shared patient equipment.

FIGURE 3.3 Standard precautions

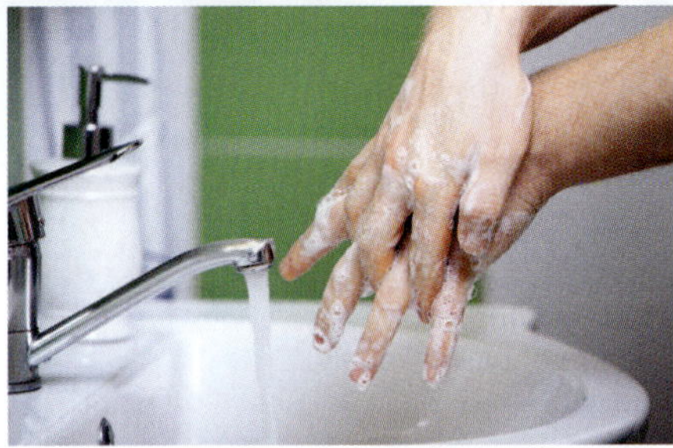

Maintain hand hygiene — before and after any patient contact.

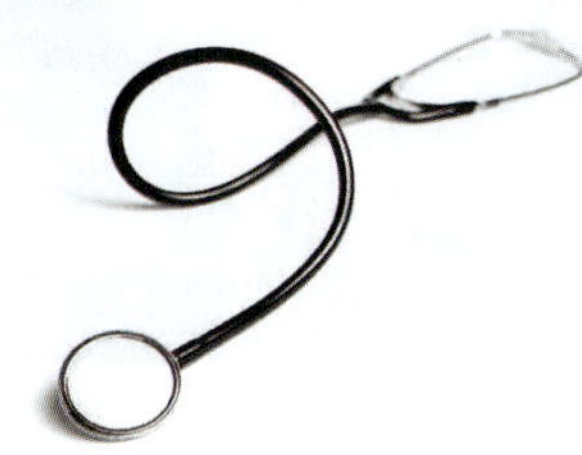

Ensure any shared patient equipment is routinely cleaned after use.

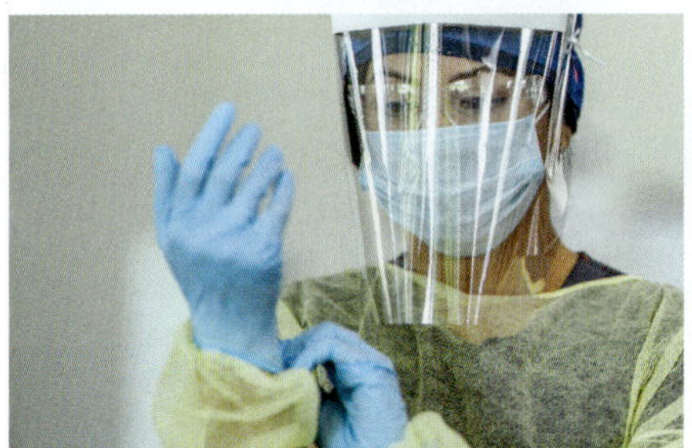

Always use PPE if coming into contact with bodily fluids.

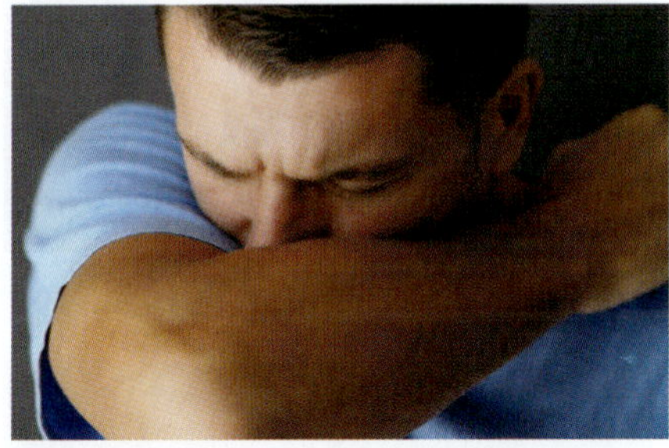

Follow respiratory hygiene and cough etiquette.

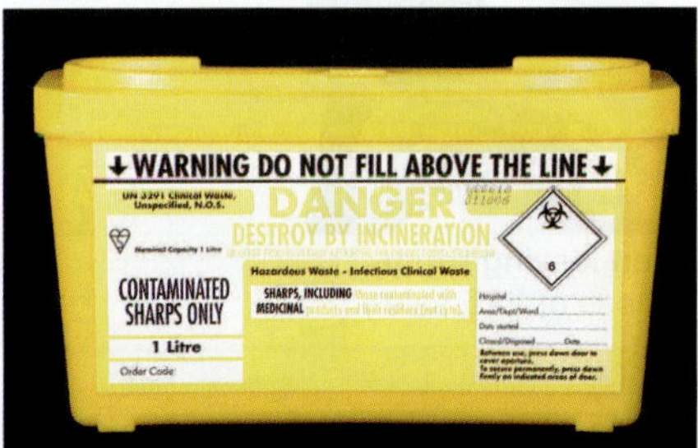

Use and dispose of sharps safely.

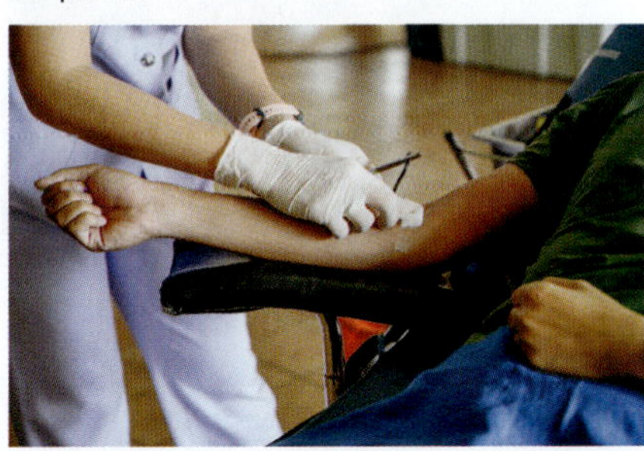

Maintain aseptic technique.

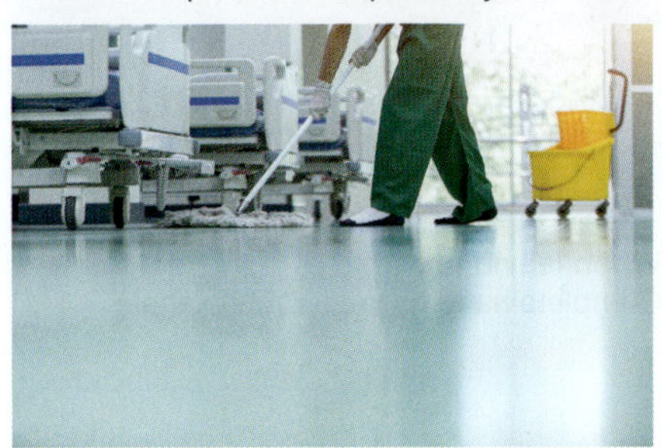

Ensure all areas undergo routine cleaning.

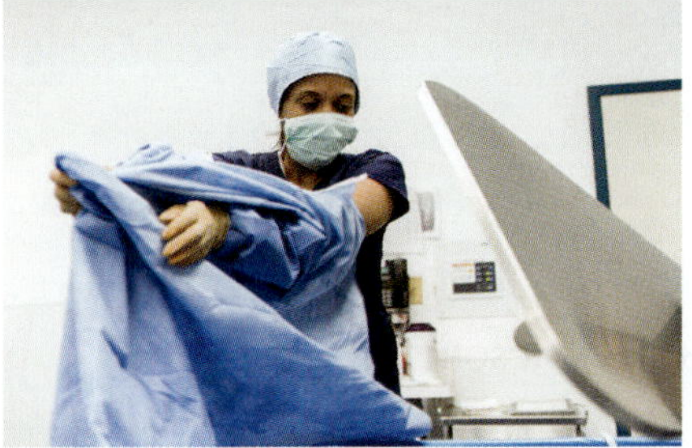

Safely dispose of waste and used linen.

Source: Adapted from ACSQHC (2012).

Contact transmission

The most common route of transmission of HAI is by direct or indirect contact (NHMRC 2019). Direct transmission occurs when a pathogen is transferred by body fluids to another person. For example, when a healthcare provider has contact with a patient's blood through a cut on the skin. Indirect transmission takes place when the pathogen is transferred to a contaminated intermediary. An example of this is when a healthcare provider transmits the pathogen from one patient to the next due to poor hand hygiene practices. Pathogens that are easily transmitted via contact are *Clostridioides difficile* and norovirus, and highly contagious skin infections/infestations such as impetigo and scabies. Contact precautions are part of the standard precautions for infection control (see figure 3.4).

FIGURE 3.4 Contact precautions in addition to standard precautions

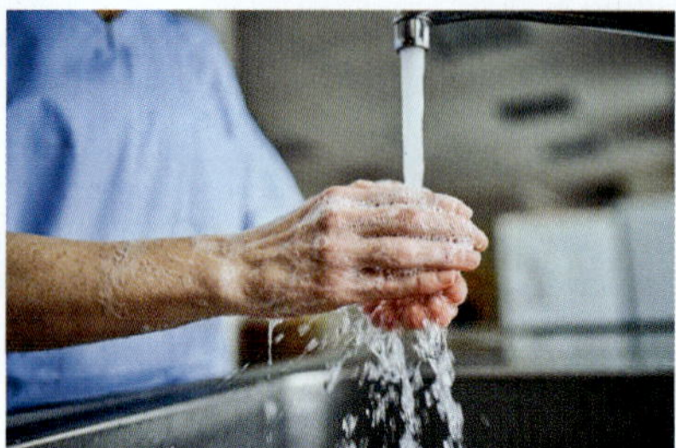

Before entering room
Complete hand hygiene routine.

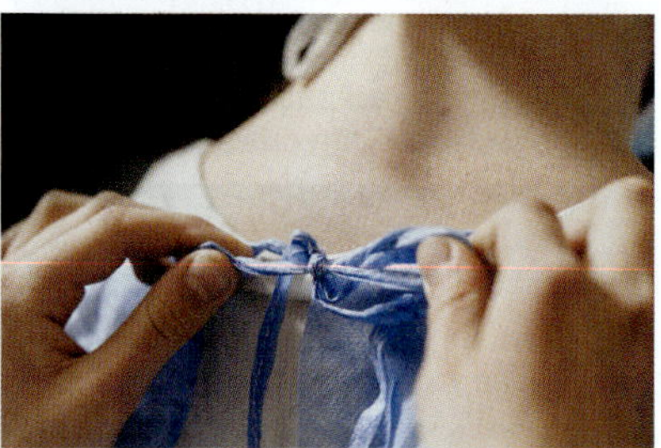

Before entering room
Put on PPE — gown or apron.

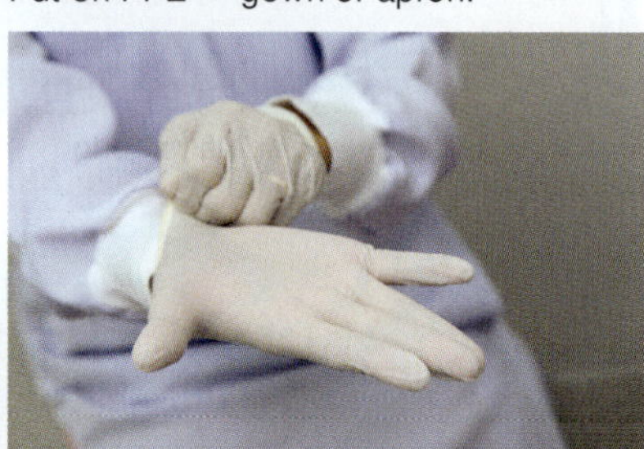

Before entering room
Put on PPE — gloves.

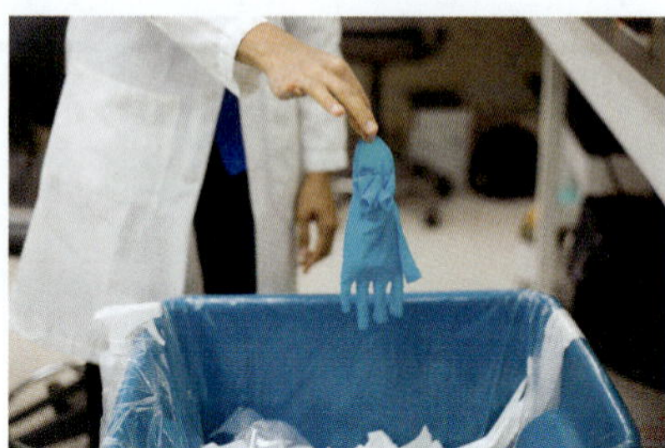

When leaving room
Dispose of gloves safely.

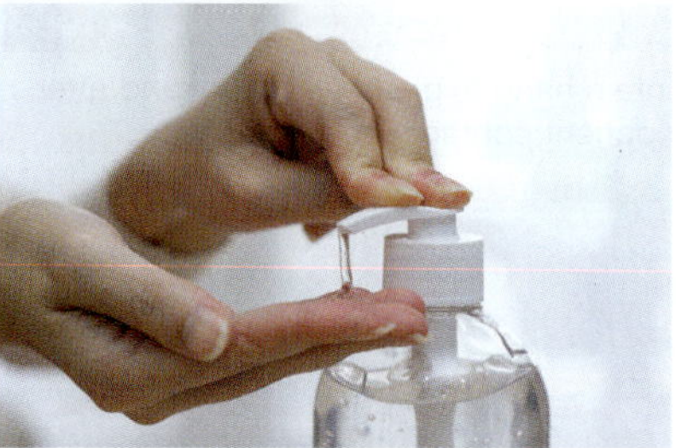

When leaving room
Complete hand hygiene routine again.

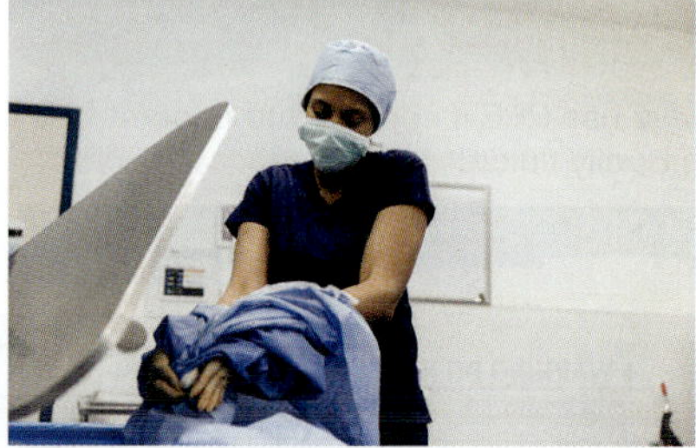

When leaving room
Dispose of PPE safely.

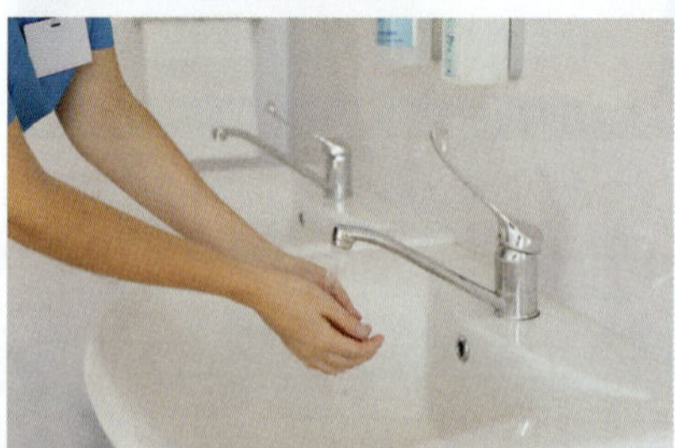

When leaving room
Complete hand hygiene routine again.

Source: Adapted from ACSQHC (2012).

Droplet transmission

A number of infectious agents are transmitted through respiratory droplet (i.e. large-particle droplets >5 microns in size), generated by a patient who is coughing, sneezing or talking (NHMRC 2019). The infected droplets travel directly from the infected person's respiratory tract to nasal, conjunctival or oral mucosal surfaces of another person. Droplet transmission is limited by the force of expulsion and gravity, and takes place when people are less than1 meter apart (WHO 2020c). COVID-19 caused by the SARS-CoV-2 virus is an example of a virus that spreads via droplet transmission when an infected person is in close contact with another person. Other examples of droplet transmission are the influenza virus and meningococcal infection. Droplet precautions are part of the standard precautions for infection control (see figure 3.5).

FIGURE 3.5 Droplet precautions in addition to standard precautions

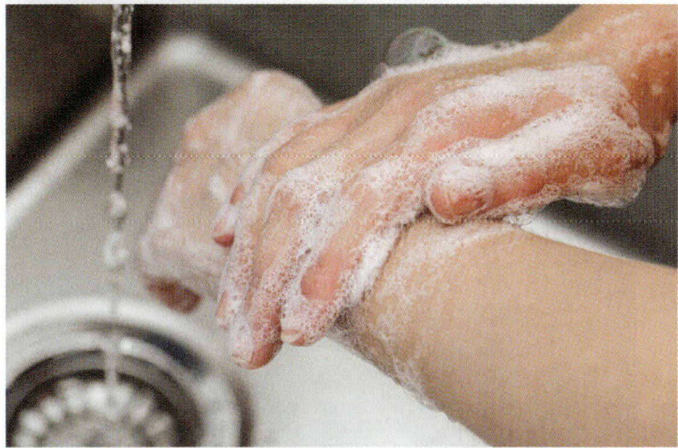

Before entering room
Complete hand hygiene routine.

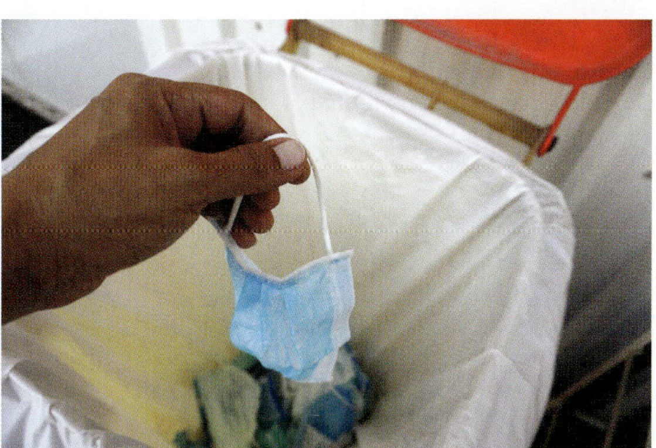

When leaving room
Dispose of surgical mask safely.

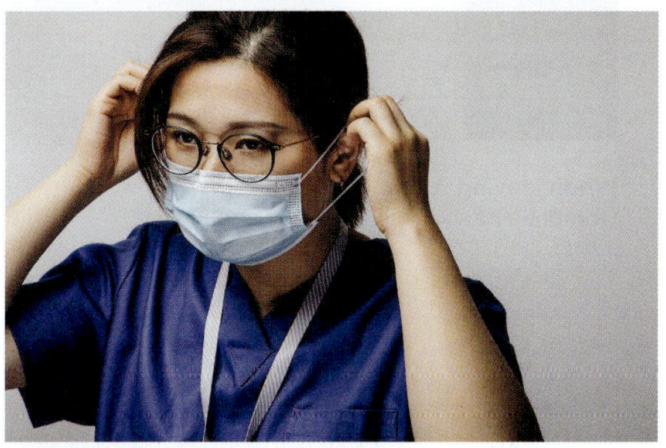

Before entering room
Put on surgical mask.

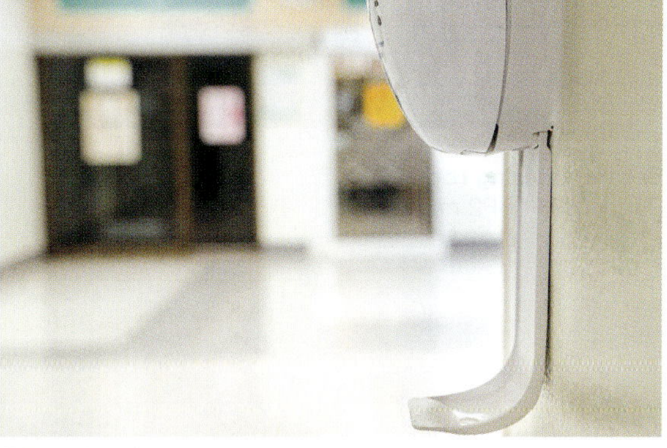

When leaving room
Complete hand hygiene routine again.

Source: Adapted from ACSQHC (2012).

Airborne transmission

Airborne transmission occurs when particles containing pathogens that remain infective over time and distance are transmitted from person to person (NHMRC 2019). These particles are often smaller than 5 microns and are generated by breathing, talking, coughing, sneezing or by the evaporation of larger droplets in low humidity (Atkinson et al. 2009). Aerosols containing pathogens can also be spread over longer distances by ventilation or air conditioning systems, such as *Legionella pneumophila*, *Mycobacterium tuberculosis* and *Measles morbillivirus*. Airborne precautions are part of the standard precautions for infection control (see figure 3.6).

FIGURE 3.6 Airborne precautions in addition to standard precautions

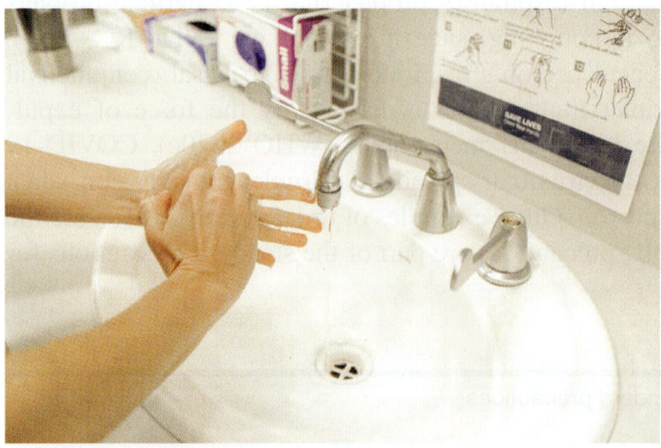

Before entering room
Complete hand hygiene routine.

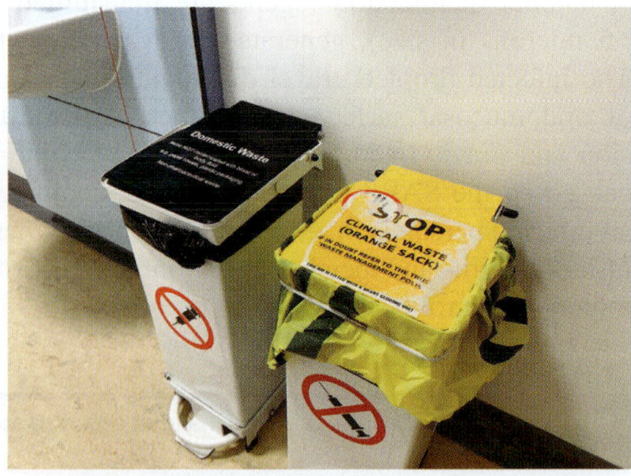

When leaving room
Dispose of mask safely.

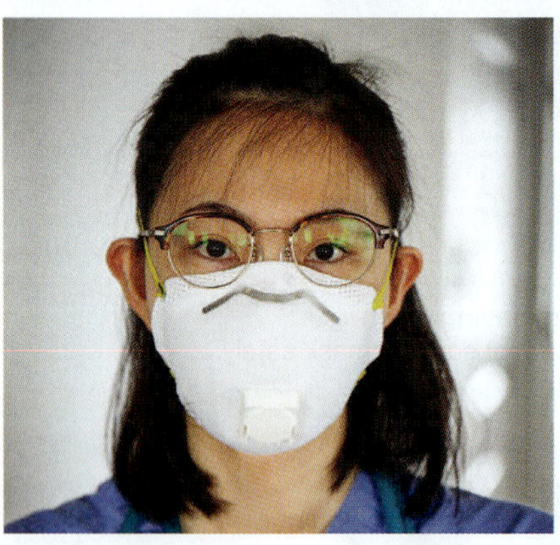

Before entering room
Put on N95 or P2 mask.

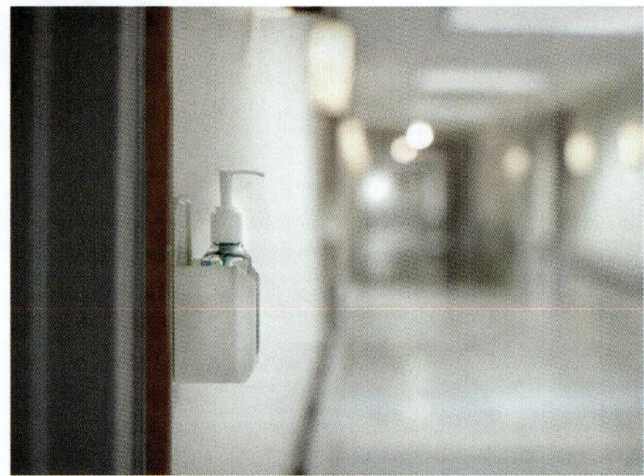

When leaving room
Complete hand hygiene routine again.

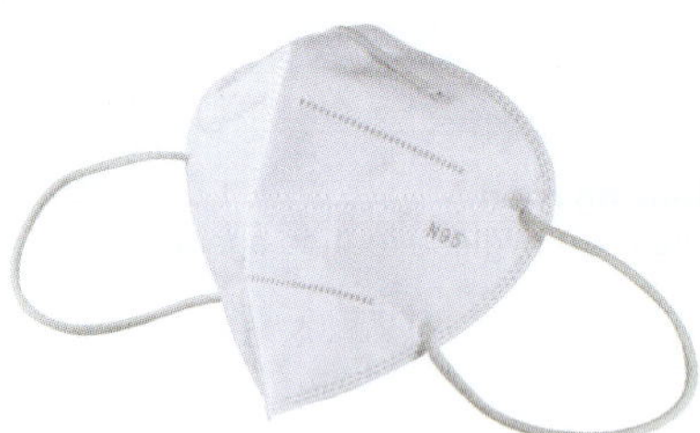

Before entering room
Perform a fit check on the mask.

Source: Adapted from ACSQHC (2012).

3.3 Antimicrobial resistance

LEARNING OBJECTIVE 3.3 Identify the role of the nurse in reducing and preventing antimicrobial resistance.

Antimicrobial resistance (AMR) is one of the top ten public health threats facing humanity globally (WHO 2020a). The WHO (2020a) is confident that AMR inhibits countries' development. Inappropriate and overuse of **antimicrobials** is one of the main causes of the development of drug-resistant pathogens. Without effective antimicrobials, our ability to treat infections, including during major surgery and cancer chemotherapy, would be at increased risk. In 2013, the Australian Commission on Safety and Quality in Health Care (ACSQHC) established a national system for surveillance of AMR and the use of antimicrobials in the healthcare system. Their work has led to the establishment of a National Alert System for Critical Antimicrobial Resistances (CARAlert) and the Australian Passive AMR Surveillance (APAS) system (ACSQHC 2019a). AMR infections are a significant challenge for delivering safe and effective healthcare (Australian Government, Department of Health 2017).

It is essential that as healthcare providers, we:

1. apply best-practice infection prevention and control
2. consider safe alternatives before prescribing antibiotics
3. prescribe using therapeutic guidelines
4. use diagnostics to inform treatment decisions
5. talk with patients about the importance of using antibiotics appropriately and the dangers of antibiotic resistance
6. provide patients with advice on how to manage symptoms without antibiotics
7. talk to patients about prevention of infections through vaccinations, hygiene and handwashing.

3.4 Clinical protocols for infection control

LEARNING OBJECTIVE 3.4 Apply the established clinical protocols that protect patients and staff in healthcare settings.

Hand hygiene

Effective hand hygiene cannot be overestimated in the control and prevention of infection. It is the most critical procedure that healthcare providers can undertake to support infection prevention and control. Healthcare providers' hands are the most common transmission of healthcare-acquired infections (HAI) (Benson & Powers 2011). A microorganism can be transmitted by contact, or droplets can be transmitted by touch. In recognition of the importance of hand hygiene the 'My 5 Moments for Hand Hygiene' (figure 3.7) was developed by the WHO, sets out when healthcare providers and healthcare workers must perform hand hygiene. Hand Hygiene Australia adopted the program and offered online training. Now that the ACSQHC has taken over the training, it is an annual competency for nurses and nursing students in most healthcare and educational settings. This program is an evidence-based, field-tested, user centred approach. It is designed to be logical, easy to understand and learn, and easy to apply across a wide range of settings.

The My 5 Moments for Hand Hygiene approach consists of the following.

1. Before touching a patient.
2. Before clean/aseptic procedures.
3. After body fluid exposure/risk.
4. After touching a patient.
5. After touching patient surroundings.

The Australian National Hand Hygiene Initiative

Poor hand hygiene practices by healthcare providers have a strong link to HAIs, yet compliance remains poor (ACSQHC 2018). The ACSQHC launched a National Hand Hygiene Initiative to promote the education and training in infection control and prevention, increase compliance to hand hygiene to reduce the numbers of HAIs related to lack of compliance (ACSQHC 2019b).

Some of the barriers to hand hygiene that have been reported include the following.

- Hand hygiene agents cause skin dryness and irritation.
- There is a lack of sinks, or they are inconveniently located.
- The misunderstanding that if you use gloves, you do not have to wash your hands.
- High workloads and patient care taking precedence over hand washing.

- Lack of education and training.
- Wearing jewellery and wristwatches on duty.
- Long fingernails, nail polish and artificial nails.

FIGURE 3.7 My 5 Moments for Hand Hygiene

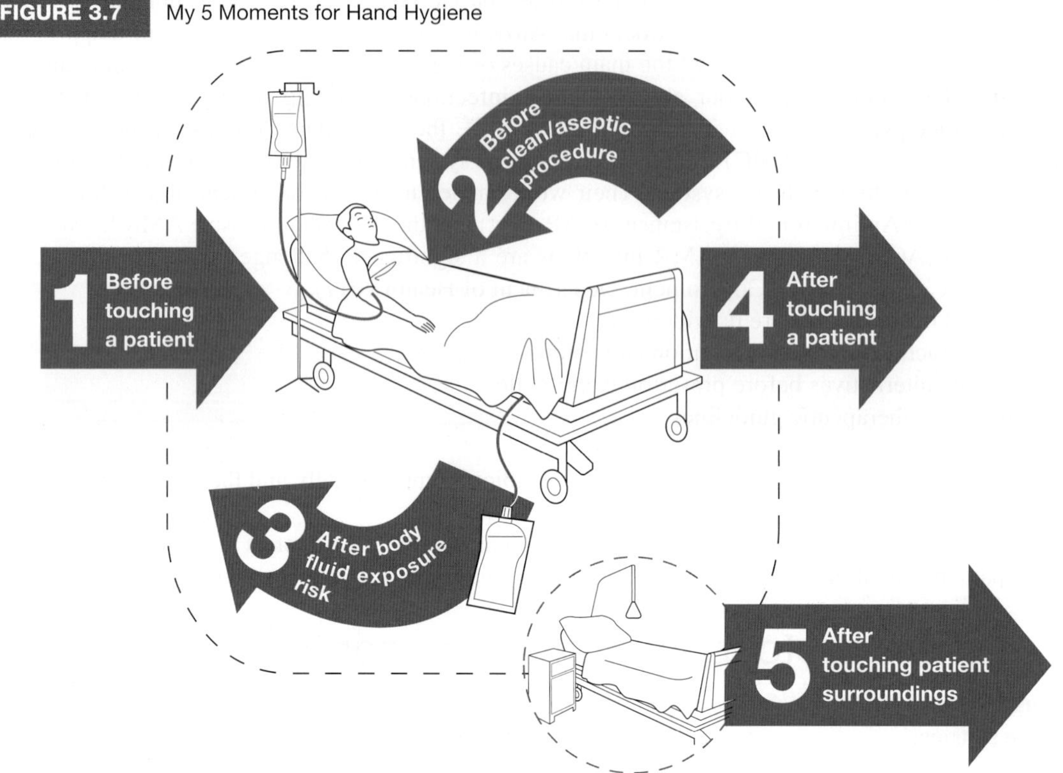

Source: WHO (2020d).

Understanding hand hygiene practices is essential for compliance. Education and training for hand hygiene is an established practice for healthcare providers. As part of the Australian National Hand Hygiene Initiative, nurses, including students, are required to complete an online hand hygiene program annually. Tips for healthcare providers include:

- regular soap is as effective as antibacterial soap
- remember to carry alcohol-based hand sanitiser for ease of access
- cough or sneeze into a tissue or your elbow
- wear disposable gloves before handling bodily fluids
- to support a 20-second hand wash; sing the Happy Birthday song to yourself twice
- take care of your hands, use moisturiser and be conscious of skin irritation (Ausmed Education Pty Ltd. 2020a).

Alcohol-based handrub (ABHR)

Alcohol-based handrub (ABHR) should be available at all points of care in the healthcare setting (Wigglesworth 2019a). Community nurses should carry their own ABHR. Hands that have visible dirt or organic material should be washed with soap and water. The preparation for the use of handrub and for handwashing are:

1. expose forearms (note that nurses are always expected to be bare below the elbows)
2. remove all rings, wristwatches or jewellery
3. ensure fingernails are short and clean
4. artificial nails or nail products are should be not worn
5. any cuts or abrasions are covered with a waterproof dressing.

The sequence for decontaminating hands using ABHR is as follows (also, see figure 3.8).

1. Apply a palmful of hand rub in a cupped hand and cover all surfaces of the hands.
2. Rub palms together.
3. Interlace hands and rub the back of each hand with the palm of the other hand.
4. Rub palms of hands interlaced.
5. Rub back of fingers with fingers interlocked.

6. Rub each thumb clasped in the opposite hand using a rotational movement.
7. Rub tips of fingers in the opposite palm in a circular motion.
8. Allow hands to dry.

FIGURE 3.8 How to use handrub

How to Handrub?

RUB HANDS FOR HAND HYGIENE! WASH HANDS WHEN VISIBLY SOILED

Duration of the entire procedure: 20-30 seconds

1a 1b

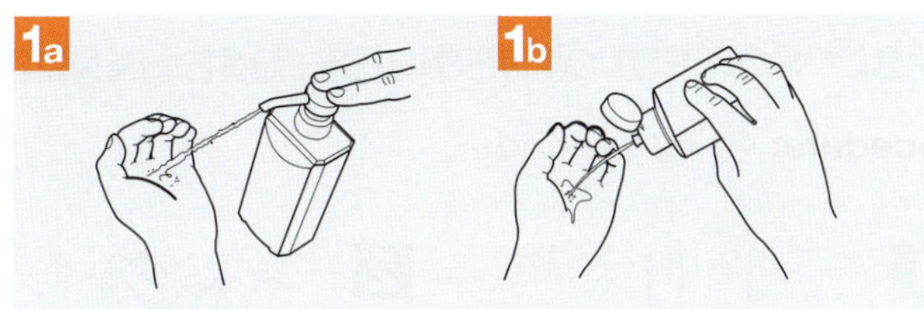

Apply a palmful of the product in a cupped hand, covering all surfaces;

2

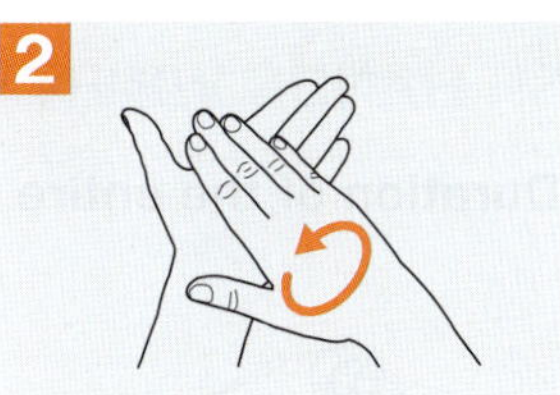

Rub hands palm to palm;

3

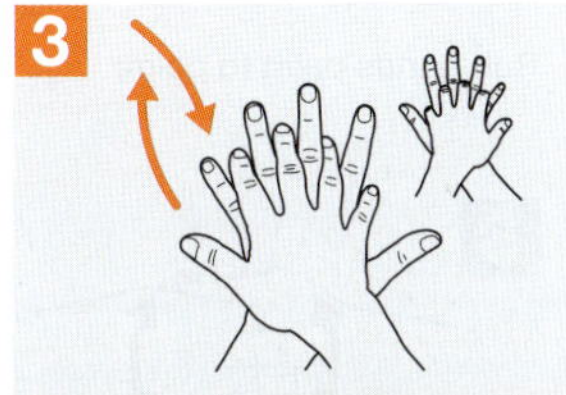

Right palm over left dorsum with interlaced fingers and vice versa;

4

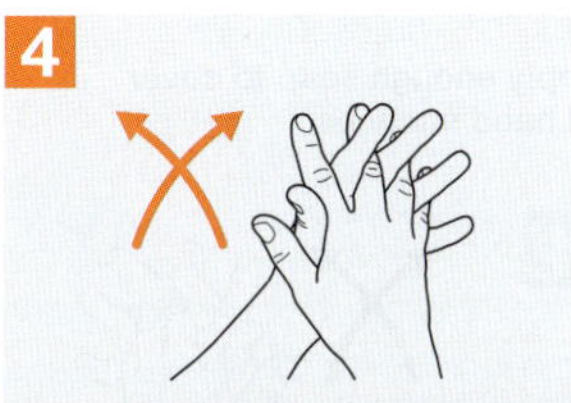

Palm to palm with fingers interlaced;

5

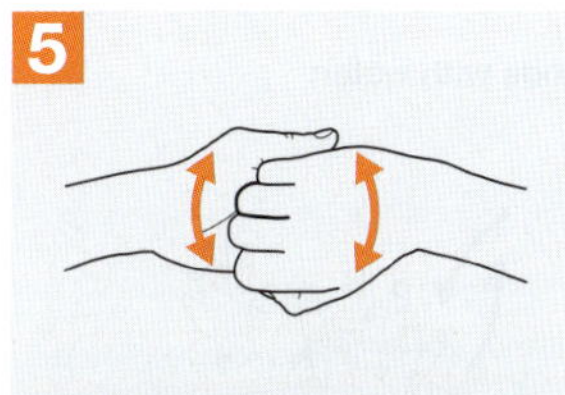

Backs of fingers to opposing palms with fingers interlocked;

6

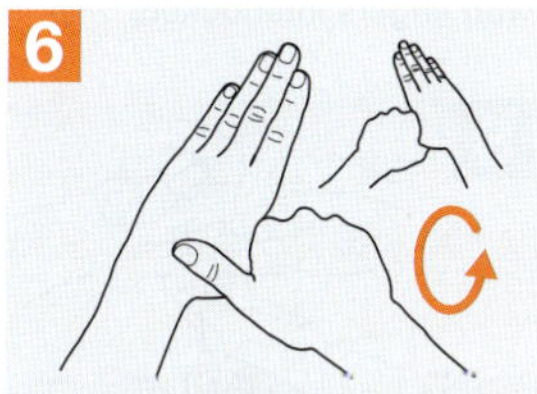

Rotational rubbing of left thumb clasped in right palm and vice versa;

7

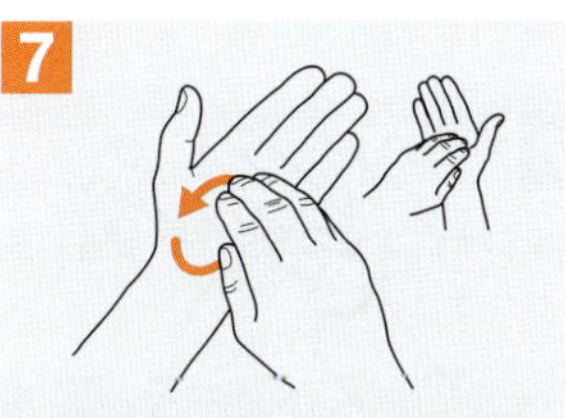

Rotational rubbing, backwards and forwards with clasped fingers of right hand in left palm and vice versa;

8

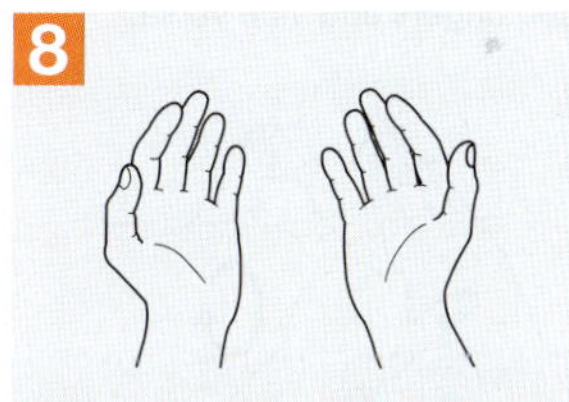

Once dry, your hands are safe.

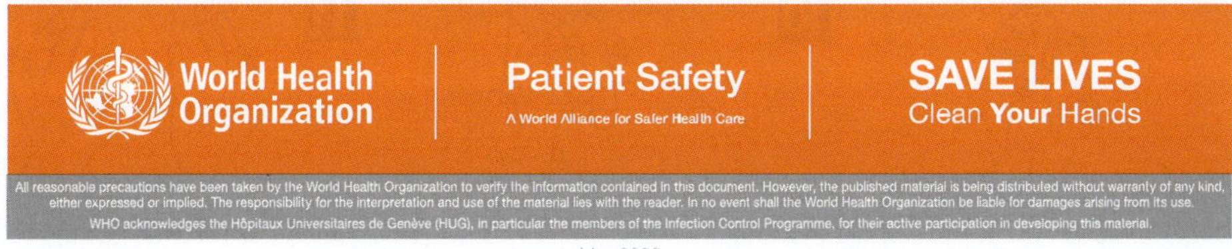

May 2009

Source: WHO (2020d).

Handwashing with soap and water

Handwashing using the soap and water procedure involves preparing, washing, rinsing and drying and should take 40–60 seconds (Wigglesworth 2019b). This handwashing procedure is used when there is visible dirt or grime on hands. The steps for handwashing are outlined below and in figure 3.9.

1. Wet hands under tepid running water.
2. Apply soap to cover all surfaces.
3. Rub hands palm to palm.
4. Rub back of each hand with the palm of other the hand with fingers interlaced.

5. Rub hands with fingers interlaced.
6. Rub with back of fingers to opposing palms with fingers interlocked.
7. Rub each thumb clasped in the opposite hand using a rotational movement.
8. Rub tips of fingers in the opposite palm in a circular motion.
9. Rinse hands thoroughly with tepid running water.
10. Use tissue to turn off tap.
11. Dry thoroughly with single-use towel.

FIGURE 3.9 How to handwash

How to Handwash?

WASH HANDS WHEN VISIBLY SOILED! OTHERWISE, USE HANDRUB

Duration of the entire procedure: 40-60 seconds

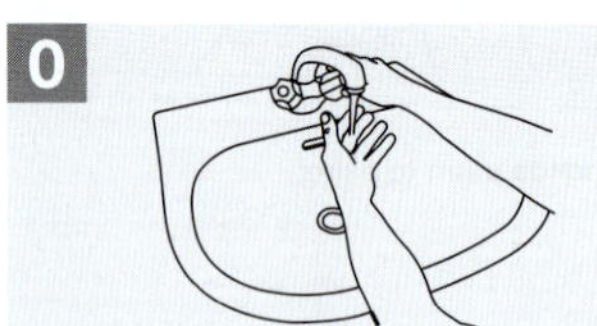

Wet hands with water;

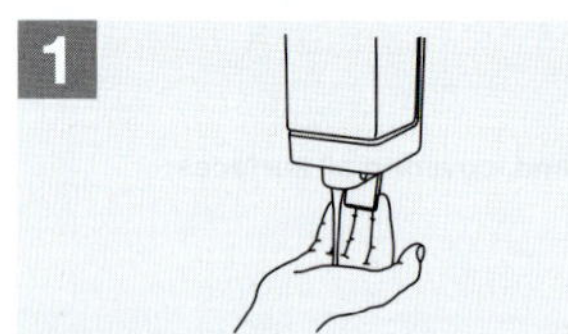

Apply enough soap to cover all hand surfaces;

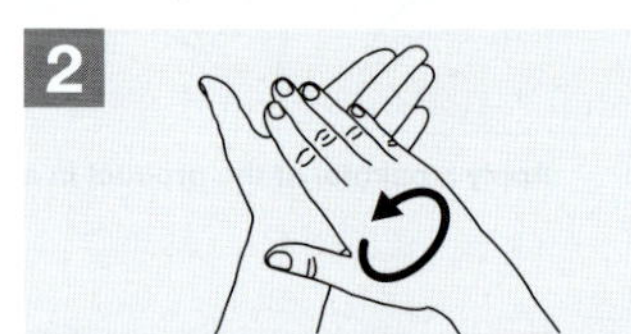

Rub hands palm to palm;

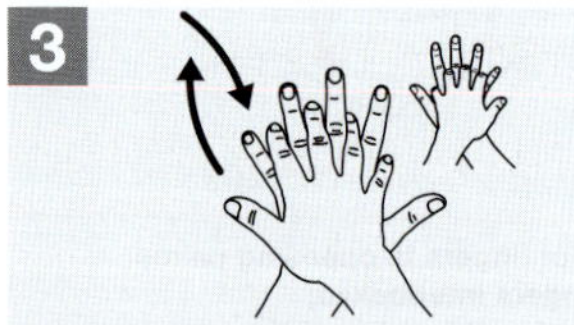

Right palm over left dorsum with interlaced fingers and vice versa;

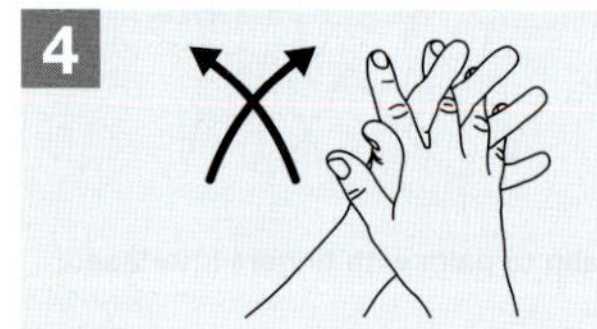

Palm to palm with fingers interlaced;

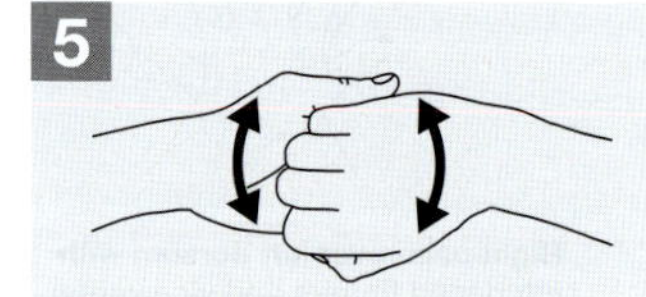

Backs of fingers to opposing palms with fingers interlocked;

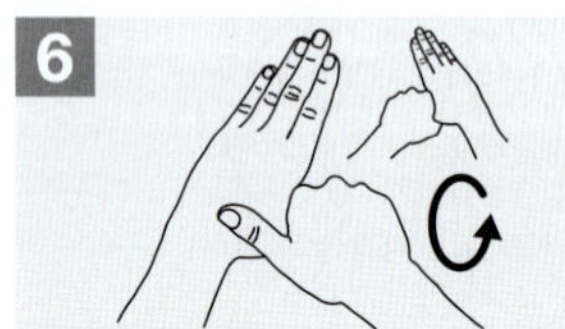

Rotational rubbing of left thumb clasped in right palm and vice versa;

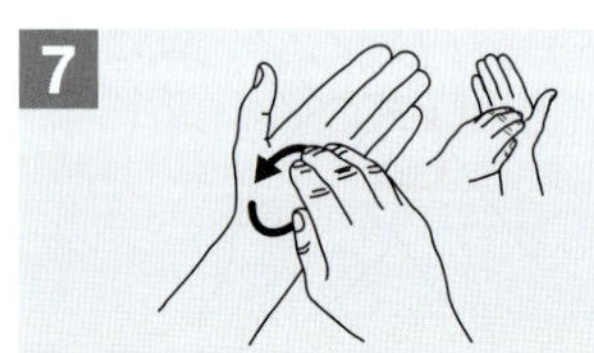

Rotational rubbing, backwards and forwards with clasped fingers of right hand in left palm and vice versa;

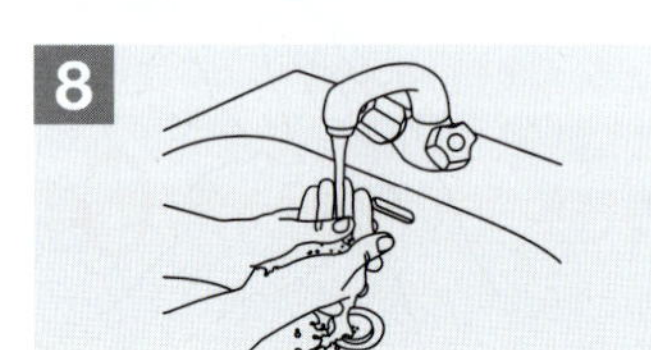

Rinse hands with water;

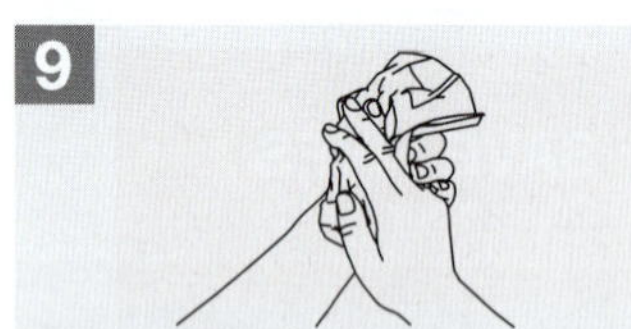

Dry hands thoroughly with a single use towel;

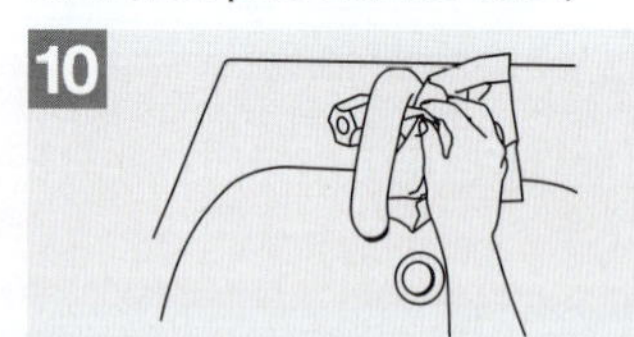

Use towel to turn off faucet;

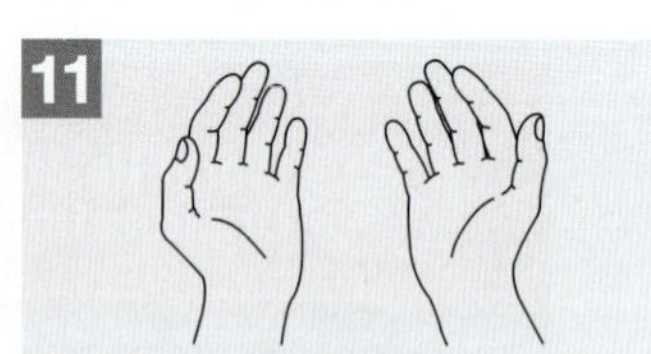

Your hands are now safe.

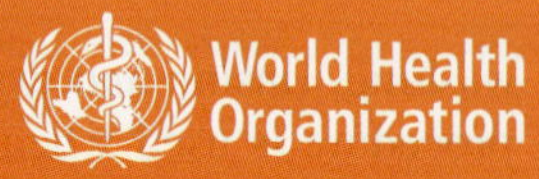

Patient Safety
A World Alliance for Safer Health Care

SAVE LIVES
Clean **Your** Hands

WHO acknowledges the Hôpitaux Universitaires de Genève (HUG), in particular the members of the Infection Control Programme, for their active participation in developing this material.

May 2009

Source: WHO (2020d).

Aseptic Non-Touch Technique (ANTT®)

Aseptic Non-Touch Technique (ANTT®) is a unique clinical practice framework for aseptic technique that is used internationally (figure 3.10). Originated by Rowley (2001), and overseen by the Association for Safe Aseptic Practice, it is based upon the unique concept of Key-Part and Key-Site Protection. The framework helps educate and support healthcare workers to practice aseptic technique safely and efficiently (Rowley 2001). Dependent upon risk assessment, there are two approaches designed for all invasive clinical procedures.

1. *Surgical-ANTT.* All Key-Parts are managed collectively upon a single critical aseptic fields. Sterile gloves are essential.
2. *Standard-ANTT.* Key-Parts are managed individually using non-touch technique and micro critical aseptic fields.

Following are the underlying principles of ANTT.

- The aim of ANTT is always asepsis/aseptic.
- Take appropriate standard precautions always including hand cleaning.
- Protect Key-Parts and Key-Sites at all times using the appropriate combination of aseptic fields and non-touch technique.
- Key-Parts must only touch other aseptic Key-Partsand Key-Sites.

ANTT Key-Sites and Key-Parts are as follows.

- Key-Sites are any body portal of entry for pathogens. This includes open wounds, insertion and puncture sites.
- Key-Parts are the parts of procedure equipment that will come in contact with other Key-Parts or the patient. For example, IV cannulas, needle tips, sterile gauze to clean wounds and dressings.

Performing Surgical-ANTT®

1. Gain consent from the patient for the procedure.
2. Perform hand hygiene.
3. Clean the trolley or work surface with detergent and water or detergent wipe. Start at the top of the trolley and work from the inside to the outside of the trolley. Clean the sides and the bottom of the trolley.
4. Clip a waste bag to the trolley.
5. Identify and gather equipment required for procedure.
6. Perform hand hygiene.
7. Prepare critical aseptic field:
   - Open procedure pack using the corners and ensuring you to not touch the contents.
   - Carefully drop sterile equipment into sterile field.
8. Perform hand hygiene.
9. Prepare your patient — use non-sterile gloves where appropriate such as when removing a dressing as you may contact body fluids.
10. Remove gloves, perform hand hygiene and apply new gloves.
11. Perform procedure ensuring all Key-Parts/components are protected:
    - Sterile items are used once and disposed into waste bag.
    - Only sterile items contact the Key-Site.
    - Sterile items do not come into contact with non-sterile items.
12. Remove gloves and perform hand hygiene.
13. Clean trolley/work surface after use and perform hand hygiene.
14. Dispose of contaminated materials in appropriate container.

Source: Adapted from Government of Tasmania (2015).

Bundles of care

A bundle of care is a set of three to five evidence-based practices and procedures that when used together and when consistently and reliably performed by all healthcare providers, have been shown to improve patient outcomes. Bundles of care reduce infection risk (The Institute for Healthcare Improvement [IHI] 2020). 'Care bundles empower nurses to make changes for the better through a scale-up approach that supports cultural change with long-term benefits for all involved' (Proops 2019). The bundles are an integrated approach that includes hand hygiene, ongoing healthcare provider education, and follow and review of infection rates (Wasserman & Messina 2018). Examples of the types of bundles that support infection prevention and control are discussed next.

FIGURE 3.10 The ANTT-Approach

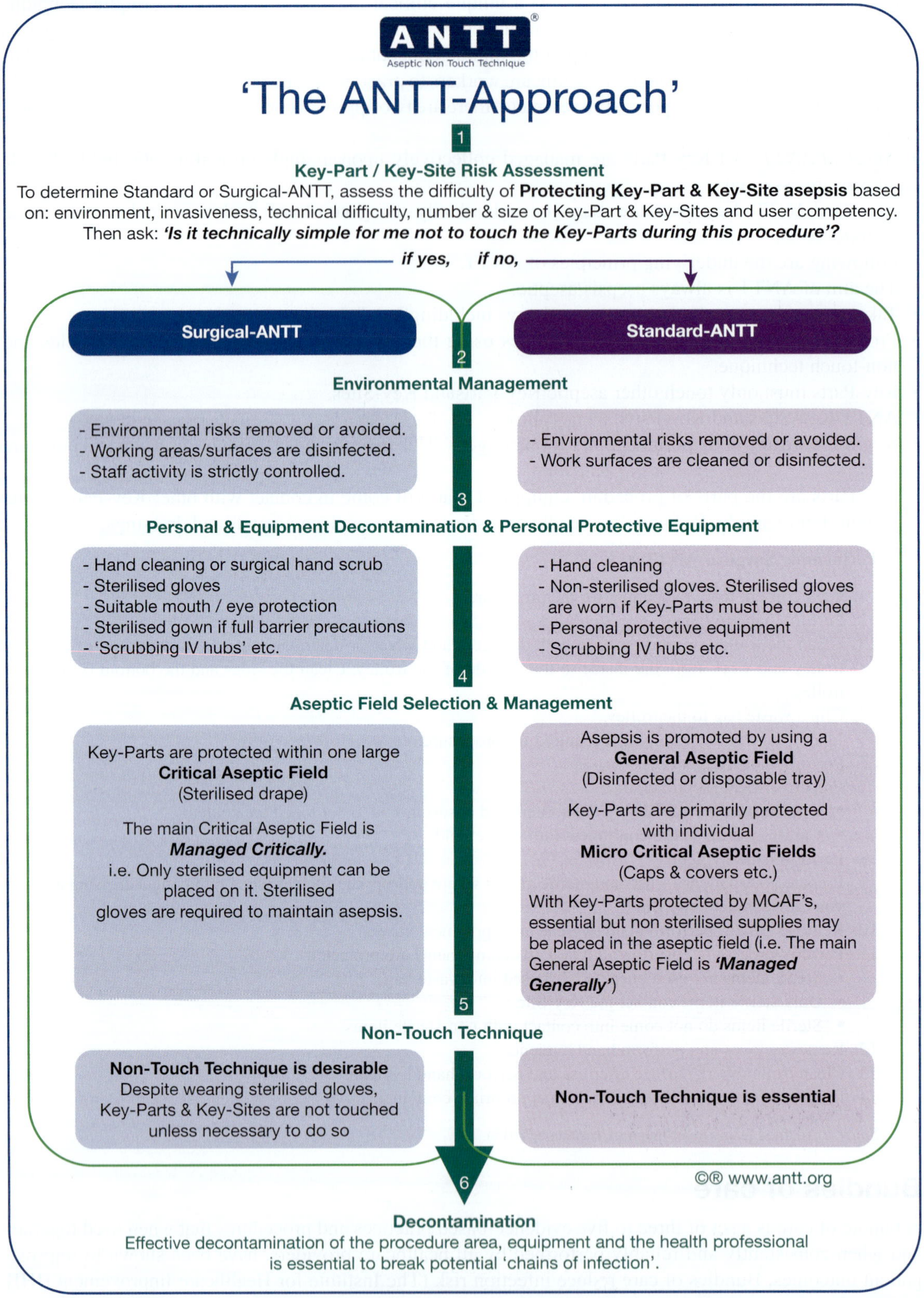

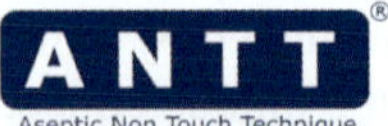

'The ANTT-Approach'

Source: Rowley (2001).

Bundle for the prevention of surgical site infection

Surgical site infections (SSIs) are infections that can occur after surgery. SSIs result in increased lengths of stay and increased healthcare costs. It has been estimated that around half of SSIs are preventable with appropriate care. Following the established set of procedures in a SSI bundle during surgery and post-operatively has been shown to reduce SSI (Wasserman 2018).

Bundle for the prevention of ventilator-associated pneumonia

Ventilator-associated pneumonia (VAP) is a lung infection that occurs within 48 hours of endotracheal intubation and occurs in up to 20 per cent of patients who are being mechanically ventilated. Endotracheal intubation is when a tube is placed into the windpipe (trachea) through the mouth or nose to support breathing. This procedure can be done in a controlled environment, such as an operating theatre. It can also be done as an emergency procedure in a trauma situation. A VAP is a serious hospital-acquired infection associated with increased mortality and morbidity, the need for increased antibiotic use, increased length of hospitalisation and a resultant increased cost to the healthcare system. Research has shown that more than 50 per cent of VAP cases are preventable using a ventilator bundle (Wasserman 2018).

Bundle for the prevention of catheter-associated urinary tract infections

Catheter-associated urinary tract infections (CAUTIs) are urinary tract infections in a patient with a current urinary catheter (IDC) or has had an IDC in the past 48 hours. CAUTI is the most common HAI globally and, like other infections, increases morbidity, length of hospital stay, costs to the healthcare system and reduced patient satisfaction. Most CAUTI are avoidable by implementing a bundle of care that include appropriate use, early removal of the IDC, aseptic insertion and ongoing care. Nurses play a significant role in reducing CAUTI and improving patient experience.

Bundles for the prevention of central line-associated bloodstream infections

Central lines are commonly used in intensive care units (ICUs), dialysis units, intraoperatively and oncology patients. Central line-associated bloodstream infections (CLABSIs) increase mortality and morbidity, prolong hospital stays and increase healthcare system costs. Bundles of care for CLABSI include an insertion and maintenance bundle. The bundles are integrated with a multi-modal approach, including hand hygiene, clinician and nurse education, and review of CLABSI rates (Wasserman 2018).

All healthcare providers should have bundles of care in place and provide ongoing education and training for staff along with programs that monitor outcomes and provide continuous quality improvement.

Personal protective equipment (PPE)

The use of appropriate PPE is fundamental to healthcare providers and their patients' safety and has assumed greater importance with the COVID-19 global pandemic created by the spread of the SARS-CoV-2 virus (Singh, Naik, Soni & Puri 2020).

PPE refers to any equipment employed to reduce the risk of harm to the health and safety of workers (Safe Work Australia n.d.). In healthcare settings, PPE is used to reduce the risk of touching, transmitting or being exposed to pathogens spread by airborne, contact or droplets (MedlinePlus 2019). Basic PPE is outlined in figure 3.11. PPE that is not donned and doffed correctly leads to a high risk of contamination for the healthcare provider, the patient and the greater community (Pyrek 2018).

FIGURE 3.11 Basic personal protection equipment

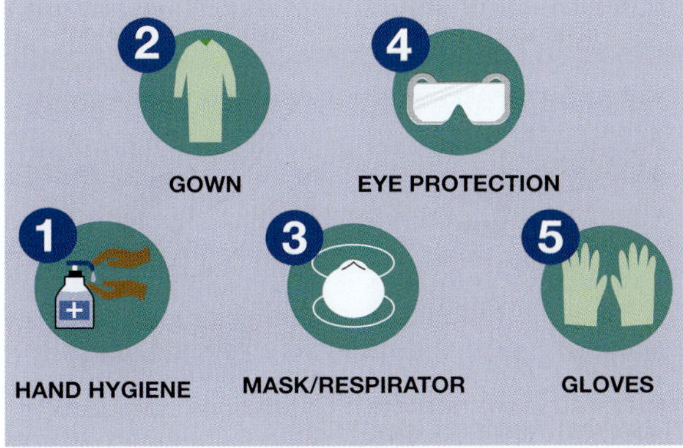

There are several special considerations when using PPE.

- Always remember to engage with your patient. It will be confronting for them not to see your face and they are likely to feel insecure in this situation. Explain that the PPE is standard hospital procedure to reduce infection risk for the patient and you.
- Always consult and follow the healthcare facility policy and procedure.
- If goggles and masks are worn for extended lengths of time, they can cause pressure injuries to your face. Ensure you protect bony prominences and, if possible, change your PPE frequently. Take regular breaks if you can.
- P2 or N95 respirators are mandatory PPE when there is a high probability of airborne transmission.
- Healthcare facilities must ensure that healthcare providers receive appropriate training on donning and doffing and for performing a fit check for all types of P2 and N95 particulate respirators.

Gloves

Gloves protect both patients and healthcare providers from exposure to pathogens (NHMRC 2019).

Gloves are used to prevent contamination of healthcare providers when they are:

- anticipating contact with bodily fluids, mucous membranes or non-intact skin such as wounds
- handling visibly or potentially contaminated equipment or surfaces.

Gloves are single-use items and must be discarded after use. They should not be washed or have ABHR applied to them. The correct use of gloves is outlined in table 3.1 and figure 3.12.

TABLE 3.1 Use of gloves in the healthcare setting

Use of non-sterile gloves	Use of sterile gloves
Potential exposure to body fluids Contact with broken skin Contact with mucous membranes Performing venepuncture Emptying a urinary catheter bag Performing nasogastric aspiration Vaginal examination Dental examination Care of minor cuts and abrasions	Potential exposure to blood, body substances, secretions or excretions in a sterile environment. Contact with sites or clinical devices where sterile conditions must be maintained. Dental procedures requiring a sterile field. Procedures that require surgical aseptic technique, e.g.: • urinary catheter insertion • complex dressings • central venous line insertion site dressing • lumbar puncture • clinical care of surgical wounds or drainage sites.

Source: Adapted from WHO (2009).

FIGURE 3.12 Removing gloves safely

HOW TO REMOVE GLOVES SAFELY

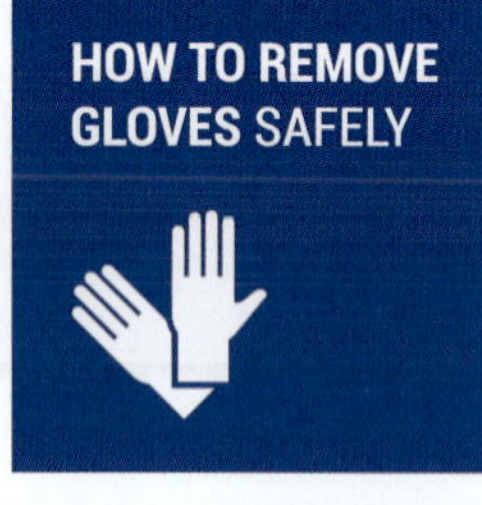

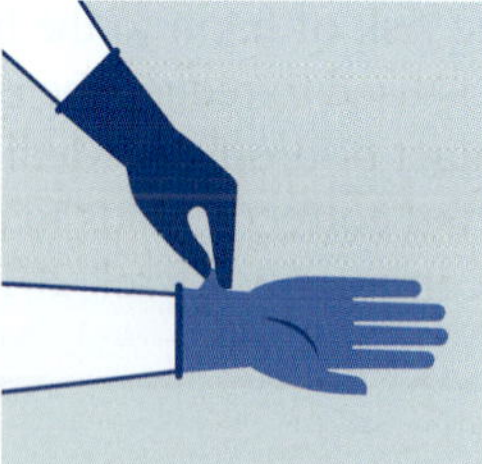

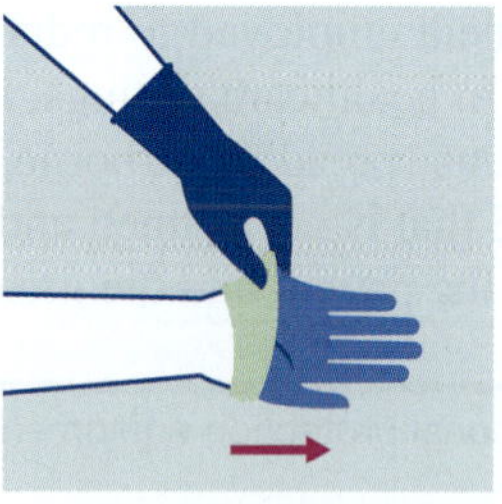

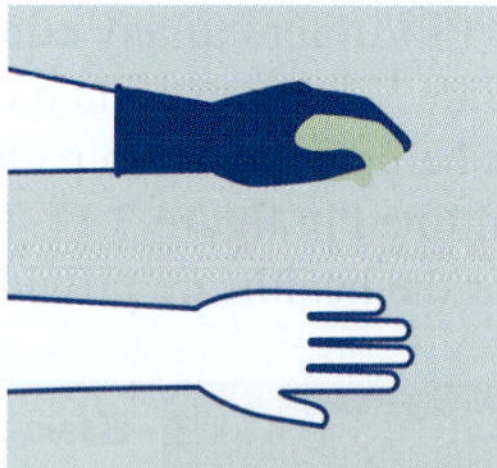

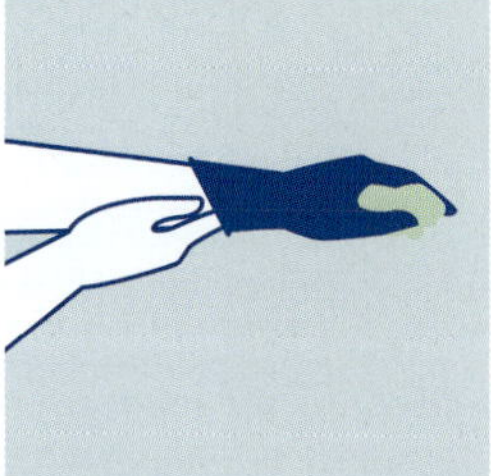

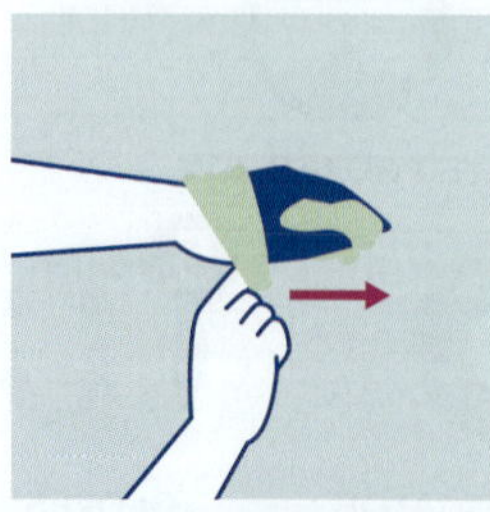

DISPOSE THE GLOVES SAFELY

WASH YOUR HANDS

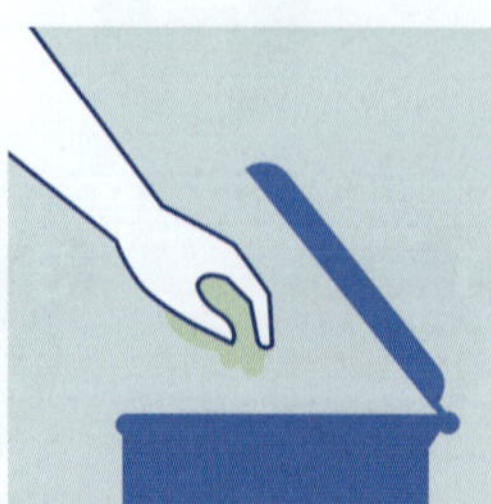

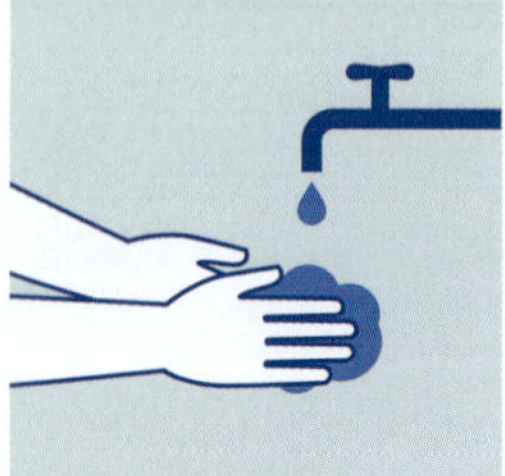

Masks, goggles and face shields

The mucous membranes of the mouth, nose and eyes are high-risk portals for pathogens (NHMRC 2019). Face and eye protection reduce the risk of healthcare workers' exposure to splashes or sprays of bodily fluids. They are an essential part of maintaining standard and transmission-based precautions. Table 3.2 outlines the situations in which masks are required and their appropriate use. Considerations when using a surgical mask include the following.

- Masks must be changed between patients.
- Masks must be changed when they are soiled or wet.
- Once masks have been removed, they must be discarded and never reused.
- Masks should not be left dangling around the neck.
- Avoid touching the front of the mask when it is worn, as this area can be contaminated.
- Hand hygiene must be performed upon touching or discarding a used mask.

TABLE 3.2 Appropriate use of masks, goggles and shields in the healthcare setting

Required use of masks/goggles/shields	No required use of masks/goggles/shields
When a patient is on droplet precautions (surgical mask) or airborne precautions (P2/N95 particulate respirator)	Routine care, routine observations, and general examination when no contact with bodily fluids is likely
All procedures that have the potential to generate splashes or sprays	
Dental procedures	
Nasopharyngeal aspiration	
Emptying wound or catheter bag	
Suctioning and other procedures that involve the respiratory tract including the mouth	
Oral or nasopharyngeal intubation	

Source: Adapted from WHO (2020).

Gowns and aprons

It should be noted that washable fabric gowns provide no protection from body substances and hence are not considered PPE for infection prevention and control. Gowns or aprons of impermeable material must be worn:

- where there is a likelihood of contacts with body fluids
- when entering an isolation room, if contact with the patient or the patient's environment is likely, and removed before or immediately after exiting the room
- as a protective layer under a sterile gown not made of impermeable material.

Other clothing

Neckties and lanyards should be avoided as evidence has shown that these may facilitate infection transmission (NHMRC 2019). Footwear should be appropriate to the healthcare setting and the care being provided. It must minimise the risk of injury from dropped sharps and exposure to bodily fluids (closed-toe). Uniforms are recommended for clinical areas due to the risk of cross-transmission of pathogens. Healthcare providers must wear a clean uniform each shift and should be washed separately from other items. Ideally, the uniform should not be worn outside the healthcare facility.

Donning (putting on) sequence

Donning PPE is important in maintaining your safety from pathogens when you are performing a procedure or caring for a patient with an infection. Donning is done outside the patient's room. These steps must be followed in strict order.

1. Complete hand hygiene.
2. Don the gown:
   a. Tie at the back.
   b. Fasten at the back of your neck and waist.
   c. The gown should:
      i. allow you to move freely without gaping
      ii. cover your body from your neck to knees and your arms including the wrists.

3. Don the surgical mask or particulate respirator (P2/N5 mask):
   a. Fasten the ties or elastic bands at the middle of the head and neck.
   b. Fit the flexible band across the bridge of your nose:
      i. Fit the mask snug to your face and below your chin.
      ii. Fit check the respirator according to the manufacturer instructions.
4. Don the protective goggles or face shield:
   a. Place over eyes/face and adjust to fit.
5. Don the gloves:
   a. Ensure the gloves cover the wrist of your gown.
   b. If at any point your gloves become contaminated, you must dispose of them, perform hand hygiene, and then replace them with new gloves.

Source: Adapted from Ausmed Education Pty Ltd (2020b).

The sequence for donning PPE is outlined in figure 3.13.

FIGURE 3.13 Sequence for putting on PPE

Put on PPE before patient contact and generally before entering the patient room

HAND HYGIENE

- Wash hands or use an alcohol based hand rub.

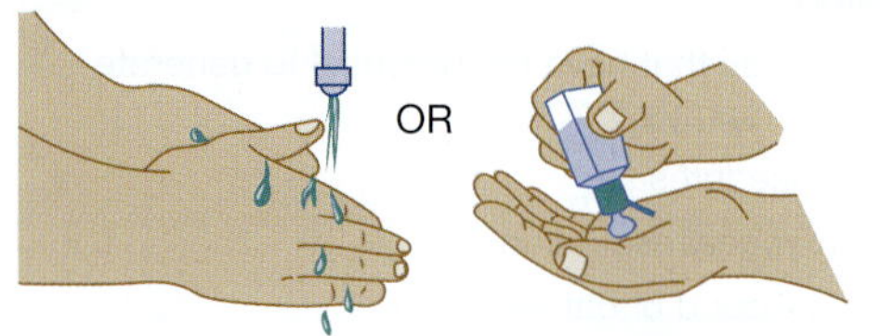

GOWN

- Fully cover torso from neck to kness, arms to end of wrists, and wrap around the back.
- Fasten at the back of neck and waist.

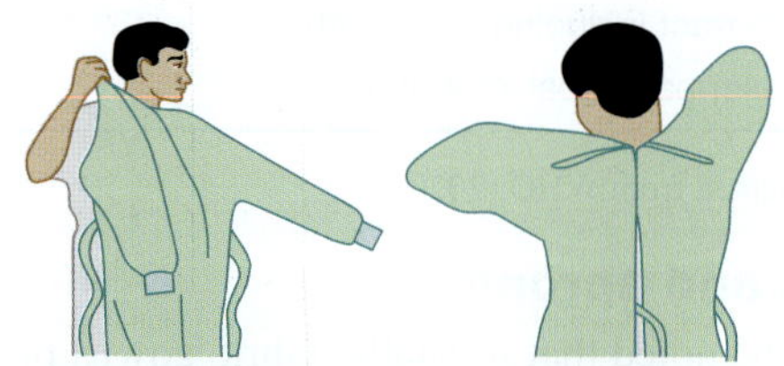

MASK

- Secure ties or elastic bands at middle of head and neck.

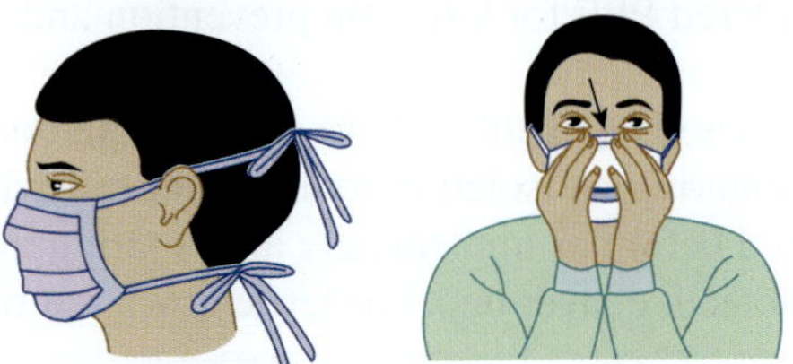

PROTECTIVE EYEWEAR OR FACE SHIELD

- Place over face and eyes and adjust to fit.

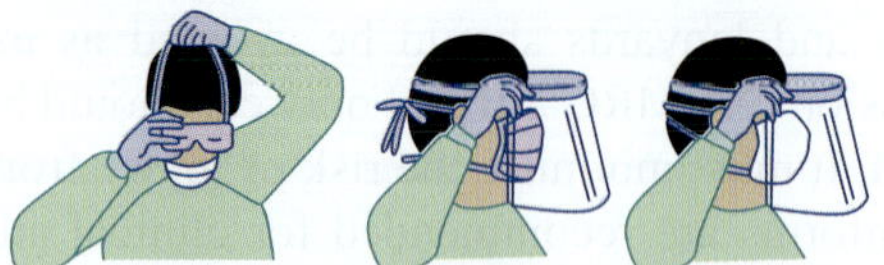

GLOVES

- Extend to cover wrist of isolation gown.

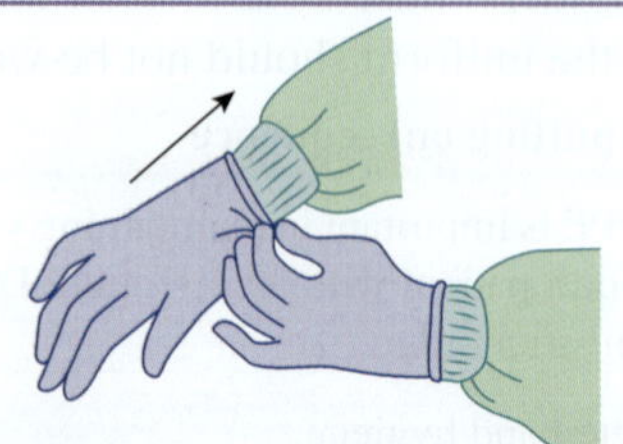

Source: NHMRC, Australian Guidelines for the Prevention and Control of Infection in Healthcare (2019).

Fit checking

Fit checking should be performed every time you put on a P2 and N95 particulate respirator. Check to see that there is a good seal over the bridge of your nose and mouth, and there are no gaps between the mask and your face. Do not provide patient care until you have undertaken a fit check and a satisfactory fit has been achieved. How to perform an appropriate fit check of a P2 and N95 mask is outlined in figure 3.14. Check the manufacturer's instructions to support safe, effective fit testing (Queensland Health 2020).

Doffing (taking off) PPE

Doffing PPE is a high-risk procedure and the most important step in preventing the transmission of pathogens. Correct doffing is a crucial step in the use of PPE. The correct order must be followed. All PPE is contaminated after it has been used. When doffing PPE you must continue to protect your clothing, skin and mucous membranes from the pathogens on the outside of the PPE. You must perform hygiene immediately after each step in the doffing procedure.

Doffing is done before you leave the patient area, or if provided, in the anteroom.

1. Remove your gloves following the correct steps:
   a. Using one hand, grasp the palm of the other hand and peel off the first glove.
   b. Hold the removed glove in the gloved hand.
   c. Slide fingers of the un-gloved hand under the remaining glove at the wrist and peel it off over the first glove.
   d. Discard gloves in a waste container.
2. Perform hand hygiene.
3. Remove your gown:
   a. Unfasten the ties whole making sure that the sleeves of the gown do not contact your body.
   b. Pull the gown away from your neck and shoulders ensure that you are only touching the inside of the gown.
   c. Turn the gown inside out so that the contaminated outside of the gown will be away from you.
   d. Fold or roll the gown into a bundle.
   e. Discard gown into the contaminated waste container.
4. Perform hand hygiene.
5. Exit the patient's room and close the door.
6. Remove your goggles or face shield:
   a. Remove from the back of your head by lifting the earpieces or the headband.
   b. If the goggles or face shield are reusable, then place in the designated reprocessing receptacle.
   c. If the goggles or face shield are NOT reusable, then place in the contaminated waste container.
7. Perform hand hygiene.
8. Remove mask or particulate respirator (P9/N95):
   a. Grasp the bottom ties/elastics, then the top ones, and remove them carefully without touching the front of the mask.
   b. Discard in the contaminated waste container.
9. Immediately perform hand hygiene

Note: PPE must be disposed of in the appropriate containers unless it is clearly marked for reuse.

Source: Adapted from Ausmed Education Pty Ltd (2020b).

Staff health and safety

Healthcare providers are exposed to many different hazards in the healthcare setting. As healthcare providers, it is vital to care for ourselves as we care for others.

Vaccinations

An integral part of the infection prevention and control program in the healthcare setting is protection for the healthcare providers (Australian Technical Advisory Group on Immunisation (ATAGI) 2018). This includes staff health screening policy, promoting **immunisation** and extra protection for specific situations such as pregnancy to reduce healthcare workers' risk. As healthcare providers, we also have a responsibility to protect ourselves and ensure we do not put our colleagues or our patients and families at risk of infection. In Australia, healthcare providers are required to be vaccinated in accordance with the recommendations in the Australian Immunisation Handbook. The vaccinations recommended for Australia's healthcare providers are outlined in table 3.3.

FIGURE 3.14 Principles of fit checking

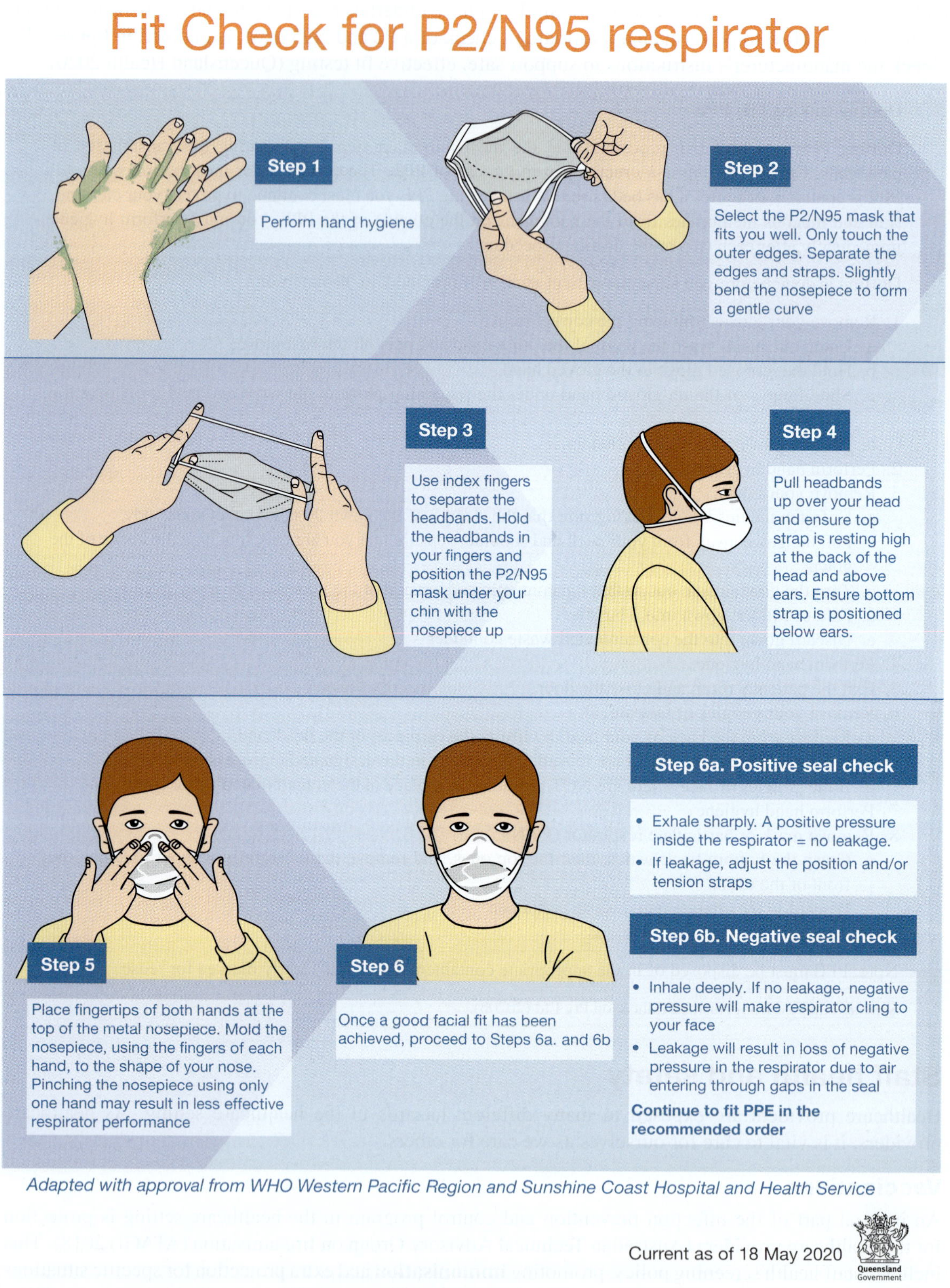

Fit Check for P2/N95 respirator

Step 1

Perform hand hygiene

Step 2

Select the P2/N95 mask that fits you well. Only touch the outer edges. Separate the edges and straps. Slightly bend the nosepiece to form a gentle curve

Step 3

Use index fingers to separate the headbands. Hold the headbands in your fingers and position the P2/N95 mask under your chin with the nosepiece up

Step 4

Pull headbands up over your head and ensure top strap is resting high at the back of the head and above ears. Ensure bottom strap is positioned below ears.

Step 5

Place fingertips of both hands at the top of the metal nosepiece. Mold the nosepiece, using the fingers of each hand, to the shape of your nose. Pinching the nosepiece using only one hand may result in less effective respirator performance

Step 6

Once a good facial fit has been achieved, proceed to Steps 6a. and 6b

Step 6a. Positive seal check

- Exhale sharply. A positive pressure inside the respirator = no leakage.
- If leakage, adjust the position and/or tension straps

Step 6b. Negative seal check

- Inhale deeply. If no leakage, negative pressure will make respirator cling to your face
- Leakage will result in loss of negative pressure in the respirator due to air entering through gaps in the seal

Continue to fit PPE in the recommended order

Adapted with approval from WHO Western Pacific Region and Sunshine Coast Hospital and Health Service

Current as of 18 May 2020

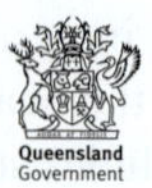

Source: © The State of Queensland (Queensland Health) 1996–2021.

Australia is a global leader in publicly-funded immunisation programs (ATAGI 2018). The program is comprehensive, and all **vaccines** available in Australia are evaluated by the Therapeutic Goods Administration (TGA) and meet strict safety guidelines before they are approved for use.

TABLE 3.3 Vaccinations recommended for healthcare providers

Healthcare providers	Vaccinations
All healthcare providers, including students directly involved with patient care or the handling of human tissues, blood or body fluids.	Hepatitis B Influenza Pertussis (dTpa) MMR (if non-immune) Varicella (if non-immune)
Healthcare workers, including students who work with remote Indigenous communities in the Northern Territory, Queensland, South Australia and Western Australia.	Hepatitis B Influenza Pertussis (dTpa) MMR (if non-immune) Varicella (if non-immune) Hepatitis A
Healthcare providers, including students who are at high risk of exposure to drug-resistant cases of tuberculosis dependent on State or Territory guidelines.	Hepatitis B Influenza Pertussis (dTpa) MMR (if non-immune) Varicella (if non-immune) Plus consider Bacillus Calmette-Guérin (BCG) vaccine.

Source: Adapted from NHMRC (2019).

Safe environments

The healthcare environment should be a clean, safe place for staff, patients and their families. Healthcare organisations are responsible for providing and implementing infection prevention and control programs across the healthcare facility (NHMRC 2019), run by dedicated, educated and trained teams. All healthcare providers must be provided with the education and training to improve healthcare-acquired infections (HAI) knowledge, antimicrobial resistance and organisation policies and procedures on cleaning and disinfection. The programs should support ongoing quality improvement for facility-based HAI surveillance to include feedback, reporting and strategies to address HAI prevention. There should be infection prevention and control policies and procedures based on evidence-based practice from the national and state/territory governments. Regular monitoring and review of healthcare practices to ensure policies and procedures are implemented correctly should be facilitated. There should also be ongoing evaluation of potential hazards and effectiveness of disinfectants, products and equipment. These programs are responsible for ensuring that healthcare environments are clean and that the appropriate materials and equipment are available to support infection prevention and control procedures. In turn, healthcare providers have a responsibility to follow and support organisation approved infection prevention and control policies, bundles of care, ANTT and policies applicable to specific areas in the healthcare setting.

Care equipment is easily contaminated with pathogens by contact with bodily fluids and skin contact. These pathogens can be easily transferred during delivery of care. To minimise these risks, we must adhere to decontamination practices within the healthcare setting. Routine decontamination of reusable non-invasive care equipment must be carried out following the manufacturers' instructions (Wigglesworth 2019c). Routine cleaning between every use after visible contamination by bodily fluids must take place. In addition, it should also be cleaned at predefined intervals dictated by policy and prior to inspection, routine servicing and repair. There are three decontamination levels for care equipment. The level of decontamination depends on the level of risk associated with the equipment and its use.

- Level one: Cleaning. Clean the equipment with neutral detergent and water or use disposable wipes to remove dust, soiling, organic matter and some microorganisms.
- Level two: **Disinfection**. Disinfection requires the use of heat and or chemicals. Disinfection is used if the equipment is contaminated with bodily fluids or has been in contact with mucous membranes. Disinfection is required when a patient with a known or suspected infection or colonisation of **multi-resistant pathogens** has used the equipment.

- Level three: **Sterilisation**. Sterilisation uses heat and, in some instances, chemicals to remove visible microorganisms, including bacterial spores and viruses. Sterilisation is used for reusable invasive equipment such as surgical instruments.

As nurses, we should undertake these activities only after receiving approved training on the processes, being supervised in our practice, and having our competency assessed and approved. All cleaning must be performed be in accordance with the policies and protocols of the healthcare organisation and manufacturers recommendations.

3.5 The clinical reasoning cycle and infection control

LEARNING OBJECTIVE 3.5 Reflect on the clinical reasoning cycle and its application to infection prevention and control.

The clinical reasoning cycle is described by Levett-Jones et al. (2009) as 'a process by which nurses collect cues, process the information, come to an understanding of a patient problem or situation, plan and implement interventions, evaluate outcomes, and reflect on, and learn from the process'. Effective use of the clinical reasoning cycle is dependent on following the stages:

- consider the patient situation
- collect information
- process gathered information
- identify the problem
- establish goals
- act
- evaluate
- reflect (European Heart Association 2018).

These steps are as important in preventing and controlling infections as they are in all other facets of healthcare. To prevent and control infection, we must consider the patient, the situation, the possible infection risks, the location and the procedure that will take place. As nurses, we collect all the information on the patient and the required care, process that information, identify any problems and establish our care goals for each event. We then provide the care, evaluate it and reflect it.

As an example, if we apply this to the provision of a basic dressing for a patient, we need to ask the following questions.

- Are we in an appropriate area to provide the dressing? Will we be able to ensure privacy and safety?
- What do the notes or the dressing chart say about the wound we will be dressing?
- What does the patient have to say about the wound? Are they in pain? Are they agreeable to have the wound dressed now? Do they have any further information for you?
- Are there any problems associated with the dressing? We need to treat the pain prior to providing the dressing.

In this example, the goal is to change the patient's dressing, maintain asepsis and document the care and any changes to the wound's condition. We will then evaluate the care and reflect on anything that should have been performed differently.

Employing the clinical reasoning cycle to infection prevention and control just as we do to all other patient care gives us a guideline to support quality patient-centred care.

3.6 Patient-centred care in infection prevention and control

LEARNING OBJECTIVE 3.6 Discuss the importance of patient-centred care in infection prevention and control.

The Australian Commission on Health Care and Safety (ACSQHC) recommend that a patient-centred approach is essential in preventing and controlling infections in the healthcare setting and providing high-quality patient care (ACSQHC 2019).

Nurses must provide patients with the education and support required to be fully informed and involved in their care. To support an inclusive approach to infection control:

- patients should be considered stakeholders in their care, and their perspectives included when developing policies and procedures

- patients should be familiarised with the healthcare facility's strategies to protect themselves, their families and the facility from infections and are encouraged to take an active role in hand hygiene
- infection risks and procedures should be discussed with patients and their families
- healthcare providers should encourage patients to disclose any healthcare risks that may be a potential hazard to other patients and healthcare providers
- healthcare providers should encourage patients to express concerns about their care.

Nurses spend more time with patients than any other healthcare provider. It is incumbent on us to ensure that the above recommendations are followed so that patients are partners in maintaining a safe care environment.

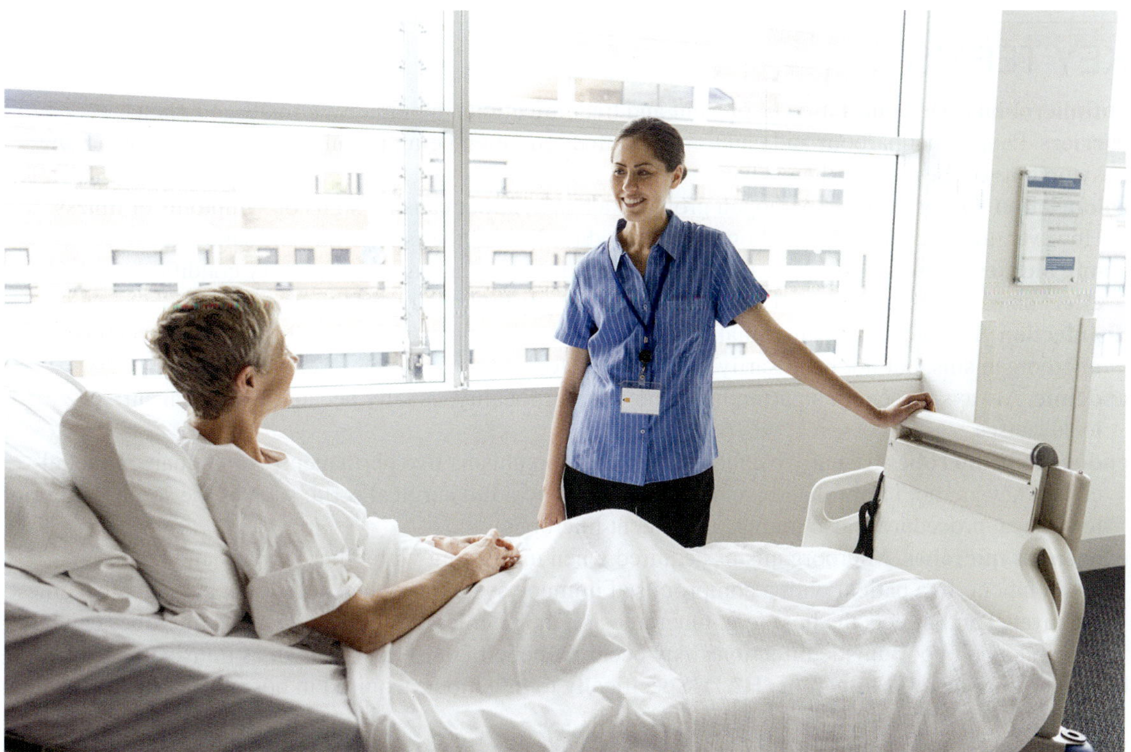

SUMMARY

Infection control and prevention is a fundamental responsibility of all healthcare providers. This chapter has provided a comprehensive summary of relevant microbiology, pathology and risks associated with infection in hospitals, including HAIs, infection prevention and control, hand hygiene, PPE and the language of infection control. Nurses are leaders in practising infection prevention and controlling the spread of infection. The prevention and control of infection is a fundamental element of nursing practice. Nurses have a clear responsibility to adhere to evidence-based guidelines in order to control infection in the clinical setting.

KEY TERMS

antimicrobials Medicines used to prevent and treat infections in humans, animals and plants.

carriers People that harbour and can transmit infection, often being immune or without showing any symptoms of the disease themselves.

colonisation Occurs when a pathogen grows in a host without causing signs or symptoms of illness. However, they may become pathogenic if introduced to another site within the same person.

comorbidities Presence of one or more conditions that occur alongside a primary condition and have an effect on each other. These can be physiological or psychological conditions.

disinfection The process of microbial inactivation that eliminates virtually all recognised pathogenic microorganisms, but not necessarily all microbial forms (e.g. spores).

endemic Always present in a particular community or locality, usually because of permanent local causes.

endogenous microbes Usually bacteria, these microorganisms live permanently on human epithelial cells. They are not harmful and are only eliminated by a full surgical scrub such as the scrub used prior to surgical procedures (also known as resident microbes).

exogenous microbes Microorganisms acquired when interacting with other humans and the environment. In a patient with a compromised immune system or when a dormant pathogen becomes reactivated and infects the host (e.g. tuberculosis), the interaction with endogenous microbes can be harmful, and opportunistic infections may occur (Mitchell 2018) (also known as transient microbes).

healthcare-associated infection (HAI) Specifically to infections acquired in hospital and not present on presentation for healthcare (ACSQHC 2018).

host Human or other entity that that provides a home for an organism.

immunisation The process by which a person becomes protected against a disease through vaccination. The term is often used interchangeably with vaccination or inoculation (CDC 2018).

infection A pathogen invades the host's tissues and causes signs and symptoms of illness.

locus The specific site in the body where an infection originates.

microorganism Any organism that is too small to be viewed without a microscope. Examples are bacteria, protozoa, some fungi and algae.

pathogen Or infective agents are organisms capable of causing disease when they enter the body (Imedpub.com 2020).

standard precautions Work practices that must be adopted by all healthcare workers to provide a first-line approach to infection prevention and control in the healthcare environment (ACSQHC 2019c).

sterile Free from or the complete absence of microorganisms including bacteria, fungus and their spores (Wound, Ostomy and Continence Nurses Society (WOCN) Wound Committee & Association for Professionals in Infection Control and Epidemiology, Inc. (APIC) 2000 Guidelines Committee 2012).

sterilisation The use of physical or chemical procedures (heat, irradiation, pressure etc.) to destroy all microbial life, including large numbers of highly resistant bacterial endospores (ACSQHC 2019c).

vaccines Products that act to stimulate the immune system to produce immunity to a specific disease, hence protecting the person from that disease (CDC 2018).

REFERENCES

ACSQHC. (2018) Health care associated infections. www.safetyandquality.gov.au/sites/default/files/migrated/SAQ7730_HAC_Factsheet_HealthcareAssociatedInfections_LongV2.pdf

ACSQHC. (2019a) Antimicrobial Use and Resistance in Australia Surveillance System (AURA) 2019. www.safetyandquality.gov.au/our-work/antimicrobial-resistance/antimicrobial-use-and-resistance-australia-surveillance-system/aura-2019

ACSQHC. (2019b) National Hand Hygiene Initiative. www.safetyandquality.gov.au

ACSQHC. (2019c) *Infection Prevention and Control Workbook 2019* www.safetyandquality.gov.au/publications-and-resources/resource-library/infection-prevention-and-control-workbook-2019

Aseptic No Touch Technique. (2019) The ANTT-Approach. www.antt.org/ANTT_Site/ANTT-Approach.html

Atkinson, J., Chartier, Y., Pessoa-Silva, C. L. et al. (Eds.). (2009) Natural ventilation for infection control in health-care settings. Geneva: World Health Organization. Annex C, Respiratory droplets. www.ncbi.nlm.nih.gov/books/NBK143281

Ausmed Education Pty Ltd. (2020a) Hand hygiene 101. www.ausmed.com/cpd/articles/hand-hygiene-101

Ausmed Education Pty Ltd. (2020b) Donning and doffing PPE correctly. www.ausmed.com/cpd/articles/donning-doffing-ppe

Australian Commission on Safety and Quality in Health Care (ACSQHC). (2012) Resource library. www.safetyandquality.gov.au/publications-and-resources/resource-library?resource_search=approach

Australian Government, Department of Health. (2017) Antimicrobial resistance. www.amr.gov.au/what-you-can-do/hospitals

Australian Technical Advisory Group on Immunisation (ATAGI). (2018) *Australian Immunisation Handbook*. Australian Government Department of Health, Canberra. https://immunisationhandbook.health.gov.au

Benson, S. & Powers, J. (2011) Your role in infection prevention. *Nursing Made Incredibly Easy*. 9(9): 36–41. doi: 10.1097/01.NME.0000395995.78267.c9

Burnett, E. (2018) Effective infection prevention and control: the nurse's role. *Nursing Standard*. doi: 10.7748/ns.2018.e11171

Caresearch. (2020) People at high risk for severe infection. www.caresearch.com.au/caresearch/tabid/5985/Default.aspx

Centers for Disease Control and Prevention (CDC). (2016) How infections spread. www.cdc.gov/infectioncontrol/spread/index.html

Centers for Disease Control and Prevention (CDC). (2018) Immunization: The basics. www.cdc.gov/vaccines/vac-gen/imz-basics.htm

Department of Health & Human Services. (2020) Antibiotic resistant bacteria. Better Health Channel. State Government of Victoria, Australia. www.betterhealth.vic.gov.au/health/conditionsandtreatments/antibiotic-resistant-bacteria

Doenges, M. E., Moorhouse, M. F. & Murr, A. C. (2019) *Nurse's Pocket Guide: Diagnoses, prioritized interventions, and rationales*, 14 ed. Philadelphia: F.A.Davis.

European Heart Association. (2108) The Clinical Reasoning Cycle: The 8 phases and their significance. www.heartassociation.eu/the-clinical-reasoning-cycle-the-8-phases-and-their-significance

Government of Tasmania. (2015) Aseptic non-touch technique — a guide for healthcare workers. Department of health and Human Services, Tasmania. www.dhhs.tas.gov.au/__data/assets/pdf_file/0017/86120/ANTT_V2_2015_B_and_Wprint.pdf

Levett-Jones, T., Hoffman, K., Dempsey, J., Jeong, S., Noble, D., Norton, C., Roche, J. & Hickey, N. (2009) The 'five rights' of clinical reasoning: An educational model to enhance nursing students' ability to identify and manage clinically 'at risk' patients. *Nurse Education Today*. 30: 515–520. 10.1016/j.nedt.2009.10.020

MedlinePlus. (2019) Personal protective equipment. *MedlinePlus*. https://medlineplus.gov/ency/patientinstructions/000447.htm

Mitchell, E. (2018) Endogenous vs. exogenous infections: It's all about crowd control. http://blog.eoscu.com/blog/endogenous-vs.-exogenous-infections-its-all-about-crowd-control

National Health and Medical Research Council (NHMRC). (2019) Australian guidelines for the prevention and control of infection in healthcare. Australian Government.

Nova Biologicals Team. (2018) Understanding the difference between sterile and clean. www.novatx.com/uncategorized/understanding-difference-sterile-clean

Proops, E. M. (2019) Implementing a surgical site infection care bundle: Implications for perioperative practice. *Journal of Perioperative Nursing*. 32(2). doi: https://doi.org/10.26550/2209-1092.1045

Pyrek, K. M. (2018) PPE donning and doffing reveals gaps in knowledge and practice. *Infection Control Today*. 13 July. www.infectioncontroltoday.com/personal-protective-equipment/ppe-donning-and-doffing-reveals-gaps-knowledge-and-practice

Queensland Health. (2020) Aseptic technique. State of Queensland. www.health.qld.gov.au/clinical-practice/guidelines-procedures/diseases-infection/infection-prevention/standard-precautions/asepti[illegible]=Aseptic%20technique%20protects%20patients%20during,and%20control%20healthcare%20associated%20infections

Rowley, S. (2001) Aseptic Non Touch Technique. *Nursing Times* (Infection Control Supplement). 97(7): V1–V111.

Safe Work Australia. (n.d.) Personal protective equipment. www.safeworkaustralia.gov.au/ppe

Singh, A., Naik, B., Soni, S. & Puri, G. (2020) Real-time remote surveillance of doffing during COVID-19 pandemic: Enhancing safety of health care workers. *Anesthesia & Analgesia*. 1. doi: 10.1213/ANE.0000000000004940

The Institute for Healthcare Improvement (IHI). (2020) What is a bundle? *Improvement Stories*. www.ihi.org/resources/Pages/ImprovementStories/WhatIsaBundle.aspx

The Johns Hopkins University. (2020) Prion diseases. *Health Home Conditions and Diseases*. www.hopkinsmedicine.org/health/conditions-and-diseases/prion-diseases

Theobald, K. A. & Ramsbotham, J. (2019) Inquiry-based learning and clinical reasoning scaffolds: An action research project to support undergraduate students' learning to 'think like a nurse'. *Nurse Education in Practice*. 38(P): 59–65. https://doi.org/10.1016/j.nepr.2019.05.018

Wasserman, S. & Messina, A. (2018) Bundles in infection prevention and safety. *Guide to Infection Control in the Healthcare Setting*. International Society for Infectious Diseases. https://isid.org/guide/infectionprevention/bundles

Wigglesworth, N. (2019a) Infection control 2: hand hygiene using alcohol-based hand rub. *Nursing Times* [online]. 115(5): 24–26. www.nursingtimes.net/clinical-archive/infection-control/infection-control-2-hand-hygiene-using-alcohol-based-hand-rub-22-04-2019

Wigglesworth, N. (2019b) Infection control 6: hand hygiene using soap and water. *Nursing Times* [online]. 115(11): 37–38. www.nursingtimes.net/clinical-archive/infection-control/infection-control-6-hand-hygiene-using-soap-and-water-07-10-2019

Wigglesworth, N. (2019c) Infection control 1: decontamination of non-invasive shared equipment. *Nursing Times* [online]. 115(3): 18–20. www.nursingtimes.net/clinical-archive/infection-control/infection-control-1-decontamination-of-non-invasive-shared-equipment-02-03-2019

World Health Organization (WHO). (2020a) Antimicrobial resistance. www.who.int/news-room/fact-sheets/detail/antimicrobial-resistance

World Health Organization (WHO). (2020b) The burden of health care-associated infection worldwide. www.who.int/infection-prevention/publications/burden_hcai/en/#:~:text=Health%20care%2Dassociated%20infection%20(HAI,at%20the%20time%20of%20admission

World Health Organization (WHO). (2020c) Coronavirus disease (COVID-19): How is it transmitted? www.who.int/emergencies/diseases/novel-coronavirus-2019/question-and-answers-hub/q-a-detail/coronavirus-disease-covid-19-how-is-it-transmitted

World Health Organization (WHO). (2020d) SAVE LIVES — Clean your hands. www.who.int/campaigns/save-lives-clean-your-hands

Wound, Ostomy and Continence Nurses Society (WOCN) Wound Committee & Association for Professionals in Infection Control and Epidemiology, Inc. (APIC) 2000 Guidelines Committee. (2012) Clean vs. sterile dressing techniques for management of chronic wounds: A fact sheet. *Journal of Wound, Ostomy and Continence Nursing*. 39(2 Suppl): S30–S34. doi: 10.1097/WON.0b013e3182478e06

ACKNOWLEDGEMENTS

Figure 3.1: © Australian Guidelines for the Prevention and Control of Infection in Healthcare, page 15. Licensed under CC BY 3.0 AU.

Figure 3.3: © Melinda Nagy / Shutterstock.com; FatCamera / Getty Images; Jamie Rogers / Shutterstock.com; Tong_stocker / Shutterstock.com; Wstockphoto / Shutterstock.com; dreii / Shutterstock.com; Boy_Anupong / Getty Images; SDI Productions / Getty Images

Figure 3.4: © Stigur Mar Karlsson/Heimsmyndir / Getty Images; aire images / Getty Images; Blue Planet Earth / Shutterstock.com; AshTproductions / Shutterstock.com; krisanapong detraphiphat / Getty Images; SDI Productions / Getty Images; nata-lunata / Shutterstock.com

Figure 3.5: © r.classen / Shutterstock.com; Kilito Chan / Getty Images; Red_Shadow / Shutterstock.com; pang_oasis / Shutterstock.com

Figure 3.6: © Vicki Smith / Getty Images; RichLegg / Getty Images; AmiNiravTank / Shutterstock.com; Charlie Goodall / Shutterstock.com; David Sacks / Getty Images

Figure 3.7: © Your 5 Moments for Hand Hygience. © World Health Organization. Reproduced with permission of WHO: https://www.who.int/images/default-source/ihs/ipc/5moment-tb.png?sfvrsn=70325401_7.

Figure 3.8: © Hand Rub Poster. © World Health Organization. Reproduced with permission of WHO. https://www.who.int/docs/default-source/infection-prevention-and-control/how-to-handrub-poster.pdf?sfvrsn=f5e8bfb1_2.

Figure 3.9: © Hand Wash Poster. © World Health Organization. Reproduced with permission of WHO. https://www.who.int/docs/default-source/infection-prevention-and-control/how-to-handwash-poster.pdf?sfvrsn=8ab212f0_2.

Figure 3.10: © 'The ANTT-Approach' An International Campaign designed to promote the essential elements of safe aseptic technique. © ANTT. Reproduced with permission of Aseptic Non Touch Technique.

Figure 3.12: © elenabsl / Shutterstock.com

Figure 3.13: © Australian Guidelines for the Prevention and Control of Infection in Healthcare (2019). Retrieved from: https://www.nhmrc.gov.au/about-us/publications/australian-guidelines-prevention-and-control-infection-healthcare-2019. Licensed under CC BY 3.0 AU.

Figure 3.14: © The State of Queensland (Queensland Health) 1996–2021 https://www.health.qld.gov.au/__data/assets/pdf_file/0035/974294/p2-n95-fit-check.pdf

Figure 3.15: © Australian Guidelines for the Prevention and Control of Infection in Healthcare (2019). Retrieved from: https://www.nhmrc.gov.au/about-us/publications/australian-guidelines-prevention-and-control-infection-healthcare-2019. Licensed under CC BY 3.0 AU.

Photo 3A: © JohnnyGreig / Getty Images

Table 3.3: © Adapted from Immunisations for health care workers. Department of Health. Commonwealth of Australia.

CHAPTER 4

Principles of nursing assessment

LEARNING OBJECTIVES

After studying this chapter, you should be able to:

4.1 review the clinical reasoning cycle applied to nursing assessment
4.2 explain the foundations of nursing assessment
4.3 recognise and interpret the different types of structured nursing assessments
4.4 identify the different types of physical assessments utilised in nursing
4.5 demonstrate nursing assessments for specific body systems.

Introduction

Assessment is the key to clinical decision making and planning patient-centred care based on the physical, psychological, social and spiritual needs of the patient and their families (Mills 2017). The Australian Nursing Practice Standards Assessment states that 'RNs (registered nurses) accurately conduct comprehensive and systematic assessments. They analyse information and data and communicate outcomes as the basis for practice' (Nursing and Midwifery Board of Australia 2020, Standard 4). This is the first step in determining the patient's health and their immediate and long-term needs. As nurses, we are responsible for carrying out the initial and ongoing patient assessments, initiating interventions that take our patients and their family's needs into consideration, evaluating the effectiveness of these interventions and reflecting on our care.

A patient's assessment involves considering the patient, collecting the cues and processing the information (Levett-Jones 2013). Only after we have completed these steps can we identify the problems, take and evaluate the action and reflect on our care. The nursing assessment is key to developing a care plan tailored to meet our patient's individual needs. It is designed to identify risks such as falls risk, pressure injury risks, nutritional risks, eliminations risks and infection risks.

This chapter aims to provide the nurse with information on indications for different types of structured assessments.

4.1 The clinical reasoning cycle

LEARNING OBJECTIVE 4.1 Review the clinical reasoning cycle applied to nursing assessment.

A group of Australian nurse researchers developed the clinical reasoning cycle. The clinical reasoning cycle explains how nurses use a methodical process to make informed practice decisions that enhance patient safety. Nursing assessment has a major role in the clinical reasoning cycle. Although it is divided into stages, it is a cyclical process that continues while we gather the information required to assess a patient's health status and is repeated every time we assess a patient (see figure 4.1) (Levett-Jones 2013; European Heart Association n.d.).

The stages of the clinical reasoning cycle are:

1. consider the patient
2. collect cues/information based on assessment
3. process the information gathered from assessment
4. identify patient problems or patient issues
5. establish patient goals
6. take appropriate nursing actions based on the assessment
7. evaluate outcomes of the care
8. reflect on care provided.

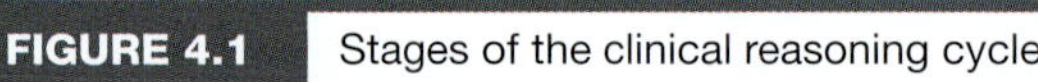

FIGURE 4.1 Stages of the clinical reasoning cycle

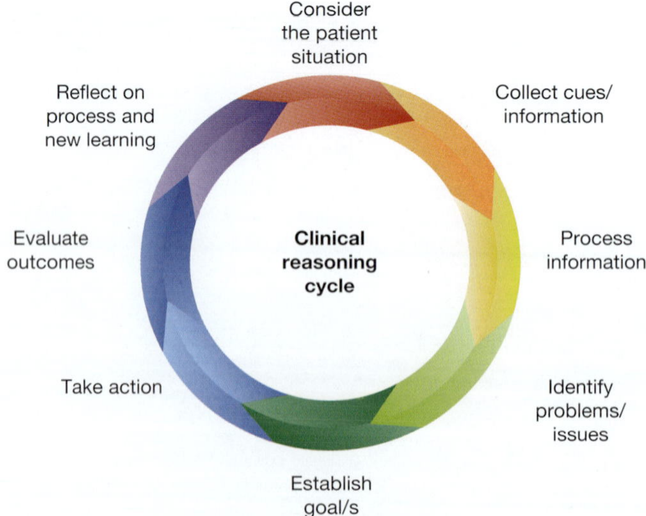

Source: Levett-Jones (2009).

The clinical reasoning cycle meets the essential elements for comprehensive patient care and clinical assessment supported by the Australian Commission on Safety and Quality in Health Care (ACSQHC). The ACSQHC states that these essential elements are:

- Element 1: Clinical assessment and diagnosis
- Element 2: Identify goals of care
- Element 3: Risk screening and assessment
- Element 4: Develop a single comprehensive care plan
- Element 5: Deliver comprehensive care
- Element 6: Review and improve comprehensive care delivery (ACSQHC 2019).

The clinical reasoning approach to nursing assessment

As nurses, we recognise that people are the experts in their life experiences (Nursing and Midwifery Board of Australia 2020, Standard 2.3). It is important that we listen to the patient and their families and do not make assumptions or allow personal bias to interfere with our assessment and care of the patient.

- *Consider* the age of the presenting patient and the needs they may have to make them comfortable and feel secure during the assessment. Elderly patients may need some assistance with hearing or mobility. Special skills are required to keep children comfortable, and it is important to enlist parents and carers help. Implement behaviours that show respect for the patient's age, gender, cultural values and personal preferences. You may need to gain the support of an interpreter to help with an assessment. The Australian Nursing Practice Standard 4 states that as nurses we conduct 'assessments that are holistic as well as culturally appropriate'. Modify your language and communication style to meet the needs of the individual. Remember to treat the patient with dignity. Standard 2 states that the RN 'communicates effectively, and is respectful of a person's dignity, culture, values, beliefs and rights'. Introduce yourself to the patient, and their family if present, to establish rapport and confidence in your ability to care for them.
- *Observe* the patient's body language, hygiene and dress. Do not judge; we must avoid bias and discrimination. Use a systematic approach to ensure that you do not miss important cues. SAMPLE (signs and systems, allergies, medications, past medical history, last meal and events leading up to presentation) is suggested as a systematic approach; however, any evidence-based approach can be used. The important thing is that we collect all available information in an orderly manner to process the information, identify problems, establish goals, take action, evaluate them and reflect on the care provided (Levett-Jones 2013).
- *Encourage* the patient and their family to voice their concerns and to ask questions. Check to see that they have understood what you have told them.

Any serious concerns should be referred to the nurse in charge or the medical team throughout the assessment process. The completed assessments should be properly documented on the appropriate documentation at the facility. Always review the facility or healthcare organisation's policies and procedures to ensure that you meet that provider's legal requirements.

4.2 Foundations of nursing assessment

LEARNING OBJECTIVE 4.2 Explain the foundations of nursing assessment.

Building your nursing assessment skills is an important part of your development as a safe, effective patient-centred nurse. You will need to use your communication skills, knowledge of anatomy and physiology and attitude towards patient confidentiality and privacy. Working within a structure that will support holistic care means that not missing important information. It takes time and energy but is fundamental in building self-confidence and patient confidence in you.

The initial assessment

In the initial nursing assessment, we start to gather data that will enable us to establish baseline data against which subsequent assessments will be compared. This assessment is performed every time we have a patient encounter. This will allow us to track the patient's ongoing status and any changes that indicate deterioration or improvement in the patient's condition. When we assess the patient, we observe (consider) the patient, collect our cues, process the information and identify problems that we will need to act on immediately. The initial assessment is where we make careful use of our observation skills.

Concerns with or changes in patient status trigger actions that need to be taken to respond to deterioration and reduce risks (ACSQHC 2019). The initial assessments also establish risks for patient safety, considering fall risk, pressure injury risk and cognitive issues that may affect care and safety in the healthcare setting.

A simple, helpful tool often used in paramedicine, but helpful for nurses to support an initial assessment of a patient, is SAMPLE, as shown in figure 4.2.

FIGURE 4.2 SAMPLE

	Health history — a tool to support initial assessment of a patient. This will help you to determine if there are any emergency issues that need immediate treatment. You will follow this assessment with a secondary assessment and a focused assessment.	
S	Signs and symptoms	Tell me what has brought you into the ED/clinic/hospital today?
A	Allergies	Do you have any allergies to medications, food, the environment, pets etc.?
M	Medications	What medications are you on? Include prescription medications, over the counter, herbal therapies.
P	Past medical history	Have you had this problem before? What medical problems do you have? Have you had any surgeries in the past?
L	Last ins/outs	When did you last have something to eat or drink? What was it and when?
E	Events	What happened to cause this issue? How did you hurt yourself?

Source: Adapted from Friese (2020); Toney-Butler (2020).

The different sections of SAMPLE are explained in more detail here.

- *Signs and symptoms.* Signs are what can be measured, such as heart rate or respiratory rate, and what can also be seen, heard and felt. Symptoms are what the patient complains about. Ask questions such as when did it start, how long has it gone on, and what things exacerbate or lessen the symptoms?
- *Allergies.* Does the patient have allergies to drugs, food or environmental factors? Ask how the patient reacts to the allergen; for instance, does it cause breathing problems, rashes or sores.
- *Medications.* What medications is the patient taking, and are they taking them as prescribed? Include over the counter medications, alternate or natural medications and illicit drugs.
- *Past pertinent medical history.* Enquire about past medical history, including chronic illnesses, surgeries, family history of heart disease, diabetes and surgical implants.
- *Last ins/outs.* This refers to the last time the patient ate, what the patient ate and how much the patient ate, and the last time they went to the toilet. This will give us valuable information if the patient must go to surgery or have a procedure done. It will also give us clues to the patient's nutritional status.
- *Events leading up to.* Events leading up to requiring care is the opportunity for the patient to share a description of what happened leading up to their illness or injury.

Admission assessment

The admission assessment is a comprehensive nursing assessment that includes the patient history, general appearance, physical examination and monitoring vital signs. As part of the admission assessment, we need to gather a history of current illness/injury such as the reason for current admission, relevant history, allergies and reactions, medications including prescription, schedule 2 and 3 medications, alternative therapies or illegal drug use. Information on immunisation status, implants, family and social history and any recent overseas travel must be documented. Again, observe the patient, collect cues, process the information and identify problems to act on. The admission assessment will be more in-depth than an initial assessment. The intent is to establish baseline data against which subsequent assessments will be compared, and to track the patient's ongoing status and changes that indicate deterioration.

Health history

Taking a health history is an essential part of patient assessment. The health history helps us gather subjective data from the patient and their family (Doyle & McCutcheon 2015). An accurate health history provides essential information required to 'identify patient problems or patient issues, establish patient goals, and taking the appropriate nursing actions' (Epstein et al. 2008). The health history supports a team approach to the care of the patient. It allows healthcare providers and the patient and their family to collaborate on a plan that will address acute health problems, avoid deterioration, minimise chronic health conditions and promote wellness.

In obtaining an accurate health history, it is important to establish a comfortable nurse–patient relationship. The patient should feel that the nurse is interested in understanding the patient's healthcare problems (Elliott 2010). It is important to put patients at ease, provide them with privacy and ensure confidentiality of information. It is also essential to recognise the importance of being sensitive to cultural differences (Tagney 2008).

Following the health history assessment performed on patient admission, a further health history should be undertaken to confirm the information in the notes and ascertain if there are any changes to the patient's condition. Patient assessments are not done in isolation. Nurses use a holistic approach to patient care. In an assessment of all systems, we include a patient interview and review of vital signs. The health history assessment can be taken as you do the vital signs and can take the form of a conversation with the patient. In the conversation, you will also be assessing ABCDE (airway, breathing, circulation, disability, environment). If the patient is talking to you, the airway is open and they are breathing. Talking to the patient will help you determine if they are orientated, and you will be able to ensure that the environment is appropriate to the situation — warm, comfortable and private.

Vital signs and **pain score** should be included in all of your assessments.

Shift assessment

The shift assessment is a concise nursing assessment that, as a minimum, is completed at the commencement and end of each shift. It involves taking and documenting vital signs. This involves reviewing, observing or considering the patient, collecting our cues, processing the information and identifying problems to act on. If a change in the patient's status occurs, such as a procedure or the assessment reveals deterioration in their condition, this assessment will be repeated more frequently. The documentation charts for patient assessment tend to stipulate the frequency of shift assessments or observations, for example, every six hours.

While often not thought of as an assessment, hourly or intentional rounding is another opportunity to undertake a patient assessment, reduce risks and support early detection of deterioration. Hourly rounding is a systematic process used by nursing to anticipate and address the patient's fundamental needs (Clinical Excellence Commission 2017). As we round on our patients, we gather information, note any changes, and provide, evaluate and plan ongoing care with our patients and their families. The information that is collected during the hourly or intentional rounds will help inform other healthcare providers in the provision of safe and effective care.

Focused assessment

A focused assessment is a detailed nursing assessment of specific body systems or systems as indicated by the presenting problem, or findings in the initial, ongoing or shift assessment. For example, if the patient states that they have abdominal pain, a focused assessment will need to be completed on the abdominal system. Likewise, if the patient is having mobility issues, a full musculoskeletal assessment will be required. The need for a focused assessment is based on the admission assessment, the shift assessment or additional assessment as required by the patient presentation.

Risk assessment

An important part of patient assessment is risk management. The aim is to identify patients 'at risk' of developing complications associated with their health problem, hospitalisation or reduced mobility (ACSQHC 2019). Key areas for risk assessment include pressure ulcers, infection, falls, malnutrition and overnutrition, dehydration, constipation, delirium and cognitive impairment, self-harm and suicide risk, aggressive and violent behaviour, and risks caused by seclusion and restraints (ACSQHC 2019). Hospital policies will include risk assessment tools as part of the admission procedure. This is supported by National Safety and Quality Health Service Standards (2019) that state 'implementing targeted, best-practice strategies can prevent or minimise the risk of these specific harms'.

Risk management tools

Table 4.1 shows some examples of risk management tools. Healthcare settings will have their own approved charts, and it is important to review and refer to healthcare provider policies on how and when to use them.

TABLE 4.1 Examples of risk management tools

Risk management tool	Use
Deterioration detection charts Adult Deterioration Detection System (ADDS) chart with blood pressure table ACSQHC. Between the Flags Eastern Health Maternity Observation Chart (health.vic 2020a) ViCTOR charts & folders (ViCTOR 2018)	The Australian Commission on Safety and Quality in Health Care (ACSQHC) has suggested track and trigger charts that provide nursing staff with guidelines for escalating care. Similar track and trigger charts are used in both private and public healthcare settings. The purpose is to provide a guide for identifying changes in status and early detection of deterioration.
Pressure injury risk tools Braden Scale Waterlow Score	Risk of pressure injury should be assessed on admission, and subsequent assessment should be dependent on the initial score. The patient is assessed as needed. It is important to remember risk areas such as tubing or cannulas resting against the skin. It is also important to recognise that if a patient has been to surgery or there is a change in status, they should be assessed again for risk of pressure injuries.
Nutrition risk tools The Malnutrition Screening Tool (MST) (health.vic 2020b) The Mini Nutrition Assessment (MNA) (health.vic 2020b) The Mini Nutrition Assessment Short Form (MNA-SF) (health.vic 2020b) The Malnutrition Universal Screening Tool (MUST) (health.vic 2020b)	Assessment of nutritional status is important for identifying a patient's nutritional risk. The recognition and treatment of malnutrition is a concern for acute, chronic and transitional healthcare settings. Nurses have the expertise and responsibility to ensure that patients' nutritional needs are being met. Nutritional screening and nutrition advice is essential to improve health outcomes. It is important to document the patient's diet to reduce malnutrition risk during admission.
Bowel charts Bristol Stool Chart	Documentation of bowel movement helps prevent constipation, urinary retention that can lead to delirium in all patients, particularly post-operative and elderly patients. The Bristol Stool Chart helps the patient indicate if they are constipated, has normal stools or has diarrhoea (Continence Foundation of Australia 2020). Charts to document bowel movements should be available in all healthcare settings.
Fluid balance charts	Fluid balance charts must be accurately completed to maintain a record of the patient's fluid intake and output and identify if dehydration or overhydration requires care (Ausmed 2020).

Distress management tools Distress Thermometer Edmonton Symptom Assessment System Canadian Partnership Against Cancer – Screening for Distress data Mini-Mental State Examination (MMSE)	The Cancer Association of Australian has led the work on monitoring screening for cancer patients' distress with validated tools and care pathways (Cancer Australia 2020). It is important to assess cognition in your patient to see if there is any indication of impairment. Tools for screening the patient can be found at Dementia Australia's website. Appropriate screening and follow up will support the healthcare provider's efforts towards safe and effective care (Dementia Australia 2020).
Pain score tools Wong Baker Faces® Visual Analogue Scale (VAS) Numeric Rating Scale (NRS) Verbal Descriptor Scale (VDS) Smiling Face Scale (SFS) Numeric Descriptor Scale (NDS)	There are several pain scoring tools available, and it is important to review and understand the use of the tool used in the clinical setting in which you are working.

Communicating and documentation

Failure to communicate and failure to document clinical information clearly and appropriately is known to result in errors in care, incorrect diagnosis and inappropriate treatments, leading to poor patient outcomes. It has been noted that communication errors contribute significantly to sentinel events in healthcare and have been identified as one of the most common underlying factors in Australian healthcare system complaints (ACSQHC 2017).

Every nurse has heard the statement, 'If it was not documented, it was not done'. A vital part of assessment is documentation. The ACSQHC (2017) Communicating for Safety Standard states 'to ensure timely, purpose-driven and effective communication and documentation that support continuous, coordinated and safe care for patients' (Intention of the Standard Para 2). Clear documentation is a recognised key to the delivery of safe, effective patient care. Poor clinical documentation undermines patient care, the healthcare facility and healthcare data (Clinical Documentation Improvement Australia Pty Ltd 2020).

Reasons for documenting healthcare include:

- communication between healthcare providers
- meeting legislative and professional standards
- research into healthcare
- legal proof of the healthcare provided (Lippincott Nursing Center 2019).

Nursing documentation is a legal document and should follow the following requirements.

- Be accurate, relevant and consistent/readable, and/or as displayed on electronic health record system screens.
- Logical, timely and sequential following the clinical reasoning cycle (Levett-Jones 2013). Document your assessment; that is, cues you have gathered, patient problems, goals established, actions taken and evaluation or outcomes of your care.
- Not be altered. *Never* use whiteout, erase, or delete an entry. If a mistake has been made, cross out the error with one line and sign it. Then write the correct information.
- Always document a patient or the family refusal to comply with a treatment or procedure or healthcare recommendations.
- Document all telephone orders including time, date, and content of the call and have the person who witnessed the call sign with you.
- Verbal orders must be co-signed by the healthcare provider giving the order.
- Never document for another healthcare provider or sign off on another practitioner's interventions.
- Do not correct or destroy another healthcare provider's documentation.
- Never document care prior to giving the care, including hourly rounding and medications (Lippincott Nursing Center 2019).

Patient assessment forms and nursing documentation are set by the healthcare facility's (or group of healthcare facilities) policy and procedures. There are standardised formats for nursing documentation and include those outlined in table 4.2.

TABLE 4.2 Assessment formats

Type	What to document
A to G	Document assessment, problems, interventions and outcomes under the following headings: • Airway • Breathing • Circulation • Disability • Exposure • Fluids • Glucose
PIE	Problem Intervention: what was done to address the problem Evaluation: what was the result of the intervention
AIR	Assessment Intervention Result of the intervention
DAR	Data or assessment, including subjective and objective information Action: what was or will be done Response: the patient's response to the action
SOAPIE	Subjective: what the patient is saying Objective: what you are observing Assessment: vital signs from head to toe Plan: your plan of care Intervention: what you did Evaluation: did it work

Handover

Handover is the process of transferring care of a patient from one healthcare professional to another. Handover of patient care is a high-risk situation (ACSQHC 2019). The risk of communication errors at these times is well documented. Structured and standardised handovers can improve patient safety (Australian Nursing and Midwifery Federation 2020).

Standard verbal communication formats are used to communicate patient information from one healthcare provider to other healthcare providers. These are:

- SBAR: Situation, Background, Assessment, Recommendation (ACSQHC 2019)
- ISBAR: Identification, Situation, Background, Assessment, Recommendation
- ISOBAR: Identification, Situation, Observations, Background, Assessment, Read back.

The nurse needs to familiarise themselves with the format used in their healthcare facility to reduce risks and provide the healthcare professional taking over the care with the information needed to support safe and effective care.

4.3 Structured nursing assessments

LEARNING OBJECTIVE 4.3 Recognise and interpret the different types of structured nursing assessments.

Structured nursing assessments support accurate nursing examination with a tool to ensure nothing is missed. A good assessment tool will support early recognition of an emergency situation, a deteriorating patient and allow for accurate verbal and written communication of the patient's status.

A to E assessment

Each patient will have an A to E assessment on every occasion the nurse has contact with them. This is a quick and basic initial assessment. However, by no means is it the only assessment performed, it is the start of a more in-depth assessment. On contact with the patient, you introduce yourself to the patient and advise them of why you are there. For example, introduce yourself and explain that you are doing an hourly round or following up on care. You are observing the patient; by looking and listening and shaking their hand you can assess the following.

- **A**irway: Is their airway open and clear? Can they speak to you in whole sentences?
- **B**reathing: What does their breathing sound like? Are there any abnormal sounds?
- **C**irculation: Do they look well perfused (is their skin colour good)?
- **D**isability: Do they have any disabilities? For instance, do they wear glasses, use a hearing aid or require a stick to walk with? Do they appear confused or disorientated?
- **E**xposure: Is there any bleeding, or does the patient have a wound, sores or a rash? Is the patient comfortable and is the environment safe? This is where you complete the environmental or bed checks. Is the area safe for the patient? Are emergency supplies ready if needed? Are the bed or chair brakes on?

This is an immediate assessment of a patient when you first meet them and very useful in an emergency. However, it does not replace the full A to G assessment or the focused assessment. It is the beginning of your full patient assessment. It provides information that you will build on or information on which you must act immediately.

A to G assessment

The A to G assessment is a structured, systematic assessment, useful in all healthcare settings (Cathala & Moorley 2020). The tool integrates the assessments to reduce morbidity and mortality with a systematic patient assessment that is useful in emergency and resuscitation and can alert nurses to patient deterioration in the hospital setting. Table 4.3 outlines the A to G assessment in detail.

TABLE 4.3	The A to G assessment

A = Airway
In a more in-depth assessment of the airways, we include the nose, mouth, larynx, pharynx, trachea and the bronchi and bronchioles (Cathala & Moorley 2020). The aim is to identify any obstruction or abnormality that will affect the patient's breathing. An indication of the condition of a patient's airway is their ability to speak in complete sentences with their usual voice (not whispered or hoarse).

B = Breathing
Breathing is the process of gas exchange wherein the air moves in and out of the lungs. Normal breathing should be effortless, with a rate of 12 to 20 breaths per minute. There should be equal bilateral chest expansion. Respirations should be quiet. Noises such as stridor, wheeze or rattle indicate abnormal [illegible]. There should be no evidence of excessive sputum.

C = Circulation
Assessment of circulation includes a review of the cardiac, hemodynamic and vascular systems. Check the peripheries and look at the hands and fingers. Are they pink and warm? Is there any sign of clubbing, indicating chronic obstructive pulmonary disease (COPD)? Check capillary refill time to ensure it is less than two seconds. Assess the pulse rate and determine the rate, regularity and strength. Complete a blood pressure check.

D = Disability
Disability should be assessed using an AVPU scale (outlined in the next section). Is the patient alert and orientated? Listen for slurred speech or signs of confusion. You should also note if the patient has glasses or a hearing aid that may make a difference to their safety during their care. Determine if the patient is in pain by completing a pain assessment.

E = Exposure
The healthcare provider will look for any signs of trauma, rashes, skin breakdown, wounds, skin turgor and consider the risk of pressure injuries. Body temperature should be taken and recorded. It is important to consider the dignity of the patient and maintain privacy and confidentiality at all times (Thim et al. 2012).

(continued)

TABLE 4.3 *(continued)*

F = Fluids Consider the fluid status of the patient (NSW Health 2020). Look at the patient's skin. Are there signs of dryness or over hydration? Does the patient have swollen ankles or hands that might suggest they are not passing fluid? If the patient is admitted to hospital, review the observation charts and their fluid intake and output balance. Is the patient complaining of being thirsty?
G = Glucose Monitoring blood glucose levels is an important part of the assessment process (NSW Health 2020; Cathala & Moorley 2020). One of the questions you will ask in an initial assessment is if the patient has a history of diabetes. If the patient does not have diabetes or has no family history of diabetes, then clinical judgement should be used. If the patient presents with signs of altered levels of consciousness, then a blood glucose level assessment needs to be completed.

AVPU scale

The AVPU (alert, verbal, pain, unresponsive) scale is a rapid assessment tool used to measure conscious state. The patient is assigned one letter to indicate their best response. The **AVPU scale** is an ideal tool in the initial assessment of a patient. It is incorporated in track and trigger charts as it is simpler than the Glasgow Coma Scale (GCS) but is not suitable for long-term monitoring of conscious state (Romanelli & Farrell 2020). The basis of the AVPU scale is based on the following criterion.

- **A**lert: The patient is aware of the environment, opens their eyes spontaneously and can track objects.
- **V**erbal: The patient's eyes do not open spontaneously. They open their eyes only when a verbal stimulus is directed at them. The patient can react to that verbal stimulus directly and in a meaningful way.
- **P**ain: The patient does not open their eyes spontaneously or to verbal stimuli. They respond to painful stimuli such as touch. If there is still no response, a trapezius squeeze is used. They may move, moan or cry out in response to the painful stimuli
- **U**nresponsive: The patient does not open their eyes spontaneously or to verbal or painful stimuli (Romanelli & Farrell 2020).

Glasgow Coma Scale (GCS)

The **Glasgow Coma Scale (GCS)** was first put forward in 1974 as a reliable, objective way of recording a person's level of consciousness. The GCS is used for both the initial and the ongoing assessment of the patient. Correctly implemented, the GCS is used to communicate patient status between healthcare providers and allows the healthcare provider to track the patient's level of consciousness. The GCS tool has withstood the test of time; however, significant research indicates a need for a clear education strategy on the tool's practical implementation (Braine & Cook 2017; Catangui 2019). Table 4.4 details the GCS.

TABLE 4.4 **Scoring for the GCS**

Eye-opening scores	Best motor response scores	Best verbal response scores
4: Spontaneously 3: To verbal command 2: To pain 1: No response	6: Obeys command 5: Localises pain 4: Flexion withdrawal 3: Flexion abnormal (decorticate) 2: Extension (decerebrate) 1: No response	5: Oriented and converses 4: Disoriented and converses 3: Inappropriate words; cries 2: Incomprehensible sounds 1: No response
Score for best eye opening + best verbal response + best motor response = GCS		

Source: Adapted from Royal College of Physicians and Surgeons of Glasgow (n.d.).

The GCS is often used to define the severity of traumatic brain injury (Royal College of Physicians and Surgeons of Glasgow n.d.). Mild head injuries are generally defined as those associated with a GCS score of 13–15. Moderate head injuries are those associated with a GCS score of 9–12. A GCS score of 8 or less defines a severe head injury. However, these definitions are not rigid and are used as a general guide to injury level. It is also important to consider situations or injuries that might affect scoring. For example, the intubated patient will not be able to speak and will be graded on eye opening and best motor response scores.

Vital signs

Vital sign monitoring is fundamental to safe, effective nursing care (Sapra, Malik & Bhandari 2020). Accurate measurement and knowledge of normal ranges for an individual patient support evaluating care outcomes and helps to detect deterioration. The quantitative data from vital signs support the ability to track client status changes and triggers actions to prevent deterioration. The initial set of vital signs provides the baseline for further assessment. Importantly it helps to establish if the patient needs urgent or emergency care on presentation.

The standard vital signs measured for all patients are temperature, pulse, respiratory rate, blood pressure, oxygen saturation, consciousness level and pain score. The National Consensus Statement states that vital signs should be monitored at least once over an eight-hour shift (ACSQHC 2019).

Normal vital signs vary with age, gender, weight, exercise capability and overall health. Normal vital sign ranges for the average healthy adult while resting are as follows. However, it is important to recognise that these are highly dependent on the individual patient (MedlinePlus 2019; Ausmed 2019).

Normal vital signs are:

- blood pressure: 100/60 mmHg to 120/80 mmHg
- respiratory rate: 12 to 18 breaths per minute
- pulse rate: 60 to 100 beats per minute
- temperature: 36.5°C to 37.3°C with an average of 37°C.

Blood pressure

Blood pressure (BP) is the force of the blood pushing against the artery walls during contraction and relaxation of the heart (Jevon 2020). The greatest pressure or systolic pressure refers to the pressure inside the artery when the heart contracts and pumps blood through the body. Once the contraction is complete and the heart is at rest, the BP drops. This lower number is called diastolic pressure. Both the systolic and diastolic pressures are recorded as millimetres of mercury (mmHg). When recording the BP measurement, it is important to document both the systolic and the diastolic rates. For example, 120/60 with the top number being the systolic pressure and the bottom number being the diastolic pressure.

Despite the increased use of automated BP devices, it is recommended that healthcare providers continue to receive training in manual BP measurement using auscultation. It is important to retain this skill for situations where automated BP devices are not available or in disaster situations where there are power failures.

High BP is recognised as a risk factor for heart attack, heart failure and stroke. With high BP, the arteries may have an increased resistance against the flow of blood. This causes the heart to work harder to circulate the blood.

Table 4.5 outlines the classifications for adult BP.

TABLE 4.5 Classification for adult blood pressure

Category	Systolic (mmHG)		Diastolic (mmHG)
Normal	<130	and	<85
High BP	130–139	and/or	85–89
Grade one hypertension	140–159	and	90–99
Grade two hypertension	≥160	and/or	≥100

Source: Unger et al. (2020).

Respiratory rate

Respiratory rate is the number of breaths a person takes each minute. It is measured when a person is at rest and is done by counting the rise and fall of the chest. The respiratory rate is counted for a full minute. The patient must not be aware you are counting their respiratory rate as there is a tendency for them to alter their respiratory rate unconsciously as you count.

Oxygen saturation (SaO_2)

The normal range of oxygen saturation for an adult is 95 per cent or greater. Like other vital signs, this must be individualised for the patient. For example, for patients with chronic COPD, the acceptable oxygen saturation for these patients may be between 88–92 per cent (Beasley et al. 2015; O'Driscoll et al. 2017). Oxygen saturation readings can be affected by nail polish, a bright light shining on the probe and interfering with the light detector, movement by the patient, cold extremities and carbon monoxide poisoning (World Health Organization [WHO] 2011).

Pulse rate

The patient's pulse rate is assessed using palpation. Peripheral pulses include the radial pulse, the femoral pulse, the brachial pulse, the popliteal pulse, the dorsalis pedis pulse of the foot and the posterior tibial pulse near the ankle (see figure 4.3). In most routine assessments, the radial pulse is usually palpated using the radial pulse. Pulse rate is recorded as beats per minute (bpm).

FIGURE 4.3 Location of pulse points

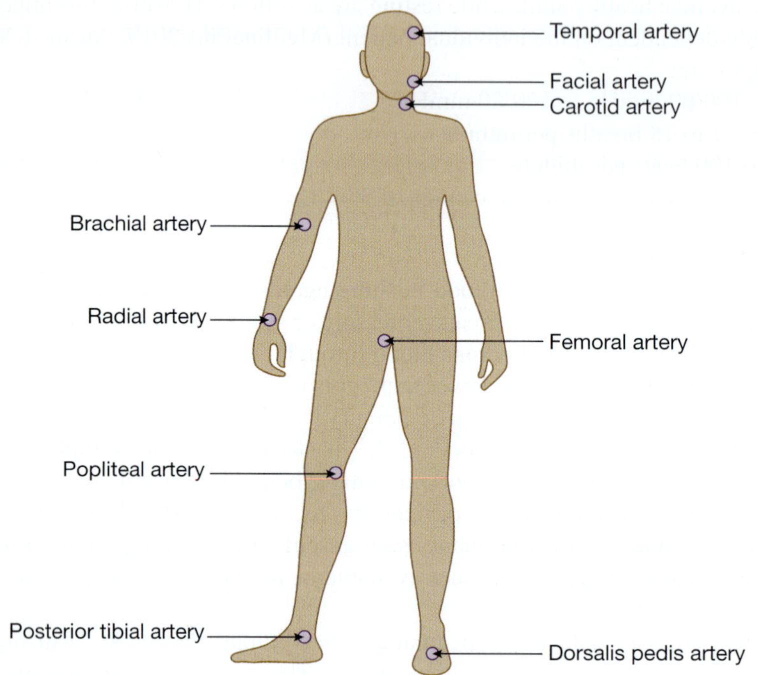

The normal parameters for pulse rates across the life span are:

- neonate: 80–180 bpm
- infant: 100–160 bpm
- toddler: 90–140 bpm
- preschool child: 80–110 bpm
- school-age child: 70–100 bpm
- adolescent: 60–100 bpm
- adult: 60–100 bpm (Healthline 2021).

Factors that may affect pulse rate are:

- age
- fitness and activity levels
- being a smoker
- cardiovascular disease
- high cholesterol levels
- diabetes
- air temperature
- body position (standing up or lying down, for example)
- emotional state
- body size
- medications (Laskowski 2020).

Temperature

Normal body temperature will vary depending on gender, activity, food and fluid consumption, time of day and stage of the menstrual cycle in females. The normal range for core temperature varies in the literature; however, 36–37.5 degrees Celsius is acceptable for a healthy adult in clinical practice (McCallum & Higgins 2012). In healthcare settings, digital, oral, axilla and tympanic thermometers are used to take a temperature. It is important to read the manufactures instructions so you are informed of the recommended use of and cleaning of equipment.

The tympanic thermometer senses reflected infrared emissions from the tympanic membrane through a probe placed in the external auditory canal. The tympanic thermometer is minimally invasive, quick and easy to perform. The Royal Children's Hospital Melbourne (RCH) recommends the tympanic thermometer for children older than six months. For children who are less than six months, the RCH recommends using a digital thermometer per axilla (RCH 2017). Poor technique and operator error have been cited as problematic in the accurate assessment of temperature. Hence, it is important to read the manufacturer's directions on the use of these thermometers to obtain accurate temperatures. Imprecise results will lead to inaccuracies in determining patient problems and the care plan, which will lead to failure to identify the patient's deterioration.

Additional measurements

Body measurements are used to assess nutritional status and help determine an accurate patient's health status. Body mass index (BMI) and risk factors associated with cardiovascular, renal and other diseases help the healthcare provider establish a full picture of the patient.

Additional measurements include:

- weight, completed on admission and weekly or/daily as clinically indicated
- height, on admission
- waist circumference
- BMI, to determine if the patient is in a healthy weight range for their height (Australian Government Department of Health 2020)
- blood glucose level (BGL), as clinically indicated.

4.4 Physical assessment

LEARNING OBJECTIVE 4.4 Identify the different types of physical assessments utilised in nursing.

Physical assessment requires mastery of four main techniques (Nursing2021 2006). These techniques are used in the same order for all body systems except the abdomen. The usual sequence is **inspection**, **palpation**, **percussion** and **auscultation**. Because palpation and percussion can alter bowel sounds, the order is changed to inspection, auscultation, palpation and percussion during an abdominal assessment (Toney-Butler & Unison-Pace 2020).

Inspection

When inspecting or observing a patient, you must use your sight, sense of smell and hearing to assess for normal and, importantly, abnormal presentations. Observe the patient's behaviour — take note of inappropriate responses and actions that can indicate neurological, metabolic, endocrine or mental health problems. Observe the overall appearance of the patient — look at their colour, centrally and peripherally. Does the patient have scars, bruising, burns, rashes, evidence of skin breakdown and are there any invasive lines such as drains or tubes present (Toney-Butler & Unison-Pace 2020)? Consider the patient's weight, height, build, posture, movements, hygiene and grooming. Look for any signs of pain or distress. Observing patients as they walk around or move between the chair to bed or getting dressed can provide important information about their mobility, balance and dexterity. Abnormal smells such as the odour of ketones on the patient's breath may indicate fasting or diabetic ketoacidosis. Information gathered from observing the patient is used with that acquired from the patient interview and physical examination to make sense of the patient's health and support clinical decision making.

Palpation

Palpation requires touching the patient with varying degrees of pressure. It is important to advise the patient that you are taking their pulse, why you are taking it and how you will take it. Informed consent for these procedures is important during all physical assessments where you are required to touch the patient.

You should palpate tender areas last. For infection control purposes, remember to wear gloves when you are palpating any areas that might require contact with body fluids such as mucous membranes. During palpation, consider bilateral symmetry of chest expansion, skin condition including temperature, turgor and moisture, capillary refill, tactile fremitus or vibrations noted in the chest wall, or the presence of subcutaneous emphysema.

Percussion

Percussion requires tapping on the body surfaces and listening to the sounds that result from the tapping (Burke 2020). You are listening to determine the presence of air, fluid or solid masses. The technique requires practice and tenderness. Direct percussion uses one or two fingers to tap directly on the patient's body (Nursing2021 2006). For indirect percussion, place the distal middle finger of your non-dominant hand on the body part you are assessing. Flex your wrist with the rest of your hand, not touching the body. Using the middle finger of your dominant hand, tap quickly over the distal part of the middle finger where it is touching the patient's body. As you percuss, ask the patient to tell you which areas are painful, and watch the patients face, being aware of body language that indicates signs of discomfort. The sounds heard with percussion are a hollow sound or resonance, a flat sound heard over bone, a booming sound called hyper and tympany, which is a drum-type sound (see table 4.6) (Burke 2020).

TABLE 4.6 Percussion notes on the posterior chest

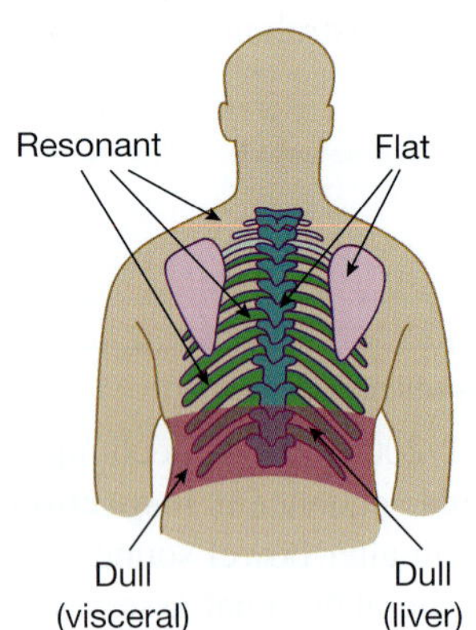

	Resonant sounds are low-pitched, hollow sounds heard over normal lung tissue.
	Flat or extremely dull sounds are normally heard over solid areas such as bones.
	Dull or thud-like sounds are normally heard over dense areas such as the heart or liver. Dullness replaces resonance when fluid or solid tissue replaces air-containing lung tissues, such as occurs with pneumonia, pleural effusions or tumours.
	Hyper-resonant sounds that are louder and lower pitched than resonant sounds are normally heard when percussing the chests of children and very thin adults. Hyper-resonant sounds may also be heard when percussing lungs hyperinflated with air, such as may occur in patients with COPD, or patients having an acute asthmatic attack. An area of hyper-resonance on one side of the chest may indicate a pneumothorax.
	Tympanic sounds are hollow, high, drum-like sounds. Tympany is normally heard over the stomach, but is not a normal chest sound. Tympanic sounds heard over the chest indicate excessive air in the chest, such as may occur with pneumothorax.

Source: RnCeus.com (2020).

Auscultation

Auscultation is a skill that, as nurses, we are likely the most familiar with. Auscultation involves using a stethoscope to listen to parts of the patient's body. The first, most likely experience with auscultation will be taking blood pressure and listening to sounds associated with turbulent blood flow, known as Korotkoff sounds (Ogedegbe & Pickering 2010). We also use auscultation to listen to bowel, lung and heart sounds. The sounds heard with auscultation are classified and described according to their duration, pitch, intensity and quality. For example, the duration of a breath sound can be described in terms of seconds of duration, or it can be described as having a longer duration of inspiration than expiration. The sound's intensity can be described as loud or soft and quiet; the pitch is described as high-pitched to a dull and low-pitched sound.

Pain score

Assessing a patient's pain can been seen as the fifth vital sign. According to Painaustralia (2020), Australia was the first to develop a national framework for pain. The National Pain Summit, held in Canberra in 2010, developed a National Pain Strategy.

The key goals of the Australian National Pain Strategy are:

- people in pain as a national health priority
- knowledgeable, empowered and supported consumers
- skilled professionals and best-practice evidence-based care
- access to interdisciplinary care at all levels
- quality improvement and evaluation
- research.

Pain is a frequent complaint of patients presenting to the emergency department (ED) (Australian Institute of Health and Welfare 2018). However, pain remains an under-investigated and underestimated problem for healthcare providers. Studies have shown that nominating pain as a fifth vital sign has led to unintentional results, including prescribed opioid addiction (Kutlutürkan 2020). However, ongoing pain management is important in gaining a holistic view of the patient's problems. According to McCaffery (1989), 'pain is whatever the experiencing person says it is, existing whenever the experiencing person says it does'. Self-reporting is considered the touchstone and most accurate measure of pain (Crozer Health 2021; Pirschel 2018). Providing a score for pain alone is not sufficient information for the provision of safe and effective care. To better understand a patient's pain, we need to collect and process information to identify problems, establish goals, take action and evaluate and reflect on care provision. The PQRST method of pain assessment helps to standardise the approach and allows the patient 'ownership' of their pain. The mnemonic PQRST (table 4.7) is a valuable tool for collecting information and assessing pain, as is a comparative pain scale chart such as the one in figure 4.4.

TABLE 4.7 PQRST pain assessment tool

Ask the patient:		
P	**Provoking/palliating**	When did it begin? How long does it last? How often does it occur?
Q	**Quality**	What does it feel like? Please describe it?
R	**Radiation**	Where is it? Where does it spread to?
S	**Severity/symptoms**	What is the intensity of your pain — on a scale of 0 to 10 with 0 being none and 10 being worst possible? Right now? At best? At worst? On average? How bothered are you by this symptom? Are there any other symptom(s) that accompany it? How does it affect your daily activities?
T	**Timing/triggers**	When does it start? How long does it last? How often does it happen?

Source: Adapted from Ausmed (2020).

FIGURE 4.4 Example of a comparative pain scale chart

0 Pain Free	1 Very Mild	2 Discomforting	3 Tolerable	4 Distressing	5 Very Distressing	6 Intense	7 Very Intense	8 Utterly Horrible	9 Excruciating unbearable	10 Unimaginable Unspeakable
No Pain	Minor Pain			Moderate Pain			Severe Pain			
Feeling perfectly normal	Nagging, annoying, but doesn't interfere with most daily living activties. Patient able to adapt to pain psychologically and with medication or devices such as cushions.			Interferes significantly with daily living activities. Requires lifestyle changes but patient remains independent. Patient unable to adapt pain.			Disabling; unable to perform daily living activities. unable to engage in normal activities. patient is disabled and unable to function independently.			

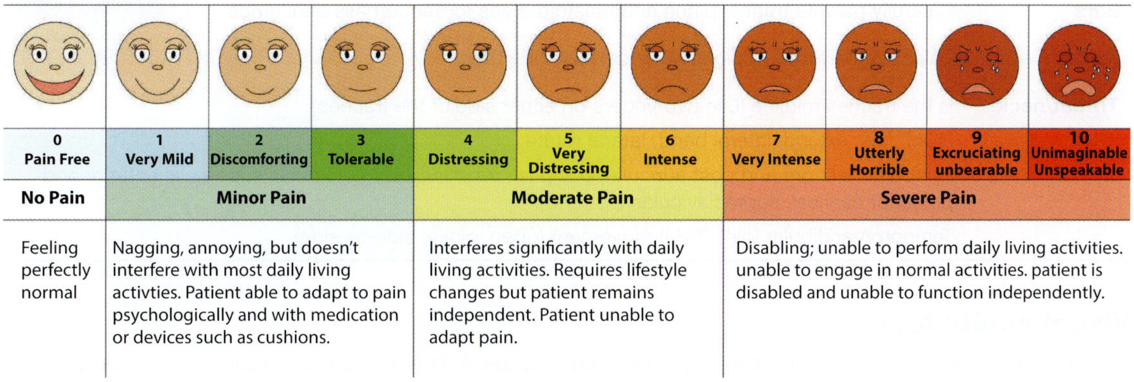

4.5 Nursing assessments for specific body systems

LEARNING OBJECTIVE 4.5 Demonstrate nursing assessments for specific body systems.

Head, ears, eyes, nose, throat (HEENT) assessment

A HEENT assessment is a focused assessment undertaken based on either the presenting complaint, prompted by the health history or your initial and secondary assessment. For example, if a patient presents with hearing difficulties or states they have a sore throat that has been reoccurring on a frequent basis, this would prompt a HEENT assessment.

Inspection

You are using your eyes, ears and sense of smell to examine the patient. You are looking for deviations from the normal.

Head	Facial symmetry: ask the patient to frown, smile, clench teeth, puff cheeks Are there any involuntary facial movements, muscle weakness, lesions, oedema or acne?
Eyes	Symmetry, alignment, position, movement Do you see any orbital oedema, inflammation, dryness, colour of sclera and conjunctiva, lacrimal apparatus (dry or teary eyes)? Use your Penlight to check PERRLA: Pupils Equal, Round, Reactive to Light and Accommodating If there is a Snellen chart or a colour blindness chart you can use them with the patient
Ears	Symmetry, position, deformities, discharge Look for internal signs of inflammation or oedema Perform a gross hearing test — hair rub and whisper test
Nose	External: review symmetry, position, deformities, discharge (colour) Internal: check for inflammation or oedema
Throat/neck	Is the trachea midline? Can you see any lesions, venous distension or an enlarged thyroid gland? What is the range of motion (ROM)? Ask the patient to move their neck from side-to-side, up and down

Palpation

You feel with the fingers or hands to examine the size, consistency, texture, location and tenderness of an organ or body part.

Head	Do you feel any lesions or lumps? Is there any oedema or tenderness? TMJ movement: ask the patient to open and close their mouth, move their chin from side-to-side and up and down (protract and retract)
Eyes	Carefully palpate tear ducts for tenderness
Ears	Carefully palpate tragus, pinna and mastoid areas for tenderness and lumps
Nose	Palpate gently for any signs of tenderness or lumps
Throat/neck	Is the trachea midline (use two fingers on either side of the trachea) ROM: flex, extend, lateral bend, lateral rotate Lymph nodes: pre and post auricular, occipital, tonsillar, submandibular, superficial anterior and posterior cervical, supraclavicular Temporomandibular joint (TMJ) movement (open, close, side-to-side)

Visual acuity test

A visual acuity test uses a standardised Snellen chart (figure 4.5) with patients standing six metres away and covering one eye and then the other eye. The patient is asked to recite the letters they can see on the chart. The last line that they can see and recite correctly denotes their level of sight and may indicate if they need glasses or contacts.

FIGURE 4.5 A Snellen chart

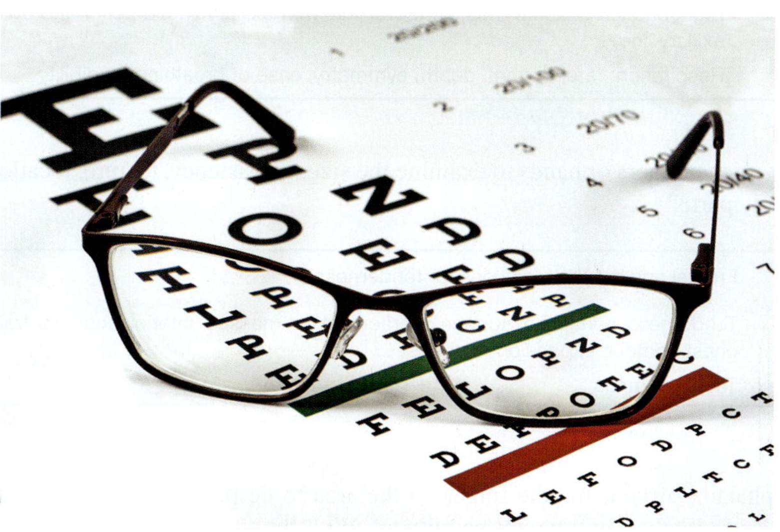

Whisper test

The whisper test is a simple, inexpensive, expedient but accurate screening test for hearing deficits.

The whisper test is conducted using the following steps.

1. Stand 0.6 m behind the patient (to prevent lip reading).
2. The opposite auditory canal is occluded by the patient or examiner, and the tragus is rubbed in a circular motion to block hearing from that ear.
3. The examiner exhales and whispers a combination of numbers and letters (example 4-K-2). *Whispering at the end of exhalation helps ensure a quiet standardised voice.*
4. If the patient responds correctly, hearing is considered normal and no further screening is necessary on that ear.
5. If the patient responds incorrectly, then repeat using a different number-letter combination.
6. If, on repeated testing, the patient can answer three out of a possible six number–letter combinations correctly, the patient passes. If they cannot answer three out of six or more, the patient fails in that ear. They will need to be referred for further hearing tests.
7. Repeat the sequence in the opposite ear using different combinations of numbers and letters. (Note: patients with memory problems may need a simplified letter/number combination to compensate for their inability to remember) (Pirozzo 2003).

Chest and thorax — respiratory assessment

During this assessment, you'll assess the thorax, identify key landmarks, and then use your stethoscope to listen to heart and lung sounds. The thorax is the chest region of the body between the neck and the abdomen. Like other assessments, this focused assessment will be prompted by the health history or the initial and secondary assessments.

Inspection

You are using your eyes, ears and sense of smell to examine the patient. You are looking for deviations from the normal.

Nose/sinuses	Colour, patency, shape, inflammation, oedema, discharge, symmetrical septum.
Mouth/throat	Lips, mucous membrane (pink, moist, lesions) Teeth, gums, halitosis, orthodontic appliances, dentures, crowns, caps, cough, sputum Tongue (midline, strength, lesions), uvula midline, gag reflex (if appropriate) Tonsils (present, removed, inflammation, oedema)

(continued)

(continued)

Thorax (anterior/ posterior)	Skin characteristics (scars / lesions) Chest: contour, shape and expansion, use of accessory muscles, presence of superficial veins, position of sternum, angle of ribs, intercostal spaces, position of scapulae Right and left scapula lines, vertebral line, mid-axillary line, anterior and posterior axillary line Respiration: rate, rhythm, depth, symmetry, ease of breathing, audibility

Palpation

You are feeling with the fingers or hands to examine the size, consistency, texture, location and tenderness of an organ or body part.

Nose/sinuses	Frontal and maxillary sinuses for tenderness.
Thorax (anterior/ posterior)	Tenderness, sensation, surface characteristics, masses anterior/posterior transverse ratio, chest contour, expansion, crepitus Tactile fremitus

Percussion

Place the distal phalanx of your middle finger on the area to be percussed, raise the second and fourth fingers so sound and vibration will be not be blunted. With the tip of your other hand's third finger, use a quick, sharp wrist motion to strike your finger. You trying to ascertain if the area under the percussed finger is air-filled (drum-like sound), fluid-filled (dull sound) or solid (flat sound). Listen for the sound produced and feel the intensity and frequency of vibrations produced.

Thorax (anterior/ posterior)	Tone: resonance to dullness commencing above the clavicles, contra laterally

Auscultation

You are listening to the internal sounds of the body, usually with your stethoscope. Auscultation can also be done with your unaided ear.

Thorax (anterior/ posterior)	Ask the patient to take slow deep breaths. Compare bilateral sounds to determine patients normal

Lung sounds are best heard with a stethoscope. Normal lung sounds occur in all parts of the chest area, including above the collarbones and at the bottom of the rib cage. Figure 4.6 shows the patter and areas for auscultating lung sounds.

FIGURE 4.6 Pattern of auscultation

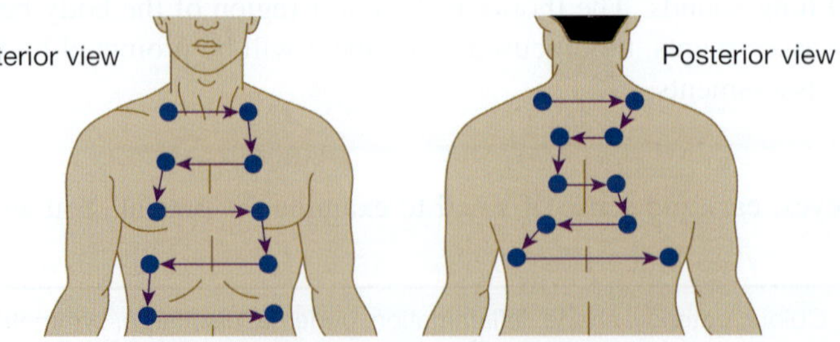

Absent or decreased sounds can mean:

- air or fluid in or around the lungs due to disease processes
- increased thickness of the chest wall
- over-inflation of a part of the lungs due to lung disease
- reduced airflow to part of the lungs.

The most common abnormal lung sounds are as follows.

- *Crackle (rales).* Small clicking, bubbling, or rattling sounds in the lungs heard on inhalation. Can be described as moist, dry, fine and course. They are believed to occur when air passes through fluid, pus or mucus.
- *Sonorous wheezes (rhonchi).* Sounds that resemble snoring. They occur when air is blocked or air flow becomes rough through the large airways. Commonly caused by pneumonia, bronchitis and cystic fibrosis.
- *Stridor (wheeze-like sound).* Usually due to a blockage of airflow in the trachea or back of the throat, and may be a sign of a life-threatening condition.
- *Sibilant wheezes (wheezes).* High-pitched sounds produced by narrowed airways heard on exhalation. Caused by asthma, bronchitis and COPD.

Wheezing and other abnormal sounds can sometimes be heard without a stethoscope.

Cardiovascular assessment

The focused cardiovascular assessment will include the heart itself and the arterial system that supports the delivery of oxygenated blood to the body. Cardiovascular disease (CVD) was the underlying cause of death for 41 800 individuals in Australia in 2018 and an associated cause of 70 600 deaths. The healthcare provider needs to complete a thorough cardiovascular assessment on their patients (Australian Institute of Health and Welfare 2020).

Inspection

You are using your eyes, ears and sense of smell to examine the patient. You are looking for deviations from the normal.

Skin characteristics (as per integumentary system)
Precordium for contours, pulsations
Examine circulatory status and hydration status of upper and lower extremities
Colour (central and peripheral): pink, flushed, pale, mottled, cyanosed, clubbing
Capillary refill time (CRT): brisk (<2 seconds) or sluggish
Presence of oedema (central and/or peripheral)
Hydration status: skin turgor, oral mucosa and anterior fontanels in infants
Jugular vein distension: ask patient to lie at a 45-degree angle, head slightly left

Palpation

You feel with the fingers or hands to examine the size, consistency, texture, location and tenderness of an organ or body part. Figure 4.7 shows the key landmark sites when palpating the heart as one of the steps of the physical assessment of the cardiovascular system.

Palpate central and peripheral pulses for rate, rhythm and volume
Skin condition: temperature, turgor and diaphoresis

FIGURE 4.7 Cardiovascular assessment palpation sites

A	Aortic valve area	Second right intercostal space (ICS), right sternal border
P	Pulmonic valve area	Second left intercostal space (ICS), left sternal border
E	Erb's point	Third left ICS, left sternal border
T	Tricuspid valve area	Fourth left ICS, left sternal border
M	Mitral valve area	Fifth ICS, left mid-clavicular line

Auscultation

You are listening to the internal sounds of the body, usually with your stethoscope. Auscultation can also be done with your unaided ear.

Heart sounds at APETM	Distinguish between Lub S1 (loudest at apex) and Dub S2 (loudest at base) Lub: tricuspid and mitral valves shut — systole begins Dub: Aortic and pulmonic valves shut — systole ends/diastole begins Auscultate the apical pulse located on the left side of the chest, fifth intercostal space at the midclavicular line 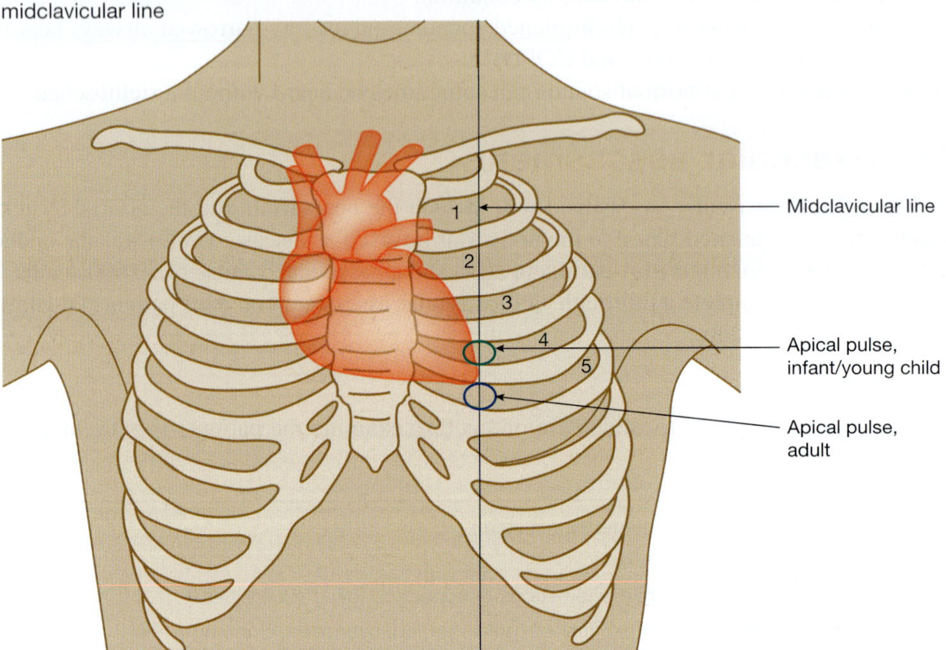 Compare peripheral pulse and apical pulse for consistency (the rate and rhythm should be similar) Auscultate the chest for heart sounds and murmurs

Neurovascular assessment

The neurovascular status assessment supports the early recognition of deterioration in the patient's sensory, motor function and peripheral circulation. Because deterioration may not be immediately detected the neurovascular observations and assessment should be repeated at regular intervals as per hospital policy or physician's request.

Inspection

You are using your eyes, ears and sense of smell to examine the patient. You are looking for deviations from the normal.

Look at skin colour and condition (review your integumentary assessment)
Compare injured left and right sides
Look at the position of extremities, are they aligned and well-formed?
Are there signs of haemorrhage, swelling, ecchymosis or skin deficits (e.g. abrasion, laceration, avulsion) present?

Palpation

You are feeling with the fingers or hands to examine the size, consistency, texture, location and tenderness of an organ or body part.

Palpate pulses and note the presence and strength of the pulse
Assess capillary refill by pressing and releasing pressure on nail, finger and/or toenail. Nail should re-colour in three seconds or less

The six Ps of neurovascular observation

The six Ps are commonly used as a neurological and neurocirculatory assessment. These are outlined in table 4.8

TABLE 4.8 **The six Ps of neurovascular observation**

Pain	Assess for pain using PQRST
Pulses	Check for pulses, assess strength and regularity Temporal artery Carotid Apical pulse Brachial Radial Femoral Popliteal artery Posterior tibial artery Pedal
Paraesthesia	Assess for numbness, tingling, or abnormal sensations. May indicate nerve damage and/or development of compartment syndrome
Paralysis	Assess for movement
Pallor	Check the colour of limbs (should be natural and well perfused)
Temperature	Check for warmth

Abdominal assessment

The abdominal assessment is vital to effective decision-making in patient care. Unlike the other body systems, you inspect first, then auscultate, percuss and palpate in an abdominal assessment. In other system assessments, you usually inspect, then percuss, palpate and auscultate. In this case, we auscultate prior to palpation as pressure on the abdomen with percussion and palpation may affect the bowel sounds. Figure 4.8 shows the quadrants of the abdomen and the organs that lie within each quadrant.

FIGURE 4.8 Abdominal quadrants

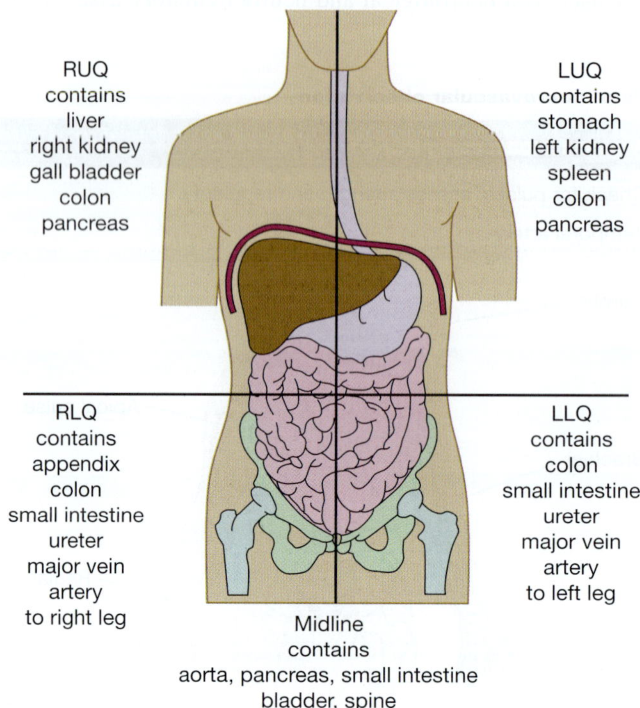

Inspection

You are using your eyes, ears and sense of smell to examine the patient. You are looking for deviations from the normal.

Abdomen	Skin characteristics refer to the integumentary system
	Shape/symmetry of the abdomen (flat, rounded, distended, scaphoid)
	Contour of the abdomen (smooth, lesions, malformations, any old or new scars)
	Distension (mild / moderate / severe / tight / shiny)
	Umbilicus (bulging, scars, piercings)
	Visible peristalsis
	Presence of NG / NGT / PEG/PEJ (indication)
	Stoma site (dressing regimen/frequency and consistency of output)

Auscultation

You are listening to the internal sounds of the body, usually with your stethoscope. Auscultation can also be done with your unaided ear.

Four quadrants	Four quadrants (RUQ, RLQ, LUQ, LLQ) for bowel motility
	Bowel sounds present (frequency/character)
	Absent bowel sounds (one or all quadrants)
	Abdominal girth measurement as clinically indicated

Palpation

You feel with the fingers or hands to examine the size, consistency, texture, location and tenderness of an organ or body part.

Abdomen	Light palpation only identify guarding, tenderness, pain (location, characteristics) Be aware of the patient's abdominal muscles' response and watch their face for signs of discomfort

Percussion

Place the distal phalanx of your middle finger on the area to be percussed, raise the second and fourth fingers so sound and vibration will be not be blunted. With the tip of the third finger of your other hand use a quick, sharp wrist motion to strike your finger. You trying to ascertain if the area under the percussed finger is air-filled (drum-like sound), fluid-filled (dull sound) or solid (flat sound). Listen for the sound produced and feel the intensity and frequency of vibrations produced.

Four quadrants	Light palpation, note guarding, inguinal lymph nodes, femoral pulses, masses Note if percussion produces pain, it may indicate and underlying inflammation Tympanic (drum-like) sounds are produced by percussing over air-filled structures Dull sounds occur when a solid structure (e.g. liver) or fluid (e.g. ascites) lies beneath the region being examined

Musculoskeletal assessment

A healthy musculoskeletal system is important for the performance of the activities of daily living. The musculoskeletal assessment is a focused assessment that will help identify not only major problems but will also help to pinpoint subtle problems that can impact on quality of life.

Inspection

You are using your eyes, ears and sense of smell to examine the patient. You are looking for deviations from the normal.

Overall appearance/first impression	Inspect overall appearance of the patient — Symmetry, body height & weight appropriate for age and gender, no structural deformities, no indication of pain Posture, spine, gait, mobility Height to weight ratio Limbs: swelling, redness and obvious deformity Joint ROM: is it passive or independent? Are limbs moving equally, is there pain on movement? Joints for redness or swelling Muscle shape, Joint contour identify obvious structural deformities, note indications of discomfort and pain
Sitting posture	Observe posture when sitting; feet should be placed firmly on the ground with toes pointing forward
Standing posture	Ask the patient to stand with feet together and observe the spatial relationship of head, torso, pelvis and limbs. Assess symmetry of shoulders, scapulae and iliac crest Normal-posture erect, upright stance with the parallel alignment of hips and shoulders; alignment of head and symmetry of extremities Abnormal-forward slouching, asymmetry
Gait	Ask patient to walk - observe gait and balance; note the base of support, foot position, stride length, arm swing. Assess if movements are smooth and coordinated; arms usually swing freely at the sides Ask the patient to walk on toes, heels, toe-to-toe (= tandem walking) Normal-evenly distributed weight, able to stand on heels and toes, movements coordinated and rhythmic, arms swing in opposition, stride length appropriate (35–45 cm), balance maintained, head and face lead body when turning Abnormal-uneven weight-bearing, cannot stand on heels or toes, limp noted, shuffles, propels forward, wide-based gait, smaller steps and wider support (older adult), feet dragging, uneven wear on shoes
Range of motion (ROM)	Ask the patient to follow your demonstration; assess the angle of joint movement, pain, limitation. Palpation and inspection are combined

Palpation

You feel with the fingers or hands to examine the size, consistency, texture, location and tenderness of an organ or body part.

Spine	Run two fingers down either side while the patient is standing and bending with arms/head falling free
Limbs	Check for muscle mass, tone and strength, pain or tenderness
Joints	Check for ease of movement, selling, pain, tenderness

Range of movement (ROM)

Ask the patient to perform range of movement (ROM) exercises to the best of their ability, but not to the point of pain.

The terminology used in a ROM assessment is outlined here. Table 4.9 outlines how to test each joint.

- Abduction: Moving away from the midline of the body.
- Adduction: Moving towards the midline of the body.
- Circumduction: The circular movement.
- Flexion: Bending the extremity at the joint and decreasing the angle of the joint.
- Extension: The opposite of flexion; a straightening movement that *increases* the angle between body parts.
- Hyperextension: joint bends greater than a 180-degree angle.
- Dorsi flexion: Flexion of the entire foot superiorly, as if taking one's foot off an automobile pedal.
- Plantar flexion: Flexion of the entire foot inferiorly, as if pressing an automobile pedal.
- Rotation: Turning of a bone on its own long axis.
  - Internal rotation: Turning of a bone towards the centre of the body.
  - External rotation: Turning of a bone away from the centre of the body.
- Eversion: Moving outwards.
- Inversion: Moving inwards.
- Pronation: Turning or facing downwards.
- Supination: Turning or facing upwards.
- Protraction: Moving forwards.
- Retraction: Moving backwards.

TABLE 4.9 Testing ROM

Spine	Flex, extend, lateral, bend, twist
Temporomandibular joint	Open, close, side-to-side
Neck	Flex, extend, lateral bend, lateral rotate
Shoulder	Shrug, flex, extend, abduct, adduct, internal/external rotation
Elbow	Flex, extend, pronate, supinate
Wrist	Flex, extend, radial deviation, ulna deviation
Hand/Fingers	Flex, extend, abduct
Hip	Flex, extend, abduct, adduct, heel to knee, internal/external rotation
Knee	Flex, extend
Ankle	Plantar/dorsiflex, inversion, eversion

Integumentary assessment

Inspection

You are using your eyes, ears and sense of smell to examine the patient. You are looking for deviations from the normal.

Skin	Integrity, colour (including variations), odour, pigmentation, scars, lesions, wounds, striae, vascularity
Scalp and hair	Lesions, colour of hair, quantity, condition, distribution, infestations Scull size, shape, contour (rounded over frontal bone and occiput), head control
Nails	Colour, cleanliness, shape, configuration

Palpation

You feel with the fingers or hands to examine the size, consistency, texture, location and tenderness of an organ or body part.

Skin	Temperature, turgor, oedema, moisture, texture
Scalp and hair	Oedema, tenderness, hair texture
Nails	Texture, consistency, capillary refill (<3 seconds)

Mole assessment

A	Asymmetry	Both sides should be the same A line in the middle would not create matching halves
B	Border	Borders should be regular Irregular, wavy, jagged border, clearly defined against surrounding skin
C	Colour	Colour should be even throughout Uneven colour: shade of tan, brown to black
D	Diameter	Less than 6 mm (the size of a pencil eraser) Size is greater than 6 mm, any growth of a mole needs to be evaluated
E	Evolution	No change in size, shape or colour The mole shape increased in size or changed in shape or changed colour, or symptoms are present such as itching, tenderness or bleeding

SUMMARY

Nursing assessment is fundamental to generating the information necessary to inform nursing actions and interventions. During the assessment process, we consider the patient, collect cues and information and process this information. This leads us to the identification of problems and issues and establishes goals for our patients. Only then can we take the necessary actions to provide safe, effective care, evaluate outcomes and reflect on the care provided. In this chapter, the principles of nursing assessment are intended to serve as a framework to guide nurses in organising their patient assessment. However, the key to nursing assessment is to listen to the patient and work towards an understanding of the nature of the healthcare problem from the patient's perspective.

KEY TERMS

AVPU scale A system to ascertain the conscious level of a patient. AVPU stands for alert, verbal, pain, unresponsive.

assessment A systematic and continuous collection of subjective and objective data to support early detection of deterioration, guide care planning and communication of patient status to other healthcare providers.

auscultation Using a stethoscope to listen to parts of the patient's body.

Glasgow Coma Scale (GCS) A commonly used scale to describe the extent of impaired consciousness in all types of acute medical and trauma patients. The scale assesses patients according to three aspects of responsiveness: eye opening, motor and verbal responses.

inspection Using all senses — eyes, ears and sense of smell — to examine the patient, looking for deviations from the normal.

pain score A tool used to assess pain, the fifth vital sign.

palpation Touching the patient with varying degrees of pressure.

percussion Tapping on body surfaces and listening to the sounds that result to determine the presence of air, fluid or solid masses.

vital signs The standard vital signs measured for all patients are temperature, pulse, respiratory rate, blood pressure, oxygen saturation, consciousness level and pain score.

REFERENCES

Ausmed. (2019) Vital signs basics. www.ausmed.com/cpd/articles/vital-signs

Ausmed. (2020) PQRST pain assessment. www.ausmed.com.au/cpd/explainers/pqrst-pain-assessment

Ausmed. (2020a) Improving fluid balance charts. www.ausmed.com.au/cpd/articles/fluid-balance-charts

Australian Commission on Safety and Quality in Health Care (ACSQHC). (2017) *National Consensus Statement: Essential elements for recognising and responding to acute physiological deterioration*, 2nd ed. Sydney.

Australian Commission on Safety and Quality in Health Care (ACSQHC). (2019) Observation and response charts. www.safetyandquality.gov.au/our-work/recognising-and-responding-deterioration/recognising-and-responding-physiological-deterioration/implementation-guide-national-consensus-statement-clinical-deterioration/observation-and-response-charts

Australian Commission on Safety and Quality in Health Care (ACSQHC). (2019a) Comprehensive Care — Element 1: Clinical assessment and diagnosis — Key actions for clinicians. www.safetyandquality.gov.au/publications-and-resources/resource-library/comprehensive-care-element-1-clinical-assessment-and-diagnosis-key-actions-clinicians

Australian Commission on Safety and Quality in Health Care (ACSQHC). (2019c) SBAR communication tool. www.safetyandquality.gov.au/publications-and-resources/resource-library/sbar-communication-tool

Australian Government. Department of Health. (n.d.) BMI calculator. Healthy weight guide. http://healthyweight.health.gov.au/wps/portal/Home/helping-hand/bmi/!ut/p/a1/04_Sj9CPykssy0xPLMnMz0vMAfGjzOI9jFxdDY1MDD0NTDzdDDzN3TwdTU0NDQ1MDYEKIoEKnN0dPUzMfQwMDEwsjAw8XZw8XMwtfQ0MPM2I02-AAzgaENIfrh-FqsTdzMsZqMTCz8LXz9Ao2NwEqgCfE8EK8LihIDc0wiDTUxEA3I8yVA!!/dl5/d5/L2dBISEvZ0FBIS9nQSEh/pw/Z7_H2EE1241I06G60IFC93LBE20G7/act/id=0/p=javax.servlet.include.path_info=QCPviewQCPbmiCalculator.xhtml/467710812763/=/#Z7_H2EE1241I06G60IFC93LBE20G7

Australian Institute of Health and Welfare (AIHW). (2018) Emergency department care 2017–18: Australian hospital statistics. Health services series no. 89. Cat. no. HSE 216. Canberra: AIHW. www.aihw.gov.au/getmedia/9ca4c770-3c3b-42fe-b071-3d758711c23a/aihw-hse-216.pdf.aspx

Australian Institute of Health and Welfare (AIHW). (2020) National mortality database. www.aihw.gov.au/reports/heart-stroke-vascular-diseases/cardiovascular-health-compendium/contents/deaths-from-cardiovascular-disease

Australian Nursing and Midwifery Federation. (2020) 5 tips to a good clinical handover. *Australian Nursing and Midwifery Journal* [online]. https://anmj.org.au/5-tips-to-a-good-clinical-handover

Australian Wound Management Association. (2012) *Pan Pacific Clinical Practice Guideline for the prevention and management of pressure injury*. WA: Cambridge Media Osborne Park.

Beasley, R., Chien, J., Douglas, J., Eastlake, L., Farah, C., King, G., Moore, R., Pilcher, J., Richards, M., Smith, S. & Walters, H. (2015) Thoracic Society of Australia and New Zealand oxygen guidelines for acute oxygen use in adults: 'Swimming between the flags'. *Resptrology.* 20(8): 1182–1191. doi: 10.1111/resp.12620

Braine, M. E. & Cook, N. (2017) The Glasgow Coma Scale and evidence-informed practice: a critical review of where we are and where we need to be. *Journal of Clinical Nursing.* 26(1–2): 280–293. doi: 10.1111/jocn.13390. PMID: 27218835

Burke, A. (2020) Techniques of physical assessment: NCLEX-RN. www.registerednursing.org/nclex/techniques-physical-assessment

Burton, T. (2013) 'Hygiene'. In J. Crisp, C. Taylor, C. Douglas & G. Rebeiro (Eds.). *Potter & Perry's Fundamentals of Nursing*, 4th ed. Chatswood, Australia: Elsevier Mosby.

Cancer Australia. (2020) Screening for distress. Cancer control continuum. https://ncci.canceraustralia.gov.au/psychosocial-care/screening-distress

Catangui, E. (2019) Improving Glasgow Coma Scale (GCS) competency of nurses in one acute stroke unit — A nursing initiative project. *Journal of Nursing Practice*. 3(1): 109–115.

Cathala, X. & Moorley, C. (2020) Performing an A-G patient assessment: a step-by-step guide. *Nursing Times* [online]. 116(1): 53–55. www.nursingtimes.net

Cleveland Clinic. (2018) Finding the way to purposeful hourly rounding. https://consultqd.clevelandclinic.org/finding-the-way-to-purposeful-hourly-rounding

Clinical Documentation Improvement Australia Pty Ltd. (2020) Home page. https://www.cdia.com.au

Clinical Excellence Commission. (n.d.) NSW Health observation charts. NSW Health. www.cec.health.nsw.gov.au/keep-patients-safe/Deteriorating-patientpatient-program/between-the-flags/observation-charts

Clinical Excellence Commission. (2017) Intentional patient rounding — Information for clinicians and health professionals. NSW Health. www.cec.health.nsw.gov.au

Continence Foundation of Australia. (2020) Bristol Stool Chart. www.continence.org.au/bristol-stool-chart

Crozer Health. (2021) PQRST pain assessment method. www.crozerhealth.org/nurses/pqrst

Dementia Australia. (2020) Cognitive screening and assessment. www.dementia.org.au/information/for-health-professionals/clinical-resources/cognitive-screening-and-assessment

Doyle, G. R. & McCutcheon, J. A. (2015) Clinical procedures for safer patient care. Victoria, BC: BC campus. https://opentextbc.ca/clinicalskills

East, L., Targett, D., Yeates, H., Ryan, E. R., Quiddington, L. & Woods, C. (2020) Nurse and patient satisfaction with intentional rounding in a rural Australian setting. *Journal of Clinical Nursing.* 29(7–8): 1365–1371. doi: 10.1111/jocn.15180

Elliott, N. (2010) 'Mutual interacting': a grounded theory study of clinical judgement practice issues. *Journal of Advanced Nursing.* 66(12): 2711–2721.

Epstein, O., Perkin, D., Cookson, J. et al. (2008) *Clinical Examination,* 4th ed. Edinburgh: Mosby.

European Heart Association. (n.d.) The Clinical Reasoning Cycle: The 8 phases and their significance. www.heartassociation.eu/the-clinical-reasoning-cycle-the-8-phases-and-their-significance

Forbes, H. (2013) 'Health assessment'. In J. Crisp, C. Taylor, C. Douglas & G. Rebeiro (Eds.). *Potter & Perry's Fundamentals of Nursing*, 4th ed. Chatswood, Australia: Elsevier Mosby.

Friese, G. (2020) How to use SAMPLE history as an effective patient assessment tool. EMS1: Lexipol. www.ems1.com/ems-products/epcr-electronic-patient-care-reporting/articles/how-to-use-sample-history-as-an-effective-patient-assessment-tool-J6zeq7gHyFpijIat

Healthline. (2021) What is a normal respiratory rate for kids and adults? www.healthline.com/health/normal-respiratory-rate#what-it-measures

health.vic. (2020a) Eastern Health maternity observation chart. Department of Health & Human Services, State Government of Victoria, Australia. www2.health.vic.gov.au/about/publications/policiesandguidelines/eastern-health-maternity-observation-chart

health.vic. (2020b) Identifying nutrition and hydration issues. Department of Health & Human Services, State Government of Victoria, Australia. www2.health.vic.gov.au/hospitals-and-health-services/patient-care/older-people/nutrition-swallowing/nutrition-and-hydration/nutrition-identifying

Jevon, P. (2020) Blood pressure 2: procedures for measuring blood pressure. *Nursing Times* [online]. www.nursingtimes.net/clinical-archive/assessment-skills/blood-pressure-2-procedures-for-measuring-blood-pressure-15-05-2020

Kutlutürkan, S. & Urvaylıoğlu, A. E. (2019) Evaluation of pain as a fifth vital sign: Nurses' opinions and beliefs. *Asia-Pacific Journal of Oncology Nursing.* 7(1): 88–94. doi: https://doi.org/10.4103/apjon.apjon_39_19

Laskowski, E. R. (2020) What's a normal resting heart rate? Mayo Clinic. www.mayoclinic.org/healthy-lifestyle/fitness/expert-answers/heart-rate/faq-20057979

Levett-Jones, T. (Ed.). (2013) *Clinical reasoning: Learning to think like a nurse.* Pearson Australia.

Lippincott Nursing Center. (2019) Nursing documentaion. www.nursingcenter.com/clinical-resources/nursing-pocket-cards/nursing-documentation

McCaffery, M. & Beebe, A. (1989) Pain. *Clinical Manual for Nursing Practice.* St. Louis: Mosby.

McCallum, L. & Higgins, D. (2012) Measuring body temperature. *Nursing Times* [online]. 108(45): 20–22.

Medical Training and Simulation LLC. (2015) Practical clinical skills. www.practicalclinicalskills.com

MedlinePlus. (2019) Vital signs. U.S. National Library of Medicine. https://medlineplus.gov/ency/article/002341.htm

Mills, I. J. (2017) A person-sentred approach to holistic assessment. *Primary Dental Journal.* 6(3): 18–23. doi: 10.1308/205016817821931006

Moyle, S. (2015) Pain assessment and management. www.ausmed.com.au/cpd/articles/pain-assessment

National Health Service (NHS). (2015) Moles: a visual guide. www.nhs.uk/Tools/Pages/Mole-slideshow.aspx

NSW Health. (2020) Recognition and management of patients who are deteriorating: policy directive. www1.health.nsw.gov.au/pds/Pages/doc.aspx?dn=PD2020_018

Nursing2021. (2006) Assessing patients effectively. https://journals.lww.com/nursing/Fulltext/2006/11002/Assessing_patients_effectively__Here_s_how_to_do.5.aspx

Nursing and Midwifery Board of Australia. (2020) Registered Nurse Standards for Practice. www.nursingmidwiferyboard.gov.au/Codes-Guidelines-Statements/Professional-standards/registered-nurse-standards-for-practice.aspx

O'Driscoll, B. R., Howard, L. S., Earis, J. & Mak, V. (2017) British Thoracic Society Guideline for oxygen use in adults in healthcare and emergency settings. *BMJ Open Respiratory Research.* 4(1). doi: 10.1136/bmjresp-2016-000170

Ogedegbe, G. & Pickering, T. (2010) Principles and techniques of blood pressure measurement. *Cardiology Clinics.* 28(4): 571–586. doi: https://doi.org/10.1016/j.ccl.2010.07.006

Painaustralia. (2020) National Pain Strategy. www.painaustralia.org.au/improving-policy/national-pain-strategy

Pirozzo, S. (2003) Whispered voice test for screening for hearing impairment in adults and children: systematic review. *BMJ.* 327(7421): 967.

Pirschel, C. (2018) Remembering Margo McCaffery's contributions to pain management. https://voice.ons.org/news-and-views/remembering-margo-mccafferys-contributions-to-pain-management#:~:text=McCaffery's%201968%20definition%20of%20pain,and%20treating%20patients%20in%20pain

Romanelli, D. & Farrell, M. W. (2020) AVPU Score. In *StatPearls [Internet].* Treasure Island (FL): StatPearls Publishing. www.ncbi.nlm.nih.gov/books/NBK538431

Royal College of Physicians and Surgeons of Glasgow. (n.d.) The Glasgow structured approach to assessment of the Glasgow Coma Scale. www.glasgowcomascale.org

Sapra, A., Malik, A. & Bhandari, P. (2020) Vital sign assessment. In *StatPearls.* Treasure Island (FL): StatPearls Publishing.

Tagney, J. (2008) Skills in taking an accurate cardiac patient history. *British Journal of Cardiac Nursing.* 3(1): 8–13.

The Royal Children's Hospital Melbourne. (2014) About Clinical Guidelines (Nursing). www.rch.org.au/rchcpg

The Royal Children's Hospital Melbourne. (2017) Fever in children. www.rch.org.au/kidsinfo/fact_sheets/Fever_in_children

Theobald, K. A. & Ramsbotham, J. (2019) Inquiry-based learning and clinical reasoning scaffolds: An action research project to support undergraduate students' learning to 'think like a nurse'. *Nurse Education in Practice.* 38(P): 59–65. doi: https://doi.org/10.1016/j.nepr.2019.05.018

Thim, T., Krarup, N. H., Grove, E. L., Rohde, C. V. & Løfgren, B. (2012). Initial assessment and treatment with the Airway, Breathing, Circulation, Disability, Exposure (ABCDE) approach. *International Journal of General Medicine.* 5: 117–121. doi: https://doi.org/10.2147/IJGM.S28478

Toney-Butler, T. J. & Unison-Pace, W. J. (2020) Nursing admission assessment and examination. In *StatPearls.* Treasure Island (FL): StatPearls Publishing.

Unger, T., Borghi, C., Charchar, F. et al. (2020) 2020 International Society of Hypertension global hypertension practice guidelines. *Journal of Hypertension.* 38(6): 982–1004. https://journals.lww.com/jhypertension/FullText/2020/06000/2020_International_Society_of_Hypertension_global.2.aspx

ViCTOR. (2018) ViCTOR charts & folders. www.victor.org.au/victor-charts

Waterlow, J. (2005) *Pressure Ulcer Prevention Manual.* London: Wound Care Society.

World Health Organization (WHO). (2011) Patient safety, using the Pulse Oximeter Tutorial 2 PPT. www.who.int/patientsafety/safesurgery/pulse_oximetry/who_ps_pulse_oxymetry_tutorial2_advanced_en.pdf

Zator Estes, M. E., Calleja, P., Theobald, K. & Harvey, T. (2013) *Health Assessment and Physical Examination*, 1st ed. South Melbourne, VIC: Cengage.

ACKNOWLEDGEMENTS

Figure 4.1: © Levett-Jones, T., Hoffman, K., Dempsey, J., Jeong, S. Y. -S., Noble, D., Norton, C. A., … Hickey, N. (2010) The 'five rights' of clinical reasoning: An educational model to enhance nursing students' ability to identify and manage clinically 'at risk' patients. *Nurse Education Today.* *30*(6): 515–520. Reproduced with permission of Elsevier.

Figure 4.4: © sunshinearts / 123RF

Figure 4.5: © Maksim Shchur / Shutterstock.com

Table 4.5: © 2020 International Society of Hypertension Global Hypertension Practice Guidelines, Volume 75, Issue 6, May 2020; Pages 1334–1357. © American Heart Association, Inc. Reproduced with permission of American Heart Association, Inc.

Extract 4.1: © Romanelli, D. & Farrell, M. W. AVPU Score. [Updated 2020 May 13]. In StatPearls [Internet]. Treasure Island (FL): StatPearls Publishing. Licensed under CC BY 4.0. https://www.ncbi.nlm.nih.gov/books/NBK538431.

Table 4.6: © Percussion, RnCeus.com. Reproduced with permission of RnCeus Interactive, LLC. https://www.rnceus.com/resp/respperc.html.

CHAPTER 5

Principles of medication administration

LEARNING OBJECTIVES

After studying this chapter, you should be able to:

5.1 describe the patient and medication-related factors that can affect drug pharmacology

5.2 describe the principles of medication administration

5.3 discuss the quality and safety considerations of medication administration

5.4 discuss the principles of safe intravenous fluid management

5.5 discuss the safe administration and management of blood and blood product transfusions.

Introduction

Medication management is one of the most common interventions provided in healthcare. Medications can include any substances used in the treatment, prevention or management of disease or illness. Despite being a common healthcare intervention, medication administration is a high-risk procedure. An estimated 250 000 people are admitted to hospital each year due to medication-related problems (Australian Commission on Safety and Quality in Health Care [ACSQHC] 2020). Medication management does not just involve the administration of medicine but is a complex process involving prescribing, dispensing, administering and monitoring (Wondmieneh et al. 2020). Mistakes can occur anywhere during this process; therefore, the National Safety and Quality Health Service (NSQHS) Standards have been developed to promote safe medication management in healthcare (ACSQHC 2020).

Nurses play an essential role in medication safety. The Australian registered nurse standards for practice state that registered nurses must 'provide safe, appropriate and responsive quality nursing practice'. The nursing practice provided is 'based on comprehensive and systematic assessment, and the best available evidence to achieve planned and agreed outcomes' (Nursing and Midwifery Board 2018, Standard 6). To meet this standard, nurses must have a sound understanding of safe medication administration principles and pharmacology, including the drug's action, indications, contraindications and possible side effects. In this chapter, we will look at the principles of safe medication administration, including intravenous therapy.

5.1 Pharmacology

LEARNING OBJECTIVE 5.1 Understand the patient and medication-related factors that can affect drug pharmacology.

Pharmacology is the science of how drugs work in the body (pharmacodynamics) and what your body does to those drugs (pharmacokinetics). Nurses must understand how different drugs work and how they affect patients. Without an understanding of pharmacology, nurses could not determine if the medications had their desired effect, monitor for possible complications and side effects or provide patient medication education, all essential to safe medication management.

Pharmacodynamics

Pharmacodynamics describes the biochemical and physiological effects medications have on the body. Most drugs apply their effect by acting on receptors usually located on the cell membrane (Currie 2018a; Neal 2016). Medications can activate or block receptors in the body and are described as:

- *agonists* — drugs that bind to the receptor and cause a maximum response
- *partial agonists* — drugs that bind to a receptor but only produce a partial response
- *antagonists* — drugs that block the receptor preventing the binding of natural transmitters.

Not everyone reacts the same way to the same medication. The effect drugs can have on the body can range from the desired effect (**therapeutic effect**) to severe complications such as allergic reactions. The body's response to medications can be influenced by the patient's age, other medications and disease processes (Edwards & Aronson 2020; Knowles, Uetrecht & Shear 2000; Smith 2013). Table 5.1 provides a brief overview of how medications may affect the body.

TABLE 5.1 Medication effects on the body

Therapeutic effect	The desired effect of the medication on the body
Adverse drug effect (ADR)	Any undesirable or harmful (adverse) responses in patients to medication. ADRs can be life-threatening and lead to severe complications. Other ADRs are milder and may not reoccur even after retaking the medication. ADRs include side effects, allergic reactions, idiosyncratic reaction and toxic reactions.
Side effect	Any effect that is not therapeutically intended and not necessarily harmful. Side effects are usually well known for the medication and are not the result of an immunological reaction. For example, nausea is a common side effect of opioid analgesics like morphine.

Idiosyncratic reaction	Any reaction to a medication that is unpredictable or unexplainable.
Toxic reactions	Reactions that occur due to a build-up of medication in the body. Medications can build up in the body for a range of reasons, including overdose, or disease processes affecting drug excretion.
Allergic reaction	A reaction that occurs due to an immunological response to the medication. Allergic reactions can be mild or life-threatening anaphylaxis.

Source: Adapted from Kramer (2003).

Pharmacokinetics

Pharmacokinetics describes the body's effect on medication and includes absorption, distribution and elimination. Pharmacokinetics are influenced by the medication itself and patient-related factors, including age, renal function, gender and weight (Currie 2018b).

Absorption

Drug absorption is the movement of the medication from the site of administration to the bloodstream. The formulation of the medication, dose, route of administration, and patient-related factors all impact the absorption process. Bioavailability describes the amount of medication that makes it into the systemic circulation. If a medication is administered intravenously, the bioavailability is 100 per cent. On the other hand, when medications are administered orally, the amount of medication that makes it to the circulation can vary greatly. Medications that enter the portal vein and are metabolised as they move through the liver (first-pass metabolism) can significantly reduce the amount of medication that makes it into the systemic circulation (Neal 2016).

Distribution

After absorption, medications enter the circulation and move around the body, entering tissues to apply their effect. This process is known as distribution. Distribution can be affected by the properties of the medication and individual patient physiology. How quickly a medication is distributed to the tissues is determined by blood flow to the area. Tissues that are more vascular such as muscle, will receive medications faster than tissues with less blood flow, such as fat. Another factor that affects distribution is how well the medication binds to plasma proteins such as albumin in the blood. Medications move around the circulation bound to plasma protein molecules and as unbound medication. The unbound portion of the medication can diffuse to the tissues or extravascular sites to work their effect. For medications to reach organs, they must cross several membranes. These membranes can act as a protective mechanism, for example, the blood–brain barrier. Only a small number of medications are able to cross the blood–brain barrier as it restricts the types of medication entering the central nervous system and cerebrospinal fluid (Neal 2016).

Metabolism

The metabolism of medication changes it into different molecules (metabolites). The liver metabolises most medications, but metabolism can occur in the lungs and gastrointestinal tract as well. When medications are metabolised, they are usually turned into less active substances, easier to excrete than the original medication. For some medications, metabolism turns them into a more active substance. These types of medications are called prodrugs. An example of a prodrug is levodopa used in the treatment of Parkinson's disease. Levodopa is metabolised into dopamine (Haddad et al. 2017).

Excretion

Most drugs are excreted by the kidneys but can be excreted by the lungs, in bile and even through breastmilk. Illness and diseases or conditions of the kidney can also affect drug elimination. If the kidney's ability to excrete medication is reduced, patients are at risk of experiencing medication toxicity. An important concept related to excretion is medication half-life. Medication half-life describes the time taken for the medication's concentration in the blood to reduce by half and is different for each medication and patient (Neale 2016).

5.2 Medication administration

LEARNING OBJECTIVE 5.2 Describe the principles of medication administration.

Medications come in many different shapes and sizes and can be administered via several routes. These are broadly categorised as enteral (administered via the gastrointestinal tract), topical (application to a surface, such as skin or mucous membranes) or parenteral (administered via routes other than the gastrointestinal route) (Shepherd & Shepherd 2020).

Enteral medication administration

Enteral medications are medications administered via the gastrointestinal tract. These medications can be administered orally or through enteral tubes. Enteral tubes can be used when patients experience a variety of problems ingesting medications, such as impaired swallowing. The enteral route is often the preferred route of medication administration due to its convenience and cost-effectiveness (Viswanathan et al. 2017).

Oral and enteral tube administration

Most medications are given orally and absorbed through the gut wall before entering the bloodstream. The absorption of most oral medications occurs in the small intestine because it has a large surface area. Drugs absorbed from the small intestine enter portal circulation (liver) before entering systemic circulation (Murakami 2017; Neal 2016). Medications administered by the oral route must tolerate a low pH and enzymes that can potentially break down the medication. Some medications such as insulin and benzylpenicillin cannot be given orally because of enzymes and acid in the gut, breaking down the medication. Patient-related factors can impact the absorption of some oral medications, such as fasting. Fasting can increase some medications' absorption, whereas eating food that slows gastric emptying can slow medication absorption (Shepherd & Shepherd 2020). Enteral tubes can be inserted nasally, or directly into the stomach through the abdominal wall (gastrostomy tube). When administering medications via an enteral tube the nurse needs to consider the size of the tube, the medication formula, and potential interactions between medications and enteral feeds. Medications can easily block enteral tubes and nurses need to check with a pharmacist if medications can be safely administered via this route. Nurses should avoid crushing medications or opening capsules and should source a suspension where possible (NSW Agency for Clinical Innovation 2014).

Topical medication administration

Topical medications are administered via absorption through the skin or mucous membranes. Topical medications can be used to treat local problems or can be absorbed into the systemic circulation. Medications administered via the topical route include eye drops, ear drops, ointments, suppositories, pessaries, inhalers, buccal and sublingual lozenges and wafers, and transdermal patches (Levette-Jones 2017). Medication administered via the topical route is not as precise, but because much of the drug does not reach systemic circulation, the risk of unwanted side effects is reduced (Shepherd & Shepherd 2020).

Buccal and sublingual administration

Buccal administration involves the medication being placed between the gums and the cheeks, whereas sublingual administration involves placing the medication under the tongue (Shepherd & Shepherd 2020). In buccal and sublingual medication administration, the drug diffuses across the vascular oral mucosa straight into the bloodstream, avoiding the gastrointestinal tract and liver (Neal 2016). This gives the medication a longer contact time with the highly vascular oral mucosa, enhancing absorption. These routes of medication administration can increase the bioavailability of medication and increase the onset of action compared to some oral medication (Neal 2016).

Inhalation drug administration

Medications can be delivered by inhaling them straight into the lungs and can be used to treat both respiratory and non-respiratory conditions. Medications are dispersed into the lungs as a fine mist and absorbed by the airway surfaces (Dolovich & Dhand 2011). These medications are administered using various devices, including metered-dose inhalers, dry-powder inhalers and nebulisation. Some of the main disadvantages of administering medications via the inhalation route include variability in the delivered dose, the need for administration equipment and the range of breathing techniques needed for patients to inhale the medication adequately (Rau 2005).

Parenteral medication administration

Parenteral medication administration is the administration of medication by any route except via the gastrointestinal or topical routes. Parenteral medication routes include intravenous (IV), intramuscular (IM) and subcutaneous (SC) (Shepherd & Shepherd 2020).

IV medication administration is the administering of medication straight into a vein and systemic circulation. This method provides rapid administration and 100 per cent absorption of the medication. IM medication is administered directly into the highly vascular muscles under subcutaneous tissues. SC medication administration is the administration of medication directly into the adipose tissue under the skin. Absorption is slower than medications administered via the IM or IV route as the adipose tissue is not as vascular.

Medication calculations

Nurses need to be able to calculate and determine correct doses for medications. Nurses are responsible for the medications they administer and must locate important information on drug doses and query any unclear prescriptions, what appears to be an unusual dose or medication contraindicated for the patient or clinical condition. Different calculations are used to determine the correct doses of oral and parenteral medications (see figure 5.1).

FIGURE 5.1 Dosage calculations

Oral medication	Parenteral medications
Number of tablets = strength required/strength in stock Volume of liquid = strength required/strength of stock solution × volume of stock solution	Volume = strength required/strength stock solution × volume stock solution
Examples 400 mg of ibuprofen has been ordered, and the hospital ward stock 200 mg tablets Tablets required = 400 mg/200 mg Tablets required = 2 tablets 500 mg of amoxycillin liquid has been ordered. The ward stocks liquid amoxycillin 250 mg/5 ml Volume = 500 mg/250 × 5 Volume = 10 ml	**Example** A patient has been ordered 20 mg of IV frusemide. The ward stocks frusemide 40 mg/2 ml Volume = 20 mg/40 × 2 Volume = 1 ml

Source: Adapted from Flinders University (2013).

5.3 Safe medication administration

LEARNING OBJECTIVE 5.3 Discuss the quality and safety considerations of medication administration.

Nurses administering medications should follow a systematic and logical process to minimise the chance of errors occurring. Most medication errors occur during the administration phase, so nurses must minimise distractions and carefully check all medications. Nurses often use the five stages or rights of medication administration to ensure the right medication is being administered to the right patient at the right time. Some resources have expanded the original five rights to include right reason and documentation (Oldham et al. 2009; Smeulers et al. 2015):

1. right patient
2. right drug
3. right dose
4. right time
5. right route
6. right reason
7. right documentation.

Documentation

In Australian hospitals, medications will be prescribed on a National Standard Medication Chart. These medication charts can be paper or electronic. In Australia, a standardised national medication chart was introduced to ensure consistent prescribing and documentation of medication management (see figure 5.2). Medication charts will have a space to document patient information, including name, date of birth, unique hospital record number, gender, allergies and adverse drug reactions (ACSQHC 2019a). The prescription section of the chart will include:

- date of prescription
- generic drug name
- route
- dose
- frequency
- prescriber name, signature and contact number.

Patient education

Patients need to be informed of the medicine they are prescribed to ensure they can make the best decisions about their healthcare and treatment. Nurses play an essential role in providing education to patients, their families and carers. Common education points include how the medications work, what they are being used for and possible side effects. When providing medication education, it is important nurses consider the individual's needs and how they will deliver the information. Education can be provided orally or in the form of written information. All information should be clear and easy for the patient to understand. Education and patient participation can reduce medication errors and help the patient safely manage their medications on discharge from the hospital (Blevins 2020).

5.4 Intravenous therapy

LEARNING OBJECTIVE 5.4 Discuss the principles of safe intravenous fluid management.

The circulatory system consists of a network of arteries and veins which move blood around the body. When administering intravenous therapy, we do so via the venous system. The venous system consists of a network of venous vessels that take deoxygenated blood from the capillary beds back to the heart. The smallest venous vessels are venules, and these join to form veins. Veins are low-pressure, high-volume vessels, which means their walls are much thinner, and the vessel lumen much wider when compared to arteries (Craft & Gordon 2014; Hobson 2008).

IV therapy administration is regularly performed in the medical-surgical setting and has become an essential healthcare intervention. It is estimated that up to 80 per cent of hospital patients will receive some form of IV therapy (Brooks 2018). The preparation and administration of medicines and fluids via the intravenous route is a high-risk procedure. The procedure often involves many steps. It is estimated over 25 per cent of all medication errors involve medicines and fluids administered via the intravenous route (ACSQHC 2015). Nurses involved in the administration and monitoring of IV therapy need to understand the theoretical, practical and legal considerations of IV therapy.

Anatomy and physiology

As can be seen in figure 5.3, veins are made up of three layers.

1. *Tunica intima.* A smooth endothelial lining that allows the passage of blood cells. If this becomes damaged, it increases the risk of thrombus formation.
2. *Tunica media.* Made up of smooth muscle and elastin, but in veins, this layer is underdeveloped and tends to be thin compared to arteries.
3. *Tunica externa.* The external layer of the vein and is the thickest. The tunica externa is made up of collagen fibres and elastic networks (Craft & Gordon 2014; Weinstein 2007; Dougherty & Watson 2011; Collins 2011).

FIGURE 5.2 Extract from the National Inpatient Medication Chart

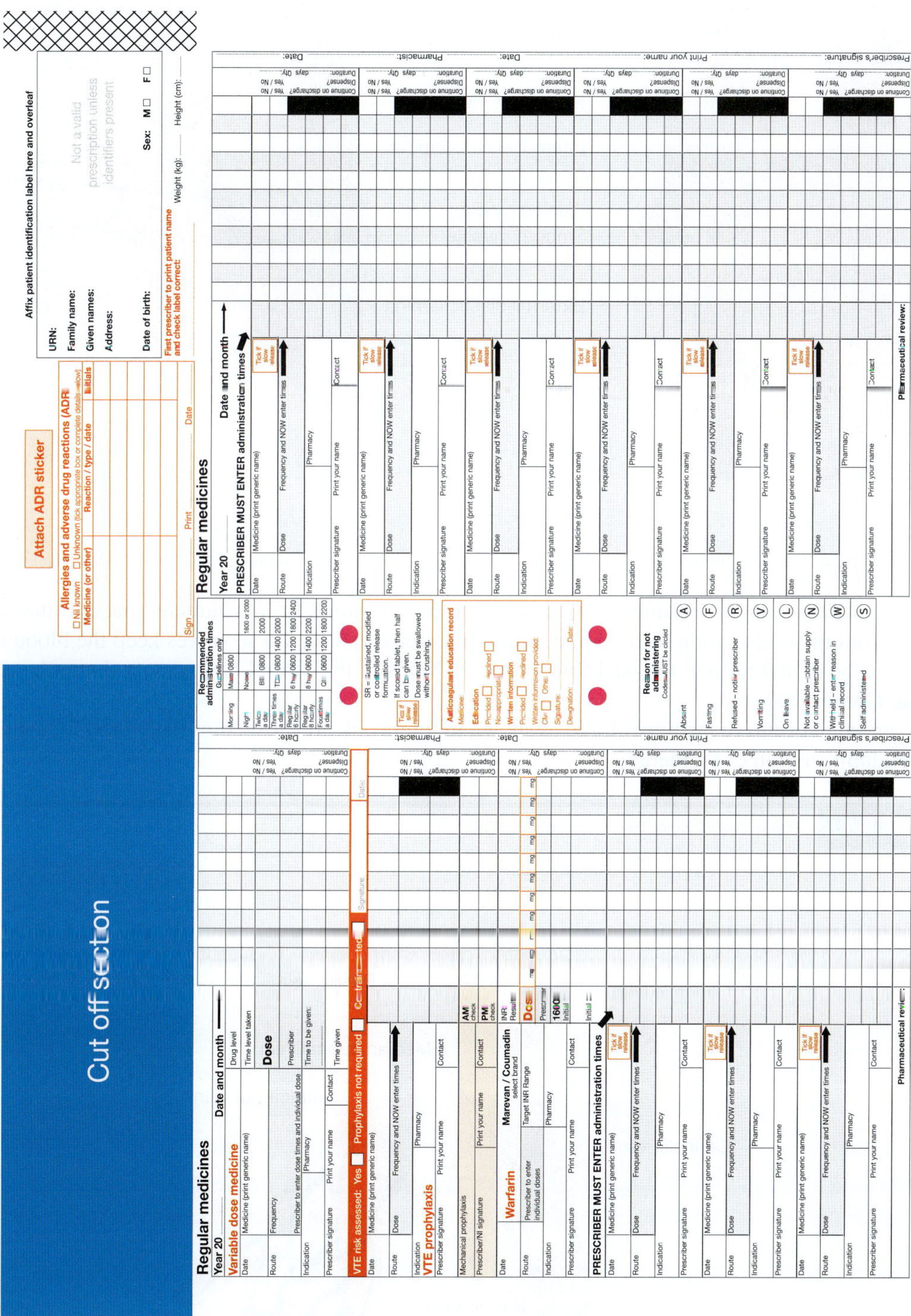

Source: ACSQHC (2019a).

FIGURE 5.3 The anatomy and physiology of the veins

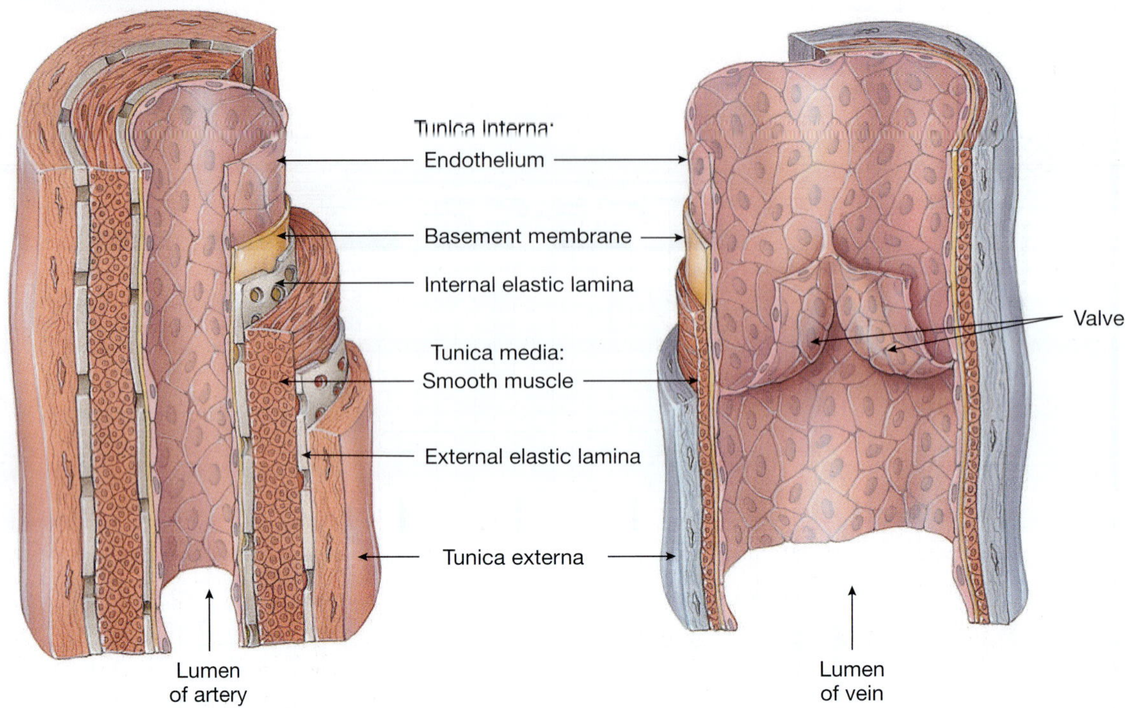

Source: Nair, M. & Peate, I. (2009) *Fundamentals of Applied Pathophysiology* with kind permission from Wiley Blackwell.

The peripheral veins of the limbs have adapted to ensure blood flow is directed back to the heart. In the tunica intima, folds within the endothelium lining create valves. These valves keep the blood moving towards the heart and prevent the backflow of blood. Veins of the central body cavity do not have valves (Craft & Gordon 2014).

The superficial veins of the upper limb, as shown in figure 5.4, are most commonly used for cannulation and the administration of IV therapy.

FIGURE 5.4 The superficial veins of the upper limb

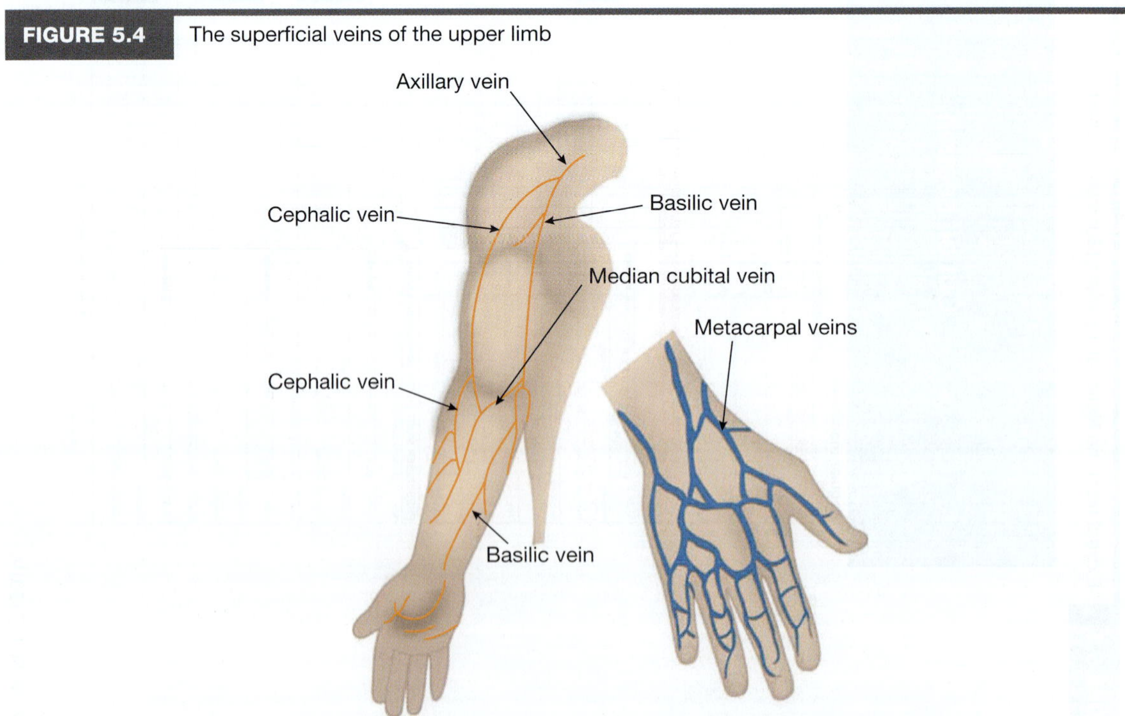

Source: Hamilton & Bodenham (2009) *Central Venous Catheters* with kind permission from Wiley Blackwell.

The main veins used are as follows.

- *Cephalic vein.* A large vein on the arm's radial side, extending past the axilla from the dorsal veins of the hand. Care needs to be taken when using the cephalic vein near the wrist as puncture of the radial nerve can occur.
- *Basilic vein.* A large vein located on the ulnar side of the forearm with numerous valves, making cannulation challenging.
- *Median cubital vein.* A large superficial vein located in the antecubital fossa.
- *Metacarpal veins.* Superficial veins located on the back of the hand that are often easily visualised and palpated. The veins in the dorsum of the hand tend to be smaller and more mobile and can make cannulation more challenging (Gabriel 2008; Hobson 2008).

Vascular access devices

Vascular access devices (VAD) are catheters that are inserted into arteries or veins and used for diagnostic (blood sampling, haemodynamic monitoring) and/or therapeutic purposes (administration of medications, fluids, blood products). VAD's can be divided into two distinct types: peripheral intravenous catheters (PIVC) and central venous access devices (CVAD).

Peripheral intravenous catheter (PIVC)

A PIVC is a small flexible device that is inserted into a peripheral vein. PIVCs are used for short-term medication and IV fluid administration. PIVCs are often referred to as cannulas and come in a range of sizes. The ideal location of insertion is the veins of the upper limbs (see figure 5.5), with PIVCs inserted into the lower limbs at a higher risk of infection (Keogh & Mathew 2019).

Central venous access device (CVAD)

CVADs are catheters where the device's tip sits in the superior vena cava, the right atrium of the heart or the inferior vena cava. As can be seen in table 5.2, CVADs come in for main types; non-tunnelled CVAD, peripherally inserted central catheter (PICC), tunnelled CVAD and implantable venous access devices (IVAD) (see figure 5.6). CVADs can be used to administer medications and fluids that are not suitable to be administered via a smaller vein, i.e. chemotherapy, or where longer-term therapy is needed (Smith & Nolan 2013). Administering IV therapy via a CVAD is a high risk procedure and requires the nurse to be adequately trained in CVAD management (NSW Agency for Clinical Innovation 2014).

FIGURE 5.5 A PIVC

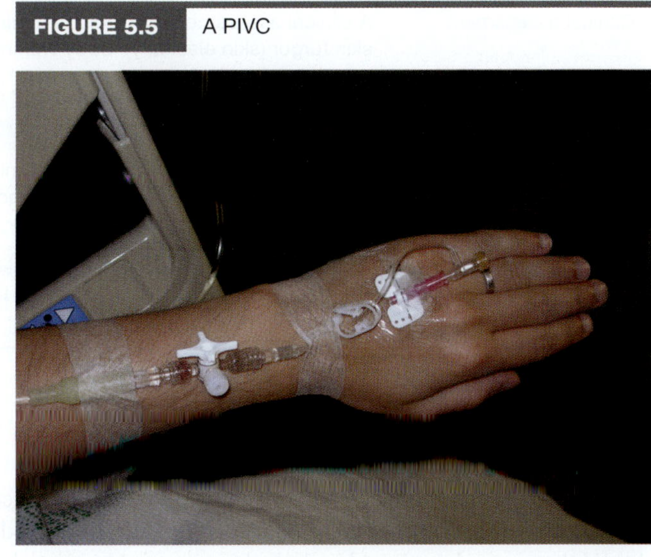

TABLE 5.2 **CVAD table**

CVAD type		Insertion sites (vein)	Duration
Non-tunnelled CVAD	CVC, central line, CVAD	Jugular, subclavian, axillary femoral	Short-term use, several days to weeks
PICC		Basilic (vein of choice) cephalic, brachial	Medium-term use, weeks to months
Tunnelled CVAD (Hickmann)		Jugular, subclavian	Long-term use, months to years
IVAD	Port, porta-cath	Jugular vein, subclavian	Long-term use, months to years

Source: Adapted from NSW Agency for Clinical Innovation (2014) and Smith & Nolan (2013).

FIGURE 5.6 PICC and IVAD

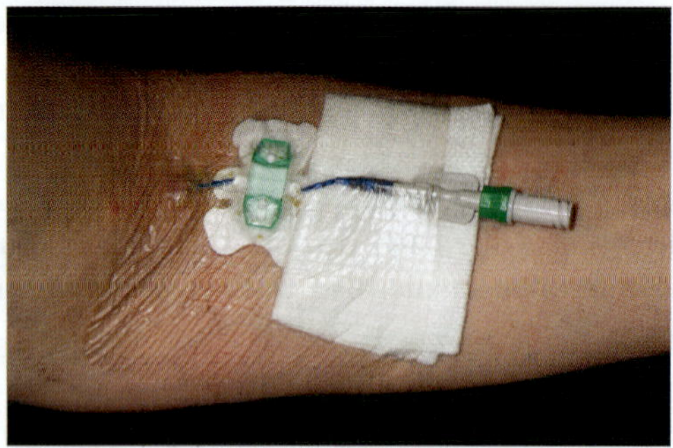

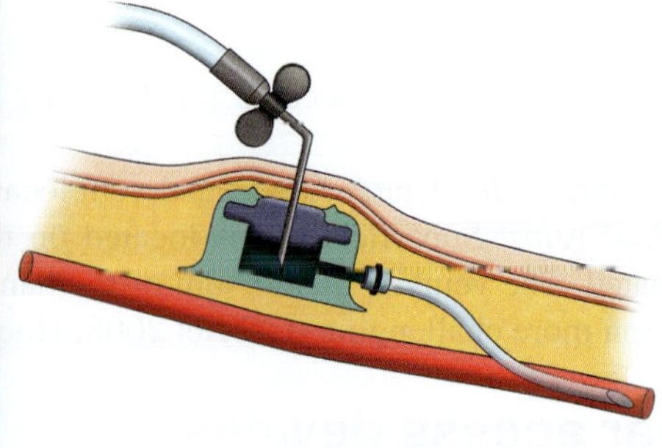

Assessment

IV therapy is administered for various reasons, including medication administration, rehydration, electrolyte replacement and resuscitation (Guest 2019). Before administering IV therapy, the nurse should conduct a thorough assessment of the patient's fluid balance and vascular access (Frost 2015; Guest 2019). Table 5.3 provides a brief overview of some of the assessments that should be performed. It is crucial for patient safety that nurses administering any IV therapy understand why the therapy has been ordered and whether following the prescription is clinically appropriate for their patient (Scales 2014).

TABLE 5.3 **Assessment table**

Clinical assessment	A clinical assessment will include a full set of vital observations, an assessment of skin turgor (skin elasticity), body weight and urine output.
Fluid balance charts	Monitoring a patient's fluid intake and out is essential in preventing dehydration or overhydration.
Laboratory tests	Monitoring electrolytes and kidney function is important to ensure adequate fluid management, and regular testing is recommended when patients are receiving intravenous fluid therapy.
VAD assessment	Assess for signs of infection, inflammation, occlusion, dislodgement and dressing integrity. Check when the device was inserted and assess if the patient is experiencing any pain or discomfort.

Source: Adapted from NICE (2017); Keogh & Mathew (2019).

Preparation

An IV therapy order must be prescribed by a competent practitioner — a doctor, nurse practitioner and in some facilities, registered nurses with specific training and education working in an extended practice role. All IV therapy orders should include the type of solution to be administered, the volume to be infused, and the rate it should be administered (Burton 2017).

All IV therapy enters the intravascular space when injected into a vein. The type and amount of fluid will influence how much enters the intracellular and interstitial compartments. There are two main types of fluids crystalloids and colloids. Colloids are aqueous solutions that contain large molecules, which do not pass easily across membranes, such as capillaries and cell membranes (Craft & Gordon 2014). Because colloids don't pass across membranes easily, the fluid tends to stay in the intravascular space longer (Lewis et al. 2018). Examples of colloids include blood products and albumin. On the other hand, crystalloids are aqueous solutions that contain smaller molecules of salt and sugars and pass more easily across membranes, moving freely between intravascular, interstitial and intracellular compartments (Frost 2015). Examples of crystalloids include normal saline and Hartmann's solution. The most common fluid used in hospitals is crystalloids solutions. Crystalloid solutions can be further categorised as isotonic, hypertonic or hypotonic (see table 5.4) (Hoorn 2017). Understanding how this fluid acts is an important consideration when administering and managing IV therapy (see figure 5.7).

TABLE 5.4 Fluid table

Isotonic fluid	Normal saline (0.9% sodium chloride) Hartmann's solution (Lactated Ringer's)	The concentration of solutes in an isotonic fluid is equal to the concentration of solutes in the cell. Water molecules move in and out of the cell at the same rate with no net gains or losses across the intracellular and extracellular spaces.	Often used to prepare intravenous medications. Also, regularly used for volume depletion.	Expands both intracellular and extracellular space monitor for fluid overload.
Hypertonic fluid	3% Saline	The concentration of solutes in a hypertonic fluid is greater than the concentration of solutes in the cell. Water moves from the intracellular compartment into the extracellular compartment causing the cell to shrink and intravascular volume to expand.	Critical conditions, critical hyponatraemia and cerebral oedema.	Vesicant to the vein – ideally administered via central line or a large-bore PIVC. Expands extracellular space. A fluid shift can cause hypervolemia pulmonary oedema/fluid overload.
Hypotonic fluid	0.45% Saline	The concentration of solutes in a hypotonic fluid is less than the concentration of solutes in the cell. Water moves from the intravascular compartment into the intracellular compartment causing the cell to expand and potentially rupture.	Put fluid into cell — diabetic ketoacidosis, hyperosmolar glycemia.	Monitor haemodynamic status — pushing blood from vascular space. Hypovolemia, vascular collapse. Don't give to patients at risk of increased ICP, or hypovolemic patients in burns and trauma.

Source: Adapted from Hoorn (2017) and Vera (2021).

FIGURE 5.7 Water molecule movement in hypotonic, hypertonic and isotonic solutions

(a) Hypotonic solution

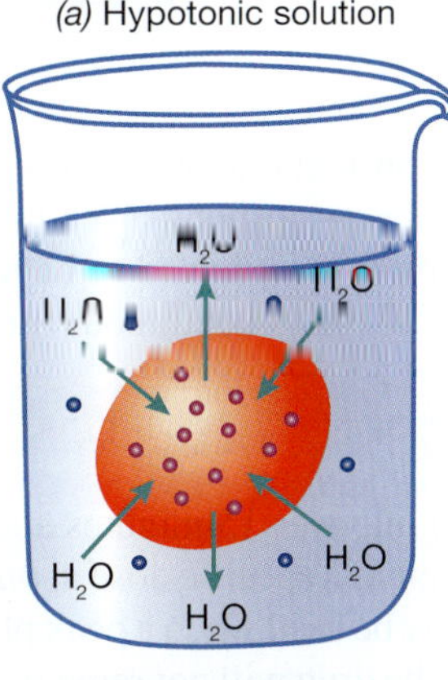

Net water gain
Cell swells

(b) Hypertonic solution

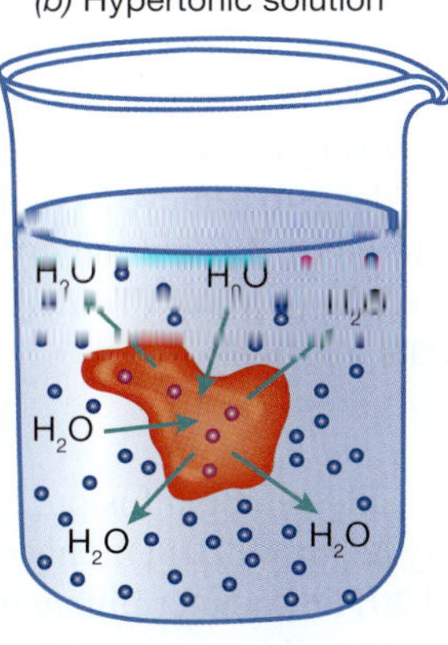

Net water loss
Cell shrinks

(c) Isotonic solution

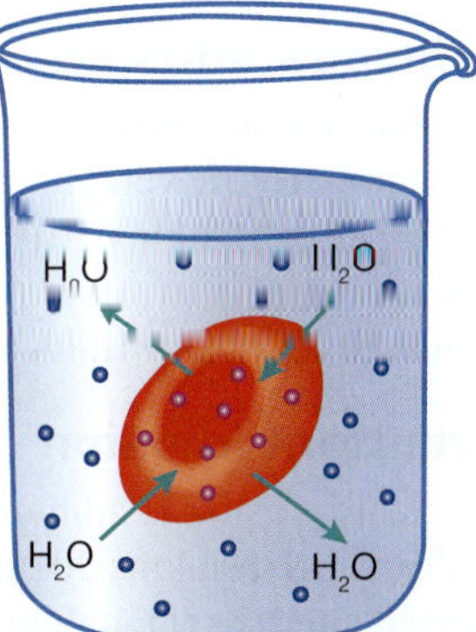

No net loss or gain

Pre-prepared IV therapies should be used wherever possible to reduce the risk of contamination and medication errors. Premixed solutions are now standard. For example, most hospitals will stock premade bags of fluids containing potassium chloride (Weinstein 2007). Intravenous fluids come prepared in different sizes ranging from 50 mL bags to 1 L bags, with the smaller bags often used for IV medication administration.

When preparing an IV infusion, sometimes additives such as medications are ordered. If an additive is needed to be mixed with an IV solution, only one additive should be added to a bag of fluid. Adding more than one additive to an infusion increases the risk of incompatibilities, putting patients at an increased risk of an adverse event (Weinstein 2007; Whittington 2008). Some fluids should not have any additives added to them at all, such as blood and blood products (Downie et al. 2003). Before adding anything to a bag of fluid, compatibility between the additive and the fluid must be checked beforehand. When preparing to administer any IV therapy, it is important to check indications, contraindications, potential incompatibilities and how the intravenous fluid should be administered, including recommended duration of infusion. Important preparation and administration information can be found in a range of reference materials, including the *Australian Injectable Drugs Handbook, Monthly Index of Medical Specialities (MIMS)* and local facility policies and procedures.

A national standard for labelling injectable medicines, fluids and lines was developed to promote safety and reduce medication error. Now all infusions that contain an additive must be labelled (ACSQHC 2015). Once an additive has been added to a fluid bag/bottle or syringe, a label should be applied immediately. Many facilities will use premade colour coded labels. Blue labels are used for intravenous therapy (see figure 5.8). IV fluid that does not have any additives does not require a user-applied label. Labels must include:

- patient name (given and family names)
- patient identifier (ID) (e.g., medical record number)
- patient date of birth (DOB)
- active ingredient/s (medicine/s) added to the bag or syringe
- amount of medicine/s added (including units)
- total volume of fluid (ml) in bag or syringe
- concentration (units/ml)
- diluent (for syringes)
- date and time prepared
- prepared by (signature)
- checked by (signature)
- route of administration (where not specified by wording and colour).

Administration

There are three methods of administering IV drugs: continuous infusion, intermittent infusion and direct intermittent injection.

Continuous infusion

Continuous infusion is defined as the IV delivery of medication of fluid at a constant rate over a prescribed time, ranging from several hours to several days, to achieve a controlled therapeutic response (Whittington 2008; Turner & Hankins 2010). It tends to be used when the drugs to be administered need to be highly diluted or maintenance of steady blood levels is required (Turner & Hankins 2010). A continuous infusion is often used to replace fluids and rehydrate a patient.

Intermittent infusion

Intermittent infusion is administering a small-volume infusion, i.e. 25–250 ml, over 15 minutes and two hours (Turner & Hankins 2010; Dougherty & Ansell 2011). This may be given as a specific dose at once or at repeated intervals (Dougherty & Ansell 2011). An intermittent infusion may be used when a peak plasma level is required. The pharmacology of the drug dictates a specific dilution. The drug will not remain stable for the time required to administer a more dilute volume, or the patient is on a restricted intake of fluids (Whittington 2008). Drugs commonly administered as an intermittent infusion include antibiotics.

Direct intermittent injection

A direct intermittent injection is also known as an intravenous push or bolus and involves injecting a drug from a syringe into an injection port of the administration set or directly into a vascular access device (Turner & Hankins 2010; Dougherty & Ansell 2011). A 'bolus' injection may be given rapidly over seconds — for example, intravenous adrenaline in a cardiac arrest emergency. Direct intermittent injections are typically given as a controlled 'push' injection over a few minutes.

FIGURE 5.8 Examples of fluid labels

National Standard for User-applied
Labelling of Injectable Medicines, Fluids and Lines

Intravenous container labels

Bags with additives (and large syringes)

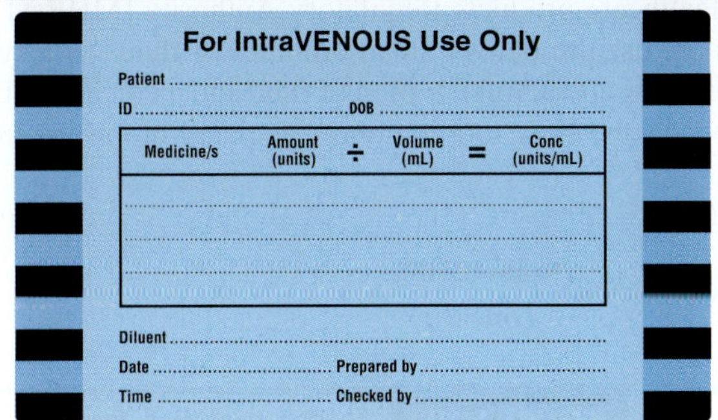
For IntraVENOUS Use Only

Patient ....

ID .... DOB ....

Medicine/s	Amount (units)	÷	Volume (mL)	=	Conc (units/mL)

Diluent ....

Date .... Prepared by ....

Time .... Checked by ....

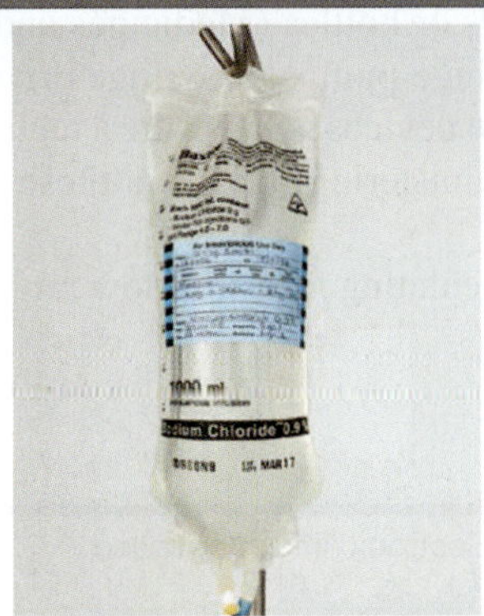

Fluid name, batch number, expiry date and bag graduations to remain visible after label placement.

Complete 'diluent' prompt if fluid name not visible.

Syringes (and small bags with additives)

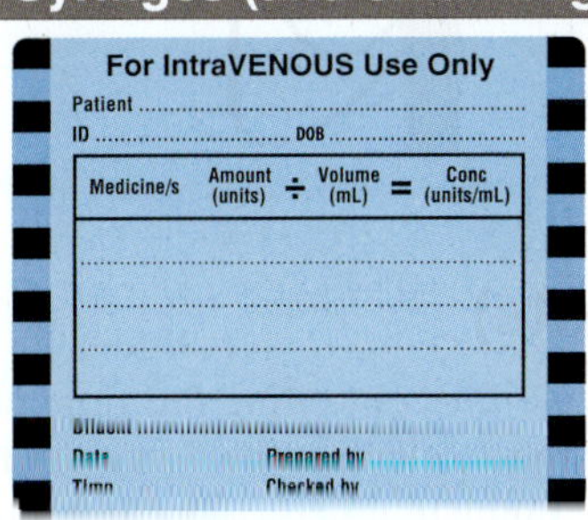
For IntraVENOUS Use Only

Patient ....

ID .... DOB ....

Medicine/s	Amount (units)	÷	Volume (mL)	=	Conc (units/mL)

Diluent ....

Date .... Prepared by ....

Time .... Checked by ....

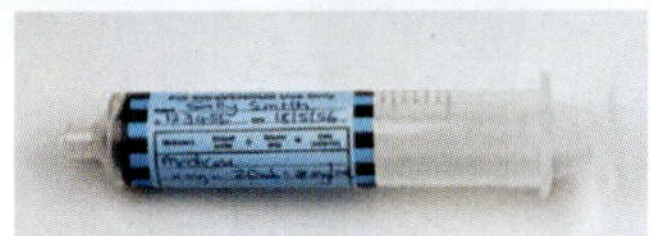

Graduations on syringe scale to remain visible after label placement.

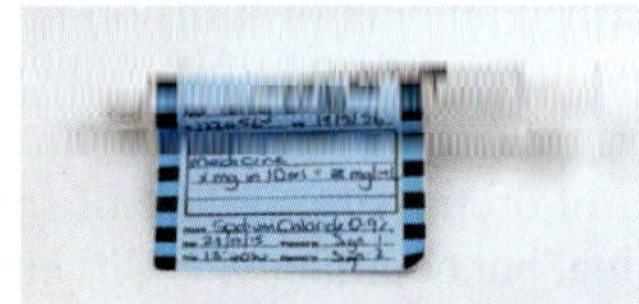

'Flag' label for smaller syringes.

Syringes with 0.9% sodium chloride for intravenous flush

Sodium Chloride 0.9%

To be read in conjunction with the National Standard for User-applied Labelling of Injectable Medicines, Fluids and Lines, 2015.

AUSTRALIAN COMMISSION ON SAFETY AND QUALITY IN HEALTH CARE

Source: ACSQHC (2015).

Infusion devices

IV fluids can be administered via an administration set via gravity or an external device such as an intravenous infusion pump or syringe driver. Gravity infusion devices consist of an administration set (containing a drip chamber and a roller clamp to control the flow) and are usually measured by counting drops (Dougherty & Ansell 2011). The indications for use are:

- the delivery of fluids without additives
- adverse effects are not anticipated, and solutions do not need to be infused with absolute precision
- the patient's condition does not give cause for concern, and complications are not anticipated (Quinn 2008).

Electronic infusion devices come in many forms, from electronic volumetric pumps (figure 5.9) to smaller syringe drivers (figure 5.10). Volumetric pumps are often used to infuse larger volumes of fluid from IV bags or bottles (Medicines and Healthcare products Regulatory Authority [MHRA] 2010; Quinn 2008). Syringe pumps or syringe drivers are used to deliver small volumes of fluid via a syringe. Electronic infusion devices help ensure a regulated flow and administration of fluid and medication (Burton 2017). When administering fluids via these devices, the flow rate is often calculated in millimetres per hour (ml/hr).

Formula for calculating infusion/flow rate per hour:

$$\text{Infusion Rate (ml/hr)} = \frac{\text{Volume (ml)}}{\text{Time (hr)}}$$

FIGURE 5.9 Electronic infusion device

FIGURE 5.10 Electronic infusion device — syringe driver

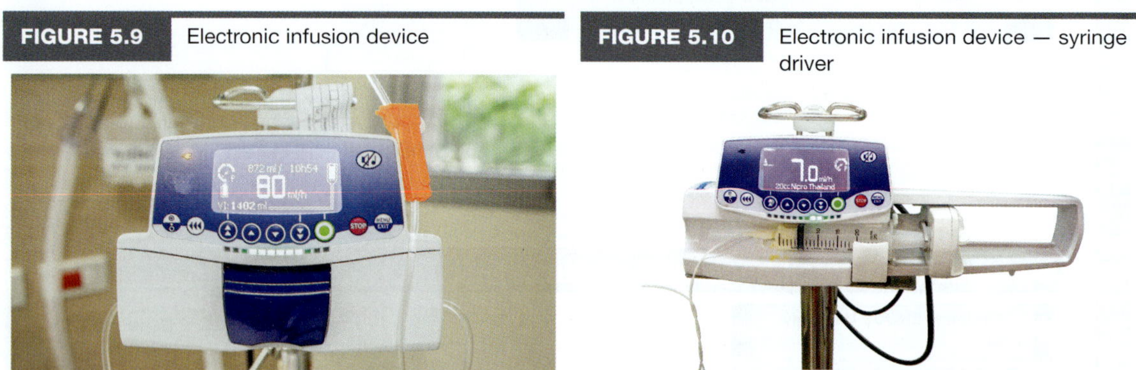

Calculating infusion rates (drops per minute)

When an infusion is administered via gravity, the nurse is responsible for controlling the flow rate. To ensure the prescribed amount of infusion is administered, the nurse must calculate the drops per minute and manually manipulate the flow rate with the roller clamp on the administration set. The drop factor of the infusion device is needed to calculate the drops per minute. Different administration sets will deliver a different number of drops per millilitre of solution (drop rate). The drop factor is printed on the infusion device's packaging, but commonly, it will either be a macrodrip set with a drop factor of 10–20 drops/ml or a microdrip set with a drop factor of 60 drops/ml (Burton 2017; Quinn 2008).

Box formula for calculation of the drop rate:

$$\text{Drops per minutes} = \frac{\text{Total volume (mls)}}{\text{Time (hrs)}} \times \frac{\text{Drop factor}}{60}$$

Complications

Complications of IV therapy can disrupt treatment and cause harm to the patient. Complications can include infection, phlebitis, infiltration, extravasation, thrombosis, circulatory overload and speed shock (Brooks 2018; Marsh 2020). Nurses need to be able to recognise potential signs of complications and respond promptly to keep patients safe from harm.

Infection

Infections can enter the circulatory system through the access device or through contaminated infusions. Signs of infection from the access device include redness and swelling, which may track along the length of the catheter. Tenderness and exudate from the insertion site may also occur. Figure 5.11 shows the consequences of an infected PIVC. Systemic signs of infection can include fevers, rigors, flushing, tachycardia, hypotension and nausea and vomiting (Brooks 2018). To prevent infections related to IV therapy administration, all staff must use the aseptic non-touch technique when preparing, administering and managing intravenous therapy (Dougherty & Ansell 2011).

FIGURE 5.11 Infected PIVC

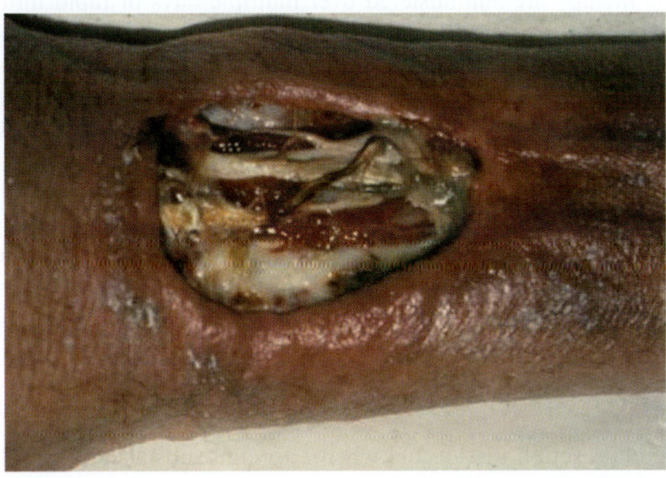

Source: Lamb & Dougherty (2008) *Intravenous Therapy in Nursing Practice* with kind permission from Wiley Blackwell.

Phlebitis

Phlebitis is inflammation of the tunica intima of the vein and can present as redness and tenderness along the vein where the cannula is inserted. Swelling along the vein can occur, making the vein look like a cord (Brooks 2018; Mermel et al. 2009). Patients will often report pain or discomfort during IV therapy administration when phlebitis is present. There are three main types of phlebitis.

1. *Mechanical.* Caused by irritation and damage to the vein by the access device. Excessive movement or leaving the device in for too long can all contribute to mechanical phlebitis.
2. *Chemical.* Caused by irritation and inflammation to the vein by medication or fluids and may include antibiotics or chemotherapy.
3. *Bacterial.* Caused by microorganisms entering the access device insertion site and can be caused by incorrect handwashing techniques and poor aseptic non touch technique (Lamb & Dougherty 2008)

Infiltration and extravasation

Infiltration is the inadvertent administration of non-vesicant therapy (medications and fluids that do not cause blisters and tissue necrosis) and is often referred to as 'tissuing'. The infiltration of large volumes of fluid can lead to compression of surrounding tissue and nerves and can lead to long-term damage (Brooks 2018; Doellmann et al. 2009; Schulmeister 2009; RCN 2010).

Extravasation is the inadvertent administration of vesicant therapy (medications of fluids that cause burns, blisters and necrosis). Vesicant therapy includes chemotherapy and potassium. Extravasation can lead to severe injury and is considered a medical emergency (Brooks 2018; Polovich et al. 2009; Schulmeister 2009).

Some patients are at greater risk of infiltration and extravasation, including children, older adults, and patients with poor venous access. Signs and symptoms of infiltration and extravasation can include localised swelling and redness to the site, and the patient may report pain during intravenous therapy administration. Sometimes the tissues surrounding the access device can begin to blanch and feel cool to touch. Early signs that something is wrong can include difficulty during the administration process with IV therapy slowing or stopping (Brooks 2018).

Management of access device complications

If a patient develops a complication related to the access device, infusions through that device should be stopped and the doctor informed. If there are signs of phlebitis or infection, the access device will be removed and re-sited, ideally to the opposite limb. The management of infiltration and extravasation will include stopping the infusion, elevating the limb and removing the access device. Close monitoring of patients and their access devices is important in the early detection and prevention of complications related to access devices.

Hypervolemia

Hypervolemia is the excess build-up of extracellular fluid and can be caused by IV therapy. When large volumes of intravenous therapy are administered over multiple days or rapid infusions administered to patients with impaired renal, liver or cardiac functioning, hypervolemia can develop (Macklin & Chernecky 2004; Lamb & Dougherty 2008). The signs and symptoms of hypervolemia can include rapid bounding pulse, distended neck veins and oedema (Dougherty & Ansell 2011). If hypervolemia is not corrected, left-sided heart failure, pulmonary oedema and, eventually, circulatory collapse and cardiac arrest can develop (Dougherty & Ansell 2011).

Management of hypervolemia

Close monitoring of all patients receiving IV therapy is crucial to the early identification of hypervolemia. If hypervolemia develops, the infusion should be stopped, and the doctor notified immediately. Treatment will depend on why the hypervolemia developed but can involve restricting the patient's fluid and salt intake and administering diuretics (Weinstein 2007).

Speed shock

Speed shock is a systemic reaction that occurs when a foreign substance is rapidly introduced into the circulation (Weinstein 2007; Perucca 2010). It can occur when IV bolus injections or large volumes of fluid are administered too rapidly, resulting in toxic concentrations (Lamb & Dougherty 2008; Perucca 2010). Toxicity may be manifested by exaggerating the drug's usual pharmacological actions or signs and symptoms specific to that drug or class of drugs. Signs and symptoms include a flushed face, headache, dizziness, chest congestion, tachycardia, hypotension, syncope, shock and cardiovascular collapse (Weinstein 2007; Perucca 2010).

Management of speed shock

The management of speed shock is dependent on the IV therapy that has been administered. The infusion should be stopped, and medical advice sought immediately. Depending on the patient's reaction, management may include stopping the infusion, administering medications to treat symptoms, or slowing the infusion. Speed shock is preventable, and all staff needs to understand the correct administration rates for all IV therapy being provided (Brooks 2018). When administering medication infusions, it is recommended to use an electronic infusion device to ensure accurate administration rates.

Principles of infection prevention

An aseptic, non-touch technique should be used to prevent infection related to the administration and management of IV therapy (see table 5.5) (Loveday et al. 2014). Regular assessment and monitoring of the PIVC is important to ensure any signs of infection are detected early. CVADs require special precautions when delivering medications and fluids (NSW Agency for Clinical Innovation 2014; Keogh & Mathew 2019).

TABLE 5.5	Infection prevention table
Inspection	The insertion site of the PIVC should be inspected for redness, swelling and pain. The use of a Visual Infusion Phlebitis (VIP) score helps to monitor and detect the development of phlebitis early.
Cleaning	Ports and hubs need to be decontaminated before the administration of intravenous fluid. The solution should be applied with friction and allowed to dry for 30–60 seconds before commencing the infusion.

Securement	PIVC need to be secured to prevent movement and dislodgement of the device. PIVC should be secured with a transparent semipermeable dressing which allows easy inspection of the insertion site.
Equipment	Changing equipment will be dependent on the type of infusion and fluid administered. Policy and procedure as well as recommendations from the manufacturer, will guide how long infusion devices can be used. A closed system should be maintained at all times with minimal disconnections.
Patency	For devices that are used regularly, the device's patency should be maintained using 0.9% sodium chloride through either regular flushes or a continuous infusion of a small amount of fluid to keep the vein open, i.e. 5 mL/hour (TKVO).

Source: Adapted from Brooks (2018); NSW Agency for Clinical Innovation (2014); Keogh & Mathew (2019).

5.5 Blood product transfusions

LEARNING OBJECTIVE 5.5 Discuss the safe administration and management of blood and blood product transfusions.

All staff have a responsibility for the safe administration and management of blood and blood product transfusions. According to the NSHQS Standards (Standard 7, blood management), any blood or blood product a patient receives should be safe and clinically appropriate (ACSQHC 2019b).

Blood transfusion indications

There are many reasons why blood or blood products may be administered to a patient, including disease symptom management and the treatment or prevention of bleeding. The most commonly administered fresh blood components are red blood cells (RBCs), platelets and plasma. Table 5.6 outlines the indications for each blood product.

TABLE 5.6 Blood product types

Fresh blood components	Indications
Red blood cells (RBCs)	Increases the oxygen-carrying capacity of the blood by increasing RBC count. Used in the treatment of anaemia due to blood loss, disease or treatment
Platelets	Prevents or stops bleeding in patients with low or dysfunctional platelets
Fresh frozen plasma (FFP)	Replaces clotting factors to prevent or stop bleeding

Source: Adapted from Australian Red Cross Lifeblood (2020)

Preparation

Before administering a blood or blood product transfusion, the nurse must adequately prepare the patient and equipment. Ensuring all the equipment and documentation are correct can reduce and prevent delays in administration and product wastage.

- Collect and check all transfusion-related equipment including electronic administration devices, approved blood administration sets and resuscitation equipment.
- Ensure valid informed consent has been obtained and appropriate documentation has been completed.
- Check blood product order making sure it is completed with all relevant information, including any special requirements, the number of units to be transfused, the time each unit is to be infused, the patient identification and relevant prescriber name and signature.
- Check the patient has IV access which is patent.
- Check the patient identification, ensuring that it matches on all documentation and ID bands. If possible, ask the patient to state their full name and date of birth, checking the spelling with the patient.
- Record a baseline set of observations within 60 minutes of the transfusion and educate the patient on the transfusion process and possible signs and symptoms of reactions.

Administration

The transfusion of blood products should only occur when clinically indicated and appropriately trained staff manage the transfusion and any potential complications. Safe administration requires the nurse to systematically prepare the patient and the transfusion (Australian Red Cross Lifeblood 2020a).

- Two staff members must independently check patient, prescription and product at the bedside.
- Prime the approved blood administration set with 0.9% sodium chloride or the blood product.
- Load the administration set into the electronic administration device and program volume and time according to the prescription. The second nurse must check the pump settings as well. All transfusions must be completed within four hours or before the component expiry.
- Monitor patient closely for the first 15 minutes and then hourly for the remainder of the transfusion. Observations need to be completed within 60 minutes prior to the transfusion, 15 minutes after the transfusion has started and then hourly at a minimum.

Complications

The close monitoring of patients is essential during the administration of blood products, so any early signs of reaction can be detected. The signs and symptoms can vary depending on the type of reaction that is occurring. Often in the early stages of a reaction, it is impossible to determine the type of reaction. Common signs and symptoms of a reaction include fevers, rashes, pruritis, tachycardia, hypotension, flank pain, nausea, chills, shortness of breath and unexplained bleeding. Patients may have one or more of these symptoms. Figure 5.12 shows a transfusion reaction card describing acute tranfusion reactions, inclusing their associated signs and symptoms, possible aetiology and the actions that should be taken by staff once a reaction is suspected. There are several different types of transfusion-related reactions ranging from mild febrile reactions to more severe reactions such as:

- severe febrile non-haemolytic transfusion reactions
- allergy and anaphylaxis
- acute and delayed haemolytic transfusion reactions
- transfusion-associated circulatory overload (TACO)
- transfusion-related acute lung injury (TRALI)
- transfusion-transmitted infection (TTI), including sepsis from bacterial contamination of blood components.

Transfusion reaction management

If a transfusion reaction is suspected, the first step is to stop the transfusion and notify senior staff. A full set of patient observations should be obtained, and local emergency procedures followed if required. The IV access should be maintained, but the blood administration set should not be flushed as this will administer blood from the line into the patient. All paperwork and products should be rechecked to ensure that no mistakes were made during the identification and checking process. Depending on the type of reaction, the transfusion service should be notified, and further test conducted, including blood and urine cultures.

FIGURE 5.12 Transfusion reaction card

Acute Transfusion Reactions

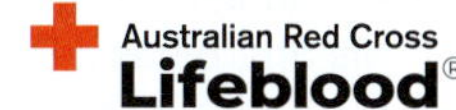

Signs and symptoms	Possible etiology	Action	Investigation
Dyspnoea, ↓O_2 saturation			
With/without hypertension, tachycardia, signs of fluid overload	TACO (transfusion associated circulatory overload)	**Stop transfusion** Sit patient upright Diuretics, O_2	Reaction form and group and save (G&S) Chest X-ray may be helpful
With/without hypotension	TRALI (transfusion-related acute lung injury) ⚠ May become a medical emergency	**Stop transfusion** Assess chest X-ray for infiltrates O_2, possible intubation, ventilation Notify lab and Lifeblood	Reaction form and G&S HLA & HNA antibodies and typing
	Bacterial contamination or acute haemolytic transfusion reaction ⚠ May become a medical emergency	**Stop transfusion** Check patient ID with label IV antibiotics if sepsis Maintain good urine output Notify lab and Lifeblood for bacterial contamination	Culture patient and product Reaction form, G&S and DAT If haemolysis suspected – FBE LDH, bilirubin, haptoglobin, coags, electrolytes, urinalysis

transfusion.com.au Version 10.0 29 August 2019

Acute Transfusion Reactions

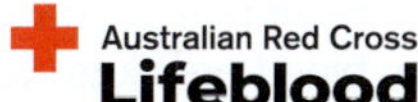

Signs and symptoms	Possible etiology	Action	Investigation
Fever (≥ 38°C and rise ≥ 1°C) and/or chills, rigors			
No other symptoms	Febrile non-haemolytic transfusion reaction	**Stop transfusion** Exclude serious adverse events Antipyretics Recommence if reaction subsides	Reaction form to transfusion lab
Other symptoms present (e.g. hypotension, tachycardia) or ≥ 39°C	Bacterial contamination or acute haemolytic transfusion reaction ⚠ May become a medical emergency	**Stop transfusion** Check patient ID with label Initiate basic life support IV antibiotics if sepsis Notify lab and Lifeblood for bacterial contamination	Culture patient and product Reaction form, G&S and DAT If haemolysis suspected – FBE, LDH, bilirubin, haptoglobin, coags, electrolytes, urinalysis
Rash or urticaria (hives)			
< 2/3 body (no other symptoms)	Minor allergic	**Stop transfusion** Antihistamine Recommence if reaction subsides	None
> 2/3 body (no other symptoms)	Severe allergic	**Stop transfusion** Antihistamine +/- corticosteroid	Reaction form
With dyspnoea, airway obstruction, angioedema, hypotension ⚠ This is a medical emergency	Anaphylaxis (consider IgA deficiency)	**Stop transfusion** Adrenaline Initiate basic life support	Reaction form Perform haptoglobin and IgA level and antibody

Source: Australian Red Cross Lifeblood (2019).

CASE STUDY 5.1

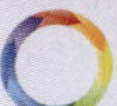

Nursing care of the patient with complex medication needs

Ms Sharp is a 19-year-old female who has been admitted to the surgical ward for an appendectomy. Ms Sharp has a history of anorexia nervosa, Wolff-Parkinson-White (WPW), depression and gastro-oesophageal reflux disease (GORD).

Ms Sharp complains of pain and redness to the PIVC and states she needs to take her morning medications. Ms Sharp is NBM for theatre, but the anaesthetist stated it was ok to administer her morning medications with a sip of water.

Ms Sharp has a PIVC in her left cubital fossa. Currently, normal saline 1 L is infusing over 6 hours.

Ms Sharp is charted for the following medications.

Medication	Dose and route	Time
Metoprolol	25 mg/PO	Twice daily
Pantoprazole 40 mg	40 mg/PO	Daily
Escitalopram	10 mg/PO	Daily
Paracetamol	1 g/PO	Every 4 hours/max 4 g

Hospital medications (ward stock)	
Medication	**Strength**
Metoprolol	50 mg tablet
Pantoprazole 40 mg	20 mg tablet
Escitalopram	5 mg tablet
Paracetamol	5 mg/ml oral suspension

Ms Sharp's vital signs were:

- temperature: 38.6°C
- heart rate: 50 beats per minute
- blood pressure: 130/70 mmHg
- respiratory rate: 16 breaths per minute
- oxygen saturation: 99% on room air
- Glasgow Coma Scale: 15.

Question

Using the information above, calculate the medication doses based on the hospital ward stock. Calculate the intravenous fluid rate at ml/hour. Based on this scenario describe what action you would take as the nurse caring for this patient. Use the clinical reasoning cycle to guide you through the process and devise a plan of care for your patient.

Answer

- *Step 1: Consider the patient.* Ms Sharp is a 19-year-old female.
- *Step 2: Collect cues/information:*. Include subjective and objective data here, including the patient's appearance and past medical history. Objective data will include measurable information such as vital signs
- *Step 3: Process information*. Separate the relevant and irrelevant data — cluster the clues together to formulate an inference about the patient. Ms Sharp has complained of redness and pain to the PIVC and is also noted to be febrile and bradycardic. All other obs are within an acceptable range, and the patient is due her medications. Ms Sharp has a history of WPW and is on a beta-blocker, and is on regular paracetamol for a known infection. The information may indicate the patient has phlebitis from her PIVC, and this warrants further investigation. The patients known beta-blocker is likely to be causing the patient to be bradycardic and stopping her HR from being elevated with the fever.
- *Step 4: Identify problems/issues*. Nursing problems or diagnosis should be listed here. Priority problems are her bradycardia, fevers and red and painful PIVC and her medications. The patient is due her beta-blocker, but she is bradycardic. The PIVC is red and painful and needs further investigation, and all the patient's morning medications are due.
- *Step 5: Establish goals*. Goals of care for Ms Sharp should focus on improving her pain and fever and establishing whether the bradycardia is normal for the patient.
- *Step 6: Take action.* The nurse should inspect the PIVC. If it is red and painful, it will need to be removed and a new one inserted for her operation today. The patient's HR and BP should be checked manually and observations compared to previous observations to identify her normal baseline. Further questions need to be asked to determine if the pain is symptomatic of bradycardia. Paracetamol should be

administered as charted, and the doctor informed of the pyrexia, bradycardia and possible need for a new PIVC.

- *Step 7: Evaluate outcomes.* The patient will need regular vital signs assessment, including pain assessment. Monitor for a resolution of pyrexia.
- *Step 8: Reflect on the process and new learning.* Reflect on any aspects of care that could have been performed in a way to achieve an improved outcome.

CASE STUDY 5.2

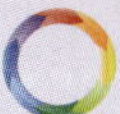

Nursing care of the patient with a blood transfusion

Mr Kumar is a 70-year-old male who has been admitted to the medical ward for a packed red blood cells (PRBC) blood transfusion after a three-day history of melaena. Mr Kumar has a history of congested cardiac failure, GORD and atrial fibrillation (AF).

The doctor prescribed the blood transfusion to run over four hours. There were 250 ml in the unit of PRBC. The transfusion is currently running at 83 ml/hr. Mr Kumar is charted for another PRBC unit once the first unit has transfused.

Mr Kumar starts to complain of shortness of breath and states he feels like he will vomit. On inspection, you can see Mr Kumar is using accessory muscle and is posturing himself in a tripod position.

Mr Kumar's vital signs were as follows:

- temperature: 36.6°C
- heart rate: 110 beats per minute
- blood pressure: 160/70 mmHg
- respiratory rate: 32 breaths per minute
- oxygen saturation: 88% on room air
- Glasgow Coma Scale: 15.

Question

Using the information above, describe what you think is wrong with the patient and what might have caused it? Describe what action you would take as the nurse caring for this patient. Use the clinical reasoning cycle to guide you through the process and devise a plan of care for your patient.

Answer

- *Step 1: Consider the patient*. Mr Kumar is a 70-year-old male.
- *Step 2: Collect cues/information*. Include subjective and objective data here, including the patient's appearance and past medical history. Objective data will include measurable information such as vital signs.
- *Step 3: Process information*. Separate the relevant and irrelevant data — cluster the clues together to formulate an inference about the patient. Mr Kumar is experiencing an increased respiratory rate, hypoxia and increased work of breathing. The patient is also tachycardic and hypertensive. The patient is receiving a blood transfusion, and when the rate is calculated, it is being administered too quickly. This information is likely to indicate the patient is reacting to the blood transfusion.
- *Step 4: Identify problems/issues*. Nursing problems or diagnosis should be listed here. The nurse needs to follow the hospital protocol for blood transfusion reaction but would stop the blood transfusion and prioritise the patients' ineffective breathing pattern and impaired gas exchange.
- *Step 5: Establish goals*. Goals of care for Ms Sharp should focus on improving oxygenation, respiratory rate and work of breathing.
- *Step 6: Take action*. The nurse needs to recognise this is a medical emergency, and the patient is likely having a blood transfusion reaction. The nurse should stop the transfusion and apply oxygen via a non-rebreather mask. The patient should be positioned upright and as comfortably as possible. Senior medical and nursing assistance should be sought. Equipment required in a medical emergency should be collected and ready, including cannulation equipment. A fresh bag of IVF should be primed and ready to be administered via a second PIVC. All blood product orders and information need to be cross-checked to ensure there has not been an administration error. The nurse needs to recognise that this can be very distressing for patients, and a calm and reassuring manner is needed.
- *Step 7: Evaluate outcomes*. Once senior help has arrived, the patient may need to be transferred to a more critical area HDU/ICU. Until this time, ensure all documentation is updated and available and stay with the patient. Observations should be performed at a minimum every 15 minutes. Close observation is required to ensure further signs of deterioration are detected early.
- *Step 8: Reflect on the process and new learning*. Reflect on any aspects of care that could have been performed in a way to achieve an improved outcome.

SUMMARY

Medication and intravenous therapy administration occur every day in the medical-surgical setting. These activities can be high risk, and all healthcare providers must ensure that all medications and intravenous therapy are administered safely. Nurses play a unique role in promoting medication safety as they are well placed to identify and intervene when something goes wrong. For nurses to safely manage medications, they must understand the indications, contraindications, potential risks and complications associated with any medication or IV fluid administered.

KEY TERMS

adverse drug effect (ADR) Any undesirable or harmful (adverse) responses in patients to medication. Serious ADRs can be life-threatening and lead to serious complications. Other ADRs are milder and may not reoccur even after taking the medication again. ADRs include side effects, allergic reactions, idiosyncratic reaction, and toxic reactions.

allergic reaction A reaction that occurs due to an immunological response to the medication. Allergic reactions can be mild or life-threatening anaphylaxis.

idiosyncratic reaction This type of reaction is an unpredictable or unexplainable reaction to a medication.

side effect Any effect that is not therapeutically intended and not necessarily harmful. Side effects are usually well known for the medication and are not the result of an immunological reaction. For example, nausea is a common side effect of opioid analgesics like morphine.

therapeutic effect This is the desired effect of the medication on the body.

toxic reactions Reactions that occur due to a build-up of medication in the body. Medications can build up in the body for a range of reasons, including overdose, or disease processes affecting drug excretion.

REFERENCES

Australian Commission on Safety and Quality in Health Care (ACSQHC). (2009) Guidelines for use of the National Inpatient Medication Chart including the paediatric version. www.safetyandquality.gov.au/sites/default/files/migrated/24380-GuidelinesForNIMC2009.pdf#:~:text=The%20National%20Inpatient%20Medication%20Chart%20%28NIMC%29%20was%20developed,medication%20chart%20standardising%20projects%20within%20their%20own%20organisations

Australian Commission on Safety and Quality in Health Care (ACSQHC). (2015) National standard for user-applied labelling of injectable medicines, fluids and lines. www.safetyandquality.gov.au/sites/default/files/migrated/National-Standard-for-User-Applied-Labelling-Aug-2015.pdf

Australian Commission on Safety and Quality in Health Care (ACSQHC). (2019a) The National Safety and Quality Health Service (NSQHS) Standards: Medication management processes. www.safetyandquality.gov.au/standards/nsqhs-standards/medication-safety-standard/medication-management-processes

Australian Commission on Safety and Quality in Health Care (ACSQHC). (2019b) The National Safety and Quality Health Service (NSQHS) Standards: Blood management standard. www.safetyandquality.gov.au/standards/nsqhs-standards/blood-management-standard

Australian Red Cross Lifeblood. (2020) Products overview. https://transfusion.com.au/products_overview

Australian Red Cross Lifeblood. (2020a) Preparing to administer a blood component including equipment. https://transfusion.com.au/transfusion_practice/administration

Blevins, S. (2020) Medication education: Preparing the patient for discharge. *MEDSURG Nursing*. 29(3): 213–214. http://search.ebscohost.com/login.aspx?direct=true&AuthType=shib&db=aph&AN=143616921&site=ehost-live&custid=s3684040

Brooks, N. (2018) Remember the risks of intravenous therapy and know how to reduce them. *British Journal of Nursing*. 27(8): S20–S21. doi: 10.12968/bjon.2018.27.8.S20

Burton, T. (2017). 'Cardiovascular nursing skills'. In B. Snyder, T. Levett-Jones, T. Burton & N. Harvey (Eds.). *Skills in Clinical Nursing* (pp. 465–545). Pearson Australia.

Collins, M. (2011) 'Anatomy and physiology'. In S. Phillips, M. Collins & L. Dougherty (Eds.). *Venepuncture and Cannulation* (pp. 44–67). Oxford: Blackwell Publishing.

Craft, J. & Gordon, C. (2014) *Understanding Pathophysiology*, 2nd ed. St. Louis, Missouri: Elsevier.

Currie, G. M. (2018a) Pharmacology, Part 1: Introduction to pharmacology and pharmacodynamics. *Journal of Nuclear Medicine Technology*. 46(2): 81–86. doi: 10.2967/jnmt.117.199588

Currie, G. M. (2018b) Pharmacology, Part 2: Introduction to pharmacokinetics. *Journal of Nuclear Medicine Technology*. 46(3): 221–230. doi: 10.2967/jnmt.117.199638

Department of Health. (2007) *Saving lives: reducing infection, delivering clean and safe care. High Impact Intervention No 1 (Central Venous Bundle) and No 2 (Peripheral IV Cannula Care Bundle)*. London: DH.

Department of Health. (2010) Peripheral cannula care and central venous catheter care — high impact interventions. http://hcai.dh.gov.uk/whatdoido/high-impact-interventions

Doellmann, D., Hadaway, L., Bowes-Geddes, L. A. et al. (2009) Infiltration and extravasation: update on prevention and management. *Journal of Infusion Nursing*. 32(4): 203–211.

Dolovich, M. B. & Dhand, R. (2011) Aerosol drug delivery: developments in device design and clinical use. *The Lancet*. 377(9770): 1032–1045. doi: 10.1016/s0140-6736(10)60926-9

Dougherty, L. (2006) *Central venous access devices: care and management*. Oxford: Blackwell Publishing.

Dougherty, L. (2008) 'Obtaining peripheral vascular access'. In L. Dougherty & J. Lamb (Eds.). *Intravenous therapy in nursing practice*, 2nd ed. Oxford: Blackwell Publishing.

Dougherty, L. (2010) Extravasation: prevention, recognition and management. *Nursing Standard*. 24(48): 48–55.

Dougherty, L. & Ansell, L. (2011) 'Medicines management'. In L. Dougherty & S. Lister (Eds.). *The Royal Marsden Hospital Manual of Clinical Nursing Procedures*, 8th ed. (Chapter 16). Oxford: Wiley-Blackwell.

Dougherty, L. & Watson, J. (2011) 'Vascular access devices'. In L. Dougherty & S. Lister (Eds.). *The Royal Marsden Hospital Manual of Clinical Nursing Procedures*, 8th ed. (Chapter 18). Oxford: Wiley-Blackwell.

Downie, G., MacKenzie, J. & Williams, A. (Eds.). (2003) 'Medicine management'. In G. Downie, J. Mackenzie, A. Willams & C. Hind (Eds.). *Pharmacology and Medicines Management for Nurses*, 3rd ed. (pp. 49–91). London: Churchill Livingstone.

Edwards, I. R. & Aronson, J. K. (2000) Adverse drug reactions: Definitions, diagnosis, and management. *The Lancet*. 356: 1255–1259. doi: 10.1016/S0140-6736(00)02799-9

Flinders University. (2013) Drug calculations (Slide 1). Flinders University Student Learning Centre. https://students.flinders.edu.au/content/dam/student/slc/drug-calculations.pdf.au

Frost, P. (2015) Intravenous fluid therapy in adult inpatients. *BMJ*. 350: g7620. doi: 10.1136/bmj.g7620

Gabriel, J. (2008) 'Long-term central venous access'. In L. Dougherty & J. Lamb (Eds.). *Intravenous Therapy in Nursing Practice*, 2nd ed. (pp. 321–351). Oxford: Blackwell Publishing.

Guest, M. (2020) Understanding the principles and aims of intravenous fluid therapy. *Nursing Standards*. 35(2): 75–82. doi: 10.7748/ns.2020.e11459

Haddad, F., Sawalha, M., Khawaja, Y., Najjar, A. & Karaman, R. (2017) Dopamine and levodopa prodrugs for the treatment of Parkinson's Disease. *Molecules*. 23(1). doi: 10.3390/molecules23010040

Hobson, P. (2008) Venepuncture and cannulation: theoretical aspects. *British Journal of Healthcare Assistants*. 2(2): 75–78. doi: 10.12968/bjha.2008.2.2.28386

Hoorn, E. J. (2017) Intravenous fluids: balancing solutions. *Journal of Nephrology*. 30(4): 485–492. doi: 10.1007/s40620-016-0363-9

Infusion Nursing Society. (2011) *Standards for infusion therapy*. Norwood, MA: Infusion Nursing Society USA.

Keogh, S. & Matthew, S. (2019) *Peripheral intravenous catheters: A review of guidelines and research*. Sydney: ACSQHC.

Knowles, S. R., Uetrecht, J. & Shear, N. H. (2000) Idiosyncratic drug reactions: the reactive metabolite syndromes. *The Lancet*. 356(9241): 1587–1591. doi: 10.1016/s0140-6736(00)03137-8

Kramer, T. (2003) Side effects and therapeutic effect. *Medscape General Medicine*. 5(1). https://www.medscape.com/viewarticle/448250

Lamb, J. & Dougherty, L. (2008) 'Local and systemic complications of intravenous therapy'. In L. Dougherty & J. Lamb (Eds.). *Intravenous therapy in nursing practice*, 2nd ed. (pp. 167–196). Oxford: Blackwell Publishing.

Levett-Jones, T. (2017) 'Medication administration'. In B. Snyder, T. Levett-Jones, T. Burton & N. Harvey (Eds.).*Skills in clinical nursing* (pp. 239–312). Australia: Pearson.

Lewis, S. R., Pritchard, M. W., Evans, D. J., Butler, A. R., Alderson, P., Smith, A. F. & Roberts, I. (2018) Colloids versus crystalloids for fluid resuscitation in critically ill people. *Cochrane Database Systematic Review*. 8: CD000567. doi: 10.1002/14651858.CD000567.pub7

Loveday, H. P., Wilson, J. A., Pratt, R. J., Golsorkhi, M., Tingle, A., Bak, A., ... Wilcox, M. (2014) epic3: National Evidence-Based Guidelines for Preventing Healthcare-Associated Infections in NHS Hospitals in England. *Journal of Hospital Infection*. 86: S1–S70. doi: 10.1016/S0195-6701(13)60012-2

Macklin, D. & Chernecky, C. C. (2004) *IV Therapy*. St Louis: Saunders.

Maki, D. G., Ringer, M. & Alvarado, C. J. (1991) Prospective randomised trial of povidone-iodine, alcohol, and chlorhexidine for prevention of infection associated with central venous and arterial catheters. *The Lancet*. 338: 339–343.

Marsh, N., Webster, J., Ullman, A. J., Mihala, G., Cooke, M., Chopra, V. & Rickard, C. M. (2020) Peripheral intravenous catheter non-infectious complications in adults: A systematic review and meta-analysis. *Journal of Advanced Nursing*.30(6):3346–3362. doi:10.1111/jan.14565

Medicines and Healthcare products Regulatory Authority. (2010) *Device Bulletin Infusion Systems DB2003 (02) v2.0 November*. London: MHRA.

Mermel, L. A., Allon, M., Bouza, E. et al. (2009) Clinical practice guidelines for the diagnosis and management of intravascular catheter-related infection: 2009 update by the Infectious Diseases Society of America. *Clinical Infectious Diseases*. 49(1): 1–45.

Mortell, M. (2019). Should known allergy status be included as a medication administration 'right'? *British Journal of Nursing*. 28(20): 1292–1298. doi: 10.12968/bjon.2019.28.20.1292

Murakami, T. (2017) Absorption sites of orally administered drugs in the small intestine. *Expert Opinion Drug Discovery*. 12(12): 1219–1232. doi: 10.1080/17460441.2017.1378176

National Institute for Health and Care Excellence (NICE). (2017) Intravenous fluid therapy in adults in hospital. www.nice.org.uk/guidance/cg174/chapter/1-recommendations

Neal, M. J. (2016) *Medical pharmacology at a glance*, 8th ed. Wiley-Blackwell.

NSW Agency for Clinical Innovation. (2014) Central Venous Access Device Post Insertion Management. https://www.aci.health.nsw.gov.au/__data/assets/pdf_file/0010/239626/ACI14_CVAD-2-2.pdf

NSW Agency for Clinical Innovation & the Gastroenterological Nurses College of Australia. (2014) Enteral medication administration guidelines Australia. https://www.aci.health.nsw.gov.au/__data/assets/pdf_file/0017/251063/gastrostomy_guide-web.pdf

Nursing and Midwifery Board of Australia. (2018) *Midwife standards for practice.* www.nursingmidwiferyboard.gov.au/codes-guidelines-statements/professional-standards/midwife-standards-for-practice.aspx

Oldham, J., Sinclair, L. & Hendry, C. (2009) Right patient, right blood, right care: safe transfusion practice. *British Journal of Nursing.* 18(5): 312–320.

Polovich, M., Whitford, J. M. & Olsen, M. (Eds.). (2009) *Oncology Nursing Society. Chemotherapy and Biotherapy Guidelines and Recommendations for Practice*, 3rd ed. Pittsburgh, PA: Oncology Nursing Press.

Quinn, C. (2008) 'Intravenous flow control and infusion devices'. In L. Dougherty & J. Lamb (Eds.). *Intravenous therapy in nursing practice*, 2nd ed. (pp. 197–224). Oxford: Blackwell Publishing.

Rau, J. L. (2005) The inhalation of drugs: advantages and problems. *Respiratory Care.* 50(3): 367–382. http://rc.rcjournal.com/content/respcare/50/3/367.full.pdf

Scales, K. (2008) 'Anatomy and physiology related to intravenous therapy'. In L. Dougherty & J. Lamb (Eds.). *Intravenous therapy in nursing practice*, 2nd ed. (pp. 23–48). Oxford: Blackwell Publishing.

Scales, K. (2014) NICE CG 174: intravenous fluid therapy in adults in hospital. *British Journal of Nursing.* 23(8): S6, S8. doi: 10.12968/bjon.2014.23.Sup8.S6

Shepherd, A. (2011) Measuring and managing fluid balance. *Nursing Times.* 107(28): 12–16.

Shepherd, M. & Shepherd, E. (2020) Medicines administration 1: understanding routes of administration. *Nursing Times.* 116(6): 42–44.

Schulmeister, L. (2009) 'Antineoplastic therapy'. In M. Alexander, A. Corrigan, L. Gorski, J. Hankins & R. Perucca (Eds.). *Infusion therapy: An evidence-based approach* (pp. 366–367). Philadelphia: Saunders Elsevier.

Smeulers, M., Verweij, L., Maaskant, J. M., de Boer, M., Krediet, C. T., Nieveen van Dijkum, E. J. & Vermeulen, H. (2015) Quality indicators for safe medication preparation and administration: a systematic review. *PLoS One.* 10(4): e0122695. doi: 10.1371/journal.pone.0122695

Smith, R. N. & Nolan, J. P. (2013) Central venous catheters. *BMJ.* 347: f6570. doi: 10.1136/bmj.f6570

Smith, W. (2013) Adverse drug reactions — allergy? side-effect? intolerance? *Australian Family Physician.* 42(1–2): 12–16. https://www.ncbi.nlm.nih.gov/pubmed/23529453

Turner, M. S. & Hankins, J. (2010) 'Pharmacology'. In M. Alexander, A. Corrigan, L. Gorski, J. Hankins & R. Perucca (Eds.). *Infusion nursing: An evidence-based approach*, 3rd ed. (pp. 263–298). St Louis: Saunders Elsevier.

Vera, M. (2021) *IV Fluids and Solutions Guide & Cheat Sheet*. Nurselabs. https://nurseslabs.com/iv-fluids

Viswanathan, P., Muralidaran, Y. & Ragavan, G. (2017) 'Challenges in oral drug delivery: a nano-based strategy to overcome'. In A. Ecaterina & M. Grumezescu (Eds.). *Micro and Nano Technologies, Nanostructures for Oral Medicine* (pp. 173–201). Elsevier.

Weinstein, S. (2007) *Plumer's principles and practices of intravenous therapy*, 8th ed. Philadelphia: Lippincott.

Whittington, Z. (2008) 'Pharmacological aspects of IV therapy'. In L. Dougherty & J. Lamb (Eds.). *Intravenous therapy in nursing practice*, 2nd ed. (pp. 117–146). Oxford: Blackwell Publishing.

Wondmieneh, A., Alemu, W., Tadele, N. & Demis, A. (2020). Medication administration errors and contributing factors among nurses: a cross sectional study in tertiary hospitals, Addis Ababa, Ethiopia. *BMC Nursing.* 19: 4. doi: 10.1186/s12912-020-0397-0

ACKNOWLEDGEMENTS

Figure 5.2: © Australian Commission on Safety and Quality in Health Care (ACSQHC). Medication chart. Retrieved from: https://www.safetyandquality.gov.au/sites/default/files/2019-08/saq8404_nimc_short stay_v3_film_nofileinfo.pdf

Figure 5.5: © Michaelberry / Wikimedia Commons

Figure 5.6: © DR P. MARAZZI / SCIENCE PHOTO LIBRARY; SCHMITT / BSIP / SCIENCE PHOTO LIBRARY

Figure 5.8: © Commonwealth of Australia

Figure 5.9: © PK289 / Shutterstock.com

Figure 5.10: © Atiwat Witthayanurut / Shutterstock.com

Figure 5.12: © Acute transfusion reactions. Resource library, Health Professionals. © Australian Red Cross Lifeblood. https://transfusion.com.au/resources/ATR

CHAPTER 6

Principles of nutritional care

LEARNING OBJECTIVES

After studying this chapter, you should be able to:

6.1 describe the effects of malnutrition and define the key elements of nutritional screening

6.2 identify current dietary guidelines

6.3 describe the implications of illness on nutrition

6.4 describe the potential impacts of surgery on nutrition

6.5 describe the different methods of nutritional support.

Introduction

Good nutrition is essential to life and health. The human race has known of the inherent importance of nutrition for millennia. Hippocrates, known as the Father of Medicine, is reputed to have said, 'Let food be thy medicine and let medicine be thy food' (Witkamp & van Norren 2018). This basic precept is as true today as it was in 400 BC. Nutrition is the process of taking in food and using it for growth, metabolism and repair (*Webster's New World Medical Dictionary* 2009). The stages of nutrition are ingestion, digestion, absorption, transport, assimilation and excretion (*Webster's New World Medical Dictionary* 2009). Good nutrition is vital for everyone, but especially those who are frail, ill or injured (National Health and Medical Research Council (NHMRC) 2017).

A balanced **diet** should provide sufficient **nutrients** in the form of energy, **protein**, fat, vitamins and minerals required to keep an individual healthy (NHMRC 2017). The ongoing absence or relative lack of some or all of these nutrients may lead to **malnutrition** (NHMRC 2017). Nutritional requirements change throughout the human lifespan. In childhood, pregnancy and advancing age, nutritional requirements differ (NHMRC 2013).

Children's nutrient and energy requirements are greater than those of adults in relation to their body weight. Children have a rapid growth rate up to age five, and the additional nutrient requirements are essential for normal growth. After the age of five, the rate of growth slows until approximately age 18. During this first 18 years of life, bodyweight increases twentyfold (this is a 1900 per cent increase). The growth rate is a fundamental indicator of nutritional status in children (NHMRC 2013).

As we age, several inevitable changes occur. Two of the most common are sarcopenia, which is the loss of muscle mass replaced with fat or connective tissue and osteoporosis, which is the loss of minerals (mainly calcium) from the bone. Both of these changes can, however, be postponed and mitigated with good nutrition. The other common change is the decrease in appetite, estimated to occur in 15–30 per cent of older people. This is complex, and the mechanism is not entirely understood, but there are two key factors. The first is the decline and production of the hormone ghrelin, which simply put stimulates appetite. (Gillie 2010) The second is the slowing of gastric emptying, which means the person will feel full longer, thus be less likely to eat as much or as often as required (Pilgrim et al. 2015).

During illness or following surgery, an individual's nutritional requirements may change. At these times, the provision of appropriate nutrition levels is vital to provide the body with ample nutrients to aid their recovery (Gillis & Wishmeyer 2019). Providing good nutritional care is essential when providing healthcare and is associated with better patient outcomes (NHMRC 2017). As nurses, we are responsible for ensuring that patients within our care receive the appropriate type and level of assistance necessary to ensure that their nutritional requirements are met via the oral, artificial enteral or parenteral routes as appropriate.

6.1 Nutritional screening and assessment

LEARNING OBJECTIVE 6.1 Describe the effects of malnutrition and define the key elements of nutritional screening.

Malnutrition is defined as 'deficiencies, excesses or imbalances in a person's intake of energy and/or nutrients' (World Health Organization (WHO) 2020). There are two broad groups of conditions that can be defined as malnutrition. The first is those who are undernourished. This includes signs of underweight — low weight for age and micronutrient deficiencies (WHO 2020). Poverty is a key factor in the prevalence of malnutrition worldwide (WHO 2020). The second group includes those who are overweight, obese or have diseases such as diabetes, heart disease and cancer (WHO 2020). The consumption of fast food has dramatically increased in the last 25 years and is associated with an excess intake of high calorie but low nutrient food (Butt 2007).

Malnutrition occurs in more than 30 per cent of patients in Australian hospitals; 30–60 per cent in acute care, 30–50 per cent in rehabilitation and 30–70 per cent in aged care (Gulgoz 2006). Some of these patients come to hospital with pre-existing malnutrition, but many become malnourished while in hospital. Those who are malnourished often experience a significantly higher incidence of complications during treatment, have longer hospital stays and have a higher mortality rate than those who are well-nourished on admission (The Australian Commission on Safety and Quality in Health Care [ACSQHC] 2018).

Nutritional screening

Nutritional screening is a process used to identify those patients at risk of malnutrition. Nutritional screening should occur within 24 hours of a patient's admission (NHMRC 2017), and the responsibility for this tends to lie with nurses as part of their admission assessment.

Nutritional screening considers an individual's current nutritional status — their weight, when they last ate and what constitutes their normal diet. This will include evidence of weight loss — unintentional weight loss, especially if rapid, is a concern in all hospital patients, regardless of their original body weight. Ask the patient about their most recent weight. If they cannot be weighed, enquire whether there are any recent changes in the way clothing or rings fit or whether dentures have become looser.

Commonly used screening tools in Australia include the:

- Mini Nutritional Assessment (MNA) (Gulgoz 2006)
- Malnutrition Screening Tool (QLD Health 2017)
- Paediatric Nutrition Screening Tool (PNST)
- Malnutrition Universal Screening Tool (MUST) (NHMRC 2017).

A basic nutrition screen may include some or all of the following.

- Measurement of height and weight on admission and calculation of body mass index (BMI). This is calculated by dividing the patient's weight in kilograms by the patient's height in metres squared (BMI = kg/m^2). This is included in the MNA and MUST.
- A history of weight gain or loss in the last three months, included in the MNA, MST and MUST.
- Decreased appetite and food intake included in the MNA and MST.

Additional useful information may include the patient's normal dietary intake, noting also medical and drug history, and an 'eyeball' assessment, which involves looking for obvious signs of weight loss or malnutrition. The initial screening acts as a baseline against which we can monitor a patient's progress or deterioration. Without this information and an ongoing review, it is difficult to determine how effective any interventions are. The documentation also acts as evidence that nutritional screening has been conducted and which nutritional care plan was implemented.

It is important to understand that the BMI values in table 6.1 should only be used as a guide and should not be used in isolation to determine whether someone is at risk of malnutrition. Malnutrition can also affect those who are in the normal and overweight categories. The BMI does not indicate body composition or the proportions of fat and lean body tissue. Therefore, some muscular individuals appear to have a higher BMI when they are not 'overweight'.

TABLE 6.1 BMI categories for adults

Underweight and at high risk of malnutrition	18.5 kg/m^2
Healthy weight	18.5–24.9 kg/m^2
Overweight	25.0–29.9 kg/m^2
Obese	≥30.0 kg/m^2

Source: Adapted from WHO (2020); NHMRC (2013)

Some population groups may have a risk of malnutrition at a lower BMI (those of Asian descent), while others may have a higher average BMI (people of Polynesian heritage, including Torres Strait Islanders, Maori, Samoans and Tongans). Indigenous people have a relatively high limb to trunk ratio and, therefore, have an increased risk of malnutrition at a lower BMI (NHMRC 2013).

Where a screening tool is not used, nurses should perform a basic nutrition screen by undertaking the actions listed above and using their clinical judgement to calculate the patient's risk of malnutrition. It is important to recognise that the screening process should not be viewed as a one-off event; nutritional screening should be ongoing and repeated weekly for inpatients (Agency for Clinical Innovation [ACI] 2017). Where the patient is a poor historian or is unconscious, information should be sought from the family or carers. Without the routine use of a screening tool, there is no clear means of checking whether patients' nutritional needs are being met and whether they are at risk of malnutrition.

Nursing action plans

When screening has been completed, and a patient has been identified as being at risk of malnutrition, they must have an appropriate care plan developed by a dietitian. Appropriate nursing action plans should be implemented without delay.

Nursing action plans may include the following.

- Recording food and fluid intake (usually for up to three days).
- Encouraging small frequent meals or providing nutritional supplements between meals.
- Ensuring enough time is taken to assist the patients who need help. Do not try to rush this procedure; it will not ultimately achieve the goal of assuring good nutrition is provided in a patient-centred manner. If the patient knows the nurse is in a hurry, they are likely to say they have had enough when they simply don't want to bother the nurse anymore.
- Offering frequent fluids, remembering that while a patient may refuse water, they may accept a cup of tea. Fluid intake is not only water but any clear fluid, including tea, coffee, soup, jelly, fruit juices, beer and soft drinks.
- Offering fluids between meals to avoid filling up on fluids at mealtimes.
- Ensuring that a high-protein, high-energy diet is ordered for the patient (Department of Health and Human Services [DHHS] 2020). This is a strategy to increase the protein and energy content of the diet to provide adequate energy for the patients' daily needs and high protein to repair and rebuild body cells that have been catabolised for energy during the time of inadequate nutritional intake.
- Recording weight regularly, at the same time of day, on the same scales (where possible) with the patient in similar clothing to help provide consistent and accurate weight trends. Please note that the weight will be a combination of their fluid weight and dry weight. In the average adult, fluid is approximately 60 per cent of body composition (Hryciw & Bonner 2019). If the patient is perceived to have had a significant weight loss or gain over 24 hours, always check their fluid status before judging this fluctuation to ensure that changes in hydration status are not assumed to be changes in actual body weight.

Appropriate and timely nutritional intervention following screening can enable many patients to meet their nutritional needs. Where there is little improvement in nutritional intake or the patient requires specialised nutritional advice, referral to another healthcare professional, such as a dietitian or a speech and language therapist, may be necessary.

Referral

Referral to a dietitian should be initiated where:

- a high nutritional risk score is present on screening, identifying an increased risk of malnutrition
- additional or specialist nutrition is required, such as enteral tube feeding or parenteral nutrition
- a more detailed nutrition assessment is required.

A speech and language therapist involvement may be initiated if the patient has swallowing problems with an oral diet or fluids. This is often the case following a cerebrovascular accident (CVA), commonly referred to as a stroke.

Nutritional assessment

A dietitian will usually take a detailed, specific and in-depth appraisal of an individual's nutritional state by identifying possible malnutrition. An individual's nutritional requirements will vary depending upon their age, gender, mobility, the presence of acute or chronic illness, the stage of that illness and their underlying nutritional state (although this list is not exhaustive). Dietary reference values guide nutritional requirements for various groups of individuals but do not consider medical conditions or factors that may affect a particular individual's nutritional requirements (NHMRC 2017).

Any person in hospital who is identified as being at risk of malnutrition must be monitored regularly, and their estimated requirements are adjusted to reflect any change in their clinical condition.

Nutritional assessment will consider the following.

- The individual's current nutritional status.
- Evidence of unintentional weight loss.
- The nutritional implications of their medical condition — surgery, intravenous fluids, pyrexia or gastrointestinal losses (through vomiting, diarrhoea and drains).
- Hydration levels of the patient — do they have sunken eyes, a dry mouth and fragile, papery skin? Are they confused?

- Evidence of fluid retention (oedema), such as swollen ankles. This may mask weight loss. Accurate fluid balance is essential so that changes in hydration status are not mistaken for changes in actual body weight.
- The severity and likely duration of their disease or illness (although this can sometimes be difficult to predict).
- Mood level — as well as being a sign of poor nutrition, poor mood may also affect appetite.
- Breathlessness — this will affect the patient's ability to eat and possibly the ability to obtain and prepare food. It may also be a symptom of anaemia.
- Evidence of pressure ulcers — these will increase the patient's nutritional requirements.
- The activity level of the individual — whether they are bed-bound or mobile around the ward. Reduced mobility may be a side effect of malnutrition. However, if an individual's mobility was already affected before hospital admission, they may have been unable to obtain, prepare or eat food for some time at home, compounding the problem.

Dietary assessment

A dietary assessment will focus on an individual's actual intake from food, oral nutritional supplements, enteral feeding or parenteral nutrition. It is sometimes difficult to obtain an accurate history from the individual, so intake charts, if completed accurately, can be particularly useful. If individuals are able, it can be helpful for them to complete their own. This will also involve the patient in their care and centres the patient in their care. It helps give the patient independence and autonomy. It may also make them more confident to speak up about any food likes and dislikes to incorporate into meal planning. Tracking any behaviour will make a person more aware, which can be used as an educational tool for the patient's ability to continue a healthier food regime after returning home (Lacey & Street 2017).

Calculating nutritional requirements

By estimating an individual's nutritional requirements, treatment aims to:

- meet their specific nutritional requirements
- ensure that nitrogen (protein) loss is minimised
- minimise or prevent the risk of weight loss or gain unless this is a desirable outcome
- ensure that sufficient vitamins and minerals are provided
- achieve an appropriate level of hydration (fluid balance).

Providing the patient with the appropriate level of nutrition prevents the loss of body fat and protein stores and the ongoing adverse effects associated with malnutrition. Overfeeding should be avoided in the short term to prevent associated biochemical derangements such as hyperglycaemia, the development of fatty liver and the additional stresses placed on the body. Long-term overfeeding should be avoided to prevent obesity.

Ongoing adverse effects of malnutrition

Adverse effects of malnutrition may be insidious and detrimental to health. These include:

- impaired immune function, placing the individual at increased risk of infections
- increased risk of tissue breakdown and pressure ulcers
- muscle wasting and weakness as the body breaks down protein and fats for energy
- delayed wound healing
- impaired mobility
- dehydration
- impaired **metabolic profile**
- apathy and depression
- increased risk of post-operative complications (ACI 2017).

6.2 Dietary guidelines

LEARNING OBJECTIVE 6.2 Identify current dietary guidelines.

The Australian Government has provided nutrition advice and guidelines to the public for 75 years, primarily through the National Health and Medical Research Council (NHMRC). The NHMRC is a statutory authority and the primary Australian Government agency responsible for medical and public research.

The Australian Dietary Guidelines have been developed to provide the best available, scientifically valid information on the different food groups, quantities of food needed for optimal nutrition and dietary patterns that promote health and wellbeing and reduce the risk of diet-related conditions and chronic disease.

The guidelines are reviewed every five years and were most recently updated in 2013. They were developed after extensive consultation with experts in food, nutrition and health from around the world. 55 000 scientific journal articles were analysed and information incorporated into the guidelines. Extensive public consultation was also undertaken, which included consideration of consumer issues, including cost and availability of foods.

There are five guidelines for eating well.

1. Achieve and maintain a healthy weight by being physically active and choosing amounts of nutritious foods and fluid to meet energy needs.
2. Eat a wide variety of foods from the five food groups daily.
3. Limit the intake of foods containing added salt and sugar, limit saturated fats and alcohol.
4. Encourage, support and promote breastfeeding.
5. Be aware of food safety; prepare food and store it safely.

The guidelines are intended to be realistic and practical. With the rising rates of obesity and type 2 diabetes, it is evident that the Australian public needs to make better dietary decisions and have the information with which to guide these choices.

The guideline resources include the following.

- Nutrient reference values, which detail the recommended macro and **micronutrients** required to avoid deficiency, toxicity and chronic disease. An example of this is the amount of iron or vitamin B12 a healthy person needs.
- A food modelling system that gives a range of computer-generated diets, describing some types, combinations and amounts of foods and examples of a healthy eating plan for different ages, genders and levels of activity and includes various dietary preferences such as vegan, vegetarian and omnivorous.
- The guide to healthy eating poster/pictorial representation of the five food groups and examples of which foods are contained within each group.
- Infant feeding guidelines.
- Companion resources, including summary booklets, an interactive website and brochures for both health professionals and consumers. These can all be found at www.eatforhealth.gov.au.

The dietary guidelines are based on whole foods and are divided into five food groups (figure 6.1):

1. grain foods (cereals) (rice, wheat, pasta, cereals and foods made from these) — 4–7 serves per day (depending on age and gender)
2. vegetables, legumes and beans — 2–6 serves per day (depending on age and gender)
3. lean meats, poultry and fish, tofu, nuts, seeds, legumes and eggs — 1–3 serves per day (depending on age)
4. fruit — 1–2 serves per day
5. dairy products and alternatives (milk, cheese and yoghurt, and calcium-enriched oat, soy and rice milks — (depending on age and gender).

Finally, drink plenty of water (NHMRC 2013).

With the exception of breast milk during the first six months of life, no single food can provide all the nutrients needed for good health. A diet with a wide variety of foods from the five food groups (grains, vegetables, fruit, dairy and alternatives, meat and legumes) is the most reliable way to ensure that nutrient requirements are met (NHMRC 2013).

There are many specific dietary guidelines for different subgroups within both hospitals and the community — for example, those with coeliac disease, diabetes, short bowel syndrome, irritable bowel syndrome, renal failure, cardiac failure, etc. Although nurses need to have a basic awareness of different dietary requirements, a dietitian will provide expert advice. Nurses should understand the concept of a healthy diet and understand the symbols on menu sheets to advise patients on foods suitable for their specific diet.

FIGURE 6.1 The Australian Guide to Healthy Eating

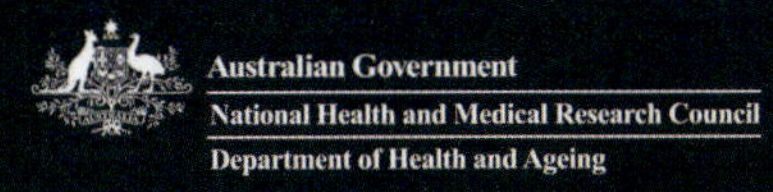

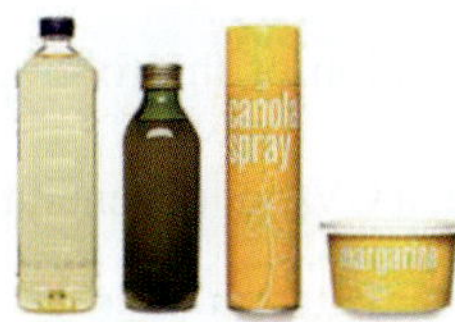

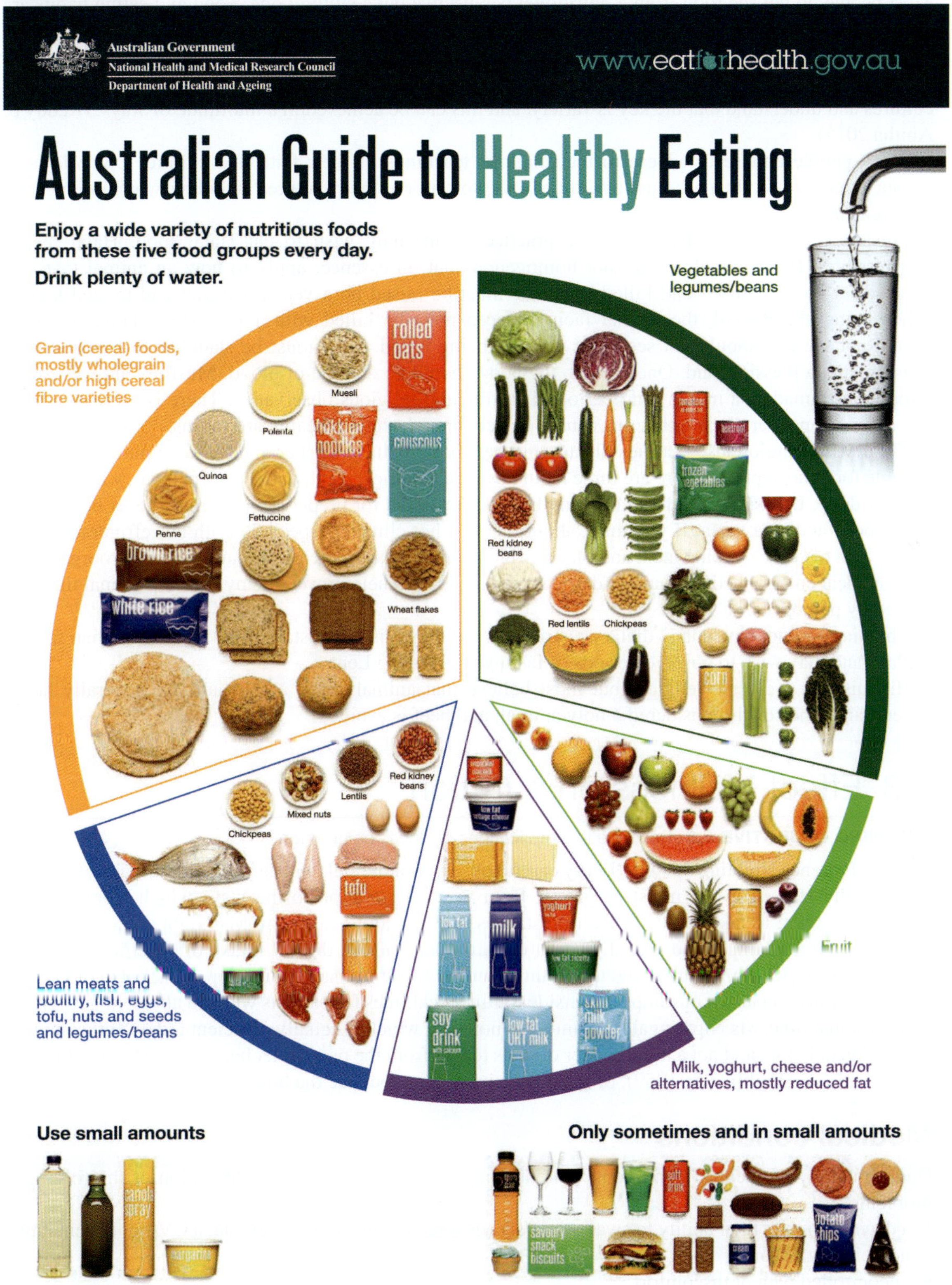

Australian Government
National Health and Medical Research Council
Department of Health and Ageing
www.eatforhealth.gov.au
Australian Guide to Healthy Eating
Enjoy a wide variety of nutritious foods from these five food groups every day.
Drink plenty of water.
Grain (cereal) foods, mostly wholegrain and/or high cereal fibre varieties
rolled oats
Muesli
Polenta
Quinoa
hokkien noodles
couscous
Fettuccine
Penne
brown rice
white rice
Wheat flakes
Vegetables and legumes/beans
tomatoes
beetroot
frozen vegetables
Red kidney beans
Red lentils
Chickpeas
corn
Fruit
peaches
Lean meats and poultry, fish, eggs, tofu, nuts and seeds and legumes/beans
Red kidney beans
Lentils
Mixed nuts
Chickpeas
tofu
baked beans
Milk, yoghurt, cheese and/or alternatives, mostly reduced fat
low fat cottage cheese
low fat milk
milk
yoghurt
low fat ricotta
soy drink
low fat UHT milk
skim milk powder
Use small amounts
canola spray
margarine
Only sometimes and in small amounts
soft drink
savoury snack biscuits
cream
potato chips

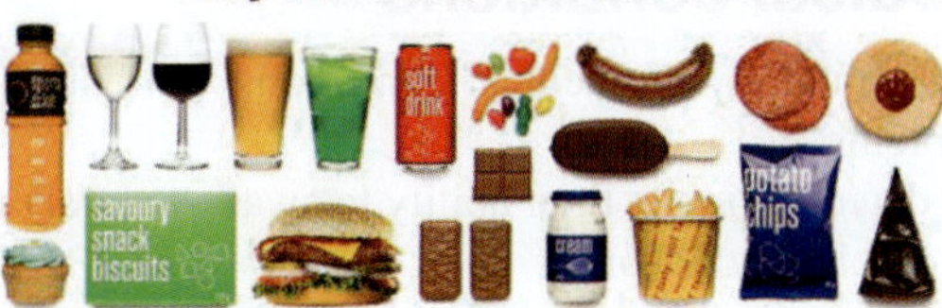

Source: NHMRC (2013).

Diet and culture

Most people do not see food from a nutritional perspective but a cultural one. Food and eating habits are deeply entrenched within a culture and as such, cannot be easily changed. In addition, food has a deeply emotional connection and is often associated with love and caring. Food rules and beliefs may have a positive or negative effect on health. In the nursing context, we need to be open to the food rules of other cultures and understand that the key is variety, and this can be achieved in a multitude of ways. (Reddy & Anitha 2015)

Many people choose to adhere to the religious teachings of their faith and culture. Our role is to do our utmost to facilitate the patient to continue to observe their culture, including worship and food requirements.

Muslim people (those that follow or practice Islam) may wish to eat Halal food. Halal means 'permissible'. Halal guidelines are not homogenous but, in essence, apply to how an animal that will be used for food is raised and killed. Animals must be raised on a vegetarian diet and treated kindly. When being slaughtered, the animal facing Mecca must be killed with a very sharp knife that they should not see and should not see other animals being killed. They must be slaughtered by hand by a Muslim, and a blessing said. Once killed, the body should be drained of blood. Muslims may also wish to observe Ramadan, a month-long period of fasting and religious observance. There is no reason from an organisational perspective that this cannot be accommodated in a healthcare setting.

The Jewish religion also outlines dietary and health guidelines. Kosher, means to be pure, proper and suitable for consumption. There are three main kosher categories: meat, dairy, and 'pareve', which are not meat or dairy. Utensils (including chopping boards, etc.) used for preparing meat must never be used for dairy foods and vice versa. If you think about this in a hot climate, especially with no refrigeration, this makes a lot of sense. Mixing meat and blood, which contain many potentially dangerous microorganisms, with an ideal culture medium such as dairy, is best avoided to help prevent many gastrointestinal illnesses caused by pathogens.

Christians do not have many dietary restrictions but may wish to abstain from meat other than fish on Fridays and may wish to observe periods of fasting, e.g. during Lent.

Hinduism is a diverse religion, but most believe that animals have a soul and are generally lacto-vegetarians. The cow is considered a holy animal, and beef is avoided.

6.3 Effect of illness on nutrition

LEARNING OBJECTIVE 6.3 Describe the implications of illness on nutrition.

In 1859, Florence Nightingale said, 'Every careful observer of the sick will agree that thousands of patients are annually starved in the midst of plenty, from want of attention to the ways which alone make it possible for them to take food'. In many instances, the attentions noted by Ms Nightingale remain the same today. For example, the non-alignment of care related to the dietary intake of specific individuals (person centring), such as frail patients and those unable to cut up their food or open packaging to access food. It may also relate to consumption outside routine mealtimes for patients who are not feeling receptive to food at that time. Ms Nightingale continued to note that which is equally prescient today 'If the nurse is an intelligent being, and not a mere carrier of diets to and from the patient, let her exercise her intelligence in these things' (Nightingale 1859), or today's lexicon 'think outside the box'.

Medical conditions

Due to underlying medical conditions, patients may experience one or a combination of the following problems:

- a deterioration in their ability to swallow safely (dysphagia) due to, for example, a CVA or degenerative neurological disorder
- uncontrolled pain or discomfort
- nausea or vomiting
- breathlessness, which will affect their ability to eat (try breathing fast and swallowing at the same time); it may also impact their ability to shop for and prepare food
- infection, resulting in discomfort, confusion and/or reduced appetite
- increased fluid losses due to diarrhoea or **malabsorption**

- being nil by mouth awaiting a swallow assessment or surgical procedure
- a change in their functional ability to care for themselves, leading to difficulties in:
  - completing a menu
  - removing wrapping from food containers, opening packaging or removing lids from bottles or cartons
  - cutting up food
  - managing a normal
  - consistent diet
  - asking for help.

Psychological status

A change in psychological status may occur due to the onset of acute illness, infection or dementia. The effects of this change can affect nutritional status and may be exhibited as:

- acute or chronic confusion or memory loss (forgetting to eat)
- poor comprehension
- poor motivation to eat
- an inability to recognise food
- the inability to eat unaided
- deterioration in swallowing, requiring purées or a soft diet.

Side effects of medication

Many drugs have unwanted side effects, and if several medications are taken simultaneously, the risk of developing side effects increases. Problems that affect nutritional status may include:

- changes in the taste and smell of food, for example, with antibiotics or chemotherapy
- changes in appetite, for example, when taking steroids or central nervous system stimulants (used to treat ADHD)
- constipation (opiates)
- diarrhoea (magnesium or vitamin C supplements)
- drowsiness (benzodiazepines)
- dry mouth (tricyclic antidepressants).

Other issues that may affect an individual's ability to eat include:

- disruption of the patient's mealtimes due to ward rounds, personal care or investigations
- being off the ward when meals are delivered
- language difficulties or a lack of understanding of the instructions given
- poor sight or hearing
- being unaware of how to order food and what is available outside patients' mealtimes poorly fitting or absent dentures
- food delivered but patient unable to reach it
- difficulties opening packaging
- psychological issues around eating, such as anorexia, autism
- medical conditions, e.g. post-operative ileus (Naithani et al. 2008; ACI 2017).

Many of these issues can be easily addressed by nursing staff at ward level, improving the patient's experience of meals and reducing the likelihood of them not receiving their appropriate nutrition in a timely manner. Other factors affecting appetite are outlined in table 6.2.

TABLE 6.2 Other problems affecting appetite

Problem	Caused by	Treatment
Constipation	Medication, e.g. opiates Lack of dietary fibre Medical conditions Reduced mobility Insufficient oral food and fluid intake	Adequate hydration Regular aperients Remember to offer the patient frequent fluids. Even if water is within reach, patients should be reminded to drink. If they don't like water, then offer a cup of tea or other suitable fluid.

(continued)

TABLE 6.2 *(continued)*

Problem	Caused by	Treatment
Nausea/vomiting, abdominal distension	Constipation Medical conditions, e.g. poor gastric emptying Side effect of other medications, e.g. antibiotics or chemotherapy	Antiemetics before food Constipation — treat as above Offer food that is appetising, well presented and in small portions Offer meals in an unhurried atmosphere Cold food may be tolerated better than hot food, due to a reduced aroma
Poor oral hygiene	Poorly fitting dentures, making eating difficult and possibly leading to mouth ulcers Oral thrush (candida), making eating painful and affecting the taste of food Mouth ulceration, making eating painful Gingivitis — as above	Check the patient's mouth, tongue and teeth at least once a shift. Ensure they are able to access necessary items to clean their teeth and rinse their mouth. If they are unable to do this themselves, then ensure they have mouth care attended to. Treatment should be specific to the route of the problem: • new dentures • antifungal treatment • vitamin B and C replacements.
Other issues including: • uraemia (high blood urea levels due to dehydration or poor kidney function) • diarrhoea • uraemia (high blood urea levels due to dehydration or poor kidney function) • medical conditions, e.g. post-operative ileus Check bowel sounds. If there are none inform a senior staff member before attempting feeding. • psychological issues around eating • increasing age • dementia • anorexia.		Ensure the patient is adequately hydrated Treatment should include: • ensuring the patient is adequately hydrated • providing small appetising meals in an unhurried atmosphere • providing assistance with eating where appropriate • stimulating appetite in stable older patients, offering a small amount of alcohol prior to a meal.

Access to food

A key and sometimes overlooked aspect of patient nutrition is that the patient can actually ingest the nutrition provided.

Historically, Matron was the head of the nursing staff and was in charge of housekeeping and kitchen staff. Nurses were responsible for delivering the meals to the patients, so there was a focus on the link between the patient and their nutrition in a very practical sense. As nurses' roles expanded and became more technical, and the acuity of the patients was increased. The roles that were deemed 'hotel services' were outsourced to private companies or otherwise attended by non-nursing staff. This meant that the patients' nutritional intake was no longer a nursing focus and malnutrition was often unrecognised (Evans 2015).

At present, food and drinks are most often delivered to the patient by the kitchen staff, who are not responsible for anything more than that. This may happen at the same time nurses are on their own meal break. Any difficulties that confront the patient in accessing their meal may go unnoticed. Check that they are willing and able to eat the food, which means it should be food they like enough to eat, it adheres to any dietary and religious guidelines, and it is cut up or presented in a form that the patient can ingest.

If the patient is frail and elderly or particularly incapacitated by their clinical condition, they may not be able to reach their food at all if it has not been placed within reach. Even if it is within reach, the packaging can be difficult to open. Even when this is achieved, the patient may not be able to cut up the food provided.

It is the nurse's responsibility to ensure the food is available to the patient and that everything has been done to facilitate the movement of food to the mouth (Evans 2015).

The process of starvation

As nutritional intake decreases, there are fewer **carbohydrates** available for energy, leading to decreased insulin concentration and an increase in glucagon levels. When immediate energy stores run low, the body uses fat and protein as an alternative energy source.

During this process:

- glycogen stores in the liver are rapidly converted to glucose
- glucose is synthesised from protein and fat (gluconeogenesis)
- fats from adipose tissue are broken down, releasing large amounts of fatty acids and glycerol, which replace carbohydrates as the main energy source.

Skeletal and cardiac muscle is also broken down (catabolised), leading to muscle weakness and an overall depletion in **electrolytes**. Electrolyte levels within cells drop, but blood serum levels may still appear within normal range. When food is reintroduced, the body switches from metabolising fat to metabolising carbohydrates, and changes from **catabolism** to protein synthesis. To enable this process, insulin levels rise and electrolytes are transferred back into cells, leaving blood serum electrolyte levels low.

If patients have received suboptimal nutrition levels for an extended period, they may develop refeeding syndrome if given uncontrolled nutrition levels reasonably quickly. If not identified or managed carefully, refeeding syndrome puts the patient at increased risk of developing cardiac arrhythmias, respiratory failure, haematological abnormalities, convulsions or even death. Refeeding syndrome can occur in patients who are fed orally, enterally or parenterally.

There is a risk of refeeding syndrome if the patient has one or more of the following:

- BMI less than 16 kg/m^2
- unintentional weight loss greater than 15 per cent within the last 3–6 months
- little or no nutritional intake for more than 10 days
- low levels of potassium, phosphate or magnesium prior to feeding.

Or, the patient has two or more of the following:

- BMI less than 18.5 kg/m^2
- unintentional weight loss greater than 10 per cent within the last 3–6 months
- little or no nutritional intake for more than 5 days
- a history of alcohol abuse or drugs including insulin, chemotherapy, antacids or diuretics (ACI 2011).

6.4 Effect of surgery on nutrition

LEARNING OBJECTIVE 6.4 Explain the potential impacts of surgery on nutrition.

Studies worldwide indicate that malnourished surgical patients have significantly worse clinical outcomes than well-nourished patients. Surgical trauma causes a state of metabolic activation called the surgical stress response. The surgical stress response initiates the retention of salt and water to maintain plasma volume, increases cardiac output and oxygen consumption to deliver nutrients and oxygen to the tissues and mobilises energy reserves to maintain energy processes, repair tissues and synthesise proteins. This response increases the metabolic rate and nutritional requirements of the patient. The surgical stress response's nutritionally relevant clinical consequences include hyperglycaemia and whole-body protein catabolism, which manifest clinically as wasting of lean tissue, including muscle.

With this in mind, the patient must be as well-nourished preoperatively as possible to enable their best recovery.

Preoperative care

Patients are admitted for surgery via one of two routes. They may have elective surgery and usually come in the night before or on the day of the scheduled surgery. The other group of patients need urgent or emergency surgery. These patients may present to the emergency department (ED) following trauma or acute and severe illness requiring surgery — appendicitis or motor vehicle accident. No matter the cause, the patient should be as well-nourished and as hydrated as possible for optimum recovery (Gilles & Wischmeyer 2019). If the surgery is urgent, there will be little time to provide premium nutrition because they are unlikely to be unable to tolerate oral intake or be fasting from their arrival due to the reason for admission. The nurse can ensure that the patient is well hydrated by ensuring that they have IV fluids administered if they are unable to take oral fluids. Malnutrition is a modifiable risk factor thus, patients should be screened preoperatively and, if malnourished, consideration should be given to perioperative nutritional support to maximise their chances of a quick and uneventful recovery (Weimann et al. 2017).

The majority of patients undergoing surgery will continue their normal food intake until six hours before surgery and continue to drink clear fluids up to two hours before surgery (ACI 2016). Historically patients were fasted (food and fluids) for eight hours prior to surgery. Generally, theatres in any hospital have a list of morning and afternoon patients due for surgery. Therefore a patient will fast for either a morning operation or an afternoon operation. Since the order of a theatre list is subject to change, all patients will usually be fasted to be ready for any time within this time frame. This has led to the practice of fasting patients for a morning list from midnight and from 6 am for those on the afternoon list.

The NSW Agency for Clinical Innovation (ACI) implemented new guidelines after consistent reports from concerned clinicians regarding extended fasting times and concern for vulnerable patients, such as elderly patients awaiting hip surgery and patients with diabetes (ACI 2016). Under the new guidelines, all patients should be able to drink clear fluids until 6 am, even if they have stopped solid intake at midnight. It is taking time to change behaviours to the new guidelines in many facilities (Gillies & Wischmeyer 2019; Weimann et al. 2017).

Prolonged fasting preoperatively

There are a number of reasons that a patient may end up fasting for several days as they await an operation. The main underlying factor is lack of theatre availability. For elderly patients awaiting surgery for a fractured hip, while painful is not generally life-threatening and patients may be fasted hoping that the theatre may become available. Unfortunately, if more urgent cases are identified (via ED admissions or an acute inpatient), the non-urgent case may not get to theatre and will be fasted again the next day. This in itself need not be detrimental to the patient if the nurses are alerted to the issue. Some patients may fast all day, and by the time the ward is notified that the surgery will not happen that day, dinner has passed, and nursing staff may not have access to more than incidental snacks. If this happens over a few days, the patient is likely to have a nutritional deficit. It is the nurse's responsibility to be aware of the patient's total food and fluid intake and take steps to ensure that if they have fasted for extended periods, they are offered nutritious food no matter what time of day or night it is. This may mean some liaison with the kitchens to ensure that food is available on the ward for this eventuality.

Extended fasting is also likely to lead to a patient becoming dehydrated so nursing staff must ensure that the patient is well hydrated between fasting periods. In some cases, the surgical team may decide to give IV fluids, but the nurse should be hyper-vigilant regarding the patient's fluid status if this is not the case.

Patients who are malnourished before surgery are at greater risk of complications. Therefore, it may be appropriate to optimise the patient's nutritional state with artificial nutritional support in the weeks before elective surgery. One option is to offer carbohydrate drinks preoperatively to improve recovery post-operatively. Most enteral feeding companies have their own specialised preoperative nutritional supplement formulation — a clear carbohydrate drink with small levels of electrolytes to aid absorption. These are significantly different from the usual oral nutritional supplements, which are not suitable for this purpose.

Post-operative care

Patients undergoing a minor operation will often start eating and drinking fairly quickly following their return to the ward. However, for those who were malnourished preoperatively, a more cautious introduction to nutrition may be necessary — using oral supplements or artificial nutrition support continuing until the patient can take sufficient nutrition orally. This will be managed in collaboration with a dietitian. If a patient develops infectious complications after surgery, artificial nutritional support is generally required (Weimann 2017). The type of nutrition support provided will depend upon the type of surgery the patient has undergone and whether their gastrointestinal tract is functioning and accessible. Patients who have had bowel surgery have historically been kept nil by mouth until bowel sounds are heard and are first given clear fluids, slowly progressing to a full diet. This extended fasting has been linked to several undesirable post-operative outcomes. Unless there are specific reasons, early enteral feeding is the best practice. Enhanced recovery after surgery (ERAS) protocols have been developed and are now standard practice in many countries, including Australia. There are a number of changes recommended under the ERAS guidelines, but a key consideration concerning nutrition is the focus on both pre- and post-operative nutrition (ACI 2016).

However, patients who have had abdominal surgery need to be carefully monitored in relation to their bowel function. Any abdominal surgery may lead to a post-operative ileus (this is an inability of the bowel to contract normally). Many factors may contribute to post-operative ileus — surgical trauma leading to oedema, the stress response, and opiates given for pain. Signs of a post-operative ileus include lack of bowel sounds, abdominal distension and pain, and an inability to pass flatus or faeces. Nursing management includes strict attention to the assessment of bowel sounds, limiting the use of opioids, liaison with the treating team to prescribe other types of analgesia and ceasing oral intake pro tem (in the short term). Chewing gum has also been shown to assist gastric motility (Lafon & Lawson 2012).

6.5 Nutritional support

LEARNING OBJECTIVE 6.5 Describe the different methods of nutritional support.

Nutritional support or artificial nutrition may be given via the oral, enteral or parenteral route and is delivered in various forms. Enteral feeding may be used when the patient has a functional gastrointestinal tract but cannot take nutrition by mouth so a tube is inserted into the stomach, duodenum or jejunum. Parenteral nutrition is given intravenously. Once the need for nutrition support has been identified, the least invasive method should be used. The least invasive method of providing nutritional support is by supplementing oral intake. Where oral intake fails to meet nutritional needs or is unsafe, the patient may need to progress to an enteral feeding tube.

Supplementing oral intake

The easiest method of supplementing the diet is to increase the number or size of meals and snacks provided although larger meals may be off-putting for some patients. Nutritious drinks such as milky coffee, milk or a milkshake between meals may be easier and more acceptable than other meals or snacks in individuals with poor appetites (Best 2008). Patients must be provided with an appropriate level of assistance to enable them to eat their meals or snacks. When necessary, antiemetics are provided before food to prevent vomiting or nausea.

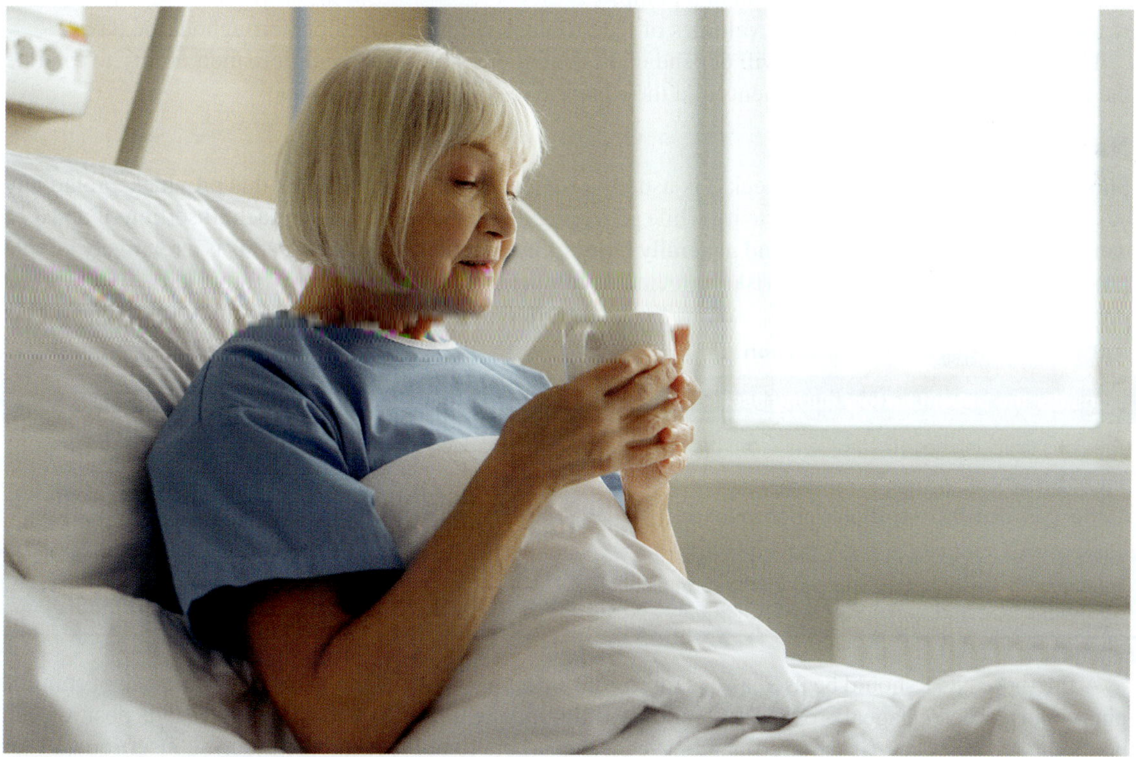

When the provision of additional food, fortified food or snacks is unsuccessful, the next step is to consider using a nutritional supplement. These supplements tend to come in the form of nutritionally complete liquids provided in a small carton or bottle — Fortisip, Ensure, Sustagen, TwoCalHN and Resource. For patients who do not like milky drinks but will eat puddings, there is Ensure pudding, FMR pudding and Sustagen pudding powder (Schneyder 2014). 'Nutritionally complete' means that if sufficient quantities of the supplement are taken each day, the patient's nutritional requirements for all vitamins and minerals, energy and protein can theoretically be met. They are not, however, nutritionally complete in one bottle or carton.

Supplements commonly come in three types: milkshake, fruit juice style or yoghurt/pudding style. In addition, some companies offer a savoury, soup-style supplement. When ill or malnourished, some people experience changes in taste perception. Nurses should be aware of this and offer patients a combination of different flavours until they find food options that suit them. Offering patients a variety of different supplements will also help to prevent taste fatigue.

Nursing responsibility for oral nutrition

Nurses are responsible for ensuring that patients and clients eat the right food at the right time with the right supervision and assistance (ACI 2017). Even when nurses are not directly involved in delivering meals to patients, they still retain the responsibility to ensure that patients in their care receive the nutrition appropriate to their needs (ACI 2017).

These responsibilities include:

- appointing a mealtime coordinator
- assessing and documenting the level of assistance that patients require at mealtimes
- minimising unnecessary interruptions
- ensuring that staff are available to provide assistance over mealtimes.

If the patient cannot be given sufficient nutrition via the oral route they may proceed to enteral nutrition.

Enteral tube feeding

Enteral tube feeding can be provided via a nasogastric tube (NGT), nasojejunal tube (NJT), gastrostomy tube (G-Tube) or jejunostomy tube (J-Tube).

A feed can be delivered through an enteral feeding tube in several ways:

- continuously via a pump providing a set rate of feed over a specified number of hours
- intermittent infusion (with or without a pump)
- using a syringe to deliver larger volumes of feed (bolus) at agreed timeslots throughout the day.

The method of administration will depend upon the patient's medical condition, their ability to tolerate the feed, their nutritional requirements and their preferences.

Nasogastric feeding

Short-term enteral feeding (2–6 weeks) is usually provided through an NGT as this provides a relatively easy means of bypassing the oral cavity while providing direct access to the stomach. Insertion of an NGT can be undertaken at the bedside and generally requires no anaesthetic. Although this is a relatively simple procedure to undertake, there are risks associated with the placement of an NGT (table 6.3).

TABLE 6.3 Risks of NGT insertion

Consider the patient history during assessment for:	Potential risks during the insertion procedure:
Previous facial injuries Facial surgery or polyps Upper gastrointestinal strictures or obstruction Base of skull fractures Patients with oesophageal varices or long-term alcohol abuse or suspected spinal fractures (ACI 2009).	Inadvertent placement in the: • bronchial tract • oesophagus • small intestine.

A fine-bore NGT should be used as it is more comfortable for the patient and reduces the risk of rhinitis, pharyngitis or oesophageal erosion. It should be radio-opaque throughout its length so that its position can be monitored on X-ray (if required), and have clear markers to aid measurement during insertion and for bedside checks (ACI 2009). The NGT is inserted via the nostril, along the nasopharynx, down through the oesophagus and into the stomach (posteriorly and inferiorly) (see figure 6.2).

FIGURE 6.2 NGT insertion

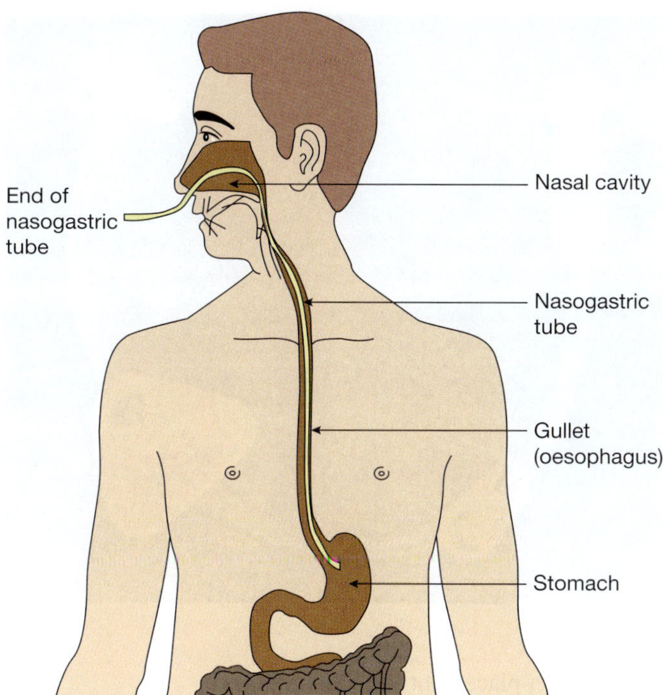

Once the tube has been inserted, its gastric positioning needs to be confirmed, which is usually undertaken using pH indicator strips, gastric placement being confirmed by a pH less than 5.5. Each test result is documented on a chart kept at the patient's bedside. If the pH is inadequate to confirm placement, an X-ray should be performed (ACI 2009).

Gastrostomy tubes

A gastrostomy provides a more permanent means of access to the stomach to enable longer-term enteral feeding (>6 weeks). It provides safe access directly into the stomach through the development of a fistula through the abdominal wall. There are four different types of gastrostomy tube (table 6.4) of which the percutaneous endoscopic gastrostomy (PEG) tube (figure 6.3) is most commonly used. In 2012, the NSW Ombudsman notified the ACI about a patient's death after a gastrostomy tube reinsertion. The ACI found no state-wide guidelines in place and, together with The Gastroenterological Nurses College of Australia (GENCA), worked on a joint project to develop these (ACI & GENCA 2015). In many hospitals, NGTs may only be inserted by a health professional [illegible]

TABLE 6.4 Types of gastrostomy tube

Type of gastrostomy tube	Rationale for use
PEG	The most common method of primary gastrostomy insertion
Radiologically inserted gastrostomy or fluoroscopically guided percutaneous gastrostomy	May be the method of choice if endoscopic placement is not available or is inadvisable
Balloon gastrostomy	May be used for primary placement or as a percutaneous replacement where further endoscopic or radiological intervention is to be avoided
Button or low-profile device	Tend to be used in younger adults and children

Figure 6.3 illustrates an example of a gastrostomy tube used for PEG feeds. Note the flange at the distal end, which ensures stabilisation of the tube after placement.

FIGURE 6.3 PEG tube

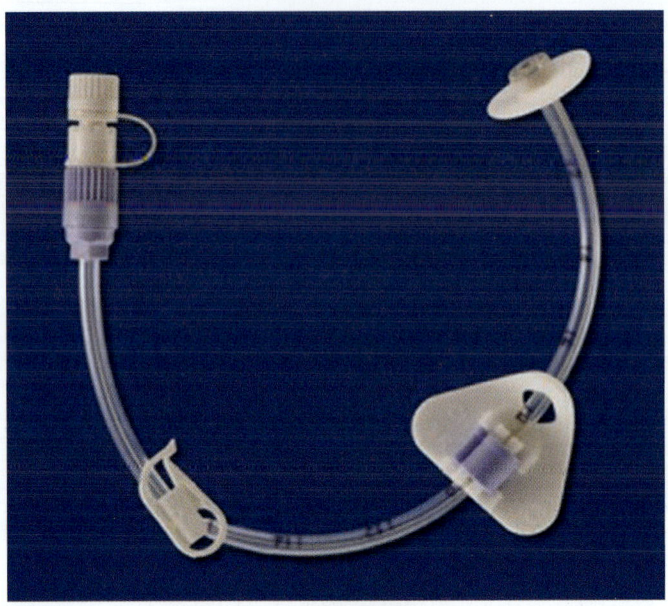

Source: Courtesy of Fresenius Kabi.

Figure 6.4 illustrates the correct placement of a PEG tube.

FIGURE 6.4 PEG tube placement

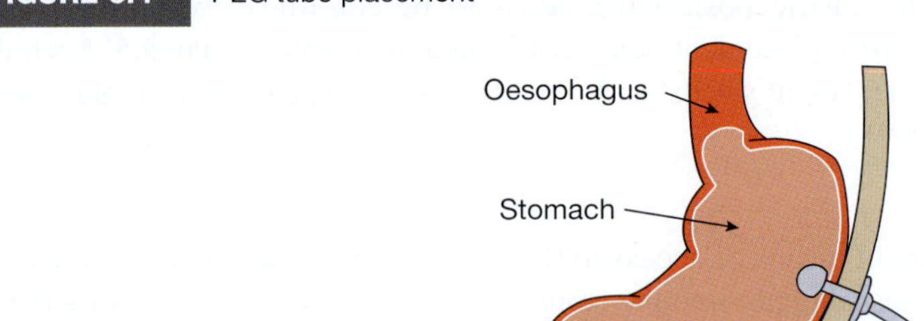

Postpyloric feeding

Postpyloric feeding may be considered for patients in whom gastric feeding is unsafe or problematic, such as patient's with gastroparesis, pancreatitis or aspiration pneumonia. The tip of the feeding tube bypasses the stomach and sits in the small intestine. Three types of tubes are used for postpyloric feeding (table 6.5).

TABLE 6.5 Enteral feeding tubes used for postpyloric feeding

Type of tube	Method of placement
Nasojejunal tube	Appears very similar to an NGT. They may be single or dual lumen Dual-lumen tubes have one gastric port for gastric decompression and one jejunal port for feeding They can be placed endoscopically, radiologically or at the bedside by specially trained healthcare professionals Some nasojejunal tubes may be assisted into the small bowel using prokinetic drugs to help stimulate gastric emptying and position the tube correctly

Percutaneous endoscopic gastrojejunostomy	Created following the placement of a PEG tube, a long small-gauge tube is passed through the lumen of the PEG and pulled down into the small intestine
Surgical jejunostomy	Placed directly into the jejunum at laparotomy May be tunnelled and secured using a Dacron cuff or held in place by sutures at the abdomen

Types of enteral tube feeds

There are many different enteral tube feeds. Some contain fibre, some provide more calories per millilitre than others, and the electrolyte level may vary between feeds. Feeds are generally presented in sterile ready-to-use containers and can hang for a maximum of 24 hours, after which any remaining feed should be discarded.

Patient monitoring

The enteral feed should be stored and administered at room temperature to avoid gastric discomfort associated with the administration of cold feed. The patient should be positioned with their head and shoulders raised to an angle of at least 30°. The patient should be monitored closely for potential side effects (as discussed above) during feeding and for at least an hour on completion of the feed. So a patient's feeding regimen can be adjusted accordingly. Nurses should check for:

- changes in weight
- changes in oral intake
- fluid balance
- electrolyte deficiencies.

If nutritional support is no longer required, there is usually a gradual reduction in feed with continued monitoring to ensure patients can maintain their nutritional status without support. In the same way nutritional support is escalated using a step-by-step approach, it is sensible to reduce it using the same approach.

Parenteral feeding

If feeding into the gastrointestinal tract is not tolerated or the gut is not available, nutritional needs must be met via the parenteral (intravenous) route. Parenteral nutrition is usually delivered through a central venous catheter (CVC) with a dedicated lumen (see figure 6.5). It may also be delivered via peripheral vein access, depending on the solution being administered. Most solutions have a high osmolarity and are only suitable to administer into a central vein. Osmolarity refers to the concentration of a solution. A high osmolarity solution will draw fluids from a low concentration to a high concentration across the cell membrane. This is likely to cause phlebitis (irritation of the vein) and may damage the vein and cause clot formation. For this reason, solutions with a high osmolarity (such as parenteral infusions) are given into large veins with high blood flow to help mitigate this effect. The main veins used for central venous access are the subclavian, internal and external jugular, cephalic and basilic veins. The tip of the CVC sits just outside the atrium in the superior vena cava. Infection control is paramount, with sepsis being the most common and serious complication of a CVC. Every aspect of care in relation to the CVC, changing of bags of feeds and insertion site care needs to be attended with strict attention to aseptic technique. If possible, a single lumen central line should be used, but if this is not possible due to the acuity of the patient, then a single lumen should be dedicated to the parenteral nutrition and labelled clearly to prevent its use for anything else. All staff involved in the care of a CVC patient should receive education and training in central venous access device (CVAD) management (ACI 2011). Placement sites for central lines are shown in figure 6.5.

Commercially premixed solutions may be used for short-term nutrition, but individualised solutions need to be mixed on-site for critically ill patients. Micronutrients and trace elements may be added to the feed, and additional electrolytes and nutrients may also be required. Due to the increased infection risks associated with using the central circulation to provide nutrition, parenteral nutrition is only used when all other nutrition options have been explored. The patient receiving parenteral nutrition will require close monitoring of bloods and fluid balance and strict aseptic care of the CVC.

FIGURE 6.5 Catheter placement

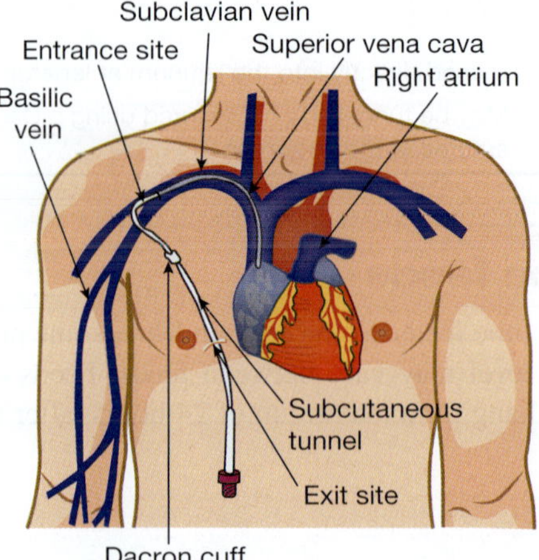

CASE STUDY 6.1

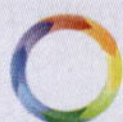

Nursing care of an elderly patient with complex nutritional needs

An 83-year-old female was brought in by ambulance following a fall at home, resulting in a fracture of the left neck of the femur (NOF). She has been stabilised in ED and has now been admitted to the orthopaedic ward.

The lady lives alone and, before her fall, was independent in her activities of daily living. She is a widow of three years, and while she misses her husband, she is pragmatic about the situation. She is generally healthy and active. She has had asthma since childhood and manages this with two puffs of Seretide (fluticasone & salmeterol) in the morning and two puffs of Ventolin (salbutamol) when necessary (PRN). She also has hypertension, which is managed with metoprolol 25 mg in the morning (mane).

Her observations are:

- temperature: 36.8°C
- heart rate: 96 beats per minute
- blood pressure: 115/75 mmHg
- respiratory rate: 20 breaths per minute
- oxygen saturation: 96% on room air
- pain score: 2/10 when resting; 7/10 on movement in bed
- blood glucose level: 3.9
- height/weight: 176 cm/60 kg
- BMI: 18.07 (underweight)
- neurovascular obs: good sensation and circulation
- IV fluids in progress N/S 0.9% at 80 ml/hr.

You perform a MNA and find she is at risk of malnutrition. She is fasting for a total hip replacement and is on bed rest. This is the third day she has fasted for her operation, but unfortunately, her surgery has been cancelled at 8 pm each day due to more acute cases being performed. She tells you she is very hungry and thirsty and feels weak.

Question

Using the information above and the track and trigger chart used in your facility (ADDS, SAGO, etc.), describe what action you would take as the nurse caring for this patient. Use the clinical reasoning cycle to guide you through the process and devise a care plan for your patient.

Answer

- *Step 1: Consider the patient.* Patient is an 83-year-old female.
- *Step 2: Collect cues/information*. Include subjective and objective data here, including the patient's appearance and past medical history. Objective data will include measurable information such as his vital signs.
- *Step 3: Process information.* Patient has a fractured NOF. Her pain is under control at the moment, and she is aware to request pain relief when necessary. While comfort is paramount, it is also important to keep pain under control as the body's response to pain may obscure other indicators of potential

problems — one response to pain is elevated blood pressure. A drop in BP due to hypovolaemia may be missed if the pain is causing the BP to be elevated.

Her general observations are within normal limits, but her respiratory rate and heart rate are slightly elevated. These signs may indicate hypovolaemia and/or anaemia. Her BGL is in the low range of normal, indicating her energy requirements need attention.

- *Step 4: Identify problems.* Identify problems related to nutrition and fluid status. She is underweight, is likely malnourished, and has now been fasting for three days. As her case has been cancelled on each occasion after the meals have been distributed there has been minimal food available to offer to her when she has been allowed to eat. Malnutrition has numerous potential problems, including slow wound healing, muscle wasting, impaired immune function and increased risk of tissue breakdown and pressure ulcers.

  As she is an older person, she is more likely to become dehydrated, and she is NBM. Her total fluid intake per IV is 1920 ml/day. This is the minimum requirement for her, and if she is dehydrated, it will not compensate for this fluid deficit.
- *Step 5: Establish goals*. Assess and if necessary improve hydration and nutritional status.
- *Step 6: Actions*. Ensure accurate documentation on the fluid balance chart. If necessary (as per findings of fluid assessment), discuss an increased IV fluid rate with the doctor.

  Commence meal chart. The degree of nutritional loss can be easily missed without documentation. Liaise with dietitian for nutrition plan and high-protein supplements. Although the patient is fasting, organise food for her that can be kept in the ward fridge so that as soon as she is allowed to eat, there is something nutritious available. Make sure other staff know it is there. Give psychological support.
- *Step 7: Evaluate outcomes.* Fluid balance chart commenced and fluids increased to 110 ml/hr to provide baseline fluids and slow rehydration.

  Meal chart commenced. It was clearly evident that her intake was significantly inadequate, high-protein supplements ordered and encouraged.

  Patient did make it to theatre at this time; however, it was noted that she had been malnourished for a significant period of time and supplementary feeds with high-protein liquids were ordered by the dietitian. Nursing staff assiduously attended supplemental feeds.

  Post-operatively this patient began to recover well, dehydration was reversed and she began to put on weight after a week.
- *Step 8: Reflect on the process and new learning.* Reflect on any aspects of care that could have been performed in a way to achieve an improved outcome.

CASE STUDY 6.2

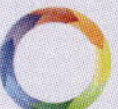

Nursing care of a young patient with complex nutritional needs

The patient is a female 19 years of age. She tripped while walking up some stairs and lacerated her left ankle. The wound is not healing well, and she has been admitted to the surgical ward for debridement and assessment of the wound. At meal times, you observe the patient has not eaten any of her vegetables. You have a conversation with her, and she says she does not like to eat fruit or vegetables. You have also observed her eating chocolate, chips and drinking soft drinks that her mother has brought in for her.

She has a medical history of depression and is on imipramine 40 mg daily.

Her vital signs are:

- blood pressure: 140/90 mmHg
- heart rate: 106 beats per minute
- respiratory rate: 20 breaths per minute
- oxygen saturation: 98% on room air
- pain: 3/10 at rest
- height/weight: 167.5 cm / 95kg
- BMI: 33.86 (obese).

Question

Using the information above and the track and trigger chart used in your facility (ADDS, SAGO, etc.), describe what action you would take as the nurse caring for this patient. Use the clinical reasoning cycle to guide you through the process and devise a care plan for your patient.

Answer

- *Step 1: Consider the patient.* Patient is a 19-year-old female, non-healing wound left ankle which has been debrided and has an intact dressing.

She is obviously overweight. She has pale skin and says she does not get outside much. She lives at home with her mother.

Her mother takes you aside and says she is worried about her daughter's weight and wants to know what might be done to help her lose weight.

- *Step 2: Collect cues/information.* Include subjective and objective data here, including the patient's appearance and past medical history. Objective data will include measurable information such as his vital signs.

  The patient says she is embarrassed about her weight and feels that it stops her from engaging in a full life but has tried to lose weight without success. You ask if she tried to lose weight with a particular plan or with the help of a professional and she says she did not.

  She says she doesn't like to cook and prefers to get food delivered. This tends to be mostly calorie-dense fast foods. Her mother works and often brings home fast food for dinner.

  Patient says she often has a dry mouth.

  You perform a MNA and find she is at risk of malnutrition.
- *Step 3: Process information.* Her vital signs are within normal limits but BP, HR and RR are high for her age. This may be related to her weight.

  Malnutrition does not only relate to people who are underweight, it also occurs in those who are overweight. Obesity and malnutrition Are detrimental to wound healing.

  She is obviously overweight to the extent that it would impact on her activities of daily living, especially in relation to her ability and desire to exercise.

  The patient is an adult, and as such, you cannot discuss her health issues with her mother without the patient's consent. If this young woman is going to lose weight successfully it will need to involve her mother.

  A side effect of imipramine (a tricyclic antidepressant) is a dry mouth.
- *Step 4: Identify problems.* Patient has a non-healing wound and difficulty mobilising. She is obese and unhappy with weight but feels helpless. Mother is enabling the daughter's unhealthy eating habits.
- *Step 5: Establish goals.* Ensure wound treatment plan is adhered to and enable better mobilisation.

  Initiate intervention to assist in weight loss goal. Involve mother to help with patient's weight loss goal. Request a drug review to see if another medication that does not cause dry mouth might be appropriate.
- *Step 6: Take action.* Ask patient if she consents to sharing information with her mother regarding her diet plans. Contact dietitian and social worker. Mother and daughter need to work together, and the social worker is best placed to assist with any services required when home.

  Go through diet plan with patient, ensuring she understands what is involved. Answer any questions and repeat information as often as is needed. Be patient and kind.

  Following dietitian consult reinforce information given to the patient. Use the Australian Dietary Guidelines to help her understand what healthy foods are and are not. Show patient the 'Eat For Health' website (www.eatforhealth.gov.au) and take time to go through any of the information with her.

  Request medication review.
- *Step 7: Evaluate outcomes*. The wound is healing well.

  Through considerate intervention the mother and daughter both feel they have been given the information and support to make a fresh start in helping their weight loss journey. They are excited at the thought of a new beginning. The mother understands that no matter how kind her intentions, unintentionally assisting her daughter's unhealthy diet is not her fault but is; however, something she can change. Mother has enrolled in a weekend course on healthy simple meal preparation.

  Medication reviewed but at this time not changed.

  The patient came to the ward six months later to bring a thank you card for the staff. She has lost 18 kilograms and says that she is feeling much happier and slimmer with the support of her mother and outpatient services. She is determined to get to a BMI of 20 and feels certain she can achieve it.
- *Step 8: Reflect on the process and new learning.* Reflect on any aspects of care that could have been performed in a way to achieve an improved outcome.

  Weight is an issue fraught with social complexity. There is a stigma attached, which can lead people to feel like outsiders in our society. This also means that people can be very defensive about any reference being made to their weight or need for weight loss, which can be difficult to overcome.

  In this case, the patient had indicated a desire to lose weight, and with delicate, factual and compassionate communication, the patient was made to feel empowered and thus able to embrace the information given to her.

SUMMARY

Many factors affect a patient's nutritional status coming into hospital, including increasing age, illness, an inability to cope, drug treatment and socioeconomic factors. As the care of health-related problems is increasingly managed in primary care settings, patients admitted to hospital are often acutely ill before admission and may already have some signs of malnutrition. Once in hospital, the risks increase due to episodes where patients are placed on 'nil by mouth' for investigations or procedures required to investigate and treat their illness or disease. In addition, appetite often decreases when a person is ill, and many patients are functionally unable to feed themselves effectively. Therefore, it is not surprising that some patients may leave hospital in a more malnourished state than when they arrived.

Providing appropriate and timely nutritional support is essential to maximise a patient's nutritional status and recovery from illness. The use of a step-by-step approach is often the safest means of progressing — from oral supplementation to parenteral nutrition. However, it is essential to consider the risks that accompany artificial nutritional support as the provision of nutritional care via enteral or parenteral feeding tubes is not without complications. Therefore the balance of risk versus benefit must be considered for each patient before nutritional support is commenced. Nurses play a central role in many of these discussions as they often have a more holistic view of the patient and any family or carers involved. Nurses must be represented within multidisciplinary teams and act as the patient's voice if and when the patient is unable to represent their own view to ensure that appropriate levels of nutrition are provided by the appropriate route.

KEY TERMS

carbohydrates Biomolecules found in sugars, starches and dietary fibre that containing carbon, hydrogen and oxygen atoms. They are converted to glucose and used by the body as an energy source.

catabolism All chemical and enzymatic reactions during which complex molecules are broken down or degraded, including proteins, sugars and fatty acids.

diet What you eat and drink. Different cultures have different diets, i.e. a different variety of foods that are ingested.

electrolytes Essential minerals such as calcium, sodium and potassium that dissolve into ions in solution (such as water) and have the ability to carry an electric charge. They are essential for a number of bodily functions including hydration.

malabsorption A disorder that occurs when people are unable to absorb adequate nutrients from their diet. This may be as a result of lactose intolerance, celiac disease or bariatric or other bowel surgery.

malnutrition Deficiencies, excesses or imbalances in a person's intake of energy and/or nutrients (WHO 2020).

metabolic profile A range of blood tests that include BGL, electrolytes (Na, K, Cl, HCO_3), liver function, renal function and iron levels (ferritin, serum iron, transferrin). Further investigations for specific anomalies may also be included, e.g. troponin levels in cardiac patients.

micronutrients Chemical elements or substances that are essential in minute amounts to sustain growth and health. Examples include vitamins and trace elements such as boron, iron, copper and molybdenum.

nutrients The chemical compounds in foods that are used by the body to maintain health and function. They include proteins, carbohydrates, fats, minerals and vitamins.

proteins Large biomolecules and macromolecules that contain amino acid residue. Proteins are involved in almost every process in the human body.

REFERENCES

Agency for Clinical Innovation (ACI). (2009) *Fine bore nasogastric feeding tubes for adults policy.* Secretary, NSW Health.

Agency for Clinical Innovation (ACI). (2011) *Parenteral nutrition pocketbook for adults.* Chatswood, NSW: NSW Health.

Agency for Clinical Innovation (ACI) & the Gastroenterological Nurses College of Australia (GENCA). (2015) *A clinicians guide: Caring for people with gastrostomy tubes and devices.* Chatswood, NSW: NSW Health.

Agency for Clinical Innovation (ACI). (2016) *Enhanced recovery after surgery.* Surgical services taskforce & anaesthesia and perioperative care network. Chatswood, NSW: NSW Health.

Agency for Clinical Innovation (ACI). (2017) *Nutrition care. Policy directive.* Secretary, NSW Health.

Australian Commission for Safety and Quality in Health Care (ACSQHC). (2018) *Hospital acquired complication 13: Malnutrition fact sheet.* www.safetyandquality.gov.au/publications-and-resources/resource-library/hospital-acquired-complication-13-malnutrition-fact-sheet

Best, C. (2008) *Nutrition: A handbook for nurses.* Chichester: Wiley Blackwell.

Butt, S., Leon, J., David, C., Chang, H., Sidhu, S. & Sehgal, A. (2007) The prevalence and nutritional implications of fast food consumption among dialysis patients. *Journal of Renal Nutrition.* 17(4): 264–268.

Department of Health and Human Services (DHHS). (2020) *What is malnutrition.* Tasmanian Government.

Evans, L. (2015) The nurses role in patient nutrition and hydration. *Nursing Times.* 111: 28–29.

Gillie, D. (2010) Overview of the physiological changes and optimal diet in the golden age over 50. *European Review of Aging and Physical Activity.* 7: 27–36. https://doi.org/10.1007/s11556-010-0058-5

Gillis, C. & Wischmeyer, P. (2019) Preoperative nutrition and the elective surgical patient. Why, how and what? *Anaesthesia.* 74(1): 27–35. doi: 10.1111/anae.14506

Gulgoz, Y. (2006) The mini nutritional assessment (MNA) review of the literature. What does it tell us? *Journal of Nutritional Health Ageing.* 10(6): 466–485.

Hryciw, D. & Bonner, A. (2019) In J. Craft, C. Gordon, S. Huether, K. McCance, V. Brashers & N. Rote (Eds.). *Understanding Pathophysiology*, 3rd ed. Elsevier.

Lacey, S. & Street, T. (2017) Measuring healthy behaviours using the stages of change model: an investigation into the physical activity and nutrition behaviours of Australian miners. *BioPsychoSocial Medicine.* 11(30). https://doi.org/10.1186/s13030-017-0115-7

Lafon, C. & Lawson, L. (2012) Postoperative ileus in GI surgical patients: Pathogenesis and interventions. *Gastrointestinal Nursing.* 10(2): 45–49.

Nutrition Education Materials Online (NEMO). (n.d.) Malnutrition screening tool. NSW Health.

Naithani, S., Whelan, K., Thomas, J., Guilford, M. & Morgan, M. (2008) Hospital inpatients' experiences of access to food. A qualitative interview and observational study. *Health Expectations.* 11(3): 294–303.

National Health and Medical Research Council (NHMRC). (2017) *Nutrient reference values for Australia and New Zealand.* Australian Government & Ministry of Health New Zealand.

National Health and Medical Research Council (NHMRC). (2013) *Australian Dietary Guidelines.* Australian Government.

Nightingale, F. (1859) *Notes on nursing. What it is and what it is not*, Dover 1969 ed. Dover publications.

Pilgrim, A., Robinson, S., Sayer, A. & Roberts, H. (2015) An overview of appetite decline in older people. *Nursing Older People.* 27(5): 27–35.

QLD Health. (2017) Malnutrition screening tools. Queensland Government. www.health.qld.gov.au/__data/assets/pdf_file/0021/152454/hphe_scrn_tools.pdf

Reddy, S. & Anitha, M. (2015) Culture and its influence on nutrition and oral health. *Biomedical and Pharmacology Journal.* 8: 613–620.

Witkamp, R. F. & van Norren, K. (2018) Let thy food be thy medicine … when possible. *European Journal of Pharmacology.* 836(5): 102–114.

Schneyder, A. (2014) Malnutrition-nutritional supplements. *Australian Prescriber.* 13: 120–123. doi: 10.18773/austprescr.2014.047

Webster's New World Medical Dictionary, 3rd ed. (2009) WebMD.

Weimann, A., Braga, M., Carli, F., Higashigushi, T., Hubner, M., Klek, S., Laviano, A., Ljungkvist, O., Lobo, D., Martindale, R., Waitzberg, D., Bishoff, S. & Singer, P. (2017) ESPEN Guideline: Clinical nutrition in surgery. *Clinical Nutrition.* 36(3): 623–650.

World Health Organization (WHO). (2020) *Malnutrition.* www.who.int/news-room/fact-sheets/detail/malnutrition

ACKNOWLEDGEMENTS

Figure 6.1: © Australian Government Department of Health, https://www.eatforhealth.gov.au/guidelines/australian-guide-healthy-eating

Photo 6A: © David Cole / Alamy Stock Photo

Photo 6B: © LightField Studios / Shutterstock.com

CHAPTER 7

Principles of geriatric nursing

LEARNING OBJECTIVES

After studying this chapter, you should be able to:

7.1 discuss the current climate around ageing and aged care in Australia

7.2 review the clinical reasoning cycle and apply it to patient centred aged care

7.3 describe the pathophysiology of ageing

7.4 reflect on the importance of the nurse in caring for the older person and our role in providing safe, effective care.

Introduction

Ageing can be described as an age-related decline of biological functions or progressive loss of function accompanied by a decrease in fertility and an increase in mortality (Libertini 2019). People do not become old or elderly at any specific age (Merck Sharp & Dohme Corp. 2020). According to the United Nations (2020), the global population is ageing, with almost all countries experiencing growth in the number and percentage of older people in their population. Work by the United Nations Department of Economic and Social Affairs, Population Division (2019) has indicated that one in every six people globally will be greater than 65 years of age by 2050. The Australian Institute for Health and Welfare (AIHW) has estimated that by 2057 there will be 8.8 million or 22 per cent of the population aged 65 years and over (Pond & Regan 2019). Longevity should bring opportunities for older people, their families, and our societies (World Health Organization [WHO] 2020a). Additional years of quality life opens the potential for further education, new careers, or the chance to follow pursuits that have been missed in younger years. The older person has a role to play in contributing their knowledge and expertise to their families and their communities. However, this is dependent on their health (Pond & Regan 2019) and our recognitions of their continued potential in our society.

The growth in the geriatric population presents challenges to the healthcare workforce (Sheets & Whittington 2012). These challenges are exacerbated by the ongoing shortage of nurses globally, especially those educated and trained to care for older persons. As nurses, we play a vital role in the health and quality of life outcomes for older people. It is essential that we, as healthcare providers, understand the ageing process, the needs of the older person and how we can offer care safely and effectively. This chapter will discuss the ageing population in Australia, factors involved in and the pathology of ageing, gerontological nursing, patient-centred care, the clinical reasoning cycle and national and nursing practice standards.

7.1 Australia's ageing population

LEARNING OBJECTIVE 7.1 Discuss the current climate around ageing and aged care in Australia.

It was estimated by the AIHW, that 70 per cent of Australia's older population considered their level of health as excellent, very good or good. Only 20 per cent stated that they experience severe or profound limitations to their **activities of daily living (ADL)**, this increased to 50 per cent of the older population by 85 years. While many older Australians are living longer and are in better health, Australia has a linguistically and culturally diverse population, and many continue to face social and economic disadvantages that affect their health. Aboriginal and Torres Strait Islander peoples are affected by age-related conditions at younger ages than non-Indigenous Australians (AIHW 2018). Other groups include persons with special needs, migrants, veterans and their families, those who live in rural and remote areas, the homeless community, and people who identify as **LGBTIQ+**.

Aged care in Australia

Aged care is defined as the support required to be provided to the older person who needs help to run their own home or who can no longer live at home and need a supportive residence. The aim is to support older people in maintaining their activities of daily living safely and satisfactorily. The activities of living listed in the *Roper-Logan-Tierney Model of Nursing* include maintaining a safe environment, breathing, communicating with others, eating and drinking, eliminating, washing, dressing, controlling temperature, mobilising, working, playing, sleeping, sexuality and death (Petiprin 2020). These activities are not a checklist but must be seen within the biological, psychological, sociocultural, environmental and political-economic framework that healthcare providers use when considering the patient situation in the clinical reasoning cycle. The biological factor considers the older person's current health, while the psychological factor considers the emotional status, cognitive abilities, belief systems and ability to understand (Petiprin 2020). With the increase in numbers of people who will require additional support, the Australian Government has recognised the need for a review of the aged care system. It has proposed reforms that will better support the older person in maintaining their individuality in society (Aged Care Quality and Safety Commission 2020). In Australia, this involves care in the individual's home, assistance with housework, shopping, cooking, social outings, personal care, supportive equipment and healthcare including nursing, physiotherapy and medical care, and includes short-term care after hospital admission and respite care. It also includes residential care in aged care homes (nursing homes).

To improve residential care, the Australian Department of Health developed a set of safety and quality standards — The National Safety and Quality Health Service (NSQHS) Standards (Aged Care Quality and Safety Commission 2020) — that residential care facilities are required to meet to be accredited as healthcare providers.

Advanced care directive is also known as a 'living will'. The advanced care directive is a legal document that states the individual's wishes regarding their healthcare and treatment should they become seriously ill or injured and reach a point where they are unable to make decisions for themselves (Services NSW n.d.).

While each Australian state and territory may have different names and differing living will policies, all Australian states recognise the advance directive and that a legally prepared and executed living will takes precedence over other estate documents (Legalvision 2021). A valid advanced care directive must be followed by healthcare providers and by family members.

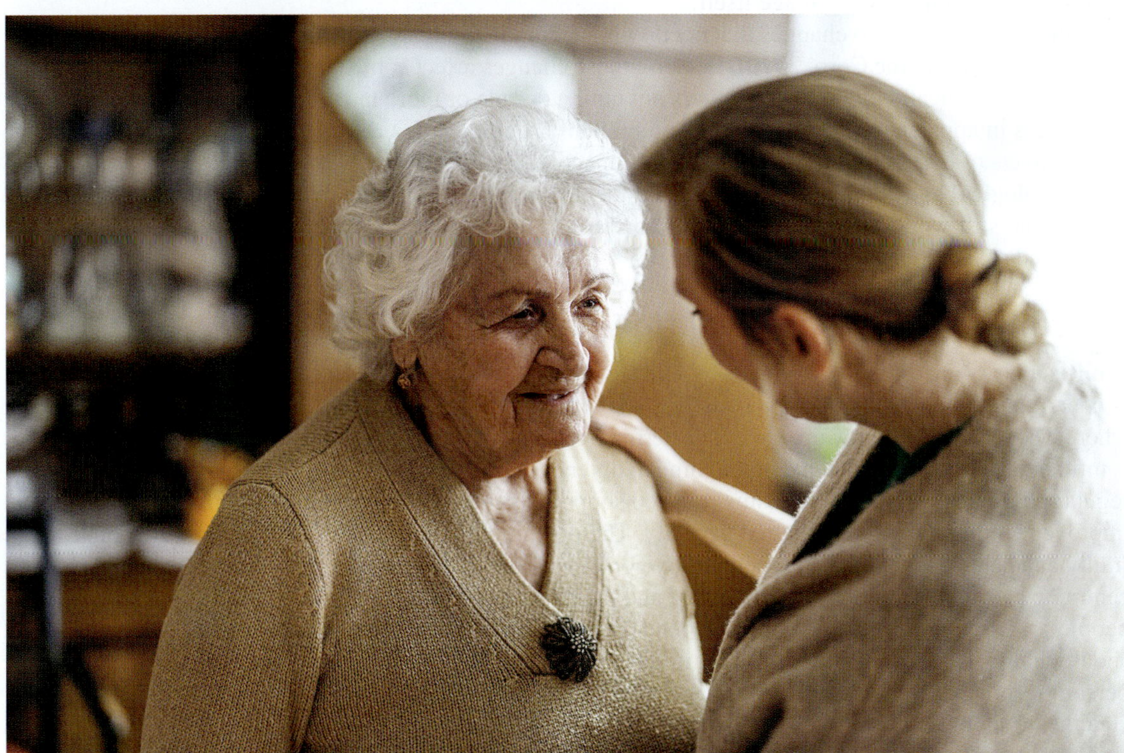

Gerontological nursing

Gerontology is the study of the physical, mental and social changes that are part of the ageing process. **Geriatrics** is the branch of medicine used to develop strategies and programs that support the appropriate care of older people (Merck Sharp & Dohme Corp. 2020). Geriatricians have studied the ageing process and are educated, trained and skilled in caring for the older person.

It is widely felt that nursing the elderly should require a specialist degree (Madigan 2018). The physiological and behavioural changes of ageing lead to a compromised ability to adapt to metabolic stress results and complex disease processes. 'Older people are complex and therefore they require specialist nurses to provide appropriate care for them' (Moyle, as cited in Madigan 2018).

As the numbers of our older people increase, there will be an increasing demand for nurses who specialise in aged care. Gerontology nurses work across many healthcare facilities, including nursing homes, residential facilities or home care services, performing various nursing tasks. They need compassion and resilience to provide day-to-day physical and mental healthcare services. The elderly care nurse requires a thorough understanding of how ageing affects the human body and mental faculties. Speciality roles in gerontological nursing include occupational therapy, mental health and oncology nursing.

What is age?

According to The Royal Australian College of General Practitioners (RACGP 2019), ageing can be defined as a failure to maintain homeostasis under psychological and physiological stress conditions.

All body systems undergo physiological ageing but at differing rates, and age-related decline varies between individuals. These age-related changes can affect the older person's ability to maintain homeostasis in times of stress and illness. There is no such thing as a 'typical' older person. While some 80-year-olds retain physical and mental capacities like much younger people, some individuals experience declines in physical and mental capacities that affect their ability to perform their daily living activities (WHO 2020a). A comprehensive public health response must address this wide range of older people's experiences and needs.

Some important definitions help to better understand what we are talking about when we discuss 'age'. **Chronological age** is a person's age in years (Merck Sharp & Dohme Corp. 2020). While chronological age has limited significance when discussing health and healthcare, we need to recognise that health problems increase with age. Health problems lead to the loss of function and independence rather than the numerical or chronological age itself.

Biological age refers to changes that occur with ageing in the body that commonly occur as people age (Merck Sharp & Dohme Corp. 2020). Because these changes affect some people sooner than others, some people are biologically old at 65 and others not until a decade or more later. However, the most noticeable differences in apparent age among people of similar chronologic age are caused by lifestyle, diet and the subtle effects of disease rather than differences in actual ageing.

Psychological age is the age people act and feel (Merck Sharp & Dohme Corp. 2020). An 80-year-old person who still works, makes plans, looks forward to future events and participates in activities can be considered psychologically young.

Factors affecting healthy ageing

While some ageing changes are genetic, some are much more due to our physical and social environments, gender, ethnicity and socioeconomic status (WHO 2020a). In combination with personal characteristics, where we are born and grow up, have long-term effects on how we age. The environment in which we live is influential in the development and ongoing maintenance of healthy lifestyle behaviours. A balanced diet, regular physical activity and not using tobacco support risk reduction of non-communicable diseases and improvement in physical and mental capacity. The potential to maintain good cognitive function, reverse frailty and delay dependency is supported by good nutrition and ongoing strength training. Good health is central to a positive experience of older age and the opportunities that ageing brings (WHO 2020c). Older people are often assumed to be frail, dependent and burdensome. As healthcare providers, we can and should address these and other ageist attitudes and provide supportive environments to enable the older person to continue to do what is important to them, despite any losses in mental and functional capacity. Healthcare should facilitate the ability of older people to participate in and contribute to their communities and society.

Ageism

The WHO has identified **ageism** as a global dilemma (Officer & de la Fuente-Núñez 2018). Ageism is the stereotyping, prejudice and discrimination towards people based on age. Ageism is the perception that individuals may be unable to do something because they are too old or too young. Ageism is prevalent in most societies; however, unlike other types of discrimination, ageism remains largely unchallenged. Ageism is considered endemic in Australian society (COTA 2020). Research has shown that behavioural discrimination is evident not only in the workplace but also in healthcare. Older people can experience ageism in the healthcare setting in the way they are addressed and undervaluing the skills, experience and earned wisdom of older people. Negative approaches are widespread in the health and social care settings where older people are most vulnerable. A 2020 report by the WHO (2020) stated that people who have negative views about their age do not recover well from disability and live approximately 7.5 years less than people with positive attitudes. Ageism also causes cardiovascular stress, lower self-efficacy and decreases in productivity. Ageism can lead to social isolation, physical and cognitive decline, lack of physical activity and economic burden. Negative attitudes around aged care also make it difficult to recruit skilled healthcare providers for the aged care sector.

Body image

Research into ageing issues has become a national priority in Australia. Body image is how people see themselves and how they feel about their physical appearance. It is closely related to self-esteem and mental health (Midlarsky 2017). While society focuses a lot on body image and self-esteem in youths, this awareness can be overlooked in older people (Baker & Gringart 2009). The relationship between body image and self-esteem does not weaken with age. A continuing issue for women (Cameron, Ward, Mandville-Anstey & Coombs 2019), the media's emphasis on health, youth, physical ability and sexual prowess also significantly affects how men view their bodies (Bennett, Hurd, Pritchard, Colton & Crocker 2020). The WHO world report on ageing and health (2015) has said that globally, healthy ageing frameworks need to move away from a disease-based curative focus to a focus on older person-centred care and recognised the importance of maintaining a positive body image in the older person.

Polypharmacy

Research by the RACGP (2020) reveals that 3 per cent of all hospital admissions are medication-related issues with a cost of $1.4 billion per year. Admissions of the older person aged 65 showed that 55 per cent of this group had been prescribed potentially inappropriate medications (RACGP 2020). **Polypharmacy** is defined as the use of multiple medications. While there is no standard for defining multiple medications, five medications is the commonly accepted threshold (Maher, Hanlon & Hajjar 2014; Parulekar & Rogers 2018). Medication use in the older person is a complex balance of managing the disease process and avoiding medication-related problems RACGP 2020). The greater the number of comorbidities leads to the greater number of medications taken, increasing the risk of interactions and adverse drug. Australia has adopted a national plan for the *Quality use of medicines to optimise ageing in older Australians* (RACGP 2020). Within this plan, there is substantial opportunity to improve the prescription and administration of medications in older people (University of Sydney 2018). Implementation of the plan can only lead to positive outcomes for the older person and Australian society. Medication safety is an essential part of the NSQHS Standards (Australian Commission on Safety and Quality in Health Care [ACSQHC] 2019).

While nurses do not prescribe medications, we administer them and have an active role in improving medication management. As registered nurses, we are responsible for being familiar with the indications, contraindications and special precautions for the drugs we administer (Durham 2015). We use our clinical reasoning to assess if the medication should be administered or withheld, given the patient's clinical status, and communicating it to their physician. We also have an essential role in educating the patient, their families and their carer on safe and appropriate medication administration. We also need to follow the rights of medication management to ensure safe medication preparation and practice our seven rights of medication administration as outlined below:

1. right patient
2. right drug
3. right dose
4. right time
5. right route
6. right reason
7. right documentation (Smeulers et al. 2015).

Elder abuse

Elder abuse is a recognised public health problem. It can be defined as 'a single, or repeated act, or lack of appropriate action, occurring within any relationship where there is an expectation of trust which causes harm or distress to an older person' (WHO 2020d). Elder abuse includes physical, psychological, sexual and financial abuse. It can also be the result of intentional or unintentional neglect. A 2017 report based on data from 52 studies in 28 countries estimated that over 15 per cent of people aged 60 years or older were subjected to abuse (WHO 2020d). With the rapid increase in the aged population, the WHO (2020d) predicate an increase in elder abuse rates. Rates of elder abuse have been found to be highest in nursing homes and long-term care facilities. Elder abuse can lead to serious physical injuries and has long-term psychological consequences for a vulnerable population. Possible causative factors for elder abuse can include:

- high levels of stress experienced by the responsible carer
- cognitive or physical limitation inhibiting the older person from stopping or reporting abuse
- location, cultural or language barriers, or health complications
- addiction problems in either the carer or older person
- dependency of either the carer or the older person, for example, financially, socially or physically (WHO 2020e).

In Australia, a national report titles *Elder Abuse—A National Legal Response* put forward some 43 recommendations to safeguard the older person, which included improvements in:

- screening of care workers
- scrutiny of restrictive practices in aged care
- building trust and confidence in advanced planning documents and tools
- protection of older people when arrangements for care fail
- regimes protecting and supporting at-risk people
- immediate response to complaints of elder abuse in residential aged care (Australian Government Australian Law Reform Commission 2017).

7.2 The clinical reasoning cycle and patient-centred aged care

LEARNING OBJECTIVE 7.2 Reflect on patient-centred aged care and how you can apply it in practice.

With the ageing process, there is a decline in physical and mental capacities. The incidence of non-communicable diseases such as cancer and chronic conditions leading to a loss of functional ability increases. The effect of ageing is influenced by personal, family, social support, financial resources and the quality of the built environment and use of assistive tools (Philp et al. 2017). To best support our ageing community, we need to take a comprehensive approach to care and integrate it with the older person's specific and stated priorities and goals. Nurses should provide patient-centred care that supports the older person's best outcomes, providing them with informed choices, allowing them to make their own decisions, respecting those decisions and allowing them to control their health and hence their lives.

The clinical reasoning cycle and care of the older person

The clinical reasoning cycle is described by Levett-Jones (2009, p. 516) as 'a process by which we as nurses collect cues, process the information, come to an understanding of a patient problem or situation, plan and implement interventions, evaluate outcomes, and reflect on, and learn from the process'. Effective use of the model is dependent on following the stages of the cyclic process:

- consider the patient situation
- collect cues/information
- process information
- identify problems/issues
- establish goal/s
- take action
- evaluate outcomes
- reflect on process and new learning (European Heart Association 2018).

These steps are necessary for the care of the older person in all healthcare settings, including acute, clinic, residential care and the community or home. To provide the best possible care for the older person, we must consider the patient and their situation, the ageing process and potential comorbidities when processing the information, identifying possible causes and establishing plans of care and achievable goals. It is important to consider the patient's personal lifestyle choices and that all decisions are made in conjunction with the patient. It is essential to evaluate and reflect on the care provided and use this process to provide ongoing care.

Patient-centred care

Patient-centredness is the hallmark of quality care (Fleming & Haney 2013). Patient-centred care recognises that we must organise care around the individual's concerns and needs to achieve the best outcomes for patients. That is even truer for older people in their healthcare. It is crucial that as healthcare providers, we reflect on our care and recognise the importance of the older person and their rights to patient-centred care and a safe and comfortable environment.

The provision of patient-centred care involves:

- treating the patient with the dignity, respect and compassion they deserve
- communicating and coordinating care between appointments and different services
- tailoring the care to suit the needs of the individual and what the individual wants to achieve
- supporting the patient and their family in learning about and understanding their health so they can make informed decisions

- helping the patient find ways to improve and sustain good health and to stay well
- always involving the patient in their healthcare decisions
- recognising that the older person has a lifetime of experience and knows their own situation
- recognising organic causes such as pain or infection before concluding that the patient is suffering from dementia (Department of Health & Human Services 2020a).

7.3 Physiology of ageing

LEARNING OBJECTIVE 7.3 Describe the pathophysiology of ageing.

Ageing is the result of molecular and cellular damage over time (WHO 2020a). These ongoing changes lead to decreased physical and mental capacity, an increased risk of disease and death. These changes are only loosely related to chronological age. In addition to biological changes, other life transitions such as retirement, relocation of homes and the death of friends and partners are related to these changes. Common health issues that can occur with ageing include:

- cardiac failure
- stroke
- respiratory diseases, including upper airway infections
- hearing loss
- cataracts
- neck and back pain
- osteoarthritis
- osteoporosis
- diabetes
- depression
- dementia.

Older age is also typified with complex health issues that affect the lifestyles of individuals and their families. These are often referred to as geriatric syndromes and include increased risk of falls, urinary incontinence, delirium and pressure injuries (WHO 2020a). These changes relate to changes in our body systems due to the ageing process.

The cardiovascular system

An efficient cardiovascular system is essential for a long, healthy life (Knight & Nigam 2017a). The cardiovascular system circulates blood throughout the body allowing for the transport of amino acids, electrolytes, oxygen, carbon dioxide, hormones and blood cells to provide the body with nourishment, temperature and disease control and maintaintaining homeostasis. As the heart's efficiency is reduced with age, it has a negative impact on all our other organ systems (see figure 7.1 and table 7.1).

The respiratory system

The respiratory system includes the airways, lungs and blood vessels that support oxygen delivery throughout the body and remove carbon dioxide (Knight & Nigam 2017b). Age-related changes in the respiratory system include loss of elasticity and decreased chest wall compliance (see figure 7.2 and table 7.2). This causes the increased work of breathing, residual volume and functional residual capacity. These changes lead to a decrease in the ability to compensate for an acute illness or respiratory failure.

The nervous system

The nervous system is the system responsible for controlling the activities of all body organs and tissues (Knight & Nigam 2017c). The nervous system is made up of the brain, spinal cord and nerves. The nervous system receives messages from the sensory organs and responds through effector organs. Due to its complexity, the brain remains a poorly understood organ. The nervous system is responsible for:

- intelligence, learning, memory, thoughts and feelings
- movement
- basic body functions such as cardiac function, respiration, digestion, sweating and shivering
- emergency response ('fight or flight' instinct)
- the senses: sight, hearing, taste, touch and smell (Healthdirect n.d.).

Like all our body systems, the nervous system goes through age-related changes that include a loss of brain cells (see figure 7.3 and table 7.3). However, we need to remember that ageing does not necessarily lead to confusion or dementia (Healthdirect n.d.).

FIGURE 7.1 Clinical changes associated with ageing and the cardiovascular system

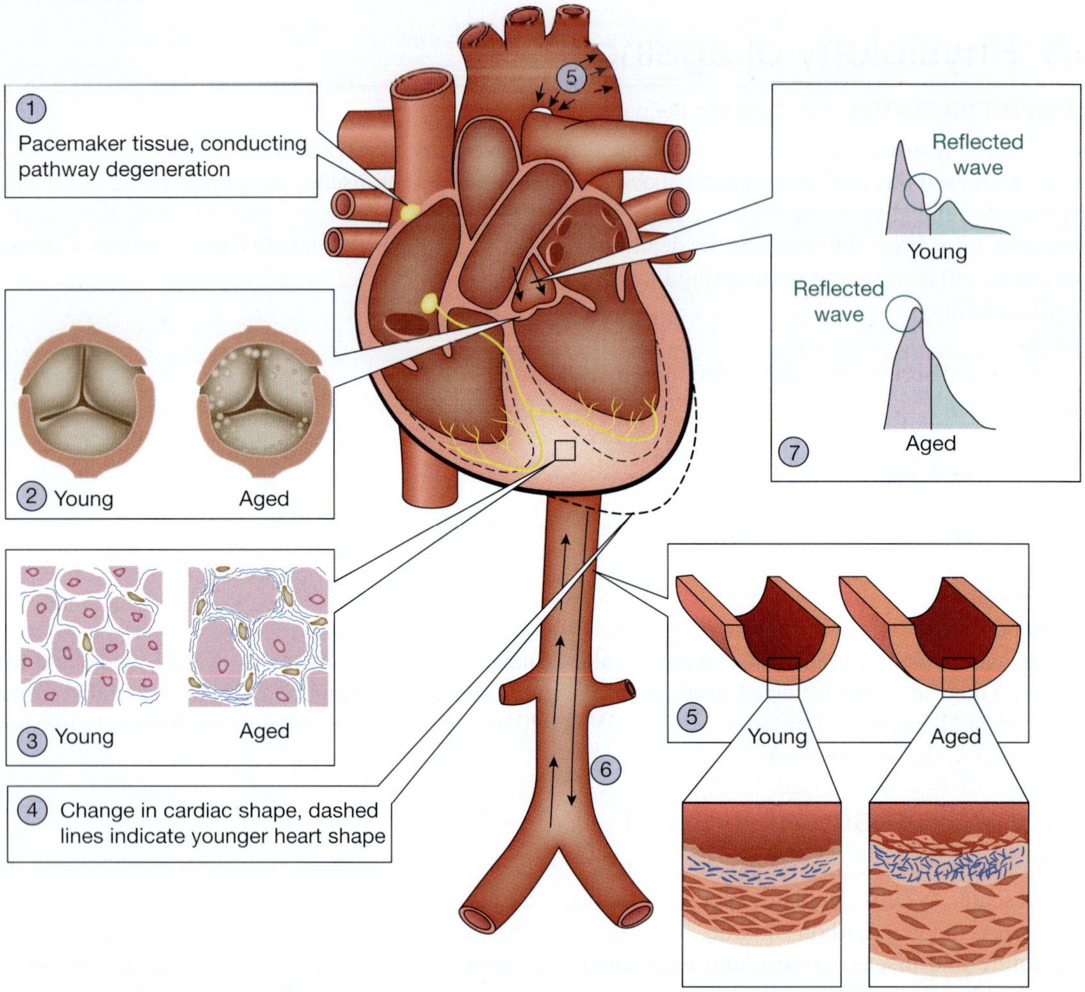

Source: Flaatten, Skaar & Joynt (2018).

TABLE 7.1 Clinical changes associated with ageing and the cardiovascular system

Clinical changes	Clinical presentations
Loss of elasticity to blood vessels, particularly arteries; the arterial walls become stiffer and thicker	Higher blood pressure (BP), including the resting BP A redistribution of heart muscle mass, which negatively affects its function
Changes in the chemical signals produced by the body contribute to restricting blood flow	Postural hypertension Bradycardia
Increase in venous stasis	Increased likelihood of atrial fibrillation
Increased pulmonary artery (wedge) pressures or the pressure that the heart needs to exert to pump blood through the pulmonary artery	Widened BP Reduced exercise tolerance Reduced response to some cardiac medications

Source: Adapted from Knight & Nigam (2017a).

FIGURE 7.2 Age-related changes to the respiratory system

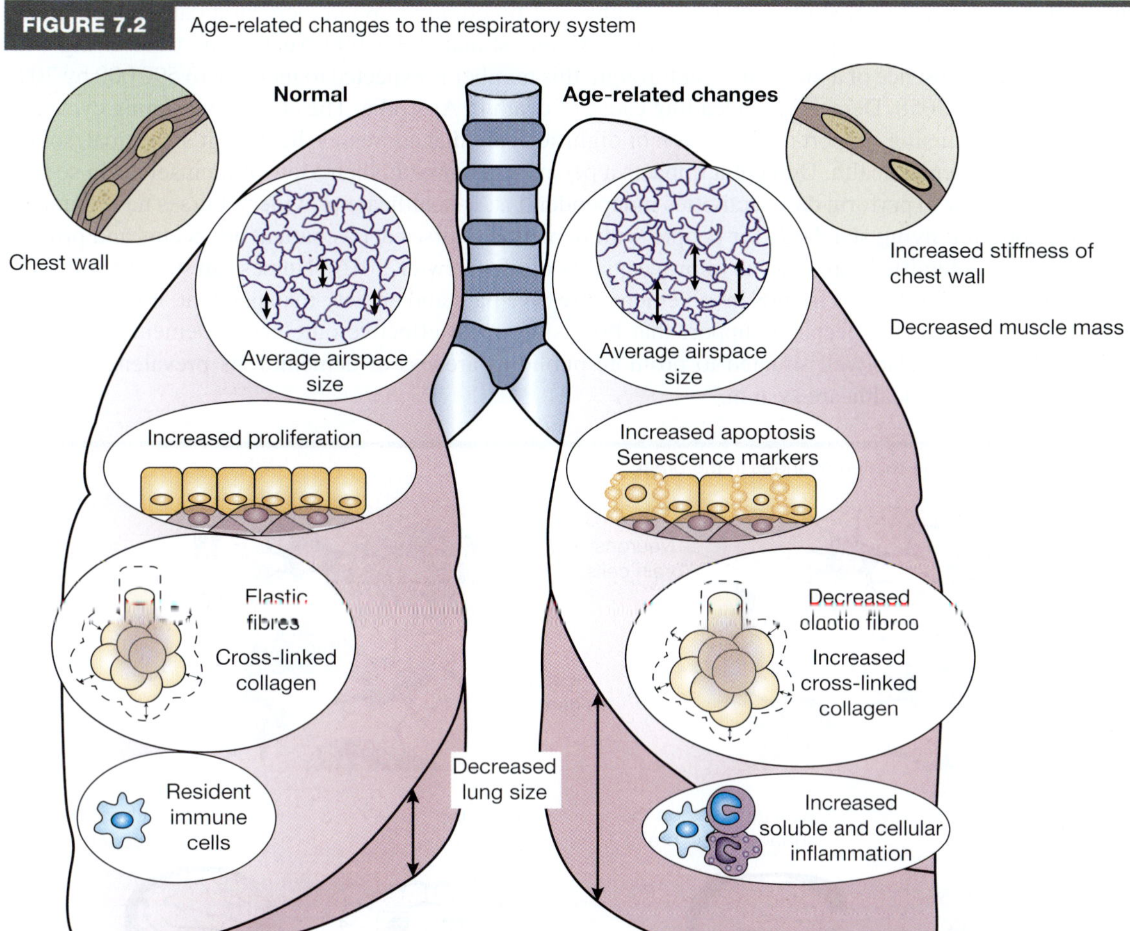

Source: Adapted from Bowdish (2019) & Winterbottom (n.d.).

TABLE 7.2 **Clinical changes associated with ageing and the respiratory system**

Clinical changes	Clinical presentations
Decreased elasticity of the alveolar surface area	Decreased ability to clear particles and mucus from: – decreased coughing reflex – decreased elasticity of lung tissue – age related emphysema.
Increased production of inflammatory mediators	Acute Respiratory Distress Syndrome (ARDS)
Increased pulmonary artery (wedge) pressures or the pressure that the heart needs to exert to pump blood through the pulmonary artery	Asthma Chronic bronchitis Emphysema Idiopathic Pulmonary Fibrosis (IPF); pleural mesothelioma Pneumonia Reduced saturations Increased risk of viruses, such as influenza, SARS, COVID-19

Source: Adapted from WHO (2020a); American Heart Association (AHA) (2020); Hicks (2018).

Dementia

Dementia is a term used to describe a group of illnesses that affect a progressive decline in functioning (Dementia Australia 2020a). Types of dementia include Alzheimer's disease, vascular dementia, frontotemporal dementia and Lewy body disease. Dementia signs and symptoms include the loss of memory, intellect, rationality, social skills and a loss of physical functioning. While dementia can happen at any age, it is more common in people over 65. In 2020, an estimated 459 000 Australians were living with dementia. In the absence of a medical breakthrough, this number is expected to increase to 590 000 by 2028 and 1 076 000 by 2058. Dementia is a leading cause of death in Australia. The clinical reasoning cycle and patient-centred nursing support the provision of dignified care that addresses the patient's physical, social, emotional and mental health. Dementia impacts a person's self-worth, their view of themselves in society and their capacity to perform daily activities independently. As healthcare providers, nurses have a unique role in improving living standards for people with dementia. Nurses act as patient advocates and provide compassionate, dignified care that can improve quality of life (Bewick 2016). Nurses can support culturally appropriate care, family and friends involvement, effective pain and anxiety management, minimal use of restraints and access to specialist support that brings the most effective outcomes (Dementia Australia 2020b). Nurses are also well situated to promote public awareness of dementia, its prevalence and the implications for the healthcare system.

FIGURE 7.3 Age-related changes in the brain

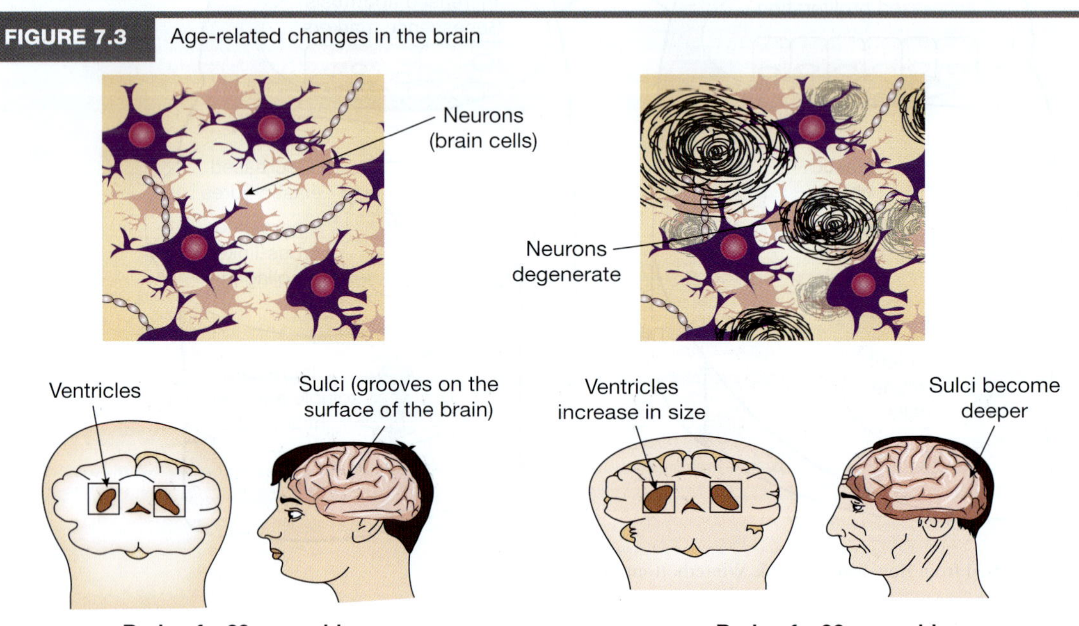

Source: Knight & Nigam (2017c).

TABLE 7.3 Clinical changes associated with ageing and the nervous system

Clinical changes	Clinical presentations
Loss of neurons and neuroglial cells most apparent in the cerebral cortex Structural changes in the frontal and parietal lobes The hippocampus (key role in memory and acquisition of new skills) loses a significant amount of neural tissue	Degenerative diseases like Parkinson's, Alzheimer's and multiple sclerosis Stroke Spinal cord injuries Seizure disorders, such as epilepsy Cancer, such as brain tumours Infections, such as meningitis Migraines
Somatic motor cortex neurons show signs of atrophy (controls the movement of muscles involved in walking, neurons in this region)	Gait problems Mobility issues
The autonomic function of the brain declines Reduction of baroreceptor responses Cerebral blood flow decreases	Compromises ability to respond quickly to internal and external environmental changes Postural hypotension
Declining production of neurotransmitters, including noradrenaline, glutamate, dopamine and serotonin	Changes in motor function

Changes to vertebrae and intervertebral discs Reduced sensory and motor conduction	Reduced muscular strength Poor balance and poor fine motor control Increased risk of injury
Changes to the peripheral nervous system	**Peripheral nerve damage**
Loss of neurons, depletion of neurotransmitters and slowing of nerve conduction	Take longer to complete tasks loss of short-term and episodic memory Increasing problems using or recalling words Slowed reaction time Depression Less prone to emotional outbursts

Source: Adapted from Knight & Nigam (2017c).

The endocrine system

The endocrine system is the glands and organs that produce and secrete hormones to control and regulate body functions (Morley 2019). Hormones are chemical substances that act as messengers controlling and coordinating activities in the body. Ageing causes changes in hormone levels, and hormone receptors become less effective; hence endocrine function declines in the older person (see figure 7.4 and table 7.4).

FIGURE 7.4 Location of many endocrine glands. Also shown are other organs that contain endocrine cells and associated structures.

FUNCTIONS OF HORMONES

1. Help regulate:
   - chemical composition and volume of internal environment (interstitial fluid)
   - metabolism and energy balance
   - contraction of smooth and cardiac muscle fibres
   - glandular secretions
   - some immune system activities.
2. Control growth and development.
3. Regulate operation of reproductive systems.
4. Help establish circadian rhythms.

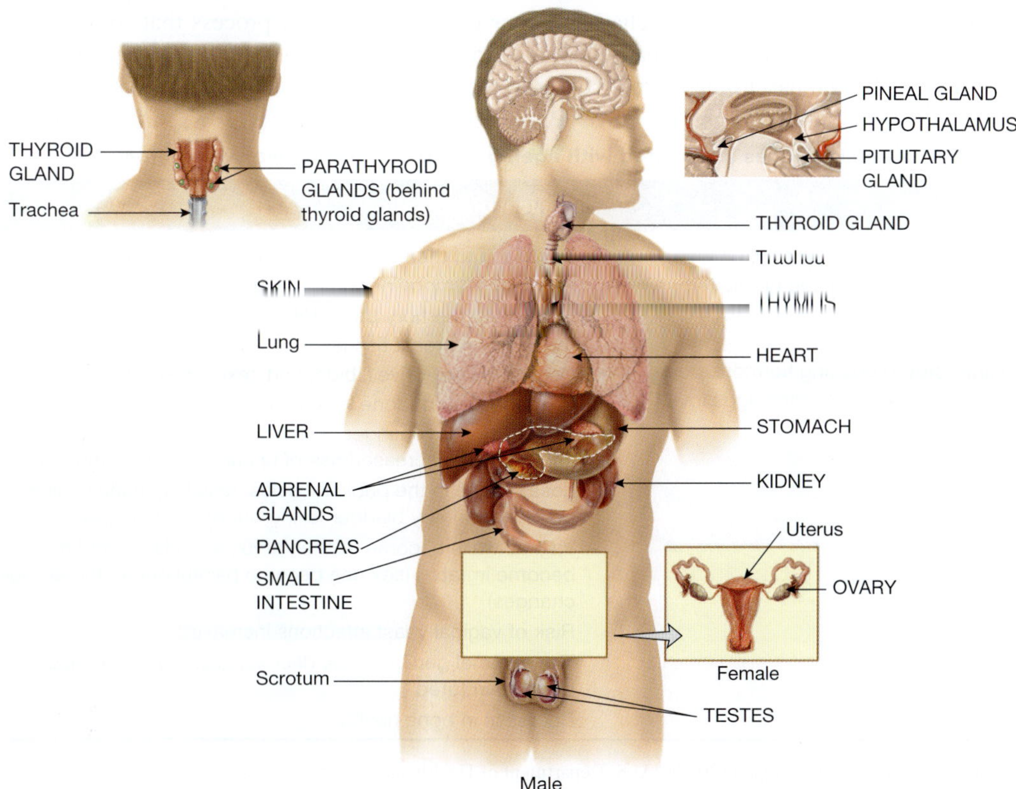

Source: Tortora et al. (2022).

TABLE 7.4 Clinical changes associated with ageing and the endocrine system

Clinical changes	Clinical presentations
Decreased levels of: • oestrogen (in women) • testosterone (in men) • melatonin the growth hormone	Women experience menopause, increased risk of cardiovascular disease and loss of bone mass Men experience decreased muscle mass and strength Increased adipose tissue, particularly abdominal fat
Remain unchanged or with minimal decrease: • cortisol • insulin • thyroid hormones	Increased risk of type 2 diabetes Alteration to circadian rhythms and reduced REM sleep
Increased levels of: • follicle-stimulating hormone (FSH) • luteinising hormone (LH) • norepinephrine • epinephrine, in the very old • parathyroid hormone	Menopause (women) Increased heart rate, BP and blood sugar levels

Source: Adapted from Knight & Nigam (2017d).

The reproductive system

During our fertile years, the testes and ovaries produce sperm and ova (Knight & Nigam 2017e; U.S. Department of Health and Human Services 2020c). With ageing, there is a gradual decline in fertility and fluctuations in the production of sex hormones. Both men and women experience changes to the reproductive system that lead to infertility (see tables 7.5 and 7.6). These changes in the ability to reproduce are due mainly to variations in oestrogen production, progesterone and testosterone. Women experience these symptoms during perimenopause and menopause (figure 7.5) and men experience physical (see figure 7.6) and psychological symptoms during andropause. While women tend to experience a major rapid decline in fertility, in men, these changes occur gradually during a process that some people call andropause. Changes for men in andropause can lead to loss of libido and erectile dysfunction. For both men and women, the changes to the reproductive system affect physical and psychological health.

TABLE 7.5 Clinical changes associated with ageing and the reproductive system (females)

Clinical changes	Clinical presentations
Perimenopause (pre-menopause) Production of oestrogen and progesterone by the ovaries slows and becomes irregular Menopause The ovaries stop producing hormones The ovaries also stop releasing eggs (ova, oocytes)	Irregular and then cessation of menstrual periods Hot flashes, moodiness, headaches, sleeping difficulties Short-term memory problems Decrease in breast tissue Decreased sex drive (libido) and sexual response Increased risk of bone loss (osteoporosis) Urinary system changes, such as frequency and urgency of urination and increased risk of urinary tract infection (UTI) Loss of tone in the pubic muscles, resulting in the vagina, uterus, or urinary bladder falling out of position (prolapse) Vaginal walls become thinner, dryer, less elastic and may become irritated (sex can become painful due to these vaginal changes) Risk of vaginal yeast infections increases The external genital tissue decreases and thins and can become irritated Decrease in bone health.

Source: Adapted from Knight & Nigam (2017e); U.S. Department of Health and Human Services (2020c).

TABLE 7.6 **Clinical changes associated with ageing and the reproductive system (males)**

Clinical changes	Clinical presentations
Mild decline of total testosterone (T) Increase of sex hormone-binding globulin (SHBG) More pronounced decline of free T Moderate increase of LH	Decreased sensitivity of the penis Decreased number of sperm in the ejaculation fluid Reduced forewarning of ejaculation Orgasm without ejaculation With orgasm, the penis becomes limp (detumescent) more quickly After orgasm there is a longer period before an erection can occur again (refractory period) The prostate gland enlarges as some of the prostate tissue is replaced with scar-like tissue leading to benign prostatic hyperplasia.

Source: Adapted from Kaufman, Lapauw, Mahmoud, T'Sjoen & Huhtaniemi (2019); Knight & Nigam (2017e).

FIGURE 7.5 Ageing of the female reproductive tract

Uterus: Loss of muscle and eventual cessation of menstrual cycle.

Ovaries: Reduction in number of ovarian follicles maturing leads to gradual decline in fertility. Levels of oestrogen begin to drop, triggering the menopause — typically around age of 51.

Fundus

Body

Cervix

Uterus

Fallopian tubes: Shrinkage in length, loss of ciliated epithelia and loss of mucosa contribute to loss of fertility.

Opening of the cervix: Reduced cervical secretions.

Vagina: Loss of elasticity, shortening in length, reduction in vaginal secretions and thinning of epithelial lining all increase risk of tears, bleeding and infection.

Source: Knight & Nigam (2017e).

FIGURE 7.6 Ageing of the male reproductive tract

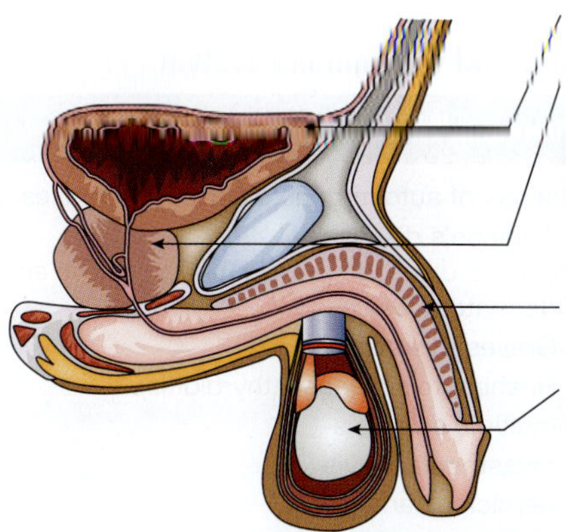

Source: Knight & Nigam (2017e).

The immune system

The immune system produces cells and antibodies that protect our body from foreign materials such as bacteria, viruses, toxins, cancer cells or blood and tissues from another person (Montecino-Rodriguez, Berent-Maoz & Dorshkind 2013; Nigam & Knight 2017a). A recognised problem of ageing is the decline in immunity (see table 7.7). The older person does not respond efficiently to new or previously encountered antigens, putting them at high risk for infection that may lead to morbidity or mortality. This was clearly demonstrated with the novel coronavirus (COVID-19) in 2019. COVID-19 is caused by a newly discovered (novel) coronavirus. The greater population infected with COVID-19 experience mild to moderate respiratory illness and do not require special treatment. However, the older population, especially those with chronic medical problems — cardiovascular disease, diabetes, chronic respiratory disease and cancer — are highly susceptible to COVID-19, often requiring hospitalisation and, in many cases, it has led to morbidity and mortality (WHO 2020b).

To reduce the risks to the older person due to ageing, healthcare providers need to help them support a healthy lifestyle, get their influenza vaccines, exercise, eat well, limit alcohol and stop smoking. We also need to investigate safety measures to prevent falls and injuries.

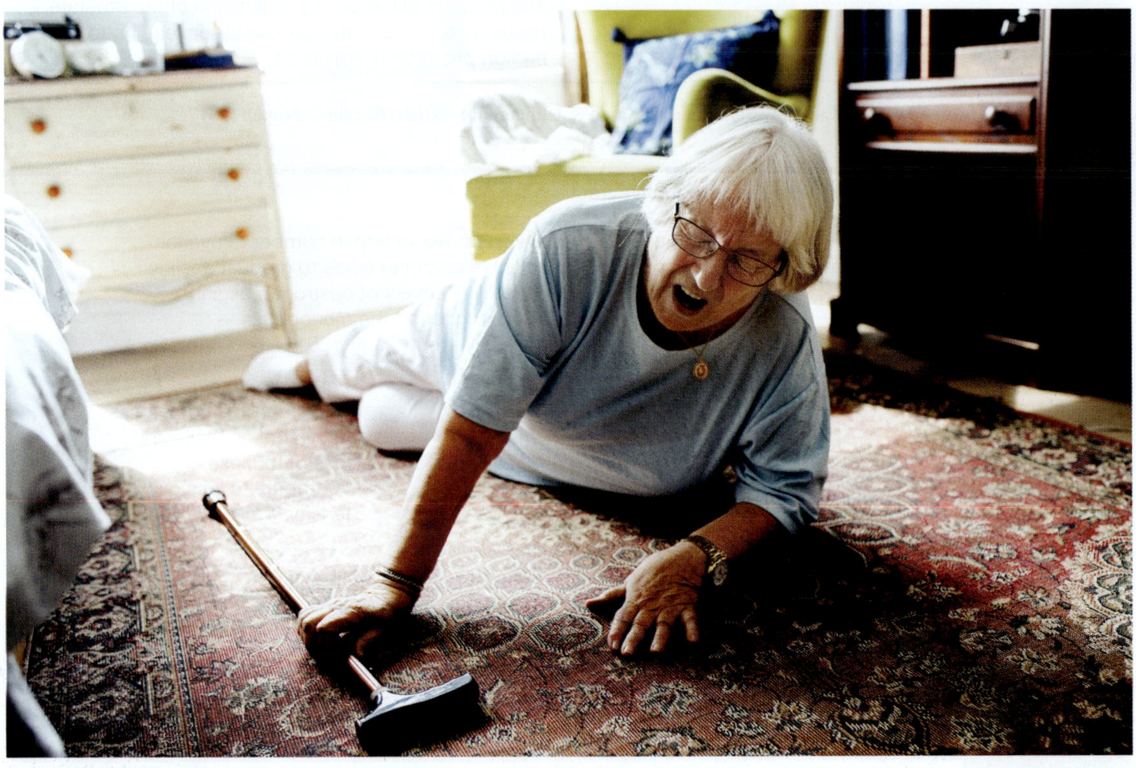

TABLE 7.7 Clinical changes associated with ageing and the immune system

Clinical changes	Clinical presentations
The immune system becomes less able to identify foreign antigens.	The risk of autoimmune disorders increases, including: • Addison's disease • coeliac disease/sprue (gluten-sensitive enteropathy) • dermatomyositis • Graves' disease • Hashimoto's disease (thyroiditis) • multiple sclerosis • myasthenia gravis • pernicious anaemia • reactive arthritis • rheumatoid arthritis • Sjögren's syndrome • systemic lupus erythematosus (SLE) • diabetes

T cells respond slower to the antigens. Reduced numbers of: • white blood cells capable of responding to new antigens • complement proteins	The body is less able to remember and defend against new antigens Reduced ability to respond to bacterial infections
The number of antibodies produced in response to an antigen is similar; however, these antibodies are less able to attach to the antigen	Vaccines are less effective Infections such as pneumonia, influenza, infective endocarditis and tetanus are more common among older people and more frequently results in mortality

Source: Adapted from U.S. Department of Health and Human Services (2020a).

The digestive system

The digestive system's role is to break down the food we eat into carbohydrates, fats and proteins that can be absorbed into our bloodstream and be utilised by the body for energy, growth and repair (Nigam & Knight 2017b). The digestive system consists of the mouth, oesophagus, stomach, small intestine, pancreas, liver, gall bladder, large intestine (colon), rectum and anus (see figure 7.7 and table 7.8).

FIGURE 7.7 The organs of the digestive system

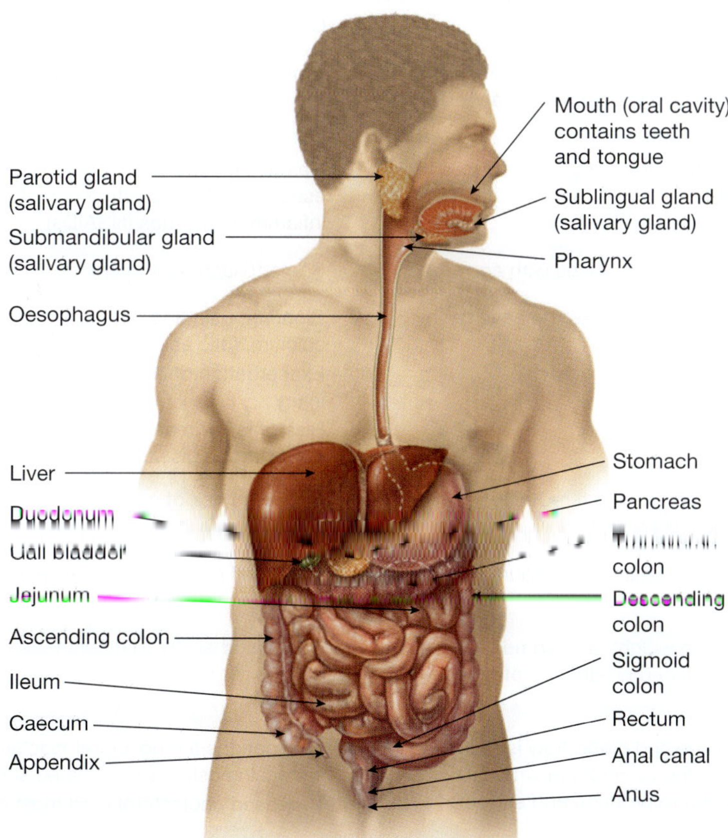

Source: Tortora & Derrickson (2011). *Principles of Anatomy and Physiology*, with kind permision of Wiley Blackwell.

TABLE 7.8 **Clinical changes associated with ageing and the digestive system**

Clinical changes	Clinical presentations
Changes to sensors in the gastrointestinal tract (GIT) that detect the presence of food and prompt the GIT to produce hormones Hormones that decrease appetite are increased, and hormones that would increase an appetite are decreased Gastric emptying slows	Decrease in appetite Malnutrition Decreased enjoyment of food Age-related anorexia
Shrinkage of the maxillary and mandibular bones > poorly fitting dentures Reduction in bone calcium content leading to the slow erosion of tooth sockets, gum recession and increased risk of root decay Loss of teeth	Difficulty chewing Chooses easy to chew food that leads to decreased fibre which may cause constipation
Muscle contractions that initiate swallowing slow down and increase the time that food passes through the pharynges	Dysphagia (difficulty swallowing and an increased risk of choking)
Changes in oropharyngeal and oesophageal motility	Dysphagia Reflux Heartburn
Stomach wall loses elasticity	Cannot accommodate as much food
Reduction in mucus-producing goblet cells, resulting in reduced secretion of protective mucus and a weakened mucosal barrier	Stomach lining becomes prone to damage
Decline in gastric bicarbonate (HCO_3^-) and mucus that protects the stomach lining	Gastro-mucosal injury such as lesions and ulcers, especially after ingesting non-steroidal anti-inflammatory drugs (NSAIDs)
Enzyme lactase production decreases with age	Prone to lactose intolerance
Bacteria that reside in the small intestine have been shown to increase:	Bloating, pain and decreased absorption of calcium, folic acid and iron Exacerbation of NSAID-induced small intestinal injury Risk of inflammatory bowel disease, diabetes and autoimmune diseases
Colonic transit slows down due to a reduction in neurotransmitters and neuroreceptors	Increased risk of constipation Haemorrhoids
Reduced cell division — digestive epithelium cannot repair and replace itself	Increased risk of colorectal cancer
Pancreases decreases in weight, and some tissues become fibrotic with reduced production of digestive enzymes	Decreased ability to digest food
The liver shrinks with age and blood flow is decreased Decrease in protein synthesis, metabolism, ability to detoxify substances and to produce and support flow of bile	Medications are no longer inactivated by the liver increasing risk of dose related side effects Increased cholesterol level most notable in women

Source: Nigam & Knight (2017b).

The renal system

The renal system filters our blood, regulates blood volume and blood pressure, controls electrolyte and metabolite levels, regulates blood pH and produces urine (Johns Hopkins Medicine 2020). Normal urine is pale straw or translucent yellow in colour. Darker urine indicates dehydration, while pink or red urine may indicate the presence of blood in the urine. The organs of the renal system are the kidneys, renal pelvis, ureters, bladder and urethra. Renal function declines gradually (see figure 7.8 and table 7.9); however, in the absence of disease, the renal system can fulfil its role throughout our lifetime. Factors that are known to decrease renal function are:

- hypertension
- smoking
- exposure to lead
- obesity
- poor diet
- increased inflammatory mediators in the blood related to critical illness, trauma, sepsis, or after surgical interventions (Andrade & Knight 2017; Terhune, Weavind & Pandharipande 2010).

FIGURE 7.8 Age-related changes to the renal system

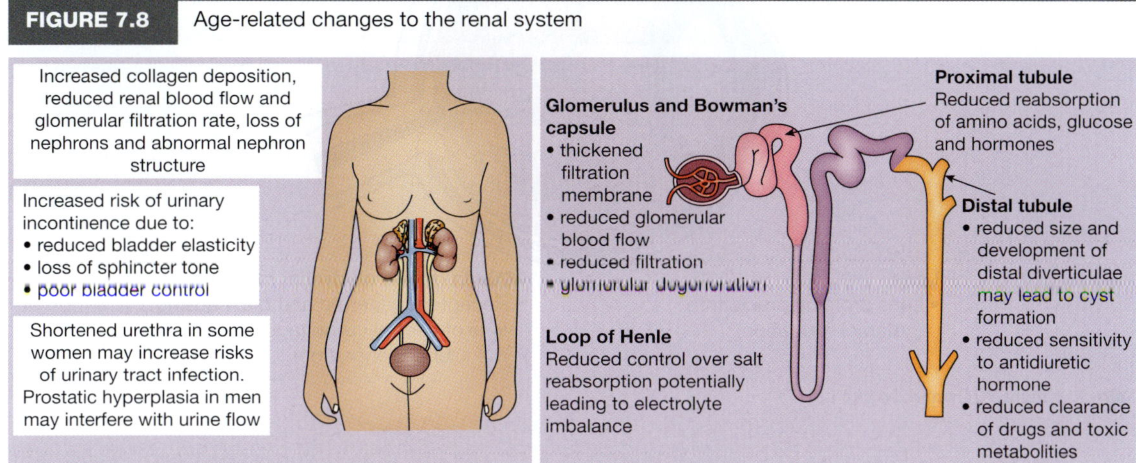

Source: Andrade & Knight (2017).

TABLE 7.9 Clinical changes associated with ageing and the renal system

Clinical changes	Clinical presentations
Kidney tissue decreases Nephrons that filter the blood decrease Blood vessels harden Renal blood flow and Glomerular filtration rates are reduced	Electrolyte imbalance Hyper or hypotension Confusion Polyuria Nocturia Reduced insulin clearance
Bladder wall elastic tissue toughens (bladder becomes less stretchy) Bladder muscles weaken	Urinary incontinence Urinary retention
In women: weakened muscles can cause the bladder or vagina to prolapse In men: the urethra can become blocked by an enlarged prostate gland	The flow of urine is blocked, causing pain and can lead to kidney damage, kidney stones and or infection

Source: Adapted from Andrade & Knight (2017); U.S. Department of Health and Human Services (2020d).

The ears and eyes

Our sight, hearing, smell, touch and balance give us a connection to the world and allow us to communicate (Knight, Wigham & Nigam 2017). The eyes, ears, nose, tongue detect information from the environment, which is relayed to the brain and processed into meaningful sensations. Stimulation is required before you become aware of a sensation, and the minimum level of sensation is called the threshold (U.S. Department of Health and Human Services 2020). Ageing raises this threshold. Older people require more stimulation to be aware of a sensation. Ageing affects all our senses; however, sight and hearing are the most affected (see figures 7.9 and 7.10). Age-related changes to the eyes and ears affect our connection with our society. Of all the age-related changes in the body, the most dramatic are seen in the eyes and ears (see tables 7.10 and 7.11). Older people should be supported with regular check-ups for hearing and sight.

FIGURE 7.9 Age-related changes to the eye

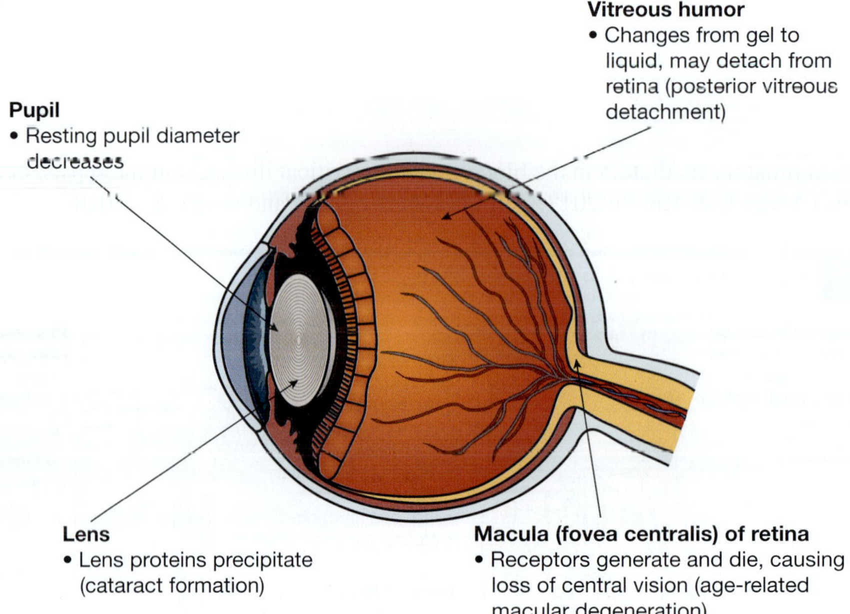

Source: Knight Wigham & Nigam (2017).

FIGURE 7.10 Age-related changes to the ear

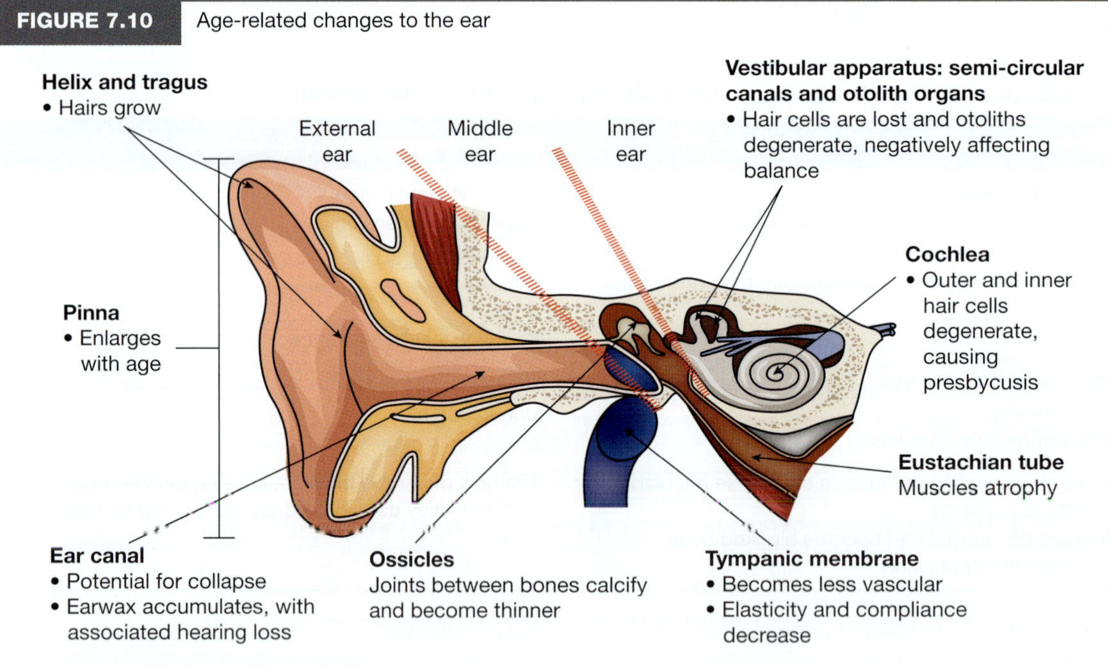

Source: Knight, Wigham & Nigam (2017).

TABLE 7.10 Clinical changes associated with ageing and the eyes

Clinical changes	Clinical presentations
The retro-orbital fat that protects and cushions the eyeball atrophies with age Atrophy causes changes to the conjunctiva lining the eyelids (tarsal conjunctiva) does sufficiently lubricate the front of the eye (cornea)	Eyeball recedes into its socket (enophthalmos) Eyelids droop (ptosis) upper field of vision can be obstructed Eyelashes can turn inwards causing irritation to the corneal surface and can cause corneal ulcers

Weakening of the eye muscles supporting the lower eyelids	Lower lids become dry and can flop away from the eyeball, causing irritation
Along with changes to the composition of the tears, the lacrimal glands produce fewer tears Stability of the tear film is reduced	Dry eye syndrome with irritation, grittiness and pain and can affect reading and watching television
Presbyopia (reduction in the ability to see close up objects)	Unable to read small print without reading glasses
Lens increase in density	Yellowing of lens Contrast sensitivity and the accurate perception of colours is affected Increased risk of cataracts
Pupils diameter decreases resulting in a reduction of light admitted	Increased risk of falls
Changes in the vitreous and aqueous humour in the hollow chambers separated by the lens of the eye	Detached retina that needs immediate medical care Increased opacities (floaters) or sheering patterns that affect vision
Photoreceptor cells in the fovea, which provide high-quality colour vision, begin to die, causing age-related macular degeneration	Pale yellow-white elevated spots appear on the retina, distorting vision and reducing visual acuity

Source: Adapted from Knight, Wigham & Nigam (2017).

TABLE 7.11 Clinical changes associated with ageing and the ears

Clinical changes	Clinical presentations
Pinna often becomes larger, dry and scaly External hair on the tragus and lower helix in men	Uncomfortable and itchy ears
Ceruminous glands produce less earwax	Dry ears prone to infection
Cartilaginous components that form the walls of the auditory meatus can lose elasticity, degrade and sometimes collapse Tympanic membrane becomes less vascular becomes thin and stiff	Reduced conduction and amplification of sound waves
Changes in blood flow in the ear Drug toxicity (from example, adverse reactions to [illegible] Muscular spasms in the ear Loss of hair cells	Tinnitus (noise such as ringing, buzzing, humming or whooshing in the ears)
The number of nerve cells and blood flow to the inner ear decreases with age	Balance problems and increased risk of falls

Source: Adapted from Knight, Wigham & Nigam (2017).

The musculoskeletal system

The skeletal system provides support and structure to the body (Knight, Hore & Nigam 2017; U.S. Department of Health and Human Services 2020b). Bones support the body, provide protection for vulnerable organs and allow for physical movement. They store fat and minerals as well as red bone marrow, responsible for the production of blood cells (Knight, Hore & Nigam 2017). Joints allow for flexibility of movement and support and cushion bones with the cartilage, synovial membranes and fluid around the joints. Muscles provide strength, force and movement for the body. Skeletal muscles allow the body to move and maintain posture. Muscles support the return of blood to the heart through the venous system and help maintain body temperature. With age, these components of the musculoskeletal system progressively degenerate, which contributes to frailty and increases the risk of falls and fractures (see figure 7.11). The musculoskeletal system is directed and coordinated by the brain. Nearly half of all Australians over the age of 75 have health issues that are related to the musculoskeletal system (see table 7.12) (Department of Health & Human Services 2020b). Research has shown that many of these issues are linked to ageing and a reduced level of or lack of activity. As healthcare providers, we need to support older people to maintain a level of physical activity that can reduce or reverse the risk of chronic disease and disability.

FIGURE 7.11 Age-related changes to the musculoskeletal system of the hand

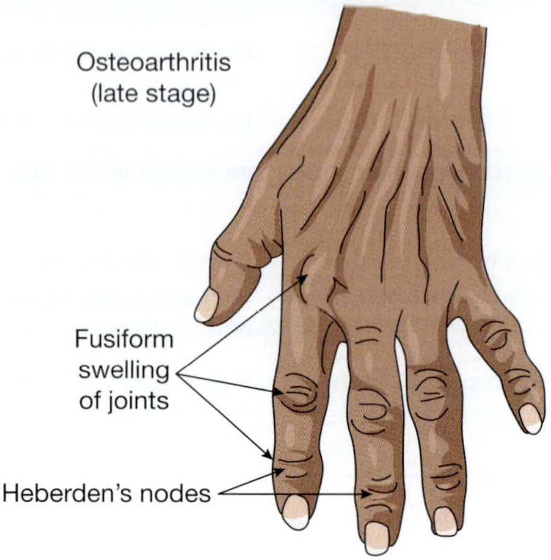

TABLE 7.12 Clinical changes associated with ageing and the musculoskeletal system

Clinical changes	Clinical presentations
Changes in the bone with ageing: • demineralisation of bones • reduced calcium absorption and vitamin D levels Reduced testosterone levels in men Reduced oestrogen levels in women Reduced growth hormone levels (somatopause) Reduced levels of parathyroid hormone	Overall height decreases Posture may become stooped Trunk and spine shorten Knees and hips may become more flexed Neck may tilt Shoulders may narrow Pelvis widens Bones become brittle Increased risk of falls and breaks
Changes in muscles include a reduction in: • blood flow to the major muscle groups • muscle growth • size and number of muscle fibres, particularly in the lower limbs • protein synthesis • number of progenitor (satellite) cells • ability of muscles to repair themselves • ability of active muscle fibres to be replaced by collagen-rich, non-contractile fibrous tissue • number of motor neurons and deterioration of neuromuscular junctions • number of mitochondria • muscle metabolism • Muscle changes are also affected by an: • increase in fat deposition at the expense of lean muscle tissue • accumulation of lipofuscin an age-related pigment	Weak or abnormal sensations Muscle contractures Reduced reflexes Reduced lean body mass Increased risk of falls and breaks Increased susceptibility to heat and cold

Chondrocytes, the cartilage-forming cells, decrease with age Joints stiffen and lose flexibility Synovial fluid may decrease Cartilage may rub together and wear away Minerals may deposit in and around some joints (calcification) Hip and knee joints lose cartilage Finger joints lose cartilage and the bones thicken slightly	Pain and inflammation Stiffness and deformity Reduced energy, easily tired Movement slows and may become limited Slowed gait Shorter steps Walking may become unsteady Arm swinging is reduced Increased risk of falls and breaks

Source: Knight, Hore & Nigam (2017).

The integumentary system

The integumentary system consists of the skin, hair, nails and exocrine glands. The skin is the largest organ in the human body (Nigam & Knight 2017c) and supports thermoregulation, storage and synthesis, sensation and protection. Because the skin covers the body and it is visible, the signs of ageing are overt (see figure 7.12 and table 7.13).

FIGURE 7.12 Age-related changes in the epidermis and dermis

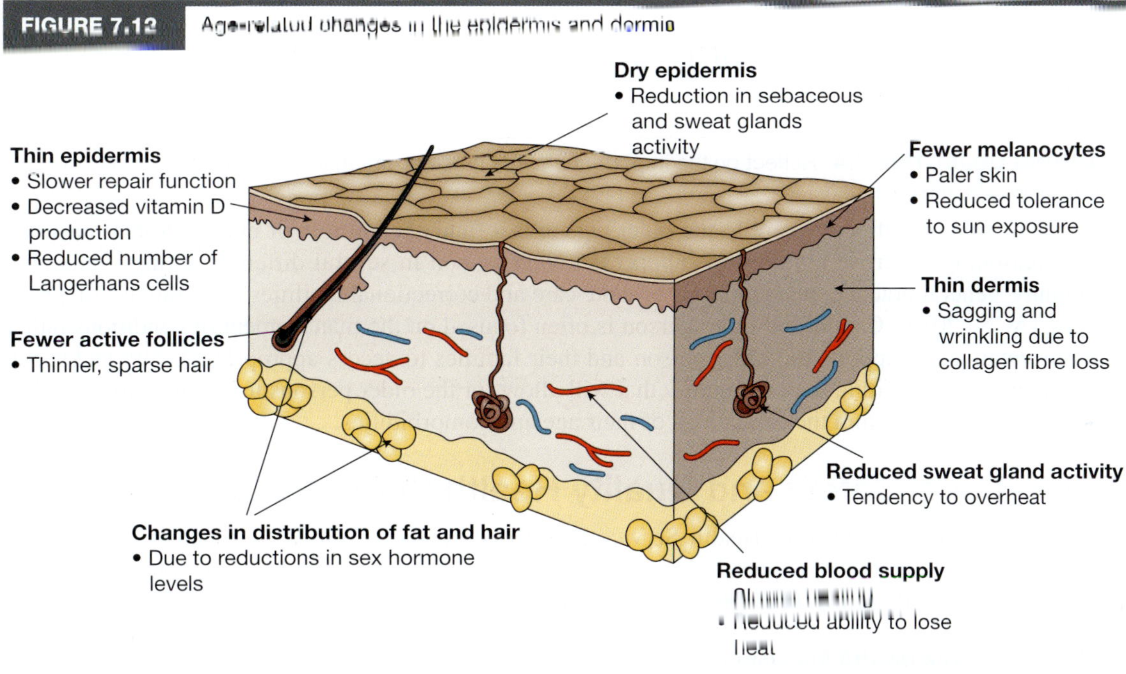

Source: Nigam & Knight (2017c).

TABLE 7.13 Clinical changes associated with ageing and the integumentary system

Clinical changes	Clinical presentations
Changes in the epidermis, dermis, hypodermis	Thin, dry and sagging skin especially notable in the facial areas
Loss of structure and integrity and ability to detect temperature and pressure changes	More disposed to trauma, tears, pressure injuries and infection Skin cancers Skin lesions Skin discolourations Skin dryness (xerosis) Pressure injuries

(continued)

TABLE 7.13 *(continued)*

Clinical changes	Clinical presentations
Loss of sensory nerve endings in the epidermis and dermis means that the older person will have a decreased ability to detect environmental changes	Less able to maintain a stable body temperature — may feel the cold and heat to a greater extent
Finger and toenails deteriorate Nails grow more slowly and become brittle	Nails become yellowed and opaque, and lines and ridges develop. Ingrown toenails become more common Thickening of the nails (mainly the toenails) Fungal infections under nails Overgrown nails that cause discomfort and pain leading to reduced mobility
Reduced melanin production in hair follicles	Causes hair to go grey and then eventually white
Strands of hair become thin and hair follicles can stop producing hair	Baldness

Source: Adapted from Nigam & Knight (2017c); Chinniah & Gupta (2014).

7.4 Providing safe and effective care for the older person

LEARNING OBJECTIVE 7.4 Reflect on the importance of the nurse in caring for the older person and our role in providing safe, effective care.

Provision of safe and effective care to the older person is a fundamental role of nurses. Nurses have the clinical reasoning expertise required to support the older person in several different settings, including community, general practice, residential care, acute care and correctional facilities (Australian College of Nursing [ACN] 2019). Care of the older person is often focused on the management of conditions rather than preventative. It supports the older person and their families to access appropriate health and social care support systems within the community that will allow for the older persons to continue to live a full and eventful lifestyle within the limitations of their age and comorbidities.

The National Safety and Quality Health Service Standards

The National Safety and Quality Health Service (NSQHS) Standards provide a coherent statement of the level of care patients can expect from health service organisations (Aged Care Quality and Safety Commission 2020). The NSQHS cover the aspects of care in the aged care sector outlined in table 7.14.

TABLE 7.14 **The NSQHS Standards**

Standard	Statement	Intent of standard
One	Consumer dignity and choice	Supports the delivery of safe, effective personal and clinical care according to the older person's needs and care preferences.
Two	Ongoing assessment and planning with consumers	Supports the ongoing assessment and planning with the older person with the input of the patient and their family.
Three	Personal care and clinical care	Requires the delivery of safe, effective personal and clinical care according to the needs, goals and preferences that enhance the health and wellbeing of the older person.
Four	Services and supports for daily living	Supports the provision of safe and effective services that provide support for activities of daily living and optimise independence, health, wellbeing and quality of life.

Five	Service environment	Supports a safe and comfortable environment to promotes older people's independence, function and enjoyment.
Six	Feedback and complaints	The older person feels safe and am encouraged and supported to give feedback and make complaints and feels listened to and that appropriate action is taken.
Seven	Human resources	Supports a workforce that is sufficient, skilled and qualified to provide safe, respectful and quality care and services, and the older person feels safe in their care.
Eight	Organisational governance	The organisation is well run, and the governing body is accountable for delivering safe and quality care and services. The older person is encouraged to partner in improving the delivery of care and services.

Source: Adapted from Aged Care Quality and Safety Commission (2020).

These quality standards aim to support the providers of aged care residential services to provide the best possible lifestyle and living conditions for the older population. The Australian Registered nurse standards for practice support these quality standards with our own seven standards to employ when caring for all patients. We are required to:

1. think critically and analyse our nursing practice
2. engage in therapeutic and professional relationships
3. maintain the capability for practice
4. comprehensively conduct assessments
5. develop a plan for nursing practice
6. provides safe, appropriate and responsive quality nursing practice
7. evaluate outcomes to inform nursing practice (Nursing and Midwifery Board 2017).

These standards are as applicable to caring for our older people in the residential healthcare or community setting as they are to our roles in acute care. A registered nurse in the residential aged care setting has the most responsibility in that facility. The registered nurse oversees all assessments and nursing care plans. Management of medical care is supervised by the registered nurse, who evaluates how the care has impacted the resident. The registered nurse provides leadership for the other nursing staff and has responsibility for clinical policies and procedures in the aged care and healthcare sector. Application of the registered nurse's knowledge and skills is paramount to providing safe and effective care for aged care facility residents.

CASE STUDY 7.1

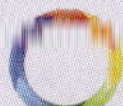

Caring for an older patient with complex respiratory needs

Mrs Rebecca Johnson is a 70-year-old female patient. Mrs Johnson has presented with a history of chronic, productive cough, breathlessness and generalised malaise. Mrs Johnson reports that she has trouble with sleeping at night due to coughing and is generally feeling unwell. She has increased difficulty with activities of daily living (ADL) due to weakness, exhaustion and breathlessness. She states she has smoked one packet of cigarettes per day since her early 20s, and she has the occasional drink. For the past 24 hours, she has been suffering from chest tightness but denies any pain. She appears to be in respiratory distress. She is noted to be sitting forward, using accessory muscles. She has a moist cough and is coughing regularly.

Personal history: The patient is a retired teacher and has been widowed for five years. She lives alone and is currently self-caring. She has two adult children who live in the same area and are supportive.

Family history: Mrs Johnson's father died from complications related to ischaemic heart disease at 58. Her mother suffered a stroke and died at age 67.

Past medical/surgical history: She has been admitted to hospital for treatment of lower respiratory tract infection (LRTI) twice in the last year. The patient has recently commenced on a low dose thiazide diuretic for hypertension. She denies any other history of cardiovascular disease, diabetes or hypercholesterolaemia.

Vital signs on admission:

- respiratory rate: 28 breaths per minute
- oxygen saturation: 90% on 3L via nasal prongs
- heart rate: 90 beats per minute
- blood pressure: 150/83 mmHg
- temperature: 37.9°C
- pain score: 0/10.

Quootion

Using the information above, describe the actions you would take as the nurse caring for this patient. Use the clinical reasoning cycle to guide you through the process and devise a care plan for your patient.

Answer

- *Step 1: Consider the patient*. Mrs Rebecca Johnson, a 70-year-old female patient. She lives alone and has two children who live in the same area. Currently self-caring. What other assessments need to be undertaken for this patient?
- *Step 2: Collect cues/information.* Include subjective data — what the patient tells you about their signs and symptoms and past medical history and objective data — what you can measure (vital signs). Include the appearance of the patient.
- *Step 3: Process information*. Separate the relevant and irrelevant data — cluster the clues together to formulate a picture of the patient. Mrs Johnson has respiratory problems and is a smoker. Currently her RR is elevated, and her oxygen saturations are 90 per cent on 3 litres via the nasal prongs. She has a low-grade temperature and is exhibiting signs and symptoms of respiratory distress secondary to infection.
- *Step 4: Identify problems/issues.* From the data gathered and the picture formulated, define your nursing problems or nursing diagnosis. Mrs Johnson's priority nursing problems are her elevated respiratory rate and her low oxygen saturations and a need for an elevated level of care.
- *Step 5: Establish goals.* Determine the short- and long-term goals of care for Mrs Jonson. Goals of care should focus on improving breathing and personal comfort.
- *Step 6: Take action.* What actions are needed, and how would you prioritise them? Contact her physician for an order to apply a Hudson/simple and a higher level of oxygen. Implement ongoing monitoring of oxygen levels and consider transfer of her care to a high level unit where she can have ongoing monitoring of her respiratory and cardiac status. Support the patient with pillows to help her maintain comfortable breathing position. Recognise the patient may be feeling extremely anxious and will need some reassurance.
- *Step 7: Evaluate outcomes*. Consider the actions you have taken to support Mrs Johnson and what the outcome of your actions was? Is the care provided meeting the short- and long-term goals that have been established?
- *Step 8: Reflect on the process and new learning*. Reflect on the care provided — what went well and what could be done to improve care? What can you do to improve your knowledge and skills to support the care of the patient?

CASE STUDY 7.2

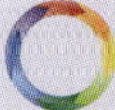

Caring for an elderly patient with complex urology needs

We are caring for James Hanson, an 82-year-old male patient. Mr Hanson has been transferred to the emergency room from the aged care facility in which he lives. The handover from the aged care staff is that Mr Hanson is confused and disorientated, and this is not his normal status. The family is concerned that their relative has dementia.

Vital signs on admission:

- respiratory rate: 25 breaths per minute
- oxygen saturation: 97% on room air
- heart rate: 150 beats per minute
- blood pressure: 130/95 mmHg
- temperature: 37.9°C
- P: Patient states it is painful to pass urine. He has a feeling that his bladder is always full
- Q: Burning sensation
- R: Back pain
- S: 6/10
- T: Several weeks now.

When collecting clues, his routine urine test shows the urine is cloudy, bloody and has an odour. You note elevated leukocytes, nitrites and is positive for blood. This leads to the order for a urine specimen to be sent to the lab to confirm a urinary tract infection (UTI) and determine the appropriate antibiotic for treatment.

Question

Using the information above, describe the actions you would take as the nurse caring for this patient. Use the clinical reasoning cycle to guide you through the process and devise a care plan for your patient.

Answer

- *Step 1: Consider the patient*. Mr James Hanson is an 82-year-old male patient. He lives alone in a local nursing home and has family who visit infrequently. Until recently, Mr Hanson has managed his own hygiene, toileting and feeding. He takes an active role in the facilities activities. He has now presented as confused and disorientated. What other assessments need to be undertaken for this patient?
- *Step 2: Collect cues/information/* Include subjective data — what the patient can tell you about their signs and symptoms and past medical history and objective data — what you observe — what you can measure (vital signs). Include the appearance of the patient.
- *Step 3: Process information.* Separate the relevant and irrelevant data — cluster the clues together to formulate a picture of the patient. Based on his pain score the clues indicate a urinary tract infection that should be confirmed with a dip stick urinalysis and followed by a specimen sent to the labs. His pain, confusion and disorientation are related to the UTI. His elevated heart rate is potentially related to the pain and discomfort.
- *Step 4: Identify problems/issues.* From the data gathered and the picture formulated, define your nursing problems or nursing diagnosis: UTI, pain, confusion and disorientation. Recognise the family are feeling extremely anxious and will need some reassurance. It would help if you also considered contacting his family to be updated about his diagnosis by the doctor.
- *Step 5: Establish goals*. Determine the short- and long-term goals of care. Goals of care should focus on safety, personal comfort and determining the reason for the change of status of the patient.
- *Step 6: Take action*. What actions are needed, and how would you prioritise them? Treat the pain and discomfort with analgesia as ordered. Complete necessary tests and relay results to the physician. Start antibiotics as/if ordered. Reassure family that the confusion and disorientation in all likelihood is related to the UTI. Maintain a safe environment and reassure the patient.
- *Step 7: Evaluate outcomes*. A routine urine test confirms that the patient has a UTI. This leads to treatment of the UTI prior to 'jumping' to a diagnosis of dementia.
- *Step 8: Reflect on the process and new learning*. Reflect on the care provided — what went well and what could be done to improve care? On reflection, we can recognise the advantage of a full assessment and collection of all clues to support the appropriate diagnosis and provide a more positive outcome for the patient. What can you do to improve your knowledge and skills to support the care of the patient?

SUMMARY

Nurses play a vital role in the health and quality of life outcomes for older people. This chapter has discussed the ageing population in Australia, factors involved in ageing and the related pathophysiology, gerontological nursing, patient-centred care and the clinical reasoning cycle and national and nursing practice standards. Care of the older person is a speciality and requires advanced knowledge and skills. Older people require assistance with their daily living activities, and aged care nurses understand the importance of patient-centred care. Both the patient and their family are encouraged to take an active role in their care, treatment and daily living plans. Gerontology nurses can adapt therapeutic communication skills to fit their patients' needs and communicate professionally with other healthcare providers to ensure that the older person receives optimum care. The gerontology nurse will be able to apply the clinical reasoning cycle to assess, plan care and detect changes in the status of the older person. Caring for the older person is a rewarding specialty and a field where the demand is growing daily.

KEY TERMS

activities of daily living (ADL) The basic ADL include ambulating, feeding, dressing, personal hygiene, continence and toileting.

aged care The support provided to the older person needing help to run their own home or who can no longer live at home and need a supportive residence.

ageism The stereotyping, prejudice and discrimination towards people based on age.

biological age A measure of how well or poorly a person's body is functioning relative to their actual calendar age and considers many lifestyle factors (also referred to as physiological age).

chronological age A person's age in years.

geriatrics The branch of medicine used to develop strategies and programs that support the appropriate care of older people.

gerontology The study of the physical, mental and social changes that are part of the ageing process.

LGBTIQ+ Lesbian, gay, bisexual, transgender, intersex, queer or questioning.

polypharmacy The use of multiple medications, more than are medically necessary.

psychological age The age a person feels and acts.

REFERENCES

Aged Care Quality and Safety Commission. (2020) Quality Standards. Australian Goverment. www.agedcarequality.gov.au/providers/standards

American Heart Association (AHA). (2020) Pulmonary Hypertension — High Blood Pressure in the Heart-to-Lung System. www.heart.org/en/health-topics/high-blood-pressure/the-facts-about-high-blood-pressure/pulmonary-hypertension-high-blood-pressure-in-the-heart-to-lung-system

Andrade, M. & Knight, J. (2017) Anatomy and physiology of ageing 4: the renal system. *Nursing Times* [online]. 113(5): 46–49. www.nursingtimes.net/roles/older people-nurses-roles/anatomy-and-physiology-of-ageing-4-the-renal-system-02-05-2017

Australian College of Nursing (ACN). (2019) *The role of nurses in promoting healthy ageing — Position Statement.* Canberra: ACN. www.acn.edu.au/wp-content/uploads/position-statement-role-nurse-in-promoting-healthy-ageing.pdf

Australian Commission on Safety and Quality in Health Care (ACSQHC). (2019) Medication Safety. www.safetyandquality.gov.au/our-work/medication-safety

Australian Government Australian Law Reform Commission. (2017) *Elder Abuse — A National Legal Response (ALRC Report 131).* www.alrc.gov.au/publication/elder-abuse-a-national-legal-response-alrc-report-131

Australian Government, Department of Health. (2020) The nervous system. www.healthdirect.gov.au/nervous- system

Australian Institute of Health and Welfare (AIHW). (2018) Older Australians at a glance. www.aihw.gov.au/reports/older-people/older-australia-at-a-glance/contents/demographics-of-older-australians/australia-s-changing-age-and-gender-profile

Baker, L. & Gringart, E. (2009) Body image and self-esteem in older adulthood. *Ageing and Society.* 29(6): 977–995. doi: 10.1017/S0144686X09008721

Bennett, E. V., Hurd, L. C., Pritchard, E. M., Colton, T. & Crocker, P. R. E. (2020) An examination of older men's body image: How men 65 years and older perceive, experience, and cope with their aging bodies. *Body Image.* 34: 27–37. doi: https://doi.org/10.1016/j.bodyim.2020.04.005

Bewick, T. (2016) Nurses can make a difference: caring for those living with dementia. *Australian Journal of Dementia Care.* https://journalofdementiacare.com/nurses-can-make-a-difference-caring-for-those-living-with-dementia

Cameron, E., Ward, P., Mandville-Anstey, S. A. & Coombs, A. (2019) The female aging body: A systematic review of female perspectives on aging, health, and body image. *Journal of Women & Aging.* 31(1): 3–17. doi: 10.1080/08952841.2018.1449586

Chinniah, N. & Gupta, M. (2014) Pruritus in the elderly — a guide to assessment and management. *Australian Family Physician.* 43: 710–713. www.racgp.org.au/afp/2014/october/pruritus-in-the-elderly---a-guide-to-assessment-and-management

Cleveland Clinic. (2020) The Structure and Function of the Digestive System. https://my.clevelandclinic.org/health/articles/7041-the-structure-and-function-of-the-digestive-system

COTA. (2020) Ageism and Discrimination. www.cota.org.au/policy/ageism-and-discrimination/#:~:text=Ageism%20is%20discrimination%20based%20on,in%20an%20older%20age%20group

Dementia Australia. (2020a) Dementia statistics. www.dementia.org.au/statistics?gclid=Cj0KCQiAlZH_BRCgARIsAAZHSBkx3UGHJpHVczokc0FookwsWxwsKgF3OhJ1KZ41AFU3MLcc0pvOpycaArPYEALw_wcB

Dementia Australia. (2020b). What is good care? www.dementia.org.au/support-and-services/families-and-friends/residential-care/what-is-good-care

Department of Health & Human Services, S. G. o. V., Australia. (2020a) Patient-centred care explained. *Better Health Channel.* www.betterhealth.vic.gov.au/health/ServicesAndSupport/patient-centred-care-explained

Department of Health & Human Services, S. G. o. V., Australia. (2020b) Ageing — muscles bones and joints. *Better Health Channel.* www.betterhealth.vic.gov.au/health/conditionsandtreatments/ageing-muscles-bones-and-joints#:~:text=Age%2Drelated%20changes%20in%20muscle,-Muscle%20loses%20size&text=Muscle%20fibres%20reduce%20in%20number,tone%20and%20ability%20to%20contract

Durham, B. (2015) The nurse's role in medication safety. *Nursing.* 45(4). doi: 10.1097/01.NURSE.0000461850.24153.8b

European Heart Association. (2018) The Clinical Reasoning Cycle: The 8 Phases and their Significance. www.heartassociation.eu/the-clinical-reasoning-cycle-the-8-phases-and-their-significance

Fleming, M. O. & Haney, T. T. (2013) An imperative: patient-centered care for our aging population. *Ochsner Journal.* 13(2): 190–193. www.ncbi.nlm.nih.gov/pmc/articles/PMC3684326

Healthdirect. (n.d.) Nervous system. Australian Government. www.healthdirect.gov.au/nervous-system

Hicks, K. (2018) The Importance of Respiratory Health in Seniors. www.aplaceformom.com/caregiver-resources/articles/respiratory-health

Johns Hopkins Medicine. (2020) Anatomy of the Urinary System. www.hopkinsmedicine.org/health/wellness-and-prevention/anatomy-of-the-urinary-system

Kaufman, J. M., Lapauw, B., Mahmoud, A., T'Sjoen, G. & Huhtaniemi, I. T. (2019) Aging and the male reproductive system. *Endocrine Reviews.* 40(4): 906–972. doi: 10.1210/er.2018-00178

Knight, J., Hore, N. & Nigam, Y. (2017) Anatomy and physiology of ageing 10: the musculoskeletal system. *Nursing Times* [online]. 113(11): 60–63.

Knight, J., Wigham, C. & Nigam, Y. (2017) Anatomy and physiology of ageing 6: the eyes and ears. *Nursing Times* [online]. 113(7): 39–42. www.nursingtimes.net/roles/older-people-nurses-roles/anatomy-and-physiology-of-ageing-6-the-eyes-and-ears-26-06-2017/?storycode=7019071&hash=888b49a0b39f8490851918756f4c301d

Knight, J. & Nigam, Y. (2017a) Anatomy and physiology of ageing 1: the cardiovascular system. *Nursing Times* [online]. 113(2): 22–4. www.nursingtimes.net/roles/older-people-nurses-roles/anatomy-and-physiology-of-ageing-1-the-cardiovascular-system-31-01-2017

Knight, J. & Nigam, Y. (2017b) Anatomy and physiology of ageing 2: the respiratory system. *Nursing Times* [online]. 113(3): 53–55. www.nursingtimes.net/roles/older-people-nurses-roles/anatomy-and-physiology-of-ageing-2-the-respiratory-system-2-27-02-2017

Knight, J. & Nigam, Y. (2017c) Anatomy and physiology of ageing 5: the nervous system. *Nursing Times* [online]. 113(6): 55–58. www.nursingtimes.net/roles/older-people-nurses-roles/anatomy-and-physiology-of-ageing-5-the-nervous-system-30-05-2017

Knight, J. & Nigam, Y. (2017d) Anatomy and physiology of ageing 7: the endocrine system. *Nursing Times* [online]. 113(8): 48–51. www.nursingtimes.net/roles/older-people-nurses-roles/anatomy-and-physiology-of-ageing-7-the-endocrine-system-31-07-2017

Knight, J. & Nigam, Y. (2017e) Anatomy and physiology of ageing 8: the reproductive system. *Nursing Times* [online]. 113(9): [illegible]–47. https://emap.com/wp-content/uploads/sites/3/2017/08/170830-Anatomy-and-physiology-of-ageing-8-the-reproductive-system.pdf

Legalvision. (2017) What is a living will? https://legalvision.com.au/what-is-a-living-will

[illegible], G. (2019) 'Aging Definition'. In D. Gu & M. E. Dupre (Eds.). *Encyclopedia of Gerontology and Population Aging* (pp. 1–10). Cham: Springer International Publishing.

Levett-Jones, T. (Ed.). (2013) *Clinical reasoning: Learning to think like a nurse.* Pearson Australia.

Madigan, N. (2018) Nursing the elderly — more than just another role. *Health Times.* https://healthtimes.com.au/hub/aged-care/2/practice/nm/nursing-the-elderly-more-than-just-another-role/3357

Maher, R. L., Hanlon, J. & Hajjar, E. R. (2014) Clinical consequences of polypharmacy in elderly. *Expert Opinion on Drug Safety.* 13(1): 57–65. doi: 10.1517/14740338.2013.827660

Merck Sharp & Dohme Corp. (2020) Overview of aging. *Older peoples health issues.* www.msdmanuals.com/home/older-people%E2%80%99s-health-issues/the-aging-body/overview-of-aging

Midlarsky, E. et al. (2017) 'Body image and aging'. In K. L. Nadal (Ed.). *The SAGE Encyclopedia of Psychology and Gender.* SAGE Publications, Inc.

Montecino-Rodriguez, E., Berent-Maoz, B. & Dorshkind, K. (2013) Causes, consequences, and reversal of immune system aging. *The Journal of Clinical Investigation.* 123(3): 958–965. doi: 10.1172/JCI64096

Morley, J. E. (2019) Effects of Aging on the Endocrine System. *MSD Manual.* www.msdmanuals.com/en-au/home/hormonal-and-metabolic-disorders/biology-of-the-endocrine-system/effects-of-aging-on-the-endocrine-system

Nikolich-Žugich, J. (2014) Aging of the T cell compartment in mice and humans: From no naive expectations to foggy memories. *Journal of Immunology.* 193(6): 2622–2629. doi: https://doi.org/10.4049/jimmunol.1401174

Nigam, Y. & Knight, J. (2017a) Anatomy and physiology of ageing 9: the immune system. *Nursing Times* [online]. 113(10): 42–45. www.nursingtimes.net/roles/older-people-nurses-roles/anatomy-and-physiology-of-ageing-9-the-immune-system-21-09-2017

Nigam, Y. & Knight, J. (2017b) Anatomy and physiology of ageing 3: the digestive system. *Nursing Times* [online]. 113(4): 54–57. www.nursingtimes.net/roles/older-people-nurses-roles/anatomy-and-physiology-of-ageing-3-the-digestive-system-27-03-2017

Nigam, Y. & Knight, J. (2017c) Anatomy and physiology of ageing 11: the skin. *Nursing Times* [online]. 113(12): 51–55. www.nursingtimes.net/roles/older-people-nurses-roles/anatomy-and-physiology-of-ageing-2-the-respiratory-system-2-27-02-2017

Nursing and Midwifery Board. (2017) Registered nurse standards for practice, www.nursingmidwiferyboard.gov.au/Codes-Guidelines-Statements/Professional-standards/registered-nurse-standards-for-practice.aspx

Officer, L. & de la Fuente-Núñez, V. (2018) A global campaign to combat ageism. *Bulletin of the World Health Organization*. WHO. www.who.int/bulletin/volumes/96/4/17-202424/en

Parulekar, M. S. & Rogers, C. K. (2018) Polypharmacy and Mobility. *Geriatric Rehabilitation*. www.sciencedirect.com/topics/medicine-and-dentistry/polypharmacy

Petiprin, A. (2020) Roper-Logan-Tierney's Model for Nursing Based on a Model of Living. *Nursing Theory*. www.nursing-theory.org/theories-and-models/roper-model-for-nursing-based-on-a-model-of-living.php

Philp, I. T. K., Hildon, Z. S., Aw, Jeon, Y. -H., Naegle, M., Michel, J. -P., Namara, A., Wang, N. & Hardman, M. (2017) Person-centred assessment to integrate care for older people. WHO. www.who.int/ageing/health-systems/icope/icope-consultation/ICOPE-Global-Consultation-Background-Paper-2.pdf

Pond, C. D. & Regan, C. (2019) Improving the delivery of primary care for older people. *Medical Journal of Australia*. 211(2): 60–62. doi: 10.5694/mja2.50236

Services NSW. (n.d.) Make an Advance Care Directive (living will). www.service.nsw.gov.au/transaction/make-advance-care-directive-living-will

Sheets, D. J. & Whittington, F. J. (2012) Gerontological Nursing: Developing the Art and Science. *The Gerontologist*. 52(6): 876–879. doi: https://doi.org/10.1093/geront/gns132

Smeulers, M., Verweij, L., Maaskant, J. M., de Boer, M., Krediet, C. T. P., Nieveen van Dijkum, E. J. M. & Vermeulen, H. (2015) Quality indicators for safe medication preparation and administration: a systematic review. *PloS one*. 10(4): e0122695–e0122695. doi: 10.1371/journal.pone.0122695

Terhune, K. P., Weavind, L. & Pandharipande, P. P. (2010) '78 — How Does One Prevent, Diagnose, and Treat Delirium in the Intensive Care Unit?' In C. S. Deutschman & P. J. Neligan (Eds.). *Evidence-Based Practice of Critical Care* (pp. 553–560). Philadelphia: W.B. Saunders.

The Royal Australian College of General Practitioners (RACGP). (2019) Physiology of ageing. *RACGP aged care clinical guide (Silver Book)*. www.racgp.org.au/clinical-resources/clinical-guidelines/key-racgp-guidelines/view-all-racgp-guidelines/silver-book/silver-book-part-b/physiology-of-ageing

The Royal Australian College of General Practitioners (RACGP). (2020) Poly-Pharmacy. www.racgp.org.au/clinical-resources/clinical-guidelines/key-racgp-guidelines/view-all-racgp-guidelines/silver-book/part-a/polypharmacy

Tortora, G. J. & Derrickson, B. (2011) *Principles of Anatomy and Physiology*. Danvers, MA: Wiley Blackwell.

Tortora, G. et al. (2022) *Principles of Anatomy & Physiology*, 2nd Asia –Pacific ed. John Wiley and Sons Ltd.

U.S. Department of Health and Human Services. (2020) Aging changes in the senses. *MedlinePlus*. https://medlineplus.gov/ency/article/004013.htm

U.S. Department of Health and Human Services. (2020a) Aging changes in immunity. *MedlinePlus*. https://medlineplus.gov/ency/article/004008.htm

U.S. Department of Health and Human Services. (2020b) Aging changes in the bones — muscles — joints. *MedlinePlus*. https://medlineplus.gov/ency/article/004015.htm

U.S. Department of Health and Human Services. (2020c) Aging changes in the female reproductive system. *MedlinePlus*. https://medlineplus.gov/ency/article/004016.htm

U.S. Department of Health and Human Services. (2020d) Aging changes in the kidneys and bladder. *MedlinePlus*. https://medlineplus.gov/ency/article/004010.htm

United Nations Department of Economic and Social Affairs, Population Division. (2019) World Population Prospects 2019. https://population.un.org/wpp/Download/Standard/Population

United Nations. (2020) Ageing. Peace, dignity, and equality on a healthy planet. www.un.org/en/sections/issues-depth/ageing

University of Sydney, i. C. w. t. A. D. N. a. N. M. (2018) *Quality Use of Medicines to Optimise Ageing in Older Australians: Recommendations for a National Strategic Action Plan to Reduce Inappropriate Polypharmacy*. Sydney, NSW. http://sydney.edu.au/medicine/cdpc/resources/quality-use-of-medicines.pdf

van den Beld, A. W., Kaufman, J. M., Zillikens, M. C., Lamberts, S. W. J., Egan, J. M. & van der Lely, A. J. (2018) The physiology of endocrine systems with ageing. *Lancet Diabetes Endocrinololgy*. 6(8): 647–658. doi: 10.1016/S2213-8587(18)30026-3

Winterbottom, F. (n.d.) The older adult patient. https://nursekey.com/the-older-adult-patient

World Health Organization (WHO). (2020a) Ageing and health. www.who.int/news-room/fact-sheets/detail/ageing-and-health

World Health Organization (WHO). (2020b) Corona virus. www.who.int/health-topics/coronavirus#tab=tab_1

World Health Organization (WHO). (2020c) The decade of healthy ageing: a new UN-wide initiative.

World Health Organization (WHO). (2020d) Elder abuse. www.who.int/news-room/fact-sheets/detail/elder-abuse

World Health Organization (WHO). (2020e) Elder abuse, what is elder abuse. www.who.int/ageing/projects/elder_abuse/en

World Health Organization, West Pacific Region (WHO). (2020) Ageing: ageism. www.who.int/westernpacific/news/q-a-detail/ageing-ageism

ACKNOWLEDGEMENTS

Figure 7.1: Flaatten, H., Skaar, E. & Joynt, G. M. Understanding cardiovascular physiology of ageing. *Intensive Care Med 44*, 932–935 (2018). https://doi.org/10.1007/s00134-018-5119-7

Figure 7.3: © Knight, J. & Nigam, Y. (2017) Anatomy and physiology of ageing 5: the nervous system. *Nursing Times* [online]; 113: 6, 55–58. © EMAP Publishing Ltd. Reproduced with permission of EMAP Publishing Ltd.

Figure 7.4: Tortora, G. J. et al., *Principles of Anatomy and Physiology*, 3rd Asia–Pacific Edition, Figure 18.1, 2021. John Wiley & Sons Inc.

Figure 7.5: © Knight, J. & Nigam, Y. (2017) Anatomy and physiology of ageing 8: the reproductive system. *Nursing Times* [online]; 113: 9, 44–47. © EMAP Publishing Ltd. Reproduced with permission of EMAP Publishing Ltd.

Figure 7.6: © Knight, J. & Nigam, Y. (2017) Anatomy and physiology of ageing 8: the reproductive system. *Nursing Times* [online]; 113: 9, 44–47. © EMAP Publishing Ltd. Reproduced with permission of EMAP Publishing Ltd.

Figure 7.7: © Tortora, G. J. et. al., *Principles of Anatomy and Physiology*, 2nd Asia–Pacific Edition, figure 24.1, 2018. © John Wiley & Sons Inc. Reproduced with permission of John Wiley & Sons Inc.

Figure 7.8: Nigam, Y. & Knight, J. (2017) Anatomy and physiology of ageing 4: the renal system. *Nursing Times* [online]; 113: 5, 46–49. © EMAP Publishing Ltd. Reproduced with permission of EMAP Publishing Ltd.

Figure 7.9: © Nigam, Y. & Knight, J. (2017) Anatomy and physiology of ageing 6: the eyes and ears. *Nursing Times* [online]; 113: 7, 39–42. © EMAP Publishing Ltd. Reproduced with permission of EMAP Publishing Ltd.

Figure 7.10: © Nigam, Y. & Knight, J. (2017) Anatomy and physiology of ageing 6: the eyes and ears. *Nursing Times* [online]; 113: 7, 39–42. © EMAP Publishing Ltd. Reproduced with permission of EMAP Publishing Ltd.

Figure 7.12: © Knight, J. et al. (2017). Anatomy and physiology of ageing 11: the skin. *Nursing Times* [online]; 113: 12, 51–55. © EMAP Publishing Ltd. Reproduced with permission of EMAP Publishing Ltd.

Table 7.3: © Knight, J. & Nigam, Y. (2017) Anatomy and physiology of ageing 5: the nervous system. *Nursing Times* [online]; 113: 6, 55–58.

Table 7.4: © Knight, J. & Nigam, Y. (2017) Anatomy and physiology of ageing 7: the endocrine system. *Nursing Times* [online]; 113: 8, 48–51.

Table 7.8: © Nigam, Y. & Knight, J. (2017) Anatomy and physiology of ageing 3: the digestive system. *Nursing Times* [online]; 113: 4, 54–57.

Table 7.10: © Nigam, Y. & Knight, J. (2017) Anatomy and physiology of ageing 6: the eyes and ears. *Nursing Times* [online]; 113: 7, 39–42.

Table 7.11: © Nigam, Y. & Knight, J. (2017) Anatomy and physiology of ageing 6: the eyes and ears. *Nursing Times* [online]; 113: 7, 39–42.

Table 7.12: © Knight, J. et al. (2017). Anatomy and physiology of ageing 10: the musculoskeletal system. *Nursing Times* [online]; 113: 11, 60–63.

Table 7.13: © Knight, J. et al. (2017). Anatomy and physiology of ageing 11: the skin. *Nursing Times* [online]; 113: 12, 51–55.

Photo 7A: pikselstock / Shutterstock.com

Photo 7B: Rawpixel.com / Shutterstock.com

CHAPTER 8

Principles of end-of-life care

LEARNING OBJECTIVES

After studying this chapter, you should be able to:

8.1 discuss the aetiology and epidemiology of death and dying specific to Australia

8.2 review the pathophysiology of death and dying and relate the pathophysiology to major physical and psychological symptoms people face towards the end of life

8.3 discuss the nature of dying and the treatment goals and expectations of palliative and end-of-life care

8.4 consider palliative and end-of-life care for specific groups in Australian society

8.5 review the principles of palliative care and the role of nurses in palliative and end-of-life care

8.6 apply the clinical reasoning cycle and patient-centred care to palliative and end-of-life patients

8.7 identify self-care strategies for nurses to help reduce the physical and psychological stressors related to palliative and end-of-life care.

Introduction

Dying and death are inevitable chapters in all our lives (Oates 2020). We must all have access to care and support when entering this final phase of life. Palliative and **end-of-life care** are to help patients through the stages of life-limiting or life-threatening illnesses with support and empathy (Department of Health & Human Services 2017). Palliative and end-of-life care help manage the symptoms of the disease process and provide comfort and assistance with activities of daily living for the patient and their families, including their emotional, mental, spiritual and social needs. They are based on needs, not the diagnosis. As healthcare providers, we must understand that the end of life is different for everyone, and needs will differ for each patient and their family. We must be prepared to provide care and support that respects the patient's and their family's dignity, privacy, confidentiality and autonomous wishes. It is also essential to understand that death and dying as well as grief affect all age groups, not just the elderly. Elizabeth Kübler-Ross (1975) said, 'Death always has been and always will be with us. It is an integral part of human existence'. While death is a part of living, it brings unique challenges for the dying person and their family. It also brings challenges for the healthcare providers who are caring for the dying person and their families. Understanding the death, dying and grieving process can help us, as nurses, prepare ourselves in supporting people through this difficult time. This chapter will discuss the aetiology and epidemiology of death in Australia, the pathophysiology of death and the nature of dying. We will discuss palliative care and palliative care nursing principles and end-of-life care for a rich and diverse society such as Australia. We will also look at voluntary assisted dying and the need for mindfulness in palliative and end-of-life care.

8.1 Palliative and end-of-life care

LEARNING OBJECTIVE 8.1 Discuss the aetiology and epidemiology of death and dying specific to Australia.

Palliative care is defined as 'the provision of physical, emotional and spiritual care for patients with life-limiting illnesses, and their families' (Palliative Care Nurses Australia 2020). It is patient and family-centred care provided to a patient experiencing advanced disease for which there is little or no prospect of cure (Australian College of Nursing 2019). The palliative patient is expected to die. Hence, the overriding goal is supporting the best possible quality of life with various physical, social and psychological supports that recognise each patient's individual needs.

End-of-life care is required for the last few weeks of life (Australian College of Nursing 2019). The patient with an active, progressive, advanced disease with little or no prospect of cure, is rapidly approaching death. The needs of patients, their families and carers are increased during this period. End-of-life care ensures quality, coordinated support across the healthcare team. This type of care includes the terminal phase and extends to bereavement care.

Palliative Care Australia is the national body that supports palliative care in Australia (Palliative Care Australia 2019). Palliative Care Australia works with patients, their families, carers and healthcare professional to provide leadership on palliative care policy and community engagement. Palliative Care Australia strives to improve the quality of palliative and end-of-life care for all Australians.

Aetiology and epidemiology

According to the Australian Institute of Health and Welfare (AIHW) coronary heart disease is the leading underlying cause of death in Australia (ANMJ Staff 2020). The second leading cause is dementia, which includes Alzheimer's disease. The top five leading causes of death in Australia in 2018, for males and females across the age range, are cerebrovascular disease, which includes stroke, lung cancer and chronic obstructive pulmonary disease (COPD) (see figures 8.1 and 8.2). There is no standardised method for grouping causes of death; however, the AIHW follows the World Health Organization (WHO) recommendations, making minor modifications to meet the needs of the Australian perspective. Currently, figures are collected for male and female genders only; however, it is expected that future statistics will include other gender identities such as non-binary and transgender groups.

In Australia, death rates have been declining since the early 1900s, falling by 73 per cent between 1907 and 2018 for males and 77 per cent for females. This is due to a reduction of infant and child deaths and an improved life expectancy from birth. A boy born in 2016–2018 will live to 80.7 years, and a girl will live to 84.9 years (AIHW 2020). Prior to the 1900s, the leading causes of death were infectious and circulatory system diseases. As our population ages, dementia (including

Alzheimer's disease), cardiovascular diseases and other chronic conditions, including cancers, are becoming the more likely causes of death.

FIGURE 8.1 Leading underlying causes of death by gender, 2018

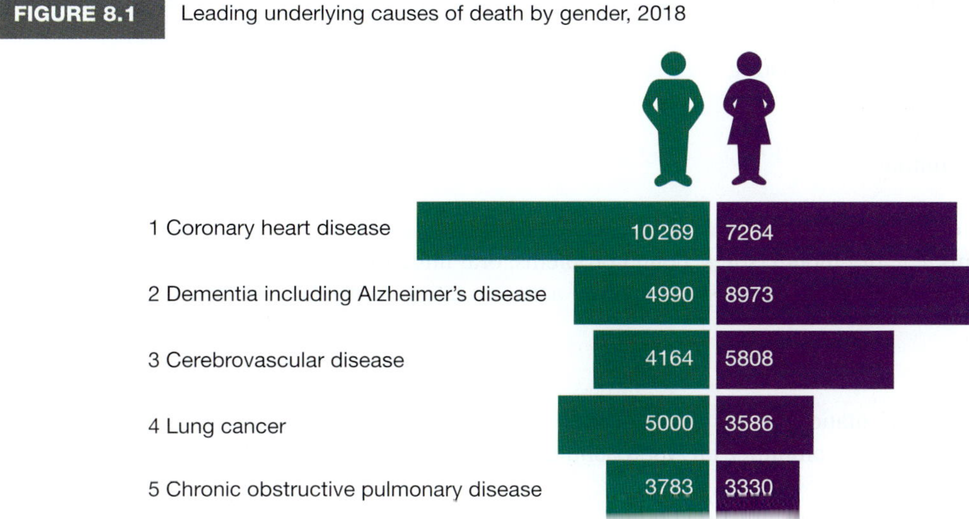

Source: AIHW National Mortality Database (2020).

FIGURE 8.2 Leading causes of death by age group, 2016–18

Age group	1st	2nd	3rd	4th	5th
Under 1	Perinatal and congenital conditions	Other ill-defined causes	Sudden infant death syndrome	Accidental threats to breathing	Cardiomyopathy
1–14	Land transport accidents	Perinatal and congenital conditions	Brain cancer	Accidental drowning and submersion	Suicide
15–24	Suicide	Land transport accidents	Accidental poisoning	Assault	Other ill-defined causes
25–44	Suicide	Accidental poisoning	Land transport accidents	Coronary heart disease	Breast cancer
45–64	Coronary heart disease	Lung cancer	Suicide	Colorectal cancer	Breast cancer
65–74	Lung cancer	Coronary heart disease	COPD	Colorectal cancer	Cerebrovascular disease
75–84	Coronary heart disease	Dementia including Alzheimer's disease	Cerebrovascular disease	Lung cancer	COPD
85 and over	Dementia including Alzheimer's disease	Coronary heart disease	Cerebrovascular disease	COPD	Influenza and pneumonia

Source: AIHW National Mortality Database (2020).

8.2 Pathophysiology

LEARNING OBJECTIVE 8.2 Review the pathophysiology of death and dying and relate the pathophysiology to major physical and psychological symptoms people face towards the end of life.

A natural death is defined as a death in which no medical, life-saving interventions have been enacted to affect the dying process (Oates 2020). Most patients who experience a natural death follow a conventional pattern of signs and symptoms leading to their death. It is important for healthcare providers to be aware of and to understand this process so we know what to expect when providing care to our patients, and so we can support their family in understanding what is happening and assist them through this period. The timeline varies for each patient. For some, their signs and symptoms may take place over 24 hours, while others may go on for several weeks. Some of the major physical and psychological symptoms people face towards the end of life are:

- pain
- reduced appetite and body wasting
- weakness and fatigue
- dyspnoea and cough
- nausea and vomiting
- dysphagia
- constipation or diarrhoea
- oral symptoms, e.g. dry mouth, sores, dental problems, oral infections
- skin symptoms, e.g. itching, dryness, chapping, acne, sweating, sensitivity to touch, pressure sores, dark spots
- lymphedema
- abdominal ascites
- confusion and disorientation
- anxiety and depression (Committee on Approaching Death: Addressing Key End of Life Issues; Institute of Medicine 2015).

These signs and symptoms can be broken into stages: early, mid- and late-stage end of life.

1. *Early stage.*
   - In the early stages of dying, there is a loss of mobility, and the patient becomes bedbound.
   - They lose interest in and the ability to drink and eat.
   - We also see an increase in sleep.
   - The patient may experience delirium, which is an acute change in the patient's level of arousal. This can be demonstrated by either a hyperactive or agitated state or a hypoactive and listless state.
   - Patients will need increased support with their activities of daily living in respect to hygiene and elimination.
2. *Middle stage.*
   - There is a further decline in mental status. The patient is slow to arouse; they have brief periods of wakefulness.
   - Respiration becomes noisy — called the 'death rattle'. This is due to a change in breathing pattern, a loss of the swallow reflex and pooling of oral secretions.
3. *Late stage.*
   - The patient falls into a comatose state.
   - They may experience a fever due to aspiration pneumonia.
   - An altered respiratory pattern known as chain stokes typified by periods of apnoea alternated with hyperpnea or irregular breathing.
   - They will have mottled extremities due to the constriction of the peripheral circulation (Oates 2020; Rudrappa 2020).

8.3 The nature of dying

LEARNING OBJECTIVE 8.3 Discuss the nature of dying and the treatment goals and expectations of palliative and end-of-life care.

Death and dying are part of life and living. In dying, there is a cascade of events that lead ultimately to death (ER services n.d.). As nurses looking after the dying patient, we continue to provide the safe, effective care we have always provided. Understanding death and dying and the grieving process (or **grief cycle**) will help us to provide that care. The five stages of grief — denial, anger, bargaining, depression and acceptance — are part of a framework that supports our understanding and making us better equipped as healthcare professional to deal with life and loss (Kessler n.d.). We need to use this framework like we do all others and understand that the process of death and dying and the grief involved is an individual experience, and our focus will be on the individual and their families.

Death, dying and grief

Swiss psychiatrist Elisabeth Kübler-Ross, was a pioneer in understanding the process of death, dying and grief (Gregory 2020). Kübler-Ross worked with terminally ill patients and established a framework for the grieving process. Kübler-Ross's work has received criticism because it was mistakenly interpreted that all people go through every stage and in the same order. It is important to note that these stages are not linear. Some people may not experience any of them, while others may experience all of them. Some people will also experience some of the stages of the cycle repeatedly. The framework's importance to healthcare providers is to help us understand what the patient and their family are going through to better support them in managing their grief. As healthcare providers, educating our patients and families about death is challenging (Roth, Mammen, Keil, Schildknecht & Latoschik 2019). The persons facing death are experiencing a difficult and stressful situation. The more we understand the experience, the more helpful we can be to our patients and their families.

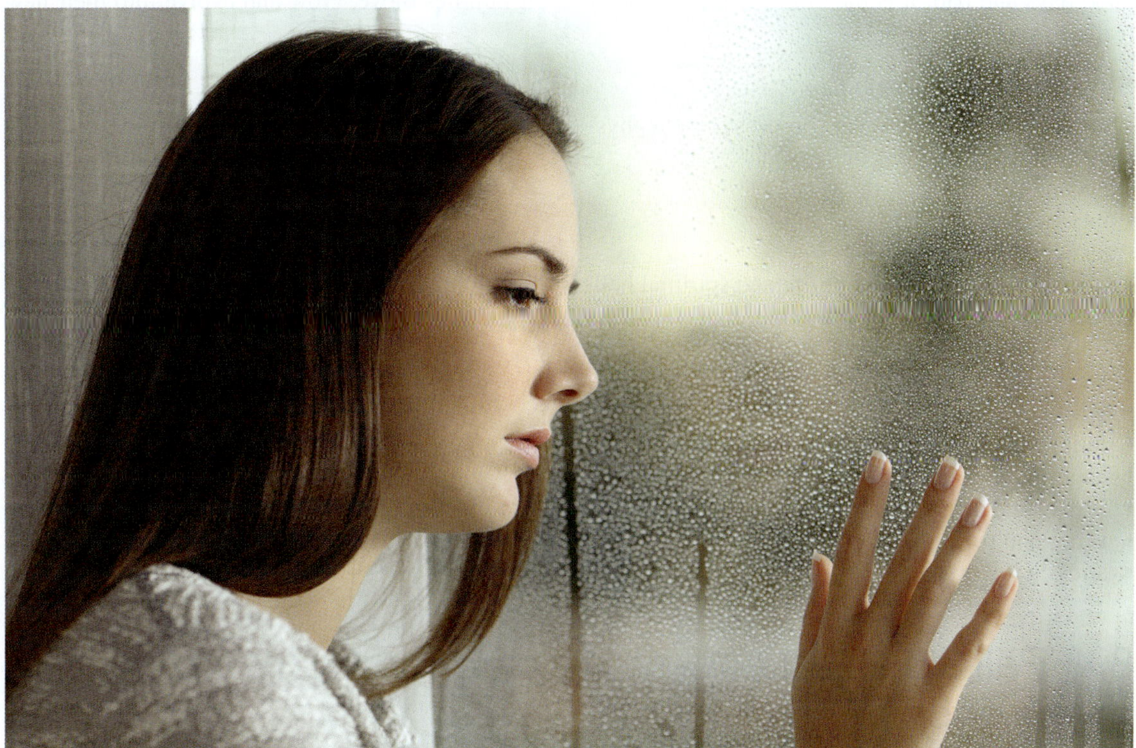

Denial

Denial is the stage when the information is denied, and many people just feel numb. People or the family of people diagnosed with a terminal disease may not believe it — someone has made a mistake (Gregory 2020, Kessler n.d.). Denial aids in pacing those intense feelings of grief. Instead of becoming completely overwhelmed, Denial helps to cushion the shock. Once the denial and shock begin to fade, the healing process can begin.

Anger

Anger is a typical stage in which the patient thinks, 'Why me? What have I done to deserve this?' (Gregory 2020). The anger may be directed at friends and family or even at the healthcare provider. Researchers and mental healthcare professionals concur that anger is a necessary stage of grief. They agree that the more the patient feels anger, the more quickly it will dissipate, and quicker they can move forward. While we are normally advised to control our anger, in the grieving stage, anger is a strength to connect the patient to the reality of the situation and an important and natural step in healing.

Bargaining

Bargaining is false hope, the patient and their family believe that they can avoid the grief through negotiation (Gregory 2020; Kessler n.d.), e.g. 'If this is not true, I promise I will be the best person I can be'. The patient and their loved ones want life back to what they knew before the grief event and negotiate to make significant life changes to reverse the diagnosis and return to the normality they knew. Guilt is a common part of the bargaining process, 'What if we had done this differently than the event would not have happened?'.

Depression

Depression has a strong association with and is a commonly accepted form of grief (Gregory 2020; Kessler n.d.). In this stage, the patient and their families will feel numb and want to withdraw. They may find it challenging to get out of bed. The patient and their families may experience suicidal thoughts during this stage.

Acceptance

The final stage of grief is acceptance (Gregory 2020; Kessler n.d.). Acceptance requires coming to terms with the new reality. It is a time of adjustment and readjustment. The patient and their families experience good days and bad. It is the time when patients and their families move, grow and evolve into their new reality.

Symptoms of grief

The symptoms of the grieving process present physically, socially or spiritually. Some of the most common signs and symptoms of grief are:
- crying
- headaches
- sleeping difficulties
- questioning the purpose of life and spiritual beliefs
- feelings of detachment and isolation from friends and family
- out of character behaviour
- worry, anxiety, frustration
- guilt
- fatigue
- anger
- loss of appetite
- aches and pains
- stress (Gregory 2020).

8.4 Palliative and end-of-life care for a rich and diverse society

LEARNING OBJECTIVE 8.4 Consider palliative and end-of-life care for specific groups in Australian society.

Culture and ethnicity make strong contributions to differences in attitudes, preferences, behaviours, perceptions and experiences in palliative and end-of-life care (American Psychological Association 2021). The age group, race, disability status, sexual orientation, gender identity, socioeconomic status, education, health status, geographic location, immigration status and religion all influence how the individual and their families approach death and dying and their expectations of the care provided at this time.

Aboriginal and Torres Strait Islander peoples

Death is a confronting certainty of life, and it varies in meaning between cultures. When we provide patient and family-centred care for our Aboriginal and Torres Strait Islander peoples, we must recognise and respect the cultural differences important to the Aboriginal and Torres Strait Islander people (Health-InfoNet n.d.). This is essential in providing safe and effective care in those final stages of life. Due to the spiritual belief of the life cycle, 'passing' is the more accepted and culturally sensitive terminology when discussing death and dying with Aboriginal and Torres Strait Islander peoples (Queensland Health 2015). We must ask our patient whom they would like to involve in discussions about their healthcare (HealthInfoNet n.d.). There may be important decision makers or spokespersons in their community who should be involved in all healthcare discussions. Aboriginal and Torres Strait Islander peoples often have customary practices before, during and after death. Such practices may be sacred and not discussed outside of the community. Requests for traditional medicine or room for multiple visitors and overnight guests need to be recognised as they are culturally significant to this group (Palliative Care Australia 2018).

Supporting people to observe their traditions at the end of someone's life can assist the person with a life-limiting illness and help their family and community with their grief and bereavement. The time surrounding the end of life is precious. Healthcare providers need to respect this and understand that there will be cultural needs that they are not aware of and that they need to approach this in a safe, responsive and culturally appropriate manner.

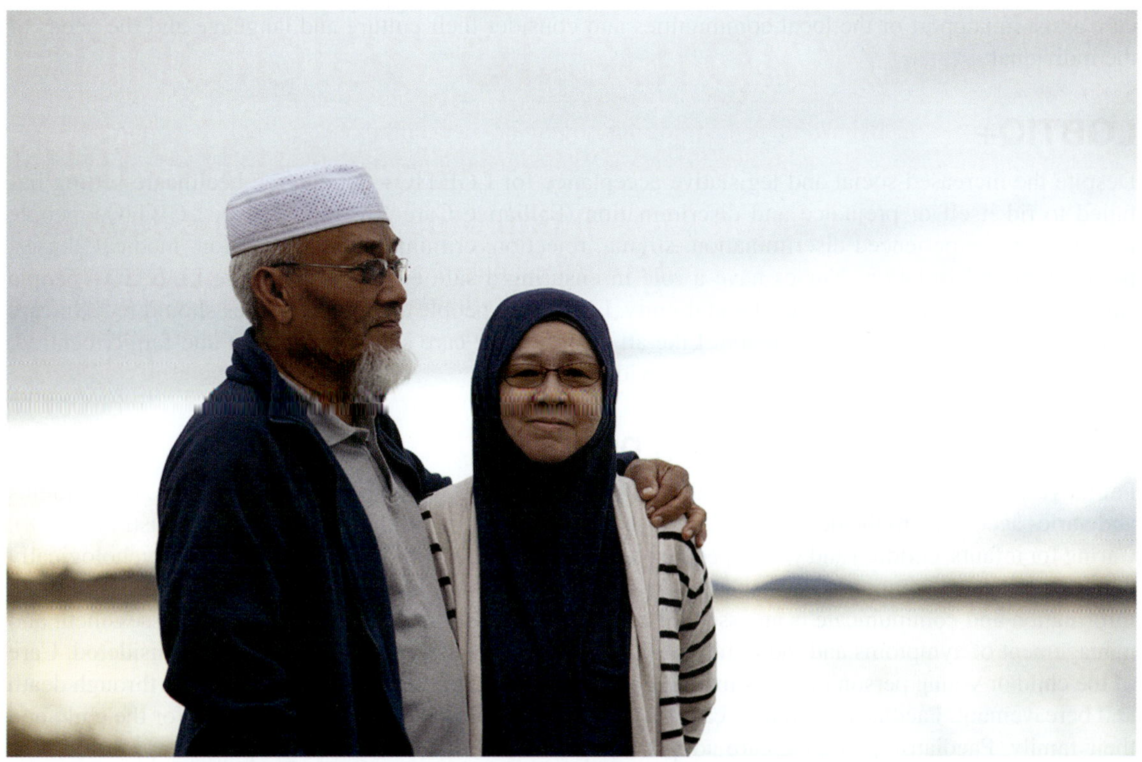

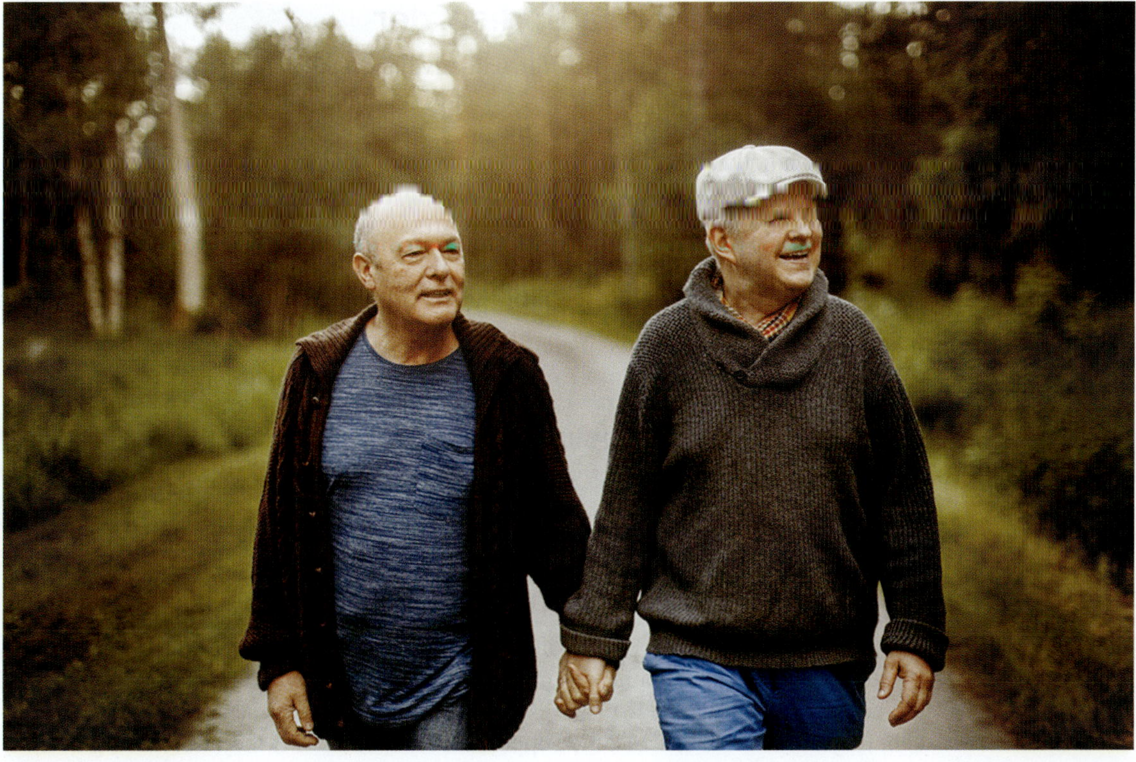

Culturally and linguistically diverse communities

Australia is a culturally and linguistically diverse nation. Quality end-of-life care must be culturally sensitive and recognise that each individual situation and expectations regarding decision-making and type of care will depend on a patient's cultural background(Palliative Care Australia 2018). As healthcare professionals, we need to ensure that our patients are familiar with the concepts of palliative care services available to them in Australia, including access to interpreters and spiritual leaders. Flexible models of care assist in support of the local communities and consider their culture and language and the needs of the individual.

LGBTIQ+

Despite the increased social and legislative acceptance for LGBTIQ+ people, the healthcare setting has failed to rid itself of prejudice and discrimination (Palliative Care Australia 2018). LGBTIQ+ people report having experienced discrimination, stigma, rejection, criminalisation, exclusion, medical abuses, persecution and isolation. Nurses have a role in ensuring a safe environment where LGBTIQ+ people can live and die with equity, respect and dignity. LBGTIQ+ people and their families should receive care free from prejudice and discrimination. Like all groups, their care should be patient and family centred, respecting their wishes and meeting their individual needs.

Infants, children and young people

Palliative and end-of-life care for or infants, children and young people differs from care for adult patients and varies according to the developmental stage and range of conditions (Palliative Care Australia 2018). Caring for infants, children and young people requires special skills and is emotionally and psychologically demanding for the family, carers and the healthcare provider. Consideration of how children process information and communicate is an essential aspect of palliative care for this group. Pain assessment and management of symptoms and their ability to participate in decision making need to be considered. Care of the child or young person involves managing symptoms, providing short breaks and care through death and bereavement. Paediatric palliative care focuses on the enhancement of quality of life for the child and their family. Paediatric palliative care adopts a physical, emotional, social and spiritual approach from diagnosis to death and beyond.

People living with a mental health disorder

People living with mental illness have special needs for palliative and end-of-life care (Palliative Care Australia 2018). Diagnosis may not come until late in the end-of-life trajectory out of fear of engaging with healthcare providers. An additional complication is the patient's capacity for making a legal decision. Palliative patients may also have a history of poorly met needs around housing, income, general medical care and social help. The best outcomes are found when partnerships between palliative care and mental health services provide patient and family-centred care for this group.

Persons living with dementia

People living with dementia may struggle to access palliative care (Palliative Care Australia 2018). Because of the lengthy unpredictable course of dementia, there are special challenges with the decision-making capacity and communication needs and wants. These issues increase if the person is culturally linguistically diverse or presents with challenging behaviours. Palliative and end-of-life care for these patients requires close attention to decision-making and delivery of care. As healthcare providers, we need to ensure that the patient and their needs are our primary focus. We need to work as a team with all other healthcare providers to give the best care of the person with dementia.

The older person and palliative and end-of-life care

The older person must be supported to receive high-quality palliative and end-of-life care in the setting of their choice. That setting might be their family home, a residential aged care facility, a hospital or a dedicated hospice service. If the older person lives in residential aged care, it is essential to recognise this as their home. As such, they are entitled to the same support they would have if they were living in their family home.

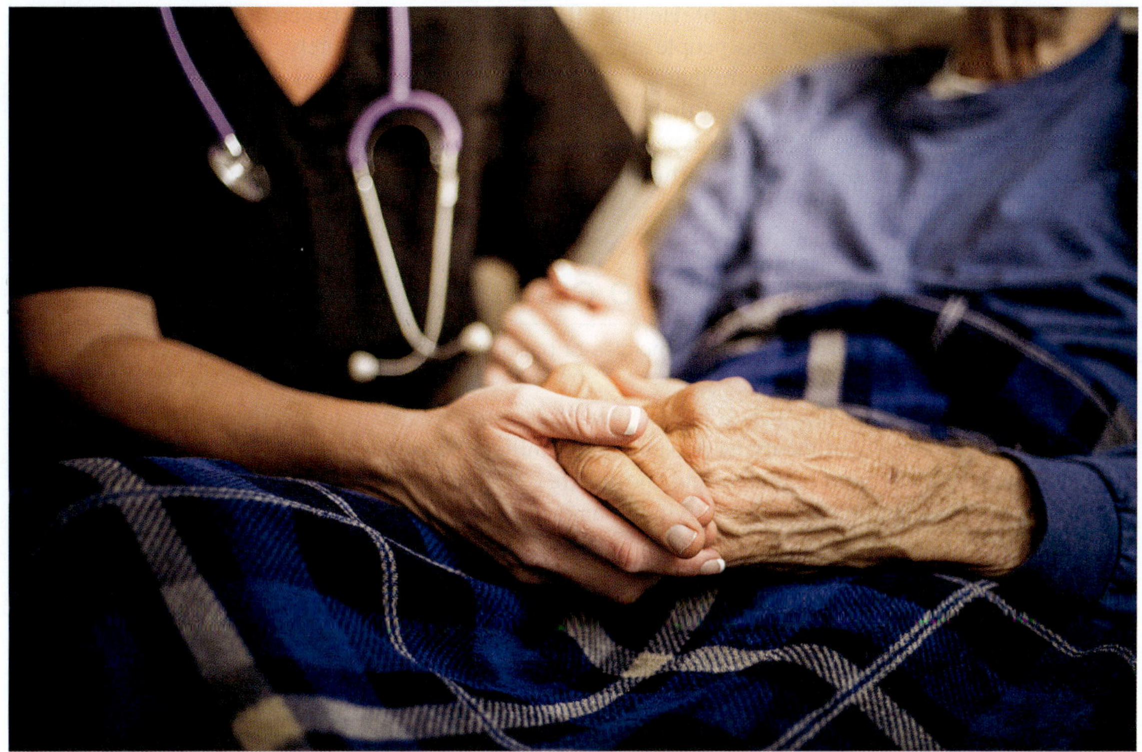

People in prison custody

People in prison have substantial and complex healthcare needs (Australian Government 2019). They have higher rates of mental health conditions, chronic disease, communicable disease, acquired brain injury, tobacco smoking, high-risk alcohol consumption and illicit drug use. In 2018, Australia's prison death rate was 0.17 deaths per 100 prisoners (Australian Government 2019). Most of these deaths were from natural causes. However, information on end-of-life and palliative care and **patient-centred care** in this setting is limited. There is a recognised need for the delivery of palliative care in prison.

People living with a disability

Provision of end-of-life and palliative care for people living in supported accommodation, such as residential disability services, requires careful coordination between disability and healthcare services. Some people living with a disability may require help to support them in understanding their diagnosis and prognosis and communicating their wishes and needs to their carers. Like all other groups in our community, we need to provide these patients with the same high quality patient centred care. This is required in addition to efforts on the part of healthcare providers and residential disability services. Palliative and end-of-life care for people living with a disability, be it physical or intellectual, needs to meet the principles of palliative care (Agency for Clinical Innovation 2021). That is, care that is patient, family or carer centred. The care provided is assessed on the need of the individual. There are local and networked services to meet the needs of the patient and their support group and the care is based on evidence and is equitable for this group as compared to the greater population.

People experiencing homelessness

People who are experiencing homelessness will live in non-conventional accommodation — sleeping rough — or they may be living in short-term, or emergency accommodation (Australian Government Department of Health 2019). Like all other sectors in our community, people who experience homelessness may require palliative care and we need to make provision for this in our society (Australian Government Department of Health 2019). As healthcare providers, we need to support care that is flexible enough to meet this underserved population's needs. Many of the homeless present directly to an emergency department and are not under the care of a general practitioner. It has also been noted that the homeless person presents only when they are at crisis point; hence, the care is reactive rather than proactive

(Australian Government Department of Health 2019). Partnerships between health and community services should ensure that homeless people's needs can be met appropriately. As healthcare providers, we must provide non-judgemental care that provides all individuals with respect, autonomy, dignity and privacy. Care of the homeless is an area that needs review and opportunities for healthcare providers to support proactive care for those persons experiencing homelessness explored. This is where the nurse can be proactive in establishing networks, partnerships, and collaborations, developing our workforce, and involving ourselves in research.

8.5 Principles of palliative care

LEARNING OBJECTIVE 8.5 Review the principles of palliative care and the role of nurses in palliative and end-of-life care.

Palliative care is not a process. It is a philosophy of care that is integrated to recognising the privacy, confidentiality and dignity of the dying person, their families and caregivers.

The principles that support palliative and end-of-life care are as follows.

- Affirmation of life and recognition of dying as a normal part of life.
- Neither hastens nor postpones death.
- Provides relief from pain and other distressing symptoms.
- Integrates psychological and spiritual aspects of care.
- Offers a support system to help patients live as fully and actively as possible until death.
- Offers a support system to help patients' families cope during the patient's illness and in their own bereavement (Hellocare Journalist Team 2020).

Palliative care nursing

Nurses spend more time with patients and families than any other healthcare provider (Schroeder & Lorenz 2018). As a result, nurses are uniquely placed to affect an improved delivery of palliative care services globally (Palliative Care Nurses Australia 2020). The needs of dying patients differ from those of other patients (Cobbs 2019). Moreover, the needs of social, economic and religious groups within our diverse society differ within the end-of-life setting. When providing palliative and end-of-life care, it is important that as healthcare providers we aim to:

- treat all people with compassion
- listen to people without preconceptions and bias
- communicate clearly and sensitively in a manner that is comprehensible to the patient and their family
- acknowledge pain, distress and anxiety and take the required action to alleviate them
- recognise when the patient is entering the end-of-life stage
- fully involve patients and their families in decisions about care and respect their wishes
- keep the patient and their families up to date with any changes in condition and care
- document a summary of conversations and decisions
- work as part of a team and seek further advice and escalate care if needed
- look after yourself and your colleagues — recognise breaking points and seek support if needed (Royal College of Nursing 2016).

Nursing and palliative care have synergy (Fitch, Fliedner & O'Connor 2015; Lynch, Dahlin, Hultman & Coakley 2011). Palliative nursing encompasses and reflects the holistic philosophy of care supported by the Registered Nurse Standards for Practice, the **clinical reasoning cycle** and patient-centred care. Like other roles that nurses undertake, palliative care nursing is an evidence-based practice that aims to relieve or reduce pain and suffering and enhance an individual's quality of life and function. As palliative care nurses, our role is to reduce the distress and uncertainties of those facing death and offer support for the individual and unique physical, social, psychological and spiritual needs of our patients and their loved ones (Schroeder & Lorenz 2018). Prior to death, patients tend to follow one of three recognised trajectories of functional decline. Some have a period of steadily progressive functional decline typical of patients with progressive cancer. For others, such as those with severe dementia, frailty or who have had a disabling stroke, there is a lengthy indeterminate period in which the patient experiences severe dysfunction. The third trajectory is typical of patients with an underlying comorbidity such as COPD or congestive heart failure. Because of these differing needs, the nursing care that is required for dying patients is specialist. Palliative care nursing embraces consideration of the patient situation, collecting the information and processing that information to identify patient problems and establish goals (Fitch et al. 2015; Levett-Jones 2017). We need to provide care that supports goals and continually evaluate, reflect on, and make any necessary changes to the care we provide. Each patient's situation will evolve around the stage of the end of the life that they are at. Our care goals will be centred around alleviating symptoms such as pain, supporting the activities of daily living and keeping the patient safe and comfortable (Schroeder & Lorenz 2018).

The Australian National Palliative Care Standards (5th edition) supports the consistent delivery of high-quality palliative care. Figure 8.3 demonstrates how the National Palliative Care Standards are divided into two categories. The first six standards refer to the systems and persons necessary to deliver high-quality clinical care. The last three standards provide the expectation for continuous quality improvement within the service providing palliative care. The intention of all nine standards are outlined in table 8.1.

FIGURE 8.3 The National Palliative Care Standards

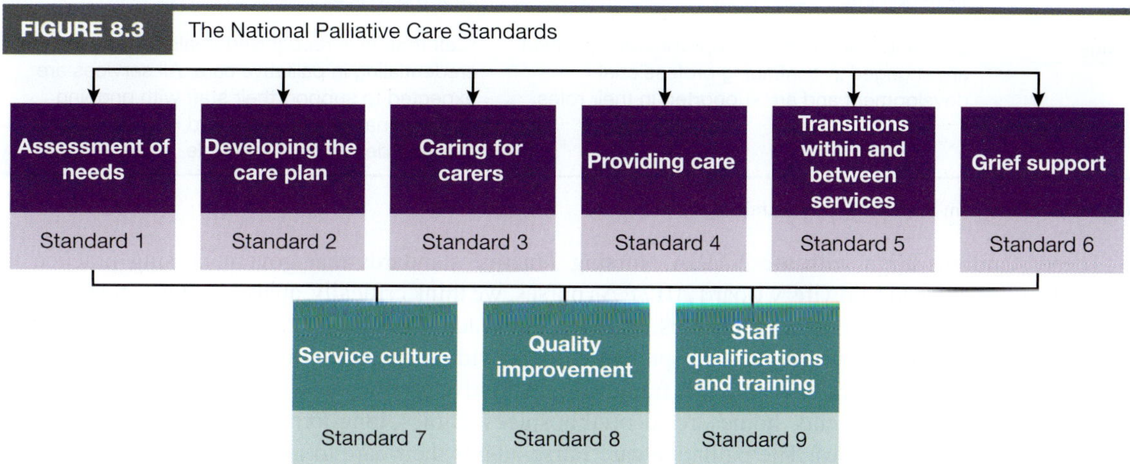

Source: Palliative Care Australia (2018).

TABLE 8.1 **National Palliative Care Standards Australia**

Standard	Statement	Intent of the statement
One	Initial and ongoing assessment incorporates the person's physical, psychological, cultural, social, and spiritual experiences and needs.	Ongoing clinical assessments are undertaken by educated and trained personnel and are patient and family centred.
Two	The person, their family and carers work in partnership with the team to communicate, plan, set goals of care, and support informed decisions about care plans.	Every individual is unique with unique needs, and their end-of-life experiences will be different. Goals of care may change over time; however, the delivery of care will always be respectful, compassionate and maintain dignity.
Three	The person's family and carers needs are assessed and directly inform the provision of appropriate support and guidance about their role.	Family and carers provide physical, emotional, social, and spiritual support and care. Healthcare providers appreciate and work with family and carers to understand the level of care that they can provide.
Four	The provision of care is based on the assessed needs of the person, informed by evidence and is consistent with the values, goals and preferences of the person as documented in their care plan.	Effective care enables the person to live as well as possible to the end of their life.
Five	Care is integrated across the person's experience to ensure seamless transitions within and between services.	Understanding and communicating the values, goals and preferences of the person, their family and carers and is necessary to support effective, person-centred care.
Six	Families and carers have access to bereavement support services and are provided with information about loss and grief.	Early identification and referral for families and carers who need support during the grieving process, including emotional and financial support.

(continued)

TABLE 8.1 *(continued)*

Standard	Statement	Intent of the statement
Seven	The service has a philosophy, values, culture, structure, and environment that supports the delivery of person-centred palliative care and end-of-life care.	Specialist palliative care services lead high-quality palliative care for people with complex needs that exceed the expertise of local care providers.
Eight	Services are engaged in quality improvement and research to improve service provision and development.	Services engage in quality improvement and lead or participate in research designed to inform practice.
Nine	Staff and volunteers are appropriately qualified, are engaged in continuing professional development and are supported in their roles.	Staff that have recognised qualifications or credentialing in palliative care. All services are expected to support their staff with ongoing professional development and in coping with the daily demands of their role.

Source: Adapted from Palliative Care Australia (2018).

These standards align with the NMBA Nursing Practice standards that govern nursing practice in Australia (Nursing and Midwifery Board 2017). As nurses, we think critically, analyse our practice, engage in therapeutic and professional relationships, maintain our practice capability and conduct comprehensive patient assessment. We develop plans for patient care, provide safe, appropriate and responsive quality care, and we evaluate that care. Within this framework, palliative care nurses work across various settings, including the palliative patients' homes, residential hospices, clinics, long-term and skilled care facilities, and acute in-patient facilities. The palliative care nurse adapts their care to meet the changing physical, emotional, social and spiritual needs of the patient and their families. Palliative care nursing, like all other nursing is a combination of art and science.

> Through the art of being present and the science of evidence-based interventions, palliative nurses assess, diagnose, and intervene to support or modify these responses in patients with acute or chronic, potentially life-limiting illnesses and their families to achieve positive patient outcomes that maximise quality of life and alleviate suffering (Lynch et al. 2011, p. 107).

The key skills of the palliative care nurse are:

- communication
- assessment and care planning
- coordination
- competence.

Communication

The first Australian Nursing Practice Standard states that the nurse will be able to communicate with respect to a person's dignity, culture, values, beliefs and rights (Nursing and Midwifery Board 2017). Effective communication takes on particular importance in palliative care or end-of-life care (Schroeder & Lorenz 2018). Patients and their families frequently seek clarity on their disease progression, the medications they have been prescribed, their plan of care and what they can expect as the disease progresses. We mustn't assume that our patients and their families understand their prognosis or recognise that death is imminent. The physician is responsible for communicating the course of disease, estimating the length of survival, and discussing the medical goals of care (Cobbs 2019). The physician will determine the need for palliative or hospice care or the need for supportive services at home with the patient and their family. However, the palliative care nurse will be instrumental in ensuring that the patient and their family fully comprehend the discussion they had with their doctor and support them in their decisions. The nurse will also help ensure that support is in place, and the patient and their family are receiving the care they need and want. As healthcare providers, we must understand these aspects of the patient's care and explain them in language the patient and their families understand and take the time to answer questions and allay concerns. Communication is key to patient-centred, safe and respectful care (Nursing & Midwifery Council NSW 2018).

8.6 Clinical reasoning cycle and patient-centred care of the end-of-life patient

LEARNING OBJECTIVE 8.6 Apply the clinical reasoning cycle and patient-centred care to palliative and end-of-life patients.

The use of the clinical reasoning cycle is as important, or even more so, with the dying patient as with the acute care patient. Effective use of the clinical reasoning cycle is dependent on following the stages of the cyclic process:

- consider the patient situation
- collect information
- process gathered information
- identify the problem
- establish goals
- act
- evaluate
- reflect (European Heart Association 2018; Levett-Jones 2017).

To provide the best possible care for the dying, we must consider the patient and their situation, spiritual and cultural beliefs and personal choices. When collecting information about our patient we need to create a calm environment that allows the patient and their family to feel safe and comfortable (Oates 2020). We need to give them enough time to answer our questions and ask their own. We need to support the opportunity for the patient, their family and their medical team to discuss their goals. Our clinical reasoning will be focused on care. Care that will keep the patient comfortable and support the family. Care that supports the needs of the patient and the family at this difficult time.

Patient-centred care

Patient-centred care has a unique role when we are caring for the dying. Death cannot be itemised as merely a medical event. Healthcare support must correspond with social, psychological and spiritual support (Institute of Medicine 2015). Healthcare providers make significant contributions to patients as they near the end of their life. We are able to relieve pain, discomfort and other symptoms of the disease or dying process. Nurses can help achieve maximum functioning, support the patient and undertake their daily living activities to keep them clean and comfortable. We can help alleviate depression and anxiety that comes with dying. Furthermore, we can ease the family and loved one's burden and enable constructive dynamics over the dying period. This can be accomplished by combining science and compassion. All patients are capable of making their own decisions and must have those decisions respected (Oates 2020).

As healthcare providers, we do not have the right to convey our values or belief systems to our patients or their families. Families who have difficulty dealing with the situation and are frightened and grieving may want their personal choices to be recognised over that of the patient. We must remember to keep the patient's goals at the centre of our care (Institute of Medicine 2015). We adjust treatments to meet the unique needs of each patient. We take the spiritual and cultural context, interests, roles and strengths of the patient and their family when providing care. Care of people nearing the end of life should be overwhelmingly patient centred.

Coordination of care

Nurses are part of a team and do not work in isolation in providing end-of-life care. The optimal model of palliative and end-of-life care is a multi-disciplinary team approach. Multi-disciplinary teams include general practitioners, specialist clinicians, nurses, pharmacists and allied health providers. Team members will depend on location, populations serviced, and the disease complexity and situation. As nurses, we play crucial roles in this team, and evidence supports nurses' work both in focused roles such as pain management or in broad roles such as case management (Schroeder & Lorenz 2018). The role of the nurse in palliative and end-of-life care is growing, and a palliative care nurse's role has developed from one of providing day-to-day care to include comfort, symptom management and support for the patient and their families.

Medications to support palliative and end-of-life care

The focus for patients at the end of life is treatment aimed at optimising comfort and dignity. Healthcare providers work as a team to support the patient with timely, appropriate and fair treatment to reduce pain and distress. Medication is an integral part of symptom management (Hellocare Journalist Team 2020). Comprehensive knowledge of the underlying pathophysiology of pain is essential for effective management. While nurses do not prescribe medications, we are responsible for administering them. As part of our role, we are required to understand the therapeutic action of medicines, including the indications, contraindications and special precautions (Australian Government Department of Health 2006). We are required to use our clinical reasoning skills to assess if medications should be administered or withheld based on the patient's clinical status. If a medication is withheld or refused by the patient, we are required to consult the prescriber of the medication or physician overseeing the patients care. Nurses have a role in educating patients, their families and carers about the safe and appropriate administration of medications. We are also responsible for following the correct medication management to ensure safe medication preparation and practice the seven rights of medication administration:

1. right patient
2. right drug
3. right dose
4. right time
5. right route
6. right reason
7. right documentation (Smeulers et al. 2015).

Pain management

Pain is recognised as one of the most distressing symptoms that a person can experience. Hence, it is crucial for healthcare providers that pain is controlled (Palliative Care Australia 2018). The essential medications for pain management are nonopioid analgesics and opioids. Some of the medications that the physician may prescribe for a patient's end-of-life care are outlined in table 8.2. If we are unsure of the role of these medications in our patients care, we must check them in a drug resource such as the Monthly Index of Medical Specialties (MIMS). MIMS contains comprehensive medication information that supports safe prescription and administration of medications. MIMS is available in hard copy and online, and most, if not all, healthcare providers have access to this validated reference.

TABLE 8.2 Standards of pharmaceutical pain management

Symptom	Medication — doses will vary according to the needs of the individual patient
Pain and discomfort	Morphine Fentanyl Hydromorphine
Anxiety or terminal restlessness	Clonazepam Midazolam
Delirium or agitation	Clonazepam Midazolam
Nausea	Metoclopromide Haloperadol
Death rattle (noisy breathing)	Hyoscine Butylbromide

Source: Government of South Australia (2019).

Non-pharmacological interventions

The role of non-pharmacological approaches to palliative care is evolving. Studies have shown that non-pharmacological and complementary therapies can work alongside pharmacological interventions to contribution to patient-centred holistic care (Caresearch 2019). There is growing evidence to support the contribution of patient education, cognitive behavioural therapy (CBT), relaxation and music. There is limited evidence to support the use of TENS and acupuncture for pain in some situations. Research on non-pharmacological approaches to pain management is important to offer effective treatments for our patients. However, patients with significant pain should be treated with the appropriate medications using an evidence-based approach. Palliative care guidelines for other symptoms commonly experienced by people with advanced disease are listed in table 8.3.

TABLE 8.3 Standards of non-pharmaceutical palliative care

Symptom	Non-pharmacological measures
Cough	Humidify room air Oral fluids Honey and lemon in warm water Hard lozenges to suck Elevate the head when sleeping
Breathlessness	Positioning is important — sit upright, legs uncrossed, let shoulders droop, keep head up Relaxation techniques Reduce room temperature A cool cloth to the face
Fever	Reduce room temperature Provide loose clothing
Management of delirium	Ensure effective communication Reorientation to time and place and person Provide reassurance for people diagnosed with delirium Consider involving family, friends, and carers to help with this Ensure adequate lighting Beware of risk to patient and others Avoid moving the location of the patient
Anxiety, distress	Keep the environment as calm and comfortable as possible Calm and reassure constantly Focus on kindness and understanding Exploring the significant fears with the patient and the family Ensure patient has constant access to a call be Offer music and items of comfort Integrate family support structures and regular contact via phone/video calls Assess need for spiritual support or counselling
Falls	Ongoing falls assessment Have a plan to prevent falls Supervision for transfers/toileting Warn persons of risk (if able to understand) Regular toileting
Constipation	Bowel charting Dietary measures
Urinary retention	Intermittent or permanent indwelling catheter
Skin integrity	Assess for risk of pressure injury Ensuring the mattress is comfortable and suitable for level of risk Regular pressure area care and repositioning Regular hygiene Skin assessments each shift — particular attention to bony prominences, sacrum, and heels Moisturise skin

Source: Association for Palliative Medicine of Great Britain and Ireland (2020).

Supporting caregivers after death

The pronouncement of death should be done promptly to reduce anxiety and stress for the family and carers. When told about death, especially unexpected death, family members and carers may be overwhelmed (Cobbs 2019). Healthcare providers need to support the psychologic needs of family members and carers providing a comfortable environment where family members can grieve together, adequate time for them to be with the body and appropriate counselling and spiritual support if needed. Nurses should ensure that all tubes, lines and signs of body fluids and odours are removed prior to the family visiting with the deceased.

Decisions around organ and tissue donation ideally should be made prior to death (Cobbs 2019). This will also depend on national and state laws regarding opt-in or opt-out legalities around organ donations. The attending physician is responsible for arranging organ donation and autopsy and other legal arrangements around autopsies.

Voluntary assisted dying

Palliative Care Australia (PCA) recognises that voluntary assisted dying legislation poses ethical, personal and professional issues for health practitioners, care workers and volunteers providing palliative and end-of-life care (Australian Centre for Health Law Research 2020; Palliative Care Australia 2019). In Victoria and Western Australia, **voluntary assisted dying (VAD)** is lawful in limited circumstances. Currently, VAD is not lawful in other Australian states and territories; however, the potential to adopt this legal process is being discussed by these state and territory governments. Where VAD remains illegal, any person, including a healthcare provider or a family member who assists someone to die, may be charged with murder, manslaughter or assisted suicide (PCA 2019).

PCA (2019) has provided a set of guiding principles for those providing care to people living with a life-limiting illness who wish to explore VAD. These guiding principles aim to support appropriate care for a person suffering from a life-limiting illness and maintain appropriate, respectful and cooperative relationships between healthcare professionals. These principles and their intentions are outlined in table 8.4.

TABLE 8.4 Principles of palliative care

Principle	Intent of the principle
Patients living with a life-limiting illness are supported and respected if they choose to access or not to access VAD	Palliative and end-of-life care supports the exploration of all available options for the patient and supports the family to identify and maintain caring networks even after death.
Patients exploring VAD will not be abandoned	A patient with a life-limiting illness, their family and carers should not feel abandoned or fear that care will be adversely affected if they want to explore VAD.
Respectful and professional behaviour towards colleagues and co-workers regardless of their views on voluntary assisted dying	While there may be different views between healthcare professionals about VAD and decisions made in an organisation that will determine the level of involvement, healthcare providers must continue to provide safe, quality and compassionate care to people living with a life-limiting illness.
Effective communication is an important part of quality care	Listening and discussion are essential for understanding preferences for care. Healthcare providers must allow space for these discussions to take place.
Ongoing development of knowledge, skill and confidence is required to provide competent and safe care to people living with a life-limiting illness	Healthcare providers need to continue professional development and education and be aware of the legislation surrounding VAD and the pathways that will allow patients to explore this possibility.
Self-care practice is a shared responsibility between individuals, colleagues and organisations	Healthcare providers need to recognise that these are stressful situations and should participate in opportunities to build resilience and facilitate supportive communication within teams.

Continue to learn from evidence and evolving practice to drive quality improvement in voluntary assisted dying	Health providers are encouraged to participate and collaborate in research related to VAD to support the implementation of best practices in this field and to act as advocates for transparency in public reporting on VAD to support patient safety.

Source: PCA (2019).

8.7 Mindfulness for palliative care nurses

LEARNING OBJECTIVE 8.7 Identify self-care strategies for nurses to help reduce the physical and psychological stressors related to palliative and end-of-life care.

While we are educated and trained caregivers, we can forget how important it is to look after ourselves (University of Texas Arlington 2016). Because of the complexity of providing palliative and end-of-life care, supporting families and the depth of emotion required, we need to remember the importance of self-awareness and self-care (Eastwood & Williams 2019). Nurses must function at high levels of physical and psychological health to deliver excellent patient care and achieve optimal outcomes for the patient and their families (Penque 2019). When we lose the ability to remember our own physical and emotional needs, we risk fatigue, burnout, health problems and making errors on the job (University of Texas Arlington 2016). This comes at a high cost to patients, ourselves and our colleagues. While no one plan suits all, some factors should not be overlooked (University of Texas Arlington 2016).

- *Diet.* Ensure that you have a diet that is nutritious and meets your energy needs. It is easy to sink into a diet of fast foods when you are busy and feel overwhelmed. Seek the help of a registered dietician or nutritionist if you find it stressful to develop an eating plan for yourself.
- *Exercise.* Exercise is vital to a healthy lifestyle. Choose activities that you enjoy and that you are likely to make a habit. Options include, but are of course not limited to, walking, running, swimming, cycling, dancing, yoga, Pilates, team sports, tennis or golf (CDC 2020).
- *Stress.* Stress reduction techniques include creative hobbies, breathing exercises, laughter, music, massage and spa therapies, meditation, visualisation, Tai Chi and pet therapy. Find an activity that you can go to help reduce your stress easily.
- *Be kind to yourself.* Take time out to be with your family, socialise with friends, read, watch movies, listen to music. Take time that is just for you.

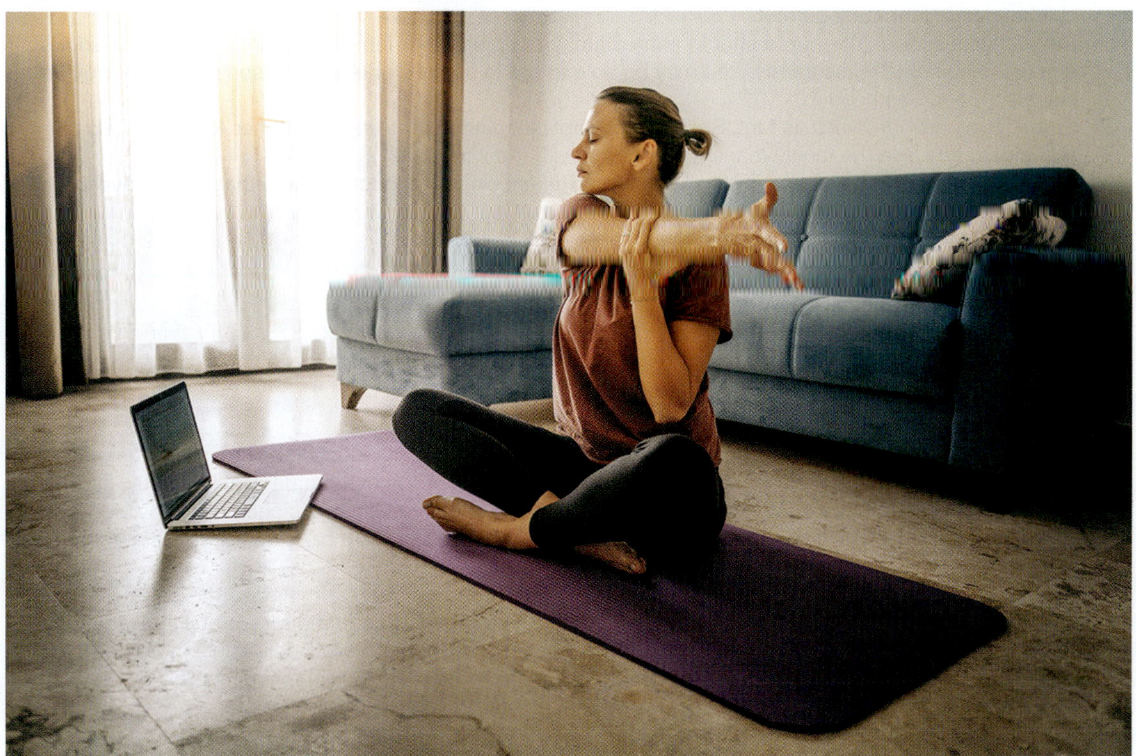

Self-care for healthcare providers is not a luxury; it is necessary for our physical, mental and emotional health and wellbeing and will benefit our patients, their families and our colleagues.

CASE STUDY 8.1

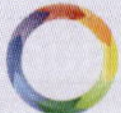

Caring for a patient with end-stage dementia

Mrs Agnus Stuart is an 87-year-old lady. Agnus has dementia diagnosed 5 years ago and is cared for in a dementia-specific unit in a RACF (RCAF). Three years ago, Agnus developed a lump in her right breast and was diagnosed with breast cancer. After discussion with the family no active treatment was commenced due to her age and her primary diagnosis of dementia. The cancerous lump has developed into a fungating wound and requires management.

Agnus is widowed and has four children who live in the local area. The children visit on a regular basis and take and active interest in her care. The oldest son is James, and he holds Enduring Power of Attorney. The other three children are Donna, Margaret and Tracy and James confers with them on decisions. The family has noted a decline in Agnus over the last 2 months. She is refusing food, takes only minimal fluids, has lost weight and her confusion has increased. She spends much of her time in a chair beside her bed.

The RCAF have called a family meeting and Agnus's doctor has advised the family that she requires palliative care and active medical interventions would be ceased and interventions will be more focused on keeping her comfortable and pain free. James agrees with the decision although the family are understandable upset.

Question

Using the information above, describe what action you would take as the nurse caring for this patient. Use the clinical reasoning cycle to guide you through the process and devise a plan of care for your patient.

Answer

- *Step 1: Consider the patient*. Mrs Agnus Stuart is an 87-year-old lady. Agnus has dementia and end stage breast cancer.
- *Step 2: Collect cues/information*. Include subjective and objective data here, including the patient's appearance and past medical history. Subjective data will be what the family tells you. Objective data will include measurable information such as the pain score, intake and output chart, nutrition chart.
- *Step 3: Process information*. Separate the relevant and irrelevant data — cluster the clues together to formulate a plan for the patient and the family.
- *Step 4: Identify problems/issues*. Nursing problems or diagnosis along with goals or desired outcomes should be listed here.
- *Step 5: Establish goals*. Goals of care for Mrs. Stuart are pain management and risk management, including management of her activities of daily living (ADL), her wound dressing and any spiritual or cultural needs that must be met.
- *Step 6: Take action*. The nurse should immediately recognise that family is feeling extremely anxious and will need some reassurance. You may be able to call in social workers or persons who can provide spiritual support as needed.
- *Step 7: Evaluate outcomes*. Is Mrs. Stuart being kept clean and comfortable with her ADL managed and she is pain free. Are the family managing to cope with the situation?
- *Step 8: Reflect on the process and new learning*. Reflect on any aspects of care that could have been performed in a way to achieve an improved outcome. What further learning do you need to undertake to better understand cases like this in the future?

CASE STUDY 8.2

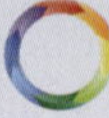

Caring for a patient with stage IV melanoma

Joseph (Joe) Sullivan is a 20-year-old male patient who has been diagnosed with stage IV metastatic melanoma. Joe has been receiving chemotherapy for treatment of the melanoma. Until recently, he was staying at home, and a community care nurse came to the home to give him his chemotherapy. Joe was studying engineering at university and has been struggling to keep up with his studies. Joe is a member of the local surfing community and has many visitors and well-wishers.

Due to the side effects of the aggressive chemotherapy, Joe has been admitted to the palliative care ward in the local hospital. His pain is increasing, and he is struggling to eat and take oral fluids. The care team have decided to start subcutaneous pain relief using a syringe driver to deliver his morphine. Joe is hesitant to start this new treatment as he does not want to be 'tied to a machine'; he feels like he is starting to lose control of the situation.

Question

Using the information above, describe what action you would take as the nurse caring for this patient. Use the clinical reasoning cycle to guide you through the process and devise a plan of care for your patient.

Answer

- *Step 1: Consider the patient.* Joe is a young male patient who has until recently been an active sportsperson and working towards a future career.
- *Step 2: Collect cues/information.* Include subjective and objective data here, including the patient's appearance and past medical history. Subjective data will be what the patient and his family tell you. Objective data will include measurable information such as his vital signs, weight, intake and output charts and so on.
- *Step 3: Process information*. Separate the relevant and irrelevant data — cluster the clues together to formulate an inference about the patient.
- *Step 4: Identify problems/issues*. Nursing problems or diagnosis should be listed here along with goals or desired outcomes.
- *Step 5: Establish goals*. Goals of care are to maintain activities of daily living (ADL).
- *Step 6: Take action*. You should recognise that Joe may be feeling anxious and will need education and reassurance. You will need to monitor intake and output, ensure his ADL are supported. He needs his medications and to remain well hydrated and supported with a diet he can tolerate. How can you best support his visitors to see him on the ward?
- *Step 7: Evaluate outcomes*. Have Joe's dignity and independence been maintained? Have his ADL been met. Has he received the necessary physical and spiritual care?
- *Step 8: Reflect on process and new learning.* Reflect on any aspects of care that could have been performed in a way to achieve an improved outcome. What further learning do you need to better understand cases like this in the future?

SUMMARY

This chapter discussed the aetiology and epidemiology of death in Australia, the pathophysiology of death, the nature of dying, and palliative care and palliative care nursing principles. It looked at palliative and end-of-life care for a diverse society such as Australia, legislation changes, and healthcare providers' role in voluntary assisted dying. It also discussed the importance of mindfulness for the palliative and end-of-life care nurse. End-of-life and palliative care are complex and require nurses caring for patients with life-limiting disease to understand the physical, psychological, social and spiritual domains within the context of palliative care and the application of patient-centred care and the clinical reasoning cycle. As nurses, we also need to be mindful of our Australian Nursing Practice standards and how they support safe and effective care for the patient. Importantly we need to be mindful of self-care to continue the high-quality care we strive to deliver.

KEY TERMS

clinical reasoning cycle A cyclic process that involves collecting cues, processing information, determining the patient problem and using this information to plan and implement interventions, evaluate outcomes and reflect on the care provided.

end-of-life care Providing physical comfort and supporting mental and emotional and spiritual needs of the individual. It does not include the initiation of care that is intended to extend life. The focus is on comfort and quality of life.

grief cycle The stages of grief, as described by Swiss psychiatrist Kübler-Ross, based on her work with terminally ill patients and their families.

palliative care Patient-centred care focused on optimising the quality of life for a patient who has little or no prospect of cure. The care focuses on managing symptoms and improving quality of life.

patient-centred care Care that aims to empower patients to become active participants in their care. Patients are treated with dignity and respect and are involved in all decisions about their healthcare.

voluntary assisted dying (VAD) A regulated voluntary intervention to provide a patient with the means to end their lives based on a fully formed consent aimed at relieving pain and suffering.

REFERENCES

Agency for Clinical Innovation. (2021) Palliative & end of life care, a blueprint for improvement. https://aci.health.nsw.gov.au/palliative-care-blueprint/the-blueprint/principles

AIHW. (2020) Causes of death. Australian Government, Canberra. www.aihw.gov.au/reports/australias-health/causes-of-death

AIHW. (2019) The health of Australia's prisoners 2018. Australian Government. www.aihw.gov.au/reports/prisoners/health-australia-prisoners-2018/contents/summary

American Psychological Association. (2021) Culturally diverse communities and palliative and end-of-life care. www.apa.org/pi/aging/programs/eol/end-of-life-diversity

ANMJ Staff. (2020) 5 tips to a good clinical handover. *The Australian and Midwifery Journal* [online]. https://anmj.org.au/5-tips-to-a-good-clinical-handover

Association for Palliative Medicine of Great Britain and Ireland. (2020) COVID-19 and palliative, end of life and bereavement care in secondary care role of the specialty and guidance to aid care. Version 4: 20 April 2020. https://apmonline.org/wp-content/uploads/2020/04/COVID-19-and-Palliative-End-of-Life-and-Bereavement-Care-20-April-2020-2.pdf

Australian Centre for Health Law Research, QUT. (2020) End of life law in Australia, euthanasia and assisted dying. https://end-of-life.qut.edu.au/euthanasia

Australian College of Nursing. (2019) Achieving quality palliative care for all: The essential role of nurses. www.acn.edu.au/wp-content/uploads/white-paper-end-of-life-care-achieving-quality-palliative-care-for-all.pdf

Australian Government Department of Health. (2006) Guiding Principle 4 — Administration of medicines in the community. www1.health.gov.au/internet/publications/publishing.nsf/Content/nmp-guide-medmgt-jul06-contents~nmp-guide-medmgt-jul06-guidepr4

Australian Government Department of Health. (2019) Exploratory analysis of barriers to palliative care issues report on people experiencing homelessness. www.health.gov.au/sites/default/files/documents/2020/01/exploratory-analysis-of-barriers-to-palliative-care-issues-report-on-people-experiencing-homelessness.pdf

Caresearch. (2019) Non pharmacological approaches. www.caresearch.com.au/caresearch/tabid/751/Default.aspx

Centers for Disease Control and Prevention. (2020) How much physical activity do adults need? U.S. Department of Health & Human Services. www.cdc.gov/physicalactivity/basics/adults

Cobbs, E. L., Blackstone, K. & Lynn, J. (2019) The dying patient. *MDF Manual, Professional version.* www.msdmanuals.com/professional/special-subjects/the-dying-patient/the-dying-patient

Committee on Approaching Death: Addressing Key End of Life Issues; Institute of Medicine. (2015) 'The delivery of person-centered, family-oriented end-of-life care'. In *Dying in America: Improving quality and honoring individual preferences near the end of life.* Washington (DC): National Academies Press (US). www.ncbi.nlm.nih.gov/books/NBK285676

Department of Health & Human Services, S. G. o. V., Australia. (2017) End of life and palliative care explained. www.betterhealth.vic.gov.au/health/servicesandsupport/end-of-life-and-palliative-care-explained

Eastwood, I. & Williams, I. (2019) Improving self-compassion and reducing burnout with mindfulness for palliative care. Helix Center. https://medium.com/helixcentre/mindfulness-for-palliative-care-dc4f9833efb0

ER services. (n.d.) Care at the time of death. https://courses.lumenlearning.com/suny-nursing-care-at-the-end-of-life/chapter/care-at-the-time-of-death

European Heart Association. (2018) The Clinical Reasoning Cycle: The 8 phases and their significance. www.heartassociation.eu/the-clinical-reasoning-cycle-the-8-phases-and-their-significance

Fitch, M. I., Fliedner, M. C. & O'Connor, M. (2015) Nursing perspectives on palliative care 2015. *Annals of Palliative Medicine.* 4(3): 150–155. http://apm.amegroups.com/article/view/7034

Government of South Australia, SA Health. (2019) Prescribing guidelines for the pharmacological management of symptoms for adults in the last days of life. www.sahealth.sa.gov.au/wps/wcm/connect/f532fc004a0f0746a22fe290d529bdaa/Prescribing+Guidelines+for+the+Pharmacological+Management+of+Symptoms+fo.._.pdf?MOD=AJPERES&CACHEID=ROOTWORKSPACE-f532fc004a0f0746a22fe290d529bdaa-niQcy60

Gregory, C. (2020) The five stages of grief, an examination of the Kubler-Ross Model. www.psycom.net/depression.central.grief.html

HealthInfoNet. (n.d.) Palliative care and end-of-life care. https://healthinfonet.ecu.edu.au/learn/health-system/palliative-care/?utm_source=google&utm_medium=cpc&utm_campaign=2019-always-on&utm_content=palliative-care

Hellocare Journalist Team. (2020) What is palliative care? The principles that you need to know. https://hellocaremail.com.au/principles-palliative-care-need-know

Kessler, D. (n.d.) The five stages of grief. https://grief.com/the-five-stages-of-grief

Kübler-Ross, E. (1975) *Death: the final stage of growth.* Simon and Schuster.

Kübler-Ross, E. (1969) *On death and dying.* Routledge.

Levett-Jones, T. (2017) *Clinical reasoning. Learning to think like a nurse.* Pearson Australia.

Lynch, M., Dahlin, C., Hultman, T. & Coakley, E. E. (2011) Palliative care nursing: Defining the discipline? *Journal of Hospice & Palliative Nursing.* 13(2): 106–111. https://journals.lww.com/jhpn/Fulltext/2011/03000/Palliative_Care_Nursing__Defining_the_Discipline_.9.aspx

Nursing & Midwifery Council NSW. (2018) Effective communications. www.nursingandmidwiferycouncil.nsw.gov.au/effective-communications

Nursing and Midwifery Board, AHPRA. (2017) Registered nurse standards for practice. www.nursingmidwiferyboard.gov.au/Codes-Guidelines-Statements/Professional-standards/registered-nurse-standards-for-practice.aspx

Oates, J. R. & Maani, C. V. (2020, Aug 30) Death and dying. *StatPearls* [Internet]. Treasure Island (FL): StatPearls Publishing. www.ncbi.nlm.nih.gov/books/NBK536978

Palliative Care Australia. (2018) Facts about morphine and other opioid medicines for pain in palliative care. https://palliativecare.org.au/facts-about-morphine-and-other-opioid-medicines-in-palliative-care

Palliative Care Australia. (2018) *National Palliative Care Standards*, 5th ed. Canberra: PCA.

Palliative Care Australia. (2019) Voluntary assisted dying in Australia. https://palliativecare.org.au/wp-content/uploads/dlm_uploads/2019/06/PCA-Guiding-Principles-Voluntary-Assisted-Dying.pdf

Palliative Care Nurses Australia. (2020) Our work. www.pcna.org.au/our-work/palliative-care-nursing

Penque, S. (2019) Mindfulness to promote nurses' well-being. *Nursing Management.* 50(5): 38–44. doi: 10.1097/01. https://journals.lww.com/nursingmanagement/Fulltext/2019/05000/Mindfulness_to_promote_nurses__well_being.9.aspx

Queensland Health. (2015) *Sad news, sorry business: Guidelines for caring for Aboriginal and Torres Strait Islander people through death and dying.* www.health.qld.gov.au/__data/assets/pdf_file/[illegible]

Roth, D., Mammen, S. V., Kell, J., Schildknecht, M. & Latoschik, M. E. (2019, Sept.) *Approaching difficult terrain with sensitivity: A virtual reality game on the five stages of grief.* Paper presented at the 2019 11th International Conference on Virtual Worlds and Games for Serious Applications (VS-Games).

Royal College of Nursing. (2016) End of life care — Fundamentals of nursing care at the end of life. https://rcni.com/hosted-content/rcn/fundamentals-of-end-of-life-care/roles-and-responsibilities

Rudrappa, M., Modi, P. & Bollu, P. C. (2020, Nov 20) Cheyne stokes respirations. *StatPearls* [Internet]. Treasure Island (FL): StatPearls Publishing. www.ncbi.nlm.nih.gov/books/NBK448165

Schroeder, K. & Lorenz, K. (2018) Nursing and the future of palliative care. *Asia-Pacific Journal of Oncology Nursing.* 5(1): 4–8. doi: 10.4103/apjon.apjon_43_17

Smeulers, M., Verweij, L., Maaskant, J. M., de Boer, M., Krediet, C. T. P., Nieveen van Dijkum, E. J. M. & Vermeulen, H. (2015) Quality indicators for safe medication preparation and administration: a systematic review. *PloS one.* 10(4): e0122695–e0122695. doi: 10.1371/journal.pone.0122695

University of Texas Arlington. (2016) Why self-care is vital for your nursing career. https://academicpartnerships.uta.edu/articles/healthcare/why-self-care-is-vital-for-your-nursing-career.aspx

ACKNOWLEDGEMENTS

Figures 8.1 and 8.2: © Australian Institute of Health and Welfare, AIHW National Mortality Database. Deaths in Australia, 07 August 2020. Retrieved from: www.aihw.gov.au/reports/life-expectancy-death/deaths-in-australia/contents/leading-causes-of-death. Licensed under CC BY 3.0.

Figure 8.3: © *National Palliative Care Standards*, 5th Edition, 2018. © Palliative Care Australia. Reproduced with permission of Palliative Care Australia. https://palliativecare.org.au/wp-content/uploads/dlm_uploads/2018/11/PalliativeCare-National-Standards-2018_Nov-web.pdf.
Photo 8A: © Antonio Guillem / Shutterstock.com
Photo 8B: © morpheuse / Getty Images
Photo 8C: © Maskot / Getty Images
Photo 8D: © LPETTET / Getty Images
Photo 8E: © Olesya Kuznetsova / Shutterstock.com

CHAPTER 9

Principles of surgical nursing

LEARNING OBJECTIVES

After studying this chapter, you should be able to:

9.1 outline the stages of a patient's perioperative journey

9.2 justify the purpose of preoperative assessment

9.3 identify and explain the primary considerations for patient safety during surgery

9.4 outline the purpose, types and stages of anaesthesia and common pharmacological agents used for anaesthesia

9.5 differentiate the anaesthetic, instrument/circulating and PACU nurse roles in the delivery of safe perioperative patient care

9.6 interpret the criteria used to identify when it is safe for a patient to return to the ward after surgery and understand the nursing care requirements for post-surgery patients.

Introduction

This chapter on **perioperative** care provides undergraduate nursing students with foundational information on perioperative nursing. Undergraduate students may have limited opportunity to experience nursing in the perioperative environment. The Australian College of Operating Room Nurses (ACORN) has a standard that governs students' expected professional behaviour in the perioperative setting, which is recognised by other professional organisations to support best practice in perioperative nursing care. Access to the complete ACORN standards can be purchased online or accessed from within the perioperative complex of the health service students are visiting.

The three stages of the patient's perioperative journey include **preoperative** (before surgery), **intra-operative** (during surgery) and **post-operative** (after surgery). The processes that support each of the phases has critical implications for the patient's surgical outcome. These stages are explored here in the context of nursing roles within the areas of perioperative practice (anaesthetic, instrument/circulating and post-anaesthetic care).

The **anaesthesia** patients receive for surgery is complex and determined by the patient's preoperative interview and assessments. The different types of anaesthesia that can be administered, the stages of anaesthesia and anaesthetic medications administered to patients will be explored in this chapter. The complex surgical considerations are also explored in the context of patient safety and surgical modalities for improved patient surgical experience and outcomes.

Once the perioperative patient has been discharged from the post-anaesthesia care unit (PACU) and arrives on the surgical ward, they are entering the final stages of their perioperative journey. Anticipating and recognising the post-operative patient's needs is fundamental to safe nursing care, and recommendations to help guide students nursing care and preparation for discharge home are also outlined in this chapter.

9.1 Stages of the perioperative journey

LEARNING OBJECTIVE 9.1 Outline the stages of a patient's perioperative journey.

For many people, their perioperative journey begins with the pre-hospital phase. In this phase, the person notices a health concern and makes an appointment to visit their general practitioner (GP). The hospital admission and aftercare phases complete the patient's journey. Table 9.1 outlines the three phases of the patient's perioperative journey.

TABLE 9.1 Three phases of the patient's perioperative journey

1. Pre-hospital phase	Person makes an appointment to see their GP. The GP assessment may refer the person for a review by a specialist surgeon; the outcome may indicate that surgery is required. The specialist surgeon will categorise the urgency of the patient's surgery, and the surgery will be booked. There can be long waiting times for booked surgery in the public hospital system. The person will then have preadmission clinic appointments/interview appointment arranged. This is known as an elective hospital admission.
2. Hospital admission	Patient is admitted to the hospital. For some patients, this will be the day before their surgery, for others, it will be on the day of their surgery. The patient will be sent to a ward where the nurse helps them change into the correct theatre attire, complete and compile documentation required for the surgery, complete patient assessments and administer medications. Some patients will stay in the hospital the night of their surgery, while others may need to stay for several nights. How long a patient stays depends on the type of surgery and the patient's recovery. If the patient is going home the day of their surgery, the nurse checks to see that the patient meets the criteria for discharge, such as having someone who is able to care for them that night.
3. Aftercare	A patient's recovery from their surgery is reviewed at the hospital, in the specialist doctors's private consulting rooms, sometimes in the GP clinic or in the patient's home. Community-based health services may also be included in the patient's care while they continue to recover from surgery.

Source: Adapted from Australian Government (2019); New South Wales Government (2020); Sutherland-Fraser, Osborne and Bryant (2016) Chapter 1, 'Perioperative Nursing' pg. 3 in Hamlin et al. *Perioperative nursing*.

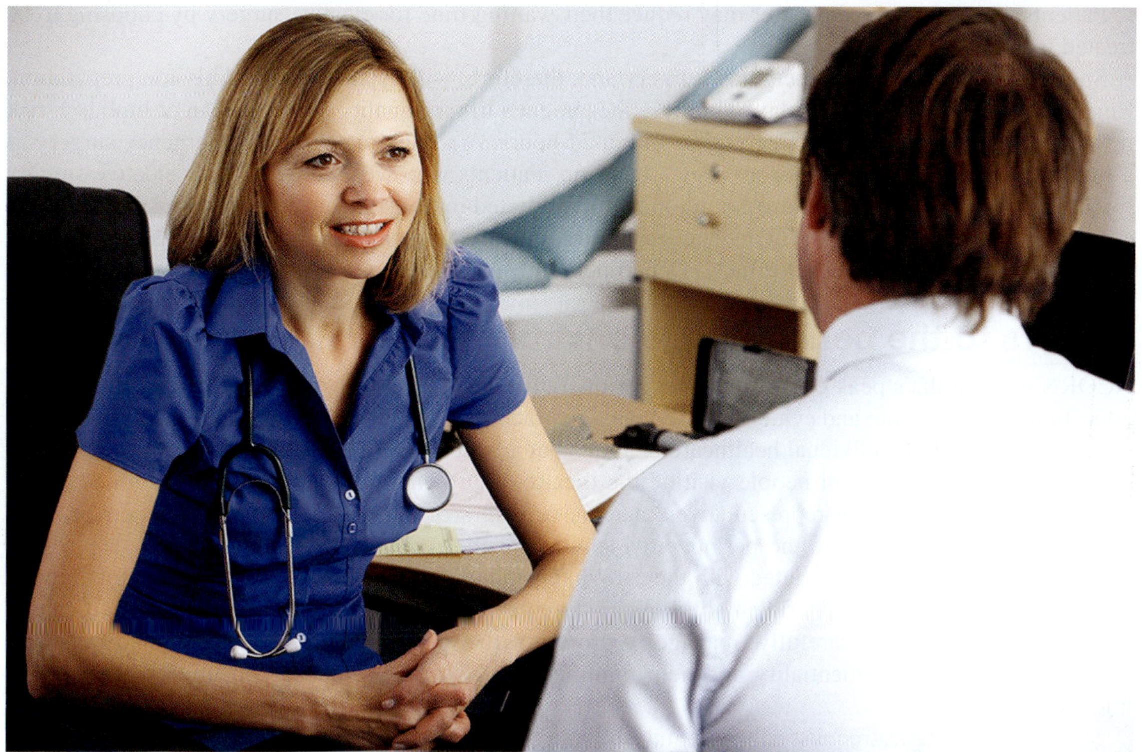

There are three overarching stages to the patient's perioperative journey. For many people, the pre-hospital phase of care begins when they visit their GP regarding one or more health concerns. The GP assessment may result in the patient being referred to a specialist surgeon for a specialist review, the outcome of which may be surgery.

A patient may need to undergo surgery for several reasons.

1. *Diagnostic.* To diagnose a condition and the degree of disease progression. Patients may undergo a biopsy or scope (endoscopy, gastroscopy, colonoscopy, bronchoscopy, arthroscopy).
2. *Curative.* To remove/repair the diseased area, such as by removing a cyst (cystectomy), lump (lumpectomy) or removing an appendix (appendectomy), or repair, such as a hip replacement.
3. *Palliation.* To reduce the symptoms of a condition the person is experiencing, such as cutting a nerve root causing pain (rhizotomy) or bypassing an obstruction.
4. *Prevention.* Removal of cancer or precancerous cells.
5. *Cosmetic improvement.* To a body area that has suffered trauma/injury, such as removing scar tissue or reconstructing the breast after cancer.
6. *Exploration.* To determine the extent of a disease (Duff 2017).

If surgical treatment is necessary, and the patient is to be treated in a public hospital, national guidelines will be used by the surgeon to assign the patient to a surgical urgency category (table 9.2). The surgery category depends on the type of surgery needed and the surgery's recommended timeframe (National Elective Surgery Urgency Categorisation 2015).

TABLE 9.2 Time-based clinical urgency categories

Urgency category	Timeframe
Category 1 URGENT	Surgery/procedure is clinically indicated within 30 days If the patient's condition is likely to deteriorate (including worsening pain, dysfunction or disability), the patient will be placed in the urgent surgery category
Category 2 SEMI-URGENT	Surgery/procedure is clinically is indicated within 90 days
Category 3 NON-URGENT	Surgery/procedure is indicated within 365 days

Source: Adapted from Australian Government (2020).

Patients with private health cover may reduce their waiting time for elective surgery by choosing to be treated in a private hospital.

Some people may require emergency surgery and, therefore, will bypass the preadmission preparation. Emergency surgery cannot be delayed because the patient's life (or quality of life), organ or limb is at risk if they do not receive surgical intervention within 24 hours. A patient may require emergency surgery as a result of trauma, head injury or an acute condition. Patients who were scheduled for elective surgery for an existing condition but whose condition has deteriorated may also receive emergency surgery. Other examples of emergency surgery include an emergency caesarean section, acute appendicitis, strangulated hernia and gastrointestinal haemorrhage (Department of Health 2012).

Visitors to the perioperative environment

ACORN is Australia's peak organisation for perioperative nurses and provides standards, guidelines and education to support safe and evidence-based nursing practice. Guidelines for visitors to the perioperative area are developed by individual healthcare facilities but are based on the ACORN standards.

There may be a variety of people visiting the theatre at any one time and may include allied health students, medical company representatives, parents or carers of children and patient support persons. ACORN standard 'Visitors to the perioperative environment' (ACORN 2020) dictates that 'any visitor in the operating suite not associated with the care that is being provided has been said to be violating the patients right to privacy and confidentiality'. As a safety measure, visitors must wear visible identification.

Health services also carefully manage visitors to the perioperative environment to maintain patient privacy and confidentiality and help minimise the risk of introducing infection to the patient undergoing surgery.

Students visiting theatre must adhere to industry and health service guidelines to 'observe' a procedure. Primarily, this requires the student to have the patients consent to observe the procedure, wear appropriate theatre attire including clearly displayed 'visitor' identification, and agree to leave an area if asked to do so at any time. Documentation of the visit is to be recorded in the visitor logbook. Students must also be supervised and instructed when observing and participating in patient care (ACORN 2020).

Surgical terminology

Words used to name surgical procedures can be complicated and technical, and understanding their meaning can be challenging. The correct interpretation of terminology is imperative for communicating the information between the multi-professional team and patient safety (Penman & Tighe 2018). Breaking down the words within the terms can explain the patient's procedure (Walker, Wood & Nicol 2017). Medical words have a combination of prefixes, word roots and suffixes.

Prefixes are at the beginning of a word root; they modify the meaning of the word root to make it more specific. For example:

- hemi- means half (hemicolectomy removal of half of the colon)
- retro- means backward/behind (retroperitoneal = behind the peritoneum)
- dys- means painful/difficult (dysmenorrhoea = painful menstruation).
- hypo- means low (hypothermia).

Word roots provide the central meaning of a word. For example:

- bronch refers to the bronchus
- gastr/o refers to the stomach
- abdomin/o refers to the abdomen
- arteri/o refers to arteries
- arthro refers to a joint
- cardi/o refers to the heart.

Suffixes are at the end of the word root and describe the condition, investigation or surgical procedure. For example:

- -ectomy = excision or surgical removal, such as adenoidectomy (removal of the adenoids), hysterectomy (surgical removal of the uterus), hemicolectomy (removal of half of the colon).
- -scope = an instrument to view, such as an arthroscope (a scope to look at joints)
- -scopy = viewing something such as colonoscopy
- -otomy = incision/cut into, such as craniotomy (cranium/head), thoracotomy (thorax/chest)
- -plasty = moulding/grafting a body part, such as an arthroplasty (to restore the function) of a hip (Walker, Wood & Nicol 2017).

The following link to American-based Stanford Healthcare provides a list of common surgical procedures with explanations to help you become more familiar with medical terminology: https://stanfordhealthcare.org/medical-treatments/g/general-surgery/procedures.html

9.2 Preoperative assessment

LEARNING OBJECTIVE 9.2 Justify the purpose of preoperative assessment.

Before surgery, the preparation patients receive is critical to thoroughly prepare them for their surgery and reduce complications during the intraoperative and post-operative stages. Preoperative assessment is a critical component of preparing a patient for surgery (Cartwright & Andrews 2017). Depending on the type of surgery, the preadmission interview can be completed a number of weeks prior to the scheduled surgery, closer to the date of surgery or on the day of surgery. The preoperative assessment also prepares patients for their stay in hospital and identifies the care and supports patients may require once they are discharged from hospital (Hea et al. 2018).

The primary goals of the preoperative assessment are to ensure patient safety by:

1. identifying if it is safe for the person to undergo anaesthesia — surgery causes immune, metabolic and hormonal responses known as the stress response, which may cause complications for the patient after the surgery (Neil 2017)
2. optimising the patient's condition before anaesthesia by identifying and stabilising chronic conditions and recommending changes to lifestyle choices that increase the surgical risk for the patient, i.e. cessation of smoking and recreational drug use (Marley & Sheets 2018)
3. establishing the most suitable anaesthetic for the patient based on their presenting condition, health history and the type of surgery they require (Neil 2017).

The majority of elective surgery patients will be admitted for their procedure as 'a day case' or '**ambulant surgery**', i.e. the patient is admitted and discharged on the same day. Patients with chronic conditions or who have complex care requirements are often admitted to hospital the day before their procedure so that a care plan can be created to accommodate their coexisting problems (McCullagh & Lee 2016).

During the preadmission interview, the nurse's role is to work as part of a multi-professional team to develop a complete health picture of the patient to create an individualised person-centred care plan (Cartwright & Andrews 2017).

Information that will be collected from the patient includes the following.

1. Patient risk factors that may cause complications or challenges for the patient prior to, during or after surgery (language barriers, genetic factors, smoking, chronic medical conditions, obesity, allergies).
2. Baseline information, including vital signs, weight, height, medical and surgical history, functional assessment/mobility, overall health, nutrition, current medication regimen and the use of recreational drugs and alcohol. Medications should include all prescription, over-the-counter (OTC) medications and herbal preparations, as some may cause immune suppression, central nervous system depression, increase the patient's risk of bleeding or prolong the effects of anaesthetic agents (McCullagh & Lee 2016). Withdrawal symptoms from recreational drugs can manifest sympathetic and parasympathetic nervous symptoms, causing hypertension, tachycardia, abdominal cramping and diarrhoea, tremors, anxiety, irritability and dilated pupils (Marley & Sheets 2018).
3. Spiritual, cultural and psychosocial needs, including support systems that are currently in place or that may need to be provided post-operatively. Any concerns or fears about the surgery/body image the patient may have and any potential impact of the surgery on relationships should also be included in the discussion (Duff 2017). Other considerations will include if the patient is a child, is pregnant, has people they provide care for, or patients with mental or physical disabilities.

The patient may undergo more detailed full-body systems assessments to determine if they are medically fit to undergo surgery and anaesthesia, or if further investigations, such as X-ray, ECG and blood tests are required (Duff 2017; McCullagh & Lee 2016). Identifying these provides baseline information for comparison after surgery, helps ensure any specialised equipment is organised in time for surgery, and if other precautions are needed to be put in place. Information provided to the patient during the preadmission assessment includes the following.

1. An explanation of the procedure and type of anaesthetic that will be used and options for alternative treatments, including the potential side effects of treatments (McCullagh & Lee 2016).

2. Specifics about the procedure and pre-surgery instructions, such as when to arrive at the hospital, fasting times (an empty stomach reduces the risk of the patient aspirating stomach contents into their lung while they are under anaesthesia), when to stop herbal preparations, anticoagulant or diabetic medications. Patient education aims to increase the patient's understanding and decrease stress and anxiety for both the patient and their family. The degree of stress patients and their family experience in response to impending surgery is individual and may depend on the patient's age, previous hospitalisations or surgical experiences. Extreme stress responses may impact the immune response and predispose the patient to infection and/or prolonged recovery (Cartwright & Andrews 2017; Duff 2017; McCullagh & Lee 2016).
3. The health service the patient will go to for the surgery, including if the patient will be admitted on the day of surgery (**DOSA**), be a short-stay patient, or if admission as an inpatient is needed (Cartwright & Andrews 2017; Duff 2017).
4. The patient will complete anaesthetic consent and surgical consent during their consultation with the anaesthetist and surgeon. This may occur as part of the preadmission assessment prior to the patient arriving in hospital, or it may occur when the patient is admitted into the health facility and is awaiting surgery (Neil 2017).

Table 9.3 summarises the goals of preadmission.

TABLE 9.3 Preadmission patient goals

The patient understands why surgery is recommended, what the outcomes may be (including risks and adverse outcomes), and what other treatment options are available to them.
The patient understands the type of anaesthetic that will be administered and the potential risks and adverse outcomes.
The patient is identified as suitable to undergo the recommended surgery and anaesthetic. The need for the patient to undergo further tests/investigations before their surgery is identified and arranged.
The patient and or their family members/carers are provided with information about the intended surgery for them to refer back to.
The patient provides informed consent for two procedures: one for the surgery and one for the anaesthetic.
The patient agrees to the recommended hospital admission for the surgery, i.e. day patient, overnight stay or inpatient.

Source: Adapted from Cartwright & Andrews (2017); McCullagh & Lee (2016); Neil (2017).

On the day of surgery, the patient will complete the final preparation for their surgery. As the theatre time gets close, many patients and their family members become anxious or scared, and the nurse's role is to provide ongoing emotional support (Cartwright & Andrews 2017).

The patient's final preparation for surgery may include a preoperative bath/shower with an antiseptic skin wash and clipping of hair at the intended surgical site to reduce the patient's likelihood of surgical site infections (SSI). The patient will wear a clean hospital gown and remove any jewellery. The nurse caring for them will complete the first check of the preoperative checklist. It is also important that the nurse know the patient's details to provide a handover to the anaesthetic nurse in the holding bay.

9.3 Patient safety considerations during surgery

LEARNING OBJECTIVE 9.3 Identify and explain the primary considerations for patient safety during surgery.

In perioperative complexes, the combination of specific design features and strict processes keeps staff and patients safe. For example, physical features to reduce infection can include the type of airflow in the operating room as well as easy to clean surfaces of the floors and walls. The flow of personnel working within the areas is also controlled to reduce the potential for infection. Therefore, some requirements dictate how staff enter operating rooms, how staff physically move about when they are inside the operating room, how they pass equipment used in the surgery, where they stand and which rooms or areas are appropriate for them to enter. Other critical considerations are the correct use of electrical, laser and radiation equipment (Sutherland-Fraser 2016). Below are a number of additional considerations that are implemented to help keep patients safe during their surgery.

Asepsis

Asepsis is the foundation of perioperative care. Asepsis is the absence of infectious organisms on living tissue (Carlile & Evans 2016).A strict aseptic technique is used to minimise the risk of contaminated hands, surfaces or equipment breaching the **aseptic field**, thereby increasing the patient risk of developing surgical wound infection (Carlile & Evans 2016). The aseptic field includes the patient, operating table, instrument trolleys, any other furniture covered in aseptic drapes and staff.

Sterile is not the same as aseptic. For example, an unopened package is considered sterile; however, it is exposed to airborne pathogens when the package is opened and can no longer be considered a sterile item.

Optimising asepsis

The area around the operating table and the patient covered in sterile surgical drapes is known as the aseptic field. Only members of the scrub team can enter this area. The instrument and circulating practitioners are relied on to demonstrate **surgical conscience** (professional honesty) by acknowledging if they break the aseptic field. For example, circulating personnel who are not wearing sterile gowns and gloves could accidentally touch the sterile drapes and possibly cause contamination of the sterile field, which would be rectified by replacing the drape with a sterile one. Other measures include complying with checking and handling processes to ensure only sterile instruments are used, reducing the risks of breaches by controlling the physical environment (movement of people into and around the theatre, appropriate adding of instruments/equipment to the aseptic field), and members of the surgical team completing a surgical hand-scrub and use of skin preparations to prepare the surgical site (Carlile & Evans 2016). Figure 9.1 identifies the aseptic field.

FIGURE 9.1 The aseptic field

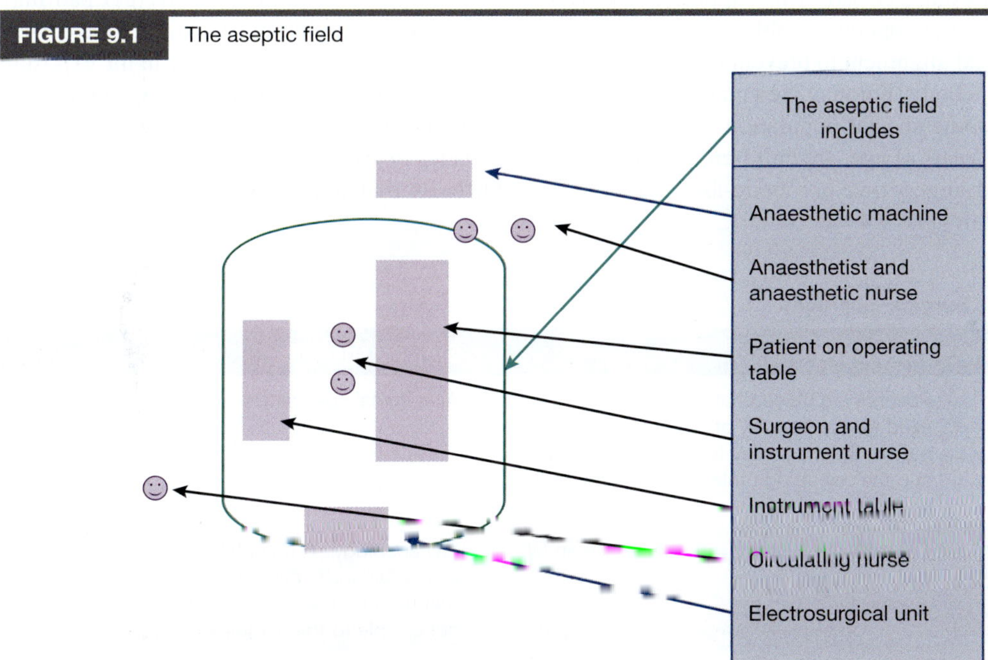

Theatre staff are the greatest avenue for the introduction of organisms into the perioperative environment. Theatre attire is provided by and laundered by health services for staff, minimising microbial shedding from key body areas such as skin, hair and the respiratory tract. Theatre attire includes hats and balaclavas covering the head and facial hair, scrub suits, warm-up jackets and cover gowns. Personal protective equipment (PPE) is also provided and should be worn according to the task. Staff must provide their own footwear that is not worn outside of the perioperative area. Fingernails must be short and polish-free. Artificial nails or acrylic nails and jewellery should be minimal and must be covered by the theatre attire (ACORN 2020).

A summary of the key elements of asepsis in the operating room is as follows.

- All materials that enter the sterile field must be sterile.
- If a sterile item comes in contact with an unsterile item, it is contaminated.

- Contaminated items are removed immediately from the sterile field. If the unsterile item is small (e.g. unopened suture), the area is marked off (i.e. covered with a sterile drape) once it is removed. If the entire field is contaminated, it should be set up again with all new materials.
- The surgical team working in the operative field must wear sterile gowns and gloves. Once dressed for the procedure, they must recognise that the only parts of the gown considered sterile are front from chest to table level and sleeves to 5 centimetres above the elbow.
- A wide margin of safety must be maintained between sterile and unsterile fields.
- Tables are considered sterile only at tabletop level. Items extending beneath this level are considered contaminated.
- The edges of a sterile package are considered contaminated once the package has been opened; their contents must be removed by methods that preserve their sterility.
- Microorganisms travel on airborne particles and will enter a sterile field with excessive air movements and currents.
- Microorganisms travel by capillary action through moist fabrics, and contamination occurs.
- Microorganisms harbour on the patient's and team members' hair, skin and respiratory tracts and must be confined by appropriate attire (Shoup & Horner 2017).

Patient positioning

Positioning the unconscious or sedated patient for surgery enables access to the site of surgery, and strategies are implemented to protect the patient from prevent pressure injury or eye injury, and skin, nerve or musculoskeletal damage that may result from poor or incorrect positioning (ACORN 2020). Pressure-dispersing gel pads will support bony prominences during surgery. A full-body gel pad may be used between the operating table and the supine patient. Patient positioning must also provide correct musculoskeletal alignment to prevent occlusion of arteries and veins and provide modesty in the exposure of the patient's body (Foran & Newman 2017). Additional positioning considerations and precautions are required for some special population groups, such as people who are underweight or obese, pregnant, older than 70 years of age, are children, people who have diabetes or vascular disease, or when there is a long-expected surgery time or robotic-assisted surgery (ACORN 2020). Commonly used surgical positions are explained in table 9.4.

TABLE 9.4 Surgical positions

Position	Description	Surgical speciality
Supine	Patients are placed flat on their back. Also used for the transfer of patients from the patient theatre trolley to the operating table, and the operating table to the patient trolley or be.	All surgical specialities
Trendelenburg	The patient is supine with a head-down tilt.	Gynaecology: The contents of the abdominal cavity fall under gravity towards the diaphragm, making the organs more accessible to the surgeon
Reverse Trendelenburg	The patient lies supine with a head-up tilt.	Head and neck and ear, nose and throat surgery
Lateral	The patient is positioned on the left or right side.	General, vascular, urology, plastic, orthopaedic, trauma and thoracic
Lithotomy	The patient lies supine with the legs raised and the feet placed in stirrups. The lower end of the operating table is removed.	Gynaecology, urology and lower bowel surgical procedures
Prone	The patient lies on his or her front.	General, urology, orthopaedic

Venous thromboembolism

Venous thromboembolism (VTE) is a potentially preventable complication when a patient develops a blood clot and pulmonary embolism, resulting in several adverse outcomes, including death. Vascular injury from surgery and venous stasis due to immobility, alterations to blood coagulability and damage to blood vessel walls are associated with the development of VTE in perioperative patients (ACSQHC 2020; Hamlin & Minton 2016).

Several other factors increase the perioperative patient's risk of developing VTE and include:

- those undergoing major surgery, especially intra-abdominal and pelvic procedures
- those undergoing surgery longer than 45 minutes and aged >40 years
- orthopaedic patients, especially those undergoing reconstructive surgery
- the elderly
- patients with an acute inflammatory condition
- smokers
- the obese
- those with a family history of thromboembolism
- major trauma victims
- those with metabolic disorders or blood dyscrasias (e.g. inherited thrombophilia disorders)
- those with certain kinds of cancer
- those on oral contraception and hormone replacement medications (Hamlin & Minton 2016).

Prevention of VTE formation can be medical (low molecular weight heparins) or intermittent pneumatic compression devices that inflate to compress the calf muscles, resulting in a passive pumping action that reduces the likelihood of venous stasis in the limb (Hamlin & Minton 2016).

Hypothermia

An anaesthetised patient cannot effectively compensate for heat loss. This is due to drug interference with their autonomic nervous system and reduction in muscle tone, preventing heat generation by shivering. Patients having open body cavity surgery (thoracic or abdominal) will also rapidly lose body heat through convection. In addition, the patient's 'central heating system', the circulatory system, will have slowed down (as shown by a decreased heart rate and blood pressure on the induction of anaesthesia) and may be cooling down due to the introduction of intravenous fluids at room temperature.

Patients with a core temperature of less than 36 degrees Celsius will receive interventions to warm up, as hypothermia has several risks to patient safety, including:

- post-operative myocardial ischaemia
- poor blood clotting times
- increased risk of wound infection
- increased post-operative pain
- delayed wound healing
- decreased metabolism and clearance of medications
- increased blood loss
- impaired immune function
- prolonged post-operative recovery time
- increased length of stay in hospital (ACORN 2020; McCullagh & Lee 2017).

Electrical safety

Electrosurgical equipment uses electricity to incise and coagulate tissue at the point it is applied. Electrosurgery has positive outcomes for surgical patients; however, risks to the patient can include burns, electric shock, explosions, fire and interference with implanted devices (ACORN 2020). Knowing how and where to correctly position the diathermy plate, which connects the patient to the ESU, is a significant safety consideration to protect the patient from injury (Foran & Newton 2017).

Specimen handling

When specimens are collected for pathology examination, errors in specimen handling can lead to delayed or misdiagnosis, delayed treatment and potentially unnecessary additional surgeries. Strict specimen collection, labelling, checking and documentation procedures guide the safe collection and transfer of specimens to pathology (ACORN 2020).

9.4 Anaesthesia

LEARNING OBJECTIVE 9.4 Outline the purpose, types and stages of anaesthesia and common pharmacological agents used for anaesthesia.

Anaesthesia is a pharmacologically induced lack of sensation and/or awareness of a specific area or the whole body. For example, local or regional anaesthesia blocks sensation to a specific body area or region. The patient will remain breathing for themselves and be lightly sedated so they do not feel anxious during the procedure

General anaesthesia

General anaesthesia (GA) affects the whole body. The patient will be unconscious and may be paralysed, which also means that they cannot breathe for themselves and will need the support of an anaesthetic machine to breathe for them (Shoup & Horner 2017).

There are three phases of GA.

1. *Induction phase*. The patient is given medications that will make them unconscious, and their airway device will be inserted.
2. *Maintenance phase*. The patient remains deeply unconscious, and their vital signs are monitored continuously. Additional anaesthetic medications are administered as needed while the surgery is performed.
3. *Emergence phase*. The patient is returned to consciousness, and any airway devices are removed when the anaesthetist deems it is safe to do so (Foran & Newman 2017).

Regional anaesthesia

Regional anaesthesia (RA) is administered into the patients back to into nerve bundles to block movement, sensation and nerve conduction to specific areas of the body, such as a limb, joint or lower abdomen (ANZCA 2020). Sometimes patients can have a regional anaesthetic block such as an epidural to control post-operative pain.

RA includes spinal, epidural and caudal analgesia. Spinal anaesthesia is a one-off injection of anaesthetic into the subarachnoid space at the level of the lumbar spine. The anaesthetic mixes with the cerebrospinal fluid (CSF) to rapidly block autonomic, sensory and motor function and causes vasodilation and hypotension. The patient may be awake or sedated but cannot feel anything or move the area that has been blocked.

An epidural block is when an anaesthetic is injected into the epidural space, working on the spinal cord's nerve roots to block sensory and or motor pathways. Epidural blocks can be used for surgery with an awake patient or in conjunction with GA. They may remain in situ post-operatively to provide the patient with ongoing pain relief (Shoup & Horner 2017).

Caudal anaesthesia is commonly used in paediatric patients and is inserted into the epidural space at the sacral level to block pain in the legs and lower body (Wiegele, Marhofer & Lonnqvist 2019).

Local anaesthesia

Local anaesthesia can be used as the sole anaesthetic in minor procedures, an adjunct to other anaesthetics, or to support post-operative pain relief. For example, local anaesthesia can be injected directly into the surgical site at the end of the surgery to help reduce post-operative pain (Foran & Newman 2017).

Sedation

Sedation helps the patient feel calm, or sleep, while other sedatives such as opioids alter the patient's sense of pain (ANZCA 2020). Sometimes sedation is used in conjunction with other types of anaesthetic or as the sole anaesthetic. When patients are sedated they are still able to breathe for themselves and respond to verbal instructions.

The anaesthetist will decide on the best type of anaesthesia for the patient, based on the type of surgery required, the preadmission patient assessment findings, the airway assessment and the availability of additional resources and equipment. The summary of types of anaesthesia can be seen in table 9.5.

TABLE 9.5 **Types of anaesthesia**

Type of anaesthesia	Effect on the patient
General anaesthesia	Loss of consciousness and all sensation, patient is unable to move, breathe for themselves or protect their airway.
Regional anaesthesia	Patient is awake and can breathe for themselves. The patient has no sensation a specific area of their body. The patient may be drowsy due to medications (sedatives, anxiolytics or analgesics) that help them feel more relaxed during the procedure.
Local anaesthetic	The patient is fully awake and can breathe for themselves. The patient has no sensation in the tissue near the area being operated on.

Source: Adapted from ANZCA (2020).

Airway devices for anaesthesia

The anaesthetist will decide to use a laryngeal mask airway (LMA) or endotracheal tube (ETT). There are significant differences between an ETT and an LMA. The anaesthetist will take the patient's anatomical and physiological condition and the length and type of surgery into consideration as well as the patient's risk of aspiration. Intubation is when an ETT is passed inserted into the patient's trachea. The ETT is passed through the patient's vocal cords. Then a balloon is inflated to seal the airway and protect against aspiration. An LMA is used on patients who have fasted for their surgery, and do not require an ETT. It is positioned to sit at the back of the patient's larynx and, therefore, does not protect the patient against aspiration of stomach contents (Walters & Kumar 2017). Table 9.6 outlines the comparison of when an ETT or LMA device is chosen.

TABLE 9.6 **Indications for endotracheal (ETT) and laryngeal mask (LMA) use**

	ETT	LMA
Patient needs	Patients who are known to be at risk of aspiration, i.e. those with: • hiatus hernia • small bowel obstruction • opiate use • pregnancy • a full stomach • trauma/emergency admission. Post-arrest — patient may need ventilating Post surgery requirements — patient may need to be ventilated	Patients who are known to have followed fasting guidelines and do not come into the category for ETT intubation Patients who are free from cardiovascular and respiratory compromise
Surgical needs	Type of surgery, i.e.: • laparoscopic surgery • with patients in particular positions • surgery lasting over 2 hours • surgery in which the surgeon needs to use a muscle relaxant, e.g. laparotomy.	Surgery that will take less than two hours Surgery in which the patient's position will not interfere with spontaneous breathing or intragastric pressure, i.e. not prone

Source: Walters & Kumar (2017).

Figures 9.2 and 9.3 show the differences between an ETT and a LMA.

Medication therapy for anaesthesia

Medications for anaesthesia include a combination of:

- intravenous (IV) medications that put the patient into an unconscious state
- inhalation medications that the patient breathes to keep them unconscious
- benzodiazepines to help alleviate patient's anxiety
- opioids for pain relief and sedation

- antiemetics to prevent vomiting while the patient is unconscious
- antibiotics (prophylactically or for treatment of infection) (Foran & Newman 2017).

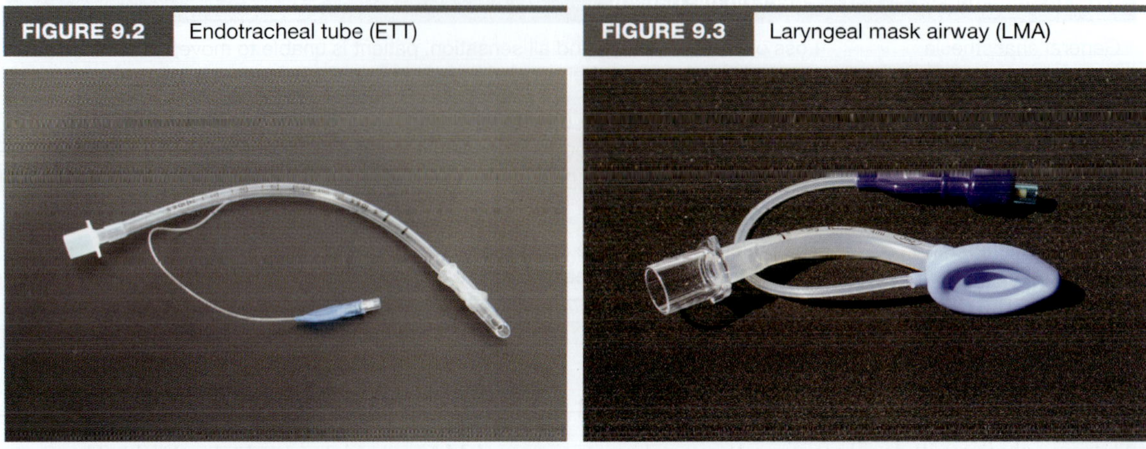

FIGURE 9.2 Endotracheal tube (ETT)

FIGURE 9.3 Laryngeal mask airway (LMA)

Commonly used medications for GA can be reviewed in table 9.7.

TABLE 9.7 Commonly used medications for GA

Medication	Example	
Induction agents	Propofol	Administered at the start of surgery to make the patient unconscious
Analgesics	Morphine	Administered throughout the surgery to provide pain relief
Muscle relaxants	Suxamethonium	Administered so the patient cannot move
Inhalation agents	Sevoflurane	The patient breaths the anaesthetic in throughout the surgery to keep them unconscious
Benzodiazepines (sedative/hypnotic medications)		Administered to cause amnesia so the patient cannot remember their surgery
Antiemetics	Droperidol	To stop the person vomiting during their surgery or to stop them feeling nauseous
Other		Medications to prevent

Source: Adapted from Australian Society of Anaesthetists (2021).

9.5 Perioperative nursing roles

LEARNING OBJECTIVE 9.5 Differentiate the anaesthetic, instrument/circulating and PACU nurse roles in the delivery of safe perioperative patient care.

There are several different nursing roles in each of the perioperative stages involved in delivering safe patient care.

The anaesthetic nurse

The anaesthetic nurse plays a pivotal role in patient care. Their role is to be a patient advocate, ensure that the patient remains the focus and that safe, high-quality care is delivered. The anaesthetic nurse provides care for patients immediately before and during surgery, when patients are at their most vulnerable (ACORN 2020).

Closer to the surgery time, the patient will be taken to the holding bay, where they will be 'checked in' for the surgery by the anaesthetic nurse. The check-in process is when the anaesthetic nurse completes the second check in the preoperative checklist to establish that the correct patient is received for the correct procedure, that consent has been completed and witnessed, and that the required processes have been followed, including:

- the patient's name and how they would like to be addressed
- checking that the patient has been sufficiently prepared for anaesthesia in terms of fasting (to reduce the risk of aspiration of the stomach contents during anaesthesia)
- surgical site marking has been completed — before the patient is taken into surgery, the surgeon will mark the operating site to avoid the potential for operating on the wrong site, such as limbs, digits, breasts, kidneys
- that any other information that may impact the patient's care is articulated, such as consent for blood use and the availability of products that have previously been requested.

An example of a preoperative checklist can be seen in figure 9.4.

FIGURE 9.4 Preoperative checklist

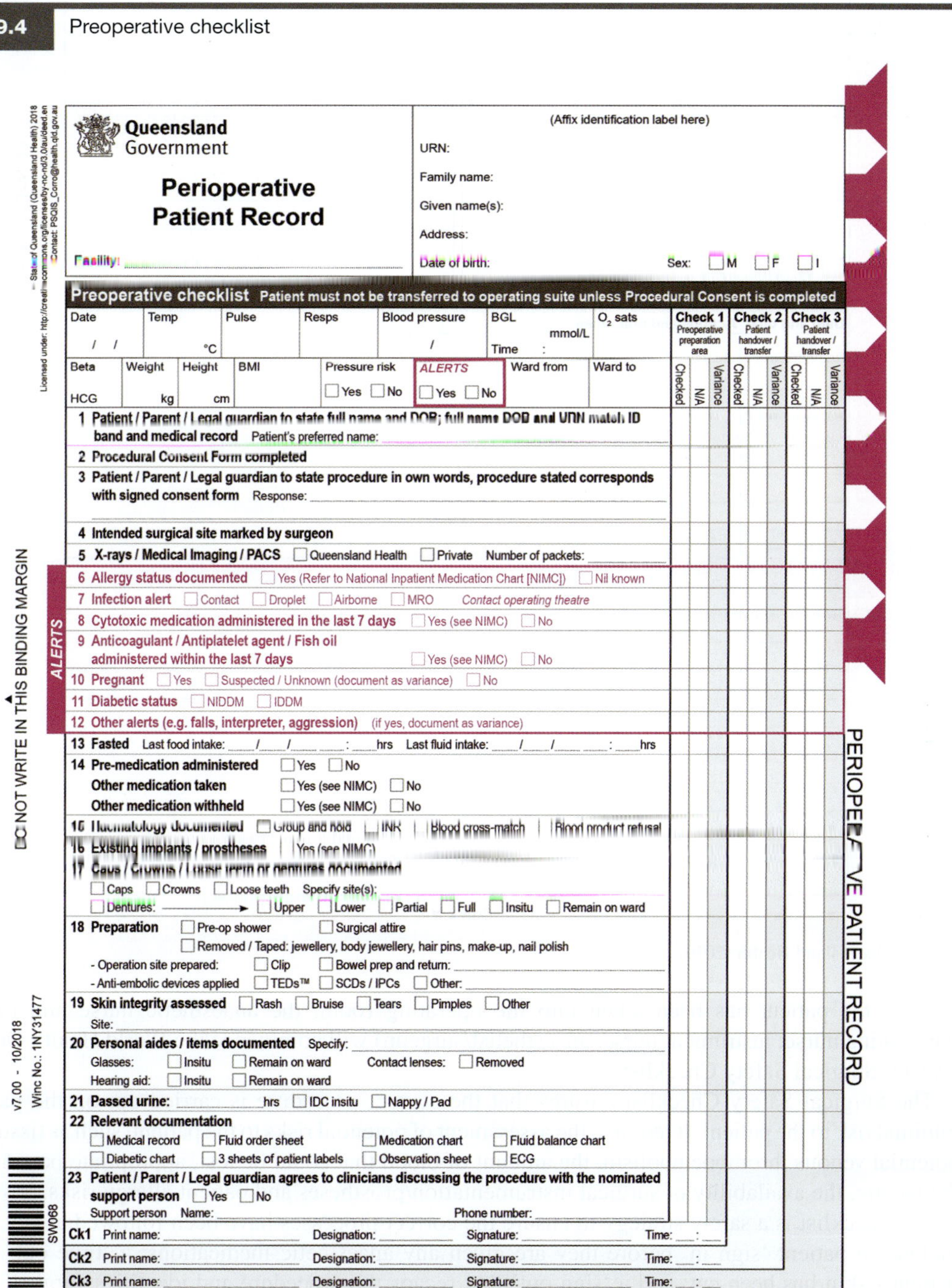

Queensland Government

Perioperative Patient Record

Facility:

(Affix identification label here)

URN:

Family name:

Given name(s):

Address:

Date of birth: Sex: ☐ M ☐ F ☐ I

Preoperative checklist Patient must not be transferred to operating suite unless Procedural Consent is completed

Date	Temp	Pulse	Resps	Blood pressure	BGL	O2 sats
/ /	°C			/	mmol/L Time :	

Beta HCG	Weight	Height	BMI	Pressure risk	ALERTS	Ward from	Ward to
	kg	cm		☐ Yes ☐ No	☐ Yes ☐ No		

Check 1 Preoperative preparation area — Checked / N/A / Variance
Check 2 Patient handover / transfer — Checked / N/A / Variance
Check 3 Patient handover / transfer — Checked / N/A / Variance

1 Patient / Parent / Legal guardian to state full name and DOB; full name DOB and URN match ID band and medical record Patient's preferred name:

2 Procedural Consent Form completed

3 Patient / Parent / Legal guardian to state procedure in own words, procedure stated corresponds with signed consent form Response:

4 Intended surgical site marked by surgeon

5 X-rays / Medical Imaging / PACS ☐ Queensland Health ☐ Private Number of packets:

ALERTS

6 Allergy status documented ☐ Yes (Refer to National Inpatient Medication Chart [NIMC]) ☐ Nil known

7 Infection alert ☐ Contact ☐ Droplet ☐ Airborne ☐ MRO *Contact operating theatre*

8 Cytotoxic medication administered in the last 7 days ☐ Yes (see NIMC) ☐ No

9 Anticoagulant / Antiplatelet agent / Fish oil administered within the last 7 days ☐ Yes (see NIMC) ☐ No

10 Pregnant ☐ Yes ☐ Suspected / Unknown (document as variance) ☐ No

11 Diabetic status ☐ NIDDM ☐ IDDM

12 Other alerts (e.g. falls, interpreter, aggression) (if yes, document as variance)

13 Fasted Last food intake: __/__/__ __:__ hrs Last fluid intake: __/__/__ __:__ hrs

14 Pre-medication administered ☐ Yes ☐ No
Other medication taken ☐ Yes (see NIMC) ☐ No
Other medication withheld ☐ Yes (see NIMC) ☐ No

15 Haematology documented ☐ Group and hold ☐ INR ☐ Blood cross-match ☐ Blood product refusal

16 Existing implants / prostheses ☐ Yes (see NIMC)

17 Caps / Crowns / Loose teeth or dentures documented
☐ Caps ☐ Crowns ☐ Loose teeth Specify site(s):
☐ Dentures: → ☐ Upper ☐ Lower ☐ Partial ☐ Full ☐ Insitu ☐ Remain on ward

18 Preparation ☐ Pre-op shower ☐ Surgical attire
☐ Removed / Taped: jewellery, body jewellery, hair pins, make-up, nail polish
- Operation site prepared: ☐ Clip ☐ Bowel prep and return:
- Anti-embolic devices applied ☐ TEDs™ ☐ SCDs / IPCs ☐ Other:

19 Skin integrity assessed ☐ Rash ☐ Bruise ☐ Tears ☐ Pimples ☐ Other
Site:

20 Personal aides / items documented Specify:
Glasses: ☐ Insitu ☐ Remain on ward Contact lenses: ☐ Removed
Hearing aid: ☐ Insitu ☐ Remain on ward

21 Passed urine: ____ hrs ☐ IDC insitu ☐ Nappy / Pad

22 Relevant documentation
☐ Medical record ☐ Fluid order sheet ☐ Medication chart ☐ Fluid balance chart
☐ Diabetic chart ☐ 3 sheets of patient labels ☐ Observation sheet ☐ ECG

23 Patient / Parent / Legal guardian agrees to clinicians discussing the procedure with the nominated support person ☐ Yes ☐ No
Support person Name: Phone number:

Ck1	Print name:	Designation:	Signature:	Time: :
Ck2	Print name:	Designation:	Signature:	Time: :
Ck3	Print name:	Designation:	Signature:	Time: :

Page 1 of 3

DO NOT WRITE IN THIS BINDING MARGIN

PERIOPERATIVE PATIENT RECORD

v7.00 - 10/2018 Winc No.: 1NY31477 SW068

Queensland Government

Perioperative Patient Record

(Affix identification label here)

URN:

Family name:

Given name(s):

Address:

Date of birth: Sex: ☐M ☐F ☐I

Allergies

Allergy	Reaction

Existing implants and prostheses

Type	Site

Variances / Other alerts / Additional notes

Date and time	Actions and outcomes

DO NOT WRITE IN THIS BINDING MARGIN

Page 2 of 3

Source: Queensland Health (2019).

Once the patient has been taken into the operating room, the anaesthetic nurse and theatre staff (circulating nurse, instrument nurse, anaesthetist/surgeon) will commence the World Health Organization (WHO) Surgical Safety Checklist.

The Surgical Safety Checklist ensures that the correct procedure is carried out on the patient, with minimal risk to the patient. It requires the assessment of potential risks to the patient, such as tissue viability, potential venous thromboembolism, the amount of blood that could be lost, appropriate personnel within the theatre, the availability of surgical instrumentation/prostheses and patient allergy risks.

The checklist is a safety strategy to ensure the correct processes have been followed at key stages and includes a patient 'sign in' before they are given any anaesthetic medications; a 'time out' before the patient's skin has been cut; and a 'sign out' that recaps the procedure and identifies surgical counts are completed and correct, specimens that have been obtained, and any concerns for the patient's recovery. The WHO Surgical Safety Checklist (see figure 9.5) has been demonstrated to dramatically reduce errors where a culture of whole-team involvement is present (ACSQHC 2019) and is used across the whole of Australia.

FIGURE 9.5 Surgical safety checklist

SURGICAL SAFETY CHECKLIST (AUSTRALIA AND NEW ZEALAND)

Before induction of anaesthesia ▶ ▶ ▶ ▶ ▶ Before skin incision ▶ ▶ ▶ ▶ ▶ ▶ ▶ ▶ ▶ ▶ Before patient leaves operating room

SIGN IN

☐ **PATIENT HAS CONFIRMED**
- IDENTITY
- SITE
- PROCEDURE
- CONSENT

☐ **SITE MARKED/NOT APPLICABLE**

☐ **ANAESTHESIA SAFETY CHECK COMPLETED**

☐ **PULSE OXIMETER ON PATIENT AND FUNCTIONING**

DOES PATIENT HAVE A :

KNOWN ALLERGY?
☐ NO
☐ YES

DIFFICULT AIRWAY/ASPIRATION RISK?
☐ NO
☐ YES, AND EQUIPMENT/ASSISTANCE AVAILABLE

RISK OF >500ML BLOOD LOSS (7ML/KG IN CHILDREN)?
☐ NO
☐ YES, AND ADEQUATE INTRAVENOUS ACCESS AND FLUIDS PLANNED

PROSTHESIS/SPECIAL EQUIPMENT:

IF PROSTHESIS (OR SPECIAL EQUIPMENT) IS TO BE USED IN THEATRE, HAS IT BEEN CHECKED AND CONFIRMED?
☐ YES
☐ NOT APPLICABLE

TIME OUT

☐ **CONFIRM ALL TEAM MEMBERS HAVE INTRODUCED THEMSELVES BY NAME AND ROLE**

☐ **SURGEON, ANAESTHESIA PROFESSIONAL AND NURSE VERBALLY CONFIRM**
- PATIENT
- SITE
- PROCEDURE

ANTICIPATED CRITICAL EVENTS

☐ **SURGEON REVIEWS:** WHAT ARE THE CRITICAL OR UNEXPECTED STEPS, OPERATIVE DURATION, ANTICIPATED BLOOD LOSS?

☐ **ANAESTHESIA TEAM REVIEWS:** ARE THERE ANY PATIENT-SPECIFIC CONCERNS?

☐ **NURSING TEAM REVIEWS:** HAS STERILITY (INCLUDING INDICATOR RESULTS) BEEN CONFIRMED? ARE THERE EQUIPMENT ISSUES OR ANY CONCERNS?

HAS ANTIBIOTIC PROPHYLAXIS BEEN GIVEN WITHIN THE LAST 60 MINUTES?
☐ YES
☐ NOT APPLICABLE

HAS THROMBOPROPHYLAXIS BEEN ORDERED?
☐ YES
☐ NOT REQUIRED

IS ESSENTIAL IMAGING DISPLAYED?
☐ YES
☐ NOT APPLICABLE

SIGN OUT

NURSE VERBALLY CONFIRMS WITH THE TEAM:

☐ **THE NAME OF THE PROCEDURE RECORDED**

☐ **THAT INSTRUMENT, SPONGE, NEEDLE AND OTHER COUNTS ARE CORRECT**

☐ **HOW THE SPECIMEN IS LABELLED** (INCLUDING PATIENT NAME)

☐ **WHETHER THERE ARE ANY EQUIPMENT PROBLEMS TO BE ADDRESSED**

☐ **SURGEON, ANAESTHESIA PROFESSIONAL AND NURSE REVIEW THE KEY CONCERNS FOR RECOVERY AND MANAGEMENT OF THIS PATIENT**

Source: Royal Australian College of Surgeons (2009).

Prior to any further intervention, the anaesthetic nurse will ensure the necessary airway equipment is set up ready for use by the anaesthetist, attach the patient to monitoring equipment such as non-invasive blood pressure, oxygen saturation probe and electrocardiograph (ECG) leads. Once baseline observations have been observed and recorded, intravenous fluids may be commenced. The anaesthetic nurse's next priority is to provide support and reassurance to the patient while assisting the anaesthetist in anaesthetising the patient and securing the patient's airway (Foran & Newton 2017).

The circulating nurse

The circulating nurse applies high levels of knowledge regarding evidence-based practice, nursing standards and principles related to a wide range of topics, including (but not limited to) risk management, asepsis and aseptic technique, infection prevention and control, documentation, anatomy and physiology, pharmacology, surgical and anaesthetic procedures, instrumentation and associated equipment, and medico-legal requirements and compliance (ACORN 2020).

The circulating nurse opens the instrument sets using an aseptic technique, and the instrument nurse opens and prepares the instruments for the surgical procedure. The instrument and circulating nurses check the swabs, needles and individual instruments as part of the instrument set against the instrument checklist. The quantities of swabs, needles and accessories are noted on the count sheet to highlight the numbers used in the surgical procedure. This is used when the wound is opened and before it is closed to ensure nothing has been left in the wound at the end of the procedure. The surgeon is told when a correct count check has been confirmed.

The instrument nurse

Instrument nurses have a highly specialised role and apply high levels of knowledge regarding evidence-based practice, nursing standards and principles related to a wide range of skills. Technical skills include (but are not limited to) recognising clinical deterioration and complications and responding by planning, implementing and evaluating nursing care. Non-technical skills include strong clinical and interpersonal communication skills that help to keep unconscious patients safe (ACORN 2020).

The instrument and circulating nurses ensure the aseptic field is not compromised, the patient is positioned correctly and that patient's privacy is maintained.

In the event of a missing item, the instrument nurse should check the sterile drapes and instrument trolley. The surgeon will check the wound, and the theatre team will check the swabs and accessories given out during the procedure, the waste and linen bags and the theatre environment. If the missing item cannot be located, an X-ray will be taken to establish whether the item is still inside the patient. If the item is not found, incident reporting is then triggered (Foran & Newman 2017).

Surgical modalities

Each surgeon has their own surgical technique and preferences, which means they will have specific instructions for post-operative care for their patients. The instructions will be handed over to the ward nurse by the **PACU** nurse and included in the surgeon's operation report. These instructions must be followed, and the surgeon notified if the nurse has any concerns for the patient's post operative recovery.

Open surgery is when a scalpel is used to make an incision large enough to perform the surgery. Open surgery is used when access to larger areas or the use of larger equipment is needed (Cole & Allanson 2016). Improved technology has allowed several modes of surgery to be developed that have improved patient outcomes.

Minimally invasive surgery (MIS) refers to surgeries that can be done laparoscopically. This approach is performed by the surgeon inserting a tiny camera and other equipment through a number of small incisions. The camera projects the images onto a video screen so that the instruments can be guided into the correct positions for surgery. MIS can take longer than open surgery; however, there is no large incision. Therefore, scars are smaller, the patient's hospital stay is shorter, there is less post-operative pain, and recovery times are faster than open surgery so the patient can resume their normal activities sooner (Ball 2018; Cole & Allanson 2016).

Robotic devices are used laparoscopically and mimic the surgeon's movements but are more precise and potentially have greater flexibility and range of motion than the surgeon. Other advantages of robotic surgery include greater visualisation of the patient's anatomy and reduced blood loss and muscle damage (Ball 2018).

Surgical dressings

Surgical drains

If fluid (blood, interstitial fluid, bile, pus) or air is allowed to collect in a wound, it compromises wound healing, impairs circulation and increases the risk of an infection developing. Surgical drain tubes are used to facilitate the drainage of fluid from the surgical site. Surgical drains are either 'passive' open drains where drainage of fluid occurs via soft tubing latex into a dressing or a collection bag, or 'active' where negative pressure creates suction that drains the fluid via a tube into a container (concertina drain, expelled bulb or re-evacuated bottle). Examples of surgical drains include the Jackson-Pratt (JP) drain and Hemovac drain (Parkman & Richardson-Tench 2016).

A description of the wound drainage is an important component of wound assessment. It can be described as sanguineous (red), serosanguinous (pink), serous (clear/yellow) or purulent (infected).

The post-anaesthesia care unit (PACU) nurse

Following surgery, all patients are admitted to the PACU, where they will be cared for in the immediate post-operative period. The PACU nurse will receive a comprehensive handover from the anaesthetist and scrub nurse that should include:

- the patient's name
- the operation or procedure that has been performed
- the type of anaesthetic delivered (spinal, epidural or general)
- the intraoperative management in terms of airway management, observations (vital signs recordings), positioning, warming devices, prophylaxis for deep vein thrombosis, and the drugs and fluids administered
- information relating to immediate post-surgery care, for example, surgical drains and wound care
- post-anaesthesia instructions for PACU
- post-operative instructions for the ward.

In PACU, care of the patient is the multi-professional responsibility of the surgeon, anaesthetist and nurse. Patients in PACU are at high risk of rapid clinical deterioration secondary to anaesthesia, surgery or pre-existing comorbidities.

The PACU nurse role requires them to work within a legal and ethical framework, apply specialist knowledge, professional standards and guidelines to recognise and respond to clinical deterioration, and assess the patient's readiness for discharge (ACORN 2020). Patients can develop a range of post-operative complications after their surgery. The PACU nurse's role is to observe, assess and document the patient's vital signs, and identify and escalate if the patient is showing signs of deterioration (Foran 2016). General comfort interventions can include:

- providing a warm blanket/warming devices
- applying pneumatic compression devices if indicated
- providing pressure area care and mouth care
- returning the patient's eye glasses/hearing aids for them to use (Foran 2016).

Figure 9.6 summarises the PACU nurse–patient assessment after surgery. The frequency of documenting vital signs depends on the type of surgery and anaesthetic the patient has had and the health service requirements but can range from between five and 30 minutes.

FIGURE 9.6 PACU patient assessments/observation

Primary survey: DR ABCDE

- D Danger
- R Response — level of consciousness, alert/oriented, pupil reaction and size
- A Airway — patent, presence of oral or nasal airway device
- B Breathing — respiratory rate and quality, breath sounds, pulse oximetry, supplemental oxygen
- C Circulation — ECG rhythm and rate, blood pressure, temperature, pulses and capillary refill
- D Disability
- E Exposure

Secondary survey and focused assessment

- Gastrointestinal system: does the patient have nausea/vomiting? — IV fluids.
- Genitourinary system: Does the patient have a urinary catheter, fluid balance chart?

- Neurological system: GCS for patients who have had neuro surgery.
- Surgical site: assess the skin around the dressing site for bruising, swelling, assess the dressing for any blood ooze from surgical wound, assess surgical drain tubes for drainage, patency, kinks in tubing and connections are connected.
- Pain assessment, including dermatome and bromage assessment if indicated by the type of anaesthetic the patient has received.
- Vascular observations for patients who have had limb surgery.

Source: Adapted from Foran (2016) 'Post-operative care', Pg. 389 in *Lewis's medical surgical nursing*.

Post-operative nausea and vomiting

Active vomiting can have a detrimental effect on the patient in terms of its being an unpleasant experience, and the physical strain can cause damage to sutured incision sites, surgical flaps and anastomosis sites. Any patient may suffer from post-operative nausea and vomiting (**PONV**), but certain factors may increase its risk, for example:

- surgical interventions
- factors related to the patient
- the type of anaesthesia
- drugs that are known to induce nausea and vomiting (e.g. opiates)
- the physiological condition of the patient in PACU.

Multimodal antiemetic regimens will involve more than one group of drugs as this offers each drug group to target a specific site of action.

Multimodal pain management

Pain management is often addressed and planned prior to surgery so that pain is managed proactively rather than reactively once the patient is out of theatre. However, patients do not always respond to pain in the same way. Hence, pain management regimens depend on effective communication skills to elicit information on how much pain patients are suffering and what type of pain it is. It is important to obtain a detailed handover to establish whether the patient has had an analgesic in theatre and what type, such as an opiate, non-steroidal anti-inflammatory drug or paracetamol.

Not all pain experienced in recovery can be attributed to surgery; other factors contributing to pain (headaches, bladder distension, pain from positioning, etc.) may need to be considered. It is important to assess the nature and cause of any pain, and several tools have been devised to establish the severity of pain, including visual and verbal pain scales. As with any drugs administered to a patient, there are a number of issues to consider, including what analgesic drugs are available, the pharmacology of these drugs, their indications and contraindications, and their interactions.

Multimodal pain relief is when more than one class of pain-relieving medication is used to treat pain. A multimodal strategy uses more than one mechanism of action to relieve pain, and lower doses of single medications are required, making it a more effective strategy (Schoenwald 2017). Unrelieved pain can have several side effects for the patient and can cause increased heart rate, blood pressure and oxygen requirements of the heart and increase respiratory rate.

9.6 Discharge and return to ward patient care

LEARNING OBJECTIVE 9.6 Interpret the criteria used to identify when it is safe for a patient to return to the ward after surgery and understand the nursing care requirements for post-surgery patients.

Discharging a patient from PACU

Once the PACU nurse thinks the patient is recovered, specific criteria are assessed to determine if the patient's condition is stable and safe to leave PACU and be cared for on the ward. Patient scoring systems assess the return of the patient's motor functions and protective reflexes by scoring the patient's limb activity/movement, respirations, circulation, skin colour and conscious state. Aldrete scoring system for patient discharge for more detailed examples.

A score of 9 or 10 is often required for a patient to be discharged from the PACU to an area of care where nurse–patient ratios are different, and the patient does not require specialist one to one nursing care (Ecoff, Palomo & Stichler 2017).

To complete the patient's journey through the theatre department, a comprehensive and succinct handover to the ward staff is necessary. This is carried out verbally as well as documented in the patient's notes. Information should be provided using the ISBAR (Identify, Situation, Background, Assessment, Recommendation) format. ISBAR is commonly used in Australian hospitals as a framework for organising important and relevant information that needs to be transferred to other health professionals (ACSQHC 2009).

Handover from the PACU nurse to the ward nurse should include the following.

- Identify: checking of the patient's name and identification band.
- Situation: the operation and type of anaesthetic administered.
- Background: patient's past medical /surgical history.
- Assessment: vital sign chart, conscious state, airway breathing circulation, wound dressings, drains, blood loss, IV infusions, urine output, patient comfort interventions, medications.
- Recommendation: instructions from the surgeon provide an opportunity for the ward nurse to ask questions and clarify information.

If the patient is leaving the day surgery unit, table 9.8 shows an example of the scoring system to ensure the patient can safely be discharged home.

TABLE 9.8 Aldrete scoring system for patient discharge

Vital signs	
Vital signs must be stable and consistent with age and preoperative baseline	
BP and pulse within 20% of preoperative baseline	2
BP and pulse 20–40% of preoperative baseline	1
BP and pulse >40% of preoperative baseline	0
Activity level	
Patient must be able to ambulate at preoperative level	
Steady gait, no dizziness, or meets preoperative level	2
Requires assistance	1
Unable to ambulate	0
Nausea and vomiting	
The patient should have minimal nausea and vomiting before discharge	
Minimal: successfully treated with PO medication	2
Moderate: successfully treated with IM medication	1
Severe: continues after repeated treatment	0
Pain	
The patient should have minimal or no pain before discharge	
The level of pain that the patient has should be acceptable to the patient	
Pain should be controlled by oral analgesics The location, type and intensity of pain should be consistent with anticipated post-operative discomfort Acceptability Yes No	 2 1
Surgical bleeding	
Post-operative bleeding should be consistent with expected blood loss for the procedure	
Minimal: does not require dressing change	2

(continued)

TABLE 9.8	(continued)
Moderate: up to two dressing changes required	1
Severe: more than three dressing changes required	0

Maximal score = 10; patients scoring ≥9 are fit for discharge.

Source: Mason & Chung (1997).

Return to ward patient care

The arrival of a post-operative patient from the PACU is a busy time for the ward nurse caring for the patient. To begin, the nurse should undertake primary, secondary and focused patient assessments, as outlined previously in figure 9.6. Additional general comfort interventions will include providing support and education to visiting family/carers and providing a post-operative wash to remove skin preparations that have remained on the skin and may cause skin irritation. Differences between the post-operative PACU assessment and ward nurse assessment will need to consider support for the patients family. The patient's vital signs will be assessed at regular intervals and as per the policies in place at the health facility. During the post-operative period, the patient is a risk of developing complications. Assessment, recognition of abnormal findings and intervention are vital components of nursing care. Post-operative complications may develop in any body system with the surgical wound or drainage devices. Table 9.9 summarises the potential post-operative complications that patients can develop when they have returned to the ward.

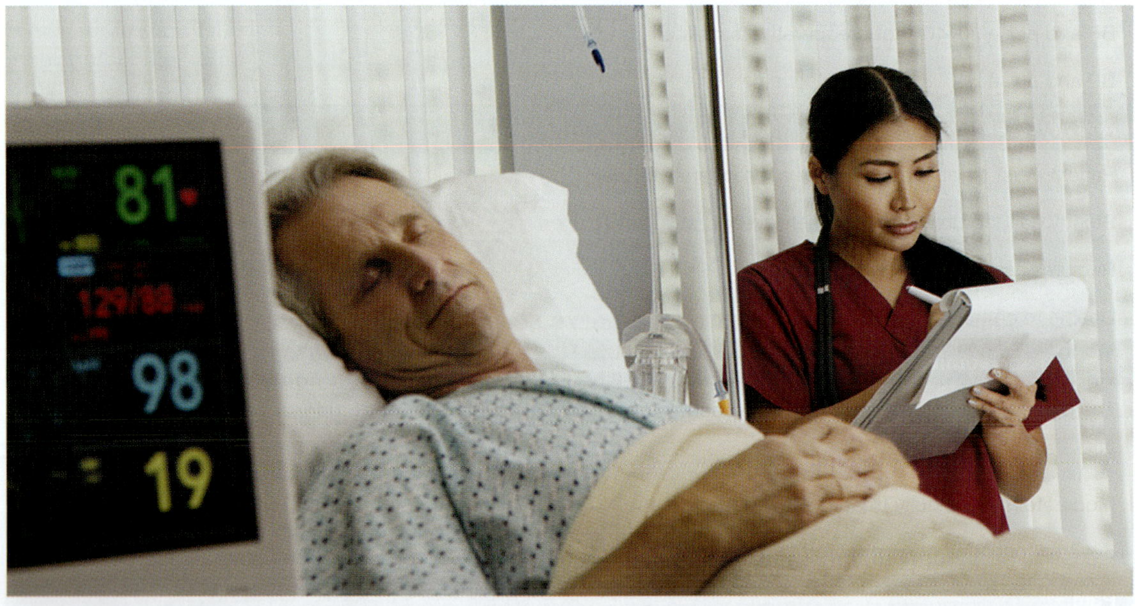

TABLE 9.9 Potential post-operative complications

Post-operative complication	Nursing intervention
Respiratory complications: 1. Strong analgesics may cause over-sedation 2. Pain (makes patients reluctant to move).	Encourage hourly deep breathing and coughing exercises to prevent alveolar collapse and move secretions for the patient to 'cough up'. Exercises have been explained to the patient during the preadmission clinic assessment and by the physiotherapist. Sometimes incentive devices such as a Triflo are used to encourage the patient.

Cardiovascular complications: 1. Hypotension 2. Haemorrhage 3. Vasovagal syncope (fainting) when the patient gets out of bed (often the first time after surgery).	1. Wound and drain tube assessment for internal/external blood loss. 2. Be with your patient the first time they are getting out of bed, get them up slowly, sitting on the edge of the bed first, make sure they do not feel dizzy/light headed before they stand up.
Deep vein thrombosis (DVT): The body's stress response to surgery contributes to hypercoagulation, venous stasis (from lying in bed for long periods, and other patient risk factors — can lead to pulmonary embolism [PE]).	1. Assess the patient for legs pain, swelling, areas of redness/heat. 2. Encourage leg exercises and use of pneumatic compression devices (foot pumps) to reduce venous stasis and encourage venous return.
Reduced urine output: Less than 0.5 ml/kg/hr indicates inadequate renal perfusion. Can occur because of the body's stress response, because the patient has had opioids or other medications that affect the patient's perception their bladder is full. Some patients also have great difficulty using urine bottles/bedpans.	Inspect patient's abdomen for bladder distention/check bladder volume with bladder scanner. Check urinary catheter for patency/kinks. Reposition patient to facilitate use of bedpan/urinal/IDC drainage. Report reduced urine output.
Paralytic ileus: A temporary deduction in bowel function due to surgery.	Is higher risk for patients who have had abdominal surgery. Assess for abdominal distention, absence of bowel sounds or constipation. The patient should have nothing orally (nil by mouth) so that the bowel can rest and IV fluids to keep the patient hydrated.
Pain: Pain is a major fear for many patients and effective pain assessment and management is a nursing priority.	Administer regular pain relief as ordered on the medication chart. Make sure the patient understands how to use their patient-controlled analgesia (PCA). Post-operative pain prolongs patient recovery time, increases the risk of the patient developing complications or DVT.
Fever: Temperature up to 38 degrees can be a normal part of the body's stress response for up to two days after surgery. A temperature over 37.7 degrees at any time may be indicating an infection/complication is developing.	Escalate findings of elevated temperature. Keep the patient comfortable with administration of antipyretics as ordered on the medication chart. Assess the patient for signs and other symptoms of infection.

Source: Adapted from Foran (2017) Chapter 17, 'Continued care of the postoperative patient in the surgical unit/inpatient ward' pp 398–406 in *Lewis's medical surgical nursing.*

After surgery, the nurse supports and encourages the patient to be as independent with their mobility and activities of daily living (ADL) as they were at prior to their surgery to be safely discharged.

Prior to the patient leaving hospital, the nurse further prepares the patient for discharge by providing patient/family education on:

- concerns/symptoms the patient may develop that will require medical review, such as fever, increases in surgical wound pain, discharge
- medications that have been prescribed (what they are for, when to take them and possible side effects)
- wound/suture care (e.g. applying waterproof dressings)
- how long the patient has restrictions on physical/recreational activities example, driving a car (People cannot drive or operate machinery or 24 hrs post-anaesthetic, and there may be further restrictions specific to the surgery)
- dietary restrictions or modifications
- where and when to return for follow-up care and appointments
- provide an opportunity for the patient and family members to ask questions about instructions or specific concerns (Foran 2017).

CASE STUDY 9.1

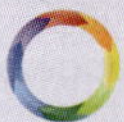

Nursing care of a young surgical patient

This morning's dental list is very big with 12 cases booked, and the staff allocated to the dental list are expecting it to be very busy. Unfortunately, the start time has been delayed and the staff are conscious that if they do not finish on time, the afternoon theatre list may also be delayed.

Rem is 19 years old and has arrived in the holding bay at 0900 hours in preparation for her dental surgery. Rem is to have an extraction of her four wisdom teeth under general anaesthetic and is very anxious. Rem is accompanied by the nurse from DOSA, who has provided you with a handover and has handed you the patient's chart to complete your section of the preoperative checklist. The anaesthetist has come to meet Rem and discusses the proposed anaesthetic for the surgery, completes the anaesthetic consent for the surgery, inserts an IV cannula, undertakes an airway assessment, and then returns to the operating room.

You commence the anaesthetic nurse check on Rem's preoperative checklist. One question on the checklist requires the nurse to ask the patient when they last had food and fluid. The first check has indicated that the last oral intake was 2400 hours on the previous night; however, Rem says she had a light breakfast of toast and coffee before leaving home early that morning at 0530. She says she was really hungry when she woke up and forgot that her surgeon told her not to eat or drink anything from midnight prior to her surgery but was too scared to say anything earlier.

The DOSA nurse asks you if they should go back to their ward to look after their other patients.

Question

Using the information above, describe what action you would take as the nurse caring for Rem. Use the clinical reasoning cycle to guide you through the process and devise a plan of care for Rem.

Answer

- *Step 1: Consider the patient.* Rem is 19 years old and has arrived in hospital for surgical extraction of four molar teeth (wisdom teeth). Rem is very anxious.
- *Step 2: Collect cues/information*. Include subjective and objective data here, including the appearance of the patient and their past medical history.
  Handover indicates that Rem's vital signs are within acceptable parameters, that all the required documentation is present (patient identification correlates with the information on the surgical list, the surgical and anaesthetic consent forms have been completed, recent dental x-rays are present), and the preoperative checklist has been completed.
  Rem has eaten a light breakfast at 0530 hrs despite the instruction provided to her by her doctor to not eat anything the morning of her surgery. This means the patient is not adequately prepared for her surgery. The time now is 0900 hrs.
- *Step 3: Process information*. Separate the relevant and irrelevant data — cluster the clues together to formulate an inference about the patient.
  The information you have about Rem is that all the relevant documentation has been completed. Rem has not completed the recommended fasting time of six hours; therefore, there is a significant risk to Rem's safety from aspiration if the surgery goes ahead at the scheduled time.
  The theatre list is running late, and staff feel very conscious of the time delay and are looking to make up time where possible. The anaesthetist has returned to the operating room to prepare for Rem's surgery. Rem has provided contradictory information regarding her last oral intake that may result in a further delay to the surgical list while the situation is resolved.
- *Step 4: Identify problems/issues*. Nursing problems or diagnosis should be listed here.
  There is a potential for airway compromise due to aspiration. Patient is anxious due to impending surgery and rescheduling of surgery. Potential for further delays to the surgery start time for the other patients on the list. The ward nurse is also waiting to know what will happen or return to DOSA to prepare other patients for surgery.
  Provide education to Rem of the safety risk with anaesthesia when fasting times are not adhered to. Discuss with the NUM where the most suitable place for Rem to wait for an outcome will be. Rem may become more anxious waiting in the holding bay for a long period, and therefore it is more appropriate to return Rem to DOSA while she is waiting.
- *Step 5: Establish goals.* Goals of care for Rem should focus on developing a solution that allows Rem to have her surgery and keeps her safe during the surgery. Rem should return to DOSA while her new surgery time is confirmed.
- *Step 6: Take action*. The nurse should alert the anaesthetist, surgeon and nurse unit manager to the surgical risk that has been identified. Tell the DOSA nurse they can return to the ward and that you will provide them with an update as soon as one is available.

Continue to reassure Rem that the situation will be resolved and that she will return to the DOSA while the situation is resolved. Discuss with Rem that she needs to remain fasting until a clear plan to manage the situation has been developed.

- *Step 7: Evaluate outcomes.* How effective have your nursing interventions been?
  Rem will understand the increased surgical risk of not adhering to the recommended fasting times. Rem's safety will be ensured by rescheduling her surgery to either later that same day or rebook for another day altogether. Rem will continue to be cared for in DOSA if her surgery is rescheduled.
- *Step 8: Reflect on the process and new learning.* Ensuring that patients have adhered to preoperative instructions is especially important on a busy surgical ward. Patient education and reassurance was especially important in this case.

CASE STUDY 9.2

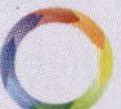 Nursing care of an elderly surgical patient

You are looking after Jeff Nguyen. Jeff is a 64-year-old gentleman who has gone to theatre to have a bowel resection under general anaesthetic. Jeff is ready to return to the ward and you are to collect him from the PACU.

In the PACU, you introduce yourself to Jeff and tell him that you will be taking him back to the ward. The PACU nurse provides a handover of Jeff's surgery and anaesthetic, specific post-operative instructions from the surgeon, and the medications that have been administered.

Jeff's vital signs are:

- temperature: 36.1C
- blood pressure: 115/80 mmHg
- pulse: 88 beats per minute
- respiratory rate: 16 breaths per minute
- pain: 6/10.

Wound assessment: abdomen is soft but is very painful on palpation, light red/purple bruising across abdomen. The drain is patent and has 45 ml of bright blood; drain tubes are open to drainage.

The nurse shows you the discharge from PACU criteria, Jeff's score is 9/10 as per the Aldrete scoring system, meaning he can move all limbs voluntarily, is able to breathe freely, BP is ±20–50% of preanaesthesia level, he is fully awake, and his SpO_2 are >92% on room air.

Question

You are preparing to take back Jeff to the ward when he asks if he can have anything for the waves of stomach pain and nausea that he has started to feel just now. Is Jeff in a stable condition to return to the ward?

Answer

- *Step 1: Consider the patient.* Jeff Nguyen is a 64 year old gentleman who has had bowel resection surgery under general anaesthetic.
- *Step 2:* [illegible]
  Jeff is 90 minutes post-operative and meets the Aldrete discharge criteria of 9/10. The PACU nurse has contacted the ward to indicate that Jeff is ready to return. You have received handover and when you are but to leave the PACU, Jeff tells you that he has pain and nausea. Jeff looks distressed.
- *Step 3: Process information*. Separate the relevant and irrelevant data — cluster the clues together to formulate an inference about the patient.
  Jeff has been in the PACU for 90 minutes. His condition has been stable. His surgical dressing is dry and intact, and his surgical drain tube is patent and has a small amount of drainage. The last time pain relief medication was administered was 30 minutes ago and is documented as morphine 2 mg IV.
  Jeff has new onset of pain and nausea, but his vital signs and wound assessments are stable and within acceptable parameters. Going to the ward will require Jeff to be pushed on the trolley through corridors, around corners and a lift ride from the 2nd to the 5th floor.
  You have basic equipment to take with you on the trip back to the ward, consisting of an emesis bag, ambu bag, oxygen cylinder with suction, 1 x Yankeur sucker, Guedels airway, Hudson mask and nasal prongs.
- *Step 4: Identify problems/issues*. Nursing problems or diagnosis should be listed here.
  Jeff has been stable, but his condition has changed in the last few minutes and there is the potential for vomiting during the return trip to the ward. The is also a potential to exacerbate pain due to inter ward

transfer and deterioration in public areas of the hospital where there are limited resources to help keep the patient safe.

- *Step 5: Establish goals*. Goals of care for Jeff should focus on relieving Jeff's pain and nausea so that he can be safely be transferred back to his ward
- *Step 6 Take action*. The nurse should prioritise Jeff's haemodynamic stability and safety. Tell the PACU nurse he would like to reassess the patient. Repeat a set of vital signs, surgical wound assessment and pain assessment.
  Observations are:
  - Temperature: 36.4°C
  - Blood pressure: 134/64 mmHg
  - Pulse: 99 beats per minute
  - Respiratory rate: 22 breaths per minute
  - Pain: 7/10
  - Surgical dressing is dry and intact, drain tubes are not kinked and clamps are open to drain
  - 55 ml of bright blood in the drain tube
  - Abdomen is guarded and is painful to palpate.

  Discuss the findings of your assessments with the PACU nurse. The findings support that Jeff requires additional pain relief and antiemetic medication prior to transferring him back to the ward. Leave Jeff in the PACU while the pain medications are administered and his condition improves.
- *Step 7: Evaluate outcomes*. How effective have your nursing interventions been?
  The PACU nurse phones you on the ward 25 minutes later. Jeff has responded well to the additional dose of pain relief and antiemetic medications and is now ready to return to the ward.
  You go the PACU and repeat the handover process and surgical wound assessments. You are satisfied that Jeff is able to be moved safely to the ward. The risk avoided is the possibility of Jeff experiencing any adverse events on the journey back to the ward.
- *Step 8: Reflect on the process and new learning*. Adverse events can include prolonged pain from lengthy delays is there is a lift malfunction, nausea and vomiting that you are not able to treat. There is the potential to exacerbate Jeff's pain and nausea by moving him, and for Jeff to become agitated and distressed in a location where you have minimal resources available to you. There is also the potential for increased anxiety for Jeff's family and members of the public seeing him in a distressed and unwell state.

SUMMARY

This chapter has explored each of the stages that patient's progress through in their perioperative journey, and identified the key factors that nurses must consider to ensure patient safety throughout anaesthesia, surgery and post-operatively. The perioperative nursing roles are diverse and require highly specialised patient assessment skills before, during and after surgery. Nurses require specialist knowledge of anatomy, physiology and pharmacology, demonstrate patient advocacy, and apply risk management strategies to achieve patient safety. Perioperative nurses further promote patients' safety and the multi-professional perioperative team by applying recognised local and international standards and guidelines to deliver care. This chapter outlined the various perioperative nursing roles as well as the primary considerations, nursing care and interventions that are expected to be delivered in each of these roles.

KEY TERMS

ambulant surgery The patient does not require an overnight stay in hospital.
anaesthesia Controlled and temporary loss of sensation or awareness for medical purposes.
asepsis The absence of infectious organisms on living tissue.
aseptic field Includes the patient, operating table, instrument trolleys, any other furniture covered in aseptic drapes and staff.
DOSA Day of surgery admission.
intraoperative During the surgery.
PACU Post-anaesthetic care unit.
perioperative Includes the pre-hospital, intraoperative and post-operative stages of the patient surgical journey.
PONV Post-operative nausea and vomiting.
post-operative After the surgery.
sterile Entirely free of germs.
surgical conscience Professional honesty by openly acknowledging if asepsis has been broken.

REFERENCES

Aldrete, A. L. (1995) The post anesthesia recovery score revisited (letter). *Clinical Anesthesia.* 7: 89. https://pubmed.ncbi.nlm.nih.gov/7772368

ANZCA. (2020) Types of anaesthesia. www.anzca.edu.au/patient-information/anaesthesia-information-for-patients-and-carers/types-of-anaesthesia

Australian College of Operating Room Nurses (ACORN). (2020) *Standards for Perioperative Nursing in Australia*, 16th ed. Adelaide. www.acorn.org.au/index.cfm?display=1021470

Australian Commission on Safety and Quality in Health Care (ACSQHC). ([illegible]) ISBAR toolkit. Identifying and Solving BARriers to effective clinical handover. Clinical Governance Hunter New England Health. www.safetyandquality.gov.au/sites/default/files/migrated/ISBAR-toolkit.pdf

Australian Commission on Safety and Quality in Health Care (ACSQHC). (2019) Surgical safety checklist resources. Australia and New Zealand edition of the Surgical Safety Checklist.

Australian Commission on Safety and Quality in Health Care (ACSQHC). (2020) Venous thromboembolism prevention. Clinical Care Standard. www.safetyandquality.gov.au/standards/clinical-care-standards/venous-thromboembolism-prevention-clinical-care-standard

Australian Government. (2020) Elective surgery media release. www.pm.gov.au/media/elective-surgery

Australian Government. (2019) Education guide. Aftercare or post-operative treatment. Information about aftercare in the Medicare Benefits Schedule (MBS). www.servicesaustralia.gov.au/organisations/health-professionals/topics/education-guide-aftercare-or-post-operative-treatment/33201

Ball, K. (2018). 'Surgical modalities'. In J. Nagelhout & S. Elisha (Eds.). *Nurse Anaesthesia*, 6th ed. (chapter 8, pp. 311–316). St Louis, Missouri: Elsevier.

Carlile, J. & Evans, M. (2016) 'Infection prevention and control'. In L. Hamlin, M. Davies, M. Richardson-Tench & S. Sutherland-Fraser (Eds.). *Perioperative Nursing: An Introduction*, 2nd ed. (pp. 128–157). Sydney: Elsevier.

Cartwright, S. & Andrews, S. (2017). 'Perianaesthesia nursing as a specialty'. In J. Odom-Forren (Ed.). *Drain's Perianaesthesia Nursing. A Critical Care Approach*, 7th ed. (pp 9–11). St Louis, Missouri: Elsevier.

Cole, S. & Allanson, A. (2016) 'Surgical intervention'. In L. Hamlin, M. Davies, M. Richardson-Tench & S. Sutherland-Fraser (Eds.). *Perioperative Nursing: An introduction*, 2nd ed. (pp. 269–302). Sydney: Elsevier.

Department of Health. (2012) *A framework for emergency surgery in Victoria*. State of Victoria.

Duff, J. (2017) 'Nursing management: Perioperative care'. In D. Brown, H. Edwards, T. Buckley & R. Aitken (Eds.). *Lewis's Medical Surgical Nursing. Assessment and Management of Clinical Problems*, 5th ed. (pp. 348–366). Chatswood, NSW: Elsevier.

Ecoff, L., Palomo, J. & Stichler, J. (2017) Design and testing of a postanesthesia care unit readiness for discharge assessment tool. *Journal of PeriAnesthesia Nursing*. 32: 389–399.

Foran, P. (2016) 'Post anaesthesia nursing care'. In L. Hamlin, M. Davies, M. Richardson-Tench & S. Sutherland-Fraser (Eds.). *Perioperative Nursing: An introduction*, 2nd ed. (chapter 12, pp. 331–357). Sydney: Elsevier.

Foran, P. & Newman, F. (2017) 'Nursing management intraoperative care'. In R. Aitken, T. Buckley, H. Edwards & D. Brown (Eds.). *Lewis's Medical Surgical Nursing*, 5th ed. (pp. 369–376). Sydney: Elsevier.

Hamlin, L. & Minton, S. (2016) 'Intraoperative patient care'. In L. Hamlin, M. Davies, M. Richardson-Tench & S. Sutherland-Fraser (Eds.). *Perioperative Nursing*, 2nd ed. (pp. 232–266). Sydney: Elsevier.

Hea, J., Gallego, B., Stubbs, C., Scott, A., Dawson, S., Forrest, K. & Kennedy, C. (2018) Improving patient flow and satisfaction: An evidence-based pre-admission clinic and transfer of care pathway for elective surgery patients. *Collegian*. 25: 149–156. doi: org/10.1016/j.colegn.2017.04.0061

Marley, R. & Sheets, S. (2018) 'Perioperative evaluation and preparation of the patient'. In J. Nagelhout & S. Elisha (Eds.). *Nurse Anaesthesia*, 6th ed. (chapter 20, pp. 311–316). St Louis, Missouri: Elsevier.

Marshall, S. & Chung, F. (1997) Assessment of 'home readiness': discharge criteria and postdischarge complications. *Current Opinion in Anaesthesiology*. 10(6): 445–450. https://journals.lww.com/co-anesthesiology/Abstract/1997/12000/Assessment_of__home_readiness___discharge_criteria.11.aspx

McCullagh, C. & Lee, T. (2016) 'Assessment and preparation for surgery'. In L. Hamlin, M. Davies, M. Richardson-Tench & S. Sutherland-Fraser (Eds.). *Perioperative Nursing*, 2nd ed. (pp. 160–192). Sydney: Elsevier.

National Elective Surgery Urgency Categorisation. (2015) Australian Health Ministers Advisory Council April 2015.

Neil, J. (2017) 'Nursing management. Perioperative care'. In D. Brown, H. Edwards, T. Buckley & R. Aitken (Eds.). *Lewis's Medical Surgical Nursing*, 5th ed. (pp. 294–311). Chatswood, NSW: Elsevier.

New South Wales Government. (2020) Going to hospital. www.health.nsw.gov.au/Hospitals/Going_To_hospital/Pages/default.aspx

Padley, A. (2015) *Westmead anaesthetic manual*, 4th ed. North Ryde: McGraw-Hill Australia.

Parkman, A. & Richardson-Tench, L. (2016) 'Wound healing'. In L. Hamlin, M. Davies, M. Richardson-Tench & S. Sutherland-Fraser (Eds.). *Perioperative Nursing: An Introduction*, 2nd ed. (pp. 304–328). Sydney: Elsevier.

Penman, J. & Tighe, J. (2018) Hold high the standard. *Australian Nursing and Midwifery Journal*. 26(1): 44.

Schoenwald, A. (2017) 'Pain management'. In D. Brown, H. Edwards, T. Buckley & R. Aitken (Eds.). *Lewis's Medical Surgical Nursing. Assessment and Management of Clinical Problems*, 5th ed. (pp. 84–114). Chatswood, NSW: Elsevier.

Shoup, A. & Horner, D. (2017) 'Nursing management intraoperative care'. In D. Brown, H. Edwards, T. Buckley & R. Aitken (Eds.). *Lewis's Medical Surgical Nursing*, 5th ed. (pp. 312–329). Chatswood, NSW: Elsevier.

Sutherland-Fraser, S., Osborne, S. & Bryant, K. (2016) 'Perioperative nursing'. In L. Hamlin, M. Davies, M. Richardson-Tench & S. Sutherland-Fraser (Eds.). *Perioperative Nursing: An Introduction*, 2nd ed. (pp. 1–29). Sydney: Elsevier.

Walker, S., Wood, M. & Nichol, J. (2017) *Mastering Medical Terminology. Australia and New Zealand*, 2nd ed. Chatswood, NSW: Elsevier.

Walters, K. & Kumar, Z. (2017) 'Patient care during anaesthesia'. In L. Hamlin, M. Davies, M. Richardson-Tench & S. Sutherland-Fraser (Eds.). *Perioperative Nursing: An Introduction*, 2nd ed. (pp. 193–231). Sydney: Elsevier.

Wiegele, M., Marhofer, P. & Lonnqvist, P. (2019) Caudal epidural blocks in paediatric patients: a review and practical considerations. *British Journal of Anaesthesia*. 122(4): 509–517. doi: 10.1016/j.bja.2018.11.030

ACKNOWLEDGEMENTS

Figure 9.2: © kevin011 / Shutterstock.com

Figure 9.3: © Michael Pervak / Shutterstock.com

Figure 9.4: © Perioperative patient record. © The Queensland Government. Reproduced with permission of The Queensland Government. www.health.qld.gov.au/__data/assets/pdf_file/0030/436845/pre-op-check-a3-11.pdf.

Figure 9.5: © Surgical safety checklist for Australia and New Zealand. © Royal Australasian College of Surgeons. Reproduced with permission of Royal Australasian College of Surgeons. www.surgeons.org/-/media/Project/RACS/surgeons-org/files/member-benefits/lst_2009_surgical_safety_check_list_-australia_and_new_zealand-.pdfrev=1bc12bd84b9944af8249055988581b0d&hash=0BC3BC836F92086751ADC838AF4A1765.

Table 9.8: © Scott, M. & Chung, F., "Assessment of 'home readiness': discharge criteria and postdischarge complications," *Current Opinion in Anaesthesiology*: December 1997: 10(6), 445–450. Reproduced with permission of Wolters Kluwer Health, Inc.

Photo 9A: © Monkey Business Images / Shutterstock.com

Photo 9B: © Rocketclips, Inc. / Shutterstock.com

CHAPTER 10

Recognising and responding to clinical deterioration

LEARNING OBJECTIVES

After studying this chapter, you should be able to:

10.1 demonstrate an understanding of NSQHS standard eight: Recognising and Responding to Acute Deterioration

10.2 demonstrate an understanding of how to recognise and respond to a patient with sepsis

10.3 demonstrate an understanding of how to recognise and respond to a patient with a surgical complication

10.4 demonstrate an understanding of how to recognise and respond to a patient with a respiratory complication

10.5 explain how to assess and monitor the critically ill patient

10.6 identify the treatment of a deteriorating patient

10.7 demonstrate an understanding of how to recognise and respond to a patient with a cardiac arrest.

Introduction

Over the last couple of decades, there has been an increase in patients suffering from chronic diseases such as diabetes and cardiovascular disease. This has led to patients presenting to hospital with increasingly complex conditions with multiple co-morbidities and medications. Consequently, nurses care for a higher acuity of patients on medical–surgical wards and need to understand how to recognise and respond to the **deteriorating patient** adequately. Vital signs are an important determinant of a patient's physiological condition. However, if these are not recorded regularly or accurately, a nurse could fail to identify the physiological deterioration of their patient. This could lead to poor patient outcomes, unplanned intensive care unit (ICU) admissions and sudden cardiac death (Bucknall et al. 2017). This chapter will discuss the importance of using a system to detect patient deterioration, highlight some of the common reasons patients deteriorate, and the associated treatment and nursing care required. The care of a patient with a cardiac arrest will be discussed, and the chapter will conclude with a case study for the consolidation of new knowledge learnt in this chapter.

10.1 Recognising and responding to patient deterioration

LEARNING OBJECTIVE 10.1 Demonstrate an understanding of NSQHS standard eight: Recognising and Responding to Acute Deterioration.

To standardise and improve clinical practice in Australian health service organisations, the Australian Commission on Safety and Quality in Health Care (ACSQHC) developed the National Safety and Quality Health Service Standards (NSQHS). Hospitals and day procedure services must meet these standards. The first edition of the NSQHS Standards was released in 2012 and was superseded by the second edition in 2017. The second edition has eight standards, including the Recognising and Responding to Acute Deterioration Standard. This standard aims to ensure that a patient's physical, mental or cognitive deterioration are promptly recognised, and there is an appropriate escalation and response (ACSQHC 2019b).

Monitoring a patient's observations and tracking changes over time is a significant factor in detecting deterioration. Acute deterioration may occur at any time during a patient's admission in any ward. If a patient's observations are recorded intermittently or inaccurately, acute deterioration may not be detected, and recognition and appropriate treatment may be delayed. This can result in serious adverse patient outcomes or death (ACSQHC 2019a).

It is the role of the nurse to record a patient's observations according to their clinical judgement; however, there are differences in individual nurse's clinical judgement and differing views on the importance of monitoring a patient's observations. Poor communication among clinical teams has also led to a delay in recognising and responding to deteriorating patients. For these reasons, a uniform standard was needed to ensure that the correct observations were taken appropriately and consistently monitored so changes could be tracked over time.

Recognising acute deterioration relies on identifying, understanding and interpreting abnormal vital signs and other observations, and escalating care appropriately. This is a complex process that requires knowledge of disease processes, pathways to deterioration and advanced clinical reasoning skills. This knowledge is developed over time, and it is often newly registered nurses that are vulnerable to making observation errors.

To ensure consistency and empower nurses to take action and improve teamwork, a nationally recognised **adult deterioration detection system** has been implemented in Australia. A core list of six vital signs was selected to be assessed every 8 hours. These are:

1. respiratory rate
2. oxygen saturation
3. heart rate
4. blood pressure
5. level of consciousness
6. temperature.

The assessment of these vital signs still requires an element of clinical judgement. Some patients may not need all of the vital signs assessed; for example, a paediatric patient may not require a blood pressure assessment. In order to assist nurses and doctors, the implementation of a standardised adult deterioration detection system must be in place in clinical settings across Australia. The system stipulates when a nurse needs to escalate the care of a deteriorating patient and to whom. Figure 10.1 shows an example of an observations chart that calculates a score based on the patient's observations falling within a coloured square.

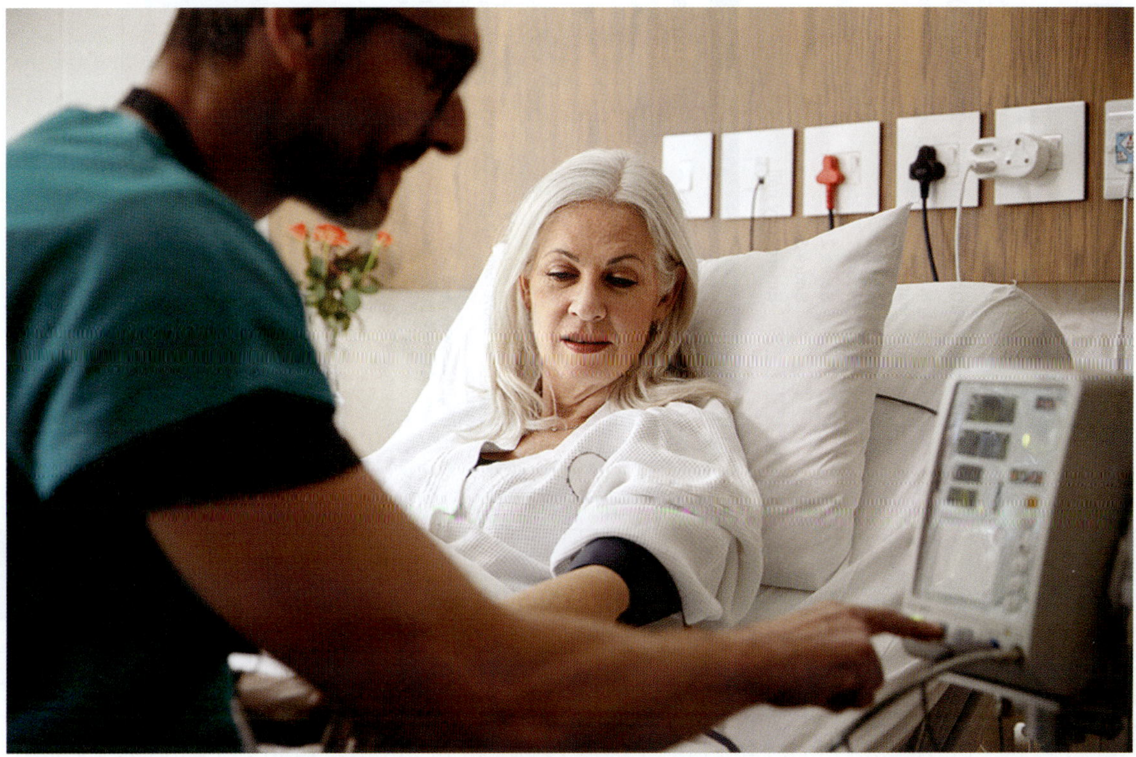

10.2 Recognising and responding to a patient with sepsis

LEARNING OBJECTIVE 10.2 Demonstrate an understanding of how to recognise and respond to a patient with sepsis.

One of the most common causes of deterioration in patients is due to **sepsis**. Sepsis occurs when there is an abnormal host response to an infection. If it is not recognised early and managed promptly, it can lead to septic shock, multiple organ failure and death (Australian Sepsis Network 2020b; Rudd et al. 2020). In 2017, there were 49 million sepsis cases and 11 million deaths globally (Rudd et al. 2020). In Australia, there were 5000 deaths due to sepsis in 2020, which is concerning given this is a largely preventable condition (Australian Sepsis Network 2020b). Death from sepsis may be preventable if patients present to hospital earlier or their deterioration is recognised and treated earlier. Anyone affected by an infection can progress to sepsis conditions. However, some vulnerable populations, such as the elderly, pregnant women, neonates, and people with HIV/AIDS, cancer, kidney disease and autoimmune diseases, are at higher risk. The Australian Sepsis Network was established to promote sepsis awareness and prompt earlier recognition and treatment of the disease (Australian Sepsis Network 2020b).

Pathophysiology

In order for sepsis to develop, microorganisms enter the body to initiate an immune response. This can be from any type of infection, but predominantly gram-positive infections from staphylococcus and streptococcus bacterium. The pathophysiology of sepsis is complex and not fully understood; however, what is known is that an abnormal immune response leads to the activation of biochemical cytokines and cellular mediators, which initiate an inflammatory response.

FIGURE 10.1 An observation chart using the adult deterioration detection system (front)

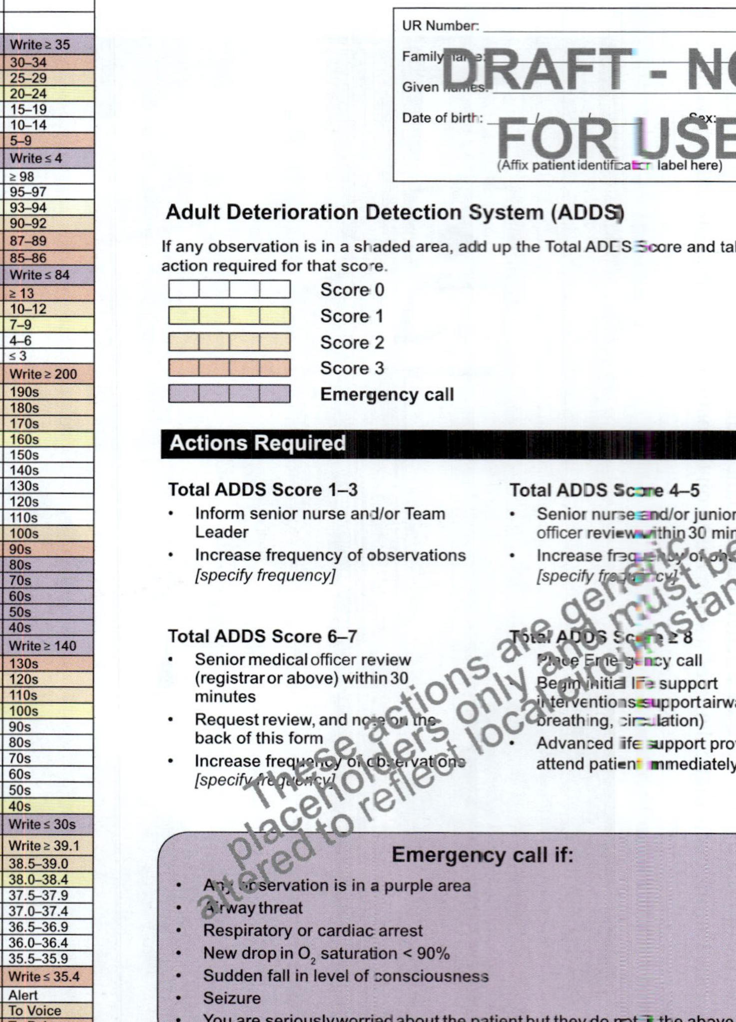

<INSERT SITE LOGO>

Adult Deterioration Detection System (ADDS) Chart

UR Number: ______
Family name: ______
Given names: ______
Date of birth: ___/___/___ Sex: ☐M ☐F
(Affix patient identification label here)

Other Observation Charts In Use

☐ Alcohol Withdrawal ☐ Insulin Infusion ☐ Pain/Epidural/Patient Controlled Analgesia
☐ Anticoagulant ☐ Neurology ☐ ______
☐ Fluid Balance ☐ Neurovascular ☐ ______

General Instructions

- You must record appropriate observations:
  - On admission
  - At a frequency appropriate for the patient's clinical state
- You must calculate a Total ADDS Score:
  - If the patient is deteriorating or an observation is in a shaded area
  - Whenever you are concerned about the patient
- When graphing observations, place a dot • (in the centre of the box which includes the current observation in its range of values and connect it to the previous dot with a straight line. For blood pressure, use the symbols indicated on the chart.
- Whenever an observation falls within a shaded area you must enter the ADDS Score for that vital sign in the appropriate row of the ADDS Scores table unless a modification has been made (see below).

Modifications

- If abnormal observations are to be tolerated for the patient's clinical condition, write the acceptable ranges below (where the ADDS Score will be 0).
- Modifications must be reviewed at least every 72 hours.
- If **any** vital sign needs further modifying, draw two diagonal lines through the entire Modification record in use and write the new acceptable ranges in the next Modification record.

	Modification 1	Modification 2	Modification 3	Modification 4
Respiratory Rate	- breaths / min	- breaths / min	- breaths / min	- breaths / min
O_2 Saturation	- %	- %	- %	- %
O_2 Flow Rate	- L / min	- L / min	- L / min	- L / min
Systolic BP	- mmHg	- mmHg	- mmHg	- mmHg
Heart Rate	- beats / min	- beats / min	- beats / min	- beats / min
Temperature	- °C	- °C	- °C	- °C
Consciousness	-	-	-	-
Doctor's name				
Signature				
Date	/ /	/ /	/ /	/ /
Time	:	:	:	:

ADDS CHART

DRAFT

DRAFT

UR Number: ______
Family name: ______
Given names: ______
Date of birth: ___/___/___ Sex: ☐M ☐F
(Affix patient identification label here)

Interventions Associated With Abnormal Vital Signs

If you administer an intervention, record here and note letter in Intervention row over page in appropriate time column.

Reference Letter	Intervention (initial if required)
a	
b	
c	
d	
e	
f	
g	
h	

Clinical Review Requests

Review requested Date ___/___ Time ___:___ ☐ Ward doctor ☐ Registrar ☐ Emergency
Specify reason ______

Review requested Date ___/___ Time ___:___ ☐ Ward doctor ☐ Registrar ☐ Emergency
Specify reason ______

Review requested Date ___/___ Time ___:___ ☐ Ward doctor ☐ Registrar ☐ Emergency
Specify reason ______

Additional Observations

Date						
Time						
Blood Glucose Level (mmol/L)						
Weight (kg)						
Bowels						
Urinalysis Specific gravity						
pH						
Leukocytes						
Blood						
Nitrite						
Ketones						
Bilirubin						
Urobilinogen						
Protein						
Glucose						

DO NOT WRITE IN THIS BINDING MARGIN

An observation chart using the adult deterioration detection system (back)

Source: ACSQHC (2012).

This inflammatory response leads to vasculature damage leading to increased cellular permeability and vasodilation. This results in decreased blood pressure, tissue perfusion, cellular hypoxia and cellular death (Belleza 2017). This response also leads to activation of the coagulation system, resulting in the development of clots, despite the lack of bleeding (Belleza 2017).

Diagnosis

Specific diagnostic criteria apply to determine whether a patient has sepsis. Sepsis is a medical emergency. However, because of sepsis's characteristics as a disease condition with multiple causative organisms and its evolving nature, patients with sepsis can present with various signs and symptoms at different times (Belleza 2017). Suspecting sepsis is the first significant step towards early recognition and diagnosis. In addition to a suspected or confirmed infection, the diagnostic criteria for sepsis include:

- temperature >38.3ºC or <36ºC (normal temperature does not exclude sepsis)
- respiratory rate >20/minute
- heart rate >90/minute
- acute confusion or decreased level of consciousness
- hyperglycaemia (blood glucose >7.7 mmol/L in patients without diabetes)
- oliguria (urine output less than 0.5 ml/kg/hour) (Australian Sepsis Network 2020a).

Sepsis can progress rapidly to septic shock if treatment is delayed. The signs of septic shock include:

- mottled or cold peripheries
- capillary refill time >3 seconds
- systolic BP <90 mmHg or MAP <60 mmHg
- purpuric rash
- arterial or venous lactate >2 mmol/L
- oliguria (urine output less than 0.5 ml/kg/hour) (Australian Sepsis Network 2020a).

Figure 10.2 outlines other signs and symptoms of sepsis as well as the common infections that can lead to this condition.

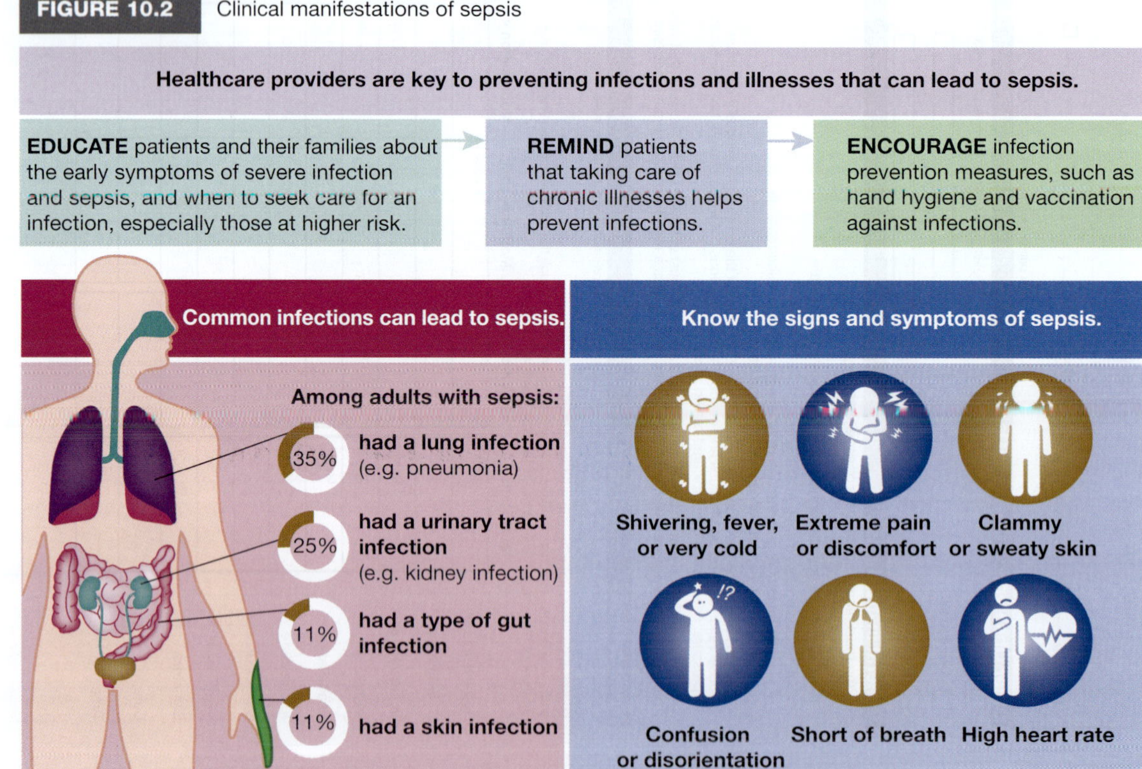

FIGURE 10.2 Clinical manifestations of sepsis

Source: CDC Vital Signs (2016).

The sepsis pathway

Treating patients with sepsis can be complex, so many facilities have adopted sepsis pathways to simplify decision making and expedite the assessment and management of the patient. Examples of sepsis pathways are pictured in figures 10.3 and 10.4.

FIGURE 10.3 The sepsis pathway

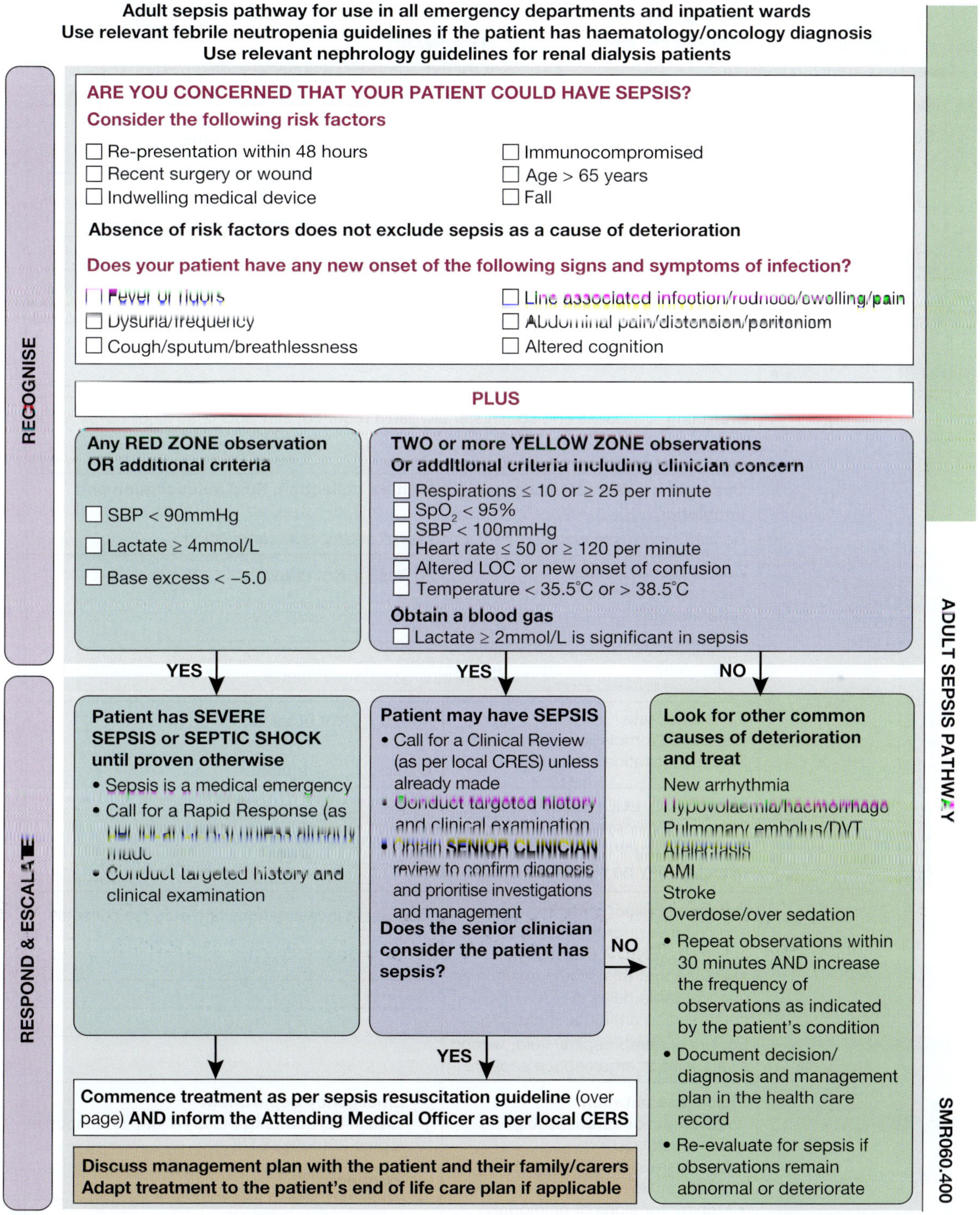

Adult sepsis pathway for use in all emergency departments and inpatient wards
Use relevant febrile neutropenia guidelines if the patient has haematology/oncology diagnosis
Use relevant nephrology guidelines for renal dialysis patients

RECOGNISE

ARE YOU CONCERNED THAT YOUR PATIENT COULD HAVE SEPSIS?

Consider the following risk factors

- ☐ Re-presentation within 48 hours
- ☐ Recent surgery or wound
- ☐ Indwelling medical device
- ☐ Immunocompromised
- ☐ Age > 65 years
- ☐ Fall

Absence of risk factors does not exclude sepsis as a cause of deterioration

Does your patient have any new onset of the following signs and symptoms of infection?

- ☐ Fever or rigors
- ☐ Dysuria/frequency
- ☐ Cough/sputum/breathlessness
- ☐ Line associated infection/redness/swelling/pain
- ☐ Abdominal pain/distension/peritonism
- ☐ Altered cognition

PLUS

Any RED ZONE observation OR additional criteria

- ☐ SBP < 90mmHg
- ☐ Lactate ≥ 4mmol/L
- ☐ Base excess < –5.0

TWO or more YELLOW ZONE observations Or additional criteria including clinician concern

- ☐ Respirations ≤ 10 or ≥ 25 per minute
- ☐ SpO_2 < 95%
- ☐ SBP < 100mmHg
- ☐ Heart rate ≤ 50 or ≥ 120 per minute
- ☐ Altered LOC or new onset of confusion
- ☐ Temperature < 35.5°C or > 38.5°C

Obtain a blood gas

- ☐ Lactate ≥ 2mmol/L is significant in sepsis

RESPOND & ESCALATE

YES →

Patient has SEVERE SEPSIS or SEPTIC SHOCK until proven otherwise

- Sepsis is a medical emergency
- Call for a Rapid Response (as per local CERS) unless already made
- Conduct targeted history and clinical examination

YES →

Patient may have SEPSIS

- Call for a Clinical Review (as per local CRES) unless already made
- Conduct targeted history and clinical examination
- Obtain **SENIOR CLINICIAN** review to confirm diagnosis and prioritise investigations and management

Does the senior clinician consider the patient has sepsis? **NO →** (Look for other common causes of deterioration and treat) **YES ↓**

NO →

Look for other common causes of deterioration and treat

New arrhythmia
Hypovolaemia/haemorrhage
Pulmonary embolus/DVT
Atelectasis
AMI
Stroke
Overdose/over sedation

- Repeat observations within 30 minutes AND increase the frequency of observations as indicated by the patient's condition
- Document decision/diagnosis and management plan in the health care record
- Re-evaluate for sepsis if observations remain abnormal or deteriorate

Commence treatment as per sepsis resuscitation guideline (over page) **AND inform the Attending Medical Officer as per local CERS**

Discuss management plan with the patient and their family/carers
Adapt treatment to the patient's end of life care plan if applicable

ADULT SEPSIS PATHWAY

SMR060.400

Source: Clinical Excellence Commission (2013).

FIGURE 10.4 The sepsis pathway (version 2)

NSW GOVERNMENT Health	FAMILY NAME	MRN
	GIVEN NAME	☐ MALE ☐ FEMALE
Facility:	D.O.B.____/____/____	M.O.
	ADDRESS	
SEPSIS KILLS ADULT SEPSIS PATHWAY	LOCATION/WARD	
RECOGNISE•RESUSCITATE•REFER	COMPLETE ALL DETAILS OR AFFIX PATIENT LABEL HERE	

Sepsis recognition Date:__ __/__ __/__ __ Time: __ __ : __ __

☐ **Emergency department** Triage category 1 2 3 4 5

☐ **Inpatient** Ward: ________________ ☐ Clinical review ☐ Rapid response

RESUSCITATE

A	**Airway** — Assess and maintain patient airway	
B	**Breathing** — Assess and administer oxygen if required; aim $SpO_2 \geq 95\%$ (or 88–92% for COPD)	
C	**Circulation - Vascular access, blood/culture collection, fluid resuscitation and antibiotics** *Consider intraosseous access after two failed attempts at cannulation*	
	Collect Blood Cultures Take two (2) sets from two (2) separate sites For patients with a central venous access device (CVAD), take one set from the CVAD plus one set peripherally	☐ Yes ☐ Not obtained
	Collect Lactate Lactate ≥ 2mmol/L after adequate fluid resuscitation is significant	☐ Yes ☐ Not obtained Lacate:__ __.__mmol/L
	Collect FBC, EUC, CRP/PCT, LFTs, coags and glucose BGL > 7.7mmol/L in the absence of diabetes may be significant	☐ Yes ☐ Not obtained BGL:__ __.__mmol/L
	Order and collect other investigations and cultures prior to antibiotics (unless a **SENIOR CLINICIAN** assesses that this would result in an unacceptable delay in commencing antibiotic therapy) Eg. Urine, cerebrospinal fluid, wound swab, joint or organ space aspirate	Document investigations and cultures collected: ________________ ________________ ________________ ________________
	Fluid Resuscitation (intravenous or intraosseous) • Use crystalloid • Aim Systolic Blood Pressure > 100mmHg • Monitor for signs of pulmonary oedema and review at risk patients more frequently	☐ **Emergency department** Give initial 20mL/kg bolus STAT, if no response repeat 20mL/kg STAT ☐ **Inpatient** Initial 250–500ml bolus STAT, if no response repeat 250–500mL STAT **If no response in SBP after 1000mL call a Rapid response**
	Consider commencement of vasopressors	

RESUSCITATE

C

Antibiotics First/new antibiotic administered Date: ___/___/___ Time: ___:___

Blood cultures (at least two sets) and other relevant cultures should be collected **PRIOR** to antibiotic administration. However in patients with severe sepsis or septic shock, if difficult to obtain cultures do not delay administration of antibiotic(s). Refer to local Antimicrobial Stewardship policies/procedures regarding antibiotic instructions.
Consult Infectious Diseases Physician or Clinical Microbiologist if required.

☐ Severe sepsis or septic shock →	Use *Therapeutic Guidelines: Antibiotic* or locally endorsed antibiotic prescribing guideline	Prescribe and administer antibiotics **within 60 MINUTES** of sepsis recognition
☐ Sepsis →	Use *Therapeutic Guidelines: Antibiotic* or locally endorsed antibiotic prescribing guideline	Prescribe and administer antibiotics promptly *in a timeframe directed by senior clinician (must be within 2 hours)*

D	**Disability - Assess level of consciousness (LOC)** using Alert, Voice, Pain, Unresponsive (AVPU)
E	**Exposure** - Re-examine the patient for other potential sources of infection to guide further investigations
F	**Fluid** - Monitor/document strict fluid input/output and consider IDC if not already inserted
G	**Check Blood Glucose Level** - Manage as per local guidelines
Monitor and Reassess	**Continue monitoring, assess for signs of deterioration and escalate as per local CERS** • Respiratory rate in the Red or Yellow Zone • SBP < 100mmHg • Decreased or no improvement in level of consciousness • Urine output < 0.5mL/kg/hour • Serum lactate level of ≥ 2mmol/L (or increasing) or no improvement after adequate fluid resuscitation may be indicative of septic shock • Consider other causes of deterioration

REFER

If no improvement Intensive Care may be required

- Update the Attending Medical Officer on the patient's condition using ISBAR ☐
- Discuss the management plan with the patient and their family/carers ☐
- Sepsis management plan documented by a medical officer in the health care record as per page 4 (over) ☐

Name: ____________ Designation: ____________ Signature: ____________

Source: Clinical Excellence Commission (2016).

10.3 The deteriorating post-operative patient

LEARNING OBJECTIVE 10.3 Demonstrate an understanding of how to recognise and respond to a patient with a surgical complication.

Patients are at a high risk of deterioration after surgery. Nurses caring for them must understand how to recognise and respond to potential post-operative complications and follow standard principles to reduce this risk. This risk has increased due to the compounding complexity of surgical procedures being performed and the increasing age of surgical patients who present with co-morbidities. Complications can arise from surgery due to infection, prolonged sedation time, bleeding from the surgical site and medication complications, such as opioid overdose (Liddle 2013).

Patient controlled analgesia

Patients undergoing surgery will require effective pain control in the post-operative period. **Patient controlled analgesia (PCA)** is often used in the post-operative period as it is highly effective at managing pain (Journal 2019). A PCA pump (figure 10.5) can allow a continuous infusion of medication, also known as the basal rate, to infuse into the patient. In addition to this, a patient can have extra medication or bolus doses when experiencing increased pain by pressing a button linked to the PCA pump (ANMF Education Team 2019).

FIGURE 10.5 A PCA pump

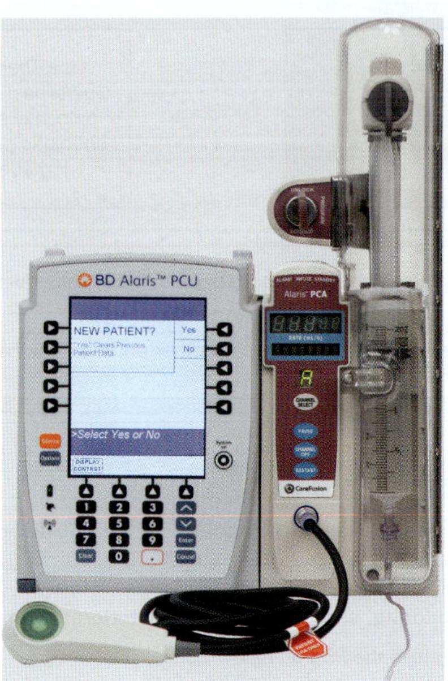

Source: Becton, Dickinson and Company (2021).

The two most common medications used in a PCA are morphine and fentanyl. These are Schedule 8 (S8) controlled medications and require stringent controls, including double-checking the medication preparation and the amount of medication administered during the previous shift. Checks are documented on a PCA observation chart. Registered nurses caring for a patient with a PCA are required to document information about their patient's pain score, attempts at pain relief (the number of times the patient has attempted to press the button) and how many attempts were successful. In order to prevent an overdose of opioids, a lockout time is usually set to only allow one dose of the medication in a 5-minute period.

PCA is now considered a gold standard of care; however, some patients that are opioid sensitive may still overdose accidentally and show signs of respiratory depression. It is essential that a nurse accurately monitors the patient's respiratory rate, so action can be taken to resolve the problem. The level and type of pain control will depend on the type of surgery performed and individual needs. Pain management can also be delivered using the following routes: oral, epidural, transdermal and intramuscular.

Another post-operative complication is the risk of bleeding. The nurse should check surgical wounds for increased or excessive bleeding each time observations are performed, which may indicate haemorrhage. Erythema to the area around the wound or sutures can also indicate infection. Surgical drains should be checked regularly to determine the volume of fluid loss and type. Frank, bright red blood indicates that there may still be some active bleeding present, and purulent discharge could indicate infection.

10.4 The deteriorating respiratory patient

LEARNING OBJECTIVE 10.4 Demonstrate an understanding of how to recognise and respond to a patient with a respiratory complication.

Patients who present to hospital with respiratory problems can deteriorate rapidly. There are many causes of respiratory failure, including chronic obstructive pulmonary disease (COPD), pneumonia, pulmonary embolism, pneumothorax, acute respiratory distress syndrome and viral illnesses such as influenza and COVID 19. Respiratory failure occurs when the lungs cannot adequately exchange gas and deliver oxygen to the tissues. It is categorised into two types according to the arterial blood gas (ABG) results:

1. hypoxaemia respiratory failure, characterised by an arterial oxygen tension (PaO_2) <60 mmHg with normal or low arterial carbon dioxide tension ($PaCO_2$)
2. hypercapnic respiratory failure is the presence of a $PaCO_2$ >45 mmHg and PaO_2 <60 mmHg.

Blood pH has to be maintained within a tight normal range to avoid cellular death and maintain homeostasis. This can be achieved by buffer mechanisms, which can be either renal or respiratory in nature. Metabolic problems require respiratory compensation, which occurs rapidly (e.g. increasing a person's respiratory rate to excrete CO_2). The faster we breathe, the more CO_2 we excrete. On the other hand, respiratory problems leading to acid–base abnormalities require renal or respiratory compensation. This process is slower; it can take up to 6 hours for the secretion of H^+ ions or reabsorption/new production of HCO_3^- ions to take place. The normal values of ABGs and reasons for common acid–base disturbances are displayed in table 10.1.

TABLE 10.1 **Acid–base disturbances in the deteriorating respiratory patient**

Uncompensated acid–base disturbances	pH	pCO_2 (mmHg)	HCO_3^- (mEq/L)	Common cause
None (normal values)	7.35–7.45	35–45	22–26	
Respiratory acidosis	<7.35	>45 mmHg	Normal	Respiratory depression (drugs, CNS trauma), COPD, pneumonia
Respiratory alkalosis	>7.45	<35 mmHg	Normal	Hyperventilation (emotions, pain)

10.5 Nursing assessment and monitoring of the critically ill patient

LEARNING OBJECTIVE 10.5 Explain how to assess and monitor the critically ill patient.

Initial assessment of the deteriorating patient should follow the A to E assessment discussed in the chapter on nursing assessment. A to E assessment, also referred to as the primary survey (figure 10.6), allows the nurse to follow a structured assessment to identify and act on any life-threatening emergencies. A nurse should always act upon a life-threatening abnormal finding before moving to the next phase of the A to E assessment. For example, if a patient's airway was obstructed with a foreign object, this would need to be actioned before the nurse assesses the patient's breathing. Failure to do this could result in the loss of the patient's life.

When caring for a deteriorating or unwell patient, the frequency of observations will need to be increased. The following six vital signs must be recorded on the observation chart:

1. respiratory rate
2. oxygen saturation (SpO_2)
3. temperature
4. blood pressure (systolic is used to determine the deterioration score)
5. heart rate
6. level of consciousness (Smith & Bowden 2017).

Once the A to E assessment has been conducted, and an initial assessment of the patient has been formed, the nurse should continue to reassess the patient to observe for signs of further deterioration (Smith & Bowden 2017). Further, more detailed assessments will need to be conducted if an abnormality is found. One example is when a patient presents with confusion — they will need to undergo a full Glasgow Coma Scale (GCS) assessment (figure 10.7). The nurse needs to recognise when to call for help and use a structured approach to handover information about the patient. ISBAR (Introduction, Situation, Background Assessment, Recommendation) is a handover communication tool used throughout Australia. A structured approach to the handover is essential to ensure that no vital information is missed (Smith & Bowden 2017). The following section will discuss assessing and monitoring a critically ill patient's airway, breathing and circulation.

FIGURE 10.6 ABCDE assessment

	Initial assessment (look, listen, feel)	Measure	Action	Consider (after initial assessment)
A Airway	**Is the airway patent — can the patient talk?** Snoring, stridor, obstruction (e.g. foreign body, vomit, blood, oedema) Cervical spine		**Non-patent airway:** - Head tilt, chin lift, jaw thrust - Suction - Naso/oropharyngeal airway **O^2 (15 L/min)**	
B Breathing	Cyanosis, use of accessory muscles, breathing depth and rhythm, tracheal position, symmetrical chest expansion Breath sounds and auscultation Chest percussion	Respiratory rate SpO^2	Positioning of patient Bag/pocket mask ventilation Decompression of pneumothorax Inhalations	ABG Chest X-ray
C Circulation	Bleeding Skin: - Colour (pale, red, mottled) - Cool/warm/dry/sweaty Auscultation	Capillary refill time Pulse Blood pressure ECG	Stop bleeding IV/IO access Fluids/blood	12-lead ECG Blood tests Urinary catheter ECHO/FAST/FATE
D Disability	AVPU Pupils (reaction, size, equal) Neck stiffness	GCS Blood glucose	Recovery position	Lumbar puncture Focused neurologic assessment Rectal examination (sphincter tonus)
E Exposure	**Head-to-toe assessment:** - Trauma, fractures, wounds, lesions - Bleeding - Infection, petechiae, rash	Temperature	Prevent hypo-/hyperthermia stabilise fracture	Blood cultures Culture from wound Antibiotics

Assess, treat as you go and re-assess

FIGURE 10.7 The AVPU and Glasgow Coma Scale

A	**The patient is alert**
V	**The patient responds to vocal stimulation**
P	**The patient responds to pain**
U	**The patient is unresponsive**

Glasgow Coma Scale

Behaviour	Response	Score
Eye opening response	Spontaneously	4
	To speech	3
	To pain	2
	No response	1
Verbal response	Oriented to time, place and person	5
	Disoriented	4
	Inappropriate words	3
	Incomprehensive sounds	2
	No response	1
Motor response	Normal, obeys commands	6
	Localises pain	5
	Withdraws from pain	4
	Abnormal flexion (decorticate)	3
	Abnormal extension (decerebrate)	2
	No response	1
Total score	Best response	15
	Threatened airway *(seek expert help — intubation?)*	≤ 8
	Worst response	3

Airway

A key aspect of the nurse's role when presented with a deteriorating patient is maintaining airway patency. If a patient is unable to maintain their own airway, they may need to be intubated (Russotto et al. 2017). A training doctor will perform intubation, and the patient will need to be cared for in the ICU so the airway can be monitored more closely. They may also have a tracheostomy in situ that may require suctioning by the nurse (Mussa et al. 2020).

Breathing

Signs of respiratory distress include tachypnoea, sweating, the use of accessory muscles and abdominal breathing (Vaporidi et al. 2020). Emergency management of breathing disorders includes early recognition and assessment, diagnosis and the administration of **high flow oxygen** therapy, with a target peripheral oxygen saturation level (SpO_2) between 92 and 96 per cent for acutely unwell patients (Beasley et al. 2015). In cases of severe chronic lung disease and other risk factors for hypercapnia, the target SpO_2 of 88 and 92 per cent should be aimed for until ABG results are available (O'Driscoll et al. 2017; Russotto et al. 2017).

ABG analysis

ABG analysis is the 'gold standard' for assessing and evaluating gas exchange and acid–base balance (see table 10.2). ABG results provide essential information about the patient's respiratory function and metabolic state. Most patients in a critical care area such as ICU or high dependency unit (HDU) will have an indwelling arterial line in place, which will give continual access to arterial blood for sampling and analysis. Alternatively, ABG samples can be taken from an arterial 'stab', normally from the radial artery (see figure 10.8) (Hill & Moore 2018). Alternatives to the radial artery include the femoral and brachial artery, which are usually used in emergency settings. A needle will be inserted into the artery so arterial blood can be drawn from the patient; this is a painful procedure, so you will need to reassure your patient during the procedure. A doctor or advanced practice nurse with extra training will take a sample of arterial blood. This is considered an advanced procedure as it is more invasive than venepuncture.

TABLE 10.2 Arterial blood gas parameters

Parameter	Normal values	Interpretation
pH	7.35–7.45	Assesses overall acid–base status of blood. Small changes can be life-threatening
$PaCO_2$	35–45 mmHg	Measures partial pressure of carbon dioxide in the blood. Reflects respiratory control of acid–base balance
PaO_2	80–100 mmHg	Measures partial pressure of oxygen in the blood. A low PaO_2 indicates hypoxaemia
HCO_3^-	22–26 mmol/L	Measures bicarbonate levels in the blood. Reflects metabolic control of acid–base balance
Base excess	−2 to +2	Reflects the quantity of acid or base required to restore the blood pH to 7.4. Negative values reflect acidosis, positive values alkalosis

Chest X-ray

A chest X-ray can provide a useful picture of any underlying pathology and evaluate the severity of disease. Important information can also be obtained about local or diffuse respiratory problems, such as local consolidation due to an infection or a tumour. Other conditions can also be easily identified on a chest X-ray, including pulmonary oedema, pneumothorax and pleural effusion (Doshi 2020). Chest X-rays also illustrate the position of the diaphragm, the size of the thoracic cavity and lung function. Portable facilities for taking X-rays are available in large hospitals as the patient may not be stable enough to be moved to the X-ray department (Doshi 2020).

FIGURE 10.8 Arterial blood sample from the radial artery

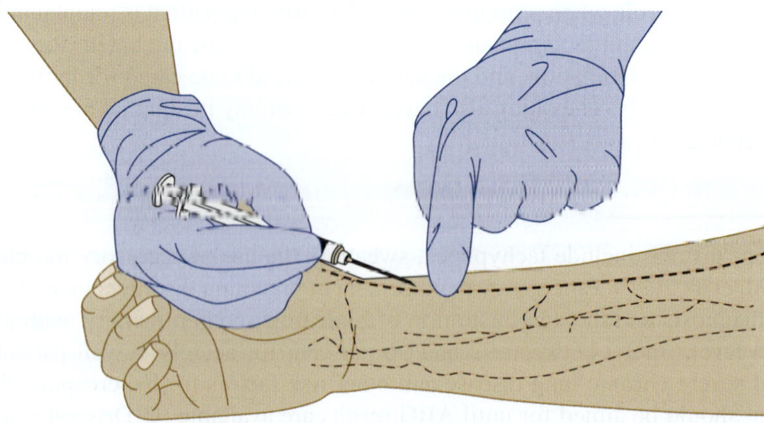

Locate artery and take a sample

Source: World Health Organization (2010).

Respiration and circulation assessment and monitoring

The respiratory rate has been an early and independent predictor of deterioration in patients, but it remains the vital sign is recorded less frequently or recorded inaccurately (Elliott 2016; Smith & Bowden 2017). An increased respiratory rate can indicate acidosis in the body, declining respiratory function, hypovolaemia, and it has also been found to increase immediately prior to cardiac arrest (Elliott 2016). So, it is imperative that nurses record this accurately. Counting the respiratory rate for 30 seconds and doubling it is sufficient for adults, whereas paediatric patients will need their respiratory rate counting for 1 minute due to their irregular breathing pattern. When recording the patient's respiratory rate, it is important to assess the rhythm, check for laboured breathing signs and listen for any audible adventitious sounds. Accurate and timely recording of vital signs is essential in order to recognise a deteriorating patient.

Alterations in the patient's cardiovascular status are also key indicators of deterioration. Cardiovascular problems can occur as a primary cause of acute illness or other disorders that compromise cardiac function. In addition to the basic cardiovascular assessment guidelines outlined in the chapter on nursing assessment, the deteriorating patient may also need an echocardiograph (ECG) recording to assess for ischaemic changes or continuous cardiac monitoring to continually assess the patient's cardiac rhythm and rate. Some facilities have cardiac monitoring facilities available on medical–surgical wards in the form of a bedside monitor or a remote monitoring device such as telemetry. Nurses need to be familiar with normal sinus rhythm and assess other common dysrhythmias such as tachycardias, bradycardias, atrial fibrillation and life-threatening rhythms, such as ventricular fibrillation, ventricular tachycardia and asystole (Currey et al. 2018). ECG interpretation is discussed in greater depth in the chapter on conditions of the circulatory system; however, some common cardiac rhythms are shown in the following figures (see figure 10.9 for normal heart rhythm for comparison).

FIGURE 10.9 A normal heart rhythm characterised by a heart rate of 60–100 bpm

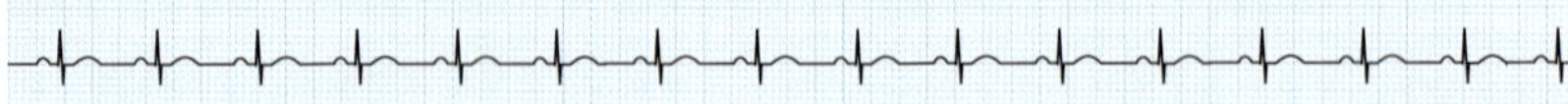

Source: Burns (2020).

Sinus tachycardia

Sinus tachycardia is when the heart beats faster than normal with a regular, rapid rate of over 100 beats per minute (figure 10.10). There are many reasons patients can develop sinus tachycardia, including during exercise, increased caffeine or alcohol intake, infection, sepsis or haemorrhage.

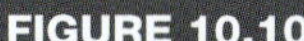

FIGURE 10.10 Sinus tachycardia

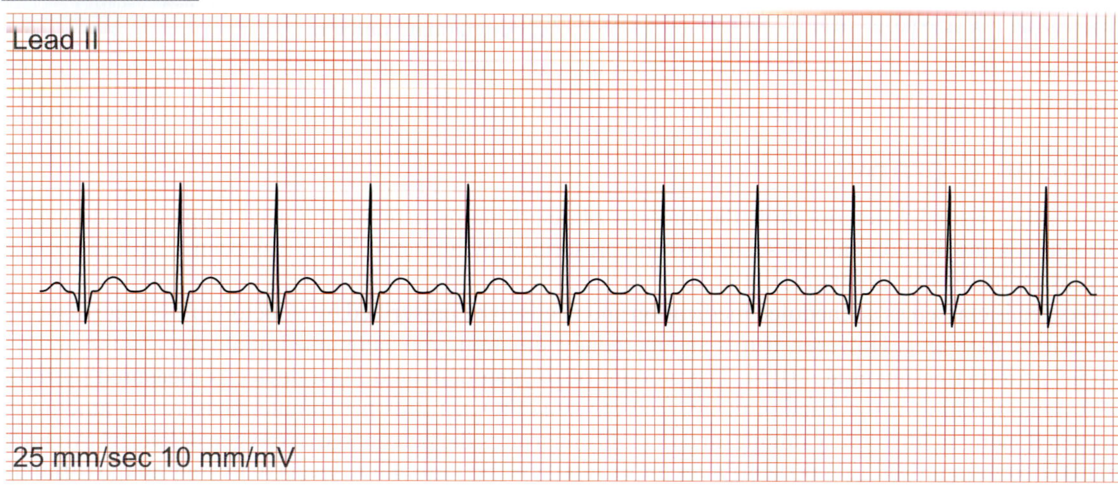

Bradycardia

Bradycardia is when the heart beats slower than normal, so the heart rate will be below 60 beats per minute (figure 10.11). This can be normal in elite athletes or during sleep. It can also occur due to medications such as beta-blockers or medical conditions such as hypothyroidism.

FIGURE 10.11 Sinus bradycardia

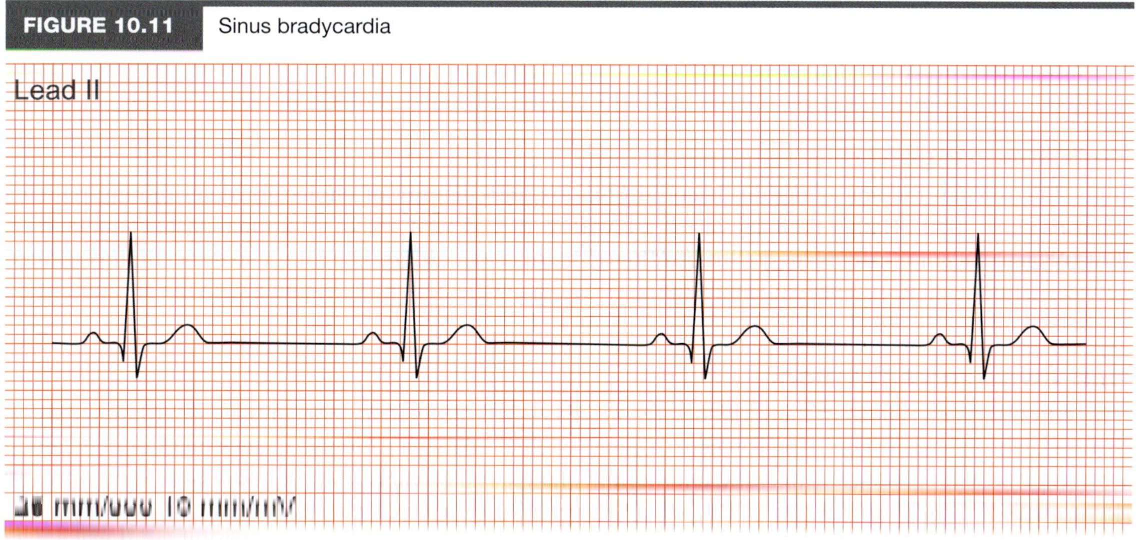

Atrial fibrillation

Atrial fibrillation is commonly referred to as 'AF'. It is the most common cardiac arrhythmia that patients present with in hospital (Proietti et al. 2020). AF is characterised by an irregular rhythm with absent P waves on a rhythm strip (see figure 10.12).

FIGURE 10.12 Atrial fibrillation

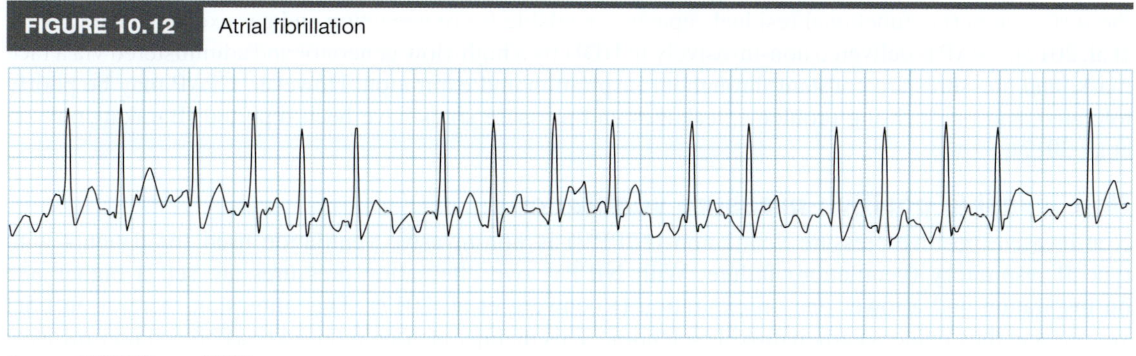

Source: ECG Library (2021).

Life-threatening cardiac arrhythmias are discussed in the cardiac arrest section of this chapter.

10.6 Treatment of the deteriorating patient

LEARNING OBJECTIVE 10.6 Identify the treatment of a deteriorating patient.

Treatment for deteriorating patients depends on the cause of deterioration. Some common interventions will now be discussed.

Oxygen therapy

Despite the reason for deterioration, the majority of deteriorating patients will need supplemental oxygen. Oxygen is a medication and, as such, must be prescribed by a doctor. There has been a shift in oxygen therapy guidelines in recent years.

Oxygen is classed as a scheduled medication and needs to be prescribed by a doctor unless a nurse works in a critical care area. However, if it is an emergency situation, you can nurse initiate oxygen therapy for a brief period (Beasley et al. 2015). The amount of oxygen delivered via a device is measured by litres per minute (L/min) or the fraction of inspired oxygen (FiO_2). Litres per minute measure the amount of oxygen flowing in litres every minute, and the FiO_2 measures the percentage of oxygen delivered. An FiO_2 of 1.0 = 100%; an FiO_2 of 0.60 = 60% an FiO_2 of 0.28 = 28% etc. FiO_2 levels delivered by the different delivery systems may vary considerably between patients and be influenced by several factors, including respiratory rate and whether the patient's mouth is open or closed. The various types of oxygen delivery devices are discussed in the chapter covering conditions related to the respiratory system.

Approximate FiO_2 values delivered by different delivery systems are that:

- standard nasal cannula can deliver an FiO_2 of 0.24–0.35 at an oxygen flow of 1–4 L/min
- Venturi masks can deliver an FiO_2 of 0.24–0.60
- high-flow nasal cannula can deliver an FiO_2 of 0.21–0.80
- a simple face mask can deliver an FiO_2 of 0.35–0.60 at an oxygen flow of 5–8 L/min
- a 100% non-rebreather reservoir mask at 12–15 L/min can deliver an FiO_2 of >0.60.

High flow oxygen

High flow oxygen therapy is rapidly becoming the oxygen therapy of choice for deteriorating patients (Sharma et al. 2020). Rather than delivering a low flow of 1–5 L/m with a traditional nasal cannula, high flow oxygen can administer up to 60 litres of flow (Sharma et al. 2020). The FiO_2 can be accurately titrated between 21 per cent to 100 per cent and administered via a wide bore nasal cannula with the air humidified via heated tubes (Ricard et al. 2020).

Non-invasive ventilation

If high flow oxygen is not sufficient for the patient's oxygen requirements, non-invasive ventilation may be required. Non-invasive ventilation is where oxygen is delivered to the patient via a face mask or hood along with some pressure. Nurses with sufficient training and expertise can manage non-invasive ventilation on some medical–surgical wards; however, non-invasive positive-pressure ventilation is most likely to be administered in the ICU. The deteriorating patient may require endotracheal intubation and mechanical ventilation if they do not respond to non-invasive ventilation.

Continuous positive airway pressure ventilation

Continuous positive airway pressure (CPAP) is non-invasive ventilation used for patients with type I respiratory (oxygenation) failure. CPAP improves oxygenation by preventing alveolar collapse and increasing the surface area (i.e. functional residual capacity) available for oxygenation and gas exchange (Rochwerg et al. 2017). CPAP is delivered non-invasively in HDU by a high-flow generator and administered via a face mask, and pressures are constant throughout inspiration and expiration. However, CPAP may be poorly tolerated, and mask fitting problems, leakages and pressure sores have been reported (Barakat-Johnson et al. 2017).

Non-invasive positive-pressure ventilation

Non-invasive positive-pressure ventilation (NIPPV) is non-invasive ventilation used for patients with type II respiratory (ventilation) failure. With NIPPV, two alternating pressures are set: a higher one on inspiration and a lower one on expiration (Rochwerg et al. 2017). This allows an increase in tidal volume and thus reduces carbon dioxide retention. This therapy is often referred to as bilevel non-invasive ventilation (Rochwerg et al. 2017).

Masks should be accurately fitted for both CPAP and NIPPV to avoid leaks (Rochwerg et al. 2017). Psychological support is also paramount as the patient can feel claustrophobic and isolated and will require time to adjust to the therapy. Some studies report a high failure of non-invasive ventilation from either refusal of therapy or ineffective treatment (Barakat-Johnson et al. 2017; Rochwerg et al. 2017).

IV fluids

Deteriorating patients may also need to be treated with intravenous (IV) fluids to maintain or increase their blood pressure. Some indications for IV fluid administration include replacing extracellular fluid volume losses, maintaining fluid and electrolyte balance, correcting existing electrolyte or acid–base disorders, and providing a source of glucose (Hoorn 2017). The types of fluids commonly administered to deteriorating patients include crystalloids, colloids and albumin (Hoorn 2017; Myles et al. 2017).

Crystalloids

Crystalloids are water with electrolytes that form a solution that can pass through semipermeable membranes and are the most common and cost-effective type of IV fluid administered to patients (Myles et al. 2017). They move rapidly from the intravascular space into the interstitial space and can remain in extracellular fluid for about 45 minutes. There are three different types of crystalloids that interact with cells and the intravascular space in different ways, including isotonic, hypertonic and hypotonic solutions (see figure 10.13).

Many patients receive crystalloids while they are fasting or during the post-operative period in order to maintain their fluid levels. Crystalloids may be the initial fluid of choice when patients show early signs of dehydration.

FIGURE 10.13 The distribution of crystalloid solutions

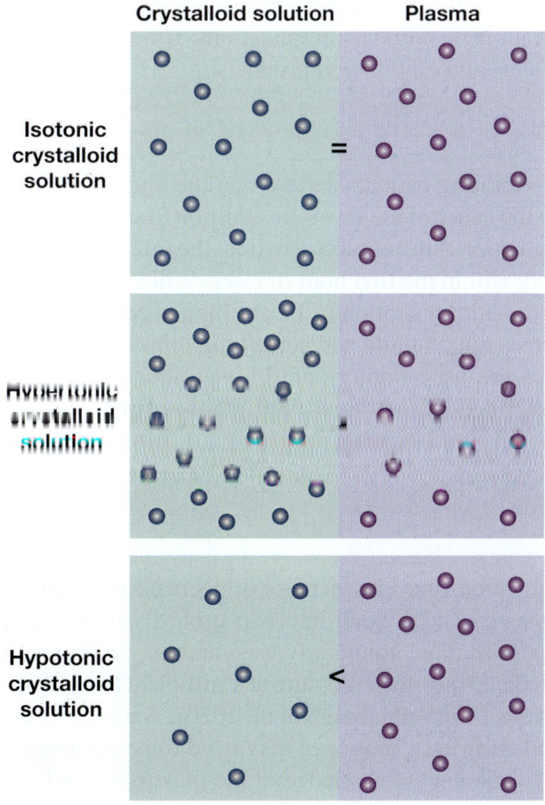

Source: CDC (2018).

Colloids

Colloids contain solutes in the form of large proteins or other similar-sized molecules and cannot pass through the walls of capillaries and into cells. They remain in blood vessels longer and increase intravascular volume by maintaining high osmotic pressure and increased vascular volume.

Colloids are administered to patients experiencing severe dehydration, shock or low albumin levels (Smith 2017). Examples of colloids are albumin, haemocoel and gelofusine (Smith 2017).

There has been an ongoing debate between medical professionals on whether crystalloids or colloids are the best fluids to use in resuscitation. A large, multi-centred randomised controlled trial was conducted to determine the best choice of fluid (Annane et al. 2013). Here is a summary of the findings:

The CRISTAL randomized controlled trial (2003–2012)

Objective: To test whether use of colloids compared with crystalloids for fluid resuscitation alters mortality in patients admitted to the ICU with hypovolemic shock.

Participants and setting: Recruitment began in February 2003 and ended in August 2012. Of 2857 sequential ICU patients treated at 57 ICUs in France, Belgium, North Africa, and Canada; follow-up ended in November 2012.

Interventions: Colloids (n = 1414; gelatins, dextrans, hydroxyethyl starches, or 4% or 20% of albumin) or crystalloids (n = 1443; isotonic or hypertonic saline or Ringer lactate solution) for all fluid interventions other than fluid maintenance throughout the ICU stay.

Conclusions and relevance: Among ICU patients with hypovolemia, the use of colloids vs crystalloids did not result in a significant difference in 28-day mortality. Although 90-day mortality was lower among patients receiving colloids, this finding should be considered exploratory and requires further study before reaching conclusions about efficacy.

Source: Annane et al. (2013)

Blood and blood products

Blood products, such as albumin, are given to increase the osmolality of the blood. This maintains intravascular fluid levels, and therefore blood pressure. Blood products are administered to patients who may have lost blood due to trauma or surgical complications. Blood products include fresh frozen plasma (FFP), packed red cells, platelets and other blood products.

Antibiotics

The initial treatment for deteriorating patients depends on the underlying cause. Sepsis and septic shock treatment focuses on treating the cause of the sepsis, in addition to supportive therapies. Patients are usually prescribed high doses of broad-spectrum antibiotics to treat the infection. Antibiotics must be administered as soon as possible, preferably within the first hour of a sepsis diagnosis, to improve the patient outcomes (Martínez et al. 2020). Delayed administration of IV antibiotics could lead to increases in mortality rates and other complications such as renal failure and acute lung injury (Martínez et al. 2020).

Broad-spectrum antibiotics are used initially until a causative organism has been identified. Broad-spectrum antibiotics are prescribed as they treat both gram-positive and gram-negative bacteria. Common broad-spectrum antibiotics used to treat infection are piperacillin-tazobactam, vancomycin and gentamycin.

Inotropes

Inotropes are a group of medications that can increase or decrease the contractility of the heart (VanValkinburgh et al. 2020). Inotropes can be divided into two groups: positive and negative (VanValkinburgh et al. 2020). Positive inotropes are more commonly used and may also need to be considered in patients with persistent hypotension to keep the blood pressure at a sufficient level to maintain perfusion and oxygen and nutrient delivery to the cells (VanValkinburgh et al. 2020). A patient will need to be cared for in ICU if they need inotropic support. However, inotropes may need to be administered during cardiac arrest, so every nurse needs to have a fundamental knowledge of the most commonly used inotrope, **adrenaline**.

Adrenaline

Indications for administering adrenaline include:

- anaphylaxis or severe allergic reaction
- cardiac arrest
- shock that is not responsive to fluid resuscitation
- bradycardia

- croup in children.

Adrenaline can be administered via a number of different routes, including:

- intravenous
- intramuscular
- inhaled (for croup)
- intraosseous (into the bone when IV access is not possible).

Emergency bedside equipment

Nurses always need to be prepared to identify and act upon their patients' clinical deterioration, no matter which clinical area they work. Adequate preparation should always start with a solid ISBAR handover from the previous nurse, a thorough initial assessment of the patient and completion of the relevant safety checks to ensure emergency equipment is available and working. On a standard medical or surgical ward, emergency bedside equipment usually consists of oxygen and oxygen therapy devices, suction, including a Yankauer sucker (see figure 10.14). A non-rebreather oxygen mask should be available as it can deliver up to 100% oxygen (see figure 10.15). Nursing care of the deteriorating patient in the initial phase requires the nurse to increase the frequency of assessment, observations and raise the alarm to senior nurses and doctors. The introduction of the observations charts inclusive of an adult deterioration detection system simplifies this process and empowers the nurse to communicate their concerns.

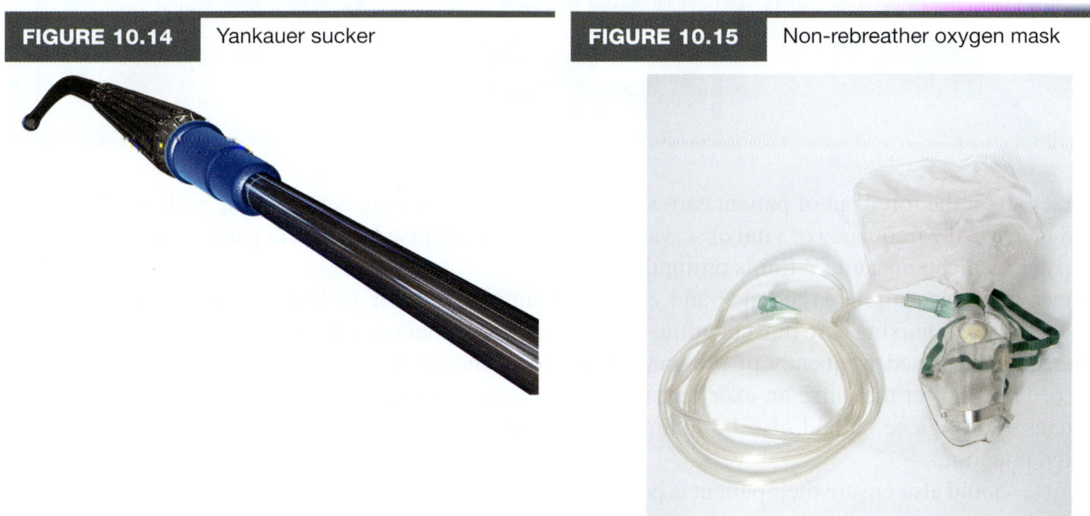

FIGURE 10.14 Yankauer sucker

FIGURE 10.15 Non-rebreather oxygen mask

At the commencement of each shift, a bedside safety check should be performed.

1. Perform the five moments of hand hygiene and adhere to infection control procedures.
2. Introduce yourself to the patient and explain what you are doing.
3. Check the patient's identification band.
4. Check both oxygen and suction are working. Wall oxygen and suction must be checked, with tubing connected. Appropriate oxygen delivery devices should be available, including a simple face mask (Hudson mask) and a non-rebreather mask. A Yankauer sucker should be connected to the suction outlet.
5. Portable oxygen and suctioning should also be located and checked in case the wall supply is not working.
6. A manual blood pressure cuff should be available as an electronic sphygmomanometer can be unreliable when recording very low blood pressures.
7. Locate the emergency trolley and automated external defibrillators (AED). Early cardiopulmonary resuscitation (CPR) and defibrillation decrease mortality rates.
8. Check all intravenous cannulas are in situ and flushing correctly. Intravenous lines that are attached to infusion pumps should be checked to ensure the correct fluid or medicine is being administered. This should be checked by both the departing and receiving nurse.
9. Ensure all drain tubes and indwelling catheters are free-flowing and remain in place.
10. Remove any clutter from the bedspace (Ausmed 2020).

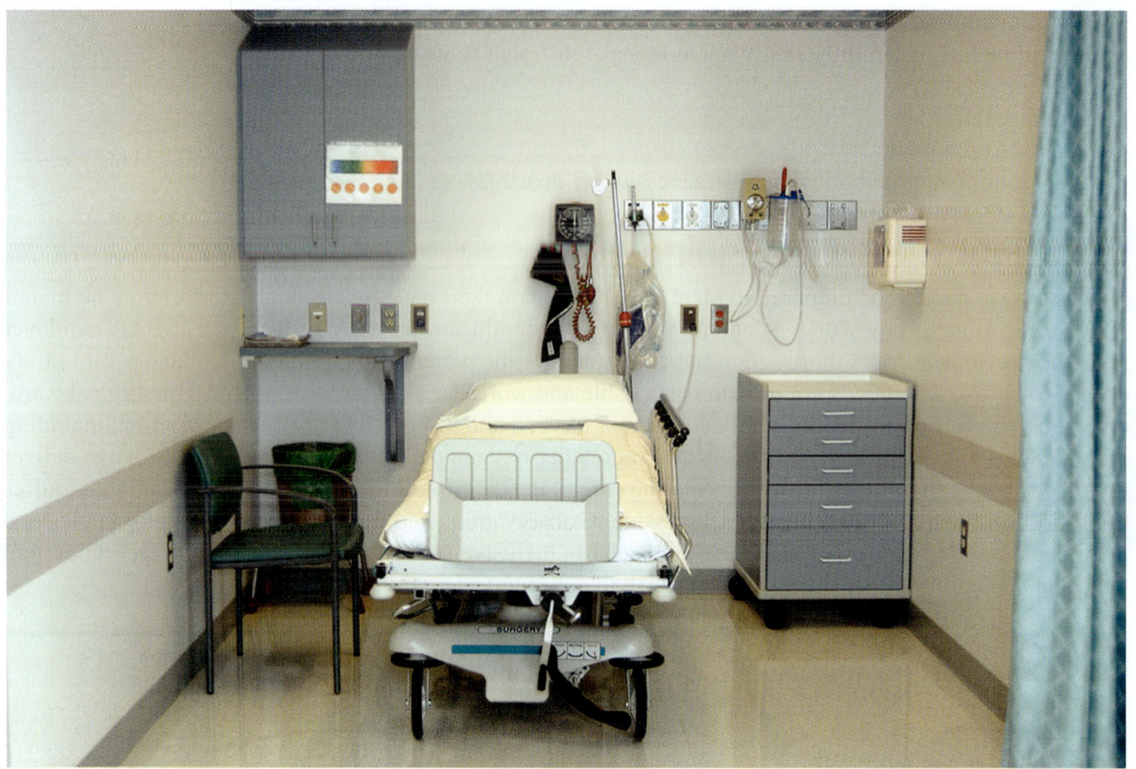

Nurses are at the forefront of patient care and are pivotal in managing deteriorating patients. The nurse should increase the frequency of vital observations, follow a recognised treatment pathway if possible, and administer medications and IV fluids promptly.

Nurses must also offer reassurance and emotional support to their patients, as they may be feeling anxious. Essential nursing care must continue in order to avoid other complications. Deteriorating patients will need an increased frequency of pressure area care as they will be bed bound for lengthy periods. Daily bed baths offer the nurse an excellent way to perform a full top-to-toe assessment of their patient. Adequate oral hygiene should also be maintained in order to avoid the risk of developing a hospital-acquired infection.

A nurse should also ensure their patient is positioned correctly. If the patient has low blood pressure, they may need to be positioned in the modified Trendelenburg position (as shown in figure 10.16) to promote blood flow to the vital organs.

FIGURE 10.16 Modified Trendelenburg position for the patient showing signs of shock

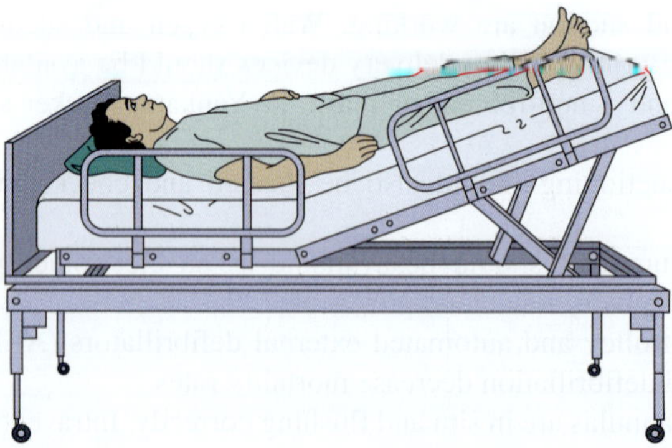

10.7 Recognise and respond to a cardiac arrest

LEARNING OBJECTIVE 10.7 Demonstrate an understanding of how to recognise and respond to a patient with a cardiac arrest.

A deteriorating patient can rapidly progress to **cardiac arrest** if action is not taken promptly. The majority of in-hospital cardiac arrests are predictable and preventable. Some patients can also suffer from a sudden cardiac arrest due to a life-threatening cardiac arrhythmia. The cause of a cardiac arrest needs to be identified so that action can be taken to reverse the cause. Irrespective of the cause of cardiac arrest, early recognition, calling for help, and appropriate management of the deteriorating patient, including early defibrillation, CPR with minimal interruption of chest compressions and treatment of reversible causes are the most important interventions. The four H's and four T's are a simple way to remember the possible causes of a cardiac arrest:

1. hypoxaemia
2. hypovolaemia
3. hyper/hypokalaemia and metabolic disorders
4. hypo/hyperthermia
5. tension pneumothorax
6. tamponade
7. toxins/poisons/drugs
8. thrombosis-pulmonary/coronary (Australian Resuscitation Council 2018).

All registered nurses in Australia must undergo basic life support (BLS) (figure 10.18) training every year to demonstrate that they can administer CPR correctly and increase their confidence in using an automatic external defibrillator. When using an AED, it is important to realise that the machine can detect both shockable and non shockable rhythms. The AED will only charge and administer a shock if the patient is in pulseless ventricular tachycardia (VT) or ventricular fibrillation (VF). When a patient is experiencing VF or pulseless VT, the electrical signal in the heart is not working as it should. This leads to uncontrolled tachycardia or fibrillation of the ventricles and inadequate pumping of blood. If a shock is administered via a defibrillator, the rhythm can be reset and blood flow restored. Non-shockable rhythms include pulseless electrical activity (PEA) or asystole. PEA shows a normal cardiac rhythm on the cardiac monitor, but the patient will not have a pulse. This can occur due to a blood clot or inadequate blood flowing to the heart. Asystole is the absence of any electrical activity or blood flow. In PEA and asystole, the cardiac rhythm cannot be shocked; CPR should be administered. Figure 10.17 shows what these different states look like on a cardiac rhythm strip.

FIGURE 10.17 Cardiac arrest rhythms

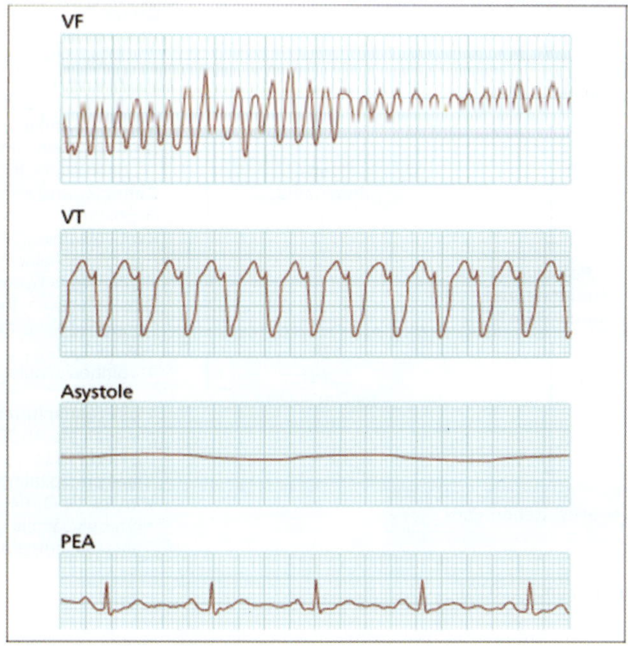

Source: Basicmedical Key (2017).

FIGURE 10.18 Basic life support response steps

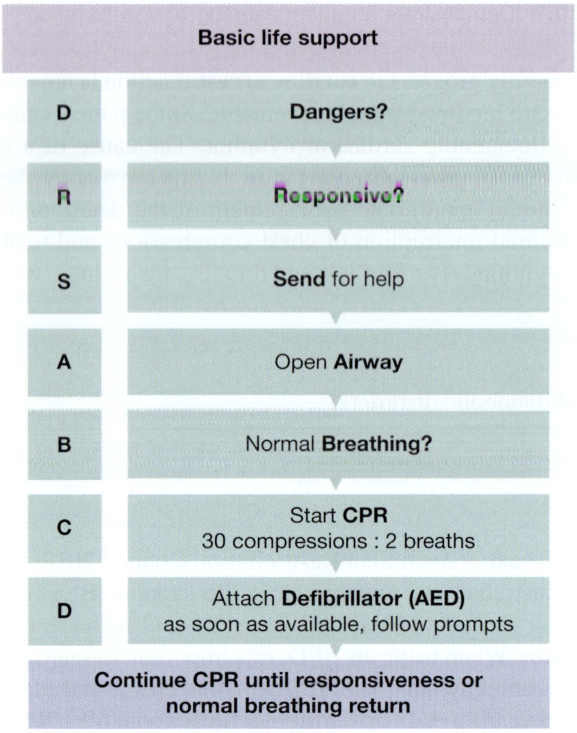

Basic life support

D	**Dangers?**
R	**Responsive?**
S	**Send** for help
A	Open **Airway**
B	Normal **Breathing?**
C	Start **CPR** 30 compressions : 2 breaths
D	Attach **Defibrillator (AED)** as soon as available, follow prompts

Continue CPR until responsiveness or normal breathing return

Source: Australian Resuscitation Council (2016).

FIGURE 10.19 Advanced life support algorithm

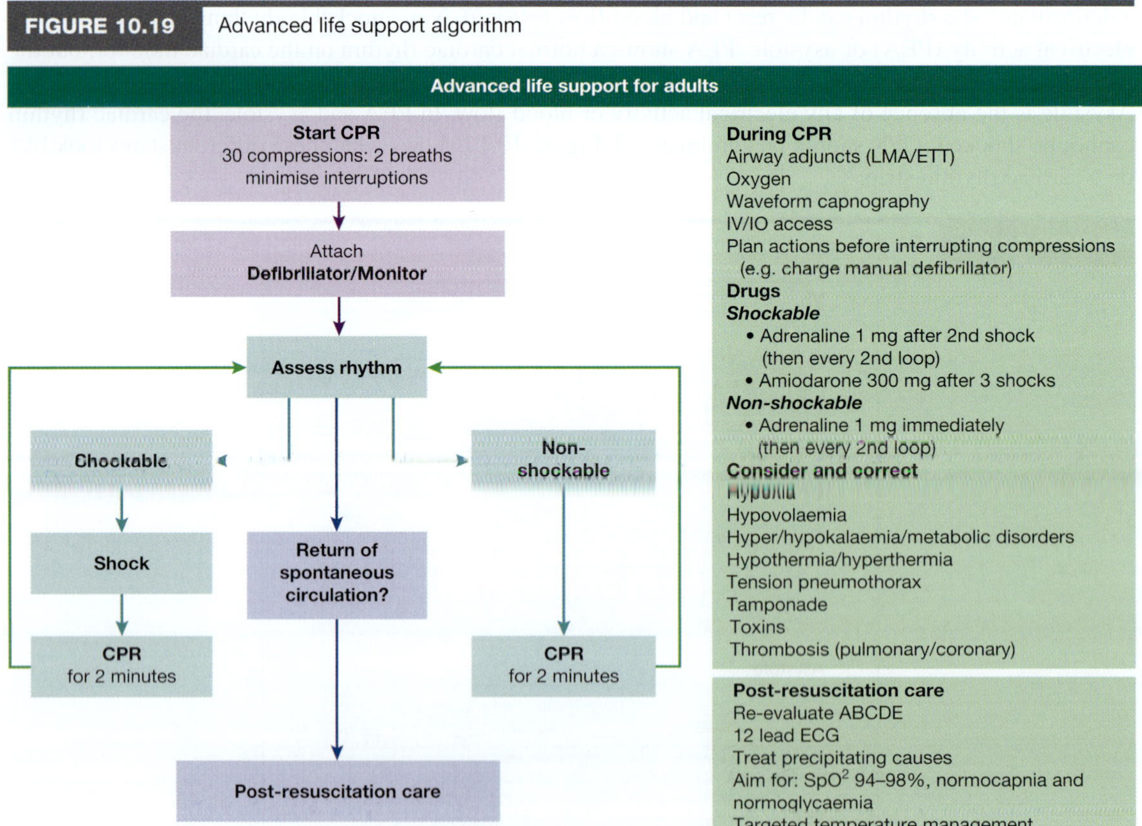

Source: Australian Resuscitation Council (2016).

CASE STUDY 10.1

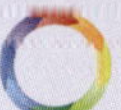

Nursing care of the patient with sepsis

Mr Kapilano is a 68-year-old Indigenous male. He has been admitted to the medical ward following a 3-day history of chest pain associated with a purulent cough. The chest pain was sharp in nature, localised to the left lower thoracic region and worse on deep inspiration. He was also complaining of nausea without vomiting. He has a past medical history of COPD, and despite his chronic cough, he verbalised that his sputum had changed to become more viscous and greener in colour. He also described his cough as more severe and frequent than usual, and he has difficulty breathing. There was no associated haemoptysis. Mr Kapilano reported that he felt feverish and had experienced chills and rigours during the preceding night.

In the emergency department, Mr. Kapilano's vital signs were as follows:

- temperature: 39.1°C
- heart rate: 140 beats per minute
- blood pressure: 90/50 mmHg
- respiratory rate: 28 breaths per minute
- oxygen saturation: 86% on room air
- Glasgow Coma Scale: 15.

On inspection, Mr Kapilano appeared to be in moderate respiratory distress, as evidenced by his inability to speak in full sentences before becoming breathless and adopting a seated tripod position. He did not appear to be peripherally or centrally cyanosed. On auscultation, Mr Kapilano's heart sounds were normal S1 and S2 with no murmur present. There was reduced air entry over the left middle-lower lung field, which accompanied coarse crackles. The assessment of other organ systems was unremarkable. Based on the history and physical examination, Mr Kapilano appeared to have an acute exacerbation of COPD secondary to pneumonia, which has led to sepsis and impending septic shock.

Question

Using the information above, describe what action you would take as the nurse caring for this patient. Use the clinical reasoning cycle to guide you through the process and devise a care plan for your patient.

Answer

- *Step 1: Consider the patient*. Mr Kapilano is a 68-year-old Indigenous male.
- *Step 2: Collect cues/information*. Include subjective and objective data here, including the patient's appearance and past medical history. Objective data will include measurable information such as his vital signs.
- *Step 3: Process information*. Separate the relevant and irrelevant data — cluster the clues together to formulate an inference about the patient. Mr Kapilano has a fever, tachycardia, hypotension, decreased oxygen saturations and an increased respiratory rate. He has also had increasing dyspnoea and purulent sputum. This information meets the criteria for sepsis with the underlying cause of acute exacerbation of COPD secondary to pneumonia.
- *Step 4: Identify problems/issues*. Nursing problems or diagnosis should be listed here. Mr Kapilano's priority nursing problems are dyspnoea, ineffective breathing pattern, impaired gas exchange and decreased cardiac tissue perfusion.
- *Step 5: Establish goals*. Goals of care for Mr Kapilano should focus on improving his oxygenation levels and blood pressure.
- *Step 6: Take action*. The nurse should immediately recognise that Mr Kapilano meets the criteria for a medical emergency call. He is extremely unwell and rapidly deteriorating, so he needs urgent treatment by the medical emergency team. As the nurse caring for Mr Kapilano, you must consider interventions, such as increased frequency of observations, gathering emergency equipment in case of sudden cardiac arrest, gathering IV fluids, ensuring the patient has two large bore IV cannulas in situ to facilitate large, rapid volumes of fluid to be administered. Ensure all IV antibiotics have been administered. Also, recognise the patient may be feeling extremely anxious and will need some reassurance. It would help if you also considered contacting his family to be updated about his deterioration by the doctor.
- *Step 7: Evaluate outcomes*. Once the medical emergency team has attended and the patient has been stabilised, they may be transferred to ICU. If they remain on the ward, then you must continually reassess the patient for signs of deterioration.
- *Step 8: Reflect on the process and new learning*. Reflect on any aspects of care that could have been performed in a way to achieve an improved outcome.

CASE STUDY 10.2

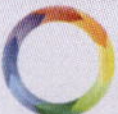

Nursing care of the post-operative patient

Mrs Jones is a 38-year-old Caucasian female. She has been admitted to the surgical ward following elective surgery for gastric banding. She has a past medical history of obesity with a BMI of 35. Her currently weight is 120 kg. She takes 10 mg atenolol daily for hypertension. Her normal systolic blood pressure is 150 mmHg. She remains nil by mouth and is complaining of feeling a little dizzy. She has IV fluids (compound sodium lactate) running at 125 ml/hr.

On return to the ward, Mrs Jones' vital signs were as follows:

- temperature: 36.5°C
- heart rate: 90 beats per minute
- blood pressure: 105/70 mmHg
- respiratory rate: 20 breaths per minute
- oxygen saturation: 96% on room air
- Glasgow Coma Scale: 15
- urine output: 90 ml in the last 4 hours.

Question

Using the information above, provide a plan of care as the nurse caring for this patient. Use the clinical reasoning cycle to guide you through the process.

Answer

- *Step 1: Consider the patient*. Mrs Jones is a 38-year-old Caucasian female.
- *Step 2: Collect cues/information.* Mrs Jones has been admitted for elective surgery for gastric banding. Her observations are within normal parameters. She has a history of hypertension and takes atenolol for this daily. She is obese, currently nil by mouth and feeling dizzy. Her urine output was 90 ml over the last 4 hours.
- *Step 3: Process information*. Despite her observations being within normal parameters, a nurse must identify that Mrs Jones normally suffers from hypertension and her regular blood pressure is 150 mmHg. Given that her current systolic blood pressure is 105 mmHg, and is complaining of feeling a little dizzy, she may be a little dehydrated due to being nil by mouth for the surgery.
- *Step 4: Identify problems/issues*. The following nursing problems are priorities for Mrs Jones: Fluid volume deficit. Risk for ineffective tissue perfusion related to decreased blood flow. Risk for impaired skin integrity related to decreased skin turgor. Nutritional imbalance. Activity intolerance related to physical weakness.
- *Step 5: Establish goals*. The main goal of care should be to restore the fluid volume deficit for Mrs Jones.
- *Step 6: Take action*. Nursing interventions would include maintaining the IV infusion, initiating and maintaining a fluid balance chart, increasing the frequency of observations and alerting the surgeon to the patient's symptom of feeling dizzy. The doctor is likely to prescribe a 'bolus' of IV fluids to slightly lift the patient's blood pressure and increase urine output.
- *Step 7: Evaluate outcomes*. An effective outcome for this patient will be that their urine output and blood pressure have increased, and her dizziness resolves.
- *Step 8: Reflect on the process and new learning:* Reflect on any aspects of care that could have been performed in a way to achieve an improved outcome. In this case, the patient may have needed more fluid during her operation.

SUMMARY

The nurse plays a critical role in recognising and responding to clinical deterioration. Accurate and timely assessment of the patient is imperative in achieving good healthcare outcomes. This chapter has reinforced the importance of vital signs monitoring, particularly the respiratory rate. It has also addressed the nursing assessment and management of the deteriorating patient, including BLS. Lifesaving care for deteriorating patients requires a team approach and structured communication. The use of multi-disciplinary treatment pathways is increasing in clinical practice and is an excellent tool to ensure adequate treatment for the patient using a multi-disciplinary approach. Caring for deteriorating patients can be very confronting and challenging for nurses, particularly if there is a negative outcome for the patient, so it is important for nurses to de-brief following stressful situations.

KEY TERMS

adrenaline An inotrope administered to increase myocardial contractility. The first-line medication to be administered in a cardiac arrest.

adult deterioration detection system An observation chart with a system that helps clinicians to identify deteriorating patients. This can range from a numbered or colour coded system.

cardiac arrest When the heart stops beating effectively.

deteriorating patient A patient who moves from a stable clinical state to a worse clinical state, increasing their risk of morbidity.

high flow oxygen Oxygen delivered via wide bore nasal prongs using a humidified circuit.

patient controlled analgesia (PCA) Analgesia delivered via the intravenous route according to the patients' needs. The patient presses a trigger when they require pain relief, so they remain in control of the amount of analgesia they receive.

sepsis A potentially life-threatening condition caused by an overwhelming immune response to infection.

REFERENCES

ANMF Education Team. (2019) Patient controlled analgesia. *Australian Nursing and Midwifery Journal.* https://anmj.org.au/patient-controlled-analgesia/#:~:text=A%20PCA%20pump%20can%20allow,linked%20to%20the%20PCA%20pump

Annane, D., Siami, S., Jaber, S., Martin, C., Elatrous, S., Declère, A. D., Preiser, J. C., Outin, H., Troché, G., Charpentier, C., Trouillet, J. L., Kimmoun, A., Forceville, X., Darmon, M., Lesur, O., Reignier, J., Abroug, F., Berger, P., Clec'h, C., Cousson, J., Thibault, L., Chevret, S. & Investigators, f. t. C. (2013) Effects of fluid resuscitation with colloids vs crystalloids on mortality in critically ill patients presenting with hypovolemic shock: The CRISTAL Randomized Trial. *JAMA.* 310(17): 1809–1817. https://doi.org/10.1001/jama.2013.280502

Ausmed. (2020) [illegible]

Australian Commission on Safety and Quality in Health Care (ACSQHC). (2019a) *Detecting and recognising acute deterioration, and escalating care.* www.safetyandquality.gov.au/standards/nsqhs-standards/recognising-and-responding-acute-deterioration-standard/detecting-and-recognising-acute-deterioration-and-escalating-care

Australian Commission on Safety and Quality in Health Care (ACSQHC). (2019b) *Standards.* www.safetyandquality.gov.au/standards

Australian Resuscitation Council. (2016) *ANZCOR Adult cardiorespiratory arrest flowchart.* https://resus.org.au/guidelines/flowcharts-3

Australian Resuscitation Council. (2018) *ANZCOR Guideline 11.2 – Protocols for adult advanced life support.* https://resus.org.au/guidelines

Australian Sepsis Network. (2020a) *Recognising sepsis.* www.australiansepsisnetwork.net.au/healthcare-providers/recognising-sepsis

Australian Sepsis Network. (2020b) *Sepsis epidemiology.* www.australiansepsisnetwork.net.au/healthcare-providers/sepsis-epidemiology

Barakat-Johnson, M., Barnett, C., Wand, T. & White, K. (2017) Medical device-related pressure injuries: An exploratory descriptive study in an acute tertiary hospital in Australia. *Journal of Tissue Viability.* 26(4): 246–253.

Beasley, R., Chien, J., Douglas, J., Eastlake, L., Farah, C., King, G., Moore, R., Pilcher, J., Richards, M., Smith, S. & Walters, H. (2015) Thoracic Society of Australia and New Zealand oxygen guidelines for acute oxygen use in adults: 'Swimming between the flags'. *Respirology.* (Carlton, Vic.). 20(8): 1182–1191. https://doi.org/10.1111/resp.12620

Becton, Dickinson and Company (BD). (2017) Alarais^{TM} PCA Model. NSW Government. www.bd.com/en-us/offerings/capabilities/infusion-therapy/infusion-system-devices/alaris-pca-module

Belleza, M. (2017) *Sepsis and septic shock.* https://nurseslabs.com/sepsis-and-septic-shock

Bucknall, T. K., Harvey, G., Considine, J., Mitchell, I., Rycroft-Malone, J., Graham, I. D., Mohebbi, M., Watts, J. & Hutchinson, A. M. (2017) Prioritising responses of nurses to deteriorating patient observations (PRONTO) protocol: testing the effectiveness of a facilitation intervention in a pragmatic, cluster-randomised trial with an embedded process evaluation and cost analysis. *Implementation Science.* 12(1): 85–85. https://doi.org/10.1186/s13012-017-0617-5

Burns, E. (2020). *Normal sinus rhythm.* https://litfl.com/normal-sinus-rhythm-ecg-library

CDC Vital Signs. (2016) Making health care safer. www.cdc.gov/vitalsigns/sepsis/infographic.html

Clinical Excellence Commission. (2016) Adult sepsis pathway. NSW Government. www.cec.health.nsw.gov.au/__data/assets/pdf_file/0005/291803/Adult-Sepsis-Pathway.PDF

Currey, J., Massey, D., Allen, J. & Jones, D. (2018) What nurses involved in a medical emergency teams consider the most vital areas of knowledge and skill when delivering care to the deteriorating ward patient. A nurse-oriented curriculum development project. *Nurse Education Today.* 67: 77–82.

Doshi, A. (2020) *Chest X-rays.* https://mindthebleep.com/2020/02/chest-x-rays.html

Elliott, M. (2016) Why is respiratory rate the neglected vital sign? A narrative review. *International Archives Nursing Health Care.* 2: 1–4.

Hill, S. & Moore, S. (2018) Arterial blood gas sampling: using a safety and pre-heparinised syringe. *British Journal of Nursing.* 27(14): S20–S26. https://doi.org/10.12968/bjon.2018.27.14.S20

Hoorn, E. J. (2017) Intravenous fluids: balancing solutions. *Journal of Nephrology.* 30(4): 485–492.

Journal, A. N. a. M. (2019) *Patient controlled analgesia.* https://anmj.org.au/patient-controlled-analgesia

Liddle, C. (2013) How to reduce the risk of deterioration after surgery. *Nursing Times.* 109(23): 16–17.

Martínez, M. L., Plata-Menchaca, E. P., Ruiz-Rodríguez, J. C. & Ferrer, R. (2020) An approach to antibiotic treatment in patients with sepsis. *Journal of Thoracic Disease.* 12(3): 1007–1021. https://doi.org/10.21037/jtd.2020.01.47

Mussa, C. C., Gomaa, D., Rowley, D. D., Schmidt, U., Ginier, E. & Strickland, S. L. (2020) AARC clinical practice guideline: management of adult patients with tracheostomy in the acute care setting. *Respiratory Care.* 66(1): 156–169.

Myles, P. S., Andrews, S., Nicholson, J., Lobo, D. N. & Mythen, M. (2017) Contemporary approaches to perioperative IV fluid therapy. *World Journal of Surgery.* 41(10): 2457–2463.

O'Driscoll, B., Howard, L., Earis, J. & Mak, V. (2017) British Thoracic Society Guideline for oxygen use in adults in healthcare and emergency settings. *BMJ Open Respiratory Research.* 4(1).

Proietti, M., Lip, G. Y., Laroche, C., Fauchier, L., Marin, F., Nabauer, M., Potpara, T., Dan, G. -A., Kalarus, Z. & Tavazzi, L. (2020) Relation of outcomes to ABC (Atrial Fibrillation Better Care) pathway adherent care in European patients with atrial fibrillation: an analysis from the ESC-EHRA EORP Atrial Fibrillation General Long-Term (AFGen LT) Registry. *EP Europace.*

Ricard, J. -D., Roca, O., Lemiale, V., Corley, A., Braunlich, J., Jones, P., Kang, B. J., Lellouche, F., Nava, S., Rittayamai, N., Spoletini, G., Jaber, S. & Hernandez, G. (2020) Use of nasal high flow oxygen during acute respiratory failure. *Intensive Care Medicine.* 46(12): 2238–2247. https://doi.org/10.1007/s00134-020-06228-7

Rochwerg, B., Brochard, L., Elliott, M. W., Hess, D., Hill, N. S., Nava, S., Navalesi, P., Antonelli, M., Brozek, J. & Conti, G. (2017) Official ERS/ATS clinical practice guidelines: non-invasive ventilation for acute respiratory failure. *European Respiratory Journal.* 50(2).

Rudd, K. E., Johnson, S. C., Agesa, K. M., Shackelford, K. A., Tsoi, D., Kievlan, D. R., Colombara, D. V., Ikuta, K. S., Kissoon, N., Finfer, S., Fleischmann-Struzek, C., Machado, F. R., Reinhart, K. K., Rowan, K., Seymour, C. W., Watson, R. S., West, T. E., Marinho, F., Hay, S. I., Lozano, R., Lopez, A. D., Angus, D. C., Murray, C. J. L. & Naghavi, M. (2020) Global, regional, and national sepsis incidence and mortality, 1990–2017: Analysis for the Global Burden of Disease Study. *The Lancet.* 395(10219): 200–211. https://doi.org/10.1016/S0140-6736(19)32989-7

Russotto, V., Cortegiani, A., Raineri, S. M., Gregoretti, C. & Giarratano, A. (2017) Respiratory support techniques to avoid desaturation in critically ill patients requiring endotracheal intubation: a systematic review and meta-analysis. *Journal of Critical Care.* 41: 98–106.

Sharma, S., Danckers, M., Sanghavi, D. & Chakraborty, R. K. (2020) 'High flow nasal cannula'. In *StatPearls.* StatPearls Publishing.

Smith, D. & Bowden, T. (2017) Using the ABCDE approach to assess the deteriorating patient. *Nursing Standard.* 32(14): 51–63. https://doi.org/10.7748/ns.2017.e11030

Smith, L. (2017) Choosing between colloids and crystalloids for IV infusion. *Nursing Times.* 113(12): 20–23.

VanValkinburgh, D., Kerndt, C. C. & Hashmi, M. F. (2020) 'Inotropes and vasopressors'. In *StatPearls.* StatPearls Publishing.

Vaporidi, K., Akoumianaki, E., Telias, I., Goligher, E. C., Brochard, L. & Georgopoulos, D. (2020) Respiratory drive in critically ill patients. Pathophysiology and clinical implications. *American Journal of Respiratory and Critical Care Medicine.* 201(1): 20–32.

ACKNOWLEDGEMENTS

Figure 10.1: © Adult Deterioration Detection System (ADDS). © Australian Commission on Safety and Quality in Heath Care. Reproduced with permission of Australian Commission on Safety and Quality in Heath Care.

Figure 10.2: © Making Health Care Safer, Centers for Disease Control and Prevention. Retrieved from: www.cdc.gov/vitalsigns/sepsis/infographic.html. Public Domain.

Figures 10.3 and 10.4: © Clinical Excellence Commission 2013, Version 2, SHPN: (CEC) 130088. © Clinical Excellence Commission. Reproduced with permission of Clinical Excellence Commission.

Figure 10.5: © BD. Reproduced with permission.

Figure 10.8: © WHO Guidelines on Drawing Blood: Best Practices in Phlebotomy. ©World Health Organization. Reproduced with permission of WHO. Retrieved from: www.ncbi.nlm.nih.gov/books/NBK138661.

Figure 10.9: © Tor Ercleve, Feb 7, 2021. Normal sinus rhythm. © Life in the Fast Lane. Reproduced with permission of Life in the Fast Lane. https://litfl.com/normal-sinus-rhythm-ecg-library.

Figure 10.10: © JY FotoStock / Shutterstock.com

Figure 10.11: © JY FotoStock / Shutterstock.com

Figure 10.12: © Tor Ercleve, Feb 7, 2021. Atrial fibrillation. © Life in the Fast Lane. Reproduced with permission of Life in the Fast Lane.https://litfl.com/atrial-fibrillation-ecg-library.

Figure 10.13: © Crystalloid Solutions. Retrieved from: www.cdc.gov/dengue/training/cme/ccm/page70749.html. Public Domain.

Figure 10.14: © Nucleus Medical Media Inc / Alamy Stock Photo

Figure 10.15: © SCIENCESOURCE / SciencePhoto

Figure 10.17: © Summary of Key Points for OSCEs, Figure 69.2. © Basicmedical Key. Reproduced with permission of Basicmedical Key.

Figure 10.18: © Basic Life Support, Australian Resuscitation Council. Retrieved from: https://resus.org.au/guidelines/flowcharts-3/. Public Domain.

Figure 10.19: © Advanced Life Support for Adults, Australian Resuscitation Council. Retrieved from: https://resus.org.au/guidelines/flowcharts-3. Public Domain

Photo 10A: © Carolina K. Smith MD / Shutterstock.com

Table 10.1: © Crown Copyright (Department of Health). Public Domain.

CHAPTER 11

Principles of paediatric nursing

LEARNING OBJECTIVES

After studying this chapter, you should be able to:

11.1 explain the primary anatomical and physiological differences at key stages in paediatric development

11.2 identify the key theories underlying paediatric care and discuss their principles

11.3 identify common conditions seen in paediatric care and discuss the underlying anatomical and pathophysiology

11.4 discuss the management of common paediatric conditions

11.5 examine the role of the nurse in the application of holistic paediatric care.

Introduction

Providing paediatric nursing care can be one of the most rewarding and challenging experiences within the profession. Because the paediatric individual may need to access all stages of the health system, paediatric care can sometimes be seen as a sub-system of the broader health system. However, this does not mean we see the **young person** as a little adult, as there are many significant differences in providing paediatric care. This chapter looks at paediatric care principles to better understand the different types of care provided in this specialty, focusing on the underlying anatomical and pathophysiological differences between the child and the adult. Fundamental assessment principles and common conditions experienced by young people will also be considered in the context of nursing.

There are many different definitions of the term paediatric, with most encompassing the age range from 0–18 years. To avoid confusion, this chapter uses the term 'young person' to refer to the paediatric individual themselves, and the term '**family**' is used to refer to the caregivers that the young person is surrounded by.

11.1 Anatomy and physiology

LEARNING OBJECTIVE 11.1 Explain the primary anatomical and physiological differences at key stages in paediatric development.

When providing care for the young person, the healthcare professional cannot simply apply adult-oriented care. There are many fundamental differences in a young person's anatomy and physiology that changes across the lifespan. Indeed, in some instances, the difference between a young person and an adult can be so significant that the applying practices from adult nursing care into paediatrics is not just ineffective, it can result in significant damage (Suris et al. 2017). Furthermore, developmental characteristics may vary significantly between young people of the same age. In fact, there may be as much as 6 years' body size (height and mass) difference between children at the chronological age of 12 years (Beunen et al. 2006). For these reasons, it is essential for the healthcare professional involved in paediatric care delivery to be aware of the underlying anatomical and physiological differences and apply this to their practice.

Major systems

To fully understand the differences in care provided to the young person compared to the adult, it is important to consider the anatomical and physiological differences. The following section will provide a brief overview of the major organ systems of the young person's body and how it can differ from adult anatomy and physiology.

Neurological

The paediatric neurological system is in a constant process of development. Indeed, the brain does not reach peak maturity until well into what is considered adulthood at 25 years of age (Somerville 2016). As such, there are several anatomical differences requiring consideration when providing paediatric care. At birth, the brain is a quarter of the size of the adult brain, doubling in size in the first year and almost reaching full growth by the age of 5 years (Holland et al. 2014). Associated with brain size is brain metabolism, which, as with most elements, develops with age. Cerebral glucose metabolism starts at around half of an adult's requirement at birth. However, it accelerates to double the adult values by age five before decreasing to adult levels through adolescence (Figaji 2017).

As well as the brain itself, there are several cranial structural changes in early life needing consideration regarding paediatric neurology. The most significant structural changes are those of the cranial vault, namely open fontanelles and unfused suture lines. The posterior fontanelle is the first to close — typically 2 to 3 months after birth — while the anterior fontanelle is generally the last to close (between 12–18 months) (Esmaeili et al. 2015). The open fontanels and unfused sutures allow for increased cerebral compliance, but only to a point. Raised intracranial pressure (ICP) is an issue as important in paediatric care as it is in adults, perhaps even more so because of the neurological system's sensitivity in the young person and the low normal ICP range (Figaji 2017).

Respiratory

The paediatric respiratory system can be divided into two major parts, the paediatric airway and the paediatric lung. The paediatric airway anatomy includes the epiglottis, glottis region, the trachea, two mainstem bronchi, bronchi and bronchioles that conduct air to the alveoli. Lung anatomy includes the lung tissue, which is subdivided into lobes and segments. While the paediatric and adult lungs' basic anatomy are the same, some important differences should not be overlooked. These differences can increase the occurrence and severity of respiratory illnesses in the young person and impact treatments and techniques that are most effective (Eber & Midulla 2013).

The most significant difference is the paediatric airway's size and shape. In general, paediatric airways are smaller and less rigid, making them more susceptible to inflammation or obstruction. In addition, infants and children tend to have a proportionally larger tongue in relation to space in the mouth. Further contributing to the risk of obstruction is the relatively large size of the young person's head compared to their body, which can cause the neck to flex when a young person is lying on their back and result in a partially obstructed airway (Gappa et al. 2009).

Moving further down the respiratory system sees some other significant differences. The ribs in infants and young children are oriented more horizontally than in adults and older children, lessening the chest movement. Rib cartilage is springier in children making the chest wall less rigid. These structural differences allow for the chest wall to retract during respiratory distress episodes and may decrease tidal volume. The intercostal muscles that run between the ribs are not fully developed until age five. This can make it difficult to lift the rib cage, contributing to respiratory difficulties when lying supine (Tomashefski & Farver 2008). Younger age is generally associated with a higher respiratory rate, resulting in the young person being more susceptible to agents in the air.

Cardiovascular

Infants and children generally have healthy cardiovascular systems. However, infants and children can only increase cardiac output by increasing their heart rate rather than stroke volume (Standing & Tuleu 2005). This means that while young people are generally effective at compensating for changes in intravascular volume, they can only maintain this to a point at which these compensatory mechanisms may begin to fail. Blood volume itself varies with age, but compared to an adult, absolute volume is smaller; thus, small amounts of blood loss can be significant and infants and children (The Royal Children's Hospital Melbourne [RCH] 2020a).

As in adults, the paediatric heart pumps blood around the body, delivering oxygen and nutrients to the tissues and returning deoxygenated blood to the lungs. However, there are significant differences in the paediatric cardiac system's many anatomical points, particularly in the neonate. The circulatory system begins to develop at approximately three weeks of gestation, with oxygen and nutrients passing from mother to embryo via the placenta (Gude et al. 2004). As the foetus develops, so does the heart and other circulatory structures. However, because the embryo receives oxygen and nutrients via the placenta, structural differences between adult and foetal heart exist. After birth, immediate changes occur in response to the umbilical cord being cut and the neonate beginning to breathe and receive oxygen. With the first breath, the neonate's lungs inflate, and the associated changes in pressure in the aorta cause the foramen ovale to close, forcing blood to flow from the right atrium to the right ventricle before moving into pulmonary circulation (Patten 1930). Another change that occurs once a baby is born is when the ductus arteriosus, connecting the pulmonary artery to the aorta, begins to close.

Parasympathetic control of the heart is predominant in the foetus and mature at birth. Sympathetic control of the heart appears after birth and is not fully mature until infancy (Yiallourou et al. 2013). As a result, neonates and infants exhibit a predominant parasympathetic response, seen as bradycardia, to noxious stimuli such as hypoxia. Due to immature compensatory mechanisms, bradycardia results in reduced output and hypotension and insufficient tissue oxygen delivery. The parasympathetic predominance in infants gradually diminishes over the first 6 months of life. However, due to autonomic tone changes, older children may exhibit heart rate variations, conduction abnormalities and various arrhythmias (Porges & Furman 2011).

Transitional circulation persists until infancy in neonates with a healthy heart. Mature circulation begins following a further fall in pulmonary vascular resistance and permanent closure of the ductus arteriosus — usually 4–8 weeks. However, the cardiovascular system remains underdeveloped until adolescence (Rogol et al. 2002). This is reflected in the variances in heart rate and blood pressure during the early years of life.

Gastrointestinal

Aside from development and growth, the gastrointestinal system does not exhibit significant anatomical and physiological changes. However, the immaturity of the gastrointestinal system does result in some differences compared to the adult. In infancy and early childhood, there is a steady movement of food through the stomach, small intestine and colon, without any definite point of delay except for very short periods in the stomach (Esposito et al. 2019). In addition, an immature biome of microflora can put the young person at increased risk of gastrointestinal infection by opportunistic microorganisms (Yankovsky et al. 2019). Chronic or pathological gastrointestinal conditions are often picked up during routine screening when the young person fails to hit growth milestones, a condition referred to as failure to thrive.

Musculoskeletal

At birth, the human body has, on average, 300 bones depending upon specific definition. These bones fuse throughout childhood development to form the 206 bones that constitute the adult body (Baker 2005). In addition to the number of bones, the main difference between the paediatric and adult musculoskeletal system is that a young person's bones are often in a growth phase, while an adult's bones have stopped growing. Bone growth happens both lengthwise and widthwise. The bone grows lengthwise in the epiphyseal plate at the ends of the long bones. Widthwise bone growth occurs on the surface of the bone (Khan et al. 2000).

Growing bone has inherent areas of weakness due to the growth process. For this reason, the young person's tendons and ligaments are strong compared to the growth plate (Benjamin et al. 2006). Therefore, when a young person experiences physical trauma, the growth plate will give way before the ligament. However, this continual growth process also means that the young person's musculoskeletal system is more elastic and can heal faster compared to adults.

Patterns of injury in the young person can be quite different due to the differences in growing bone. There are two common types of bone injuries. The first type is referred to as an acute injury, usually associated with a singular traumatic event. The second type is a chronic injury, resulting from recurring stresses applied to the bone over a prolonged period. Chronic recurring stresses are often termed overuse syndromes and include stress fractures (Iyer et al. 2012). If not managed correctly, stress fractures can result in complete fracture or lead to changes that affect the joints, causing early arthritic changes. Growth plate injuries can cause interruption of bone growth, resulting in limb-length discrepancy or altered joint mechanics (Kiuru et al. 2004). Adolescents in the peak period of bone growth, often referred to as a growth spurt, are most vulnerable to growth plate injuries. Sports involving contact and jumping carry increased injury risks.

Development

Childhood development is a biological process closely tied to cultural phenomena. For this reason, there are several ways in which to categorise the young person. This chapter uses the term neonate to refer to the period from birth to 28 days; infancy to refer to the period from 1 to 12 months; early childhood represents the period of 1 year to 4; **childhood** refers to the period of age 5 to 12, and adolescence refers to the period of age 13 to 18. Each of these different periods have developmental characteristics and set milestones. The paediatric healthcare professional needs to be aware of these milestones and provide health education when necessary.

Neonate (28 days old)

Neonatal care is often managed primarily within the maternity setting. Indeed, in some cases, a young person less the 28 days requiring inpatient care may be admitted to the maternity ward as the most appropriate setting, though this may not always be the case. Unfortunately, the lack of experience with neonatal care among the generalist healthcare setting often results in poorer outcomes.

The **neonate** has several notable anatomical differences. The immature heart is relatively small compared to the body size, meaning a higher heart rate is necessary to maintain adequate perfusion. Cardiovascular immaturity is often linked with a lack of compensatory mechanisms, with the neonate demonstrating limited ability to increase heart rate or respiratory rate (Yiallourou et al. 2013). A relatively larger head to body ratio, combined with small fat reserves, puts the neonate at increased sensitivity to the surrounding environment's temperature (Hey 1969).

An important consideration when providing care to the neonate is the increased risk of infection. The neonate's immature and ineffectual immune system combined with little vaccination coverage increases the risk of both infection and serious complications associated with infection (Chan et al. 2013). In addition, due to a difference in how the **infant** body fights an infection, the traditional signs of infection such as fever, tachycardia and tachypnoea may be lessened or absent entirely, making it difficult to assess.

Regardless of the reason for contact, it is important to recognise that a neonate is an incredibly vulnerable individual within the healthcare system.

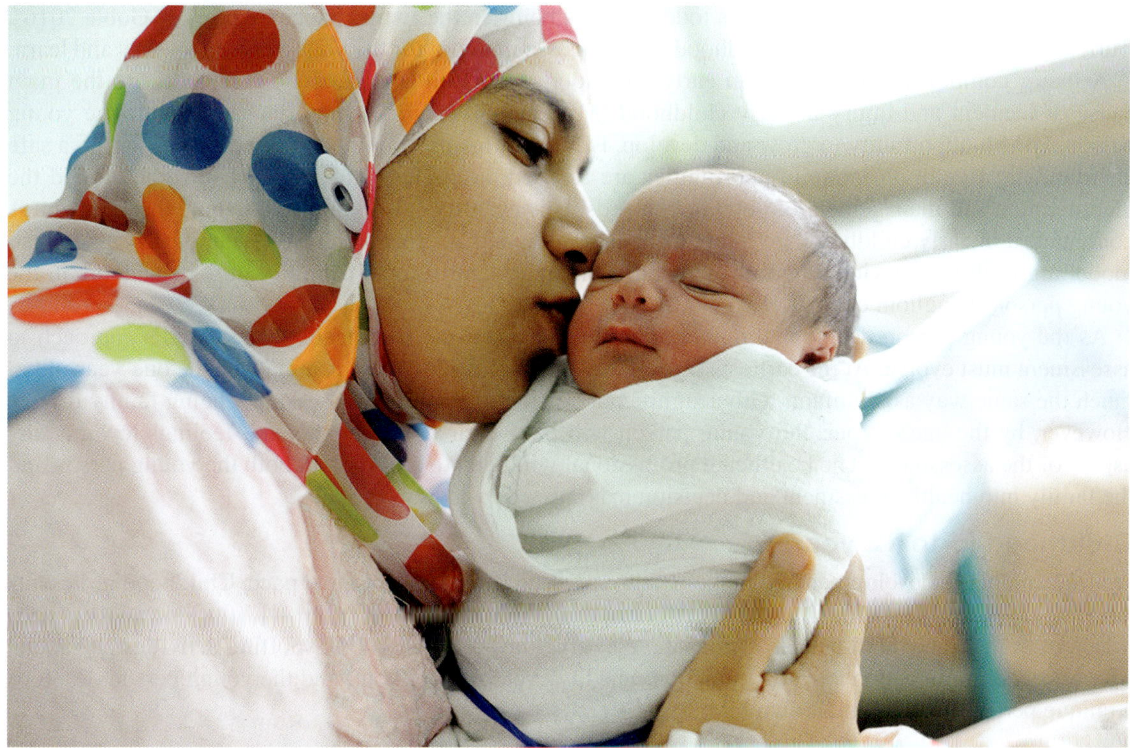

Infancy (1 month to 1 year)

Infancy represents a significant period of growth over a relatively short period. Between the ages of 1 month to 1 year, the infant will have more than tripled their birth weight, increased their height by over half, and their head circumference will have doubled (Fenton et al. 2017). The infant transforms from being a completely dependent being, unable to provide any self care, to being able to ambulate, pick up food and small objects, verbalise noticeable words, and just as importantly, play.

A significant consideration of the neonate's care is the numerous milestones they are expected to meet over the first year of life. The paediatric nurse needs to be able to assess developmental milestones as early indicators of potential concerns needing further investigation. However, it is also important to be aware of the wide variations expected of certain milestones, which may be up to a year variation in some cases. In many cases, the paediatric healthcare professional is responsible for providing the family with education around the ranges associated with specific milestones and alleviate fears that the infant may be 'falling behind'

It can be difficult to assess both the neonate and the infant due to the differing sleep cycles and characteristics. Table 11.1 provides an overview of the common terms used to describe the neonate and infant sleep/wakefulness states.

TABLE 11.1 Neonate and infant sleep/wakefulness state

Deep sleep	Eyes closed, regular breathing, little to no movement
Active sleep	Eyes closed, irregular breathing, small twitches only
Quiet awake	Eyes open, no major movement, regular breathing
Active awake	Eyes open, movement of the head, limbs and/or trunk irregular breathing
Crying and fussing	Eyes either open or closed, vigorous diffuse movement, crying and fussing sounds

Source: Adapted from Humphreys et al. (2015).

Early childhood (1 to 4 years)

Early childhood can be an eventful period for the young person and their family. Physical growth begins to slow, while psychosocial and cognitive development accelerate. Young people in the stage of early childhood are sometimes referred to as toddlers or as being in the 'why?' stage (Worley & Goble 2016). Curiosity is a key feature of early childhood and is an essential tool for the young person to grow and learn.

A major component of wellness in early childhood is environmental safety. Accidents are the main cause of incident and injury in early childhood (Manciaux 1985). It is important to provide the young person with an opportunity to grow and develop. However, this needs to be balanced with ensuring a safe environment. Health promotion opportunities are focused on emphasising family education around the identification and management of potential hazards. However, it is also important to note that behaviours commenced in early childhood are likely to remain ingrained across much of the young person's life, so modelling healthy behaviours by family members is important in establishing healthy behaviours in the young person (Scaglioni et al. 2018).

As the young person develops throughout early childhood, the healthcare professional's approach to assessment must evolve. At the earliest stages, the healthcare professional can manage the one-year-old in much the same way as an infant, with a significant portion of the health assessment being family driven. However, by the age of four, the young person will have their own thoughts and feelings towards any aspect of the assessment. The healthcare professional will need to incorporate both the young person and the family into health assessment and decision making.

Childhood (5 to 12 years)

During childhood, developmental changes occur at a slow, even and continual pace. Childhood represents a period of continual growth. The world continues to expand as the young person learns more and engages in activities that take them outside of their family structure, such as school, sporting activities and social networks. Communication and cognition continue to develop throughout, and the young person develops a unique personality with their own interests.

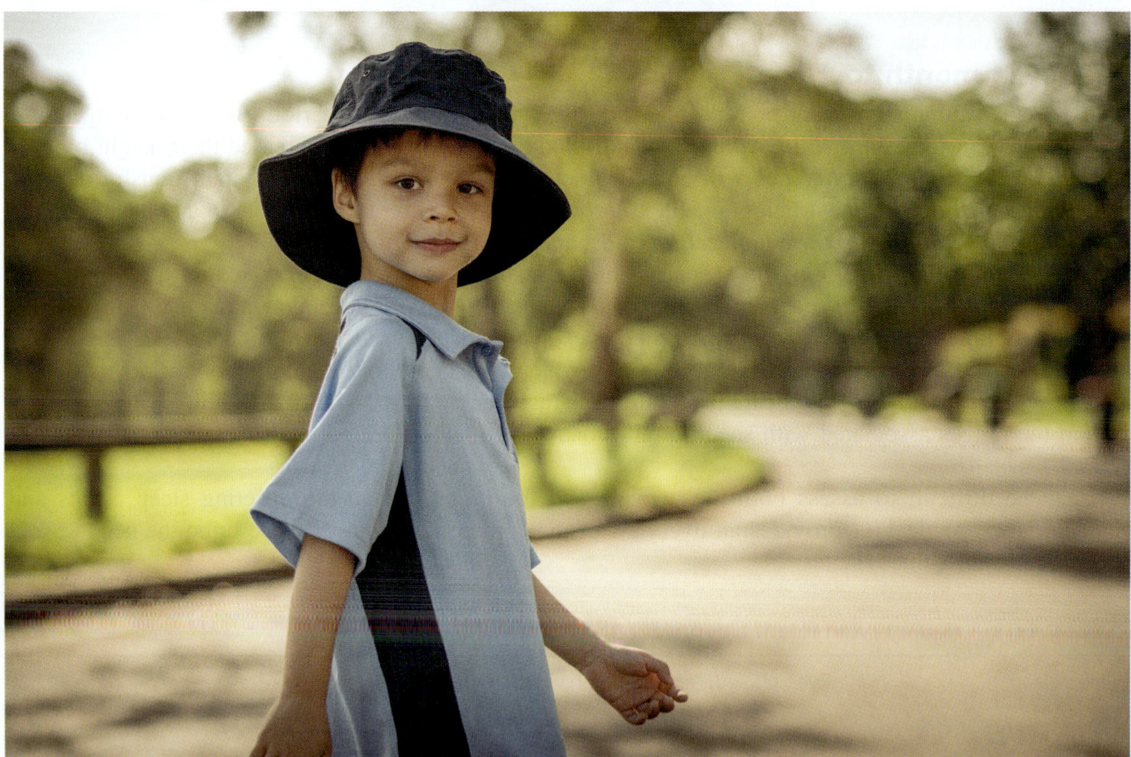

Accidents and injury remain the leading healthcare concern in childhood, with the occasional mild illness. However, many lifelong chronic illnesses such as diabetes may also be diagnosed during childhood, requiring a particular level of specialist care (LeBlanc, Goldsmith & Patel 2003). During childhood, wellness and health promotion are similar to those presented during early childhood, only at a higher level — education around road rules and healthy eating. Ongoing healthy modelling by family is essential in continuing to support the young person's healthy development. As the young person enters the late stages of childhood, they may begin to enter early stages of puberty, and supportive age appropriate education becomes essential.

As the young person grows and develops, they will take an active role in their health assessment. During childhood, there may be stages of the health assessment where the healthcare professional asks the family to leave to provide the child with privacy. However, these need to be carefully balanced with family inclusion and the young person's comfort level (Noiseux et al. 2019). Two young persons at the chronological age of twelve may be at very different physiological, psychosocial, and cognitive stages; therefore, the healthcare professional must ensure they are providing the most appropriate level of care to match the young person's needs.

Adolescence (13 to 18 years)

Adolescence is another period of significant development, specifically puberty. Hormonal changes result in the onset of secondary sex characteristics and stimulate the last significant growth stages for the young person. See figure 11.1 for an overview of puberty stages for the female-presenting and male-presenting individual. Adolescence is a difficult time for many young people as both their bodies and the world around them change. There is an expectation of increasing responsibility as many young people commence their first job and look towards making decisions for their future (Johnson & Mollborn 2009).

Health promotion and wellness in the adolescent can begin to take a more person-centred approach according to the young persons' particular needs (Hayes et al. 2020). While puberty results in inherent education around changing bodies and sexual functions, the adolescent will have various interests and health concerns that will need to focus on health promotion endeavours.

The adolescent takes centre stage in most health assessment processes. Depending on specific policy and legislation and the adolescent's age, they may have full rights of consent and confidentiality, even before the ages of 16 or 18, as is common in most settings. However, this is rarely a simple matter, and the paediatric healthcare professional needs to consider both guidelines and context when making healthcare decisions (Dove et al. 2013). For instance, in some settings, a 15-year-old may be able to give informed consent to undergo surgery; however, this does not mean that all 15-year-olds have the cognitive capacity to give informed consent.

FIGURE 11.1 Stages of puberty: male-presenting individual; female-presenting individual

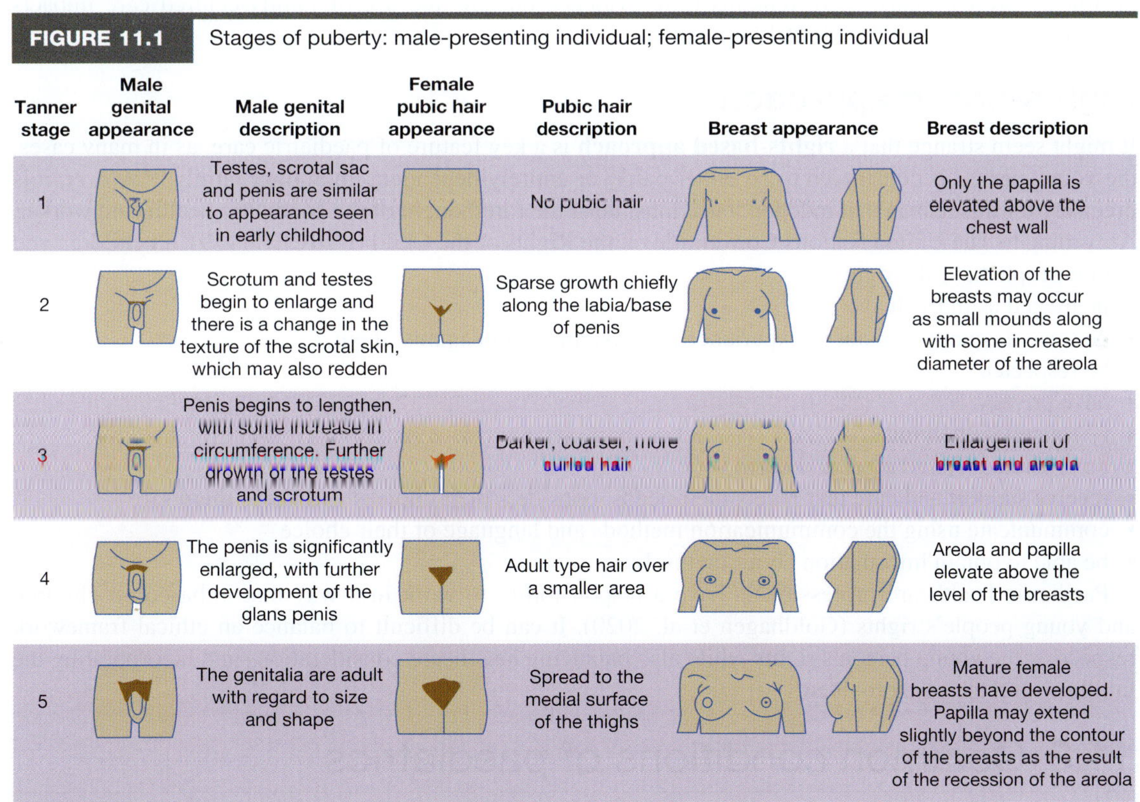

Tanner stage	Male genital appearance	Male genital description	Female pubic hair appearance	Pubic hair description	Breast appearance	Breast description
1		Testes, scrotal sac and penis are similar to appearance seen in early childhood		No pubic hair		Only the papilla is elevated above the chest wall
2		Scrotum and testes begin to enlarge and there is a change in the texture of the scrotal skin, which may also redden		Sparse growth chiefly along the labia/base of penis		Elevation of the breasts may occur as small mounds along with some increased diameter of the areola
3		Penis begins to lengthen, with some increase in circumference. Further growth of the testes and scrotum		Darker, coarser, more curled hair		Enlargement of breast and areola
4		The penis is significantly enlarged, with further development of the glans penis		Adult type hair over a smaller area		Areola and papilla elevate above the level of the breasts
5		The genitalia are adult with regard to size and shape		Spread to the medial surface of the thighs		Mature female breasts have developed. Papilla may extend slightly beyond the contour of the breasts as the result of the recession of the areola

Source: Adapted from Bradley, Lawrence, Steele & Mohamed (2020) and Feingold (1992).

11.2 Key theories in paediatrics

LEARNING OBJECTIVE 11.2 Identify the key theories underlying paediatric care and discuss their principles.

Prior to providing care to the young person, it is important to be aware of the principles that influence the context in which that care is provided. There are many ways in which care of the young person is different from the care of the adult, regardless of the setting the care occurs in.

Family-centred care

When providing care for the paediatric individual it is essential to consider their role within the family dynamic. **Family-centred care** provides paediatric nursing care in a partnership approach to care delivery and decision making (Dennis et al. 2017). Family-centred care has been recognised by healthcare systems and state and federal legislative bodies as a philosophy integral to young people's satisfaction and quality of care (McCance et al. 2016). Family-centred care is commonly used to describe achieving positive healthcare as experienced by the individual and their family. Several different approaches fall within the category of family-centred care, and they generally employ a partnership and collaborative approach with an appreciation of the expert experience of families in providing care to a young person (Irlam & Bruce 2002). The following general principles are shared among many of the family-centred care approaches.

- *Information sharing.* The exchange of information is open, objective and unbiased.
- *Respect.* The therapeutic relationship is marked by respect for diversity, culture and care preferences.
- *Partnership and collaboration.* Medical decisions that are made by all involved parties at the level they choose.
- *Negotiation.* The desired outcomes of medical care plans remain flexible.
- *Expertise.* The family has experience providing care for the young person, which should be valued.
- *Context of care.* Healthcare and decision making reflect the young within the context of their family and life.

Despite being one of the most frequently used models to enhance families' involvement within paediatric care, there are some challenges to implementing family-centred care. There have been many attempts to provide a firm definition, resulting in some confusion as to the core principles. As such, there remain fundamental misunderstandings about what family-centred care is, how to implement it best, and how to determine how family-centred the care actually is. In addition, despite having strong support from healthcare professionals, there remains little evidence on how the use of family-centred care impacts outcomes for families (Shields 2015).

Rights-based approach

It might seem strange that a **rights-based approach** is a key feature of paediatric care, as in many cases, the young person is considered to be either partly or entirely dependent upon their family. However, it is precisely for this reason that independence must be at the forethought of the paediatric health care worker. According to The United Nations Convention on the Rights of the Child (UNICEF 1989), all children and young people have the right to:

- be treated as individuals
- be treated equally and not to experience any discrimination against them
- be respected
- have privacy
- be treated with dignity
- be protected from danger and harm
- receive support and care that meets their needs, considers their choices and keeps them safe
- communicate using the communication methods and language of their choice
- be able to obtain information about themselves.

Paediatric healthcare professionals have a responsibility to work in a way that is based on children and young people's rights (Goldhagen et al. 2020). It can be difficult to balance an ethical framework respecting the young person's rights while also balancing healthcare considerations and incorporating the family within the care provided.

11.3 Common conditions of paediatrics

LEARNING OBJECTIVE 11.3 Identify common conditions seen in paediatric care and discuss the underlying anatomical and pathophysiology.

The paediatric individual is exposed to many potential sources of infection. In addition, anatomical, physiological and developmental differences mean young people experience different types of conditions compared to adults and in some ages are unable to communicate how they are feeling. Family and caregivers play an important role in effectively assessing and managing the unwell young person, and building trust with them is important in gaining trust.

Fever

Fever is a common and normal response to infection. While the exact processes dictating fever are still not fully understood, we know that infection by microorganism stimulates the release of pyrogenic cytokines that stimulate the hypothalamus to raise the body's basal temperature. This higher temperature creates an environment that may be less favourable to the microorganism while also promoting numerous immunological factors (Dalal & Zhukovsky 2006).

Fever is one of the most common reasons for paediatric presentation to the emergency department. Fever in the young person can be of significant concern to the family (Freed et al. 2015). However, in most cases, paediatric fever is mild and short-lived. Family concern is often focused on issues such as the first childhood illness, distress and pain experienced by the young person, or seeing temperature as a number that can be measured to determine how sick the young person is (Richardson & Purssell 2015). As such, the paediatric healthcare professional's primary role in treating fever is to perform an assessment, identify additional symptoms or conditions, and provide support and health education to the family.

Respiratory infection

Respiratory infections are common in young people due to immature respiratory muscles making it difficult for young people to compensate for long periods when they are sick and predisposing them to a range of respiratory illnesses ([illegible] 2017). There are a number common of microorganisms responsible for causing childhood respiratory infection, including:

- respiratory syncytial virus (RSV)
- influenza
- rhinovirus
- adenovirus
- picornavirus.

As most common respiratory infections are caused by viruses, there is little in the way of active treatment that may be needed. In most cases, a young person with a respiratory infection will be managed at home, and the healthcare professional's responsibility is to provide health advice. However, in respiratory infections with moderate to significant respiratory distress, further health support may be necessary.

Other common childhood illnesses

There are many **common childhood illnesses**, so common in fact that they are referred to as such. In addition, what is common in childhood is very dependent upon the culture and context that the young person is raised. Therefore, it is difficult to outline every illness and disease a child may develop. Most common illnesses are mild and will only cause short term discomfort; however, some can be serious. A number of these diseases have vaccines that are included in childhood immunisation schedules, for example:

- chickenpox (varicella)
- whooping cough (pertussis)
- measles
- rotavirus
- influenza
- meningococcal ACWY.

Other mild illnesses seen in childhood include:

- conjunctivitis
- ear infections
- hand, foot and mouth disease.

In general, common childhood illnesses are managed in a supportive manner and rarely require inpatient admission (Lambrechts et al. 1999). The family should be advised to support the young person and ensure their comfort. The young person should be kept home from childcare or school until no longer infectious.

11.4 The management of common paediatric conditions

LEARNING OBJECTIVE 11.4 Discuss the management of common paediatric conditions.

Fever management

Management of paediatric fever generally follows two pathways: (1) management of fever in the infant (under 3 months of age); and (2) management of paediatric fever in individuals over 3 months of age (Clinical Excellence Commission 2014).

Fevers in individuals under the age of 3 months should be treated as serious due to their immune system's immaturity making fever a late infection sign. Without an apparent focal cause of fever, a full assessment will need to be completed, including comprehensive history and investigations such as bloods (FBC, CRP, B/C), urine and stool culture if indicated. Depending upon the findings, further investigation such as radiology and lumbar puncture may be indicated. Often time's cannulation and intravenous fluids, and antibiotics will be required.

Management of fever in the individual over the age of 3 months is, by comparison, a relatively general process. If the individual is stable and compensating, management will be supportive, providing analgesia as needed and encouraging fluids. Where there is clinical concern, such as deranged vital signs, further investigations may be warranted.

As well as medical management, there are several other considerations to the management of paediatric fever. It is important to keep in mind that the child should not be over-wrapped or underdressed. Tepid sponging or cool baths are not recommended, as significant temperature changes can be detrimental (Walsh et al. 2005). Simple analgesia such as paracetamol is given according to directions; however, it is important to note that these are given to children who are in pain or distress for their analgesic effect. Medicines are given for antipyretic effects in only the most extreme cases (Walsh et al. 2006).

Febrile convulsions

Febrile convulsions are a type of seizure that can occur in any individual experiencing a fever but at more prominent in individuals under the age of 5 years (Friderichsen & Melchior 1954). While febrile convulsions are relatively common and affect up to one in twenty individuals, they must be managed as a medical emergency. There are two main types of febrile convulsions. Simple febrile convulsions are characterised by general tonic-clonic movements lasting at most 15 minutes, with little to no post-ictal period and are rarely recurrent. Complex febrile convulsions are characterised by focal movements of greater than 15 minutes, with a significant post-ictal period and are often recurrent within 24 hours (Verity et al. 1998). The exact cause of febrile convulsions is still not fully known. However, it is thought to be a combination of genetic and environmental factors in association with the relative immaturity of the paediatric neurological system resulting in increased sensitivity to temperature changes. A young person who experiences a febrile convulsion should undergo medical review as soon as possible to ensure there are no ongoing concerns.

Respiratory infection management

The management of paediatric respiratory infection is highly dependent on the needs of the young person, and in many regards, is focused primarily on support and comfort. Rarely is intense healthcare intervention required. Often, the healthcare professional will find themselves providing support and comfort to both the young person and their families within the family-centred care model (Bush & Thomson 2007). Specific types of respiratory tract infections may have formulated pathways.

Bronchiolitis

Bronchiolitis is a common respiratory tract infection in young people. Generally infectious, the causative microorganism causes inflammation and congestion in the small airways (bronchioles) of the lung. As with many respiratory conditions, the peak time for bronchiolitis is during the winter months but can occur year-round. Initial symptoms are similar to those of a common cold but progress to coughing, wheezing and increased work of breathing, with symptoms lasting several days to weeks. Most cases of bronchiolitis are managed at home. A small percentage of young people may require inpatient admission to manage bronchiolitis (O'Brien et al. 2019).

Bronchiolitis can be categorised into mild, moderate or severe, as outlined in table 11.2.

TABLE 11.2 Assessment of bronchiolitis severity

	Mild	Moderate	Severe
Activity	Normal	Intermittent irritability	Increasing irritability and/or lethargy Fatigue
Respiratory rate	Normal–mild tachypnoea	Increased respiratory rate	Marked increase or decrease in respiratory rate
Work of breathing	Nil to mild intercostal or subcostal recession	Moderate intercostal or subcostal recession. Nasal flaring	Marked intercostal or subcostal recession. Marked nasal flaring
Oxygen saturation	Oxygen saturations >92% (in room air)	Oxygen saturations 90–92% (in room air)	Oxygen saturations <90% (in room air)
Feeding	Normal	May have difficulty with feeding or reduced feeding	Reluctant or unable to feed

The primary treatment for bronchiolitis is supportive, ensuring adequate oxygenation, fluid intake and managing the young person's distress. Mild bronchiolitis will rarely require inpatient admission and is commonly managed at home with review by a general practitioner or presentation to the emergency department as needed. Moderate to severe bronchiolitis may require inpatient admission for assessment and monitoring as well as ongoing management. Dependant on the severity of symptoms, management may include oxygen administration, hydration and nutrition via medical device, with continuous monitoring (O'Brien et al. 2019). There is little evidence supporting the use of any medications such as beta2-agonists, steroids or antibiotics and antivirals in bronchiolitis (Øymar et al. 2014), though specific guidelines vary.

Bronchiolitis also rarely requires significant levels of diagnostics, with most diagnostics only occurring upon deterioration.

Asthma

Asthma is another common respiratory illness among children. Asthma is an inflammatory disease in which airways narrow and swell, producing extra mucus. Inflammation results in respiratory distress and narrowing of the airways triggering a respiratory sound referred to as a wheeze. In the young person, this is exacerbated by the inherently smaller airways. For this reason, some people are seen to 'grow out' of asthma as they age and their airways develop (Barnes 2002). While asthma is not always linked to infection, infection is a common trigger of the inflammatory process, particularly in the young person.

Like bronchiolitis, asthma can be categorised into mild, moderate and severe, as seen in table 11.3.

TABLE 11.3 Assessment of asthma severity

	Mild	Moderate	Severe
Mental state	Normal mental state	Normal mental state	Agitated/distressed
Work of breathing	Subtle or no increased work of breathing	Some increased work of breathing Tachycardia	Moderate — Marked increased work of breathing Tachycardia
Speaking	Able to talk normally	Some limitation of the ability to talk	Marked limitation of the ability to talk

Severe asthma should be treated as a medical emergency as the individual will quickly lose the ability to compensate. The presence or absence of wheeze is a poor indicator of severity, and wheeze may become entirely absent in the most severe case, a condition termed silent chest, where little to no air entry results in little breath sounds (Morgan et al. 2005).

Management of asthma focuses on addressing the inflammation in the airways. Bronchodilators are commonly administered by a metered-dose-inhaler (MDI) also called a puffer. There are a number of different bronchodilators available. They are commonly referred to as short-acting bronchodilators, with an immediate effect, and long-acting bronchodilators, given as a prophylactic or for ongoing management. In severe asthma cases, the use of systemic steroids may be required to address the inflammation (Babl et al. 2008).

Like bronchiolitis, diagnostics are used infrequently in asthma cases, with most diagnostics only occurring upon deterioration. However, a chest X-ray may be indicated to rule out other causes of respiratory distress and assess the causes of asthma not responsive to treatment. Blood gases and electrolytes may also be indicated in severe cases depending upon specific management (Hedlin et al. 2012).

11.5 Nursing management in paediatric care

LEARNING OBJECTIVE 11.5 Examine the role of the nurse in the application of holistic paediatric care.

The nursing assessment and monitoring of the paediatric patient will be highly dependent on the particular condition, the child's age and their support network, such as family. Assessing the young person can be stressful, especially for those not familiar with paediatric principles.

Comfort

It is the paediatric healthcare professional's responsibility to ensure the comfort and safety of the young person prior to commencing any assessment. This requires delicate management of the therapeutic relationship.

If performing invasive procedures in an inpatient setting, it is common practice for these to be held in a procedure room or similar, with the aim being that the young person's space is respected and kept safe (Valler-Jones & Shinnick 2005). Where possible and appropriate, the child should be included in any discussion regarding their treatment, and informed consent should be gained from both the child and parent (Lloyd et al. 2008). For unwell young persons, minimal handling is encouraged to avoid disruption; however, this needs to be balanced with regular family contact. Everyday routines should continue to be followed to allow the young person to remain in familiar territory.

Primary assessment framework

As in the adult, a primary assessment can be used to gain a quick and structured overview of the immediate healthcare needs of the young person. While the basic steps of a **primary paediatric assessment** remain the same, the young person's particular needs alter how the clinician gains essential information in each phase of the assessment.

Airway

Assessment of the paediatric airway should begin with enquiries about the child's medical history, including details of the birth and subsequent development (Adewale 2009). Previous respiratory illness should be noted, together with a history of any injuries or surgical procedures involving the airway. Specific questions should also be asked about the child's respiration, feeding and phonation, as well as the presence and nature of any cough. Information about the paediatric airway can also be obtained from the general appearance of the young person. Distressed facial expression or the presence of nasal flaring may suggest respiratory distress. Mouth-breathing or drooling often occur in the presence of enlarged tonsils or adenoids (Hallas et al. 2019).

In the neonate and infant, in particular, there may be a history of respiratory distress in relation to feeding or when the child is in a particular position. Similarly, abnormal feeding patterns may be associated with respiratory insufficiency, particularly when accompanied by choking, coughing, vomiting and other signs of aspiration (Adewale 2009).

Abnormalities within the paediatric airway are often associated with noisy breathing. Cough is a common symptom of respiratory abnormality and is often associated with upper respiratory tract infection. It may be caused by stimuli arising in the mucosa of any part of the respiratory tract. The frequency, severity and character of the cough are dependent on several factors. In a respiratory infection, the cough is usually productive and associated with nasal secretions. However, the cough does not only indicate infection. Sudden onset of cough in the absence of systemic illness suggests foreign body obstruction and requires immediate management (Hallas et al. 2019). The young person's voice and cry should be noted, as hoarseness or a weak cry may occur in the presence of airway obstruction. Stridor is a high-pitched sound that is indicative of laryngeal or tracheal obstruction. Inspiratory stridor suggests obstruction at or above the upper trachea. Expiratory stridor suggests obstruction of the lower trachea or bronchi.

Breathing

If the young person is distressed, or shows signs of respiratory distress, minimal handling should occur. Much of a respiratory assessment can be performed without touching the patient. Respiratory assessments should be conducted regularly throughout the child's stay in hospital. Like adults, a 'look, listen and feel' approach can be used.

Look. When approaching the patient, ask the parents to continue to interact with the child. Examine the child for level of consciousness — how interactive and interested they are in their surroundings — and their general appearance, including colour. In infants, assess for signs of nasal congestion, as infants are predominantly nose breathers. Ask the parents to lift clothing so the chest can be inspected, looking for increased breathing work. The respiratory rate can be counted, watching the abdomen. Assessing the work of breathing is essential in paediatric respiratory assessment. Respiratory distress can be characterised by respiratory muscle contraction, paradoxical abdominal breathing, and accessory muscle use, such as nasal flaring, head bopping and forward posturing.

Listen. Before auscultating, take time to listen to the child breathing and assess for audible sounds such as wheeze or stridor. For best results, auscultating the lungs should occur when the child is at rest or least distressed. Use a stethoscope bell auscultate the lung fields, systematically noting any adventitious breath sounds, such as wheeze, stridor, crackles or rhonchi. See figure 11.2 for further information on paediatric respiratory auscultation.

Feel. If the young person is settled, place your hand on their chest to count respiratory rate. When feeling the chest, assess for equal chest expansion as well as noting rate and depth. Regardless of the method used, paediatric respiratory rate should be counted for a full minute to ensure accuracy.

FIGURE 11.2 Paediatric chest auscultation.

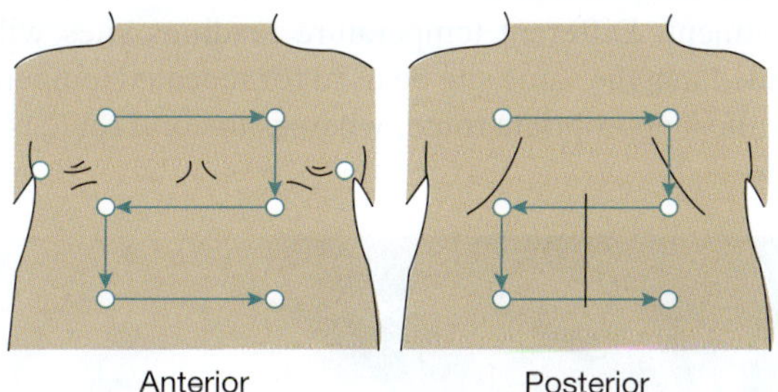

Circulation

As in adults, paediatric circulation system assessment involves assessing heart rate, blood pressure and circulation. Heart rates vary significantly across the lifespan. The location of where the heart rate is palpated will also vary depending on age. In neonates and infants, the heart sits more transverse compared to an adult, and therefore the heart rate is best auscultated using a stethoscope over the apical beat. If it is not possible to auscultate over the apical site, then the brachial or femoral artery may be used as alternative sites. In children and adolescence, the radial pulse can be palpated (Lehrer 2011). Similar to respiratory rate, the paediatric heart rate should be palpated for a full minute, noting rate and regularity.

Blood pressure varies greatly across age groups. Generally, paediatric blood pressure will be lower due to lower systemic vascular resistance (Monyeki & Kemper 2008). Due to the young person's ability to compensate for vascular volume changes, blood pressure is often a late sign of deterioration (Marlais et al. 2017). In the paediatric setting, blood pressure is often only obtained once at first contact with the healthcare professional and then only repeated as clinically indicated. Like an adult, the arm is used to obtain paediatric blood pressure; however, the thigh remains a viable option if necessary. When performing paediatric blood pressure, it is important to note correct cuff size and positioning as errors can lead to inaccurate readings. The cuff's bladder should cover 80–100 per cent of the limb's circumference and 40 per cent of the width between the shoulder and elbow.

Circulation effectiveness can be assessed through capillary refill. Changes in capillary refill can indicate serious illness and be impacted by other conditions such as fever or environmental temperature. Capillary refill should be assessed in conjunction with other vital signs. When assessing capillary refill, the skin should be inspected and palpated, assessing for changes such as mottling, pallor or cyanosis and temperature (Tibby et al. 1999). Capillary refill can either refer to central or peripheral refill. Central refill is most important and can be obtained by placing pressure on the sternum for 5 seconds, releasing and counting the seconds for the skin to return to normal colour. A central capillary refill of 2 seconds or less is considered normal.

Disability

Infants and children are prone to accidents and injuries from falling due to developmental and physiological differences. Due to the young person's head size and weight, their centre of gravity is much higher, resulting in frequent falls and an increased risk of sustaining a head injury (Figaji 2017). The assessment of neurological status is essential when assessing the paediatric patient. It includes both a primary survey approach using the AVPU tool (alert, verbal, pain, unresponsive) and a formal Glasgow Coma Scale. Paediatric versions of the Glasgow Coma Scale have been developed for use in the paediatric setting. Family and carers play an important role in detecting subtle changes in a young person's presentation and should be actively involved in the neurological assessment (Moore et al. 2009). Generally, disability assessment is also inclusive of pain assessment; however, due to the added complexities of pain assessment in paediatric care, this will be discussed in a later section.

Exposure

Assessment of exposure in the young person includes assessment of the skin and temperature. Young people differ in their thermoregulation response due to an immature autonomic nervous system, under-developed hypothalamus and larger body surface area (Rowland 2008). As such, the young person is more susceptible to changes in temperature. For example, infants undergoing surgery are more likely to experience hypothermia due to their inability to shiver in response to a decrease in temperature (Don Paul et al. 2018). Assessment of temperature requires the selection of the correct equipment for the right age group. Using inappropriate temperature assessment techniques can lead to inaccurate readings and potential under- or over-treatment. Different temperature readings sites will provide slightly different readings, and it is recommended that the same site be used for repeated temperature readings. In the infant, axillary temperatures are the most appropriate route, whereas the oral route is more appropriate for young people who can tolerate such.

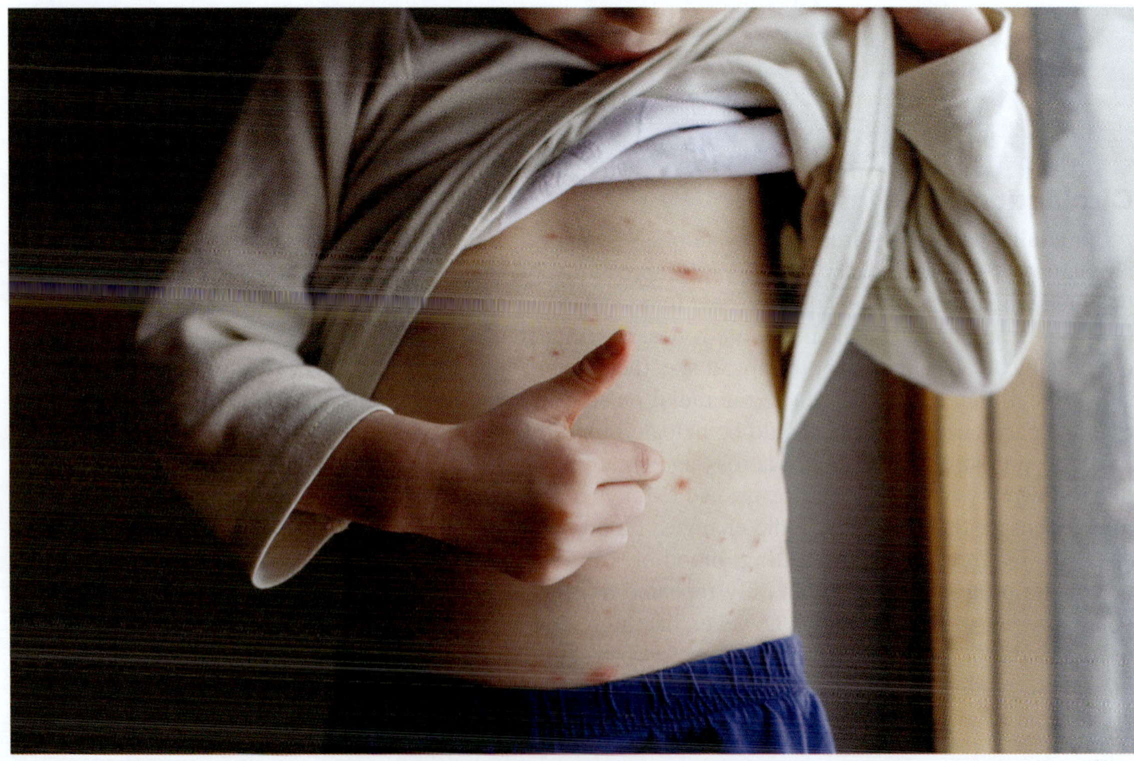

The integumentary system plays an important role in normal physiological function, from acting as a barrier between internal organs and the outside environment to thermoregulation. The intermediary system includes the skin, considered the largest organ of the body as well as its appendages, including nails, hair, sweat glands and sebaceous glands. When assessing exposure, an assessment of the whole body occurs, looking for abnormalities such as bruises, bleeding, wounds or rashes. Young people are more susceptible to alterations in the integumentary system, such as nappy rashes in the pre-continent child and injuries such as pressure injuries. One significant common finding during the assessment of exposure is that of a rash. There are several benign rashes; however, there are also rashes of significant concern.

Fluids

Young people have a smaller circulating blood volume than adults and are more susceptible to changes in intravascular volume such as haemorrhage or dehydration. The assessment of hydration is important for detecting early signs of deterioration in the young person. In infants and pre-continent children family and carers should be asked about feeding habits and how many nappies have been changed. It is important to ask specific questions such as whether the nappies feel lighter than usual, what colour is the urine, or is it darker than normal. Similar questions need to be asked if the patient is experiencing changes to their bowel motions. Inquiring as to the amount and type of stool will help determine fluid losses. Clinical signs of dehydration in the young person include sunken eyes, sunken fontanelle and dry oral mucosa and should be noted if identified during the assessment (Colletti et al. 2010).

Glucose

The young person has a higher metabolic rate compared to adults but fewer glycogen stores. This means the young person is more likely to experience fluctuations in blood glucose levels, especially in times of illness and injury. Paediatric blood glucose level (BGL) should be assessed upon the first contact with the healthcare professional and then reassessed as clinically indicated. Generally, the acceptable paediatric BGL range is the same as in adults.

Vital signs

Oxygen saturation and temperature remain relatively consistent from childhood to adulthood, the same cannot be said for the other vital signs. There is a significant range difference between different age groups, and it is essential the paediatric nurse is familiar with these ranges to ensure effective and safe assessment. See table 11.4 for further details regarding acceptable ranges of vital signs across childhood.

TABLE 11.4 **Paediatric vital sign ranges**

Age bracket	Weight (kg)	Respiratory rate (breath/minute)	Heart rate (beats/minute)	Blood pressure (systolic)
Neonate	3.5	25–60	120–185	60–95
Infant	4–8	25–55	115–180	60–105
Early childhood	10–15	20–40	105–150	70–105
Childhood	15–30	16–30	75–120	75–115
Adolescence	30+	15–25	65–115	90–120

In Australia, the Clinical Excellence Commission (2008) developed the Standard Paediatric Observation Chart (SPOC) to act as a safety net and protect patients at risk of deterioration. Like the Standard Adult General Observation (SAGO) charts, various colour-coded criteria trigger responses from increased frequency of observations to rapid review by a senior clinician. The SPOC is broken down into different age groups: under 3 months, 3 to 12 months, 1 to 4 years, 5 to 11 years and over 12 years to align with the varying vital sign limits associated with those age groups. The SPOC records:

- respiratory rate in breaths per minute
- respiratory distress: normal, mild, moderate or severe
- oxygen saturation (SpO_2)
- heart rate in beats per minute
- capillary refill
- blood pressure

- level of consciousness
- pain score
- temperature
- blood glucose level (BGL)
- weight.

Medications

Paediatric medication administration is a high-risk procedure and requires nurses to be vigilant when preparing and administering medications. As with adults, the 7 rights of medication administration apply, but as a high-risk procedure, many facilities will also require paediatric medications to be independently checked by a second nurse (National Safety and Quality Health Service Standards 2019). As standard doses of medication are based on adults, the younger person will require much smaller calculated doses based on factors such as weight, age and body surface area. Age-related consideration plays an important role in the selection of the right medication preparation. For example, young children may not be able to swallow tablets, and a liquid formulation may be needed.

Pain assessment

Pain is a common occurrence in the healthcare setting, from the pain associated with medical conditions such as a fractured bone or routine care such as vaccination. Assessing and managing a young person's pain can be challenging due to developmental factors that mean they cannot communicate where the pain is or the type of pain they are experiencing. Young people's pain often goes under assessed, and they often do not receive adequate pain relief, even when presenting with painful conditions. Failure to treat a young person's pain can lead to both short- and long-term consequences, including increased response to painful procedures, anxiety and chronic pain (Rajasagaram et al. 2009).

There is a range of pain assessment tools that can be used based on age and development. Pain assessment includes self-report, behavioural cues and physiological cues. Self-report is used for older children who can verbalise their pain and understand what is being asked. For children unable to understand what is being asked, behavioural cues are used to assess pain. Physiological cues are also used to assess pain; however, they cannot be used by themselves as they can be affected by other things such as fever and anxiety (Simons & MacDonald 2006).

The Wong-Baker FACES Pain Scale is widely used with individuals ages three and older, not limited to children. The individual must understand this self-assessment tool to choose the face and number combination that best illustrates the physical pain they are experiencing. Unlike sometimes assumed, the faces scale is not a tool to be used by a third person, parents, healthcare professionals or caregivers, to assess the patient's pain (Garra et al. 2010).

The Face, Legs, Activity, Cry, Consolability (FLACC) scale is a pain assessment tool for young people between the ages of 2 months and 7 years. It is sometimes also used in other individuals that are unable to communicate their pain. The FLACC scale has five criteria that contribute to the name, each assigned a score of 0, 1 or 2, giving a total pain score out of 10 (Merkel et al. 2002).

The Abbey pain scale is for the measurement of pain in people who cannot verbalise. It is similar to the FLACC scale in that it is largely based on behavioural and philological ques, using six criteria; vocalisation, facial expression, body language, behavioural change, physiological change and physical changes. Each criterion is ranked nil, mild, moderate or severe, corresponding to a number 0–3, giving a summative pain score out of 14 (Gregory & Richardson 2014).

Pressure injury

While generally, the younger person has a healthy integumentary system, they are still at risk of developing pressure injuries under certain circumstances. In particular, the younger person is at a higher risk due to not being able to vocalise pain or discomfort associated with the start of a pressure injury. Pressure can be caused by a range of medical devices and equipment such as oxygen tubing, peripheral intravenous cannular, splints and plasters. Like in other settings, the young person needs to be assessed regularly using a validated paediatric pressure injury assessment tool and regular skin assessments. The two most common pressure injury assessment tools used in paediatric care are the Adapted Glamorgan Pressure Ulcer Risk Assessment Scale, which is suitable from birth to age 18, and the Modified Braden Q Pressure Ulcer Risk Assessment Scale, which is suitable from birth to five years (Galvin & Curley 2012).

CASE STUDY 11.1

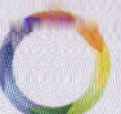

Paediatric patient with a respiratory condition

Oscar, a 6-year-old boy, is brought to the emergency department by his mother Kylie at 1700 with a cough and trouble breathing. Kylie reports Oscar began to cough 2 hours previous, but he has not been feeling well for 2 days. Past medical history is notable for respiratory concerns since infancy, with multiple prior hospitalisations for bronchiolitis and asthma. Kylie has treated Oscar with salbutamol at home, which has had little effect.

On assessment, Oscar appears to be in moderate respiratory distress, with moderate accessory muscle use. His vital signs documented on the SPOC in the emergency department and are:

- respiratory rate: 40 breaths per minute
- respiratory distress: moderate
- oxygen saturation: 93% on room air
- heart rate: 120 beats per minute.
- capillary refill: 2 seconds
- blood pressure: 115/64 mmHg
- pain score: 2/10 and alert
- temperature: 38.5°C.

On auscultation, there was widespread adventitious noises over all lung fields. Kylie's report that Oscar has had decreased oral intake, along with clinical findings of dry mucous membranes and sunken eyes, suggests that Oscar is moderately dehydrated. The assessment of other organ systems was unremarkable. Based on the history and physical examination, Oscar appears to be experiencing a lower respiratory tract infection with an acute exacerbation of asthma.

Question

Using the information above, outline the priorities in providing care to Oscar, noting the importance of physiological care and psychosocial care of the young person, and provide a rationale for each priority. Use the clinical reasoning cycle to guide you through the process and devise a plan of care for your patient.

Answer

- *Step 1: Consider the patient*. Oscar, a 6-year-old boy.
- *Step 2: Collect cues/information*. Include subjective and objective data here, including the patient's appearance and past medical history. Objective data will include measurable information such as vital signs.

  Patient has been coughing for 2 hours and has not been feeling well for 2 days. Kylie has treated Oscar with salbutamol at home, which has had little effect. Decreased oral intake.

  Past medical history of respiratory concerns since infancy, multiple hospitalisations for bronchiolitis and asthma. Moderate respiratory distress, with moderate accessory muscle use.

  Auscultation, there was widespread adventitious noises over all lung fields. Dry mucous membranes and sunken eyes,
- *Step 3: Process information*. Separate the relevant and irrelevant data — cluster the clues together to formulate an inference about the patient.
- *Step 4: Identify problems/issues*. Moderate respiratory distress and dehydration. Mild level of pain. There is a risk of deterioration.
- *Step 5: Establish goals*. Support Oscar's respiratory system to ensure adequate oxygenation until he is able to recover. Support Oscar to rehydrate and achieve adequate input throughout his admission. Ensure he is comfortable and not in pain during the admission and that there is an adequate assessment to promptly detect deterioration and activate escalation of care. Support and empower Oscar's family to enable collaborative family-centred care.
- *Step 6: Take action*. Oxygen should be commenced via an appropriate oxygen administration device to help support Oscar's respiratory system while it manages the infection. Further review may be required depending upon how Oscar responds to the oxygen administration.

  Fluid management should be commenced taking the form of strict fluid balance and encouraging small amounts of food and fluid more often. Further review may be required if Oscar is unable to tolerate any input. A pain management strategy should be considered to ensure his comfort during the management of his respiratory condition.

  Oscar needs a high level of monitoring to ensure further deterioration is able to be picked up promptly and to ensure the effectiveness of the treatment plan. Kylie needs to remain at the centre of care, provided with regular updates and kept apprised of any changes to Oscar's care. As admission is likely Kylie might benefit from a social work referral to ensure she is supported throughout the admission.

  Kylie was administering salbutamol with little effect at home. A medication review should be completed to ensure the best possible management strategy in regards to Oscar's asthma.

▶

- *Step 7: Evaluate outcomes*. Review the impacts of the implementation of care. Ask yourself:
  Has there been the expected response?
  Is there a further deterioration?
  Is there an indication for further assessment or escalation of care?
- *Step 8: Reflect on the process and new learning*. Reflect on any aspects of care that could have been performed in a way to achieve an improved outcome.

CASE STUDY 11.2

Nursing care of the febrile paediatric patient

Tara is a two-year-old girl brought to the emergency department at 1900 hours by her mother, Jane and father, Tim. Tara has been unwell all day and alternating between being drowsy and asleep and irritable when awake. She has not eaten or drunk anything all day, and her last wet nappy was this morning. Past medical history is uneventful, with a full-term pregnancy delivered vaginally. Tara was last given a dose of paracetamol 1 hour prior to presenting.

On assessment, Tara appears to be asleep in Jane's arms; however, she is easily disturbed and cries when touched. Her vital signs documented on the SPOC in the emergency department are:

- respiratory rate: 65
- respiratory distress: mild
- oxygen saturation: 92% on room air
- heart rate: 172 beats per minute
- capillary refill: 3 seconds
- blood pressure: 80/58 mmHg
- pain score: 5/10, responding to verbal stimuli
- temperature: 39.9°C.

It is identified that Tara is at significant risk of deterioration, and as she has three vital signs in the SPOC red zone, the paediatric sepsis protocol is activated.

Question

Using the information above, outline the immediate care that needs to be delivered to Tara. Use the clinical reasoning cycle to guide you through the process and devise a care plan for your patient.

Answer

- *Step 1: Consider the patient.* Tara is a two-year-old girl.
- *Step 2: Collect cues/information*. Include subjective and objective data here, including the patient's appearance and past medical history. Objective data will include measurable information such as vital signs.

  Tara has been unwell all day and alternating between being drowsy and asleep and irritable when awake. Tara appears to be asleep in Jane's arms; however, she is easily disturbed and cries when touched.

  Tara has not eaten or drunk anything all day, and her last wet nappy was this morning. Tara was last given a dose of paracetamol 1 hour prior to presenting.

  Past medical history is uneventful with a full-term pregnancy delivered vaginally.
- *Step 3: Process information.* Separate the relevant and irrelevant data — cluster the clues together to formulate an inference about the patient.
- *Step 4: Identify problems/issues*. Tara is at significant risk of deterioration. There are a number of vital signs outside of limits and a number of important issues reported within the assessment. The sepsis protocol should be activated, and Tara should undergo immediate review.
- *Step 5: Establish goals*. Care should be initiate according to the sepsis protocol with the set time lines of each stage adhered to.
- *Step 6: Take action*. Take action according to the directions on the sepsis protocol, ensuring thorough assessment and escalation of care as needed.
- *Step 7: Evaluate outcomes*. Review the impacts of the implementation of care. Ask yourself:
  Has there been the expected response?
  Is there a further deterioration?
  Is there an indication for further assessment or escalation of care?
- *Step 8: Reflect on the process and new learning.* Reflect on any aspects of care that could have been performed in a way to achieve an improved outcome.

SUMMARY

Paediatric nursing is a specialist setting with specific underlying theories and approaches to care that influence the context in which we practice. The paediatric healthcare professional needs to have familiarity with the underlying concepts of paediatric care to be successful.

This chapter discussed differences in the young person's developing body when compared with the adult pathophysiology. In some cases, these differences may significantly change how the young person responds to certain stimuli that a change in practice is required. There is a need for a generalist healthcare professional to be aware of the common conditions seen in paediatric care and the underlying anatomy and pathology that influence the assessment and management of the young person experiencing these conditions.

Paediatric management is a specialty care that has a number of common approaches. The nurse has a responsibility to provide holistic care to the healthcare consumer. In the paediatric setting, this takes on additional meaning as the application of paediatric care is broader than simply focusing upon the patient.

KEY TERMS

adolescence The period of life between 13–18 years.
bronchiolitis A common respiratory infection in the young person with a variety of causative microorganisms.
childhood The period of life between 5–12 years.
common childhood illnesses Any of the commonly mild illnesses experienced by a child within a particular demographic.
early childhood The period of life from 1–4 years.
family The main non-healthcare caregivers of a young person.
family-centred care An approach to providing care to a young person which recognises their role within the family dynamic and places value on the knowledge and experience of the family as the care givers.
infant A young person between the ages of 1–12 months.
neonate An individual between the ages of 1–28 days old.
primary paediatric assessment A structured approach to performing the initial health assessment of a young person.
rights-based approach An approach to providing care to a young person that respects their vulnerability and places emphasis upon their rights to ensure these are not otherwise forgotten.
young person A person under the age of 18 years who are the focus of paediatric care.

REFERENCES

Adewale, L. (2009) Anatomy and assessment of the pediatric airway. *Pediatric Anesthesia.* 19: 1–8.

Babl, F. E., Sheriff, N., Borland, M., Acworth, J., Neutze, J., Krieser, D. & Francis, P. (2008) Paediatric acute asthma management in Australia and New Zealand: practice patterns in the context of clinical practice guidelines. *Archives of Disease in Childhood.* 93(4): 307–312.

Baker, B. J., Dupras, T. L. & Tocheri, M. W. (2005) *The osteology of infants and children* (Vol. 12). Texas A&M University Press.

Barnes, P. J. & Drazen, J. M. (2002) *Pathophysiology of asthma. Asthma and COPD.* pp. 343–359. Elsevier.

Benjamin, M., Toumi, H., Ralphs, J. R., Bydder, G., Best, T. M. & Milz, S. (2006) Where tendons and ligaments meet bone: attachment sites ('entheses') in relation to exercise and/or mechanical load. *Journal of Anatomy.* 208(4): 471–490.

Beunen, G. P., Rogol, A. D. & Malina, R. M. (2006) Indicators of biological maturation and secular changes in biological maturation. *Food and Nutrition Bulletin.* 27(4_suppl5): S244–S256.

Bush, A. & Thomson, A. H. (2007) Acute bronchiolitis. *BMJ.* 335(7628): 1037–1041.

Chan, G. J., Lee, A. C., Baqui, A. H., Tan, J. & Black, R. E. (2013) Risk of early-onset neonatal infection with maternal infection or colonization: a global systematic review and meta-analysis. *PLoS Medicine.* 10(8): e1001502.

Clinical Excellence Commission. (2008) *Deteriorating patient program: between the flags.* www.cec.health.nsw.gov.au/keep-patients-safe/deteriorating-patient-program/between-the-flags

Clinical Excellence Commission. (2014) Paediatric sepsis pathway. www.cec.health.nsw.gov.au/keep-patients-safe/deteriorating-patient-program/sepsis/Paediatrics

Colletti, J. E., Brown, K. M., Sharieff, G. Q., Barata, I. A., Ishimine, P. & ACEP Pediatric Emergency Medicine Committee. (2010) The management of children with gastroenteritis and dehydration in the emergency department. *The Journal of Emergency Medicine.* 38(5): 686–698.

Dalal, S. & Zhukovsky, D. S. (2006) Pathophysiology and management of fever. *The Journal of Supportive Oncology.* 4(1): 9–16.

Dennis, C., Baxter, P., Ploeg, J. & Blatz, S. (2017) Models of partnership within family-centred care in the acute paediatric setting: a discussion paper. *Journal of Advanced Nursing.* 73(2): 361–374.

Don Paul, J. M., Perkins, E. J., Pereira-Fantini, P. M., Suka, A., Farrell, O., Gunn, J. K. & Tingay, D. G. (2018) Surgery and magnetic resonance imaging increase the risk of hypothermia in infants. *Journal of Paediatrics and Child Health.* 54(4): 426–431.

Dove, E. S., Avard, D., Black, L. & Knoppers, B. M. (2013) Emerging issues in paediatric health research consent forms in Canada: working towards best practices. *BMC Medical Ethics.* 14(1): 1–10.

Eber, E. & Midulla, F. (Eds.). (2013) *ERS Handbook of paediatric respiratory medicine.* European Respiratory Society.

Esmaeili, M., Esmaeili, M., Sharbaf, F. G. & Bokharaie, S. (2015) Fontanel size from birth to 24 months of age in Iranian children. *Iranian Journal of Child Neurology.* 9(4): 15.

Esposito, F., Di Serafino, M., Mercogliano, C., Ferrara, D., Vezzali, N., Di Nardo, G. & Zeccolini, M. (2019) The pediatric gastrointestinal tract: ultrasound findings in acute diseases. *Journal of Ultrasound.* 22(4): 409–422. doi: 10.1007/s40477-018-00355-0

Fenton, T. R., Chan, H. T., Madhu, A., Griffin, I. J., Hoyos, A., Ziegler, E. E. & Ehrenkranz, R. A. (2017) Preterm infant growth velocity calculations: a systematic review. *Pediatrics.* 139(3): e20162045. doi: 10.1542/peds.2016-2045.

Feingold, D. (1992) *Atlas of Pediatric Physical Diagnosis* 2nd ed. W. B. Saunders.

Figaji, A. A. (2017) Anatomical and physiological differences between children and adults relevant to traumatic brain injury and the implications for clinical assessment and care. *Frontiers in Neurology.* 8: 685.

Freed, G. L., Gafforini, S. & Carson, N. (2015) Age distribution of emergency department presentations in Victoria. *Emergency Medicine Australasia.* 27(2): 102–107.

Fridcrichscn, C. & Melchior, J. (1954) Febrile convulsions in children, their frequency and prognosis. *Acta Paediatrica.* 43: 307–317.

Galvin, P. A. & Curley, M. A. (2012) The Braden Q+ P: a pediatric perioperative pressure ulcer risk assessment and intervention tool. *AORN Journal.* 96(3): 261–270.

Gappa, M., Noël, J. L., Severin, T., Baraldi, E., Bush, A., Carlsen, K. H. & Paton, J. (2009) Paediatric HERMES: a European syllabus in paediatric respiratory medicine. *Breathe.* 5(3): 236–247.

Garra, G., Singer, A. J., Taira, B. R., Chohan, J., Cardoz, H., Chisena, E. & Thode Jr, H. C. (2010) Validation of the Wong-Baker FACES pain rating scale in pediatric emergency department patients. *Academic Emergency Medicine.* 17(1): 50–54.

Goldhagen, J., Clarke, A., Dixon, P., Guerreiro, A. I., Lansdown, G. & Vaghri, Z. (2020) Thirtieth anniversary of the UN Convention on the Rights of the Child: advancing a child rights-based approach to child health and well-being. *BMJ Paediatrics Open.* 4(1): e000589.

Gregory, J. & Richardson, C. (2014) The use of pain assessment tools in clinical practice: A pilot survey. *Journal of Pain and Relief.* 3(2): 140–146.

Gude, N. M., Roberts, C. T., Kalionis, B. & King, R. G. (2004) Growth and function of the normal human placenta. *Thrombosis Research.* 114(5-6): 397–407.

Hallas, H. W., Chawes, B. L., Rasmussen, M. A., Arianto, L., Stokholm, J., Bønnelykke, K. & Bisgaard, H. (2019) Airway obstruction and bronchial reactivity from age 1 month until 13 years in children with asthma: a prospective birth cohort study. *PLoS Medicine.* 16(1): e1002722.

Hayes, D., Edbrooke-Childs, J., Martin, K., Reid, J., Brown, R., McCulloch, J. & Morton, L. (2020) Increasing person-centred care in paediatrics. *The Clinical Teacher.* 17(4): 389–394.

Hazinski, M. F. (2012) *Nursing Care of the Critically Ill Child-E-Book.* Elsevier Health Sciences.

Hedlin, G., Konradsen, J. & Bush, A. (2012) An update on paediatric asthma. *European Respiratory Review.* 21(125): 175–185.

Hey, E. N. (1969) The relation between environmental temperature and oxygen consumption in the new-born baby. *The Journal of Physiology.* 200(3): 589–603.

Holland, D., Chang, L., Ernst, T. M., Curran, M., Buchthal, S. D., Alicata, D. & Dale, A. M. (2014) Structural growth trajectories and rates of change in the first 3 months of infant brain development. *JAMA Neurology.* 71(10): 1266–1274.

Humphreys, K. L., Zeanah, C. H. & Scheeringa, M. S. (2015) Infant development: The first 3 years of life. *Psychiatry.* 1: 134–158.

Irlam, L. K. & Bruce, J. C. (2002) Family-centred care in paediatric and neonatal nursing-a literature review. *Curationis.* 25(3): 28–34.

Iyer, R. S., Thapa, M. M., Khanna, P. C. & Chew, F. S. (2012) Pediatric bone imaging: Imaging elbow trauma in children. A review of acute and chronic injuries. *American Journal of Roentgenology.* 198(5): 1053–1068.

Johnson, M. K. & Mollborn, S. (2009) Growing up faster, feeling older: Hardship in childhood and adolescence. *Social Psychology Quarterly.* 72(1): 39–60.

Khan, S. N., Bostrom, M. P. & Lane, J. M. (2000) Bone growth factors. *Orthopedic Clinics.* 31(3): 375–387.

Kiuru, M. J., Pihlajamäki, H. K. & Ahovuo, J. A. (2004) Bone stress injuries. *Acta Radiologica.* 45(3): 317–326. doi: 10.1080/02841850410004724.

Lambrechts, T., Bryce, J. & Orinda, V. (1999) Integrated management of childhood illness: a summary of first experiences. *Bulletin of the World Health Organization.* 77(7): 582.

LeBlanc, L. A., Goldsmith, T. & Patel, D. R. (2003) Behavioral aspects of chronic illness in children and adolescents. *Pediatric Clinics.* 50(4): 859–878.

Lehrer, S. (2011) *Understanding pediatric heart sounds.* Steven Lehrer.

Lloyd, M., Law, G. U., Heard, A. & Kroese, B. (2008) When a child says 'no': Experiences of nurses working with children having invasive procedures. *Nursing Children and Young People.* 20(4).

Manciaux, M. R. G. (1985) Accidents in childhood: from epidemiology to prevention. *Acta Paediatrica.* 74(2): 163–171.

Marlais, M., Lyttle, M. D. & Inwald, D. (2017) Ten concerns about blood pressure measurement and targets in paediatric sepsis. *Intensive care medicine.* 43(3): 433–435.

McCance, T., Wilson, V. & Kornman, K. (2016) Paediatric International Nursing Study: Using person-centred key performance indicators to benchmark children's services. *Journal of Clinical Nursing.* 25(13-14): 2018–2027.

Merkel, S., Voepel-Lewis, T. & Malviya, S. (2002) Pain control: pain assessment in infants and young children: the FLACC scale. *The American Journal of Nursing*. 102(10): 55–58.

Monyeki, K. D. & Kemper, H. C. G. (2008). The risk factors for elevated blood pressure and how to address cardiovascular risk factors: a review in paediatric populations. *Journal of Human Hypertension*. 22(7): 450–459.

Moore, M. H., Mah, J. K. & Trute, B. (2009). Family-centred care and health-related quality of life of patients in paediatric neurosciences. *Child: Care, Health and Development*. 35(4): 454–461.

Morgan, W. J., Stern, D. A., Sherrill, D. L., Guerra, S., Holberg, C. J., Guilbert, T. W. & Martinez, F. D. (2005) Outcome of asthma and wheezing in the first 6 years of life: follow-up through adolescence. *American Journal of Respiratory and Critical Care Medicine*. 172(10): 1253–1258.

National Safety and Quality Health Service Standards. (2019) Medication Safety Standard. www.safetyandquality.gov.au/standards/nsqhs-standards/medication-safety-standard

Noiseux, J., Rich, H., Bouchard, N., Noronha, C. & Carnevale, F. A. (2019) Children need privacy too: Respecting confidentiality in paediatric practice. *Paediatrics & Child Health*. 24(1): e8–e12.

O'Brien, S., Borland, M. L., Cotterell, E., Armstrong, D., Babl, F., Bauert, P. & Paediatric Research in Emergency Departments International Collaborative (PREDICT) Network, Australasia. (2019) Australasian bronchiolitis guideline. *Journal of Paediatrics and Child Health*. 55(1): 42–53.

Øymar, K., Skjerven, H. O. & Mikalsen, I. B. (2014) Acute bronchiolitis in infants, a review. *Scandinavian Journal of Trauma, Resuscitation and Emergency Medicine*. 22(1): 1–10.

Patten, B. M. (1930) The changes in circulation following birth. *American Heart Journal*. 6(2): 192–205.

Porges, S. W. & Furman, S. A. (2011) The early development of the autonomic nervous system provides a neural platform for social behaviour: A polyvagal perspective. *Infant and Child Development*. 20(1): 106–118.

Rajasagaram, U., Taylor, D. M., Braitberg, G., Pearsell, J. P. & Capp, B. A. (2009) Paediatric pain assessment: differences between triage nurse, child and parent. *Journal of Paediatrics and Child Health*. 45(4): 199–203.

Royal Children's Hospital Melbourne [RCH]. (2020a) Trauma Service. How are children different. www.rch.org.au/trauma-service/manual/how-are-children-different

Richardson, M. & Pursell, E. (2015) Who's afraid of fever? *Archives of Disease in Childhood*. 100(9): 818–820.

Rogol, A. D., Roemmich, J. N. & Clark, P. A. (2002) Growth at puberty. *Journal of Adolescent Health*. 31(6): 192–200.

Rowland, T. (2008) Thermoregulation during exercise in the heat in children: old concepts revisited. *Journal of Applied Physiology*. 105(2): 718–724.

Scaglioni, S., De Cosmi, V., Ciappolino, V., Parazzini, F., Brambilla, P. & Agostoni, C. (2018) Factors influencing children's eating behaviours. *Nutrients*. 10(6): 706.

Shields, L. (2015) What is 'family-centred care'? *European Journal for Person Centered Healthcare*. 3(2): 139–144.

Simons, J. & MacDonald, L. M. (2006) Changing practice: implementing validated paediatric pain assessment tools. *Journal of Child Health Care*. 10(2): 160–176.

Somerville, L. H. (2016) Searching for signatures of brain maturity: what are we searching for? *Neuron*. 92(6): 1164–1167.

Standing, J. F. & Tuleu, C. (2005) Paediatric formulations—getting to the heart of the problem. *International Journal of Pharmaceutics*. 300(1-2): 56–66.

Suris, J. C., Larbre, J. P., Hofer, M., Hauschild, M., Barrense-Dias, Y., Berchtold, A. & Akre, C. (2017) Transition from paediatric to adult care: what makes it easier for parents? *Child: Care, Health and Development*. 43(1): 152–155.

Tibby, S. M., Hatherill, M. & Murdoch, I. A. (1999) Capillary refill and core–peripheral temperature gap as indicators of haemodynamic status in paediatric intensive care patients. *Archives of Disease in Childhood*. 80(2): 163–166.

Tomashefski, J. F. & Farver, C. F. (2008) 'Anatomy and histology of the lung'. In *Dail and Hammar's pulmonary pathology* (pp. 20–48). Springer, New York, NY.

UNICEF. (1989) Convention on the rights of the child. https://www.unicef.org/child-rights-convention/convention-text#

Valler-Jones, T. & Shinnick, A. (2005) Holding children for invasive procedures: preparing student nurses. *Paediatric Nursing* 17(5): 20.

Verity, C. M., Greenwood, R. & Golding, J. (1998) Long-term intellectual and behavioral outcomes of children with febrile convulsions. *New England Journal of Medicine*. 338(24): 1723–1728.

Walsh, A. M., Edwards, H. E., Courtney, M. D., Wilson, J. E. & Monaghan, S. J. (2005) Fever management: paediatric nurses' knowledge, attitudes and influencing factors. *Journal of Advanced Nursing*. 49(5): 453–464.

Walsh, A. M., Edwards, H. E., Courtney, M. D., Wilson, J. E. & Monaghan, S. J. (2006) Paediatric fever management: continuing education for clinical nurses. *Nurse Education Today*. 26(1): 71–77.

Worley, L. E. & Goble, C. B. (2016) Enhancing the quality of toddler care: Supporting curiosity, persistence, and learning in the classroom. *YC Young Children*. 71(4): 32.

Yankovsky, D. S., Shirobokov, V. P. & Dyment, G. S. (2019) The role of microbiome in the formation of child health (literature review). *Modern Pediatrics Ukraine*. 5(101): 64–111.

Yiallourou, S. R., Witcombe, N. B., Sands, S. A., Walker, A. M. & Horne, R. S. (2013) The development of autonomic cardiovascular control is altered by preterm birth. *Early Human Development*. 89(3): 145–152.

ACKNOWLEDGEMENTS

Photo 11A: © ZouZou / Shutterstock.com

Photo 11B: © noBorders - Brayden Howie / Shutterstock.com

Photo 11C: © Ternavskaia Olga Alibec / Shutterstock.com

CHAPTER 12

Nursing care of conditions related to the integumentary system

LEARNING OBJECTIVES

After studying this chapter, you should be able to:

12.1 describe the structure and function of the skin

12.2 explain about diagnostic investigation used in skin disorders

12.3 discuss the key components in skin assessment of patients with altered skin integrity

12.4 explain the management of commonly encountered dermatological disorders

12.5 demonstrate an understanding of the pathophysiology and management of skin infections

12.6 demonstrate wound assessment and management.

Introduction

This chapter provides an overview of the anatomy, physiology and related disorders of the skin. The nursing assessment, diagnosis and management of skin disorders are also outlined. Case scenarios relating to skin disorders are provided to enhance learning through reflection and discussion.

12.1 The anatomy and physiology of the integumentary system

LEARNING OBJECTIVE 12.1 Describe the structure and function of the skin.

The **integumentary system** includes the skin, hair, oil and sweat glands, nails and sensory receptors. The skin is the largest organ of the body in weight; hence, this chapter will focus on the skin. The skin is composed of two distinct parts — a superficial layer, the **epidermis**, and a deeper layer, the **dermis** (figure 12.1).

FIGURE 12.1 Sectional view of skin and subcutaneous layer

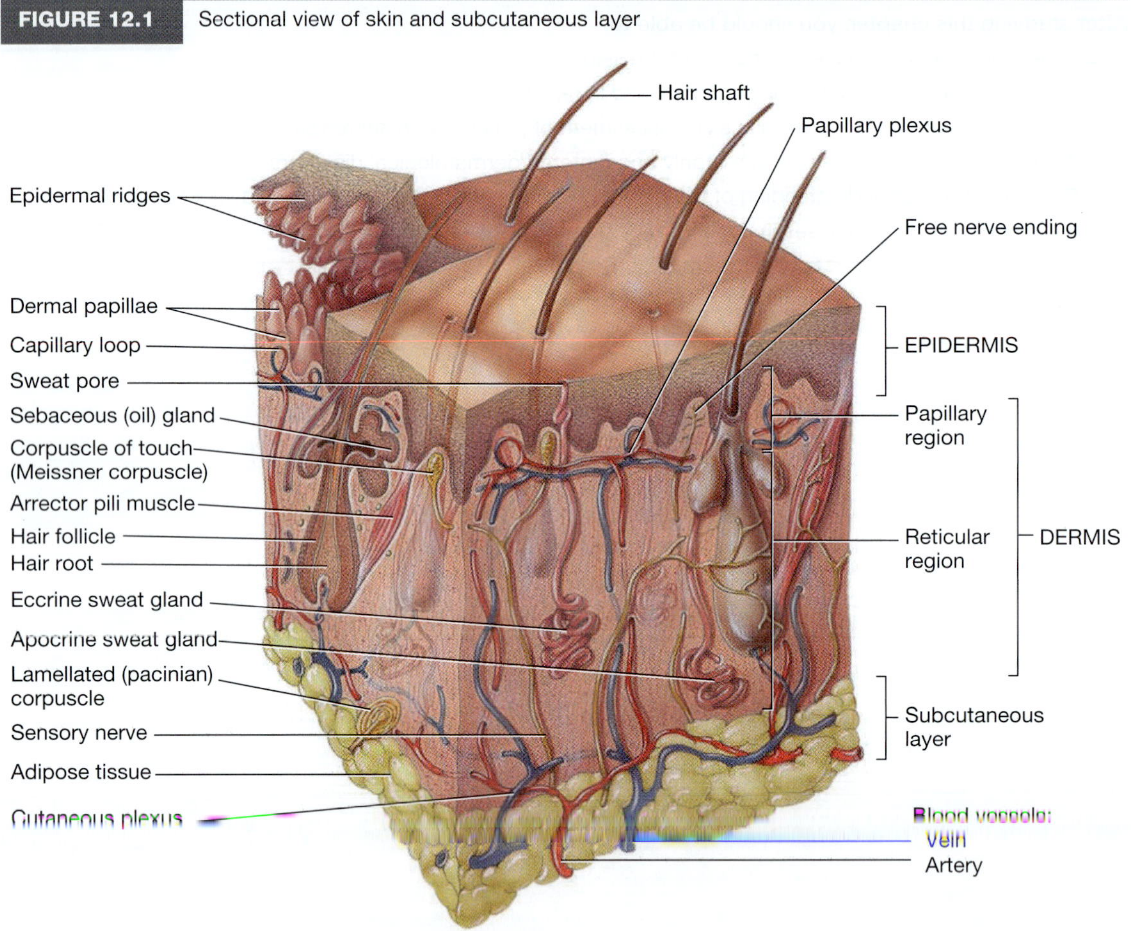

Source: Tortora & Derrickson (2011) *Principles of Anatomy and Physiology*, with kind permission of Wiley Blackwell.

The epidermis provides a physical barrier and tissue strength. The thickness of the epidermis differs across the body, with the soles of the feet and the palms of the hands displaying the thickest layers. The epidermis is avascular and consists of five layers in areas where the skin is thick: stratum basale, stratum spinosum, stratum granulosum, stratum lucidum and stratum corneum. Stratum lucidum appears to be absent in thin skin. The four principal cells of the epidermis are keratinocytes, melanocytes, intraepidermal macrophages and tactile epithelial cells. Melanin produced by melanocytes contributes to skin colour and, most importantly, absorbs damaging ultraviolet light. The deepest layer of the epidermis is the stratum basale. Stem cells in stratum basale undergo continual cell division to produce new keratinocytes. Hence, new skin cannot regenerate if a large area of the stratum basale and its stem cells are destroyed (Tortora

& Derrickson 2011). A protective barrier function is achieved by keratin, a fibrous protein produced by keratinocytes.

The dermis is made up of connective tissue composed of fibroblasts, dermal dendrocytes, mast cells, lymphocytes and macrophages, and blood vessels and lymphatics (Tortora & Derrickson 2011). Collagen and elastin fibres, essential for wound healing, are produced by fibroblasts. Collagen fibres prevent penetration of the dermis from minor jabs and scrapes (Marieb & Hoehn 2018).

Please watch the video explaining the different layers of skin here: www.youtube.com/watch?v=yKAzVC0WcmI.

Subcutaneous tissue that lies beneath the dermis is not part of the skin. It is made up of loose connective tissue and fat, which provides padding and protection of the bony prominences.

The skin's primary functions are barrier and immune defence, sensation, storage, absorption, excretion, thermo-regulation and vitamin D synthesis (Mitchell 2020). Skin serves as a barrier and protects underlying tissues from microbes, chemicals and physical trauma (Bohjanen 2017). Sensory nerve endings and special receptors in the skin are responsible for sensing pain, heat and cold, touch, pressure and vibration. The skin contributes to the body's thermo-regulation through **perspiration** and regulation of blood flow in the skin by vasodilation or vasoconstriction. Vitamin D precursor cells in the epidermis layer are responsible for vitamin D synthesis. Skin is also an effective medium for delivering medications.

12.2 Diagnostic interventions

LEARNING OBJECTIVE 12.2 Explain about diagnostic investigation used in skin disorders.

Some of the commonly used investigations used for skin conditions are outlined in the following sections.

Dermoscopy

Inspection of the skin using dermatoscope is called dermoscopy. A dermatoscope allows the visualisation of skin structures in the epidermis and papillary dermis such as melanin and blood vessels. It is most commonly used to diagnose melanocytic lesions, basal and squamous cell carcinomas and benign tumours (Bohjanen 2017).

Please watch the following YouTube clip explaining the dermoscopy procedure: www.youtube.com/watch?v=dHXOwNU4tYY.

Patch test

A skin patch test is used mainly for allergy testing. The test kit consists of common allergens and allergen mixes in a gel coating on polyester sheeting. It is applied to patient's back and left on for 48 hours (figure 12.2). Skin of the area is inspected for any reaction such as erythema, papules or vesicles at 48, 72 and 96 hours after application.

Wood's light examination

A Wood's lamp emits ultraviolet light at a certain wavelength. The examination takes place in a dark room, and the lamp is held about 10 to 30 centimetres from the skin. Fluorescence (coloured glow) is noted in areas affected.

Punch biopsy

A punch biopsy is a procedure where a skin lesion is excised using a punch device. The site is cleaned, and the location of the lesion is marked. A photo is then taken of the lesion. A local anaesthetic is injected around the lesion, and the punch device is then applied directly over the lesion. The specimen is extracted using forceps. The small wound is then closed using a suture. For superficial or raised lesions, a shave biopsy can be used. Instead of using punch device, a scalpel blade is used to excise or shave the skin lesion.

FIGURE 12.2 Patch tests; (a) Test patches in place; (b) Patches being removed after 48 hours; (c) Positive patch test reactions

(a)

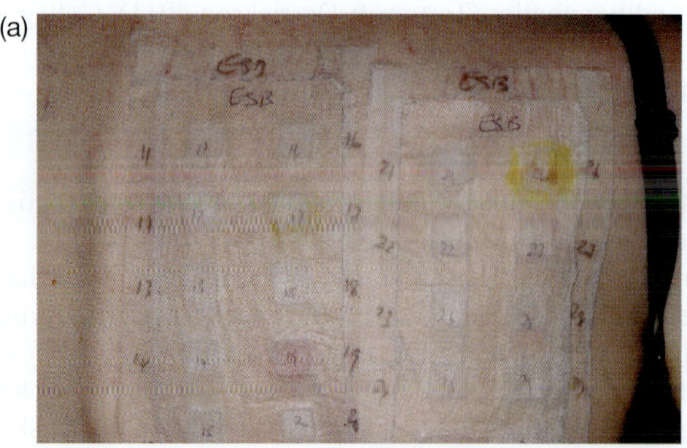

(b)

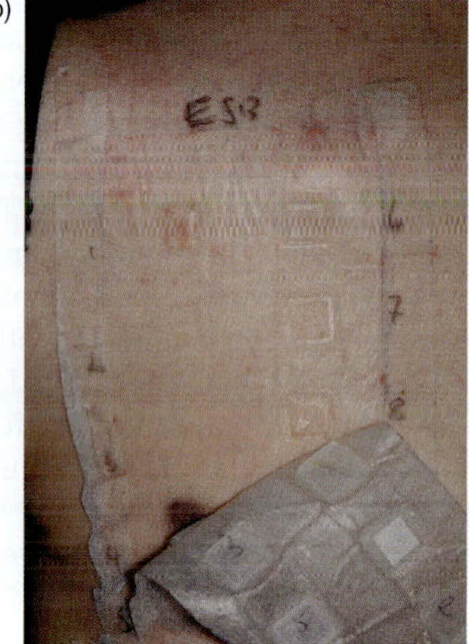

(c)

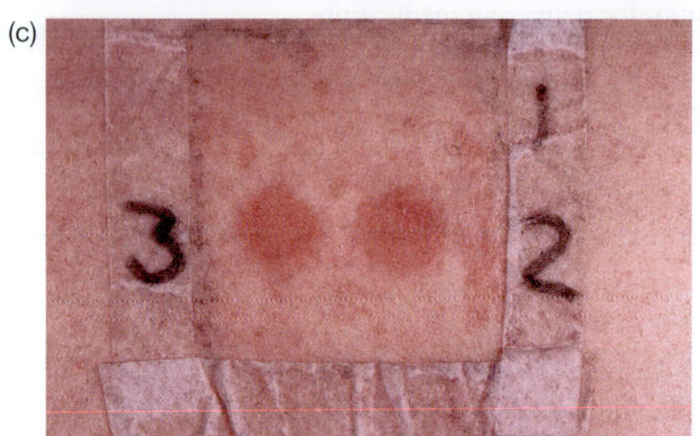

Source: Morris-Jones (2019) *ABC of Dermatology*. 7th ed., Wiley Blackwell.

12.3 Skin assessment

LEARNING OBJECTIVE 12.3 Discuss the key components in skin assessment of patients with altered skin integrity.

As with any other systems' assessment, physical examination and patient history are also important in skin assessment. Skin lesions may be the first indicator of an underlying disease (Morris-Jones 2019). For example, blistering of the elbow may be the initial presentation for a patient with underlying coeliac disease. Genetics, occupation, recent travel, environment and social habits should all be factored in when collecting history. Hence, it is important to take a thorough history, ask about any other symptoms and examine the entire patient as part of skin assessment.

The following points must be included when collecting history:

- *demographic information* — age, gender, ethnicity, marital status, occupation, education and religion
- use of the 'OLD CARTS' mnemonic to note the onset, location, duration, characteristics, associated symptoms, relieving factors, timing and severity of the condition
- *past medical history* — skin cancer or other disorders, allergies to medications, food, pollens
- *family history* — skin cancer, psoriasis, autoimmune diseases or any disorder similar to presenting skin problem
- *the patient's social history* — alcohol, tobacco, recreational drugs, diet, exercise, exposure to toxins and sun, tanning bed use, hobbies and sexual habits
- *travel* — any domestic and international travel in the past year
- *the patient's occupation* — this may relate to contact dermatitis
- *children* — notification about any communicable disease condition from school or child care centre
- *the skin care routine usually followed* — hygiene, the use of soaps, oils and home remedies, and sunscreen
- *hair and nail care* — when assessing the hair, note the texture, colour, brittleness, hair loss and presence of parasites; when assessing the nails, note the length, colour, symmetry, thickness and hygiene, as well as deformities, pitting and splinter haemorrhages.

Physical examination

The room should be warm and bright, and have fluorescent lighting to determine changes in the skin. A flexible metric ruler, a small torch and a magnifying glass should be available.

The initial assessment before a head-to-toe assessment is as follows.

- Scan the skin tone looking for changes such as pallor, jaundice, cyanosis or flushing.
- Feel for any variations in skin temperature and or increased sweating.
- Pinch the skin over the dorsal hand or forearm and quickly release it to check the turgor and elasticity. Normal skin should quickly return to its normal shape.

A head-to-toe skin assessment should follow after the initial assessment and includes the following areas.

- *Head, face and neck.* Look at the hair's texture, the pattern of hair loss, and include a visual inspection of the scalp by parting hair at regular intervals. Inspect the face and neck for sun damage (Soutor 2017).
- *Hands.* Examine all surfaces, including web spaces. Observe nail bed for any colour change.
- *Chest, abdomen and inguinal area.* In females, breast tissue must be lifted to check the skin underneath. Axilla should be examined as part of skin assessment of chest. For obese patients, skin fold must be lifted and spread for proper skin assessment. Fungal infection can commonly occur in inguinal areas.
- *Legs and feet.* Knees and popliteal surface are common areas for the involvement of psoriasis and atopic dermatitis. The legs' arterial and medial surfaces are common sites for melanoma in women (Soutor 2017). Check toe webs as they are common sites for fungal infections.
- *Back and perianal area.* Ask the client to lie face down or sidewise to examine the back, gluteal cleft and perianal area.

The head-to-toe examination should include checking the skin for colour, texture, temperature, moisture, erythema (redness), integrity, sensation, lesions, tattoos and needle track marks. The following terminologies are commonly used to document skin colour changes.

- *Erythema.* Intense red colour of the skin due to excess blood in the dilated superficial capillaries.
- *Pallor.* Whitish skin colour due to the loss of red-pink tone from oxygenated haemoglobin exposing the colour of collagen.
- *Cyanosis.* Bluish mottled colour due to inadequate supply of oxygenated blood.
- *Jaundice.* Yellow discolouration due to elevated bilirubin (Jarvis 2019).

If lesions are found, it is important to record their size, shape, location and distribution. Distribution of lesions is documented using terminologies such as generalised, localised, grouped, asymmetrical (unilateral distribution), discrete (separate), etc. (Jarvis 2019). Note other features such as itching, burning, scaling or blisters, whether the lesions are raised (papular) or flat (macular), ulcerated or pigmented, and whether the edges of the lesions are well defined (Brown 2019). Any association with blood vessels and any odour should also be noted. Observation of the lesions for plaques, crusts, scabs, wheals, bullae, pustules, cysts or vesicles should also occur. Swabs can be taken over exuding areas and sent for culture and sensitivity to treat local infections.

An additional video resource for dermatology examination can be accessed here: www.youtube.com/watch?v=qI4E9JDs2Tw.

12.4 Management of common dermatological disorders

LEARNING OBJECTIVE 12.4 Explain the management of commonly encountered dermatological disorders.

Dermatitis

It is a common term used for inflammation of the skin due to an overreaction of the immune system's non-specific defences. Inflamed, dry, occasionally scaly and vesicular skin rashes are the main characteristics of dermatitis (see figure 12.3). Atopic dermatitis, allergic dermatitis, irritant dermatitis and photodermatitis are some of the common forms of dermatitis (see figure 12.4). Allergic, irritant and photodermatitis come under contact dermatitis. Some of the characteristics of allergic contact dermatitis include previous exposure to the substance, delay of 48 to 86 hours between contact and development of skin changes, activation of previously sensitised sites by contact with an allergen at a distant skin site and persistence of allergy for many years (Morris-Jones 2019). Common allergens include fragrances, **topical** antibiotics, hair dye, latex, etc.

FIGURE 12.3 Contact dermatitis to iodine

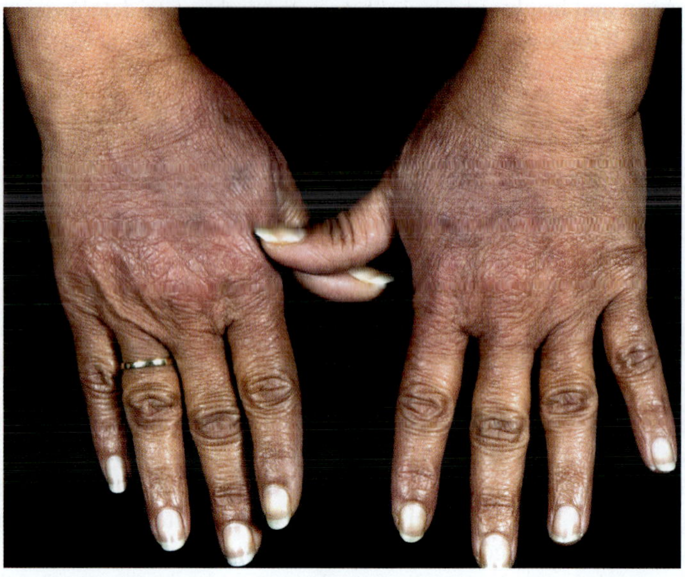

Source: Morris-Jones (2019). *ABC of Dermatology*. 7th ed., Wiley Blackwell.

FIGURE 12.4 The inflammatory pathways of atopic and contact dermatitis

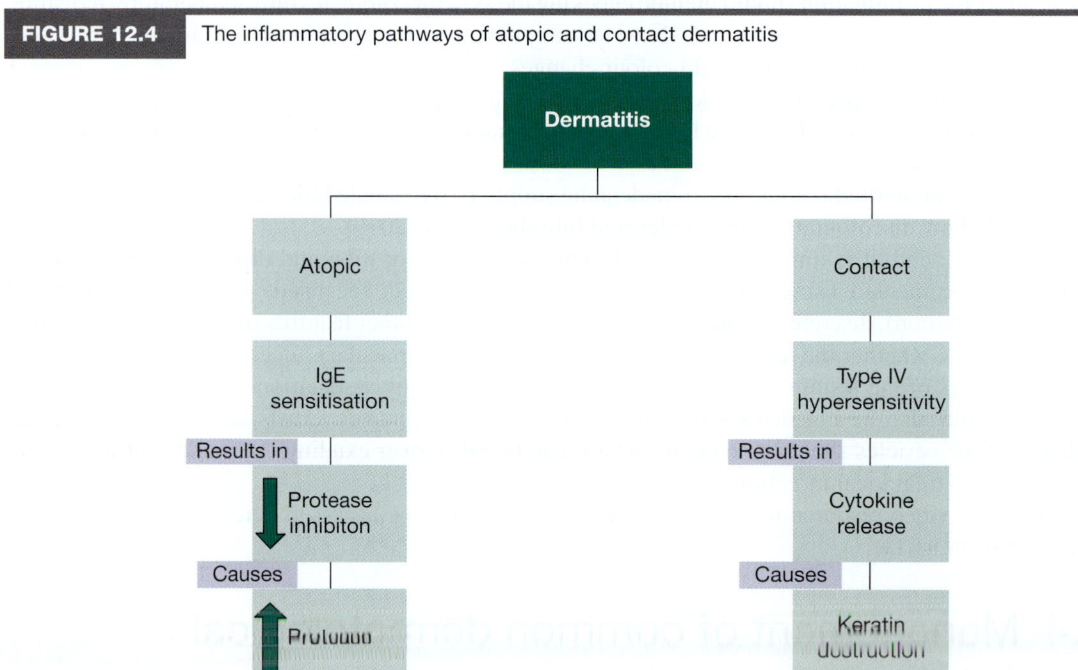

Source: Adapted from Bullock & Hales (2019) *Principles of Pathophysiology*. 2nd Ed. Melbourne: Pearson Education Australia.

Irritant dermatitis can develop immediately or following multiple exposures to the skin over time. The dermis and epidermis are damaged by the denaturing of keratin along with the release of cytokines (Bullock & Hales 2019). This damage depends on the strength of the irritant, duration of exposure and contact location. Photodermatitis is when there is a reaction on the skin as a result of interaction between ultraviolet radiation and substances that have been applied to the skin.

Atopic dermatitis is a chronic inflammatory skin condition with intermittent acute episodes or 'flare-ups' (Bullock & Hales 2019). **Pruritis**, eczematous skin lesions and dry skin are the main characteristics of atopic dermatitis. It commonly occurs in children under five years of age. Relapse can occur in adolescence. Family history of asthma and hay fever are risk factors for developing atopic dermatitis.

Pathophysiology

Atopic dermatitis is an inflammatory skin disease with multifactorial pathophysiology involving alterations in cell-mediated immune response, IgE mediated hypersensitivity and environmental factors. Cleaning products that raise skin pH can cause increased endogenous proteases (Bullock & Hales 2019), leading to a disruption of the dermal barrier. Certain bacteria such as *Staphylococcus aureus* and dust mites can produce exogenous proteases. An overproduction of IgE and cytokines contribute to the inflammatory cascade of erythema, pruritis and oedema. Filaggrin is a key protein essential for the normal skin barrier. Mutation to this protein is seen in patients with atopic dermatitis. Loss of filaggrin results in poorly formed stratum corneum, increasing water loss and resulting in pruritis. There is no specific pathology test to diagnose atopic dermatitis. Cutaneous manifestation includes erythematous scaly lesions over the scalp, cheeks, peripheries and trunk with pruritis (figure 12.5).

FIGURE 12.5 Facial atopic dermatitis

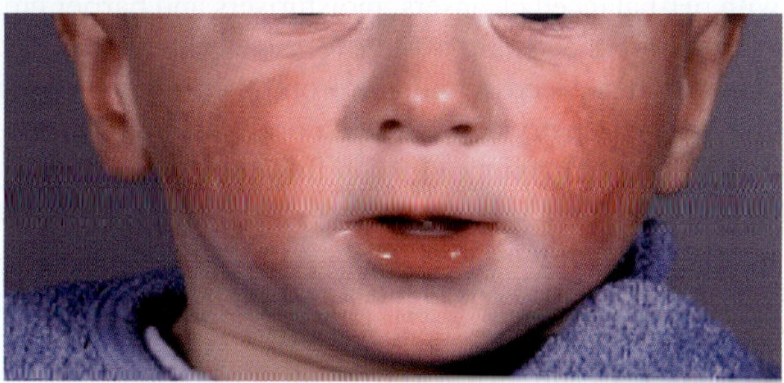

Source: Morris-Jones (2019). *ABC of Dermatology*. 7th ed., Wiley Blackwell.

An additional video resource on atopic dermatitis can be viewed here: www.youtube.com/watch?v=46ebVEAvs9o

Treatment for dermatitis

Emollients

Emollients (moisturising creams/lotions) help reduce itching and restore the skin's barrier function (Morris-Jones 2019). They should be applied after bathing and repeated two to three times throughout the day to restore and preserve the stratum corneum barrier. Lotions with a high water content may not be suitable because of drying due to evaporation (Simpson et al. 2019). Thicker emollients with high lipid content can be more effective. However, these are not well tolerated in some people as they can interfere with the function of sweat ducts, causing itching. It is not recommended to use pure oil products, such as coconut oil, as they can dry the skin and increase transepidermal water loss (Wollenberg et al. 2018). Propylene glycol should not be used in children younger than two years of age due to its toxicity.

Topical anti-inflammatory agents

Topical glucocorticosteroids are first-line anti-inflammatory treatment of choice (Wollenberg et al. 2018). Ultrahigh-potency glucocorticoids should be used daily or twice daily for short periods (usually for two weeks) due to their potential side effects (Simpson et al. 2019).

Mid-potency glucocorticoids can be used for longer periods to treat chronic atopic dermatitis. Prolonged daily use of topical corticosteroids can cause steroid withdrawal symptoms on discontinuation. Severe erythema, swelling and burning are some of the characteristics of this symptom. Topical corticosteroids can cause adrenal suppression in infants and young children (Simpson et al. 2019).

Topical calcineurin inhibitors

Treatment using topical calcineurin inhibitors has been effective in managing atopic dermatitis. Proactive tacrolimus ointment therapy has been used for up to one year in reducing the number of flare-ups in both children and adults (Wollenberg et al. 2018).

Phototherapy

Phototherapy involves treating the affected area by exposing it to non-ionising radiation. This involves the delivery of distinct wavelengths of ultraviolet radiation to skin lesions. Equipment must be checked and safety standards maintained when delivering phototherapy. Photoadaptation may be decreased in the elderly secondary to decreased epidermal turnover, melanocyte number and tanning response (Jaleel, Pollack & Elmets 2019). It is important to initiate phototherapy at a lower dose and increase slowly to avoid phototoxic events in elderly. Phototherapy should be avoided in patients who have had arsenic exposure. Patients should be supported with lifestyle modification to avoid trigger factors.

Nursing management of dermatitis

Some patients require hospitalisation and systemic medications for the treatment of atopic dermatitis. Family support may need to be organised for parents of kids with atopic dermatitis who need long term management.

Management can occur in different settings (primary, secondary, etc.) depending on the severity of the condition. Disease assessment, structured education and emotional support must be addressed in nurse–patient consultation. Identification and avoidance of triggers (food, environment, occupation) are essential for effective management. Hence, a thorough history is essential (refer to the section at the beginning of the chapter for history taking). The skin should be assessed at least daily. Skin cleansing should be carried out at frequent intervals with pH-balanced cleansers, moisturisers and barrier creams to aid skin integrity. Care should be taken when washing the skin to avoid excessive rubbing and when repositioning patients to avoid shearing and friction. Hygiene needs should be promptly attended to if incontinence is present — extremes of temperature that may cause drying of the skin or excessive moisture should be avoided.

Penetration of topical medication is maximised when the stratum corneum is soft. Soaking hydration during a shower softens the stratum corneum layer; hence, it is ideal to use topical applications immediately after bathing. Rehydrate skin using emollients to restore skin barrier and avoid breakdown. In some cases, patients should be taught self-administration of subcutaneous injections and wet wrap technique. Wet wrap therapy is used in some patients to apply emollients or topical corticosteroids, which are then covered by a layer of wet bandages and then further by a layer of dry clothing. Individualised information on self-management should be provided to promote active participation and shared decision making.

Incontinence-associated dermatitis

Incontinence-associated dermatitis is an inflammatory skin condition characterised by erythema and exudation that predominantly affects the perineum, gluteal region, lower abdomen and thigh.

Nursing management of incontinence-associated dermatitis

Routine skin assessment is essential in the management of incontinence-associated dermatitis. Skin cleansing must be performed using warm, clean water or no-rinse liquid skin cleanser with a pH similar to normal skin after each defecation (Yates 2018). Disposable non-woven towels or alcohol-free wet tissue should be used for cleaning. Care should be taken to avoid aggressive cleansing technique using regular wash clothes as it can increase the frictional force and abrade the skin. Incontinence pads should be changed before getting saturated. Skincare should be performed with each change by gently cleaning the perineal area, moisturisation and application of skin protectant cream. If absorbent pads are used, talc, ointments that are petroleum-based or creams that are thick should be avoided as they can interfere with the pad's absorbency. Depending on the cognitive ability of the patient, bladder control education should be provided. Containment devices (condom catheter, flexiseal) could be used to avoid maceration of skin from urine or faeces. Reversible causes of incontinence such urinary tract infection should be treated promptly. Some medications can increase incontinence frequency and should be substituted if appropriate. It is also important to maintain the nutritional status of the patient. Pain is usually associated with skin damage, and appropriate analgesics should be administered prior to cleaning the skin if possible.

Moisture-associated skin damage

Moisture-associated skin damage (MASD) refers to a spectrum of skin damage resulting from frequent exposure to moisture such as sweat, urine, saliva, etc. (Voegeli 2019). Identifying the moisture source, such as disease conditions causing incontinence, excessive perspiration or body fluid loss over the skin surface, is the first step in managing MASD. Different forms of MASD are given codes in the 11th revision of the *International Statistical Classification of Diseases and Related Health Problems (ICD-11)* (Voegeli 2019) and include intertriginous dermatitis, periwound moisture-associated dermatitis, peristomal moisture-associated dermatitis and incontinence-associated dermatitis.

Inflammation of the skin because of skin on skin friction due to moisture trapped in skin folds is termed **intertrigo** or intertriginous dermatitis. Predisposing factors in adults include obesity, hyperhidrosis, diabetes mellitus, urinary and/or faecal incontinence, poor hygiene and immunocompromised conditions. Babies and infants can develop intertrigo in the neck folds because of their short neck, flexed postures and drooling. Restrictive clothing and tightfitting shoes can also cause intertrigo.

Erythema and maceration of peristomal skin due to prolonged exposure to output from a stoma is termed as peristomal MASD (Burch 2019).

Nursing management of MASD

Patient education on caring for skin folds and keeping them clean and dry is the first step in preventing intertrigo. Advice should be given on managing predisposing factors such as obesity and diabetes mellitus. Loose, light clothing made from absorbent natural fabric is ideal for preventing intertrigo. A pH-balanced cleanser should be used for cleaning the skin, and alkaline soaps should be avoided if possible. An alternate option is to use emollient based soap substitutes (Metin et al. 2018). Skin barrier products can be used to protect the skin from moisture and reduce friction. Intertrigo must be adequately managed to prevent the development of secondary infection. Topical antibacterial or antifungal preparations should be used if there is a secondary infection. Application of moisture wicking textiles on skin folds are used in some countries. These textiles wick moisture away, allowing it to evaporate, keeping the skin fold dry — some contain broad spectrum antimicrobial silver (Voegeli 2019).

People with ileostomy, colostomy and urostomy have stomal bags to collect the exudate. Wear time of stoma bags is important in preventing skin damage. In general, the stoma bag should be changed between once a day and three times a week (Burch 2019). This depends on the stomal output as well as the product used. Output from the stoma can damage the skin if the collection bag is left for too long. Hence, it is important to empty the bag and or change the bag appropriately. For some products, it is only necessary to change the bags while the base plates remain attached to the skin for several days. The aperture of the base plate should be an appropriate size to cover the stoma. A bigger aperture may expose unnecessary peristomal skin to the corrosive output, causing skin damage. It would be useful to use filler paste or seals if the stoma output is in contact with skin because of skin creases (Burch 2019).

If the source of moisture is from a wound, dressings should be carefully chosen for maximum absorption of the leakage. Dressings should be checked frequently and changed before getting saturated. Use skin barrier ointment or paste to protect periwound skin. Wound care is described in detail later in this chapter.

Psoriasis

Psoriasis is a common chronic inflammatory skin condition resulting from complex interactions between genetic, environmental and immunological factors. There can be an early peak between ages 20 and 30 and a late peak between 50 and 60 of the incidence of psoriasis (Nicol 2015). Psoriasis increases the risk of painful arthritis and cardiovascular morbidity. Clinical presentation of psoriasis includes a well-demarcated, raised red plaque with a white scaly surface. Scalp, elbow, knees, hands, feet, trunk and nails are the most commonly affected sites (Gudjonsson & Elder 2019). Psoriasis lesions usually occur bilaterally. Pruritis is common in severe psoriasis, and most patients have a history of joint pain and swelling, especially in the fingers and toes (Zlotoff, Keck & Padilla 2017). Nail dystrophies associated with psoriasis include pitting, nail plate separation, yellow-orange discolouration and thickening. Inflammatory arthritis associated with psoriasis is known as psoriatic arthritis. Distal interphalangeal joints are most commonly affected, and the arthropathy is usually asymmetrical (Morris-Jones 2019).

Pathophysiology

Dysregulation of cell-mediated immune response is the primary cause of psoriasis (Zlotoff, Keck & Padilla 2017). The plaques present in psoriasis arise due to the hyperproliferation of epidermal cells, which leads to thickening of the skin as a result of trying to replace itself too quickly (see figure 12.6). The capillaries become dilated, and the white blood cells infiltrate the cells. This stimulates the T cells to release chemokines and cytokines, which cause keratinocyte hyperproliferation. Stressful life events, low humidity, human immunodeficiency virus, streptococcal pharyngitis, skin trauma, medications, cold and obesity can trigger the disease condition (Zlotoff, Keck & Padilla 2017). Beta-blockers, antimalarials and lithium can exacerbate psoriasis (Lyons & Ousley 2014). A punch biopsy may be considered if the diagnosis is unclear based on clinical findings, and uric acid serology is needed in some cases to differentiate psoriatic arthritis from gout.

FIGURE 12.6 Generalised plaques

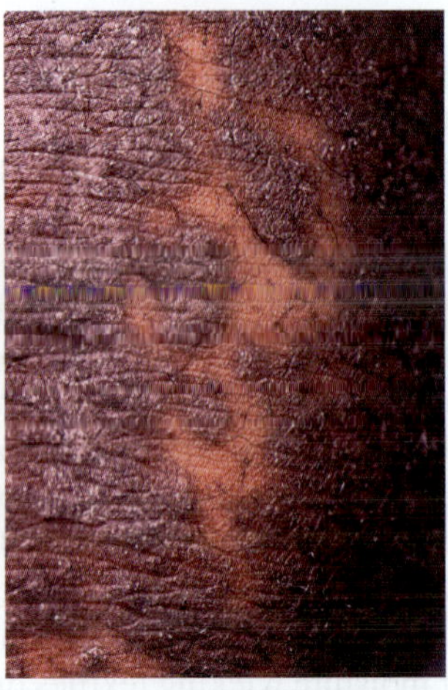

Source: Morris-Jones (2019). *ABC of Dermatology*.7th ed., Wiley Blackwell.

An additional video resource on psoriasis can be accessed here: www.youtube.com/watch?v=aYNgLQNpA6E.

Treatment of psoriasis

Treatment of psoriasis comprises topical preparations, phototherapy, photochemotherapy, and systemic therapy (tablets, S/C, IV). The first line of treatment for localised, stable plaques includes tar preparations, vitamin D, salicylic acid preparations and topical steroids. Mild to moderate potency topical steroids are used for facial psoriasis. Pustular psoriasis of hands and feet are treated with moderate potency topical steroids and propylene glycol. Inpatient management may be required for acute erythrodermic unstable generalised pustular psoriasis.

Nursing management of psoriasis

The psychosocial burden associated with psoriasis can affect a person's relationships, social activities and emotional wellbeing. To prevent social isolation and maintain psychosocial health, nurses should encourage the patient to engage in enjoyable activities, refer the patient to support groups, promote healthy eating and exercise. Patient education on self-management of the condition is also important and should focus on identifying and avoiding triggers, adhering to treatment regimens and appropriate skincare. Nurses should also discuss follow-up visits. Patients on systemic medications should have frequent follow-ups with lab investigations every three to six months. Patients should be educated on signs and symptoms of psoriatic arthritis so treatment can be initiated early. Patients should also be advised to seek medical care if there are signs of infections such as pus, fever or increased pain. Smoking is associated with the increased severity of psoriasis; hence, patients should be educated on smoking cessation and referred to a support group if needed.

Acne

Acne is an inflammatory disease of the pilosebaceous follicles commonly affecting adolescents (Rocha & Bagatin 2018). Acne pathophysiology is multifactorial — immune-mediated and androgen triggered (Rocha & Bagatin 2018). There is an increase in sebum production, a blockage of the follicles, inflammation and altered shedding of the skin's outer layers. Androgenic hormones are mainly responsible for the increase in production of sebum. Thickening of the keratin lining and subsequent obstruction of the sebaceous duct results in closed comedones (whiteheads) or open comedones (blackheads) (Morris-Jones 2019). Some conditions such as polycystic ovarian syndrome (PCOS), virilising tumours, congenital adrenal hyperplasia and Cushing's syndrome can contribute to acne. Medications such as oral contraceptives, phenytoin, barbiturates, isoniazid, lithium, and topical and systemic steroids can also cause acne. Stress induces inflammation in the pilosebaceous unit also results in acne (Morris-Jones 2019).

Acne can range from mild to severe. In mild acne, there are no inflammatory lesions and scarring is unlikely. Severe acne, however, involves pustules on the face, back and underarms, and scarring is highly likely.

Nursing management of acne

A key concern in the treatment of acne is to lessen the disease's duration and severity, reducing the risk of scarring and enhancing the individual's psychosocial welfare. Both topical and systemic therapies are used, such as antibiotics, anti-inflammatory agents and hormonal therapies. Other treatments include laser therapy and chemical peels. Topical retinoid, azelaic and salicylic acid are used as first-line treatments (Morris-Jones 2019). Topical preparations should be chosen carefully depending on skin type. For dry, sensitive skin, creams are ideal. Solutions or gels are suitable for oily skin, and lotions are well tolerated in hair-bearing sites.

Bullous pemphigoid

Bullous pemphigoid is an autoimmune disorder characterised by blistering and most often affects the elderly. The appearance of blisters may be preceded by pruritic urticaria or oedematous lesions for months. The lesions are commonly seen over the lower abdomen (figure 12.7), groin and flexor surface of the extremities (Yates 2018). **Biopsy** and direct immunofluorescence examination are used for diagnosis.

FIGURE 12.7 Immunobullous and other blistering disorders

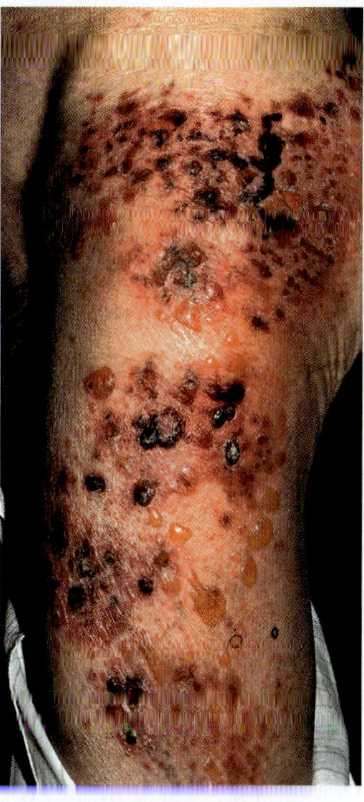

Source: Morris-Jones (2019). *ABC of Dermatology*. 7th ed., Wiley Blackwell.

Nursing management of bullous pemphigoid

For mild conditions, an ultrapotent topical corticosteroid may be adequate. Systemic steroid therapy may be required in widespread conditions (Papadakis, McPhee & Bernstein 2020). Other treatments include methotrexate, cyclophosphamide, mycophenolate mofetil and rituximab (Morris-Jones 2019). Patients should be educated to enhance their ability to live with the condition. It is important to stress that this is not a contagious condition.

Skin cancer

Australia has one the highest skin cancer rates in the world. An imbalance in cell homeostasis and excessive cell proliferation resulting from cancer-associated gene mutations, such as skin proto-oncogenes and tumour suppressors within the skin cells, are responsible for causing skin cancer (Sajadimajd et al. 2020). Cutaneous melanoma and non-melanoma are the main classes of skin cancer based on cell type.

Non-melanoma can be further classified into basal cell carcinoma and squamous cell carcinoma. The head and neck are the common sites for basal cell carcinomas (Bullock & Hales 2018). Basal cells grow upwards and outwards, and it is unusual for basal cell carcinomas to metastasise. Surgical excision is the most appropriate treatment for basal cell carcinomas. Squamous cell carcinomas are associated with an increased risk of malignancy. The most common area for squamous cell carcinoma is the face, especially the lips, ears, nose, cheek, eyelids, and can spread to lymphatic nodes. They appear as erythematous papules in the beginning and may have a degree of hyperkeratosis. These lesions may ulcerate, bleed and cause discomfort after a period. Surgical excision remains the primary mode of treatment. Radiotherapy may be needed for persistent or recurrent squamous cell carcinomas.

Melanoma

Melanoma is the most dangerous and aggressive form of cancer. It is an invasive malignant type of cancer affecting the melanocytes. The highest melanoma incidence is found in Australia and New Zealand (Curti, Leachman & Urba 2018). Sun exposure and genetics are the most important risk factors for melanoma. The DNA damaging, carcinogenic, inflammatory and immunosuppressive properties of ultraviolet (UV) radiation contribute to the initiation, progression and metastasis of primary melanoma. The pathogenesis of different melanoma types depends on the type and amount of UV radiation exposure, genetic makeup and oncogene mutations in each individual. Risk factors for melanoma include unprotected sun exposure, history of childhood tanning and sunburn, short, intense periods of exposure to UV radiation, increased number of unusual moles, depressed immune systems, family history of melanoma in a first-degree relative, fair skin, a tendency to burn rather than tan, freckles, light eye colour, light or red hair colour and previous melanoma or non-melanoma skin cancer (Cancer Council 2021). An additional video resource showing melanoma animation can be viewed here: www.youtube.com/watch?v=1vJSsJdSosU.

Superficial spreading melanoma is the type of skin cancer where melanoma cells spread superficially in the epidermis and become invasive after months or years. Commonly affected areas include the back for men and legs for women. Nodular melanoma presents as a dark nodule from the start and is in a vertical growth phase (figures 12.8 and 12.9). Hence the prognosis is poor. This is more common in men than in women, usually in their 50s and 60s. Acral melanoma occurs on the palms, soles and near or under the nails (figure 12.10).

Diagnostics

Skin examination under optimal lighting should be performed for the early diagnosis of melanoma. ABCDE is a well-known acronym used in melanoma detection.

- A = asymmetry (one half not identical to the other half)
- B = border (irregular, notched or poorly defined border as opposed to smooth straight edges)
- C = colour (varying shades from one area to another)
- D = diameter (greater than 5 mm)
- E = evolution (changes in the lesion over time).

Additional video resource for ABCDE assessment for melanoma can be seen here: www.youtube.com/watch?v=pmfPDt7GnW8 (RegisteredNurseRN.com, 15 July 2019).

Other diagnostic tools used in the diagnosis of melanoma include:

- contact dermoscopy: the lesion is examined through a film of liquid using non-polarised light
- noncontact dermoscopy: the lesion is examined under polarised light without a contact medium
- sequential digital dermoscopy: the lesion is captured by successive dermoscopic images, separated by an interval of time to detect suspicious change (helps to improve early detection of melanoma)
- biopsy (incisional, punch or shaved) sent for histological examination
- blood investigation for tumour makers
- regional skin and lymph node ultrasound to detect nodal metastases
- CT scan of the chest, abdomen and pelvis if distance spread is suspected.

Treatment of skin cancer

Surgical removal of melanoma with at least one to two centimetres of normal skin around the site is required to treat early-stage melanoma. Draining lymph nodes may also need to be removed.

For advanced melanoma, where it has spread to lymph nodes, internal organs or bones, management involves surgery, radiation therapy, targeted therapy and immunotherapy. Targeted therapy drugs attack specific genetic mutations that allow melanomas to grow and spread while minimising harm to healthy cells. Immunotherapy stimulates the body's immune system. Ipilimumab, nivolumab and pembrolizumab are some of the commonly used immunotherapy drugs for treating advanced melanoma.

FIGURE 12.8 Melanoma with a pale area of regression around it

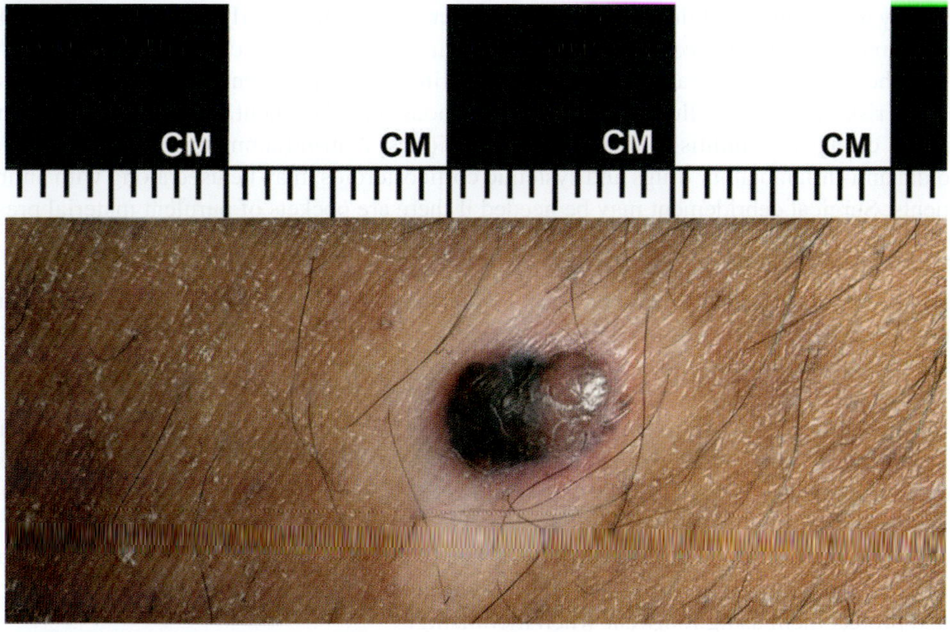

Source: Morris-Jones (2019). *ABC of Dermatology*. 7th ed., Wiley Blackwell.

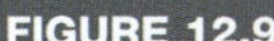

FIGURE 12.9 Nodular melanoma

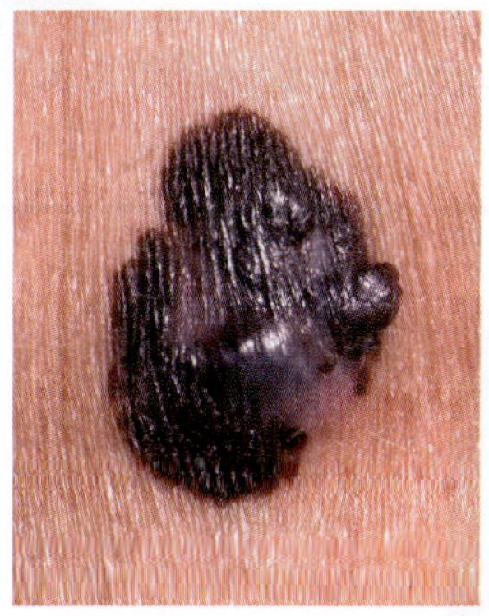

Source: Morris-Jones (2019). *ABC of Dermatology*. 7th ed., Wiley Blackwell.

FIGURE 12.10 Acral melanoma

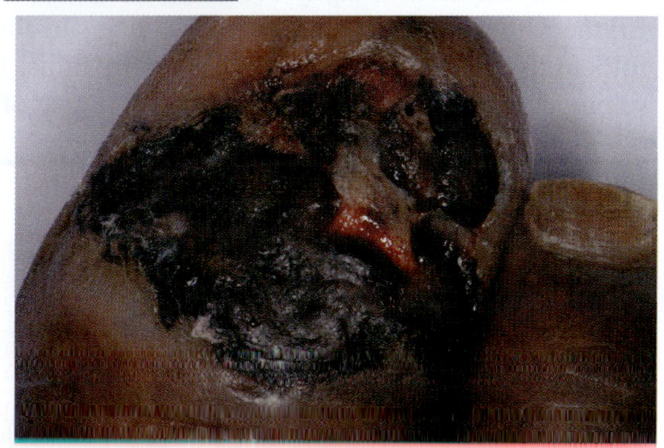

Source: Morris-Jones (2019). *ABC of Dermatology*. 7th ed., Wiley Blackwell.

12.5 Skin infections

LEARNING OBJECTIVE 12.5 Demonstrate an understanding of the pathophysiology and management of skin infections.

Any break in the continuity of the skin will provide organisms with a portal for entry. Infection will develop depending on the immune status of the patient and the virulence of the organism. Infections in the skin can range from mild to severe and may be caused by fungi, bacteria or viruses.

Cellulitis

Cellulitis is an infection of the subcutaneous tissue commonly caused by bacteria (Pearson & Margolis 2019). Symptoms include inflammation, swelling, pain and redness over the affected skin. Systemic signs include high temperature, general malaise and regional adenopathy. Lower extremities are the most commonly affected sites in adults. In the majority of cases, cellulitis presents unilaterally. It typically occurs near surgical wounds and cutaneous ulcers. Sepsis is suspected if there is haemodynamic instability associated with cellulitis and treatment should start immediately. *Staphylococcus aureus* and *Streptococcus pyogenes* are the most common bacteria causing cellulitis (Pearson & Margolis 2019). Atypical organisms are more likely to be found in children, immunocompromised and the elderly (Sutherland & Parent 2017).

It is important to treat predisposing factors such as lymphoedema, toe web infections, local skin barrier defects, peripheral vascular disease, etc., to prevent primary and recurrent cellulitis episodes. Some of the iatrogenic risk factors for cellulitis include intra venous line placement, surgical site intervention and post-radiation changes. Cellulitis is treated with antibiotics. Anti-inflammatory medications, including non-steroidal anti-inflammatory drugs and systemic corticosteroids, may be used along with antibiotics in some patients. Surgical debridement may be needed if there are pockets of purulent material present.

Nursing management of cellulitis

A thorough history of the patient should be taken and include time, site, the evolution of lesions, cutaneous symptoms such as burning and pruritis, precipitating factors, treatment (including self-treatment), occupation, hobbies, family history and close contact exposure to similar symptoms. Inspect the skin and mark the edges of the area affected. A swab specimen should be sent for investigation if there is an ulcer or skin tear present. A blood specimen is often sent to check C-reactive protein (CRP) level and white cell count. Skin scrapings and nail clippings are sent if a fungal infection is suspected. Antibiotics and analgesics may be prescribed. Keeping the affected extremity elevated may hasten recovery. Skincare should be attended by washing and applying emollients depending on the skin condition. A zinc paste bandage may be applied to sooth, prevent evaporation of topical medications and inhibit the accumulation of oedema (Sutherland & Parent 2017). For cellulitis on the lower extremities, advise the patient to keep the feet and toes clean and dry and protect them using footwear when mobilising.

Folliculitis

Folliculitis is the inflammation of hair follicles and can be caused by mechanical factors and bacterial or fungal infections. Staphylococcus aureus is the most common organism causing bacterial folliculitis. Erythematous, dome-shaped papules that surround the hair follicle, are the primary lesion seen in folliculitis (see figure 12.11). Diabetes mellitus, obesity, malnutrition, immunodeficiency and chronic staphylococcal infections are all risk factors for folliculitis.

FIGURE 12.11 Bacterial folliculitis

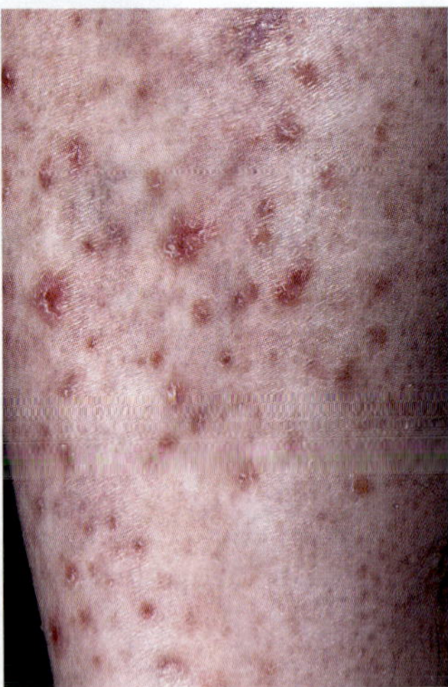

Source: Morris-Jones (2019). *ABC of Dermatology*. 7th ed., Wiley Blackwell.

Candidiasis

Candidiasis is a fungal infection caused by Candida species (most commonly, *Candida albicans*). Diabetes, obesity, pregnancy, HIV, use of broad-spectrum antibiotics, corticosteroids or immunosuppressive medications are considered risk factors for candidiasis (Ahronowitz & Leslie 2019). Oral candidiasis (thrush) presents with white patches over the tongue (see figure 12.12). Antifungal topical formulations such as clotrimazole, miconazole, nystatin are used for treating candidiasis.

FIGURE 12.12 *Candida albicans* stomatitis

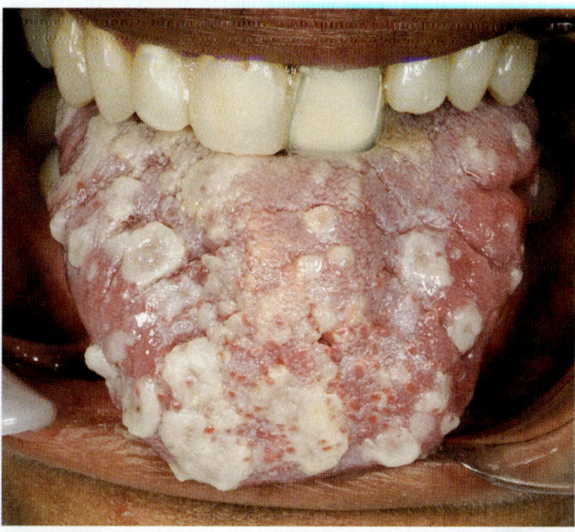

Source: Morris-Jones (2019). *ABC of Dermatology*. 7th ed., Wiley Blackwell.

Herpes zoster (shingles)

Herpes zoster or **shingles** is a viral rash that consists of macules and papules that develop into vesicular lesions (figure 12.13). Shingles is caused by the reactivation of *Varicella zoster* (the virus that causes chickenpox) in a dorsal root ganglion. Pain, fever and malaise may precede the rash in shingles (Morris-Jones 2019). The rash may take two to four weeks to heal.

Treatment with an antiviral agent can be used if the rash is diagnosed within the first 72 hours (Stein 2020). Soaks and topical antipruritics might be useful in managing the symptoms of shingles.

Scabies

Scabies is an infestation of the skin by mites called *Sarcoptes scabiei* (figures 12.14 and 12.15). Pruritis typically appears four to six weeks after initial infestation, and burrows can be seen in the affected areas. Excoriations and eczematous dermatitis are present commonly in interdigital webs, sides of fingers, elbows, axilla, scrotum, penis, labia and areola in women (Wheat, Burkhart, Burkhart & Cohen 2019). Elderly patients may have fewer cutaneous lesions but may have intense itching.

Diagnosis is made by microscopic identification of mites or eggs from skin scrapings. Crusted scabies is more severe and the load of mite infestation is much higher. It is characterised by hyperkeratotic plaques over the infested area. Scabies is highly contagious and is transmitted by person to person contact.

Treatment for scabies

First-line treatment is with 5 per cent permethrin cream applied from the neck downwards in adults and all over the skin in babies and infants (Morris-Jones 2019). The cream is left overnight and two applications at seven days interval is the minimal requirement. The second line of treatment is the application of 0.5 per cent malathion lotion. Ivermectin can be given to an immunocompromised patient and those with crusted scabies. Menthol cream is helpful in relieving pruritis associated with scabies.

Nursing management of scabies

Strict contact precaution using appropriate personal protective equipment should be practised while looking after infected scabies patient. Topical creams should be applied appropriately, ensuring sufficient coverage of the body surface. It should be thoroughly massaged into body crevices as well as under the fingernails. Keep the patient environment clean by vacuuming regularly due to the shedding of skin lesions. The patient's clothing and linen need to be washed in hot water and dried in hot driers. Close contacts with the patient should also be treated simultaneously. Visitors should be restricted to a minimum. Pruritis may persist for weeks after the treatment has finished. Nails should be kept short to avoid skin damage from scratching.

FIGURE 12.13 Herpes zoster in a dermatome

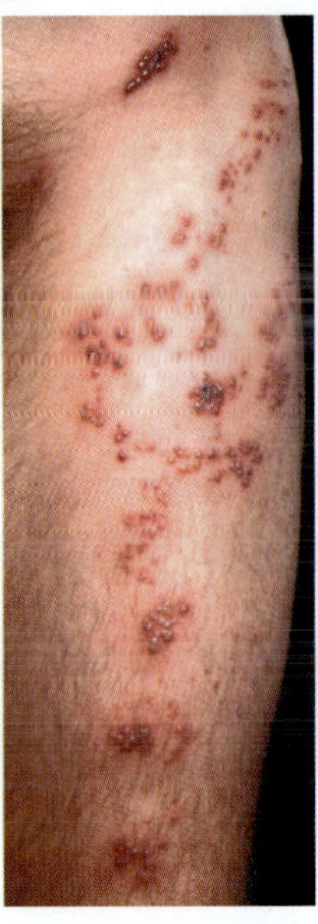

Source: Morris-Jones (2019). *ABC of Dermatology*. 7th ed., Wiley Blackwell.

FIGURE 12.14 Scabies nodules in a child

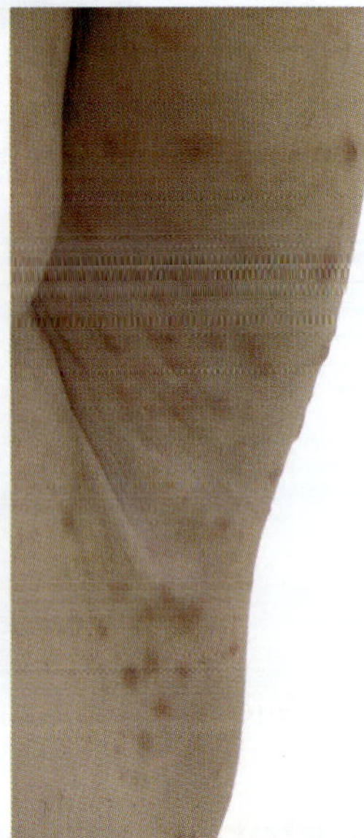

Source: Morris-Jones (2019). *ABC of Dermatology*. 7th ed., Wiley Blackwell.

FIGURE 12.15 Crusted scabies on buttocks

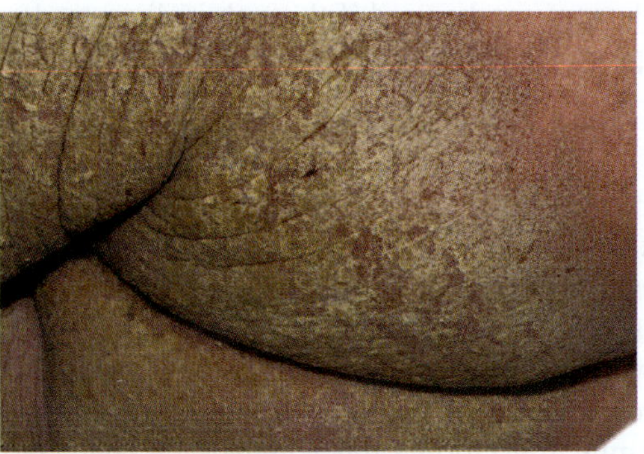

Source: Morris-Jones (2019). *ABC of Dermatology*. 7th ed., Wiley Blackwell.

12.6 Wound assessment and management

LEARNING OBJECTIVE 12.6 Conduct wound assessment and management.

A cut or break in the continuity of any tissue caused by injury or operation is called a wound (Morris-Jones 2019). This may consist of a tear, cut, erosion, puncture or ulcer where the skin's top layer is breached.

Assessment

Holistic patient assessment is essential to identify causative factors, plan interventions and design person-centred care (Mitchell 2020). To identify intrinsic and extrinsic factors that could impact wound healing, nurses need to interview the patient. This should include age, history and duration of the wound, past medical/surgical history, family history, allergies, skincare routines, dietary habits, socioeconomic circumstances, pain and medications.

It is necessary to do accurate and timely wound assessment for effective clinical decision making, type of product to be used, reducing morbidity and costs associated with wound care (Mitchell 2020). Anatomical location and dimensions of the wound should be documented along with the type of wound (skin tears, venous leg ulcers, pressure injuries, diabetic foot ulcers, etc.), colour of wound bed, wound edges, extent of tissue involvement (epidermis, dermis, fascia, muscle, bone, etc.), odour from wound, characteristics of exudates, pain and discomfort. Length, width and depth measured at the longest and deepest part of the wound should be included when recording wound dimension (Wound Australia 2016). It is also important to document any undermining edges or sinus tracking. Depending on the type of wound, risk assessment for **pressure injury**, falls, skin tear, etc., should also be included in ongoing wound management.

Wound edges and wound bed

Assessing the colour of the wound bed and wound edges can help to indicate the physiological processes occurring within the wound. A wound can be classified into different types based on the appearance of wound bed and surrounding tissues (see figure 12.16). **Necrotic** wounds consist of dead ischaemic tissue, which usually appears as black, brown or dark. Sloughy wounds appear mostly yellow due to the accumulation of cellular debris, fibrin, serous exudate, leucocytes and bacteria on the wound surface (Morris-Jones 2019). Slough is yellow or white in appearance and adheres firmly to the wound bed. Granulating wound appear as bright red in colour as a result of new blood vessel growth, connective tissue or dermal cells. Epithelialising wounds appear as pink translucent tissue in the wound as a result of epidermal regrowth. TIME is a popular acronym used in wound bed preparation, and stands for tissue (T), infection or inflammation (I), moisture (M) and edge (E).

FIGURE 12.16 Wound classifications

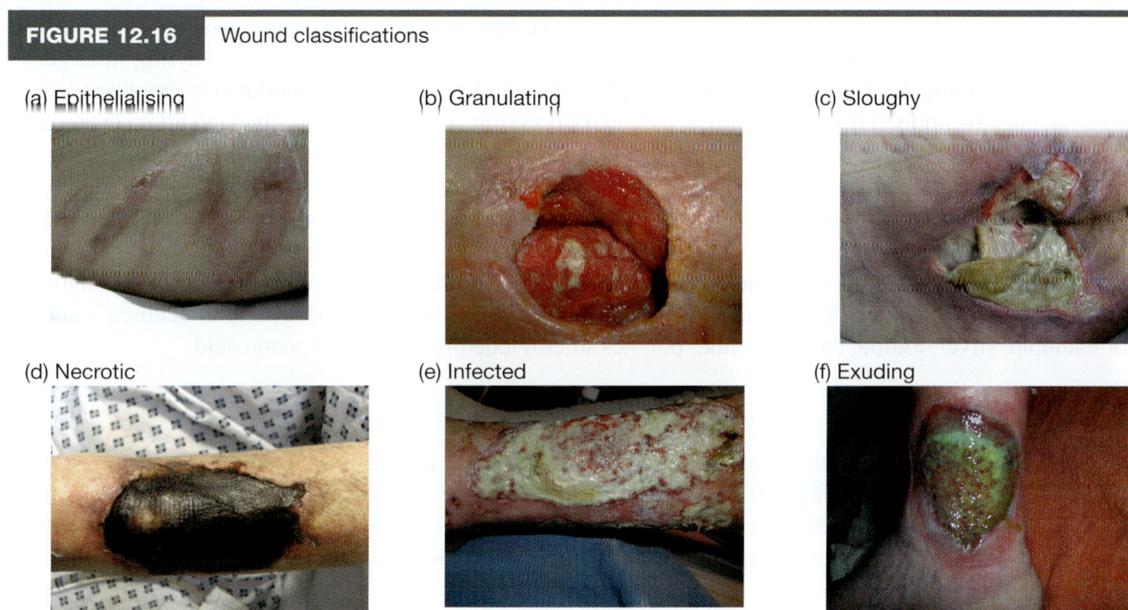

Source: Morris-Jones (2019). *ABC of Dermatology*. 7th ed., Wiley Blackwell.

Nature of wound drainage

An estimation of the nature and amount of wound fluid will help judge wound healing progression and enable the practitioner to make an appropriate wound dressing selection. The amount, colour and viscosity of the wound exudate should be recorded (Alavi & Kirsner 2019). Clear, straw-coloured exudate with thin watery consistency is described as serous. Serosanguinous exudate is clear, pink in colour with a slightly thicker consistency than water. Reddish thin exudates are described as **sanguineous** . Purulent exudates are viscous and sticky in consistency with opaque, milky, yellow or brown or sometimes green. Haemopurulent exudates are reddish, milky in colour and viscous. Both purulent and heamopurulent exudate suggest that the wound is infected. Fibrinous exudates are thin, watery and cloudy in colour. Haemorrhagic exudates are dark red and viscous (Mitchell 2020). Some dressings may affect the amount and type of fluid produced.

The presence of malodour of the wound is often a very distressing experience for the patient. The nature and severity of any malodour should be recorded as this may provide an indication of wound deterioration.

Pain and discomfort

Location, character, severity and duration of pain, including any exacerbating factors, should be recorded as part of initial and ongoing wound management using a validated pain assessment tool. The impact of pain on daily living and the effectiveness of treatments needs to be included in this assessment to develop a more effective management program.

Wound dressing

When wounds are kept moist, they have been shown to heal more rapidly, with a faster epithelialisation rate than when they are left to dry out. Some of the factors to be considered when selecting an ideal dressing for a wound are providing a moist environment for the wound bed, absorption of excess wound exudate, protecting against pathogenic invasion, maintaining constant wound interface temperature, reducing pain and promoting autolytic debridement. Depending on their composition and structure, modern dressings are either passive or interactive (Morris-Jones 2019). Passive dressings do not stick to the wound bed. They are generally used on small, lightly exuding superficial wounds. These dressings allow exudate to pass through to secondary dressing, maintain wound bed moisture, and reduce dressing change trauma. Some of the products include Melonin, Opsite, paraffin gauze, etc. Dressings that actively interact with the wound surface are called interactive dressing. Some of the products include hydrogels, hydrocolloids, alginate, etc. Hydrogel dressings consist of insoluble polymers, which can absorb excess fluid or produce a moist environment at the wound surface. These dressings need to be changed daily to every three days. Hydrocolloid dressings form a gel when it comes in contact with wound exudate, thereby promoting new blood vessels, rehydrating dry slough and necrosis. These dressings can be left in place for up to seven days. Both these dressing cannot be used on highly exuding wounds. **Alginate** consists of alginic acid extracted from brown seaweed (Morris-Jones 2019). Fibres in alginate dressing create hydrophilic gel in the presence of exudate. They have haemostatic properties and can be used on moderately exuding wound. Alginate must be applied dry and require a secondary dressing, and it should be changed after seven days. Negative pressure wound therapy is when negative pressure is applied to the wound bed using a foam dressing with tubing connected to a device.

The decision to use a topical antimicrobial agent should be based on assessing both the patient and the wound. The use of newer formulation topical antimicrobials, particularly silver- and iodine-containing products, is increasingly recommended as one component of managing wounds with a problematic or increased bacterial burden. Several antimicrobial choices are available if the wound is deemed suitable, for example, silver, iodine, chlorhexidine, polyhexamethylene biguanide and acetic acid.

Surgical wounds

According to Australian Institute of Health and Welfare data, one in four hospitalisations involved a surgical procedure in Australia in 2016–17. Surgical site infection is a serious post-operative complication resulting in significant morbidity, mortality and increased health-related costs. It is reported to be the third most commonly reported hospital-associated infection (Stryja, Riha & Szkatula 2020). Nurses have an important role in preventing surgical wound infections.

Surgical wounds may heal by primary intention, in which the edges are drawn together with sutures, staples or clips (Gillespie et al. 2020). Alternatively, the wound may be left open to heal by secondary intention, where the wound bed fills with granulation tissue to replace the tissue that has been lost. Wounds may also heal from a skin graft or tissue flap, depending on the amount of tissue loss.

Pressure ulcer or injury

Localised skin and tissue injury as a result of sustained pressure and or shear applied to the skin and underlying tissue results in pressure injury (EPUAP, NPIAP & PPPIA 2019). The most common locations in adults are the bony prominences over the hip and sacral regions and to a lesser extent in lower extremities especially the heels. Although it is uncommon, pressure injuries can occur in the neonate and paediatric population, and one of the common sites is the occiput. Pressure injuries remain a significant problem in hospitals and long-term care facilities.

Stages of pressure injury

According to the National Pressure Ulcer Advisory Panel Staging System, there are six stages of pressure injury. It is important to clean the wound bed for better visualisation before staging the pressure injury (Mervis & Phillips 2019).

- Stage 1: Non blanchable erythema with skin intact.
- Stage 2: Partial thickness skin loss with exposed dermis.
- Stage 3: Full-thickness skin loss. Adipose tissue is visible under the ulcer bed.
- Stage 4: Full-thickness skin and tissue loss. Fascia, muscle, tendon, ligament, cartilage or bone may be exposed (see figure 12.17).

- Unstageable pressure injury: Extent of tissue damage within the ulcer is obscured by slough or eschar and cannot be determined.
- Deep tissue pressure injury: Persistent, non-blanchable deep red, maroon or purple discolouration.

FIGURE 12.17 A stage 4 pressure ulcer

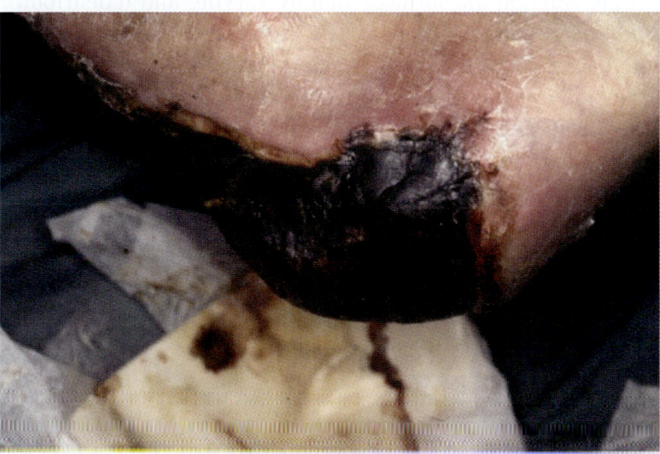

Source: Courtesy of Dr Zena Moore.

Pathophysiology

Sustained pressure, shear, friction and moisture are the main contributing factors for pressure injury development. Sustained pressure on the skin and subcutaneous tissue over the bone from the patient's own body weight or from an external medical device inhibits blood flow and causes tissue hypoxia (Mervis & Phillips 2019). Reperfusion injury occurs due to the return of blood after a period of ischaemia from the formation of increased reactive oxygen species and triggering an inflammatory response. The highest pressure is often experienced at the interface between bone and muscle. The effect of tissue hypoxia is initially greatest at the muscles, then the subcutaneous tissue and the skin. Hence, it is important to remember that extensive tissue damage at the deeper tissues would have already occurred when skin ulcer occurred. When lying at an incline, internal organs such as bones and muscles are displaced downwards due to gravity, while the skin remains immobile as it is in contact with the external surface. This shearing force can compress or distort the blood vessels between bones and skin surface, resulting in decreased blood flow and tissue hypoxia. Excess moisture can macerate the skin resulting in an increased risk of skin break down.

Nursing management of pressure wounds

Risk assessment using a standardised tool (e.g. Braden, Waterlow, Norton) is the first step in pressure injury prevention and management (Latimer, Chaboyer & Gillespie 2016). The purpose of these assessments is to identify some of the factors that could cause sustained pressure, friction and moisture. Patients with impaired mobility and sensation are more susceptible to pressure injuries as they either fail to sense the need to reposition or are not physically able to reposition themselves to avoid sustained external pressure to specific body parts over the bony prominences. Incontinent patient and excessive perspiration can lead to skin maceration due to moisture. External medical devices especially plaster casts, bandages and arm boards can all cause pressure injuries due to excessive pressure on skin surfaces. Nutritional status is important, as it influences collagen deposition and synthesis needed for tissue strength. Poor nutrition also leads to increased muscle wasting and soft tissue loss, increasing the prominence of bony points. Skin changes associated with ageing such as dermal and epidermal thinning, decreased epidermal turnover, loss of dermal papillae makes it more susceptible to shear forces causing pressure injuries. Braden scale assesses sensory perception, activity, mobility, nutrition, shear and friction to predict the risk of pressure injury development. Sex, age, continence, mobility, nutrition, body mass index and a visual assessment of the skin are aspects included in the Waterlow scale.

Repositioning is one of several key ways nurses can prevent pressure ulcers among those who cannot reposition themselves. Although the exact degree of tilt and frequency remain inconclusive, 30 degrees lateral tilt position with three hourly repositioning may help to reduce the incidence of pressure injuries over bony prominences (Chew, Thiara, Lopez & Shorey 2018). The use of pressure-relieving devices should be used when there is an increased risk of pressure injury.

Pressure redistributing support surfaces redistribute the mechanical load imposed on body parts and tissues and thereby reduce pressure damage (Serraes et al. 2018). A wide variety of support surfaces are currently available such as integrated bed systems, mattresses, overlays, cushions, etc. Air mattresses cyclically inflate and deflate cells on the surface, thereby varying and redistributing the pressure exerted by the surface on the body parts (Serraes et al. 2018). A pressure redistribution cushion should be used when the patient is sitting out of bed. Protective dressing (Mepilex) over the heels and sacrum has shown to reduce pressure injury incidence. It is also important to keep the skin clean and prevent maceration from moisture, especially in the incontinent. Barrier creams could be used to protect the skin from the damaging effects of moisture. Adequate nutrition is also important to maintain skin integrity. Hence, nurses should assess the patient's nutritional status by checking weight, food and fluid intake, and so on..

CASE STUDY 12.1

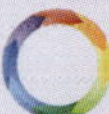

Nursing care of a child with atopic dermatitis

Helena is a 14-year-old girl who presented with pink scaly plaques on her cubital fossa and wrists of both arms and increasing pruritis and oedema to the upper extremities. Symptoms have worsened in the past two days preceding the visit. Her medical history was unremarkable. She has been using over the counter emollients over the plaques with not much effect. She denied any history of insect bites or injury to the limbs. She received treatment for atopic dermatitis at age three. Helena is not allergic to any medication or food. There was no report of communicable skin disease at the school.

Vital signs on presentation were:

- height: 142 cms
- weight: 52 kg
- temperature: 37.1°C
- heart rate: 106 beats per minute
- respiratory rate: 20 breaths per minute
- oxygen saturation: 98% on room air
- blood pressure: 110/70 mmHg.

On examination, the area over the upper limbs was warm and tender to touch. There was no open wound on the body. She has two younger siblings aged 11 and 5 and lives with her mother (single parent). There is a family history of asthma. Helena attends school regularly and plays basketball on Saturdays. A diagnosis of atopic dermatitis was made by a clinician.

Question

Using the information above, describe what action you would take as the nurse caring for this patient. Use the clinical reasoning cycle to guide you through the process and devise a care plan for your patient.

Answer

- *Step 1: Consider the patient*. Helena, 14-year-old schoolgirl.
- *Step 2: Collect cues/information*. Include subjective and objective data here, include the appearance of the patient and their past medical history. The patient has pink scaly plaques on both arms, pruritis, oedema to upper extremities, warm and tender upper limbs. Objective data will include measurable information such as vital signs.
- *Step 3: Process information*. Separate the relevant and irrelevant data — cluster the clues together to formulate an inference about the patient — scaly plaques, pruritis, oedema, tenderness and warmth to upper extremities associated with the skin condition. Tachycardia may be related to stress experienced from the condition.
- *Step 4: Identify problems/issues*. Nursing problems or diagnosis should be listed here. Helena's main problems are pruritis, oedema, tenderness and scaly plaques of upper extremities, tachycardia associated with stress and low self-esteem due to altered body image.
- *Step 5: Establish goals*. Goals of care for Helena should reduce pain, itchiness and oedema. The second goal is to reduce scaly plaques on the cubital fossa and wrist. Helena is 14 and may have concerns about body image due to the skin condition. Provide psychological support to alleviate fear and anxiety about the disease condition. Promote emotional wellbeing by alleviating concerns associated with altered body image.
- *Step 6: Take action*. Analgesics should be administered for pain relief, topical application of emollients and anti-inflammatory agents, patient education regarding the use of soap and skincare products, and a referral to the school nurse or school counselling service. Her mother may need support from a social worker.

- *Step 7: Evaluate outcomes*. Decreased oedema, tenderness and pruritis, minimal scaly plaques, normal heart rate, active participation in school activities and sports.
- *Step 8: Reflect on the process and new learning*. Reflect on any aspects of care that could have been performed to achieve an improved outcome.

CASE STUDY 12.2

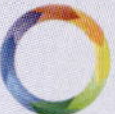

Nursing care of a male patient with severe itching

Gerald is a 29-year-old man who presents to the clinic with severe itching on his hands and feet. He does not have any known allergy and is not on any medications. On close examination, multiple burrows are visible on his hands and feet. Medical and surgical history is unremarkable. No family history of illnesses.

Vital signs on presentation were:

- height: 178 cms
- weight: 72 kg
- temperature: 36.8°C
- heart rate: 76 beats per minute
- respiratory rate: 16 breaths per minute
- oxygen saturation: 95% on room air
- blood pressure: 120/70 mmHg.

Gerald smokes four packets of cigarette a week and consumes around 12 glasses of whisky weekly. He has worked on a cattle farm for the past three years and lives with his wife and son in a cottage on the property. No other family member report itching.

Question

Using the information above, describe what action you would take as the nurse caring for this patient. Use the clinical reasoning cycle to guide you through the process and devise a care plan for your patient.

Answer

- *Step 1: Consider the patient*. Gerald, a 29-year-old farmer.
- *Step 2: Collect cues/information*. Include subjective and objective data here, include the appearance of the patient and their past medical history. Itching on hands and feet with multiple burrows, smoker, alcohol abuse. Objective data will include measurable information such as his vital signs.
- *Step 3: Process information.* Separate the relevant and irrelevant data — severe itching and multiple burrows in hands and feet, smoker, alcohol abuse.
- *Step 4: Identify problems/issues*. Nursing problems or diagnosis should be listed here. Pruritus is the main problem. Smoking and alcohol abuse is another issue and the potential for spreading the infection to family members.
- *Step 5: Establish goals*. Reduce pruritis by commencing treatment for scabies, prevent transmission to staff by maintaining contact precaution, prevent contamination of patient surrounding prevent transmission to family members, patient education about reducing consumption of alcohol and quit smoking.
- *Step 6: Take action*. Topical application of medications for scabies, regular cleaning of surface areas, linen and floors to avoid contamination from skin shedding, commence prophylactic scabies treatment for family members, refer to alcohol and other drugs services and smoking cessation services.
- *Step 7: Evaluate outcomes*. No itching, healthy skin with no burrows, no signs of scabies infection for family members, patient maintaining a healthy lifestyle with minimal consumption of alcohol and cigarettes.
- *Step 8: Reflect on the process and new learning*. Reflect on any aspects of care that could have been performed in a way to achieve an improved outcome.

SUMMARY

The skin is the largest organ in the body and provides the key functions of protection, heat regulation, absorption, sensation and storage. Due to the diverse nature, aetiology and variety of skin disorders encountered, assessment, diagnosis and management require a systematic, rigorous and holistic approach. The patient's history and lifestyle, and a physical examination, are the main factors in diagnosing and effectively managing skin conditions. Fundamental aspects of nursing management are ensuring patient dignity, warmth, comfort and effective management of symptoms including pain, skin irritation and exudates.

KEY TERMS

alginate Type of wound dressing.
atopic dermatitis Chronic inflammatory skin condition due to alteration in cell-mediated immune response, IgE-mediated hypersensitivity and environmental factors.
biopsy Tissue specimen for investigation.
bullous pemphigoid An autoimmune disorder characterised by blistering.
dermis Layer of the skin underneath epidermis.
emollients Type of topical application to moisturise skin.
epidermis First layer of the skin.
integumentary system Body system which involves, skin, hair, oil and sweat glands, nails and sensory receptors.
intertrigo Inflammatory skin disorder associated with friction and moisture.
melanoma Type of cancer affecting melanocytes.
necrotic Ischaemic dead tissue which is black, brown or dark.
perspiration Excretion of sweat through the skin surface.
phototherapy Treatment using ultraviolet rays.
pressure injury Localised skin and tissue injury as a result of sustained pressure and or friction.
pruritis Itching of the skin.
sanguineous Reddish coloured wound exudate that is thin in consistency.
scabies Hyperkeratotic skin lesion caused by mites.
shingles Skin lesion caused by Herpes zoster virus.
topical Over the skin.

REFERENCES

Ahronowitz, I. & Leslie, K. (2019) 'Yeast infections'. In S. Kang, M. Amagai, A. L. Bruckner, A. H. Enk, D. J. Margolis, A. J. McMichael & J. S. Orringer (Eds.). *Fitzpatrick's Dermatology*, 9th ed. New York, NY: McGraw-Hill Education.

Alavi, A. & Kirsner, R. S. (2019) 'Wound healing'. In S. Kang, M. Amagai, A. L. Bruckner, A. H. Enk, D. J. Margolis, A. J. McMichael & J. S. Orringer (Eds.). *Fitzpatrick's Dermatology*, 9th ed. New York, NY: McGraw Hill Education.

Beeckman, D., Serraes, B., Anrys, C., Van Tiggelen, H., Van Hecke, A. & Verhaeghe, S. (2019) A multicentre prospective randomised controlled clinical trial comparing the effectiveness and cost of a static air mattress and alternating air pressure mattress to prevent pressure ulcers in nursing home residents. *International Journal of Nursing Studies.* 97: 105–113.

Bohjanen, K. (2017) 'Structure and functions of the skin'. In C. Soutor & M. K. Hordinsky (Eds.). *Clinical Dermatology.* New York, NY: McGraw-Hill Education.

Bullock, S. & Hales, M. (2018) *Principles of Pathophysiology*, 2nd ed. Melbourne: Pearson Education Australia.

Brown, D. (2019) *Lewis's Medical-Surgical Nursing*, 5th ed. Australia: Elsevier.

Burch, J. (2019) Peristomal skin care considerations for community nurses. *British Journal of Community Nursing.* 24(9): 414–418.

Cancer Council. (2021) Melanoma. www.cancer.org.au/cancer-information/types-of-cancer/melanoma

Chew, J. H. -S., Thiara, E., Lopez, V. & Shorey, S. (2018) Turning frequency in adult bedridden patients to prevent hospital-acquired pressure ulcer: A scoping review. *International Wound Journal.* 15(2): 225–236.

Curti, B. D., Leachman, S. & Urba, W. J. (2018) 'Cancer of the skin'. In J. L. Jameson, A. S. Fauci, D. L. Kasper, S. L. Hauser, D. L. Longo & J. Loscalzo (Eds.). *Harrison's Principles of Internal Medicine*, 20th ed. New York, NY: McGraw-Hill Education.

European Pressure Ulcer Advisory Panel (EPUAP), National Pressure Injury Advisory Panel (NPIAP), & Pan Pacific Pressure Injury Alliance (PPPIA) (Eds.). (2019) *Prevention and treatment of pressure ulcers/injuries: clinical practice guidelines*, 3rd ed. EPUAP, NPIAP & PPPIA.

Gillespie, B. M., Walker, R., Lin, F., Roberts, S., Nieuwenhoven, P., Perry, J. & Chaboyer, W. (2020) Setting the surgical wound care agenda across two healthcare districts: A priority setting approach. *Collegian.* 27(5): 529–534.

Gudjonsson, J. E. & Elder, J. T. (2019) 'Psoriasis'. In S. Kang, M. Amagai, A. L. Bruckner, A. H. Enk, D. J. Margolis, A. J. McMichael & J. S. Orringer (Eds.). *Fitzpatrick's Dermatology*, 9th ed. New York, NY: McGraw-Hill Education.

Hsiu Hui, W., Chih-Ling, H., Wen-Pei, H. & Hsiu-Chin, C. (2020) Development of an incontinence-associated dermatitis prevention bundle using an evidence-based framework. *World Council of Enterostomal Therapists Journal.* 40(3): 37–42.

Jaleel, T., Pollack, B. P. & Elmets, C. A. (2019) 'Phototherapy'. In S. Kang, M. Amagai, A. L. Bruckner, A. H. Enk, D. J. Margolis, A. J. McMichael & J. S. Orringer (Eds.). *Fitzpatrick's Dermatology*, 9th ed. New York, NY: McGraw-Hill Education.

Jarvis, C. (2019) *Physical examination and health assessment*, 8th ed. Elsevier.

Latimer, S., Chaboyer, W. & Gillespie, B. (2016) Pressure injury prevention strategies in acute medical inpatients: an observational study. *Contemporary Nurse.* 52(2–3): 326–340. doi: 10.1080/10376178.2016.1190657

Lyons, F. & Ousley, L. (2014) *Dermatology for the Advanced Practice Nurse.* New York, NY: Springer Publishing Company.

Marieb, E. N. & Hoehn, K. (2018) *Human Anatomy & Physiology, Global Edition.* Harlow, United Kingdom: Pearson Education Limited.

Mervis, J. S. & Phillips, T. J. (2019) Pressure ulcers: Pathophysiology, epidemiology, risk factors, and presentation. *Journal of the American Academy of Dermatology.* 81(4): 881–890. doi: 10.1016/j.jaad.2018.12.069

Mitchell, A. (2020) Assessment of wounds in adults. *British Journal of Nursing.* 29(20): S18–S24. doi: 10.12968/bjon.2020.29.20.S18

Morris-Jones, R. (2019). *ABC of Dermatology.* UK: Wiley Publishing.

Metin, A., Dilek, N. & Bilgili, S. G. (2018) Recurrent candidal intertrigo: challenges and solutions. *Clinical, cosmetic and investigational dermatology*. 11: 175–185. https://doi.org/10.2147/CCID.S127841

Nicol, N. (2015) *Dermatologic Nursing Essentials: A Core Curriculum.* Hagerstown, USA: Wolters Kluwer Health.

Papadakis, M. A., McPhee, S. J. & Bernstein, J. (2020) 'Bullous pemphigoid'. In *Quick Medical Diagnosis & Treatment 2021*. New York, NY: McGraw-Hill Education.

Pearson, D. R. & Margolis, D. J. (2019) 'Cellulitis and erysipelas'. In S. Kang, M. Amagai, A. L. Bruckner, A. H. Enk, D. J. Margolis, A. J. McMichael & J. S. Orringer (Eds.). *Fitzpatrick's Dermatology*, 9th ed. New Yok, NY: McGraw-Hill.

Rocha, M. A. & Bagatin, E. (2018) Adult-onset acne: prevalence, impact, and management challenges. *Clinical, Cosmetic and Investigational Dermatology.* 11: 59–69. https://link.gale.com/apps/doc/A574178440/AONE?u=dixson&sid=AONE&xid=596df8bc

Sajadimajd, S., Bahramsoltani, R., Iranpanah, A., Kumar Patra, J., Das, G., Gouda, S. & Xiao, J. (2020) Advances on natural polyphenols as anticancer agents for skin cancer. *Pharmacological Research.* 151: 104584. doi: https://doi.org/10.1016/j.phrs.2019.104584

Serraes, B., van Leen, M., Schols, J., Van Hecke, A., Verhaeghe, S. & Beeckman, D. (2018) Prevention of pressure ulcers with a static air support surface: a systematic review. *International Wound Journal.* 15: 333–343. doi: http://dx.doi.org/10.1111/iwj.12870

Simpson, E. L., Leung, D. Y. M., Eichenfield, L. F. & Boguniewicz, M. L. (2019) 'Atopic dermatitis'. In S. Kang, M. Amagai, A. L. Bruckner, A. H. Enk, D. J. Margolis, A. J. McMichael & J. S. Orringer (Eds.). *Fitzpatrick's Dermatology*, 9th ed. New York, NY: McGraw-Hill Education.

Soutor, C. & Hordinsky, M. K. (2017) *Clinical dermatology.* New York, NY: McGraw-Hill Education.

Stein, S. (2020) 'Varicella zoster virus [VZV] (Herpes zoster/shingles)'. In S. D. C. Stern, A. S. Cifu & D. Altkorn (Eds.). *Symptom to Diagnosis: An Evidence-Based Guide*, 4th ed. New York, NY: McGraw-Hill Education.

Stryja, J., Riha, D. & Szkatula, J. (2020) A silver-based antimicrobial dressing for the prevention of surgical site infection — a pilot study. *European Wound Management Association Journal.* 21(1): 41–48.

Sutherland, M. & Parent, A. (2017) Cellulitis: assessment, diagnosis and management. *Dermatological Nursing.* 16(4): 24–28.

Tortora, G. J. & Derrickson, B. (2011) *Principles of Anatomy and Physiology*, 2nd Asia Pacific ed. Melbourne: Wiley.

Voegeli, D. (2019) Prevention and management of moisture-associated skin damage. *Nursing Standard.* doi: 10.7748/ns.2019.e11314

Wheat, C. M., Burkhart, C. N., Burkhart, C. G. & Cohen, B. A. (2019) 'Scabies, other mites, and pediculosis'. In S. Kang, M. Amagai, A. L. Bruckner, A. H. Enk, D. J. Margolis, A. J. McMichael & J. S. Orringer (Eds.). *Fitzpatrick's Dermatology*, 9th ed. New York, NY: McGraw-Hill Education.

Wollenberg, A., Barbarot, S., Bieber, T., Christen-Zaech, S., Deleuran, M., Fink-Wagner, A. & Specialists, t. E. U. o. M. (2018) Consensus-based European guidelines for treatment of atopic eczema (atopic dermatitis) in adults and children: part I. *Journal of the European Academy of Dermatology and Venereology.* 32(5): 657–682.

Wound Australia. (2016) *Standards of wound prevention and management*, 3rd ed. www.woundsaustralia.com.au/Web/Resources/Publications/Publications_Users_Only/Standards_for_Wound_Prevention_and_Management__Third_Edition___2016_.aspx

Yates, A. (2018) Incontinence-associated dermatitis: what nurses need to know. *British Journal of Nursing.* 27(19): 1094–1100.

Zlotoff, B., Keck, L. E. & Padilla, R. S. (2017) 'Psoriasis and other papulosquamous diseases'. In C. Soutor & M. K. Hordinsky (Eds.). *Clinical Dermatology.* New York, NY: McGraw-Hill Education.

ACKNOWLEDGEMENTS

Figures 12.2, 12.4, 12.5, 12.6, 12.7, 12.8, 12.9, 12.10, 12.11, 12.12, 12.13, 12.12, 12.15, 12.16: © Morris-Jones (2019). *ABC of Dermatology*, 7th ed. Wiley Blackwell.

CHAPTER 13

Nursing care of conditions related to the respiratory system

LEARNING OBJECTIVES

After studying this chapter, you should be able to:

13.1 describe the structure and function of the respiratory system
13.2 explain the physiological processes involved in respiration
13.3 describe the techniques involved in respiratory system assessment
13.4 identify the diagnostic investigations used in respiratory conditions and explain the findings related to pathophysiology
13.5 describe the different respiratory conditions based on their pathophysiology and the nursing management of these conditions
13.6 explain the common nursing interventions for respiratory conditions.

Introduction

Chronic respiratory illnesses are often associated with a negative impact on the quality of life in terms of physical function, anxiety, depression and social isolation. Nurses are well placed to address the complex care needs required to enhance these patients' quality of life.

This chapter provides an overview of respiratory conditions that dominate hospital care, including infections such as pneumonia and tuberculosis (TB), diseases that affect the airways such as **asthma**, chronic obstructive pulmonary disease (COPD), **respiratory failure** and bronchiectasis, **cystic fibrosis** (CF) and lung cancer. The chapter will discuss the respiratory system's anatomy and physiology, steps involved in conducting respiratory assessment and common diagnostic interventions for respiratory conditions. It will also touch on the pathophysiology, treatment and nursing management of common respiratory conditions.

13.1 The function of the respiratory system

LEARNING OBJECTIVE 13.1 Describe the structure and function of the respiratory system.

The respiratory system's function is to exchange gases, assist in regulating blood pH and maintain acid–base balance.

The respiratory tract consists of the nose, pharynx, larynx, trachea and two lungs (see figure 13.1). The lungs are covered by the parietal and visceral **pleura** and contain bronchi, bronchioles and **alveoli**. Each lung is subdivided into lobes (see figure 13.2). The pulmonary vascular system facilitates gas exchange in the alveoli.

13.2 The physiology of respiration

LEARNING OBJECTIVE 13.2 Explain the physiological processes involved in respiration.

Respiration consists of a cycle of inspiration, expiration and rest, through which gas exchange occurs (figure 13.3).

The control of respiration

Respiration is controlled by a complex set of processes involving an interplay between the cerebral cortex, respiratory centre, chemoreceptors, proprioceptors and stretch receptors (figure 13.4). Rate, rhythm, depth and effort all change to meet the demands of the body and maintain normal levels of PaO_2 (the partial pressure of oxygen in the blood: 80–100 mmHg), $PaCO_2$ (the partial pressure of carbon dioxide in the blood, which reflects respiratory control of the acid–base balance: 35–45 mmHg) and pH (7.35–7.45) (Chaboyer, Marshall & Aitken 2015). The following are involved in the control of respiration.

- *Respiratory centre*. Respiration is controlled by the medulla oblongata and the pons in the brainstem.
- *Chemoreceptors*. Monitor the levels of CO_2, O_2 and hydrogen ions (H^+). Hypercapnia (too high CO_2 level) causes an increase in the level of H^+ and causes hyperventilation, thus increasing the level of O_2 and decreasing CO_2:

$$\uparrow CO_2 \leftrightarrow \uparrow H^+ (\downarrow pH) \leftrightarrow Hyperventilation \leftrightarrow \uparrow O_2 and \downarrow CO_2$$

In contrast, hypocapnia (too low CO_2 level) causes H^+ levels to fall, which increases pH, but does not cause a change in respiration:

$$\downarrow CO_2 \leftrightarrow \downarrow H^+ (\uparrow pH)$$

Hypoxaemia (too low O_2 level) initially stimulates breathing, although not as powerfully as **hypercapnia**. However, extreme hypoxaemia can cause respiratory depression.

- *Stretch receptors and the inflation reflex*. Stretch receptors in the bronchi and bronchioles cause breathing to stop when they are overstretched, leading to expiration.
- *Proprioceptors*. Stimulation of proprioceptors in the muscles and joints increases the rate and depth of breathing.

FIGURE 13.1 (a) The upper respiratory tract (b) The lower respiratory tract

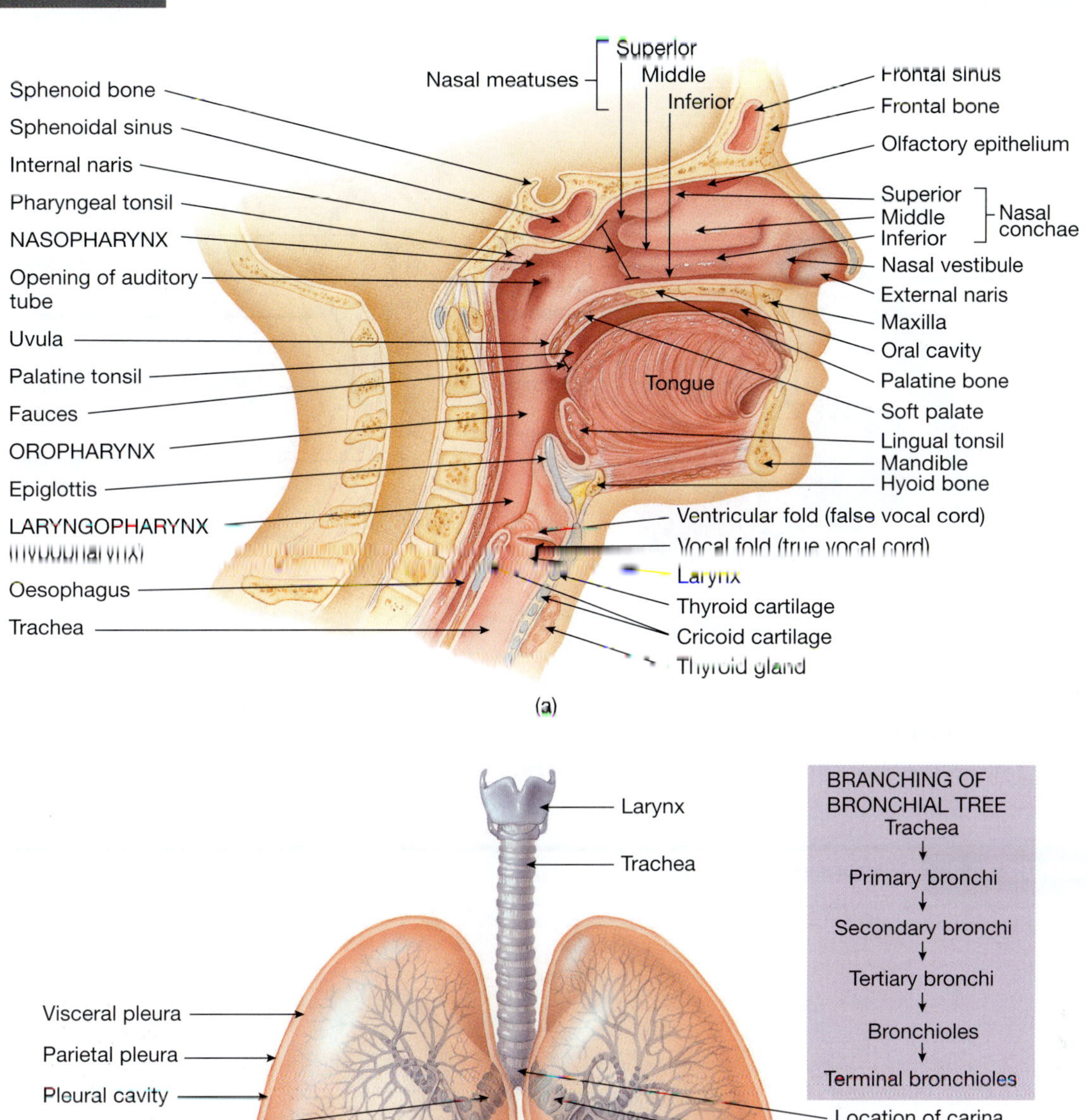

Source: Tortora & Derrickson (2011) *Principles of Anatomy and Physiology*, with kind permission of Wiley Blackwell.

Gas exchange

In the alveoli, oxygen from the atmosphere is taken up into the pulmonary capillaries to meet the tissues' needs. At the same time, carbon dioxide, a waste product of metabolism, is excreted by expiration (figure 13.5).

FIGURE 13.2 Microscopic anatomy of a lung

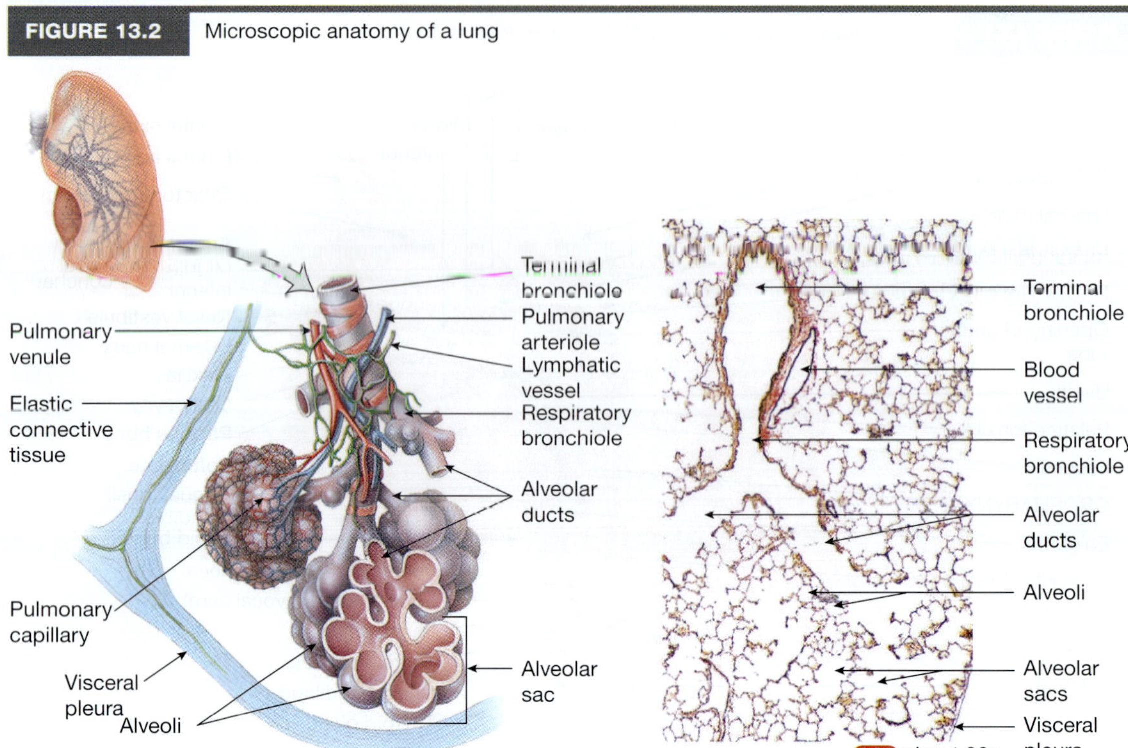

Source: Tortora & Derrickson (2011) *Principles of Anatomy and Physiology*, with kind permission of Wiley Blackwell.

FIGURE 13.3 Mechanics of respiration

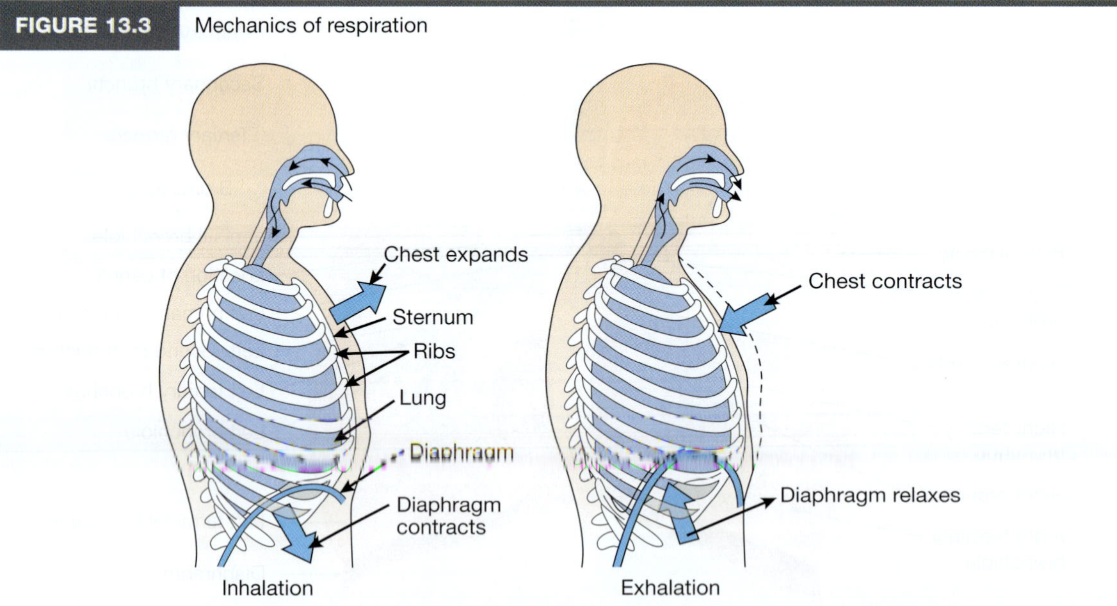

Source: Nair & Peate (2009) *Fundamentals of Anatomy and Physiology*, with kind permission of Wiley Blackwell.

Transport of oxygen

Oxygen is almost entirely transported bound to haemoglobin in the blood (98.5 per cent), with 1.5 per cent dissolved in the plasma (figure 13.5). At rest, only 25 per cent of the oxygen is used by the tissues (Tortora & Derrickson 2011).

Transport of carbon dioxide

Carbon dioxide is carried in the blood in three forms: approximately 70 per cent as bicarbonate ions (HCO_3^-), approximately 23 per cent as carbamino compounds, and about 7 per cent as dissolved carbon dioxide (figure 13.6).

FIGURE 13.4 Factors influencing the rate and depth of breathing

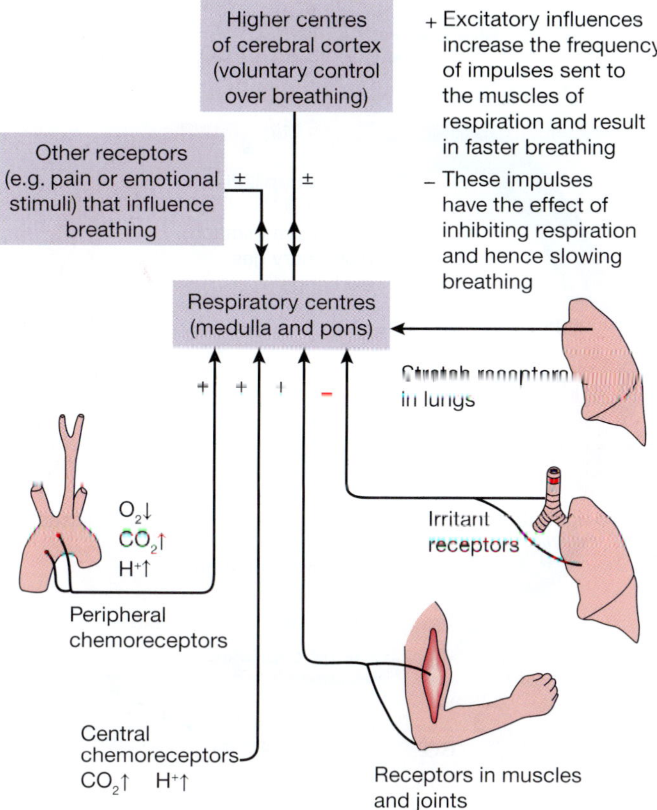

Source: Dougherty & Lister (2011) *The Royal Marsden Hospital Manual of Clinical Nursing Procedures*, with kind permission from Wiley Blackwell.

Regulation of pH

The respiratory system contributes to acid–base balance via the regulation of pH and H^+ associated with carbon dioxide transport. Carbon dioxide diffuses into the red blood cells and binds with water to form a weak acid: carbonic acid (H_2CO_3), which in turn dissociates into H^+ and HCO_3^-:

CO_2	+	H_2O	↔	H_2CO_3	↔	H^+	+	HCO_3^-
Carbon dioxide	+	Water	↔	Carbonic acid	↔	Hydrogen ion	+	Bicarbonate ion

The free H^+ is buffered by binding with haemoglobin, thereby changing its structure and releasing oxygen to the tissues. Similarly, the build-up of lactic acid during exercise causes a release of oxygen to the tissues.

Ventilation, perfusion and V/Q ratio

Ventilation (V) refers to the flow of air throughout the lungs, whereas perfusion (Q) refers to the flow of blood in the pulmonary capillaries. In ideal circumstances, the two are matched, and their relationship is expressed as the V/Q ratio. V/Q imbalance occurs when there is inadequate ventilation and/or perfusion (figure 13.7). V/Q imbalance can result in shunting, in which the blood is not oxygenated and remains high in carbon dioxide. The imbalance may be the result of one or a combination of different factors (table 13.1).

FIGURE 13.5 Gas exchange

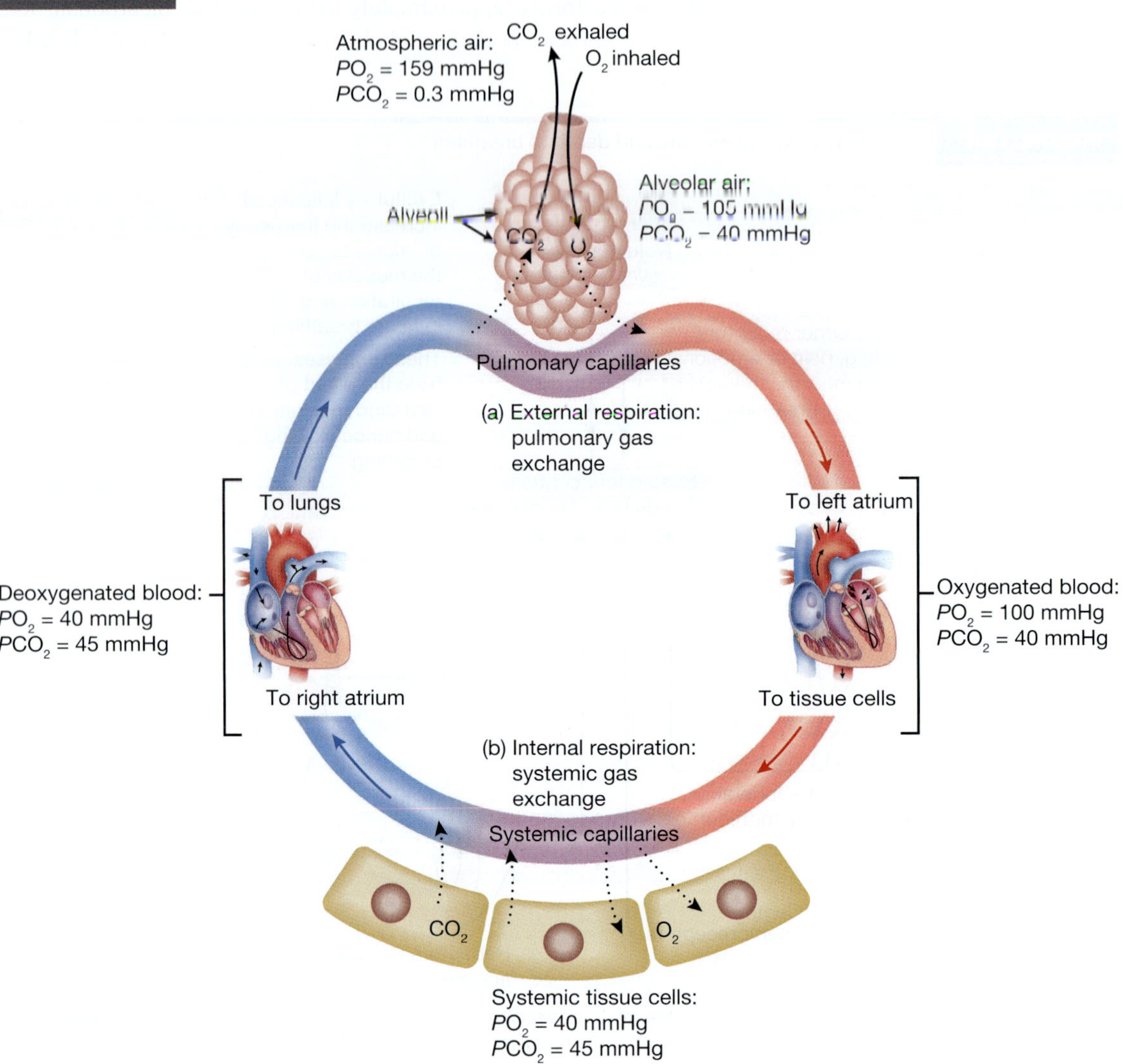

Source: Tortora & Derrickson (2011) *Principles of Anatomy and Physiology*, with kind permission of Wiley Blackwell.

TABLE 13.1 Causes of V/Q imbalance

Inadequate ventilation	Inadequate perfusion
Airway blockages	Increased alveolar pressure
Low compliance	Increased pulmonary artery pressure
Increased airway resistance	Gravity
Pulmonary oedema	Pulmonary embolism
Atelectasis (collapse of an area of lung tissue that has not ventilated by normal breathing)	

FIGURE 13.6 Transport of oxygen and carbon dioxide in the blood

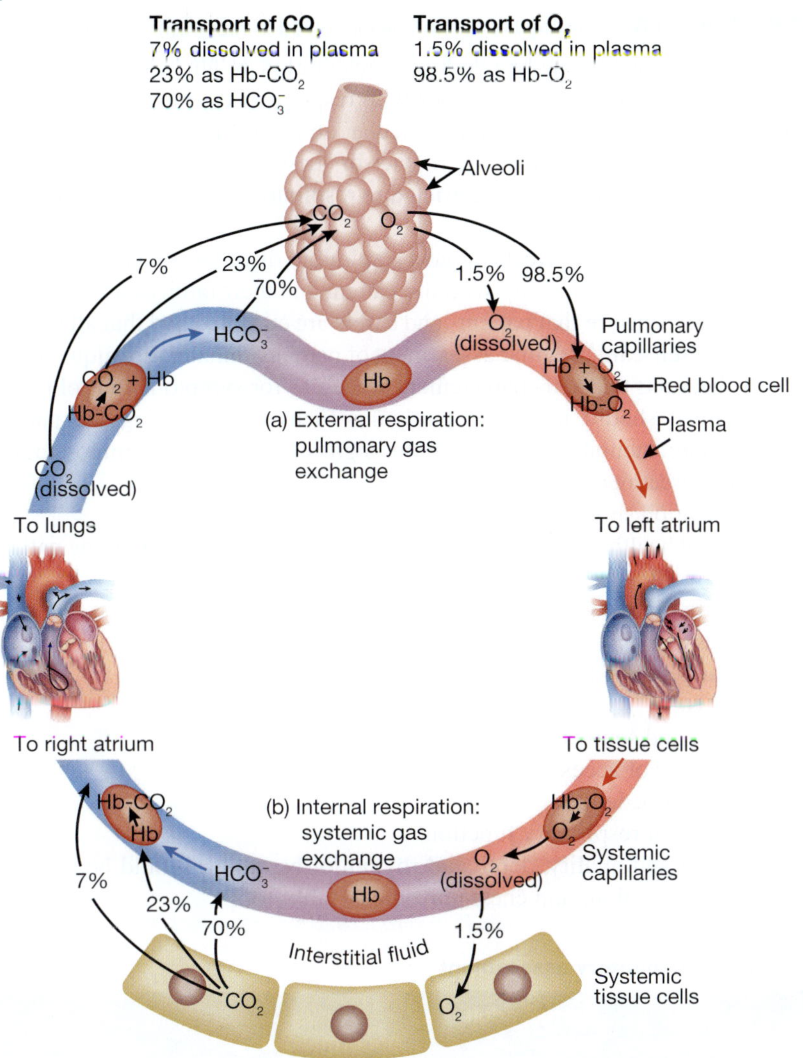

Source: Tortora & Derrickson (2011) *Principles of Anatomy and Physiology*, with kind permission of Wiley Blackwell.

FIGURE 13.7 V/Q ratio

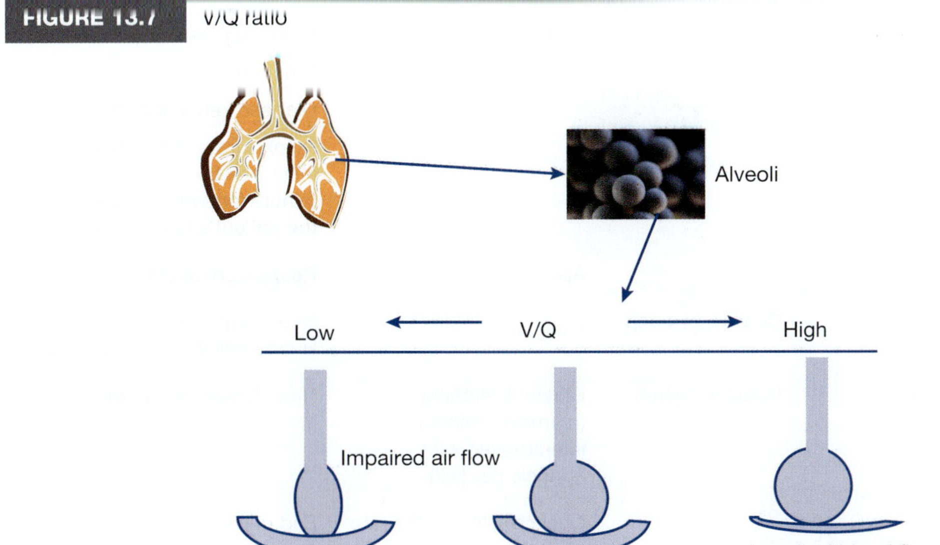

13.3 Respiratory assessment

LEARNING OBJECTIVE 13.3 Describe the techniques involved in respiratory system assessment.

The nursing assessment of a patient in relation to respiration is an essential aspect of nursing care. Abnormal breathing patterns are not synonymous with respiratory disorders. They can present in cardiac disease, diabetes, head injury, anaemia and muscular and neurological disorders. Initial assessment involves identifying health problems and the impact of these on the patient's function and wellbeing. Similarly, respiratory interventions are not restricted to respiratory conditions and are necessary for every acutely ill patient.

Due to the chronicity and adverse effects of most respiratory disorders on health and wellbeing, building a therapeutic and long-lasting relationship with the patient and their family/carer is critical.

Care needs to be taken to ensure that patients and carers are educated and that all resources and supports are in place to maximise self-care. Regular assessment of patients' inhaler technique if applicable and their understanding of medications and self-management strategies for symptom control is imperative.

Respiratory assessment should include a particular focus on observing the patient's temperature, respiration, blood pressure, mentation and hydration. Signs of confusion are important markers of disease severity and response to treatment.

The following information should be collected during the assessment:

- patient history: general health and the development of symptoms, along with the patient's social history
- recent weight loss or gain
- recent experience with night sweats, fevers and/or reflux
- anxiety and/or depression
- colour of the skin, fingernails, lips, etc.
- level of consciousness
- respiratory rate, effort and sounds
- ability to talk and the use of accessory muscles
- the presence of cough or oedema
- physiological measures of respiratory function.

Respiratory rate, effort and quality, depth and rhythm of breathing should be assessed in conjunction with observing the patient's colour and chest movement (table 13.2).

TABLE 13.2 **General respiratory assessment**

Focus	Observe	Normal adult values	Abnormalities	Indications
Respiration	Quality, rate	Rate: 12–18 per minute	Bradypnoea <10 breaths per minute	Head injury Narcotic overdose
			Tachypnoea	Following exertion Pneumonia Diabetic ketoacidosis Pyrexia (rate of breathing increases by 7 breaths per minute for every 10°C rise in the patient's temperature)
			Apnoea	Respiratory arrest
	Depth	Shallow or deep		Hyperventilation Hypoventilation (hypercapnia)
	Rhythm	Regular rhythm	Cluster breathing (normal breathing interspersed with apnoeic pauses)	Neurological disorders
			Cheyne–Stokes (the rate changes with increasing periods of apnoea)	End of life

	Effort		Unable to complete a sentence Use of accessory muscles Muscle retraction (intercostal and suprasternal muscles) Nasal flaring	Pneumonia Airway inflammation/obstruction Emphysema Trauma
Colour	Skin colour: check skin, nail beds, lips, tongue, ears and nose		Cyanosis (central or peripheral)	Central: hypoxaemia Peripheral: perfusion abnormality
Chest	Shape	Symmetrical	Barrel chest	Emphysema
	Movement		Pigeon chest	Rickets
			Asymmetrical	Pneumothorax (air trapped in the pleura) [illegible] atelectasis

Dyspnoea

Dyspnoea, or difficulty breathing, is common to many respiratory disorders. Nursing assessment should include the questions below, which will provide a comprehensive outline of the patient's condition.

- Is the breathlessness episodic or persistent?
- Is it associated with seasonal change, exposure to environmental irritants, anxiety, emotion?
- Is it associated with any other symptoms: cough/wheeze/stridor?
- Does it occur at rest or on exertion? Is there nocturnal dyspnoea? Or orthopnoea?
- What is the exercise tolerance? For example, how does it affect daily activities such as washing, dressing or walking?
- Is it associated with chronic fatigue?
- How does the dyspnoea affect social activities with family and friends?
- Does the dyspnoea make the patient feel anxious or depressed?
- What is the patient's perception of the severity of their dyspnoea?

Cough

The presence, nature and trigger (acute or chronic) of cough should be assessed (table 13.3). Cough can be characterised as paroxysmal, barking, hacking, harsh or hoarse, and classified as effective or ineffective and dry or productive.

TABLE 13.3 Assessment of productive cough

Characteristic	Monitor	Observe	Indication/action
Effective or ineffective	Breath sounds Fatigue	Improvement, lack of improvement or deterioration in condition Signs of decreased effort without clinical improvement	Increase respiratory support as necessary to avoid respiratory failure
Productive or dry	Amount	Teaspoon/tablespoon/cup	Record amount
	Colour	Clear	Non-infective
		Yellow	Infection
		Green Brown	Send sample for culture and sensitivity

(continued)

TABLE 13.3 *(continued)*

Characteristic	Monitor	Observe	Indication/action
		White — frothy	Pulmonary oedema: monitor fluid intake and output, restrict intake, give diuretics Pulmonary TB — send a sample for isolation of acid fast bacilli Lung cancer — send a sample for cytology
		White or pink-tinged; frothy sputum	Pulmonary oedema Lung cancer
	Consistency	Watery	Easy to expectorate
		Thick and tenacious	Difficult to expectorate Give warmed humidified inhalations, keep the patient well hydrated
	Smell	Purulent	Infection

Haemoptysis

Haemoptysis refers to coughing up blood or bloody sputum. It is associated with pneumonia, abnormalities of the pulmonary blood vessels, pulmonary embolism, TB, bronchiectasis, epistaxis, forceful coughing, cardiac disease and lung cancer. It may also occur as a result of anticoagulant use. The amount produced is assessed using terms such as 'teaspoon', 'tablespoon' and 'cup'.

Chest pain

Chest pain with a respiratory origin may be related to painful coughing, pleural inflammation, pulmonary embolism or lung cancer. It may be persistent, dull and aching, which is associated with lung cancer, or sharp and stabbing, as with pleural inflammation and pulmonary embolism. Pleuritic pain is typically felt on inspiration and often results in the client taking only shallow breaths, which leads to a worsening of pleural inflammation and any associated respiratory tract infection. The pain may be musculoskeletal in origin, sharp or dull, and may result from traumatic injury.

Abnormal breath sounds

Breath sounds are an essential part of respiratory assessment and are usually assessed by the respiratory team (table 13.4).

TABLE 13.4 **Breath sounds**

Sound	Characteristic	Signs of
Wheezing	Whistling sound, generally heard on expiration	Asthma and airway obstruction
Stridor	Snoring sound heard on inspiration	Typical of obstruction, sputum plug or foreign body, anaphylactic reaction
Crackles	A crackling or popping sound	Collapsed alveoli popping open on inspiration
Rhonchi	Snoring or rattling sounds	Fluid partly blocking the bronchi; generally heard on expiration
Pleural friction	A grating or rubbing sound heard on inspiration and expiration	Indicative of pleural inflammation

Non-respiratory signs of respiratory illness

It is essential to assess the patient's general health and look for non-respiratory signs of respiratory-related illness such as the following.

- *Clubbing of the fingers.* Found with persistent hypoxia, as in chronic respiratory disease and lung cancer.
- *Tremor.* Associated with salbutamol use, which also causes tachycardia and cardiac arrhythmias. Flapping of the wrists when the arms are held outstretched is indicative of carbon dioxide retention. Warm, red skin and hands with a bounding pulse and headache are also indicative of hypercapnia.
- *Pitting oedema.* Associated with heart failure when seen in dependent areas, such as the ankles, sacrum and lower arms.

Smoking history

It is essential to check whether the patient smokes and assess their smoking history, including their exposure to passive smoking. Previous attempts at smoking cessation should be explored, and the level of success and facilitators and barriers should be identified.

Medications

Determine whether the patient receives any medications or treatments, including oxygen and non-invasive ventilation (NIV). Note the drug, dose, frequency, effectiveness and side effects, if any. Patient education is imperative to ensure that patients are competent to manage their medications, adjust the dosage and medicate as necessary to best manage their condition. The use of symptom diaries or measures of function should be encouraged to gain an accurate picture of the impact of the disease. Oxygen use should be assessed in relation to the amount and the duration of use. Assessing patients' technique when using inhalers or **nebuliser** preparations is essential to maximise the treatment's benefit.

13.4 Respiratory function testing

LEARNING OBJECTIVE 13.4 Identify the diagnostic investigations used in respiratory conditions and explain the findings related to pathophysiology.

Peak expiratory flow

Peak expiratory flow (PEF) measures maximum expiratory flow following a forced expiration (figure 13.8); it can provide a crude record of respiratory function over time if a diary of the results is kept. Morning and evening daily monitoring of PEF rate for two to four weeks can identify variability in airflow limitation for diagnosis and monitoring.

FIGURE 13.8 Measurement of peak flow

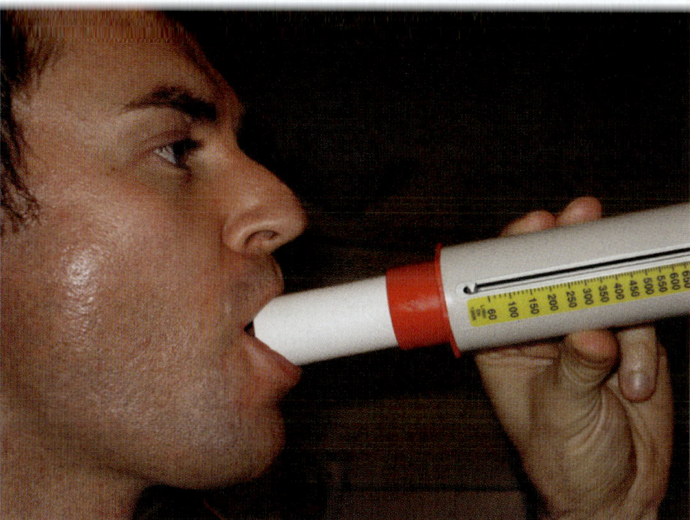

Source: Dougherty & Lister (2011) *The Royal Marsden Hospital Manual of Clinical Nursing Procedures*, with kind permission from Wiley Blackwell.

Pulse oximetry

Pulse oximetry is a non-invasive device (figure 13.9) used to measure the oxygen saturation of haemoglobin in arterial blood in the peripheral circulation. This is very useful to identify respiratory deterioration early. The probe for measuring saturation is commonly placed on the fingers, but it can be placed on a toe, earlobe or forehead. Cold peripheries, artificial nails, nail polish and external light (fluorescent light and heat lamps) can interfere with the light on the probe and give false readings. For adults, saturation should be above 95 per cent. A lower threshold of above 92 per cent is accepted for patients with chronic obstructive pulmonary disease. A **pulse oximeter** cannot differentiate between oxyhaemoglobin, carboxyhaemoglobin and methaemoglobin. Carbon monoxide poisoning can show falsely elevated saturation due to high carboxyhaemoglobin.

FIGURE 13.9 Pulse oximetry

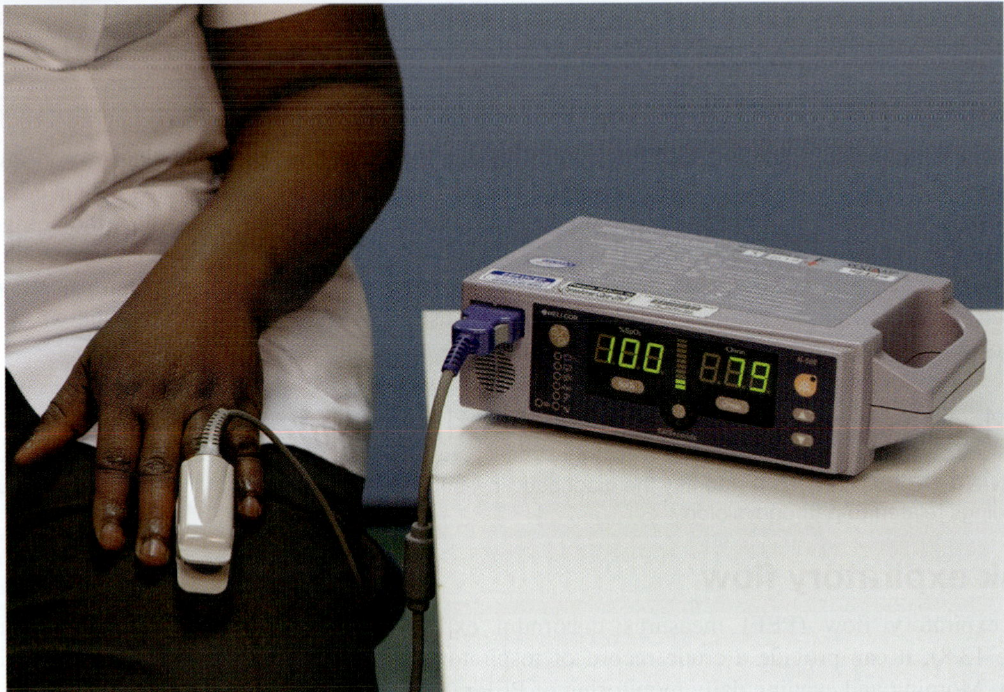

Source: Dougherty & Lister (2011) *The Royal Marsden Hospital Manual of Clinical Nursing Procedures*, with kind permission from Wiley Blackwell.

Spirometry

Spirometry is used to diagnose patients as well as monitor disease progression and the response to medication. Measures include forced expiratory volume in 1 second (FEV_1), forced vital capacity (FVC), lung capacity and FEV_1/FVC ratio, a measure of the amount of air in the full lungs that has been expired after 1 second.

Radiological investigations

Radiological investigations are used for diagnosis and monitoring. They include chest X-ray, computed tomography (CT) and magnetic resonance imaging.

Chest X-ray remains one of the most commonly used investigations for diagnosing respiratory conditions. This is either done at the bedside or in the radiology room. It is vital to make sure that jewellery, cloth hooks, oxygen tubing, ECG leads, etc. are not in the field of radiation while X-raying. Position the patient appropriately to avoid rotation of the body. ABCDE is a common acronym used to evaluate chest radiograph.

- A = Airway (trachea and main bronchi) — check the trachea's position in the midline. Deviation to one side can be a sign of tension pneumothorax.
- B = Breathing (lungs) — compare the different zones and apices of the lungs. Lung margins should be traced to the peripheries to identify the presence of pneumothorax.

- C = Circulation (heart and mediastinum) — cardiac silhouette and mediastinum is evaluated for size and shape. A cardiac silhouette larger than 50 per cent of the chest diameter indicates cardiomegaly. Pneumomediastinum or Pneumopericardium is suspected if there is abnormal lucency within the mediastinum or surrounding cardiac silhouette. Mediastinum should not be more than 8 centimetres in width.
- D = Diaphragm — right hemidiaphragm is slightly higher than the left due to the presence of the liver. The costophrenic angle is the angle where the diaphragm meets the ribs. Costophrenic angles can be blunted by fluid commonly seen in pleural effusion.
- E = Evaluate everything else such as bony skeleton, soft tissues, foreign bodies, lines, tubes, etc. The nasogastric tube should be within the stomach below the left hemidiaphragm. Bony structures should be examined to identify fractures.

Bronchoscopy

Bronchoscopy is used to directly visualise the lungs. A fibreoptic camera is passed into the patient's trachea and lungs. The lungs can then be assessed for signs of disease. Samples can be taken for histological and cytological examination.

Arterial blood gas (ABG) readings

Arterial blood gases (ABGs) indicate the level of functioning of the lungs. Normal ABG measures are presented in table 13.5 .Arterial blood is taken to measure PaO_2, $PaCO_2$ and pH . ABG values demonstrate the level of functioning of the lungs and are used to diagnose, assess and monitor critically ill patients. Arterial blood gas provide information about oxygenation and ventilation status (PaO_2, $PaCO_2$, SaO_2), acid–base balance (pH, bicarbonate, base excess), electrolyte imbalance (potassium, sodium and chloride), haemoglobin level (Hb) and blood glucose level.

TABLE 13.5 **ABG normal values**

Parameters	Normal values
Oxygen (PaO_2)	80–100 mmHg (10.7–13.3 kPa)
Acid–base status (pH)	7.35–7.45
$PaCO_2$	35–45 mmHg (4.7–6.0 kPa)
Bicarbonate (HCO_3^-)	22–26 mmol/L
Base excess	−3 to +3 mmol/L
SaO_2[a]	95–100%

[a] SaO_2, arterial oxygen saturation.

Source: Adapted from Chaboyer, Marshall & Aitken (2015) *ACCN's Critical Care Nursing* 3rd ed. Elsevier, Chatswood, NSW, Australia

Skin prick testing

Skin prick testing is used to test for specific allergies that can aggravate asthma or rhinitis. Various potential allergens are tested, for example, house dust mite, animal dander and grass pollen.

13.5 The pathophysiology of specific respiratory conditions

LEARNING OBJECTIVE 13.5 Describe the different respiratory conditions based on their pathophysiology and the nursing management of these conditions.

Pneumonia

Pneumonia is an infection of the lungs involving an acute inflammatory response that impairs the alveoli and interferes with ventilation. Pneumonia can be caused by bacteria, viruses, fungi or other pathogens.

Non-infectious cause includes inhalation of volatile or irritating substances or the aspiration of gastric contents (Bullock & Hales 2019). Pneumonia is manifested when the alveolar macrophages' capacity to kill or ingest bacteria is exceeded (Mandell & Wunderink 2018). This triggers a host inflammatory response. Fever occurs due to the release of inflammatory mediators such as interleukin 1 and tumor necrosis factor. Chemokines, such as interleukin 8 and granulocyte colony-stimulating factor, stimulate the release of neutrophils. Purulent secretion occurs as a result of their attraction to the lungs. The localised advanced alveolar-capillary leak in the initial stages of pneumonia is due to the inflammatory mediators released by macrophages and newly recruited neutrophils.

Pneumonia can be classified as:

1. community-acquired pneumonia
2. hospital-acquired pneumonia (ventilator-associated pneumonia)
3. aspiration pneumonia.

The clinical manifestations of pneumonia are:

- fever
- pleuritic chest pain
- tachypnoea (25–45 breaths per minute) and possibly orthopnoea
- tachycardia
- a productive cough with purulent, blood-stained sputum
- general symptoms including anorexia, headaches and muscle pains
- on auscultation, there may be reduced breath sounds, **crackles** or dullness.

Diagnosis

The following investigations are used in diagnosing pneumonia:

- chest X-ray
- blood analysis for white cell count, c-reactive protein, procalcitonin, urea, etc.
- pulse oximetry
- arterial blood gas analysis
- blood and sputum for culture and sensitivity
- polymerase chain reaction (PCR) test of nasal swabs for diagnosing respiratory viral infection.

Nursing assessment and management

Assessment of severity is important to determine the patient's management with pneumonia, and the CURB65 score can be used for this. This scores one point for each of the following criteria:

- C = confusion
- U = blood urea >7 mmol/L
- R = respiratory rate: >30/min
- B = blood pressure: systolic <90 mmHg, diastolic <60 mmHg
- 65 = >65 years of age.

Medical management includes the prompt administration of intravenous antibiotic therapy, oxygen and intravenous fluids to correct the fluid balance. If oxygen saturation of more than 92 per cent is not achieved using oxygen, NIV may be considered. The patient may require pain relief and management of dyspnoea. A high semi-Fowler's position can relieve dyspnoea. The patient's position should be alternated to enhance oxygenation and sputum clearance. Oxygen should be humidified and the patient well hydrated to facilitate sputum clearance. Pulse oximetry should be monitored closely, and any abnormalities treated promptly. Breathing and coughing exercises and mobilisation as tolerated can be used to maximise expectoration. Supportive care is necessary, so manage pyrexia, assist with hygiene needs, alternate rest with activity and encourage a high-protein, high-calorie diet as far as the patient can tolerate it.

Patients admitted to the intensive care unit on mechanical ventilation may develop ventilator-associated pneumonia. Oral care is extremely important in this situation. Improved oral hygiene can decrease the concentration of oral pathogenic microorganisms, decrease the build-up of dental plaque, and reduce bacterial pneumonia risk. In unconscious patients who are intubated, cleaning the teeth with a toothbrush and toothpaste is required every two hours. Suctioning of the oral cavity, including the back of the throat, using a flexible suction tube, should also be performed to prevent aspiration. Endotracheal tubes need to be suctioned as required to clear the lungs of secretions without contaminating the suction cannula. Ensure the cuff of the endotracheal tube is sufficiently inflated so that there is no leak between the tube and trachea, preventing aspiration of contents into lower respiratory tract.

Tuberculosis

Tuberculosis (TB) is an infectious disease that, in humans, is caused by *Mycobacterium tuberculosis* (Doucette & Cooper 2015). Mycobacteria are transmitted from person to person by droplet infection through coughing or sneezing. The response to infection can result in latent or active TB (Stern 2020). Prevention requires the rapid identification of new cases, effective treatment and contact tracing.

Pathophysiology

TB can affect any organ, but the focus here is on pulmonary TB. Extrapulmonary or disseminated TB occurs when there is an infection in the blood or lymphatic system. Alveolar macrophages ingest tubercle bacilli that reach the alveoli. However, in some individuals, invading bacteria that are engulfed in alveolar macrophages can evade intracellular killing. These bacteria replicate without limitation, spreading to regional lymph nodes and silently disseminating haemotogenously (Doucette & Cooper 2015). The adaptive cellular immune response is initiated after a few weeks, and once stimulated, T lymphocytes release cytokines, including interferon gamma (measured for diagnosing TB in lab investigation), triggering intracellular mycobacteria killing. In some individuals, initial mycobacterial replication is not controlled, and it progresses to primary TB. This is particularly common in immunocompromised individuals.

In most persons with intact cell-mediated immunity, T-cells and macrophages surround the organism in granulomas limiting their multiplication and spread. The organism is contained but not eradicated, and they can remain dormant within the granulomas for years. Individuals with latent tuberculosis infection do not have active disease and cannot transmit the organism. However, reactivation of the disease may occur if the host immune defence is compromised.

Clinical manifestations of TB can include:

- a persistent cough, possibly with haemoptysis, that may initially be dry but can become productive with blood-streaked sputum
- weight loss
- low-grade fever with night sweats
- loss of appetite
- dyspnoea
- on blood sample analysis, usually anaemia and a raised erythrocyte sedimentation rate and lymphocyte count.

Diagnosis

Investigations for diagnosis can include:

- sputum for mycobacterial culture — early morning sputum specimen on three consecutive days is ideal
- chest X-ray and CT scan
- interferon gamma release assays in blood
- tuberculin skin testing, commonly referred to as the **Mantoux test**, is used for screening purposes and can detect those infected or have received vaccination (BCG) but do not have active disease.

Nursing assessment and management

TB therapy aims to interrupt transmission, relieve symptoms and prevent drug resistance and future relapse and mortality (Doucette & Cooper 2015). A standard course of treatment involves a 6-month regimen of a combination of anti-TB medications. This regimen is extended to 9 months in certain circumstances, including persistent positive sputum cultures and resistance of the organism to pyrazinamide.

Multi-drug-resistant (MDR) TB is an increasing problem, with risk factors including a history of TB treatment prior to the current diagnosis, contact with known MDR TB, HIV infection and birth in a country where the World Health Organization (WHO) has reported a high incidence of MDR TB. Treatment is complex and needs to be directed by a specialist respiratory infectious diseases physician.

The risk of healthcare-associated transmission is increased during aerosol-producing procedures, including suctioning, bronchoscopy, endotracheal intubation, open abscess irrigation and autopsy. Patients should be advised to avoid unnecessary contact with people from outside their household for the first two weeks of treatment and until the patient has three negative Acid-fast bacilli (AFB) sputum cultures and feels better to prevent community transmission (Smith 2019).

Directly observed therapy is a recognised approach to enhancing adherence to TB therapy. It involves a health worker meeting with and observing the patient taking the medication. This demands daily or weekly visits as required by the treatment regimen. Although it is resource-intensive, directly observed therapy has been shown to be a key mechanism for the control of TB (Smith 2019).

Breathing and coughing exercises, with close attention to infection control and hygiene needs, can be used to facilitate expectoration. Supportive care with the management of pyrexia and assistance to manage night sweats may be necessary. Ensure the patient is well hydrated and alternate rest with activity. A high-protein, high-calorie diet and oxygen as necessary can be used to manage appetite loss, weight loss and any consequent fatigue. Monitoring for side effects of the medication is important — hepatitis is one of the side effects. Anorexia, nausea, right upper-quadrant pain, unexplained malaise should be immediately reported. Blood investigation for liver function should be done if side effects are reported. Common TB medications and their side effects are outlined in table 13.6.

TABLE 13.6 TB medication and possible side effects

Medication	Common side effects
Isoniazid	Peripheral neuropathy, hepatitis, rash, mild CNS effects
Rifampicin	Hepatitis, fever, rash, flu-like illness, gastrointestinal upset, bleeding problems, kidney failure
Pyrazinamide	Hyperuricemia, hepatotoxicity, rash, gastrointestinal upset, joint aches
Ethambutol	Optic neuritis (reversible on discontinuation of the drug), rash

Source: Chesnutt, Chesnutt, Prendergast & Prendergast (2021). 'Pulmonary tuberculosis'. In Papadakis, McPhee & Rabow (Eds.), *Current Medical Diagnosis & Treatment*. McGraw-Hill

In-patient nursing management of TB patients

Patients should be in a negative pressure isolation room with a toilet and bathroom to minimise infection spread. To maintain droplet precaution, healthcare staff should wear full personal protective equipment (PPE), including gown, gloves, mask and goggles. Surgical masks are insufficient in preventing transmission; hence, it is important to use appropriate fit-tested respirators while providing care to TB patients. If a healthcare worker cannot be fitted with an appropriate respirator, a powered air-purifying respirator should be made available for use. Always keep the room closed. Frequent visits to the room should be minimised by clubbing the procedures to specific time slots. Masks should only be removed outside the room after the door is closed, and hand hygiene must be performed after removing PPE. The movement and transport of the patient from the room should be limited to essential purposes only. The patient must wear a surgical mask if transport from the room is necessary. Cough inducing (suctioning, bronchoscopy) and aerosol-generating procedures (nebulisation) should also be minimised. The patient should be taught about covering the nose and mouth with a tissue while coughing, discarding it properly and washing hands immediately after the episode. For intubated patients, it is ideal to use a closed inline suction tube to suction the endotracheal tube. It is also essential to avoid accidental disconnection of the endotracheal tube from the ventilator circuit.

In performing a respiratory assessment, place the patient in an upright position to facilitate breathing. Observe the respiratory rate, depth, pattern and saturation level. Auscultate the lungs for any adventitious lung sounds. An X-ray should be done bedside if possible, to avoid transporting the patient outside the room. Frequent arterial blood gas analysis may be required in acutely unwell patients. Collect and send sputum specimen for investigation.

Asthma

Asthma is a chronic inflammatory disease of the airway. It is characterised by airflow obstruction due to airway hyperresponsiveness that is often reversible either spontaneously or with treatment. One in nine Australians had asthma diagnosed by a doctor or nurse in 2017–18 based on self-reported survey data (AIHW 2020a).

Common triggers for asthma symptoms and exacerbations include exercise, changes in weather (cold air, thunderstorms), strong odours, perfume, rhinosinusitis, medications (ACE inhibitors, beta antagonist, NSAIDs, especially aspirin) and stress.

Other risk factors include:

- a familial predisposition
- atopy (an inherited trait in which the immune system is highly responsive to allergens)
- exposure to allergens and irritants (fungi, pollens)
- smoking
- frequent respiratory tract infections, such as with respiratory syncytial virus
- parasitic infections.

Pathophysiology

Airway inflammation, with associated airway hyperresponsiveness, is the underlying feature of asthma irrespective of whether symptoms are triggered by exposure to allergy, irritants or a combination of both. Two distinct phases exist in allergy induced asthma: early phase and late phase. Bronchoconstriction, vasodilation of the airway vasculature, hyperaemia and vascular congestion occurs in the early phase due to the release of histamines, leukotrienes and cytokines. This increases capillary permeability, resulting in airway oedema. Late phase occurs approximately four hours later and can last up to 24 hours. Eosinophils are mainly responsible for the late phase reaction as they exaggerate the airway's inflammatory response, causing more bronchoconstriction and impairing mucociliary function. Airway hyperresponsiveness results from the presence of inflammatory mediators in the airway and the failure of neuroregulation. Airflow limitation in asthma is mainly from bronchoconstriction, inflamed airways and mucus hypersecretion.

The following video explains the pathophysiology of asthma: www.youtube.com/watch?v=rgphaHmAC_A.

Clinical manifestations of asthma include:

- breathlessness with wheezing and/or cough
- chest tightness
- symptoms that are usually worse at night and in the early morning
- cyanosis and abnormal ABGs
- respiratory effort marked by nasal flaring and the use of accessory muscles
- wheezing that may be absent on auscultation, indicating that the airways are too constricted for air to flow
- in very severe attacks, respiratory failure — PaO_2 (on air) will be <60 mmHg and $PaCO_2$ >45 mmHg.

Diagnosis

Diagnosis involves:

- patient history
- physical examination
- blood investigation for IgE and eosinophils
- skin test for allergy
- chest X-ray
- ABG analysis (only in critically ill patients)
- lung function tests.

Spirometry is the most common lung function test and is recommended to diagnose and assess asthma severity by measuring airflow limitation and reversibility. Reversibility of airflow limitation is confirmed by measuring forced expiratory volume in one second (FEV_1) before and after **bronchodilator** use. Expiratory airflow limitation is confirmed when FEV_1/FVC< lower limit of age. The diagnostic pathway for asthma diagnosis in adults is outlined in figure 13.10.

Monitoring of PEF every morning and evening for 2–4 weeks can identify any variability in airflow limitation for diagnosis and monitoring. Greater than 10 per cent (great than 13 per cent in children) diurnal variation in PEF rate with twice-daily readings averaged for one week suggests a diagnosis of asthma (National Asthma Council Australia 2020).

COVID-19 and asthma

Systematic reviews have not shown an increased risk of COVID-19 in people with asthma (GINA 2020a). People with asthma should continue to use their inhaled asthma controller medications during the COVID-19 pandemic (GINA 2020a). Spirometry or PEF should not be performed on asthma patients who have symptoms consistent with COVID-19 (National Asthma Council Australia 2020). Nebulisers should not be used unless it is unavoidable. Pressurised metered-dose inhaler (puffer) and spacer with a tightly fitting face mask should be used, especially in children who cannot seal lips tightly around the mouthpiece. If nebulisation cannot be avoided, strict infection control measures must be followed. The patient should be in a negative pressure room if available. If not available and there is no alternative, use a single room with the door closed. Staff administering nebulisers should wear full PPE against airborne exposure (gloves, gowns, N95 or P2 masks and protective eyewear). These precautions should be maintained for at least 30 minutes after the nebuliser treatment.

FIGURE 13.10 Steps in the diagnosis of asthma in adults

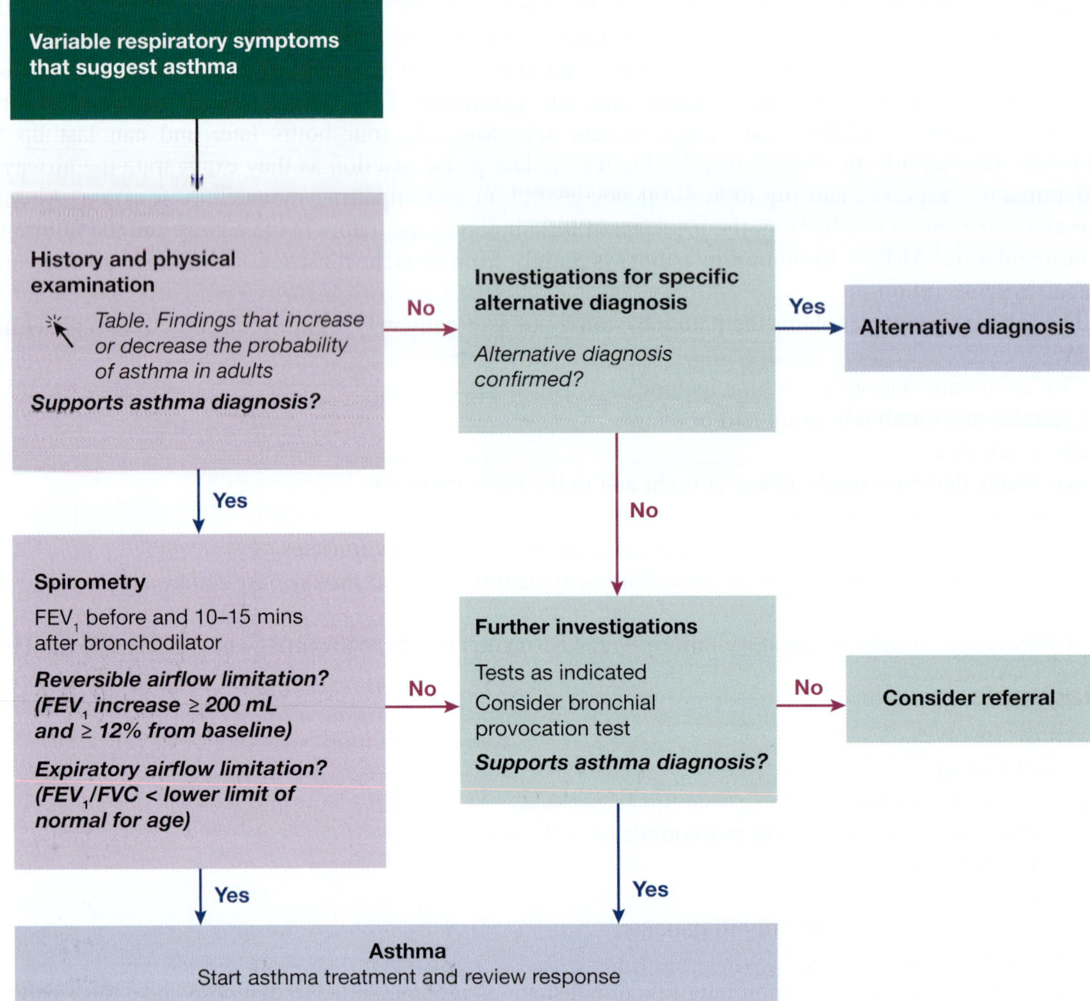

Source: National Asthma Council Australia (2020).

Nursing assessment and management

Assessment of the patient's clinical condition, level of control and risk of exacerbation are essential aspects of the nurse's role, including educating and supporting patients to manage their treatment.

A thorough history must be taken to identify trigger factors on the first visit. Questions should include lifestyle, smoking, occupation, medications, family history, exercise, medical conditions, etc. The patient or parent should be encouraged to keep a diary of asthma episodes to explore further if trigger factors could not be properly identified during the initial visit. Prevention should be the priority in asthma management; hence, trigger factors should be avoided by making lifestyle modifications, changing cleaning practices, pet care, etc.

In severe asthma attack episodes, the patient may need to be admitted to hospital for treatment. Continuous observation of respiratory rate and oxygen saturation is essential. Auscultation for adventitious lung sounds, such as **wheeze**, will help to monitor the effectiveness of treatment. The patient should be placed in a sitting position to facilitate breathing. Supplemental oxygen with a mask or nasal prong should be initiated and adjusted according to the patient's condition. Bronchodilators are given either as puffs or nebulisers. Patients should be educated about the correct use of puffers.

Please check the National Asthma Council Australia website for videos demonstrating the correct use of various types of inhalers www.nationalasthma.org.au/health-professionals/how-to-videos.

In severe cases, patients may need to be admitted to critical care units for advanced respiratory management. Such patient may need regular arterial blood gas analysis.

Shortness of breath in asthma is relieved by the use of medication as it is a reversible condition. Hence medications should be promptly restocked so they are readily available in asthma episodes. This is especially important for children. Teachers and care coordinators should be well aware of the asthma management plan for each child. Teachers and carers should be extra cautious when taking children for outdoor activities such as camping trips (exposure to triggers).

Asthma medication is categorised into two groups: **controllers** and relievers.

Controllers are usually anti-inflammatory medications taken daily on a long-term basis to maintain clinical control. Controllers include inhaled glucocorticosteroids taken alone or in combination with long-acting beta-2-agonists. Secondary agents, including anti-leukotrienes and glucocorticosteroids, can be used in addition if necessary. Glucocorticosteroids work by reducing oedema and airway spasm. Anti-leukotrienes work by blocking the action of leukotrienes, which attract inflammatory-promoting eosinophils to the airway mucosa.

Relievers or rapidly acting beta2-agonists are bronchodilator medications that stimulate beta-adrenergic receptors to dilate the airways. Beta2-agonists are taken on an as-needed basis to reverse the bronchoconstriction and relieve symptoms. Ideally, relievers should not be required if the asthma is well controlled. Increased use of reliever medication is a sign of deteriorating control and increased inflammation.

Asthma treatment can be administered in inhaled, oral or injectable forms. The wide range of inhaler devices allows greater choice in meeting patients' preferences and maximising adherence to treatment. However, all inhalers require coordination, training and skill for effective use. Poor inhaler technique results in inadequate delivery of medication to the airways and increased deposition of medication in the mouth, resulting in poor symptom control. Deposition of glucocorticoids in the mouth can also lead to oral candidiasis.

Guidelines for the management of exacerbations of asthma provide a step-wise management program based on the symptoms and the response to beta2-agonists, involving a combination of controllers and relievers to relieve the symptoms and reduce inflammation (see www.ginasthma.org for up-to-date international management guidelines).

Self-management is extremely important; hence nurses should educate patients on managing the condition at home as part of discharge planning. Patient education should include identifying and avoiding trigger factors, symptom monitoring, inhaler technique, treatment adherence as per the individualised management plan, and regular follow-ups. It is essential to educate not only the patient but the family members as well. Immediate medical management should be sought if the patient is experiencing severe breathing problems, rapid worsening of symptoms, little or no effect of reliever medication, difficulty saying sentences, blue lips, drowsiness, etc. Parents should be advised on maintaining proper oral health of children to reduce the risk of dental caries (with inhaled beta2-agonists) and oropharyngeal candidiasis (with inhaled corticosteroids). Rinsing and spitting after using these inhaler medications via the oral route should be practised.

Effective management relies on developing a partnership between the patient and the healthcare professional; knowledge, skills and self-care confidence are essential to this partnership (GINA 2020b). Guided self management reduces asthma morbidity (GINA 2020b) and features:

- education
- joint goal-setting
- regular review
- a written action plan
- self-monitoring.

By demonstrating and checking, the nurse must ensure that all patients use their inhalers correctly as poor inhaler technique is associated with deteriorating asthma. It is important to regularly check the inhaler and PEF technique in the ward, clinic and emergency department. Information on inhaler devices and techniques is also provided on the GINA website (www.ginasthma.org).

A guided self-management can reduce morbidity with a personalised written asthma action plan to adjust the treatment in response to changes in asthma control (GINA 2020b).

Chronic obstructive pulmonary disease (COPD)

Chronic obstructive pulmonary disease (COPD) is a preventable and treatable disease presenting with persistent respiratory symptoms such as dyspnoea, cough and airflow limitation due to airway and or alveolar abnormalities usually caused by noxious particles or gases, especially cigarette smoke (Global Initiative for Chronic Obstructive Disease [GOLD] 2020). Other risk factors include exposure to significant air pollutants.

The main risk factors for COPD include:

- age (COPD is more common as people age)
- genetic predisposition
- lower socioeconomic status
- tobacco and marijuana smoke
- occupational exposure to dust, chemicals and fumes
- air pollution (indoor and outdoor)
- alpha-1-antitrypsin deficiency
- asthma and airway hypersensitivity
- any factor affecting lung growth during gestation and childhood (GOLD 2020) e.g. smoking during pregnancy affects lung growth and development in utero, increasing COPD risk for the child.

COPD is characterised by airflow obstruction that is not fully reversible and is usually progressive. In Australia, COPD was the fifth leading cause of death in 2018 (AIHW 2020b). The prevalence of COPD among Indigenous Australians was 2.3 times higher than non-Indigenous Australians after adjusting for age (AIHW 2020b).

COPD is a treatable and preventable disease that is also associated with extrapulmonary effects that can, in some patients, contribute to the severity of their condition. The extrapulmonary effects of COPD include weight loss, skeletal muscle dysfunction and nutritional abnormalities. In addition, COPD is associated with an increased risk of myocardial infarction and angina, osteoporosis, anxiety and depression, respiratory infections, lung cancer, diabetes and anaemia (GOLD 2020). The two main conditions associated with COPD are chronic **bronchitis** and **emphysema** (Bullock & Hales 2019).

The Global Initiative for Chronic Obstructive Disease (GOLD) classified COPD into four stages reflecting the degree of severity — mild, moderate, severe and very severe — with the FEV_1 ranging from 80 per cent or more to less than 30 per cent. Although mild COPD generally remains undiagnosed, severe and very severe COPD have a significant impact on quality of life, with fatigue and frequent exacerbations commonplace. Very severe COPD may also involve respiratory and cardiac failure with life-threatening exacerbations (GOLD 2020).

Pathophysiology

COPD pathophysiology can be explained on the basis of two discrete conditions: chronic bronchitis and emphysema.

Bronchitis is inflammation of the bronchi causing shortness of breath, cough and increased mucus production. When these symptoms persist for more than three months to a year over a period of two consecutive years, it is classified as chronic bronchitis (Bullock & Hales 2019). Increased mucus production, decreased ciliary function to clear the secretion and, most importantly, inflammation of the bronchial lining are the main pathophysiological changes in chronic bronchitis. The normal ciliated pseudostratified columnar epithelium is frequently replaced by patchy squamous metaplasia as a consequence of the chronic inflammation. Mucociliary clearance function is diminished due to the absence of normal ciliated epithelium and an increase in mucus secretion due to hyperplasia of mucosal glands. These pathological changes can be arrested but not reversed following smoking cessation.

Emphysema is a disease of the lung parenchyma. Destruction of terminal respiratory units, loss of alveolar capillary bed and loss of elastic containing connective tissue are three important physiological changes occurring in emphysema. Smoking activates alveolar proteases and elastases. These enzymes can digest the alveolar walls decreasing the area for gas exchange and, in late stages, contribute to the loss of capillary network. This also damages the elastic fibres of distal airways and results in the premature collapse of these airways during exhalation causing gas to trap within the alveoli.

Inflammation, fibrosis (structural changes) and exudate in small airways correlate with a reduced FEV_1 and FEV_1/FVC ratio, while destruction of the lung tissue results in decreased gas transfer. As a consequence of destruction at the alveolar level and loss of airway recoil, air trapping occurs, resulting in hyperinflation — abnormal gas exchange results in hypoxaemia and hypercapnia. Hypoxic vasoconstriction of the small pulmonary arteries can result in the development of pulmonary hypertension late in COPD.

Clinical manifestations of COPD include:

- increasing breathlessness
- a breathing pattern that involves a long expiration phase using pursed lips
- a prolonged forced expiratory phase may extend to longer than five seconds in advanced disease
- an increased use of the accessory muscles during respiration

- the patient visibly leaning forward
- cough with production of sputum
- a wheeze
- weight loss
- fatigue
- hyperinflation of the lungs and a 'barrel-shaped' chest
- **Hoover's sign** (flattening of the diaphragm and pulling in of the lower ribs on inspiration)
- jugular vein distension, liver enlargement and peripheral oedema indicating right-sided heart failure associated with pulmonary hypertension.

Diagnosis

Investigations for diagnosis can include the following.

- Chest X-ray — findings include increased lung volume with relatively depressed diaphragm consistent with hyperinflation; cardiac size may be increased, suggesting right heart volume overload (Sisson, Claar, Chesnutt & Prendergast 2019).
- A CT scan is not routinely recommended, but it may be required in some cases for differential diagnosis where concomitant diseases are present.
- Pulmonary function test — FEV_1, FVC and the FEV_1/FVC ratio reduced.
- Arterial blood gas analysis — hypoxaemia and hypercapnia present.
- Blood investigation — elevated haematocrit because of chronic hypoxaemia.
- Alpha-1 antitrypsin deficiency (AATD) screening.
- Exercise testing (e.g. paced shuttle walk).
- The BODE (body mass index, obstruction, dyspnoea and exercise) method — measures the severity of the disease condition and is a better predictor of survival than any single component (GOLD 2020).

Nursing assessment and management

Assessment is aimed at determining the level of airflow limitation, its impact on patient health status and the risk of future events such as exacerbations, hospital admission or death. Proper assessment and documentation of symptoms are essential. Various symptom measurement tools such as Modified British Medical Council Questionnaire, Chronic respiratory questionnaire, St. George's respiratory questionnaire, COPD assessment test and the COPD control questionnaire are all used in measuring symptoms of COPD.

The overall aim of COPD management is to relieve symptoms, assess severity, improve exercise capacity and health status, prevent disease progression, and prevent and treat complications and exacerbations (GOLD 2020). Bronchodilator medications form the basis of symptom relief and improvement of exercise tolerance. Commonly used medications in COPD include short- and long-acting beta2-agonists, anticholinergic agents, methylxanthines, phosphodiesterase-4 inhibitors and mucolytic agents. Beta2-agonists relax the airway's smooth muscle resulting in bronchodilation. Regular and as-needed use of short acting beta2-agonists (SABA) improves FEV_1 and symptoms (GOLD 2020). Inhalation treatment is preferred both for its effectiveness and to minimise side effects. Long-term inhaled anticholinergics reduce the rate of exacerbations and improve the effectiveness of **pulmonary rehabilitation**. Regular assessment of inhaler technique is essential.

An acute exacerbation of COPD is identified by an increase in respiratory symptoms beyond everyday variations that possibly requires hospitalisation (GOLD 2020). Antibiotic therapy is usually prescribed as well as a course of oral corticosteroids to reduce inflammation. However, this has to be balanced against the risk of complications from their regular use. Oxygen therapy is indicated for hypoxaemia management (oxygen saturation of over 90 per cent is acceptable). ABG analysis is essential to detect carbon dioxide retention. Rapid assessment units, early discharge and hospital-at-home programs are increasingly being developed to support the treatment of patients with acute exacerbations at home.

A care plan for the nursing assessment and management of COPD is shown in table 13.7.

TABLE 13.7 **COPD care plan**

Assessment and management	Action	Outcome
Dyspnoea	Monitoring of respiratory rate and pattern, oximetry, mental state and orientation	Prompt recognition of and response to deteriorating respiratory function, anxiety and distress

(continued)

TABLE 13.7 *(continued)*

Assessment and management	Action	Outcome
	Positioning the patient in an upright position	An upright position enables breathing
	Spirometry	Establishes respiratory function status
	Administering medication	Inhaled or nebulised bronchodilators relax bronchial smooth muscle
	Monitoring inhaler and nebuliser technique	Ensure optimum deposition of medication and minimise unwanted side effects such as tremor and tachycardia
Oxygenation saturation	Oximetry	Prompt recognition of and response to desaturation
	Monitoring ABGs	Prompt recognition and treatment of hypoxemia and carbon dioxide retention
	Administering oxygen therapy as prescribed when saturation is <90%	Avoidance of suppression of respiratory drive
Cough and mucous clearance	Encouraging an effective coughing technique	Effective clearance while conserving energy
	Encouraging fluid intake	Adequate hydration to help thin secretions
	Oral care	Removal of mucus deposits in the mouth
Anxiety	Remaining with the patient who is experiencing increased dyspnoea	Minimising anxiety and its effects on an increasing sense of breathlessness
		Reduction in risk of panic attacks associated with severe dyspnoea
	Enhancing the environmental impact on dyspnoea-related anxiety: provide care in a calm and reassuring manner; reduce the impact of noise; position the patient near a window or door if possible	Minimise the sense of suffocation and feeling of being trapped in an enclosed area
	Encouraging deep breathing and relaxation exercises	Enhance self-care
Activity and exercise tolerance, fatigue	Monitoring dyspnoea and oxygenation	Prompt recognition of and response to activity-related desaturation
		Conservation of energy
	Planning exercise activity, increasing exercise tolerance and returning to the (pre-exacerbation) baseline activities of daily living	Synchronisation of exercise with administration of medication for maximum benefit
	Seeking physiotherapy support	Redress and improve exercise tolerance and management of dyspnoea
	Assisting patients with a gradual return towards (pre-exacerbation) baseline activities of daily living	Minimise loss of overall health status and independence
	Supporting and teaching the patient about energy conservation through pacing activities, alternating high and low-energy activities; pursed-lip breathing	Minimise loss of overall health status and independence while also enhancing self-care in the longer term
	Support patient to identify priorities	Energy is focused on priorities

Nutritional status	Monitoring the patient's weight	Prompt recognition of and response to changes in both fluid retention and nutritional status Small frequent meals is better tolerated as it prevents breathlessness associated with full stomach
	Seeking the nutritionist's support	Dietary support in terms of high-protein and low-carbohydrate meals
Emotional, social and psychological wellbeing	Opening a conversation with the patient and carer about illness experiences	Prompt recognition of and response to signs of depression; address fears and concerns about the future
	Providing information on community support groups	Help to minimise the risk of increased social isolation
	Seeking an occupational therapist, social worker and/or psychologist for information and support	Optimisation of the capacity to self-care and remain independent; ensuring access to social benefits and supports
Palliative care needs	Communication — prognosis and fears	Open communication between the patient, family and carers
	Providing a supportive environment	The patient and family feel supported
	Establishing priorities	The patient and family focus on the patient's identified priorities
	Establishing a plan for advanced care, use of opiates and ventilation	Patients' and families' wishes in relation to management are adhered to where possible

Bronchiectasis

Bronchiectasis is an obstructive lung condition in which there is destruction and widening of the large airways and abnormal bronchial wall thickening due to a recurring cycle of infection and inflammation. Bronchiectasis is usually localised to one lung segment or lobe but may spread over time to other parts of the same lung as a result of unresolved infections. Exacerbations are associated with infections.

Pathophysiology

Bronchiectasis is associated with airway epithelial remodelling characterised by mucus cell metaplasia and decreased ciliated cell (Barker & Brody 2015). There is intense infiltration of the bronchial wall with neutrophils, lymphocytes and monocytes. Affected bronchi show polypoidal appearance due to underlying granuloma formation and lymphoid [illegible] smooth muscle hypertrophy and plugging due to dilated mucus glands.

Several conditions lead to bronchiectasis, including infection, bronchial obstruction caused by tumour, enlarged lymph nodes etc., aspiration/inhalation airway injury, CF, primary ciliary dyskinesia, alpha-1 antitrypsin deficiency, allergic bronchopulmonary aspergillosis, inflammatory disorders such as rheumatoid arthritis, chronic ulcerative colitis and immune deficiency diseases (Barker & Brody 2015).

Signs and symptoms include:

- a productive cough
- breathlessness with chest pain
- increased sputum production, possibly with haemoptysis
- fatigue
- clubbing of the fingers in severe cases.

Diagnosis

Diagnosis of bronchiectasis will involve:

- chest X-ray
- high-resolution CT
- spirometry and demonstration of a reduced FEV_1 and reduced FEV_1/FVC ratio
- sputum for microscopic culture and sensitivity study.

Nursing assessment and management

Management of bronchiectasis is directed at infection control, improvement in secretion clearance and bronchial hygiene. Antibiotics are prescribed depending on the type of pathogen identified. Hydration, mucolytic administration, bronchodilators, chest physiotherapy and hyperosmolar agents are all used to enhance secretion clearance. Anti-inflammatory therapy using glucocorticoids may be used depending on the aetiology responsible for bronchiectasis.

Management is similar to that of COPD; however, the main aim is to facilitate the clearance of secretions to improve breathing. Hence chest physiotherapy should be performed on patients to help with mucus clearance. Humidified oxygen and/or air should be used to prevent the drying of the mucosa. The patient should be sufficiently hydrated with oral and or intravenous fluids to prevent sputum retention.

Cystic fibrosis

Cystic fibrosis (CF) is a life-threatening, inherited multisystem disease that results from a genetic mutation of the CF transmembrane conductance regulator (CFTR) protein found in epithelial surface of the airways, pancreatic and sweat gland ducts. In Australia, one in 2500 babies are born with CF each year (Cystic Fibrosis 2020).

Pathophysiology

Defective CFTR mainly affects chloride ion transport from the cells. This results in decreased chloride secretion and increased reabsorption of sodium and water, causing the mucus to become thick and eventually diminishing ciliary movement. Mucociliary dysfunction encourages bacterial colonisation, infection and initiation of the inflammatory process (Bullock & Hales 2019). Structural damage to the parenchyma occurs due to the release of antiprotease chemicals by neutrophils. *Pseudomonas aeruginosa* and *Staphylococcus aureus* are the most common pathogens causing infection in CF in Australasia (Bullock & Hales 2019). The abnormal gene is subject to autosomal recessive inheritance. Parents who are carriers of CF have a 25 per cent chance of having a child with CF with each pregnancy. Dyspnoea, tachypnoea, paroxysmal cough, wheezing, mucoid or purulent rhinorrhoea or sputum and nasal obstruction are some of the common respiratory clinical manifestations. Digital clubbing due to hypoxia is a late sign of CF.

Other common clinical manifestations include:

- a positive sweat test (Pilocarpine iontophoresis test showing high chloride in sweat)
- typically, a patient who is small in stature and underweight, and has finger clubbing
- failure to thrive in infants
- steatorrhoea
- respiratory symptoms
- infertility in males.

Watch this video which explains the pathophysiology of CF: www.youtube.com/watch?v=6IbP1ASGv9w

Diagnosis

Diagnostic tools used in the diagnosis of CF include:

- chest X-ray and CT scan
- pulmonary function test
- newborn screening — neonatal blood spot to determine the concentration of immunoreactive trypsinogen (Voynow, Mascarenhas, Kelly & Scanlin 2015).

Nursing assessment and management

As a consequence of the multisystem involvement, patients require management of gastrointestinal, pancreatic and hepatic complications in addition to respiratory problems. Poor secretion clearance from the airways results in recurrent infections, damage to the bronchi, the development of bronchiectasis and respiratory failure. With bronchiectasis and as a result of exacerbations, there is progressive scarring of the lungs and colonisation with pathogens. The respiratory tract is colonised with bacteria that must frequently be treated with combinations of antibiotics. Management of exacerbations requires a microbiologist's involvement to explore treatment options as antibiotic resistance is a significant challenge.

Treatment with mucolytic agents such as N-acetylcysteine effectively dissolves mucin components and reduces the viscosity of sputum. Inhaled hypertonic saline therapy may help in airway surface hydration and improve airway clearance (Voynow, Mascarenhas, Kelly & Scanlin 2015). Bronchodilators and anti-inflammatory agents are used in the treatment of CF. Their use should be individualised as some patients experience deterioration in lung function following the use of bronchodilators.

A specialist multidisciplinary CF team should provide care, but where this is not possible, a shared care approach involving specialist team support is necessary. Historically, CF was a disease of childhood. However, over the past decade, early diagnosis and significant advances in treatment have resulted in more patients surviving early adulthood. Consequently, new challenges have emerged in terms of care transition from paediatric to adult care and the emerging complications of CF, including diabetes, in adult life.

The patient's nutritional status should be checked regularly, as should their weight, to calculate BMI. Calories may need to be increased in patients with chronic lung disease. For aggressive nutritional rehabilitation, nocturnal nasogastric feeds may be required for short term management. Patients with feeding intolerance and poor weight gain from standard formula may benefit from hydrolysed formulas. Pancreatic enzyme doses may be required in some cases. This usually comes in enteric-coated capsules and contains amylases, proteases and lipases. Patients with pancreatic insufficiency are also at increased risk of fat-soluble vitamin deficiency; hence vitamin D supplementation may be needed if levels are low. A high-energy, high-protein diet is a cornerstone of CF management. As respiratory symptoms increase with the loss of lung function, intensive nutritional support is needed. Physiotherapy support for help with airway clearance, maintenance of exercise capacity and management of dyspnoea is a key component of care in CF.

CF patients are prone to infection, and strict infection control measures should be followed by avoiding visiting infected people and environments and vaccinating against respiratory infections such as influenza. Nurses should practice reverse barrier precaution when caring for CF patients. Sharing of equipment should be avoided, and patients should be cared for in a single room if possible.

When respiratory failure and end-stage lung disease develop, patients are assessed for lung transplant, but many do not meet the criteria. Patients approaching end-stage disease experience loss of lung function and oxygen dependency, and may require NIV.

The emotional, social and financial wellbeing of the patient and family should be part of holistic management. Patient and family should be referred to appropriate support groups to deal with some of these issues. Young adults with CF may have difficulty forming intimate relationships due to body image disturbances, decreased mobility and lack of opportunity to meet suitable partners. Patient's should be educated about reproductive issues such as male infertility, genetic inheritance of CF etc. Genetic counselling may be needed for couples considering having children. Premature death of a carrier parent is a real possibility, and hence this should be part of the discussion. Advocacy, support and education, assessment and the transition from paediatric to adult care are some of the important roles of nurses in CF management.

The Cystic Fibrosis Australia website (cysticfibrosis.org.au) has important resources to maintain psychological health and build resilience for both patients and caregivers. Cystic Fibrosis Foundation is another useful website (www.cff.org/Life-With-CF/Daily-Life/Emotional-Wellness/Coping-While-Carin g-for-Someone-With-Cystic-Fibrosis).

Respiratory failure

When the lungs fail to maintain sufficient arterial oxygenation or carbon dioxide elimination, respiratory failure can occur. Respiratory failure is defined as a PaO_2 <8 kPa (<60 mmHg) or a $PaCO_2$ >7 kPa (>55 mmHg).

Pathophysiology

Carbon dioxide retention from insufficient ventilation results in hypercapnia or respiratory **acidaemia** — the $PaCO_2$ rise above the normal limits of 35–45 mmHg. Low amounts of carbon dioxide as a result of hyperventilation result in hypocapnia or respiratory **alkalaemia**.

Respiratory failure may be type I (hypoxaemic) respiratory failure or type II (hypercapnic) respiratory failure (table 13.8). In type I respiratory failure, hypoxaemia is present, but there is no associated hypercapnia. This may be caused by a reduction in inspired oxygen pressure (high altitude), hypoventilation, impaired diffusion or ventilation-perfusion mismatch. Type I respiratory failure occurs in clinical settings such as sepsis, gastric aspiration, pneumonia, near-drowning, multiple blood transfusion and pancreatitis (Kress & Hall 2018). In type II failure, both hypoxaemia and hypercapnia are present. This failure is caused by alveolar hypoventilation, where the respiratory effort is not sufficient to allow the adequate exchange of oxygen and carbon dioxide. This may be caused by a condition that affects respiratory drive, such as neuromuscular disease (Guillain-Barré syndrome), chest wall trauma, severe airway diseases (e.g. asthma or COPD) and medications such as opiates.

TABLE 13.8 Respiratory failure and ABG values

ABG parameter	Normal values	Values in type I respiratory failure	Values in type II respiratory failure
pH	7.35–7.45	7.35–7.45	<7.35–7.45
PaO_2	12–14 kPa	<8 kPa	<8 kPa
$PaCO_2$	4.6–6.0 kPa	4.6–6.0 kPa	>6 kPa
SaO_2	>95%	<92%	<92%

Nursing assessment and management

Nursing care needs to include observations with a particular emphasis on respiration and the signs of hypoxaemia and hypercapnia, mentation, the ability to tolerate an increased work of breathing, ABGs and oxygen saturation levels. The management of dyspnoea, airway clearance and impaired gas exchange are essential. Administration of bronchodilators, corticosteroids, **diuretics** and possibly opiates and anxiolytics should be as prescribed.

Type I respiratory failure is managed by oxygen therapy and treatment of the underlying condition. The concentration of prescribed oxygen varies from patient to patient but may be as high as 60–100 per cent. However, oxygen therapy should be reduced as the patient shows clinical improvement.

Type II respiratory failure may develop over some time. These patients may have developed compensatory mechanisms for hypercapnia. Patients' respiratory drive depends on their degree of hypoxia rather than the usual dependence on hypercapnia.

Thus, in type II respiratory failure, oxygen must be used with caution and is usually commenced at low levels of 24–28 per cent. Monitoring of ABG analysis is important in type II respiratory failure and guides the titration of oxygen therapy.

The use of medications depends on the underlying cause of respiratory failure. Medications commonly prescribed in respiratory failure include steroids, bronchodilators, antibiotics and analgesics. NIV is preferred over invasive ventilation to treat acute respiratory failure in patients hospitalised for acute exacerbation of COPD (GOLD 2020).

COVID-19

Since COVID-19 is a recent phenomenon, the information presented here should be treated with caution, as knowledge of this disease is constantly evolving.

Pathophysiology

COVID-19 (coronavirus disease 2019) is caused by coronavirus from the betacoronavirus family (Chu et al. 2020). It is closely related to the SARS-CoV-1 virus responsible for the 2004 SARS epidemic and has therefore been named severe acute respiratory syndrome coronavirus 2 (SARS-CoV-2).

The COVID-19 virus has surface receptors that attach to the ACE2 receptor on human epithelial cells in the mouth, nose and airways. Humans are infected by contact with surfaces or aerosol droplets. During the first week of infection, symptoms are relatively mild, typically sore throat, cough and fever, and smell and taste alterations. Some carriers, especially children, may be asymptomatic. Virus shedding appears to peak 24 to 48 hours before symptom onset. Hence pre-symptomatic transmission is likely to occur, complicating efforts to prevent or control the spread of infection. The risk of COVID-19 increases with age. Other risk factors include chronic kidney disease, COPD, type 2 diabetes, obesity, smoking, severe cardiac conditions, sickle cell disease, etc. Residents of nursing homes and long-term care facilities are also at high risk of acquiring the infection. Complications of the disease include acute respiratory distress syndrome, septic shock, acute kidney injury, myocardial injury, multiorgan failure, thrombotic events and Guillain-Barré Syndrome. There are numerous variants of SARS-CoV-2 circulating globally.

Watch this video which explains the structure of COVID-19: www.youtube.com/watch?v=GQUCCkI1NjN8 — Video resource: Viral structure & Pathogenesis

Diagnosis

Diagnosis of COVID-19 requires the following investigations:

- PCR test of upper respiratory tract specimen
- antigen testing only for emergency use (these tests are less sensitive than PCR)
- chest X-ray
- CT scan
- ultrasonography.

Nursing assessment and management

There are not enough data to suggest an effective treatment of COVID-19 with particular medications. Remdesivir is a commonly used antiviral medication to treat hospitalised patients. Antiviral and monoclonal antibodies may be effective when used early in the course of infection. Casirivimab and imdevimab are two recombinant human monoclonal antibodies. Combining these two drugs blocks the binding of the receptor-binding domain of SARS-CoV-2 to the host cell. This combination may be used in patients with mild to moderate COVID-19 who are at high risk of progressing to severe disease and or hospitalisation (Grishaw 2020). Corticosteroids such as dexamethasone may be helpful for hospitalised patients who require supplemental therapy. Patients may require oxygen via a high-flow device, NIV, mechanical ventilation or extra-corporeal membrane oxygen, depending on hypoxaemia severity.

COVID-19 vaccines are now available. The Pfizer-BioNTech COVID-19 vaccine is a lipid nanoparticle formulated, nucleoside-modified mRNA vaccine encoding the prefusion spike glycoprotein of SARS-CoV-2. This vaccine is administered in two separate intramuscular doses 21 days apart. The AstraZeneca vaccine is also given as two intramuscular doses 28 days apart. Moderna's COVID-19 vaccine is also available. This vaccine is also administered in two intramuscular doses, one month apart.

Please check the Agency for Clinical Innovation website for more information about vaccines: https://aci.health.nsw.gov.au/covid-19/critical-intelligence-unit/covid-19-vaccines

Lung cancer

Lung cancer refers to malignancies that originate in the airways or pulmonary parenchyma. It is the most common cause of cancer-related death worldwide. Lung cancer is associated with late diagnosis and poor prognosis.

Tobacco smoking is the most important modifiable risk for lung cancer (Dela Cruz, Tanoue & Matthay 2015). Other factors that play an important role in lung cancer risk include underlying acquired lung disease, such as COPD or pulmonary fibrosis and environmental exposure to agents such as asbestos and radiation.

Symptoms of lung cancer include cough, haemoptysis, chest pain and/or shortness of breath. Breathlessness may be a consequence of airflow obstruction or pleural effusion. More general symptoms include weight loss and fatigue. Symptoms of metastatic lung cancer depend on the site(s) of metastasis. Haemoptysis in lung cancer is associated with vascular invasion by the tumour. Breathlessness may be accompanied by stridor due to the tumour pressing on the trachea or main bronchi. Chest pain may typically be central and persistent.

Diagnosis

A chest X-ray or CT scan is indicated for patients with suspicious symptoms such as haemoptysis, persistent central chest pain, hoarseness or stridor.

Diagnostic procedures include:

- bronchoscopy
- sputum analysis
- cytology
- positron emission tomography
- CT-guided biopsy
- mediastinoscopy
- autofluorescence bronchoscopy.

Nursing assessment and management

Nursing management should focus on the patient's understanding of the diagnosis and treatment options and respond to the support needs for coping with what is often devastating news and complex information. Once a diagnosis of lung cancer has been confirmed, the patient faces uncertainty, and possibly extensive and radical medical treatment, with all its intended and unintended consequences.

Therefore, nursing assessment is of significant importance in developing a care plan that can anticipate needs and offer support. Symptoms of dyspnoea, recurrent infection, fatigue, pain and weight loss should be explored with the patient. Family history, smoking and occupational history should be recorded. Assessment and care should determine the available support at home and in the community for dealing with the condition and its effects in the short, medium and longer term, including the effects of treatment regimens.

Patients with small cell lung cancer are treated with chemotherapy in combination with thoracic radiotherapy. Patients with non-small cell lung cancer may be assessed for surgical resection followed by chemotherapy. Immune checkpoint inhibitors used alone or in combination with chemotherapy could be effective. Bronchoscopic laser therapy, photodynamic therapy and airway stenting are some of the treatment modalities used in lung cancer. Palliative radiotherapy may also be offered for symptom relief.

Early involvement of the palliative care team facilitates communication and the exploration of treatment options with the patient and family while also enabling a discussion about advanced care planning and discussion about the patient's fears.

13.6 Common nursing interventions to improve oxygenation and prevent respiratory complications

LEARNING OBJECTIVE 13.6 Explain the common nursing interventions for respiratory conditions.

Positioning

Positioning can help patients to maximise their lung function. The high side-lying position facilitates maximum lung expansion while the patient in bed (figure 13.11a). The tripod position (figure 13.11b) increases the potential for thoracic expansion with minimal effort; in this, the patient leans forward with their arms on a table. Chest clearance can be enhanced with the use of postural drainage. Relaxed sitting (figure 13.11c), forward-lean standing (figure 13.11d) and relaxed standing against a wall (figure 13.11e) also provide support for the body by minimising the use of postural muscles and reducing oxygen requirements. Alternating positions in critically ill and immobile patients can help to prevent and treat atelectasis and pneumonia.

FIGURE 13.11 Optimal positions to reduce breathing effort

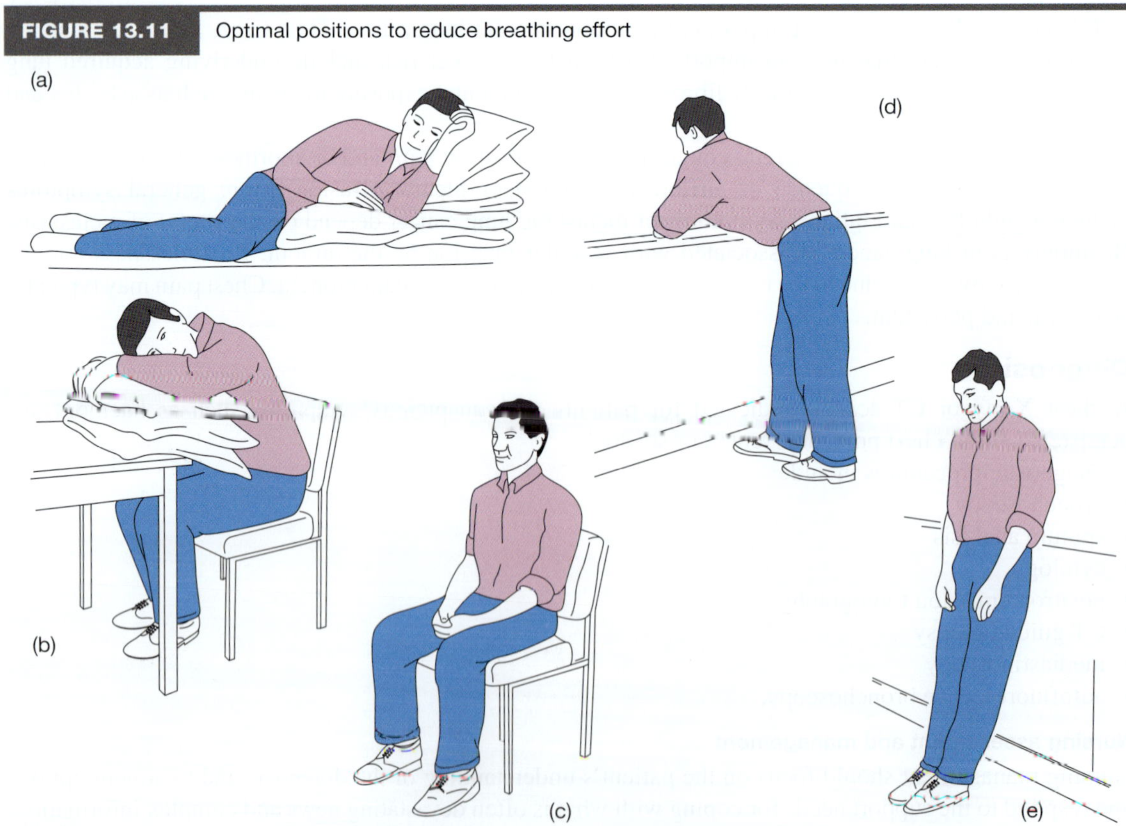

Source: Dougherty & Lister (2011) *The Royal Marsden Hospital Manual of Clinical Nursing Procedures*, with kind permission from Wiley Blackwell.

Oxygen administration

Oxygen can be administered via a nasal cannula (figure 13.12), oxygen mask (figure 13.13) or mask with Venturi valve (figure 13.14) to enhance the amount of oxygen delivered to the tissues. Oxygen can be humidified to offset its drying effects and loosen secretions. This is particularly useful for patients with tenacious sputum. Showers and baths or steam inhalation in the home setting also help to liquefy secretions, aiding expectoration. Nebulisers can be used to moisten the air and deliver medications to the respiratory tract.

FIGURE 13.12 Nasal cannula

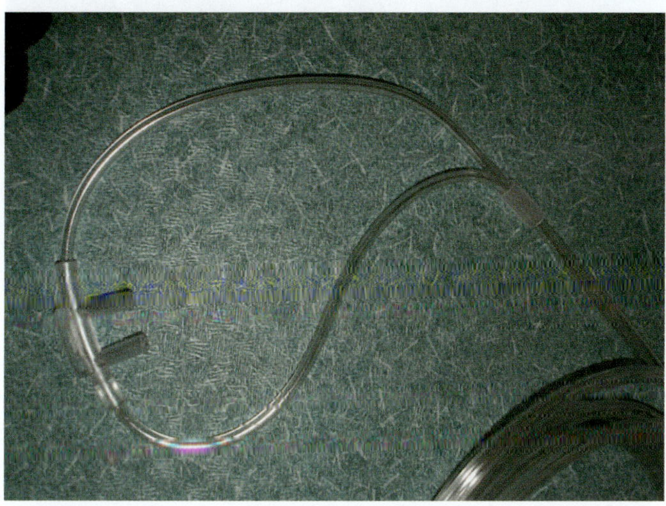

Source: Dougherty & Lister (2011) *The Royal Marsden Hospital Manual of Clinical Nursing Procedures*, with kind permission from Wiley Blackwell.

FIGURE 13.13 Oxygen mask

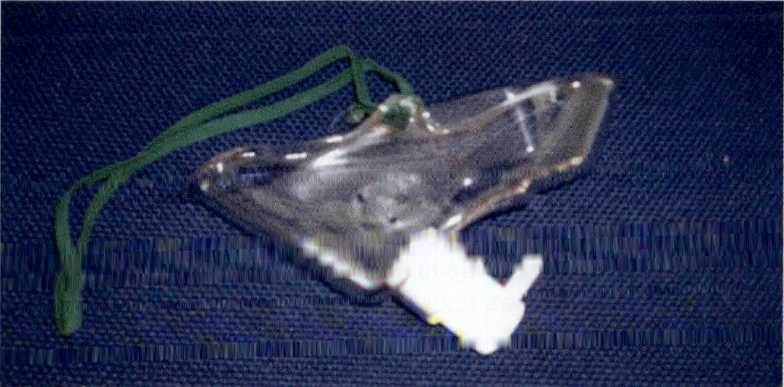

Source: Dougherty & Lister (2011) *The Royal Marsden Hospital Manual of Clinical Nursing Procedures*, with kind permission from Wiley Blackwell.

Prolonged exposure to high concentrations of oxygen can result in oxygen toxicity. Presence of excess highly reactive oxygen free radicals (ROS) such as superoxide (O_2^-), hydrogen peroxide (H_2O_2) and the hydroxyl radical (OH^-) are responsible for oxygen toxicity. When there is an imbalance between ROS and antioxidant defences, it may result in either adaptation or cellular injury and cell death. Clinical manifestations of oxygen toxicity include substernal distress (ache or burning sensation behind the sternum), respiratory distress with decreased vital capacity, nausea, vomiting, restlessness, tremors, twitching, paraesthesias, convulsions and a dry, hacking cough. Excessive oxygen supplied to preterm infants to treat respiratory distress syndrome can cause blindness. Hence oxygen therapy should be titrated according to targeted saturation level, and oxygen should be discontinued once the patient's condition is stabilised.

FIGURE 13.14 Mask with Venturi valve

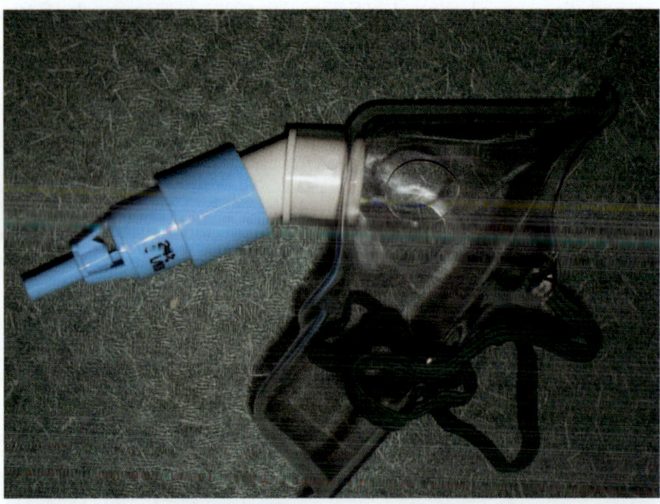

Source: Dougherty & Lister (2011) *The Royal Marsden Hospital Manual of Clinical Nursing Procedures*, with kind permission from Wiley Blackwell.

Breathing exercises

Breathing exercises help patients to manage their breathlessness and maximise the amount of oxygen delivered to the tissues. Pursed-lip breathing, in which the lips are pursed on exhalation to slow breathing, prevents airway collapse in emphysema. Practising huffing and coughing clear lung secretions. Incentive spirometry can be used to increase inspiratory volume and induce coughing.

Mobilisation and exercise

Mobilisation, especially early mobilisation following surgery, is essential in maximising chest clearance. A passive range of movement exercises will stimulate deep breathing and effectively reduce atelectasis and respiratory tract infections in immobile patients.

CASE STUDY 13.1

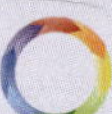

Nursing care of a child with chest pain

Archie, a 10-year-old boy, was brought in to the emergency department with respiratory distress. He was diagnosed with asthma at the age of nine. His mother reports that he developed nasal congestion, cough and sore throat 24 hours prior. Over the past 2 hours, Archie has complained of chest pain and has been breathing rapidly. His mother administered a dose of albuterol and another dose 5 minutes later with no improvement. He appears drowsy and uses accessory muscles to breathe. Faint inspiratory wheeze is heard on chest auscultation.

Vital signs taken in the emergency department are:

- temperature: 38.4°C
- blood pressure: 120/70 mmHg
- heart rate: 120 beats per minute
- respiratory rate: 40 breaths per minute
- oxygen saturation: 88% on 10 litres of oxygen via non-rebreather mask
- Glasgow Coma Scale: 13 E4V4M5
- capillary refill: 4 to 6 seconds.

Question

Using the information above, describe what action you would take as the nurse caring for this patient. Use the clinical reasoning cycle to guide you through the process and devise a care plan for your patient.

Answer

- *Step 1: Consider the patient*. Archie is a 10-year-old boy. Since he is a paediatric patient, it is important to consider the family while caring for the patient.
- *Step 2: Collect cues/information*. Include subjective and objective data here. Include the appearance of the patient, investigation results and their past medical history (asthma). Objective data will include

measurable information such as vital signs. Subjective data include nasal congestion, sore throat, cough, chest pain.

- *Step 3: Process information.* Separate the relevant and irrelevant data — cluster the clues together to formulate an inference about the patient.
- *Step 4: Identify problems/issues*. Impaired gas exchange, as evidenced by low oxygen saturation. Ineffective breathing, as evidenced by tachypnoea and use of accessory muscles. Impaired tissue perfusion, as evidenced by capillary refill (4–6 seconds). Impaired haemodynamic status, as evidenced by tachycardia and poor capillary refill. Suspected infection, as evidenced by high temperature.
- *Step 5: Establish goals.* Improving oxygenation and haemodynamic status should be the priority as Archie's condition is critical.
- *Step 6: Take action*. Archie is in imminent danger of cardiac arrest; hence the medical emergency team should be called immediately. The nurse should initiate interventions to relieve dyspnoea, such as sitting the patient upright, administering bronchodilators, continuously using a nebuliser and providing high-flow oxygen. Prepare for advanced airway management. Place arrest trolley close to the patient. Dedicate a staff member to update the family about what is happening at the bedside. IV fluid bolus should be given and antibiotics should commence.
- *Step 7: Evaluate outcomes.* Check whether the respiratory rate has come down and the patient is breathing normally. Check whether the saturation level is consistently above 95 per cent. Heart rate returned to normal, skin is warm and well perfused with normal capillary return.
- *Step 8: Reflect on the process and new learning*. Reflect on any aspects of care that could have been performed in a way to achieve an improved outcome.

Once Archie has recovered from the critical stage, education should be provided to both Archie and his mother about identifying and avoiding trigger factors and using preventer and reliever medications. A comprehensive asthma management plan should be prepared before discharge.

CASE STUDY 13.2

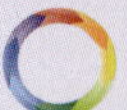

Nursing care of a patient with shortness of breath

Ibrahim Salah is a 34-year-old man brought into the emergency department from the local refugee centre with increasing shortness of breath, night sweats and productive cough. His history was collected with the help of an interpreter. He mentioned a loss of appetite for a week and generalised lethargy. A chest X-ray revealed patchy, localised consolidation in the right mid and lower zone of the lungs. AFB was detected in the sputum specimen. The patient is admitted to the ward from the emergency department.

The patient's vital signs in the emergency room were as follows:

- temperature: 37.9°C
- blood pressure: 110/70 mmHg
- heart rate: 86 beats per minute
- respiratory rate: 28 breaths per minute
- [illegible]
- Glasgow Coma Scale: 15
- height: [illegible] cm
- weight: [illegible] kg

Question

Using the information above, describe what action you would take as the nurse caring for this patient. Use the clinical reasoning cycle to guide you through the process and devise a care plan for your patient.

Answer

- *Step 1: Consider the patient.* Mr. Ibrahim Salah is a 34-year-old male. He is a refugee and needs the help of an interpreter to communicate.
- *Step 2: Collect cues/information.* Include subjective and objective data here, include the appearance of the patient, investigation results and their past medical history. Objective data will include measurable information such as vital signs. Subjective data include loss of appetite, generalised lethargy, shortness of breath, productive cough, night sweats. Investigations show consolidation in lungs, sputum positive for AFB.
- *Step 3: Process information*. Separate the relevant and irrelevant data, cluster the clues together to formulate an inference about the patient — Mr Salah has decreased oxygen saturation and an increased respiratory rate. He also had increasing dyspnoea and purulent sputum.
- *Step 4: Identify problems/issues*. Nursing problems or diagnosis should be listed here — Mr Salah's priority nursing problems are: dyspnoea, ineffective breathing pattern, impaired gas exchange and risk of infection transmission.

- *Step 5: Establish goals.* Goals of care for Mr Salah should focus on relieving his dyspnoea, improving his oxygenation levels and prevention of bacterial transmission
- *Step 6: Take action.* The nurse should initiate interventions to relieve dyspnoea, such as sitting the patient upright, administering bronchodilators, etc. Oxygen flow should be increased to maintain saturation above 95 per cent. The patient should be transferred to a closed negative pressure room to prevent the spread of infection, and airborne precaution should be initiated.
- *Step 7: Evaluate outcomes.* Check whether the respiratory rate has come down and the patient is breathing normally. Check whether the saturation level is consistently above 95 per cent.
- *Step 8: Reflect on the process and new learning.* Reflect on any aspects of care that could have been performed in a way to achieve an improved outcome.

SUMMARY

Patients presenting with respiratory issues are common in healthcare settings. Hence, nurses should be familiar with accurate respiratory assessment and interventions to relieve breathing difficulty and maintain optimal respiratory status. This chapter provides an overview of the anatomy and functions of the respiratory system. Pathophysiological changes and diagnostic intervention specific to individual disease conditions are mentioned in this chapter, as this information is essential in providing appropriate nursing management strategies. The treatment and nursing care discussed addresses physical and psychological issues that can have a negative impact on a patient's quality of life. Knowledge gained from this chapter will help provide holistic nursing care to both acute and chronic respiratory conditions across various settings.

KEY TERMS

acidaemia Blood pH below 7.35.
alkalaemia Blood pH above 7.45.
alveoli Tiny sacs within the lungs where gas exchange takes place.
asthma A chronic inflammatory disease due to hyperresponsiveness of the airway.
bronchitis Inflammation of bronchi.
bronchodilator A group of medications that relax the bronchial smooth muscle and dilates the bronchi.
controllers A group of medications used to control asthma attacks.
crackles Abnormal lung sound heard on auscultation when air passes through secretions or collapsed alveoli pop open.
cystic fibrosis (CF) A genetic condition affecting the chloride ion transfer of cells in the epithelial lining.
diuretics Medications given to increase urine output.
dyspnoea Difficulty in breathing.
emphysema A disease characterised by the destruction of terminal respiratory units.
haemoptysis Coughing up blood or bloody sputum.
Hoover's sign The flattening of the diaphragm and pulling in of the lower ribs on inspiration.
hypercapnia A condition in which partial pressure of carbon dioxide in arterial blood is above the normal range.
hypoxaemia Condition in which partial pressure of oxygen in arterial blood is below the normal range.
Mantoux test A diagnostic intervention to detect tuberculosis.
nebuliser A device used to vaporise liquid medications for inhalation.
pleura The outside layer covering the lungs.
pulmonary rehabilitation A program of education and exercise for self-management of dyspnoea associated with chronic lung conditions.
pulse oximeter A device used to measure the percentage of oxygen bound haemoglobin molecules.
respiration The process that involves inhalation, exhalation and the exchange of gases between the alveoli and tissues.
respiratory failure A condition in which PaO_2 <8 kPa (<60 mmHg) or a $PaCO_2$ >7 kPa (>55 mmHg) in arterial blood.
wheeze A whistling sound heard on lung auscultation.

REFERENCES

Australian Institute of Health and Welfare (AIHW). (2020a) Asthma. www.aihw.gov.au/reports/chronic-respiratory-conditions/asthma/contents/asthma

Australian Institute of Health and Welfare (AIHW). (2020b) Chronic obstructive pulmonary disease (COPD). www.aihw.gov.au/reports/chronic-respiratory-conditions/copd/contents/copd

Barker, A. F. & Brody, S. L. (2015) 'Bronchiectasis'. In M. A. Grippi, J. A. Elias, J. A. Fishman, R. M. Kotloff, A. I. Pack, R. M. Senior & M. D. Siegel (Eds.). *Fishman's pulmonary diseases and disorders*, 5th ed. McGraw-Hill.

Bullock, S. & Hales, M. (2019) *Principles of pathophysiology*, 2nd ed. Melbourne: Pearson Education Australia.

Bilton, D. & Jones, A. L. (2011) Bronchiectasis: epidemiology and causes. *Bronchiectasis: European Respiratory Society Monograph.* 52: 1–10.

Cystic Fibrosis, Australia. (2020) *What is CF?* www.cysticfibrosis.org.au/about-cf/what-is-cf

Chaboyer, W., Marshall, A. & Aitken, L. (2015) *ACCN's Critical Care Nursing*, 3rd ed. Chatswood, NSW: Elsevier.

Chesnutt, A. N., Chesnutt, M. S., Prendergast, N. T. & Prendergast, T. J. (2021) 'Pulmonary tuberculosis'. In M. A. Papadakis, S. J. McPhee & M. W. Rabow (Eds.). *Current Medical Diagnosis & Treatment 2021.* McGraw-Hill.

Chu, D. K. W., Pan, Y., Cheng, S. M. S., Hui, K. P. Y., Krishnan, P., Liu, Y., Daisy, Y. M. N., Carie, K. C. W., Peng, Y., Quanyi, W., Malik, P. & Poon, L. L. M. (2020) Molecular diagnosis of a novel coronavirus (2019-nCoV) causing an outbreak of pneumonia. *Clinical Chemistry.* 66(4): 549–555. doi: 10.1093/clinchem/hvaa029.

Dela Cruz, C. S., Tanoue, L. T. & Matthay, R. A. (2015) 'Epidemiology of lung cancer'. In M. A. Grippi, J. A. Elias, J. A. Fishman, R. M. Kotloff, A. I. Pack, R. M. Senior & M. D. Siegel (Eds.). *Fishman's pulmonary diseases and disorders*, 5th ed. McGraw-Hill.

Doucette, K. & Cooper, R. (2015) 'Tuberculosis'. In M. A. Grippi, J. A. Elias, J. A Fishman, R. M. Kotloff, A. I. Pack, R. M. Senior & M. D. Siegel (Eds.). *Fishman's pulmonary diseases and disorders*, 5th ed. McGraw-Hill.

Dougherty, L. & Lister, S. (2011) *The Royal Marsden Hospital manual of clinical nursing procedures*, 8th ed. Oxford: Wiley Blackwell.

Global Initiative for Asthma (GINA). (2020a) GINA guidance about COVID-19 and asthma. https://ginasthma.org/wp-content/uploads/2021/04/21_04_26-GINA-COVID-19-and-asthma.pdf

Global Initiative for Asthma (GINA). (2020b) GINA patient guide. https://ginasthma.org/wp-content/uploads/2020/02/GINA-Patient-Guide-PRINT-Pocket-Guide-final.pdf

Global Initiative for Chronic Obstructive Lung Disease (GOLD). (2020) 2021 global strategy for prevention, diagnosis and management of COPD. https://goldcopd.org/2021-gold-reports

Grishaw, J. (2020) *COVID-19 treatment.* McGraw-Hill Education. www.accessmedicinenetwork.com/posts/covid-19-treatment?channel_id=2610-accessmedicine-covid-19-central

Kress, J. P. & Hall, J. B. (2018) 'Approach to the patient with critical illness'. In J. Jameson, A. S. Fauci, D. L. Kasper, S. L. Hauser, D. L. Longo & J. Loscalzo (Eds.). *Harrison's principles of internal medicine*, 20th ed. McGraw-Hill.

Mandell, L. A. & Wunderink, R. (2018) 'Pneumonia'. In J. Jameson, A. S. Fauci, D. L. Kasper, S. L. Hauser, D. L. Longo & J. Loscalzo (Eds.). *Harrison's principles of internal medicine*, 20th ed. McGraw-Hill.

Nair, M. & Peate, I. (2009) *Fundamentals of Applied Pathophysiology.* Wiley Blackwell.

National Asthma Council Australia. (2020) *COVID-19 and your asthma patients.* www.nationalasthma.org.au/news/2020/covid-19-and-your-asthma-patients

Sisson, T. H., Claar, D., Chesnutt, M. S. & Prendergast, T. J. (2019) 'Pulmonary disease'. In G. D. Hammer & S. J. McPhee (Eds.). *Pathophysiology of disease: An introduction to clinical medicine*, 8th ed. McGraw-Hill.

Smith, M. A. (2019) 'Tuberculosis'. In R. P. Usatine, M. A. Smith, E. J. Mayeaux, Jr. & H. S. Chumley (Eds.). *The color atlas and synopsis of family medicine*, 3rd ed. McGraw-Hill.

Stern, S. C. (2020) 'Tuberculosis (tb)'. In S. C. Stern, A. S. Cifu & D. Altkorn (Eds.). *Symptom to diagnosis: An evidence-based guide,* 4th ed. McGraw-Hill.

Tortora, G. J. & Derrickson, B. (2011) *Principles of anatomy and physiology*. Danvers, MA: Wiley Blackwell.

Voynow, J. A., Mascarenhas, M., Kelly, A. & Scanlin, T. F. (2015) 'Cystic fibrosis'. In M. Grippi, J. A. Elias, J. A. Fishman, R. M. Kotloff, A. I. Pack, R. M. Senior & M. D. Siegel (Eds.). *Fishman's pulmonary diseases and disorders*, 5th ed. McGraw-Hill.

ACKNOWLEDGEMENTS

Figure 13.10: © Australian Asthma Handbook v2.0 asset ID: 4. Reproduced with permission of National Asthma Council Australia. https://d30b7srod7pe7m.cloudfront.net/uploads/2020/08/Figure_Steps-in-the-diagnosis-of-asthma-in-adults_web.pdf

CHAPTER 14

Nursing care of conditions related to the circulatory system

LEARNING OBJECTIVES

After studying this chapter, you should be able to:

14.1 describe the basic anatomy and physiology of the heart and circulatory system

14.2 demonstrate how to complete a cardiovascular patient assessment

14.3 identify common diagnostic investigations of the cardiovascular system

14.4 understand the presentation of and treatment options for a patient with coronary artery disease

14.5 explain the nursing care of a patient with acute coronary syndrome

14.6 recognise other cardiac conditions such as valvular disease, rhythm problems and heart failure

14.7 outline the management of a patient with a vascular disorder

Introduction

Cardiovascular disease is one of the major causes of death in Australia. There were 41 800 deaths from cardiovascular disease (CVD) in Australia in 2018, which accounts for 1 in 4 deaths (Australian Institute of Health and Welfare [AIHW] 2020). Indigenous Australians death rate for cardiovascular disease was 1.7 times higher than non-Indigenous Australians (AIHW 2020). The largest number of deaths in all cases comes from coronary heart disease (42 per cent), followed by stroke (20 per cent) and heart failure and cardiomyopathy (10 per cent) (AIHW 2020). This chapter explores the anatomy and physiology, assessment, diagnosis, clinical management and nursing care of individuals with cardiovascular disease.

14.1 The anatomy and physiology of the circulatory system

LEARNING OBJECTIVE 14.1 Describe the basic anatomy and physiology of the heart and circulatory system.

The circulatory or cardiovascular system consists of two main components: the heart and the blood vessels. The heart is a muscular pump that provides the pressure necessary to propel blood throughout the body. The blood vessels are a closed system of tubes that carries blood away from the heart, transports it to body tissues and returns it to the heart.

The heart

The heart is a hollow, four-chambered organ that rests on the diaphragm near the midline of the thorax, between the lungs. It is surrounded by a protective membrane called the pericardium. The walls of the heart are composed of a thick layer of cardiac muscle known as the myocardium. The myocardium is covered externally by the epicardium and internally by the endocardium. The heart is divided into four chambers: two upper atria and two lower ventricles (figure 14.1). The two atria and two ventricles are separated by the septum (Tortora & Derrickson 2011).

FIGURE 14.1 The heart: internal structures

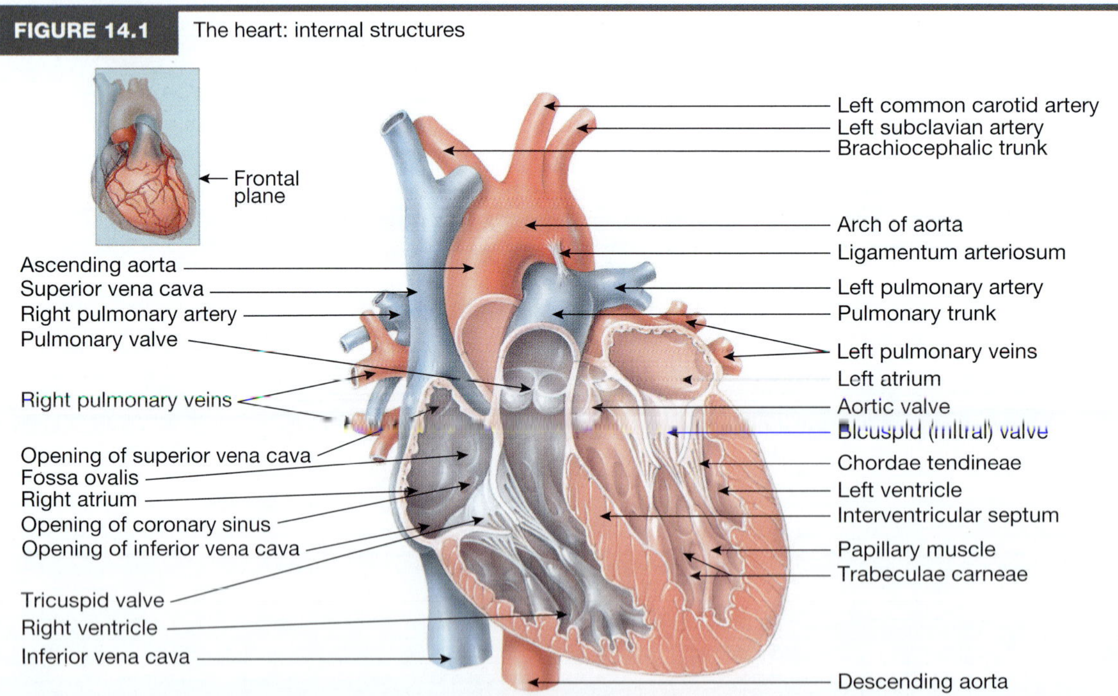

Source: Tortora & Derrickson (2011) *Principles of Anatomy and Physiology*, with kind permission of Wiley Blackwell.

The heart contains four valves (figure 14.1) that open and close in response to pressure changes during contraction and relaxation. The atrioventricular valves are located between the atria and ventricles on both sides of the heart. The tricuspid valve is located on the right-hand side, and the bicuspid, often called the mitral valve, is located on the left. The other two valves are located where the aorta (aortic valve) and pulmonary artery (pulmonary valve) join the heart and are referred to as the semilunar valves. The purpose of heart valves is to ensure that the blood flows through the heart in one direction by opening to let blood flow through and then closing to prevent it from flowing backwards.

The heart requires a constant supply of blood to maintain its cellular activity. This is delivered via the coronary arteries. Two coronary arteries arise from the aorta immediately above the aortic valve, each of which has several branches (figure 14.2).

FIGURE 14.2 The heart: coronary circulation

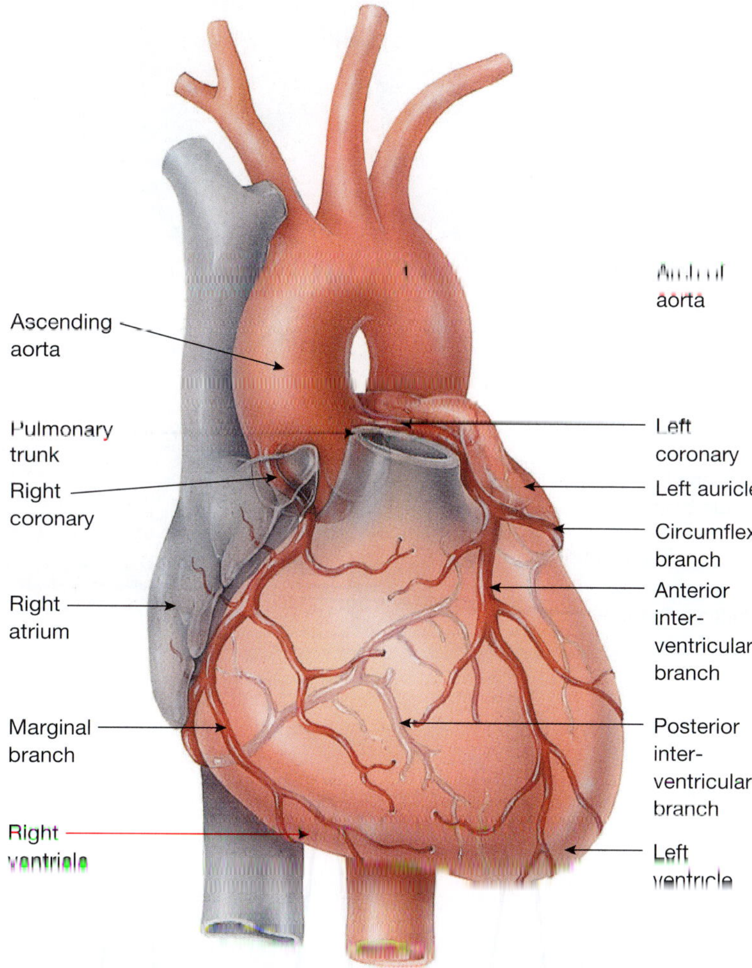

Anterior view of coronary arteries

Source: Tortora & Derrickson (2011) *Principles of Anatomy and Physiology*, with kind permission of Wiley Blackwell.

The heart contains a small proportion of specialised muscle fibres that are self-excitable, meaning that they are able to generate an electrical impulse spontaneously. These cells form the conduction system (figure 14.3). In normal circumstances, the impulse is generated in the sinoatrial node (the pacemaker). The impulse travels down the rest of the conduction system and then to different regions of the heart, producing a coordinated contraction of the four chambers of the heart (Tortora & Derrickson 2011). The sequence of electrical events can be captured and recorded on an **electrocardiogram (ECG)**.

Blood flow through the heart

Deoxygenated blood enters the heart's right atrium via the inferior and superior venae cavae and coronary sinus (figure 14.4). Blood then flows to the right ventricle through the tricuspid valve. The ventricle is stimulated to contract, pumping blood to the lungs through the pulmonary valve and pulmonary arteries, at which point gaseous exchange occurs. Carbon dioxide is exchanged for oxygen. Oxygen-rich red blood cells are then transported back to the heart (left atrium) to be distributed to the rest of the body. Blood flows through the mitral valve into the left ventricle. Oxygenated blood is then pumped into the aorta via the aortic valve to be transported around the body. Deoxygenated blood returns to the right atrium, and the process is repeated.

FIGURE 14.3 The heart: conduction system

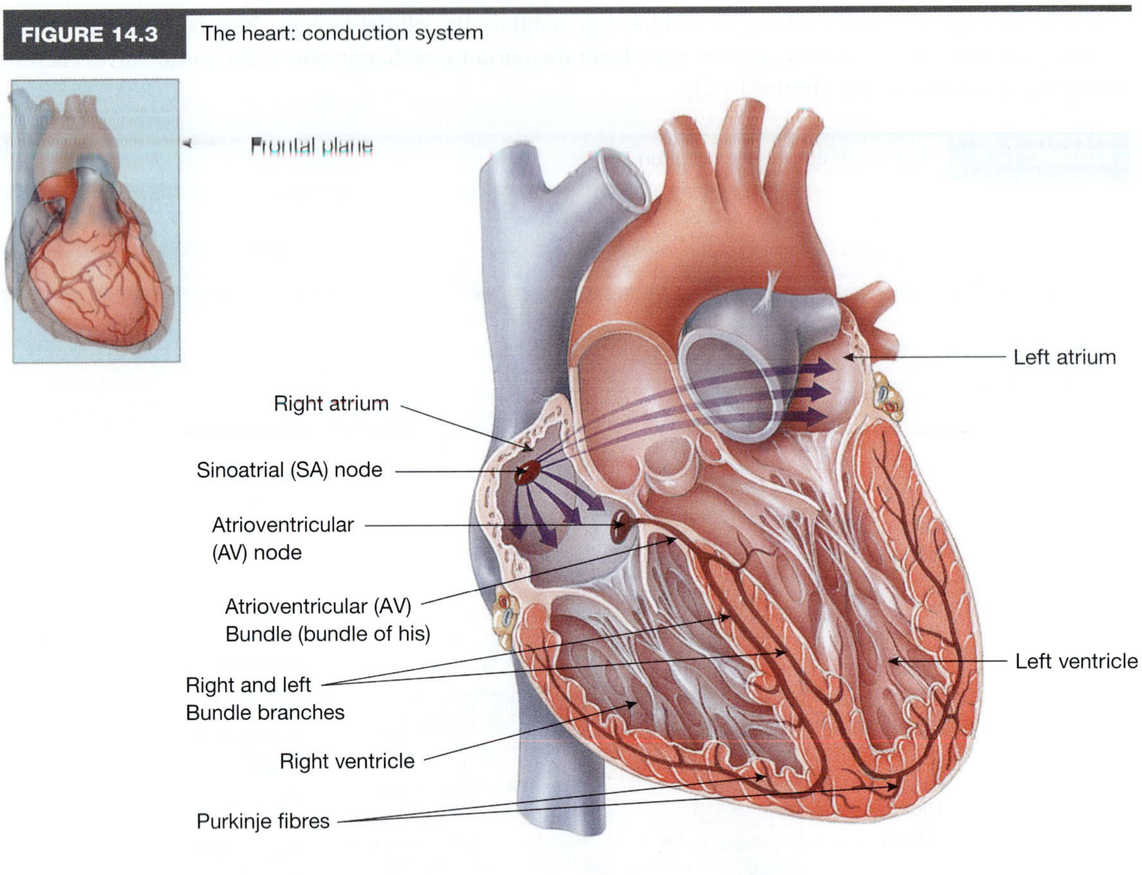

(a) Anterior view of frontal section

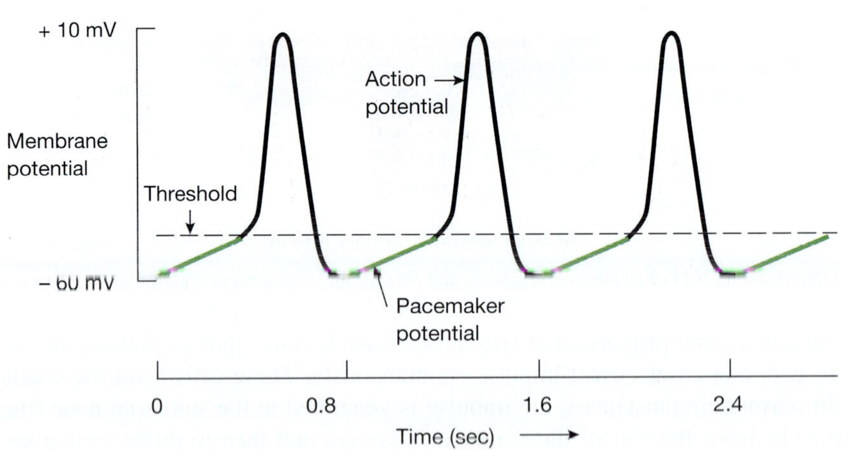

(b) Pacemaker potentials and action potentials in autorhythmic fibres of SA node

Source: Tortora & Derrickson (2011) *Principles of Anatomy and Physiology*, with kind permission of Wiley Blackwell.

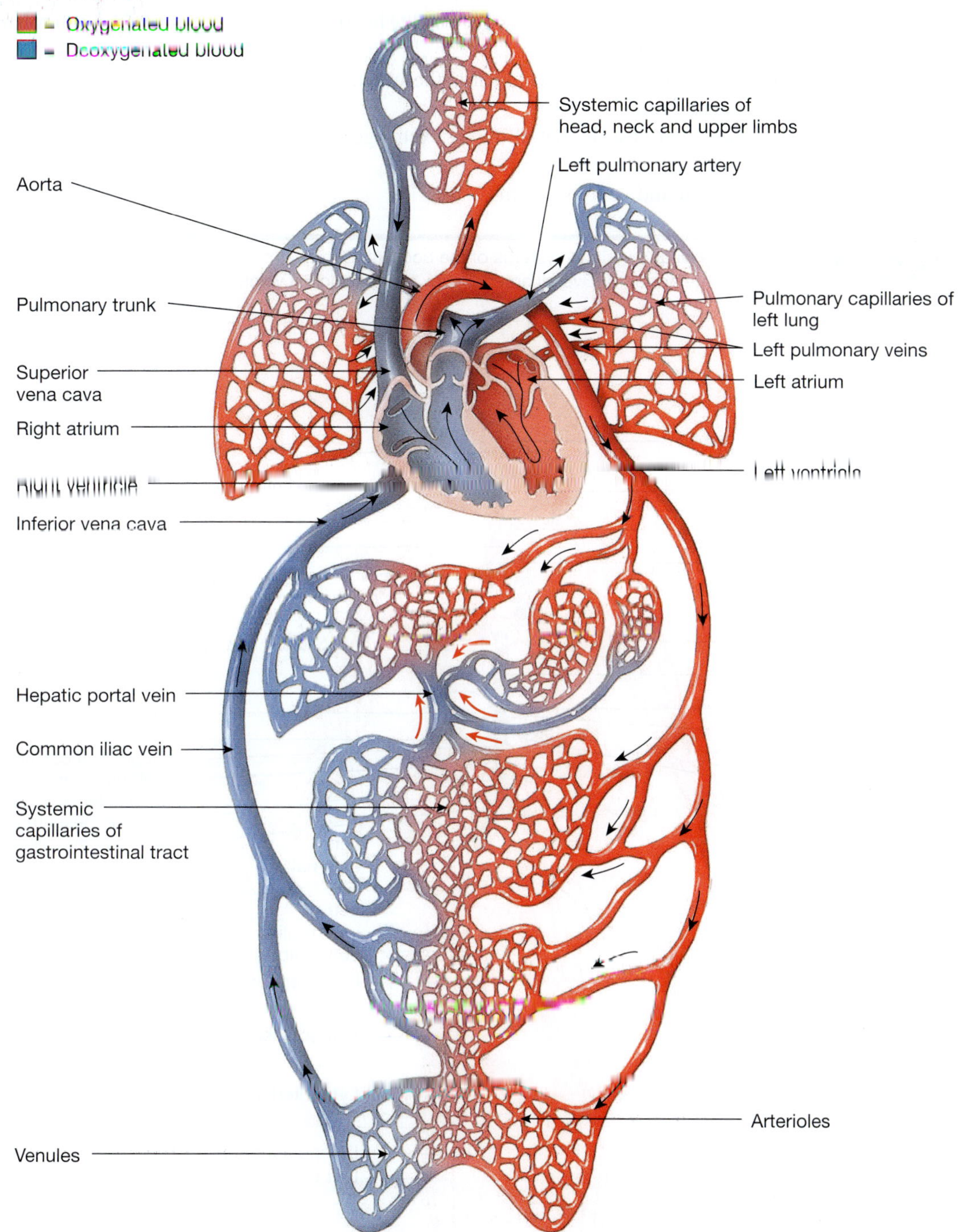

FIGURE 14.4 Blood flow through the heart

Source: Tortora & Derrickson (2011) *Principles of Anatomy and Physiology*, with kind permission of Wiley Blackwell.

Regulation of the heart

The sinoatrial node is responsible for initiating the impulse and the heart rate. However, the heart rate may be influenced by the autonomic nervous system. The sympathetic nerve supply is responsible for increasing the heart rate, whereas the parasympathetic (vagus) nerve decreases the heart rate. The nerve supply originates in the cardiorespiratory centre, located in the medulla oblongata. Other factors that affect the heart rate include hormones, stress, drugs, body temperature, electrolyte imbalance and circulating blood volume.

Blood vessels

There are several types of blood vessels within the body.

- **Arteries** and arterioles carry oxygenated blood away from the heart, with the exception of the pulmonary artery, which carries deoxygenated blood.
- **Veins** and venules carry deoxygenated blood towards the heart, with the exception of the pulmonary vein, which carries oxygenated blood.
- **Capillaries** are tiny, thin-walled vessels that allow an exchange of substances between the blood and body tissues.

  Figure 14.5 depicts the arterial and venous sytems.

FIGURE 14.5 The main arterial and venous systems of the body. (a) Overall anterior view of the principal branches of the aorta. (b) Overall anterior view of the principal veins.

(a)

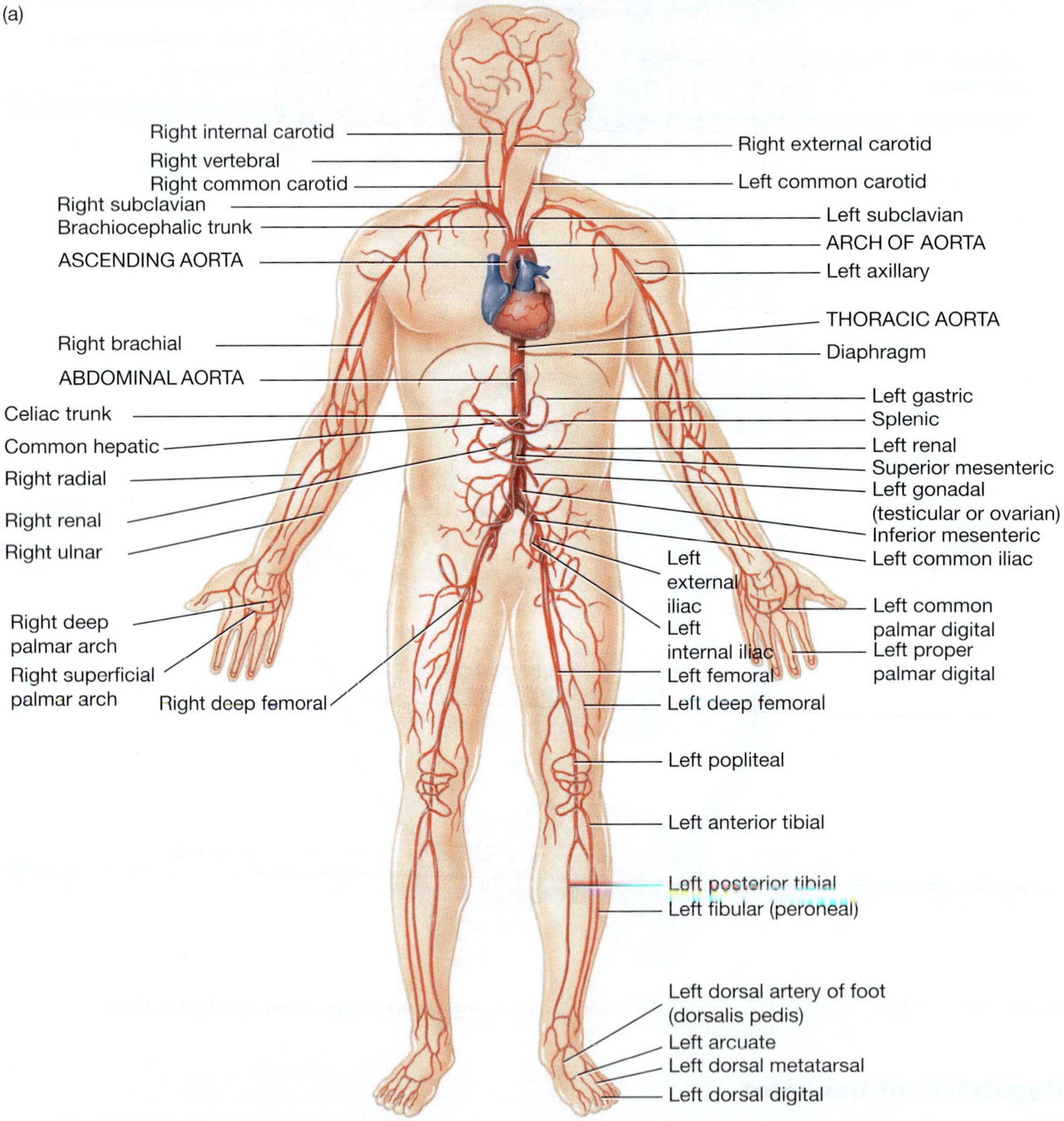

Right internal carotid
Right vertebral
Right common carotid
Right subclavian
Brachiocephalic trunk
ASCENDING AORTA
Right brachial
ABDOMINAL AORTA
Celiac trunk
Common hepatic
Right radial
Right renal
Right ulnar
Right deep palmar arch
Right superficial palmar arch
Right deep femoral
Right external carotid
Left common carotid
Left subclavian
ARCH OF AORTA
Left axillary
THORACIC AORTA
Diaphragm
Left gastric
Splenic
Left renal
Superior mesenteric
Left gonadal (testicular or ovarian)
Inferior mesenteric
Left common iliac
Left external iliac
Left internal iliac
Left common palmar digital
Left proper palmar digital
Left femoral
Left deep femoral
Left popliteal
Left anterior tibial
Left posterior tibial
Left fibular (peroneal)
Left dorsal artery of foot (dorsalis pedis)
Left arcuate
Left dorsal metatarsal
Left dorsal digital

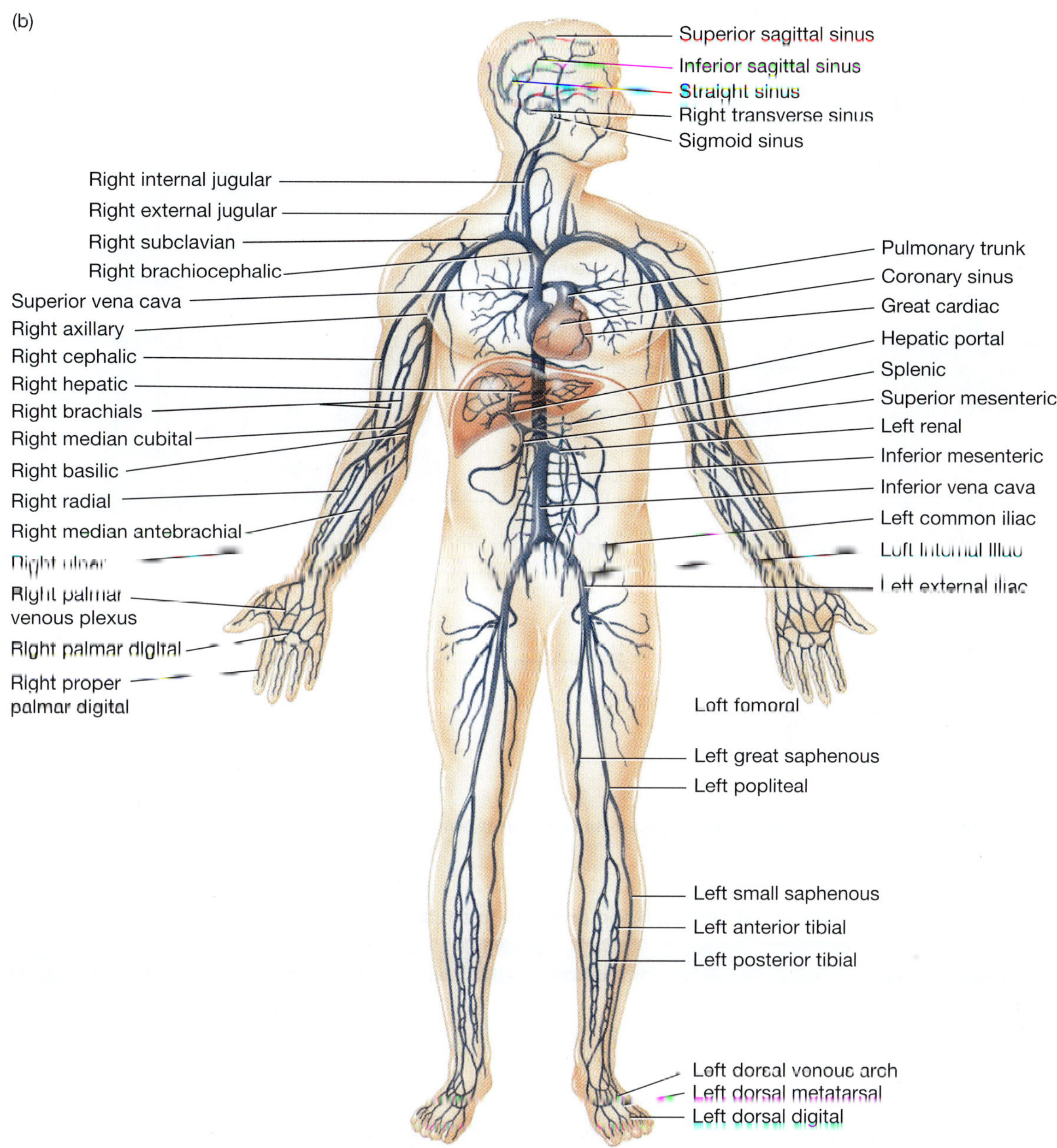

Source: Tortora & Derrickson (2011) *Principles of Anatomy and Physiology*, with kind permission of Wiley Blackwell.

With the exception of the capillaries, blood vessels are composed of three layers of the vessel wall (figure 14.6) surrounding a central lumen through which blood flows (Tortora & Derrickson 2011). The layers are:

1. the tunica intima — the epithelial lining
2. the tunica media — the middle layer of smooth muscle and elastic connective tissues
3. the tunica externa — a connective tissue outer covering with a plentiful nerve supply.

Blood pressure

As blood is pumped out of the left ventricle into the aorta, the circulating blood exerts pressure on the blood vessel walls, referred to as blood pressure (Nicol et al. 2008). Blood pressure varies in different vessels, and in clinical practice, the systemic arterial pressure is measured. Blood pressure varies throughout the day. It is often lower during sleep and higher during periods of activity. Several factors affect blood pressure, including cardiac output, circulating blood volume, peripheral resistance, stress, hormones and drugs. The Heart Foundation of Australia has produced clinical guidelines for diagnosing and managing hypertension in adults in Australia and has indicated an optimal blood pressure of 120 mmHg systolic and 80 mmHg diastolic (Gabb et al. 2016). Other categories of hypertension range from high-normal to grade three and are displayed in table 14.1.

FIGURE 14.6 Structure of a blood vessel

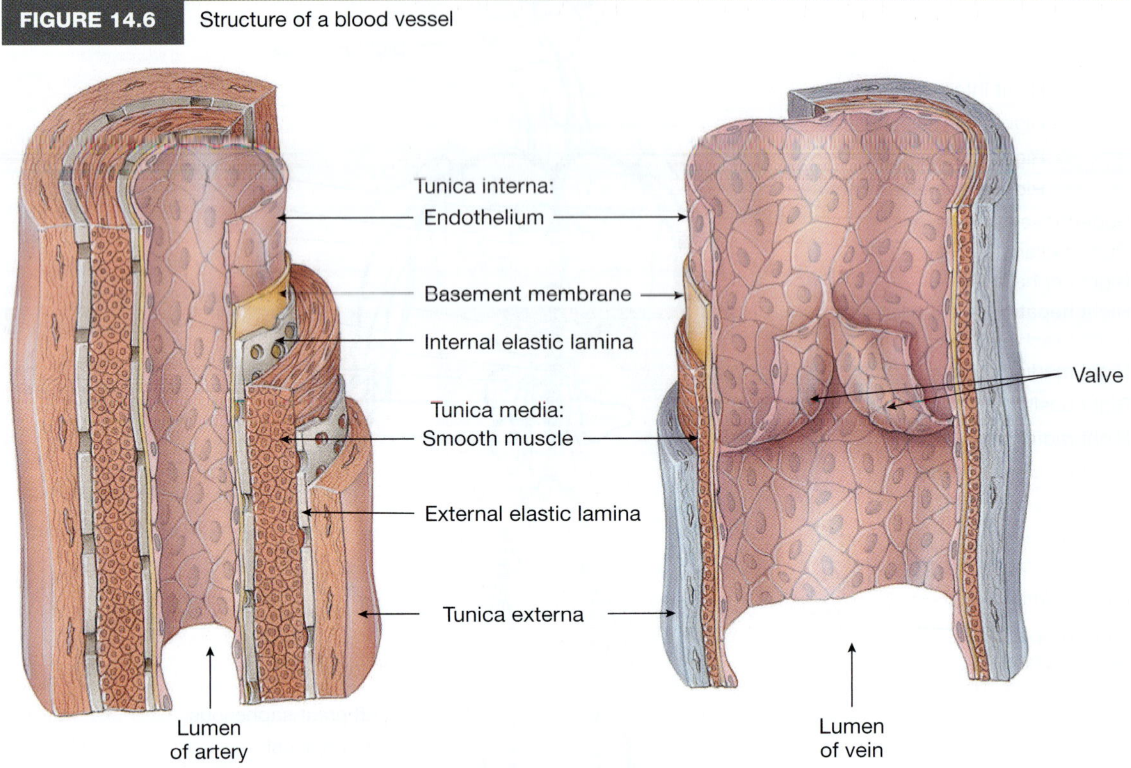

Source: Nair & Peate (2009) *Fundamentals of Applied Pathophysiology*, with kind permission from Wiley Blackwell.

TABLE 14.1 Classification of clinical blood pressure in adults

Diagnostic category	Systolic (mmHg)		Diastolic (mmHg)
Optimal	<120	and	<80
Normal	120–129	and/or	80–84
High-normal	130–139	and/or	85–89
Grade 1 (mild) hypertension	140–159	and/or	90–99
Grade 2 (moderate) hypertension	160–179	and/or	100–109
Grade 3 (severe) hypertension	≥180	and/or	≥110
Isolated systolic hypertension	≥140	and	<00

Source: Adapted from Gabb et al. (2016).

14.2 Cardiovascular nursing assessment

LEARNING OBJECTIVE 14.2 Demonstrate how to complete a cardiovascular patient assessment.

Effective and accurate cardiovascular assessment should be systematic and requires good communication skills. The assessment includes:

- the patient's current and previous medical and surgical history, including medications
- assessment of the presenting complaint, including symptoms, aggravating and relieving factors, and duration, for example:
  - dizziness and/or syncope
  - chest pain (location, type and intensity)

- palpitations
- fatigue
- heartburn
- shortness of breath
- nausea and vomiting

• social history — social isolation can be an important factor in determining mortality and morbidity following a cardiovascular event, and is also useful to know in terms of discharge planning
• family history — any incidence of CVD, diabetes or hyperlipidaemia in close family members should be noted.

Physical assessment

Physical assessment starts with recording the vital signs, including temperature, pulse, blood pressure, respiration and peripheral oxygen saturation. The nurse should pay careful attention to the patient's general appearance, such as pallor, positioning and increased work of breathing. Other areas of assessment include:

• urine output and urinalysis
• height, weight and body mass index
• waist circumference
• allergies
• pain assessment (see the section on angina for assessment tools)
• blood glucose monitoring (if appropriate) (Johnson & Rawlings-Anderson 2007).

The assessment needs to be documented carefully, and reassessment should take place as the patient's condition dictates.

If the patient is acutely unwell, the ABCDE approach may be used (figure 14.7).

FIGURE 14.7 The ABCDE approach to assessment

Assess the patient using the ABCDE approach.

- Assess the patient for a response.
- Airway: check patency.
- Breathing: check respiratory rate, expansion, effort, percussion, breath sounds, SpO_2.
- Circulation: check pulse, blood pressure, capillary refill, urine output.
- Disability: assess conscious level (AVPU, GCS) and pupils, measure blood glucose.
- Exposure: temperature, assess the whole patient, look for evidence of haemorrhage, rashes, etc.

Source: Australian Resuscitation Council (2016).

Assessment of cardiovascular risk factors

CVD risk factors can be divided into non-modifiable, modifiable, behavioural and psychosocial (table 14.2).

TABLE 14.2 **Risk factors for CVD**

Modifiable risk factors	Non-modifiable risk factors	Related conditions
Smoking status	Age and gender	Diabetes
Blood pressure	Family history of premature CVD	Chronic kidney disease (albuminuria ± urine protein, eGFR)
Serum lipids	Social history includingcultural identity, ethnicity and socioeconomic status	Familial hypercholesterolemia
Waist circumference and body mass index (BMI)		Evidence of atrial fibrillation (history, examination, electrocardiogram)
Nutrition		

(continued)

TABLE 14.2 *(continued)*

Modifiable risk factors	Non-modifiable risk factors	Related conditions
Physical activity level		
Alcohol intake		

Source: Adapted from National Heart Foundation (2012).

The probability of an individual developing the disease can be estimated using a cardiovascular risk assessment tool such as the Heart Foundation Absolute CVD Risk Calculator. This is available at www.heartfoundation.org.au/health-professional-tools/cvd-risk-calculator.

During a risk assessment, the nurse should ensure that the patient understands the nature of the risk and the likelihood that behavioural change may need to occur. Health promotion interventions can then be tailored to this.

14.3 Diagnostic investigations of the cardiovascular system

LEARNING OBJECTIVE 14.3 Identify common diagnostic investigations of the cardiovascular system.

Several diagnostic interventions can identify problems with the cardiovascular system, ranging from non-invasive tests such as an electrocardiogram (ECG) or an echocardiogram to the more invasive test of coronary angiography. These will now be explored in more detail.

Blood tests

Biochemical markers are particularly important to help diagnose acute coronary syndromes (ACSs). Myocardial necrosis (death of heart muscle) results in, and can be recognised by, the appearance of different proteins in the blood released into the circulation from the damaged myocytes, including cardiac troponin T, cardiac troponin I, creatine kinase and lactate dehydrogenase. Cardiac troponins are now considered the gold standard biochemical marker for myocardial necrosis. The measurement of troponin levels has largely superseded the measurement of creatine kinase and lactate dehydrogenase. Troponin is detectable in the bloodstream within four to eight hours of the onset of an ischaemic injury, peaks at around 18–24 hours and remains elevated for 10 days (Nickson 2020). Other routine blood tests include urea and electrolytes, clotting, glucose and lipids.

Electrocardiography

The ECG is a graphic representation of the electric current generated by the wave of depolarisation that progresses through the atria and ventricles (the P wave and QRS complex), followed by the wave of ventricular repolarisation (the T wave) (Huszar 2007). The electrical current is detected by electrodes placed on the patient's body and amplified through the electrocardiography machine (see figure 14.8 for details of electrode placement and how to record a 12 lead ECG). The image is displayed on a cardiac monitor or recorded on ECG paper.

Cardiac monitoring provides continuous information relating to the heart rate and rhythm, whereas the 12-lead ECG provides a 'snapshot' of multiple surfaces of the heart. The 12-lead ECG is an essential tool in the diagnosis of ACS. It also has a role in detecting atrial or ventricular enlargement and certain electrolyte imbalances.

Ambulatory monitoring

Outpatient ambulatory ECG devices, such as Holter monitors and patient-activated devices allow patients to be monitored while carrying out their everyday activities. They are often used to determine the cause of intermittent symptoms thought to be due to a cardiac arrhythmia. The data retrieved are interpreted retrospectively and cannot be viewed in real time. Alternatively, intermittent monitoring may be preferred, for example, if the patient's symptoms are infrequent. Patients are required to activate the recorder when they experience symptoms. Patients should ideally be asked to record their activities and any symptoms to determine whether there is any correlation with an arrhythmia.

FIGURE 14.8 Electrocardiographic anatomy of the thorax and 12-lead ECG electrode placement

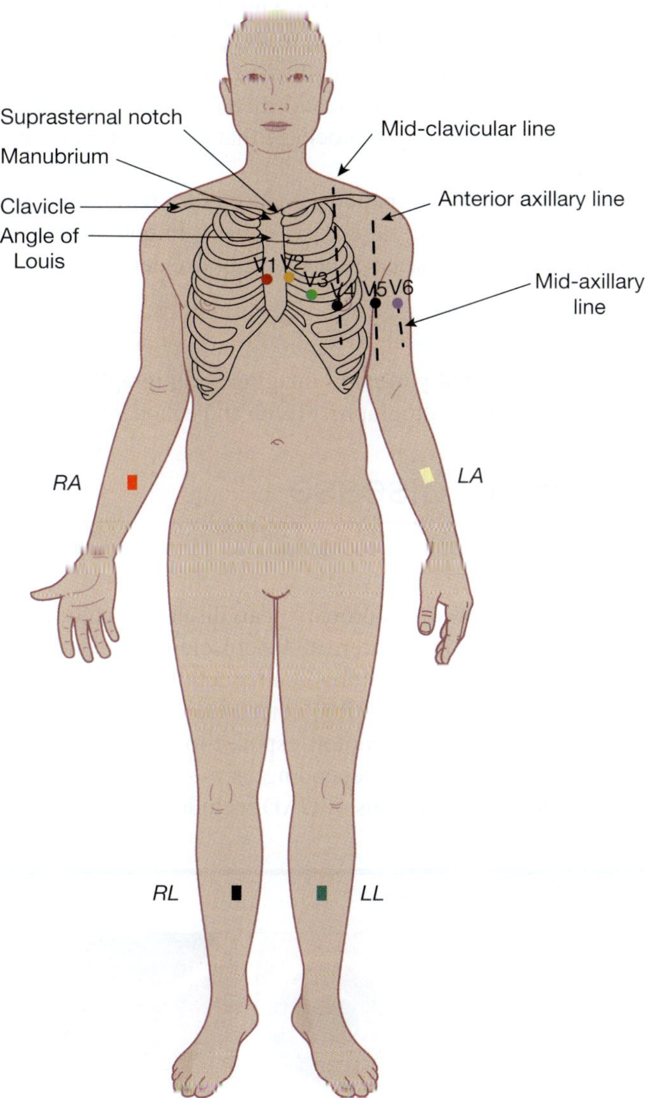

Source: Australia Resuscitation Council (2016).

CT calcium scoring

CT calcium scoring is a non-invasive test using CT scanning to detect and measure the number of calcified plaques within the coronary arteries (Chua et al. 2020). The plaques are formed by the build-up of substances such as fat in the coronary arteries' inner layers. Calcification of this substance is known as atherosclerosis. The amount of calcium evident on the cardiac CT scan is converted to a calcium score, which correlates with the blockage's severity. Measuring coronary artery calcium deposits using a CT scan has played an increasingly important role in diagnosing, managing and risk stratification of patients with coronary artery disease (CAD) (Chua et al. 2020).

Echocardiogram

An echocardiogram uses ultrasound technology to provide information on the anatomy and physiology of the heart and great veins. It assesses structural and functional abnormalities such as left ventricular failure and valve disease, and can visualise the flow of oxygenated and deoxygenated blood moving through the heart.

Coronary angiography

Coronary angiography is an invasive test used to diagnose the presence or absence of CAD. The procedure involves the insertion of a specially shaped catheter into the coronary arterial system. This is performed under fluoroscopic X-ray guidance. The catheter is advanced through the arterial system until it reaches the ostium (opening) of the coronary arteries. Contrast is then injected into each coronary artery, allowing visualisation of the lumen and any narrowing or blockage that exist. Arterial access may be achieved via the femoral, brachial or radial artery.

Nurses have an important role in caring for patients undergoing angiography, particularly with physical and psychological preparation. Post-procedural care is equally important to ensure that complications related to arterial access and systemic or disease-related events are detected as early as possible.

Other tests

Other diagnostic tests include myocardial perfusion imaging (scintigraphy), cardiac magnetic resonance imaging (MRI), transoesophageal echocardiography (TOE) and echocardiogram (ECHO).

14.4 Coronary artery disease

LEARNING OBJECTIVE 14.4 Understand the presentation of and treatment options for a patient with coronary artery disease.

Coronary artery disease (CAD), also known as coronary heart disease, is characterised by the development of atherosclerotic plaques within the coronary arteries. Atherosclerosis is a thickening or hardening of the arteries. It is a slow and progressive disease resulting in a reduction of blood flow to the myocardium and the development of angina (figure 14.9). In addition, atherosclerotic plaques result in endothelial injury and dysfunction, which affects the normal vasomotor response to changes in myocardial oxygen demand (Sertic 2021). The development of CAD varies depending on the individual's risk factors (see table 14.2) and the coronary arteries affected. Manifestations of CAD include stable angina and ACS.

FIGURE 14.9 The development of atherosclerosis

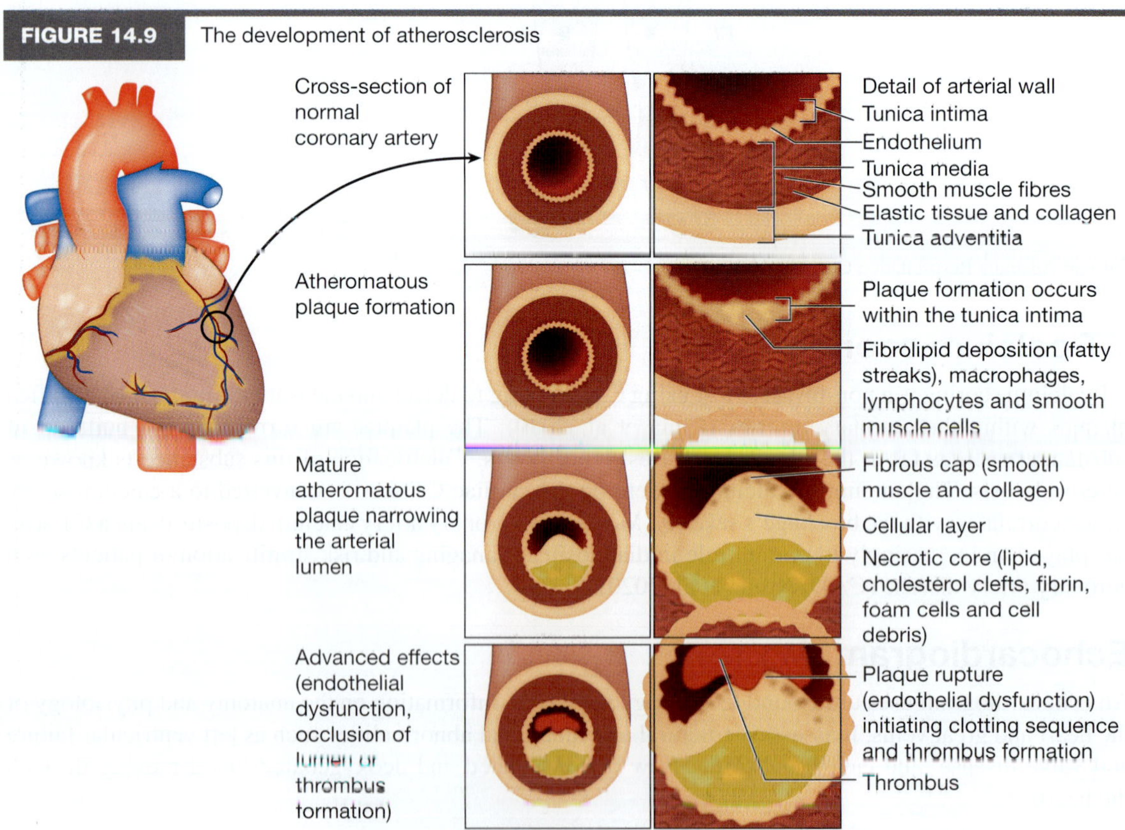

Source: Peter Lamb, HFS Imaging.

Stable angina

Angina is the most common manifestation of CAD. It is a symptom describing the pain or discomfort resulting from a transient, reversible reduction in blood supply to the myocardium. It is often associated with exertion and relieved by rest. Angina is regarded as stable if it has been recurring over several weeks without any major deterioration.

Angina develops when the atherosclerotic plaque within the affected coronary artery causes an obstruction of at least 70 per cent. When the myocardium requires an increased oxygen supply, for example, the vessel cannot meet this demand during exercise because the plaque is severely limiting the coronary blood flow. In addition, the plaque damages the endothelium, resulting in an inability of the vessel to control the blood flow by local vasoconstriction or vasodilatation.

The diagnosis of angina may be based on clinical assessment alone, as outlined above, but further diagnostic investigations are often required. Angina is diagnosed when the pain is described as tight or heavy in the chest, neck, shoulders, jaw or arms (National Heart Foundation n.d.). Angina can be described as stable if it caused by physical exertion and is relieved by rest or glyceryl trinitrate (GTN) within five minutes, or unstable if the pain develops at rest (Atherton et al. 2018).

The PQRST chest pain assessment tool is useful for ensuring that adequate information is obtained relating to the characteristics of chest pain (table 14.3).

TABLE 14.3 The PQRST chest pain assessment tool

P	Precipitating factors: What brought on the chest pain? What were you doing when the chest pain started? Is there anything that worsens the pain? (Position, medication, relaxation?)
Q	Quality: Can you describe what the pain feels like in your own words? Sharp? Dull?
R	Region and radiation: Can you show me where the pain is? Do you have pain anywhere else?
S	Severity: On a scale of 0 (no pain) to 10 (worst pain ever experienced), how would you rate your pain?
T	Timing: When did the pain start?

Source: Adapted from Australian Nursing Federation (2018).

Patients presenting with chest pain must be assessed to determine whether they are experiencing ACS or another life-threatening condition (Atherton et al. 2018). The Australian Triage Scale recommends patients presenting with chest pain be assessed within 10 minutes of presentation (Atherton et al. 2018).

Clinical and nursing management of CAD

The main treatment options for CAD include:

- medical management and modification of risks
- revascularisation by percutaneous coronary intervention (PCI) or coronary artery bypass grafting (CABG).

Patients with stable angina do not usually require hospitalisation. Instead, their GP may refer them to a chest pain clinic where they are often assessed by specialist nurses. Clinical and nursing management is aimed at improving patients' prognosis and minimising their symptoms. Secondary prevention of cardiac events achieves this: medication is prescribed to reduce the risk of death or ACS and often includes a nitrate, antiplatelet agent (aspirin or clopidogrel), statin, beta-blocker and calcium-channel blocker.

14.5 Nursing care for acute coronary syndromes

LEARNING OBJECTIVE 14.5 Expain the nursing care of a patient with acute coronary syndromes.

Acute coronary syndrome (ACS) is a life-threatening manifestation of atherosclerosis induced by a ruptured atherosclerotic plaque, which causes a sudden complete or critical occlusion or rupture of the coronary artery leading to a reduction in blood flow to the myocardium and subsequent ischaemia (Vergallo et al. 2021). ACS is an umbrella term that encompasses unstable angina and myocardial infarction (MI).

The definition of, and distinction between, ACS is based on clinical presentation (table 14.4), serial ECGs and biochemical markers of necrosis. If ACS is suspected after the initial assessment of signs and symptoms (table 14.5), an ECG is conducted. Following the ECG, patients will be categorised as having an ST elevation myocardial infarction (**STEMI**) or a non-ST elevation myocardial infarction (NSTEMI). This is an important distinction to make as treatment options are initially based on the patient's symptoms and ECG changes (Marshall 2011).

TABLE 14.4 ACS at a glance

ECG	ST segment elevation	ST segment depression, T wave inversion	
Troponin		+	–
Diagnosis	STEMI	NSTEMI	Unstable angina

TABLE 14.5 Signs and symptoms of ACS

Signs	Symptoms
Pallor	Chest pain (see below)
Cool and clammy peripheries	Shortness of breath
Blood pressure may be lower than normal (reduced cardiac output) or higher than normal (pain and anxiety)	Nausea
Heart rate may be normal or outside normal parameters depending on several factors such as pain, ischaemia of the conduction system and arrhythmias	Sweating
	Dizziness
	Fear and anxiety

Chest pain is the most common symptom of ACS. It is often described as a tightness ('vice-like'), pressure, heaviness or crushing, and is often mistaken for indigestion. It is usually located in the central chest but often radiates to the arms, jaw, back and/or shoulder.

Non-ST elevation myocardial infarction

NSTEMI, also known as non-ST elevation acute coronary syndrome (**NSTEACS**), is a type of infarction resulting in the formation of a thrombus that does not cause a sustained complete occlusion of the coronary artery. These patients usually present with prolonged chest pain. Biochemical markers (via a blood test) will be elevated outside the normal parameters, and a diagnosis of NSTEMI will be made. If the ischaemia does not result in myocardial cell necrosis, biochemical markers will not be elevated, and a diagnosis of unstable angina is made.

ST elevation myocardial infarction

STEMI is also known as ST elevation acute coronary syndrome (**STEACS**). STEMI results in the formation of a fixed and persistent clot that causes a complete sustained occlusion of the affected coronary artery and subsequent cellular necrosis and damage to the cardiac muscle. These patients usually present with prolonged (more than 20 minutes) chest pain and persistent ST segment elevation. Urgent revascularisation is required.

Immediate clinical and nursing management of patients with ACS

All patients with confirmed or suspected ACS will initially be managed in the emergency department. Emergency departments in Australia should follow an ACS pathway to ensure evidenced-based treatment is administered. These pathways are based on clinical guidelines provided by the Heart Foundation of

Australia (Atherton et al. 2018). Although there are some distinct differences in the treatment of ST elevation ACS and non-ST elevation ACS, all patients require the following.

- Continuous cardiac monitoring to observe for any arrhythmias.
- Vital signs should also be monitored closely to detect any changes in the patient's condition and life-threatening complications such as:
  - cardiac arrest
  - cardiac arrhythmias
  - heart failure
  - hypoxia
  - cardiogenic shock
  - myocardial rupture
  - pericarditis (Jones et al. 2020).
- Bed rest to reduce myocardial oxygen demand.
- Oxygen therapy may only be given with caution. Current recommendations dictate that oxygen should not be given routinely, and that the oxygen saturation (SpO_2) levels should be monitored and used to guide oxygen therapy. Oxygen should only be administered if the patient's SpO_2 levels are less than 93 per cent in patients without chronic obstructive pulmonary disease (COPD) and between 88 and 92 per cent in those with COPD (Atherton et al. 2018).
- Venous access and blood tests.
- A 12-lead ECG should be recorded on admission and frequent intervals such as when the patient is experiencing symptoms and following every chest pain episode when the symptoms have subsided.
- Pain relief. Pain is associated with sympathetic activation, which causes vasoconstriction and increases the workload of the heart. The administration of morphine or fentanyl relieves pain as well as anxiety (Atherton et al. 2018). An antiemetic should also be given.
- Sublingual GTN every five minutes if the patient's systolic blood pressure is greater than 90 mmHg.
- Antiplatelet agents – 300 mg aspirin (chewed or dissolved) should be administered as soon as possible.
- Revascularisation options should be considered and tailored to the individual patient, and should include conservative management, PCI or CABG.

Cardiac arrest rhythms

The cessation of effective pumping of the heart will result in cardiac arrest. Once cardiac arrest has been established, cardiopulmonary resuscitation should be commenced immediately. A cardiac monitor should be attached at the earliest opportunity to determine the cardiac rhythm as this will determine the appropriate treatment. Rhythms encountered during a cardiac arrest include the following.

- *Shockable rhythms.* The definitive treatment for the following rhythms is defibrillation by an appropriately trained practitioner.
  - *Ventricular fibrillation.* This is the only rhythm that does not require systematic interpretation. It is characterised by its chaotic appearance without any distinguishable complexes.
  - *Ventricular tachycardia.* This rhythm appears as a regular, fast rhythm with broad QRS complexes. The patient in ventricular tachycardia may or may not have a pulse.
- *Non-shockable rhythms.* Defibrillation is not effective in the treatment of the following rhythms.
  - *Asystole.* No electrical activity is present, and there is an absence of identifiable waveforms.
  - *Pulseless electrical activity.* This term is used when there is a clinical absence of cardiac output despite electrical activity seen on the monitor (Australian Resuscitation Council 2018).

Cardiac arrest rhythms, including nursing care and treatment, are discussed in the chapter on special nursing care (including emergency).

Percutaneous coronary intervention

Percutaneous coronary intervention (PCI) is a term that collectively describes a group of procedures that aim to restore or improve the blood flow to the myocardium following a period of ischaemia or injury. PCI includes percutaneous transluminal coronary angioplasty (PTCA) and intracoronary stenting. It is often performed electively in patients who continue to have symptoms of angina despite medication. PCI may also be performed urgently as a treatment option for patients presenting with MI.

PTCA involves widening a coronary artery from within using a balloon catheter to increase the blood supply to the myocardium. The catheter is inserted into the artery (femoral, radial or less commonly brachial) and guided through the arterial system under X-ray guidance. A contrast medium is injected into the coronary artery to determine the size and location of the atherosclerotic plaque(s). The balloon is then advanced and inflated to compress the plaque against the arterial wall, resulting in widening of the coronary artery.

Stents are thin mesh wire structures that act as 'scaffolding' to keep the artery open. The Heart Foundation of Australia's *Clinical Guidelines for the Management of Acute Coronary Syndromes* suggests that stents should be used routinely if PCI is clinically appropriate (Atherton et al. 2018). In addition to the pre-procedural care discussed for coronary angiography, unfractionated heparin or enoxaparin is required in patients undergoing primary PCI (Atherton et al. 2018). Following the procedure, frequent observations are taken to ensure that complications related to arterial access and systemic or disease related events are detected as early as possible. Complications are listed in table 14.6.

TABLE 14.6 PCI complications

Recurrent chest pain	Abrupt closure of the artery
Non-STEMI/STEMI	In-stent re-stenosis
Arrhythmias and conduction disturbances	Cerebrovascular complications
Vagal reaction	Bleeding at the puncture site
Occlusive thrombus at the puncture site	Coronary artery dissection

14.6 Other cardiac conditions

LEARNING OBJECTIVE 14.6 Recognise other cardiac conditions such as valvular disease, rhythm problems and heart failure.

Cardiac arrhythmias

An arrhythmia is any cardiac rhythm that is not normal sinus rhythm at a normal rate. There is a deviation from the normal pattern of electrical activity in which the heart beats too slowly (bradycardia), too fast (tachycardia) or irregularly. Symptoms experienced with an arrhythmia include:

- palpitations
- dizziness
- a feeling of faintness (pre-syncope)
- shortness of breath
- chest pain
- anxiety
- reduced exercise tolerance.

If a **cardiac arrhythmia** is suspected, a 12-lead ECG should also be obtained as soon as possible. This will provide documented evidence of the arrhythmia and enable a more detailed interpretation by an appropriately experienced practitioner. Continuous cardiac monitoring may also be necessary. Adverse events from cardiac arrhythmias include:

- hypotension (systolic blood pressure <90 mmHg)
- syncope
- signs of heart failure
- chest pain or signs of ischaemia on the ECG
- an extreme heart rate: >150 beats per minute or <40 beats per minute.

Tachyarrhythmias

A tachyarrhythmia is an arrhythmia with a heart rate of more than 100 beats per minute. It does not include sinus tachycardia, which is a normal pattern of electrical activity with an abnormally high heart rate, often due to an alternative physiological or pathological state, for example, exercise, anxiety or fever. Tachyarrhythmias are often categorised by (and treated according to) the width of the QRS complex — narrow or broad.

Narrow complex tachycardias usually originate in the atria and include the following.

- *Atrial fibrillation (AF).* This is the most common arrhythmia encountered in clinical practice. It is recognised by ineffective atrial activity and an irregular rhythm. The heart rate may be slow, normal or fast. P waves will be absent from the ECG and the rhythm will be irregular.

- *Atrial flutter.* This rhythm is characterised by its unique atrial activity — often described as a 'sawtooth' pattern. Ventricular activity is often normal. The heart rate is dependent on the degree of blockage at the atrioventricular node; a ratio is used to describe this, for example, 4:1, meaning the atria are activated four times for each ventricular activation.
- *Supraventricular tachycardia (SVT).* This rhythm is fast, usually over 160 bpm and characterised on an ECG by absent P waves and a regular narrow complex QRS.

Figure 14.10 shows how atrial arrhythmias present on an ECG rhythm.

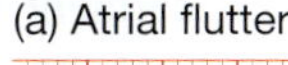

FIGURE 14.10 Atrial arrythmias

(a) Atrial flutter

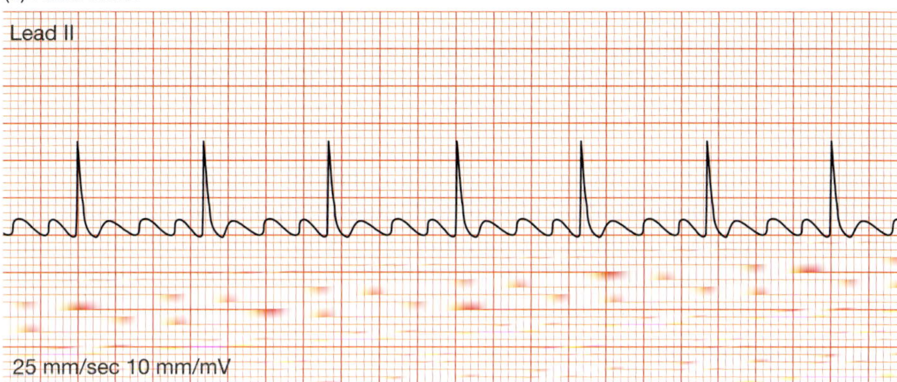

(b) Atrial fibrillation (AF)

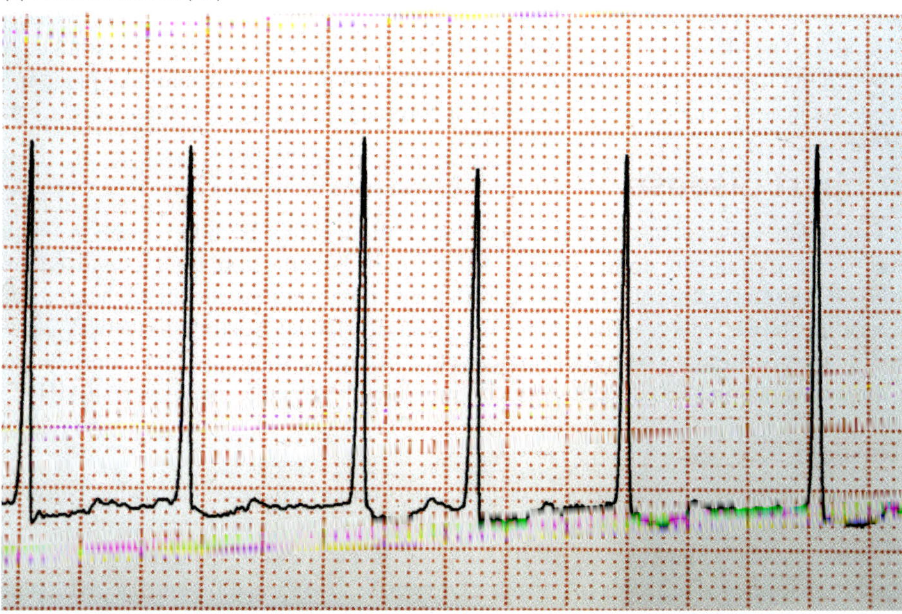

(c) Supraventricular tachycardia (SVT)

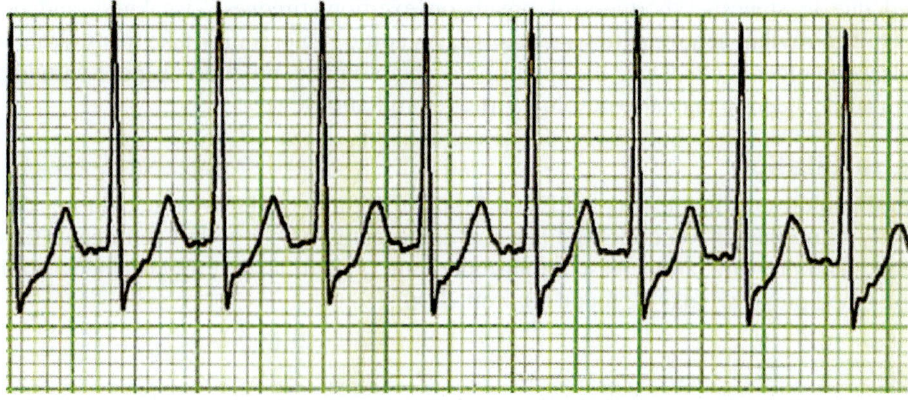

Broad complex tachycardias are any rhythm with a fast heart rate and a broad complex. The most common broad complex tachycardia is ventricular tachycardia. The patient may be asymptomatic, symptomatic and haemodynamically compromised or pulseless. The patient's condition determines treatment. Always treat the patient and not the monitor or the rhythm.

Clinical and nursing management

Treatment aims to either control the heart rate (rate control) or restore sinus rhythm (cardioversion). Generally speaking, if the patient is stable during the arrhythmia, pharmacological agents are preferred over electrical intervention. Amiodarone is a common antiarrhythmic medication for both narrow and broad complex tachycardias, and adenosine is often given to treat SVT.

If the patient is unstable or displaying adverse signs, DC cardioversion is the treatment of choice. This is the process of delivering an electric current, in a controlled manner, externally to the heart via a defibrillator. Anaesthesia or sedation is usually administered to the patient. Alternative electrical therapies for arrhythmias include ablation and implantable cardioverter defibrillator implantation.

Bradyarrhythmia

A bradyarrhythmia is an arrhythmia with a heart rate of less than 60 beats per minute. It does not include sinus bradycardia, which is a normal pattern of electrical activity with an abnormally slow heart rate, as in seen in athletes, during sleep or as an effect of medication such as beta-blockers. Bradyarrhythmias usually develop because the conduction from the atria to the ventricles is either slowed or blocked, resulting in an atrioventricular block. There are three degrees of heart block: first, second and third degree.

Clinical and nursing management

Treatment options for bradyarrhythmia include the following.

- *Pharmacological management*. Intravenous atropine is administered as a first-line treatment to patients who are displaying adverse features
- *Cardiac pacing*. The delivery of a small electrical current to the heart to stimulate myocardial contraction. Pacing may be required temporarily or permanently. This would take place in specialised clinical areas such as the emergency department, a coronary care unit or an intensive care unit.

Valvular heart disease

Any of the four heart valves can develop a problem, although this is more common on the left side of the heart — the mitral and aortic valves. Valves may become too tight (stenosis) or may leak (regurgitation). A common cause of valvular heart disease in Australia is rheumatic heart disease (RHD), which disproportionately affects Aboriginal and Torres Strait Islander Australians (AIHW 2019). In 2013–2017, 322 Indigenous Australians with RHD underwent 350 cardiac surgeries. Over three-quarters of those were under the age of 45, and 12 per cent were children aged between 5 and 14 years (AIHW 2019).

Aortic stenosis

The aortic valve has three semilunar cusps. Aortic stenosis may result from narrowing below the cusps in the left ventricular outflow tract (subvalvular) or constriction of the aorta (supravalvular).

Although there may be acute cases of aortic stenosis, in most cases, the cusps stiffen over time and movement becomes limited. This leads to concentric hypertrophy of the left ventricle, which increases the myocardial oxygen demand. Oxygen supply may be limited by compression of the coronary epicardial vessels, which can lead to angina. Other symptoms are syncope on exertion as the cardiac output is decreased due to stenosis, shortness of breath on exertion, tiredness, weakness and occasionally palpitations due to rhythm abnormalities such as AF. As aortic stenosis may take many years to develop, it is mainly seen in older adults. Once the condition is symptomatic, prognosis is poor without treatment. Patients with aortic stenosis may also develop aortic regurgitation.

Aortic regurgitation

Aortic regurgitation results in a leakage of blood from the aorta to the left ventricle during diastole. This will eventually cause the left ventricle to dilate and can eventually lead to left ventricular failure. When recording the blood pressure, an increase in pulse pressure (a significant difference between the systolic and diastolic blood pressure) may be found (Barrett 2006).

Mitral valve prolapse

Mitral valve prolapse can occur as a result of Marfan's syndrome, pregnancy or a hereditary condition. It does not usually require treatment unless symptomatic mitral regurgitation develops.

Mitral valve regurgitation

In mitral valve regurgitation, blood leaks back into the left atrium during systole. This leads to an increase in left ventricular volume, a decreased afterload and eventually left ventricular dilatation and left ventricular remodelling. Mitral valve regurgitation can be due to abnormalities of the valve leaflets, annulus, chordae tendineae or ventricle. Symptoms include shortness of breath, AF (in around a third of patients), night cough, fatigue and signs of right heart failure such as peripheral oedema.

Mitral stenosis

The mitral valve is usually affected by RHD. As the orifice narrows, the pressure in the left atrium will increase. The walls will stretch, leading to pulmonary oedema and, eventually, signs of right ventricular failure.

Symptoms will develop slowly but include shortness of breath, cough, frothy sputum (if pulmonary oedema is present), atrial arrhythmias and fatigue.

Investigations

Investigations for valvular heart disease include:

- ECG
- echocardiogram
- chest X-ray
- coronary angiogram
- heart sounds.

Clinical and nursing management of valvular heart disease

While patients are asymptomatic, their condition is monitored regularly. Once symptoms develop, the patient will be considered for surgery (see below), as in some cases, the prognosis is poor. Therefore, management will be tailored to the symptoms the patient is experiencing. For example, those with aortic stenosis should be advised to avoid excessive activity as this may cause syncope or possible collapse. Arrhythmias are treated with an appropriate antiarrhythmic and an anticoagulant such as warfarin if there is a risk of thrombotic events.

Where valvular conditions lead to heart failure, the patient will be managed in the same way with diuretics and other appropriate pharmacological therapy.

Surgery

Valves may be repaired or replaced. Valvular surgery was traditionally performed via a sternotomy with the patient on cardiopulmonary bypass. However, in the last few years, new minimally invasive techniques have been developed, such as thoracoscopically assisted mitral valve surgery and transcatheter aortic valve implantation (Goldstone & Woo 2016). These techniques are particularly good for those who are at high risk with traditional surgery.

Types of valve replacement include mechanical valves, homografts (human) and bioprosthetic valves (tissue valves derived from bovine (cow) or porcine (pig) tissue) (Goldstone et al. 2017).

Heart failure

Heart failure is a generic term for the heart's inability to pump blood to meet the body's requirements (Atherton et al. 2018). The type of heart failure will determine the symptoms exhibited and the subsequent management. However, heart failure is usually characterised by shortness of breath (dyspnoea), fluid retention, effort intolerance, fatigue and eventually death. The causes of heart failure are outlined in table 14.7.

TABLE 14.7 Causes of heart failure

Right ventricular failure	Left ventricular failure
Right ventricular MI	ACS
Pulmonary disorders	Ischaemia

(continued)

TABLE 14.7 *(continued)*

Right ventricular failure	Left ventricular failure
Valvular disease	Valve disease
COPD	Hypertension
Congenital defect	Cardiomyopathy
	Arrhythmias

Source: Atherton et al. (2018).

Left ventricular failure

If the left ventricle is not functioning properly, some blood will remain at the end of the systole. This will initially lead to an increase in left ventricular size and pressure. However, as time goes on, there will be a backflow of blood into the left atrium, causing an increase in pulmonary pressure, resulting in fluid entering the alveoli, leading to pulmonary oedema.

Right ventricular failure

Right ventricular failure is less common than left ventricular failure. It can occur on its own or as a consequence of left ventricular failure. Right ventricular failure leads to peripheral oedema, most commonly in the lower limbs, and abdominal ascites.

Signs and symptoms of heart failure

The patient may exhibit any of the following signs and symptoms depending on the origins of the heart failure and whether it is acute or chronic:

- shortness of breath on exertion
- frothy white sputum
- paroxysmal nocturnal dyspnoea
- swollen ankles
- abdominal discomfort and ascites
- fatigue
- cough
- tachycardia
- jugular vein distension.

Diagnosis and investigations

Heart failure diagnosis is usually based on the patient's history and symptoms and is confirmed by an echocardiogram. The patient will also have an ECG, chest X-ray and blood tests. In addition, an assessment needs to be made of the patient's cardiac output, heart rhythm, cognitive function, nutritional status and functional capacity.

Clinical and nursing management of heart failure

The management of heart failure depends on whether the patient is suffering from ongoing chronic heart failure or presenting acutely unwell with acute heart failure. These will both be discussed in more detail.

Acute heart failure

Acute heart failure is usually rapid in onset and can result from an acute MI, cardiac arrhythmias or pulmonary embolism (Atherton 2018). Alternatively, it may be an exacerbation of chronic heart failure. Acute heart failure can deteriorate into cardiogenic shock if not treated quickly and appropriately. Cardiogenic shock is a medical emergency; therefore, patients would be cared for in a critical care area.

A patient with acute heart failure may become hypotensive and could develop cardiac arrhythmias (Atherton 2018). These could lead to decreased cardiac output. Patients' with acute heart failure can also develop acute pulmonary oedema, a condition where fluid builds up on the lungs due to the ineffective pumping mechanism of the heart. Therefore, patients need monitoring, including continuous cardiac monitoring, blood pressure, respiratory rate, SpO_2 and, in some cases, central venous pressure monitoring. Invasive monitoring of blood pressure and central venous pressure can only be done in critical care areas.

Patients should be nursed upright, supported by pillows in either a bed or a chair. Supplemental oxygen is given if patients have an SpO_2 below 93 per cent. If the SpO_2 cannot be maintained with oxygen therapy, the patient may require non-invasive ventilation either via high flow nasal prongs, continuous positive airway pressure or bilevel positive airway pressure (Atherton 2018). Regular oral hygiene needs to be given to combat the effects of humidified oxygen. The oxygen demand on the myocardium needs to be minimised as much as possible, so patients will need assistance with activities of living. The patient and family may be very distressed and anxious; therefore, reassurance and psychological care are very important.

Pharmacological care aims to reduce both preload and afterload using a combination of intravenous vasodilators and diuretics. Other therapies that may be indicated include inotropes or even the insertion of an intra-aortic balloon pump or left ventricular assist device. However, these last two therapies should only be considered a bridge to cardiac transplantation or if recovery is likely and only conducted in critical care areas (Atherton 2018).

Chronic heart failure

A number of pharmacological therapies can be used to help alleviate symptoms and improve prognosis in those with chronic heart failure. Current pharmacological guidelines are:

- angiotensin-converting enzyme inhibitors
- beta-blockers
- diuretics
- angiotensin receptor blockers
- aldosterone antagonists
- digoxin (Atherton 2018).

The current guidance means that patients could be on at least six different medications a day, which may cause problems with both medication interactions and patient compliance. Nurses have a critical role in helping patients understand what each of the medications is for and the importance of taking them as prescribed.

14.7 Vascular disorders

LEARNING OBJECTIVE 14.7 Outline the management of a patient with a vascular disorder.

The management of patients with vascular disorders varies according to the type of vascular disorder they may be suffering from. The following section will outline the management of the most common types of vascular disorders.

Aortic aneurysm

An aneurysm is defined as a permanent dilation of a blood vessel. An abdominal aortic aneurysm (AAA) is dilatation of the abdominal section of the aorta (Australian and New Zealand Society for Vascular Surgery n.d.). Aneurysms can occur in one area or along a length of the aorta and may be completely circumferential (known as fusiform) or a pouch out from a weakened area (known as saccular). Please refer to figures 14.11 and 14.12 for a visual representation of the location and type of aneurysm.

Causes of aneurysm include:

- hypertension
- male gender
- Marfan's syndrome
- increasing age
- coarctation of the aorta
- trauma
- intra-aortic balloon pump
- pregnancy
- atherosclerosis
- infection, for example, syphilis.

An aneurysm may be asymptomatic initially or may mimic other problems. They are often an incidental finding when conducting clinical examinations or tests for other conditions (Theivendran & Chuen 2018). An AAA may cause a pulsatile bulge in the abdomen when the patient is lying flat. Although there is a high morbidity and mortality rate when an aneurysm ruptures, there is no official screening program in Australia like there is in the UK and Europe. Instead, patients are screened on an individual basis if their medical practitioner believes the patient is a high risk (Theivendran & Chuen 2018). The clinical manifestations of symptomatic AAA may include back pain, often described as sudden in onset and a sharp, stabbing type pain. The signs and symptoms of a thoracic aneurysm will depend on the location. Pressure on other structures such as the oesophagus may lead to problems. If the aneurysm ruptures, patients are likely to feel intense tearing pain. They may also experience neurological or renal problems if the blood supply to these areas is affected. Signs of a low cardiac output will be found, and peripheral pulses may be lost. Blood pressure recordings may be different for the two arms.

FIGURE 14.11 Abdominal aortic aneurysm

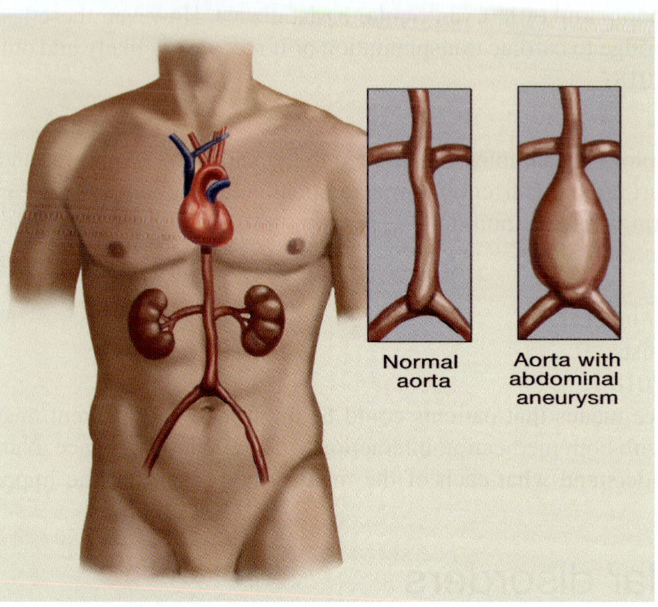

FIGURE 14.12 Abdominal aneurysm types

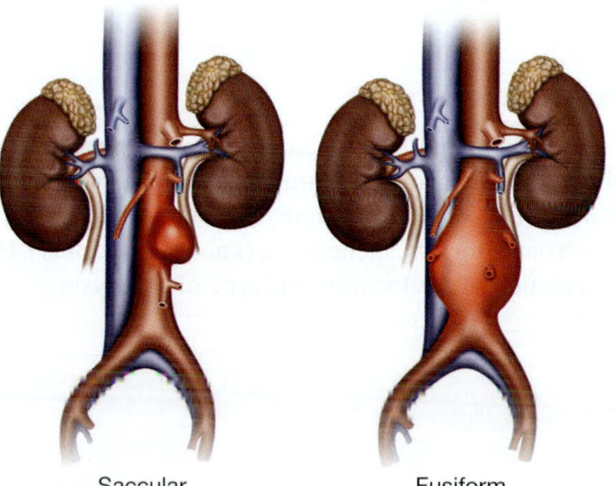

Clinical and nursing management of aortic aneurysm

The size, type and location of the aneurysm will determine the treatment given. Investigations will include ultrasound, MRI and CT scans.

Either major abdominal surgery may repair abdominal aortic aneurysms with a graft inserted or a procedure called an endovascular aneurysm repair (EVAR), in which catheters are inserted into both groins and stents are placed at the site of the aneurysm. There has been a significant EVAR preference in recent years due to fewer post-operative complications (Thievendran & Chuen 2018).

If a ruptured aneurysm is suspected, the patient will need to be cared for in a critical care area with close monitoring. Intravenous opiates may be given to control pain, and intravenous vasodilators or beta-blockers may be required if the patient is severely hypertensive. The patient and family may be extremely anxious, so excellent psychological care is paramount. Urgent surgery is usually required, and the post-operative care is similar to that of cardiac surgery

Peripheral vascular disease

Arterial and venous disease can occur alone or together. Many of the risk factors for heart disease will be the same for vascular disease.

Atherosclerosis can occur within the peripheral arteries, and plaques may form. As this happens over a period of time, collateral circulation may develop, providing a blood supply to the extremities. Symptoms may therefore progress slowly over a number of years.

Clinical manifestations

The patient may experience intermittent claudication with peripheral vascular disease — when patients suffer from intermittent pain related to exercise. This may start as fairly mild but can be very severe and will initially be relieved by rest. However, as the disease progresses, pain may be experienced at rest. The distance a patient can walk on the flat before pain occurs is a good indicator of the progress of the disease.

Investigations

Peripheral vascular disease is assessed by evaluating the patient's pulses, skin colour, skin temperature and sensation. The tibial, popliteal and femoral pulses are assessed as the dorsalis pedis pulse may not be present in all people, it is not a reliable indicator. The presence or absence of the pulse and its strength should be compared between the two legs. As occlusion progresses, the toes may become quite bluish and mottled in appearance. If the legs are elevated, the feet will become extremely pale, with colour only resuming once they have been lowered again.

Other investigations include X-ray, doppler ultrasonography (including an ankle brachial pressure index), helical computed tomography and arteriograms. Exercise testing will indicate how far the patient can walk without pain.

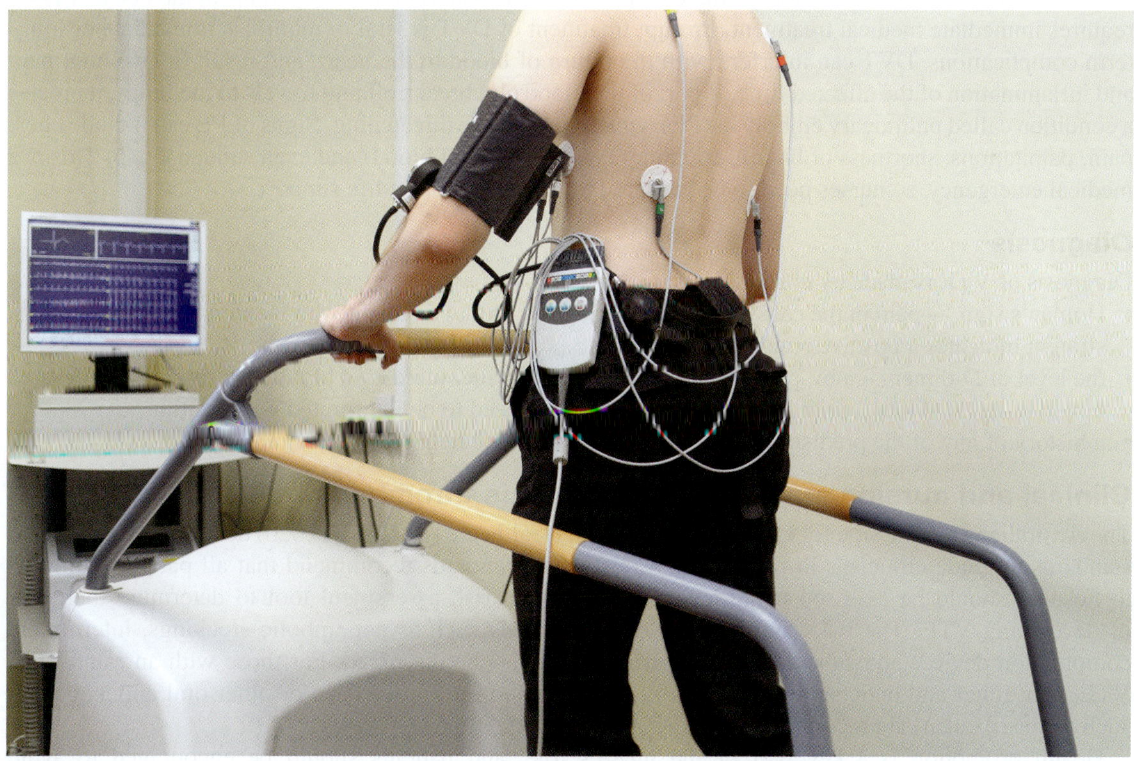

Clinical and nursing management of peripheral vascular disease

The patient should be advised to avoid extremes of temperature and tight clothing. Lack of sensation means that they can be at risk of burns, so their lower limbs should be kept away from direct heat sources such as hot water bottles, and they should avoid sitting close to a fire or soaking their feet in hot water. Ill-fitting shoes also need to be avoided. Exercise should be encouraged where possible.

Treatment includes aspirin or antiplatelet agents, percutaneous transluminal balloon angioplasty or even a femoral popliteal bypass. An embolectomy may be performed for a localised embolus. In extreme cases, an amputation may be performed if gangrene is present.

Venous thromboembolism

Valvular incompetence or an obstruction can lead to venous disease such as thrombus. A thrombus is more likely to form when there is a decrease in blood flow, for example, with an obstruction, stasis or damage to the endothelial wall. Venous thromboembolism (VTE) is more likely to occur in the deep veins of the legs (deep vein thrombosis), but if a section of the thrombus dislodges, it can travel to the lungs and cause a **pulmonary embolus (PE)**, which can be fatal.

Factors predisposing to VTE are:

- thrombophilia
- obesity
- trauma
- pregnancy
- contraceptive agents
- dehydration
- cancer
- long-haul travel
- varicose veins
- hormone replacement therapy
- immobility
- central venous catheters (Scottish Intercollegiate Guidelines Network 2010).

Symptoms usually include a hot, tender and swollen calf (although more than 25 per cent of patients with deep vein thrombosis have no symptoms).

Deep vein thrombosis (DVT) is the development of a blood clot in a deep vein. Although the deep veins of the legs are most commonly affected, a DVT can also affect other deep veins in the body. A DVT requires immediate medical treatment. Prompt treatment of DVT is vital to minimise immediate or long-term complications. DVT can interfere with the return of blood to the heart, and result in swelling, pain and inflammation of the affected limb. If part of the blood clot breaks off and travels to the lungs, it creates a condition called pulmonary embolism (PE), which may be life threatening. Signs of PE can include chest pain, palpitations, shortness of breath, coughing (with or without blood) and even sudden death. This is a medical emergency, so nurses need to be prepared to administer basic life support.

Diagnosis

Diagnosis of VTE is made by considering:

- Homan's sign — pain in the calf when dorsiflexing the foot of a patient who is lying flat with their legs straight indicates a positive result
- the level of D-dimer — a by-product of fibrin production measured by a blood test; this can be elevated due to other conditions, so the results of the blood test need to be interpreted with caution
- a history of any of the predisposing factors, which will also help reach a diagnosis.

Clinical and nursing management of venous thromboembolism

The Australian Commission for Quality and Safety in Healthcare [ACQSH] (2020) developed clinical care standards to guide clinicians in preventing VTE. These standards recommend that all patients admitted to hospital should be assessed using a locally developed risk assessment tool to determine their risk of developing VTE. The risks and benefits of prophylaxis such as antiembolic stockings, intermittent compression devices and subcutaneous heparin should also be discussed. For those with an established VTE, pain relief and anticoagulants (heparin infusion followed by warfarin or other oral anticoagulant, such as rivaroxaban) are recommended.

Health promotion is a key part of the nurse's role, and patients should be encouraged to avoid dehydration, external pressure and immobility. Awareness of risk factors such as smoking and the contraceptive pill also needs to be raised.

Varicose veins

Varicose veins occur when valves in the veins become incompetent and tortuous. They are usually found in those who stand for long periods. Other causes include pregnancy, obesity and genetic predisposition. Thrombophlebitis may also lead to an increase in venous pressure as well as the destruction of valve tissue.

Valves become incompetent and veins dilate. Eventually, patients may complain of aching legs. Although there are not usually serious complications of varicose veins; discomfort or cosmetic reasons cause people to seek treatment. Varicose veins can also lead to venous ulcers.

Clinical and nursing management

A number of treatment options are available depending upon the size and location of the varicose veins and the symptoms a patient may be experiencing. Ultrasonography may be carried out to assess the veins. Support stockings may initially be recommended.

Traditionally, surgical removal of the veins by ligation and stripping was the primary treatment. This involved a general anaesthetic, and patients would have several small cuts in their leg. There are now less invasive procedures such as radiofrequency ablation, laser therapy or the injection of a sclerotherapy agent. These can all usually be carried out under local anaesthetic, but they may not be suitable for all patients, and the long-term effects of some of these treatments are not yet known.

Whatever treatment is used, patients are usually only in hospital for one day and are normally required to wear compression stockings for a period afterwards. Patients may have some tenderness and swelling after the procedure. They can usually drive one week afterwards and return to work after one to three weeks.

Cardiovascular medication management

Patients with cardiovascular disease may be on a number of medications depending on their presenting complaint. Table 14.8 highlights some of the common medications that you will come across in clinical practice.

TABLE 14.8 Common cardiovascular medications

Drug family	Common medications	Mechanism of action	Nursing considerations
Cardiac glycoside	Digoxin	Increases the force of contraction (positive inotropism) and alters the heart's electrophysiological properties by slowing the HR.	Ensure heart rate >60 before administering. Patient may need digoxin levels checking.
Antiarrhythmic drugs	Amiodarone Verapamil	Act on various parts of the electronic pathways in the heart to restore a normal cardiac rhythm.	Observe for cardiac arrhythmias.
Beta blockers	Metoprolol Bisoprolol Atenolol	Block the effects of adrenaline to reduce blood pressure.	Ensure patient's systolic blood pressure is above 90 mmHg before administration.
Diuretics	Furosemide Spironolactone	Aids in the excretion of fluids from the body by increasing water excretion in the kidneys.	Ensure patient's systolic blood pressure is above 90 mmHg before administration. Monitor patient's fluid status. Furosemide can reduce potassium levels.
Anticoagulants	Heparin Warfarin Rivaroxaban	Act on various parts of the coagulation pathway to prevent thrombosis. Heparin can be given intravenously or subcutaneously.	Patients on warfarin will need their INR levels checked. Rivaroxaban is a new oral anticoagulant and increasing in popularity as patients do not need regular INR checks.

Cardiac surgery

CABG may be performed for patients who have triple vessel disease and/or left main stem stenosis not suitable for PCI and stent insertion. Grafts are used to bypass the patient's diseased coronary arteries and therefore improve the blood supply to the myocardium, alleviate the symptoms of angina and improve quality of life (Gallo et al. 2020). A patient may have several bypass grafts (usually between three and six) depending on their disease process. One end of the graft is attached to the aorta, and the other end is attached beyond the diseased area. Veins such as the long saphenous vein from the leg may be used as grafts, as may arteries such as the radial artery or internal mammary artery.

During surgery, the patient's heart is stopped, the body temperature is lowered, and a cardiopulmonary bypass machine carries out the work of the heart and lungs. Combining the effects of the cardiopulmonary bypass and the sternotomy approach can lead to complications (figure 14.13). Although this method is still widely used, more minimally invasive techniques and beating heart surgery have become common.

FIGURE 14.13 Potential complications of cardiac surgery

- Cardiovascular: bleeding, arrhythmias, conduction problems, hypertension, hypotension, left ventricular failure, anaemia
- Respiratory: pulmonary oedema, pleural effusion, atelectasis, basal collapse
- Renal: decreased urinary output
- Neurological: stroke, memory loss, confusion
- Gastrointestinal: nausea and vomiting, loss of appetite
- Other: pain, wound infection

Preoperative nursing management

Many patients will attend a preadmission clinic where they are psychologically and physically prepared for surgery. As well as the nurse and surgeon, they may also be assessed by an anaesthetist and physiotherapist.

Tests include:

- ECG
- chest X-ray
- echocardiography (for those having valve surgery)
- blood tests
- dental clearance to reduce the risk of developing endocarditis, particularly required for Indigenous Australians or those with a poor level of oral hygiene
- baseline observations
- height and weight.

Other comorbidities that may affect the outcome of surgery are assessed. A discussion of what the surgery entails and the recovery afterwards will also be included. In some cases, patients may be shown the intensive care or high-dependency area to prepare them and their families for this. Issues affecting discharge should also be assessed. Some medications, such as digoxin, diuretics, beta-blockers, warfarin and aspirin, have to be stopped prior to surgery, and patients should be advised of this.

Patients are then usually admitted the day before surgery. Hair removal (if necessary) is carried out, and the patient will also have a shower using surgical soap. They will be nil by mouth in line with the usual hospital policy.

Post-operative nursing management

Post-operative objectives include cardiovascular monitoring and support, pain relief, detection and management of complications, fluid management, respiratory support, wound care, assistance with everyday activities, psychological support and discharge preparation.

Some patients will remain intubated following surgery and may stay on a ventilator in intensive care for a few hours. In order to perform the surgery, the patient is put into a hypothermic state to protect the myocardial cells. The patient is then slowly warmed using warming blankets. There will usually be two or three chest drains, a catheter, one or more central lines and an arterial line *in situ*. Central venous pressure, heart rhythm, peripheral oxygen saturation and arterial blood pressure are continuously monitored. Urine output and blood loss in the drains will be checked carefully. Intravenous antibiotics are also given (Johnson & Rawlings-Anderson 2007).

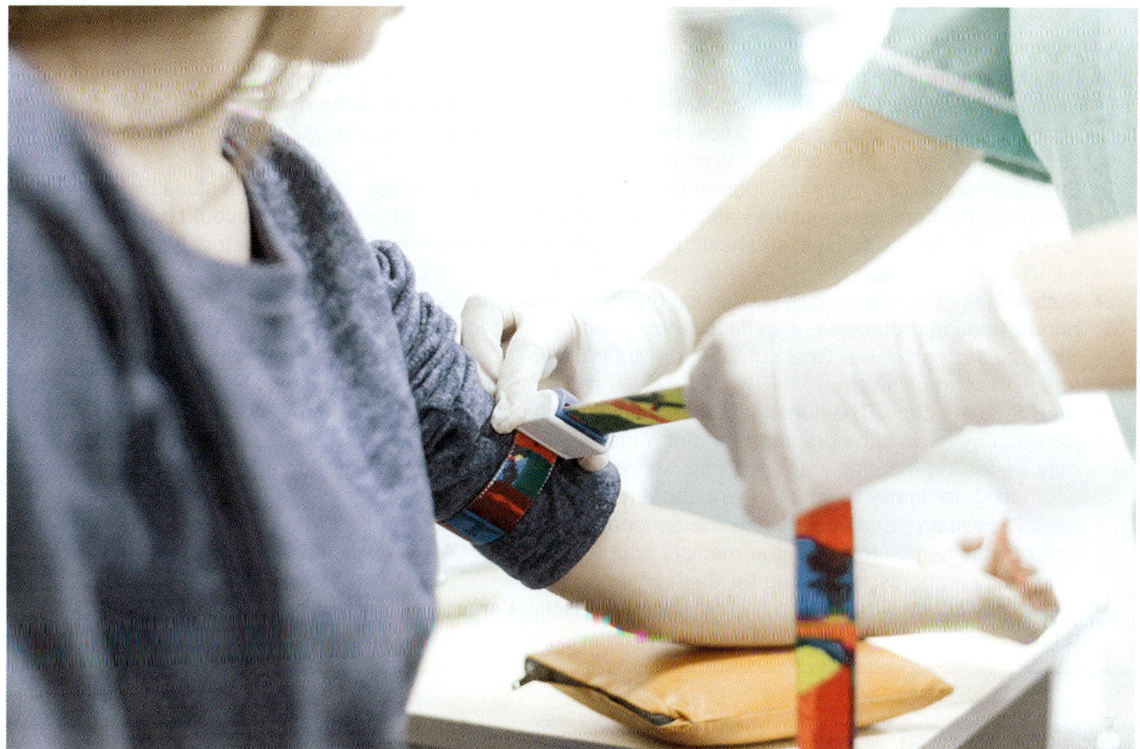

Once patients are awake and removed from the ventilator and ICU, they are usually transferred to a high-dependency unit where their cardiovascular status is still carefully monitored. Fluids will be titrated to urine output and blood pressure. Approximately one-third of patients may develop AF, so close monitoring to detect this is important. An intravenous infusion of morphine may initially control pain, but this will be replaced by patient-controlled analgesia once the patient is awake.

In the following days, drains will be removed, infusions including patient-controlled analgesia will be discontinued, and the catheter will also be removed. Oxygen is discontinued, and the patient is encouraged to mobilise. Physiotherapists will also assess to check for chest infection signs and encourage the patient to breathe deeply and cough. The patient will usually be discharged five to seven days after surgery. In some cases, they may be invited to attend a cardiac rehabilitation program six weeks after discharge.

CASE STUDY 14.1

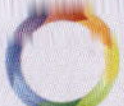

Nursing care of an Indigenous Australian patient with leg pain

Mrs Wurramara is a 36-year-old Indigenous female who has presented to her local rural hospital with cramping pain to her right leg with some associated swelling and erythema. She lives with her husband, and she is 32 weeks pregnant with her third child. She is otherwise fit and healthy. On examination, the patient's observations are within normal parameters, and she is afebrile. Unilateral oedema is evident to the right lower leg with erythema. The patient describes a 'heavy, cramping' pain to the affected limb.

Her vital signs in the emergency department are:

- temperature: 37°C
- heart rate: 89 beats per minute
- blood pressure: 126/76 mmHg
- respiratory rate: 16 breaths per minute
- oxygen saturation: 98% on room air
- pain score: 4/10.

Question

What could be the presenting problem and why? Using the information above, describe what action you would take as the nurse caring for this patient. Use the clinical reasoning cycle to guide you through the process and devise a plan of care for your patient.

Answer

- *Step 1: Consider the patient.* Mrs Wurramara, a 36-year-old Indigenous female.
- *Step 2: Collect cues/information.* Include subjective and objective data here. Include the appearance of the patient and their past medical history. She describes cramping pain in her right lower leg. Observations are normal, and she is afebrile.
- *Step 3: Process information.* Separate the relevant and irrelevant data — cluster the clues together to formulate an inference about the patient. The unilateral swelling, erythema and pain could be an indicator of a DVT. Despite being fit and healthy, she is pregnant, which is one of the risk factors for developing a DVT.
- *Step 4: Identify problems/issues.* Nursing problems or diagnosis should be listed here. Mrs Wurramara's priority nursing problems are ineffective tissue perfusion and acute pain.
- *Step 5: Establish goals.* Goals of care for Mrs Wurramara should focus on improving tissue perfusion and managing pain.
- *Step 6: Take action.* The nurse should administer anticoagulants need when they are prescribed. The patient may need to be prepared for clot retrieval surgery or thrombolysis. Also, recognise the patient may be feeling extremely anxious and will need some reassurance. The nurse should also consider contacting her family to update them about her status.
- *Step 7: Evaluate outcomes.* Once the anticoagulants have been prescribed, the patient will need to be continually monitored on the medical ward for signs of DVT complications. A DVT can lead to a pulmonary embolus, which can be life threatening.
- *Step 8 Reflect on the process and new learning.* Reflect on any aspects of care that could have been done better.

CASE STUDY 14.2

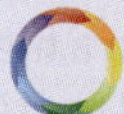

Nursing care of a male patient with chest pain

Mr Jolly is a 66-year-old Caucasian man who presented to the hospital due to severe, crushing chest pain lasting 12 hours. The patient has a medical history of being hypertensive and was a smoker. Without any prior symptoms, he complained of a sudden onset of chest pain and sought emergency medical care after about 12 hours due to the pain increasing.

A physical examination and observations revealed the following vital signs:

- temperature: 36.9°C
- heart rate: 90 beats per minute
- blood pressure:110/70 mmHg
- respiratory rate: 20 breaths per minute
- oxygen saturation: 94% on room air
- pain score: 10/10
- Glasgow Coma Scale: 15
- lung examination showed no alterations
- the initial ECG showed sinus rhythm, with ST elevation in leads V1 to V6.

Question

Using the information above, describe what action you would take as the nurse caring for this patient. Use the clinical reasoning cycle to guide you through the process and devise a plan of care for your patient.

Answer

- *Step 1: Consider the patient.* Mr Jolly, a 66-year-old Caucasian man.
- *Step 2: Collect cues/information.* Include subjective and objective data here. Include the appearance of the patient and their past medical history. He described increasing, persistent crushing chest pain. Objective data will include measurable information such as his vital signs.
- *Step 3: Process information.* Separate the relevant and irrelevant data — cluster the clues together to formulate an inference about the patient. Mr Jolly has central crushing chest pain that is worsening, and ST elevation in his anterior leads on his ECG. He has a past medical history of hypertension and smoking, which places him at a higher risk of MI. This information meets the criteria for STEMI, a medical emergency, and he needs urgent treatment to reduce the damage to his myocardium.
- *Step 4: Identify problems/issues.* Nursing problems or diagnosis should be listed here. Mr Jolly's priority nursing problems are ineffective tissue perfusion: cardiac, ineffective breathing pattern, impaired gas exchange and acute pain.
- *Step 5: Establish goals.* Goals of care for Mr Jolly should improve his cardiac tissue perfusion.

- *Step 6: Take action*. The nurse should immediately recognise that Mr Jolly meets the criteria for a medical emergency call. He could suffer from a life-threatening cardiac arrhythmia at any time. Urgent treatment by the medical emergency team, including thrombolysis or PCI if available, is needed to avoid any further damage to the patient's heart. As the nurse caring for Mr Jolly, you must consider interventions such as increased frequency of observations, gathering emergency equipment in case of sudden cardiac arrest, ensuring the patient has two large-bore IV cannulas in situ to facilitate large, rapid volumes of fluid to be administered (in case of cardiac arrest). Ensure an ACS pathway has been initiated and the patient is connected to continuous cardiac monitoring. Also, recognise the patient may be feeling extremely anxious and will need some reassurance. You should also consider contacting his family so they can be updated about his deterioration by the doctor.
- *Step 7: Evaluate outcomes*. Once the medical emergency team has attended and the patient has been stabilised, they may need to be prepared to go to the cardiac catheter lab for PCI or transferred to the coronary care unit.
- *Step 8: Reflect on the process and new learning*. Reflect on any aspects of care that could have been done better.

SUMMARY

CVD is one of the major causes of death in Australia. Therefore nursing students must understand the assessment and treatment of conditions related to the cardiovascular system, such as valvular disease, rhythm problems, vascular disorders, coronary heart disease and venous thromboembolism. As nurses are at the forefront of patient care, they must have the skills required to perform a cardiovascular assessment and act upon any abnormal findings to prevent any patient deterioration. This chapter has explored the assessment and diagnosis of common cardiovascular conditions and discussed the nursing management of the same. High-quality nursing care before, during and after cardiac/vascular investigation and treatment is essential in ensuring a good outcome for patients.

KEY TERMS

arteries Carry oxygenated blood away from the heart, with the exception of the pulmonary artery, which carries deoxygenated blood.

capillaries Thin-walled vessels that allow an exchange of substances between the blood and body tissues.

cardiac arrhythmia An abnormal conduction of the electrical impulses in the heart.

deep vein thrombosis (DVT) The development of a blood clot in a deep vein.

electrocardiogram (ECG) A graphic representation of the electric current generated by the wave of depolarisation that progresses through the atria and ventricles (the P wave and QRS complex), followed by the wave of ventricular repolarisation (the T wave) (Huszar 2007).

NSTEACS Non-ST elevation acute coronary syndrome.

NSTEMI Non-ST elevation myocardial infarction.

pulmonary embolus (PE) A clot of blood(s) travel from the legs, pelvis, abdomen or heart, through the veins, and cause a sudden blockage of blood flow in the arteries that supply the lungs.

STEACS ST elevation acute coronary syndrome.

STEMI ST elevation myocardial infarction.

veins Carry deoxygenated blood towards the heart, with the exception of the pulmonary vein, which carries oxygenated blood.

REFERENCES

Atherton, J. J., Sindone, A., De Pasquale, C. G., Driscoll, A., MacDonald, P. S., Hopper, I., Kistler, P. M., Briffa, T., Wong, J. & Abhayaratna, W. (2018) National Heart Foundation of Australia and Cardiac Society of Australia and New Zealand: guidelines for the prevention, detection, and management of heart failure in Australia 2018. *Heart, Lung and Circulation*. 27(10): 1123–1208.

Australian and New Zealand Society for Vascular Surgery. (n.d.) Aortic aneurysm. www.anzsvs.org.au/patient-information/aortic-aneurysm

Australian Institute of Health and Welfare (AIHW). (2020) Cardiovascular disease. www.aihw.gov.au/reports/heart-stroke-vascular-diseases/cardiovascular-health-compendium

Australian Institute of Health and Welfare (AIHW). (2019) Acute rheumatic fever and rheumatic heart disease in Australia, 2013–2017. www.aihw.gov.au/reports/indigenous-australians/acute-rheumatic-fever-rheumatic-heart disease

Australian Nursing Federation. (2018) Chest pain assessment and management. *Australian Nursing and Midwifery Journal*. 26(3). 30–33. https://search.proquest.com/openview/71a7a4c3be96078086b5ff5a1560d3d7/1?pq-origsite=gscholar&cbl=33490

Australian Resuscitation Council. (2016) The ABCDE approach to assessment guidance. https://resus.org.au/?s=assessment

Australian Resuscitation Council. (2018) ANZCOR Guideline 11.2 – Protocols for adult advanced life support. https://resus.org.au/guidelines

Barrett, D. (2006) 'Valve disease, cardiomyopathy and inflammatory disorders'. In Barrett, D., Gretton, M. & Quinn, T. (eds), *Cardiac care. An introduction for healthcare professionals*. Chichester: John Wiley & Sons.

Chua, A., Blankstein, R. & Ko, B. (2020) Coronary artery calcium in primary prevention. *Australian Journal for General Practitioners*. 49: 464–469. www1.racgp.org.au/ajgp/2020/august/coronary-artery-calcium-in-primary-prevention

Gabb, G. M., Mangoni, A. A., Anderson, C. S., Cowley, D., Dowden, J. S., Golledge, J., Hankey, G. J., Howes, F. S., Leckie, L. & Perkovic, V. (2016) Guideline for the diagnosis and management of hypertension in adults— 2016. *Medical Journal of Australia*. 205(2): 85–89.

Gallo, M., Blitzer, D., Laforgia, P. L., Doulamis, I. P., Perrin, N., Bortolussi, G., Guariento, A. & Putzu, A. (2020) Percutaneous coronary intervention versus coronary artery bypass graft for left main coronary artery disease: A meta-analysis. *The Journal of Thoracic and Cardiovascular Surgery*. https://doi.org/https://doi.org/10.1016/j.jtcvs.2020.04.010

Goldstone, A. B., Chiu, P., Baiocchi, M., Lingala, B., Patrick, W. L., Fischbein, M. P. & Woo, Y. J. (2017) Mechanical or biologic prostheses for aortic-valve and mitral-valve replacement. *New England Journal of Medicine*. 377(19): 1847–1857 https://doi.org/10.1056/NEJMoa1613792

Goldstone, A. B. & Woo, Y. J. (2016) Is minimally invasive thoracoscopic surgery the new benchmark for treating mitral valve disease? *Annals of Cardiothoracic Surgery*. 5(6): 567–572. https://doi.org/10.21037/acs.2016.03.18

Huszar, R. J. (2007) *Basic dysrhythmias: Interpretation and management*. 3rd ed. St Louis: Mosby.

Johnson, K. & Rawlings-Anderson, K. (2007) *Oxford Handbook of Cardiac Nursing*. Oxford: Oxford University Press.

Jones, D. E., Braun, M. & Kassop, D. (2020) Acute coronary syndrome: Common complications and conditions that mimic ACS. *FP Essent*. 490: 29–34.

Marshall, K. (2011) Acute coronary syndrome: diagnosis, risk assessment and management. *Nursing Standard*. 25(3): 47–57.

Nair, M. & Peate, I. (2009) *Fundamentals of Applied Pathophysiology*. Wiley Blackwell.

National Heart Foundation. (n.d.) What is angina. www.heartfoundation.org.au/conditions/angina

National Heart Foundation. (2012) Guidelines for the management of absolute cardiovascular disease risk. www.heartfoundation.org.au/getmedia/4342a70f-4487-496e-bbb0-dae33a47fcb2/Absolute-CVD-Risk-Full-Guidelines_2.pdf

Nickson, C. (2020) Troponin in critical illness. https://litfl.com/troponin-in-critical-illness

Nicol, M., Bavin, C., Cronin, P. & Rawlings-Anderson, K. (2008) *Essential Nursing Skills*, 3rd ed. London: Mosby Elsevier.

Scottish Intercollegiate Guidelines Network. (2010) Prevention and management of venous thromboembolism. SIGN 122. www.sign.ac.uk/guidelines/fulltext/122

Sertic, F. (2021) 'Chapter 6 — Endothelial signaling in coronary artery disease'. In S. Chatterjee (Ed.), *Endothelial Signaling in Vascular Dysfunction and Disease* (pp. 59–67). Academic Press. https://doi.org/https://doi.org/10.1016/B978-0-12-816196-8.00022-9

Theivendran, M. & Chuen, J. (2018) Updates on AAA screening and surveillance. *Australian Journal of General Practice*.

Tortora, G. J. & Derrickson, B. H. (2011) *Principles of Anatomy and Physiology*. Danvers, MA: John Wiley & Sons.

Vergallo, R., Jang, I. K. & Crea, F. (2021) New prediction tools and treatment for ACS patients with plaque erosion. *Atherosclerosis*. 318: 45–51. https://doi.org/10.1016/j.atherosclerosis.2020.10.016

ACKNOWLEDGEMENTS

Figure 14.10(a): © JY FotoStock / Shutterstock.com

Figure 14.10(b): © DR P. MARAZZI / SCIENCE PHOTO LIBRARY

Figure 14.10(c): © James Heilman, MD / Wikimedia Commons / CC BY-SA 3.0.

Figure 14.11: © SPENCER SUTTON / SCIENCE PHOTO LIBRARY

Figure 14.12: © ilusmedical / Shutterstock.com

Table 14.1: National Heart Foundation of Australia. Guideline for the diagnosis and management of hypertension in adults — 2016. Melbourne: NHFA, 2016.

Photo 14A: © Pavel L Photo and Video / Shutterstock.com

Photo 14B: © Romanets / Shutterstock.com

CHAPTER 15

Nursing care of conditions related to the digestive system

LEARNING OBJECTIVES

After studying this chapter, you should be able to:

15.1 describe the anatomical structures of the digestive system

15.2 describe the elements required to perform a comprehensive nursing assessment of the digestive system

15.3 describe all the essential components of routine nursing care for gastrointestinal patients

15.4 identify the key features of the care of pre- and post-operative gastrointestinal patients

15.5 identify the investigations that may be necessary to aid diagnosis

15.6 recognise the common presenting symptoms of gastrointestinal tract disorders

15.7 detail common disorders of the gastrointestinal tract

15.8 identify the components of the biliary system and their function

15.9 discuss the epidemiology of obesity and available operative treatments.

Introduction

This chapter provides an overview of disorders affecting the digestive system. The specific nursing care of individuals with disorders of the digestive system is presented, alongside the related anatomy and physiology where appropriate. Nursing priorities when assessing individuals with disorders of the digestive system are then addressed, followed by a consideration of the nursing care required from both a conservative and a surgical approach as indicated. The aetiology, pathophysiology, investigations, diagnosis and clinical treatment of these conditions are outlined.

15.1 The anatomical structures of the digestive system

LEARNING OBJECTIVE 15.1 Describe the anatomical structures of the digestive system.

The digestive system extends from the mouth through the pharynx, oesophagus, stomach, duodenum and small and large intestines, terminating in the anal canal and rectum. The digestive system's accessory organs include the teeth, salivary glands, liver, pancreas and gallbladder (figure 15.1). The digestive system's primary functions (including both the main and the accessory organs) include the ingestion, **mastication** and digestion (mechanical and chemical) of food, absorption of nutrients, and the elimination of the waste products of digestion.

FIGURE 15.1 Organs of the digestive system

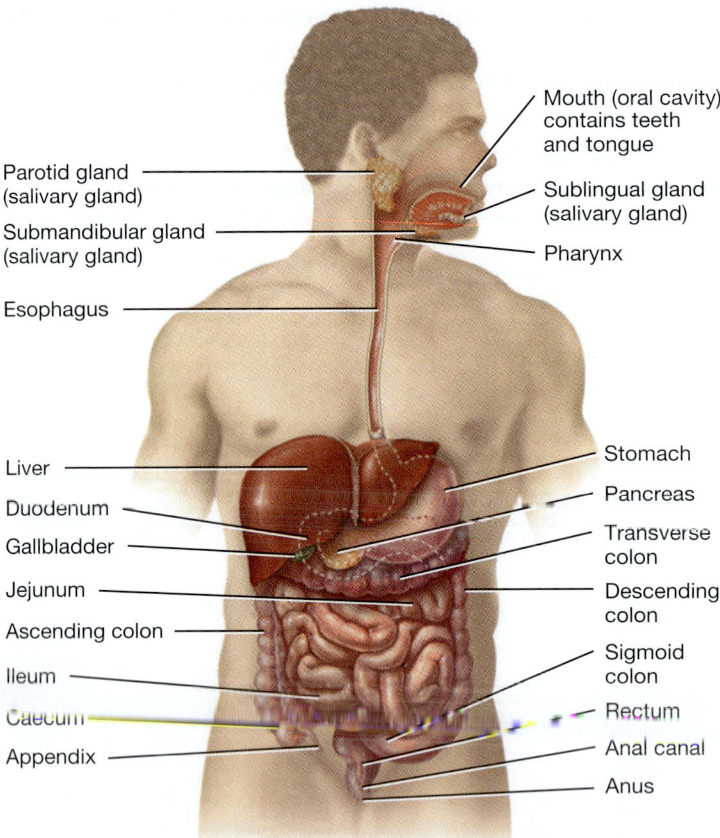

Source: Tortora & Derrickson (2011) *Principles of Anatomy and Physiology*, with kind permission of Wiley Blackwell.

15.2 Routine nursing assessment for the gastrointestinal patient

LEARNING OBJECTIVE 15.2 Describe the elements required to perform a comprehensive nursing assessment of the digestive system.

A detailed assessment is essential in determining an appropriate nursing care plan for all individuals with conditions affecting the digestive system. Assessment should include, but is not limited to, the following key areas:

- a general observation of the patient, including the vital signs
- the patient's medical, surgical and social history
- identification of the presenting signs and symptoms.

The principles of nursing assessment chapter covers nursing assessment in detail; however, this chapter addresses specific observations and clinical features of conditions related to the digestive system. These observations should include:

- general appearance, including:
  - skin — dehydration, pallor, jaundice, bruising, itching
  - eyes — sunken eyes, yellow sclera, pale conjunctivae
  - mouth — halitosis; lips (dry, chapped, pale, presence of sores); tongue (dry and coated, ulcerations); condition of the gums and teeth
  - weight — current weight in addition to any recent unexplained changes in weight
- vital signs — blood pressure, temperature, pulse, respiration and pain score
- diet — any changes in dietary habits or appetite, altered bowel pattern, food intolerances
- medical/surgical history — any pre-existing conditions or previous surgery
- medication history — usual medications, any recently commenced medications, drug allergies
- social/personal history — any recent international travel, use of recreational drugs including alcohol and smoking, significant life events, occupation
- symptoms — the presence or absence of any of the following specific symptoms:
  - nausea and vomiting — note the onset, duration and triggers of vomiting in addition to the characteristics of any vomitus
  - dyspepsia (indigestion)
  - **dysphagia** (difficulty swallowing)
  - abdominal pain — note the site, onset, nature and severity, the course and any precipitating and relieving features
  - bowel sounds — present or absent
  - **haematemesis** (the presence of blood in the vomitus)
  - diarrhoea — note the onset, duration and frequency, the characteristics of the stools and any exacerbating or relieving features
  - constipation — note the onset and duration, the characteristics of the stool, whether the condition is chronic or irregular, and whether there is any associated pain or discomfort
  - **melaena** (a black tarry stool resulting from bleeding in the upper gastrointestinal tract)
  - palpable lump(s) — note the site, onset and characteristics.

It is imperative to ascertain from the patient the characteristics of specific symptoms, including their onset, nature, severity and duration, to make a comprehensive nursing assessment and provide an accurate and prompt medical diagnosis.

15.3 Routine nursing care for the gastrointestinal system

LEARNING OBJECTIVE 15.3 Describe all the essential components of routine nursing care for gastrointestinal patients.

A systematic approach to planning and implementing nursing care will ensure that an individual's needs are comprehensively addressed. Appropriate nursing care is outlined here.

Communication

It is crucial to have clear person-centred communication at all times in order to establish trust and a good nurse–patient relationship. This should ensure that patients' needs are identified and met quickly and effectively to maximise patient outcomes.

Observations

In addition to the signs and symptoms outlined previously, the patient should be monitored closely for any deterioration in condition. The vital signs (blood pressure, temperature, pulse, respiration and pain score) should be monitored regularly, the frequency of readings being determined by the patient's condition and medical advice. Any deviation from baseline observations should be documented and reported immediately.

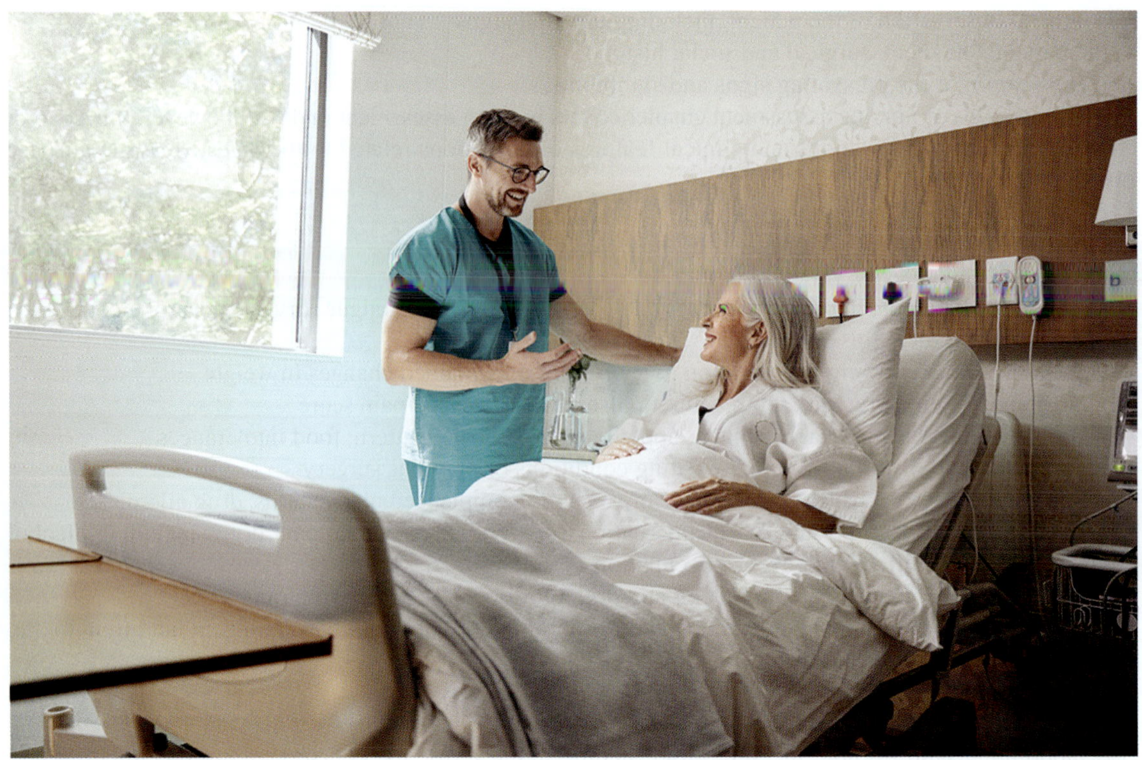

Nutrition and hydration

It is imperative to ensure that any patient with a digestive disorder is adequately hydrated at all times. If, as is frequently the case with this patient group, oral intake is not permitted due to the presenting symptoms, intravenous access must be established and hydration facilitated by an intravenous infusion. A strict fluid balance record must be maintained. In addition, meticulous attention to oral hygiene is a priority when oral intake is prohibited or inhibited.

Where oral intake is possible, a balanced nutritional intake should be encouraged. It helps enlist the hospital dietitian's assistance, who can provide appropriate dietary advice and guidance. Symptoms such as dyspepsia, dysphagia, nausea and loss of appetite are likely to interfere with the patient's nutritional intake, and such symptoms should be reported, investigated and managed appropriately. The management of these symptoms may be conservative, for example, the prescription of antacids such as calcium carbonate; histamine (H_2) receptor antagonists such as ranitidine; or proton pump inhibitors such as omeprazole in the case of dyspepsia (Bryant, Knights, Darroch & Rowland 2019), but further interventions may also be required. It is essential to provide adequate patient education on the actions, side effects and potential interactions of any medications.

Elimination

Common presenting features of digestive disorders include nausea, vomiting, diarrhoea and constipation. As already mentioned, it is important to observe the nature, course and characteristics of these symptoms to get a clear insight into the patient's condition and determine the best treatment course. An accurate record of the patient's output (vomitus, diarrhoea and urinary output) is essential to determine hydration needs and prevent dehydration. A patient experiencing frequent diarrhoea should, where possible, be located close to the bathroom in order to maintain their privacy and dignity during elimination and hygiene needs. Ensure a bedpan is in place so that output can be measured. Stool samples should be obtained for investigations, including faecal occult blood and culture and sensitivity of any organisms present.

Pain relief

Patients with a digestive disorder are likely to experience varying degrees of pain. An accurate pain assessment using a recognised pain assessment tool is integral to adequate pain management and should include observation of verbal and non-verbal cues. The nurse needs to act promptly to any complaints of pain the patient may have. It may be necessary to establish a definitive diagnosis in specific emergencies before pain relief can be administered. In these cases, it is important to communicate this clearly to patients and reassure them that the situation will be resolved as quickly as possible. All efforts should also be made to maximise the patient's comfort. Clear reporting and documenting of the patient's pain, prescription medication(s), and administration and evaluation of pain relief are paramount in diagnosis and management. Any drug allergies must be ascertained prior to administering any medication.

Preparation for investigations

A variety of investigations may be necessary to make a diagnosis. Specific examples include X-rays, ultrasound, gastroscopy, barium swallow, colonoscopy and laparoscopy (see figure 15.4 and 15.5). Some of these require no particular preparation. However, investigations such as colonoscopy and laparoscopy require very specific preparation, including bowel clearance and/or fasting in advance. Local policy regarding the preparation for such investigations must be adhered to.

If the patient is to have a colonoscopy, it should be explained to the patient that their bowel needs to be completely clean so no faecal material will obstruct the camera lens, ensuring a successful procedure. Bowel preparation is found to be ineffective in 25 per cent of cases. It is linked to missed diagnoses of bowel cancers during screening. This increases costs to the health system and adds to the patient's distress as they will need to be rebooked for the procedure and have to go through the bowel prep again. Be aware that the commonly used bowel preps generally work by causing an osmotic shift of fluid into the bowel. Thus, the patient is at risk of dehydration and electrolyte shifts. Care must be taken to ensure adequate hydration. Patients with renal disease or cardiac conditions should be administered hyperosmotic bowel prep with care and careful monitoring (Lichtenstein 2009).

Mobilisation

The patient's mobility may be limited. It is important to encourage active mobilisation if the patient's condition permits to prevent complications of prolonged bed rest, such as chest infection, constipation, pressure ulcer development and deep vein thrombosis. Anti-embolism stockings or sequential compression devices may also be needed for this purpose. Otherwise, active limb exercises, repositioning and deep breathing exercises should be encouraged.

Psychosocial support

Hospital admission can be traumatic and frightening for the patient and indeed for their family members. This anxiety may be compounded by a fear of any impending diagnosis and treatment. A friendly approach and clear, regular communication can help to reassure the patient and their family. Keeping the patient (and where appropriate, the next of kin) informed on their progress with prompt updates regarding any test results and care plan can alleviate unnecessary worry. It is also imperative to ask for the patient's social history, including their next of kin and any social support network, as such information is vital for optimal discharge planning.

15.4 Patients undergoing gastrointestinal surgery

LEARNING OBJECTIVE 15.4 Identify the key features of the care of pre and post-operative gastrointestinal patients.

Surgery on the digestive system can range from laparoscopic ('keyhole') surgery to open abdominal surgery (figure 15.2). It can be for the purpose of:

- investigation (e.g. laparoscopy)
- excision (e.g. appendix, gallbladder or intestine)
- repair (e.g. hernia)
- transplantation (liver or pancreas).

Surgery may be elective (planned) in nature or carried out as an emergency. In some cases, it may have life-changing consequences, such as the formation of a stoma, as in the case of an ileostomy or colostomy.

FIGURE 15.2 Gastrointestinal surgery

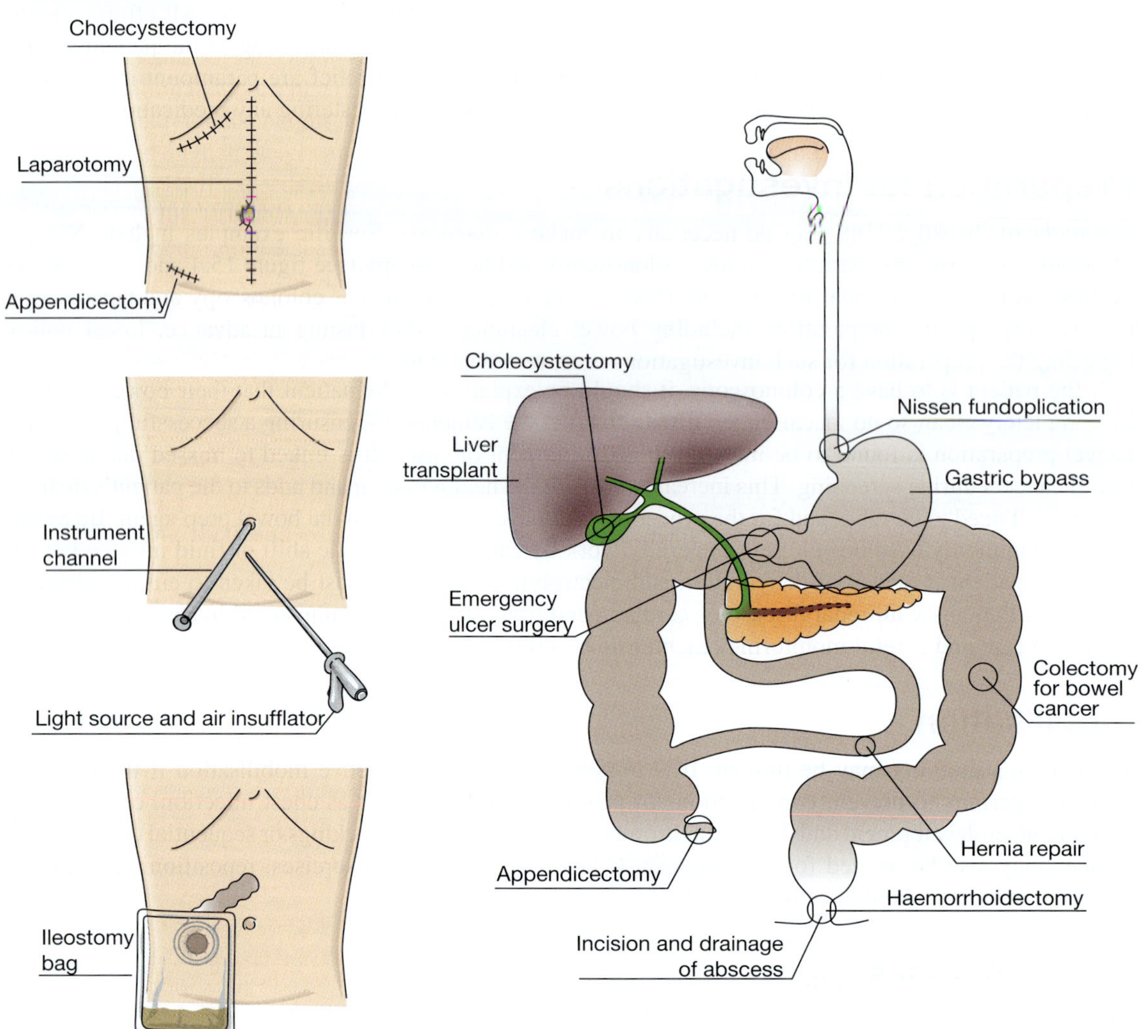

Source: Keshav & Baily (2012). *Gastrointestinal System at a Glance*, 2nd ed. with kind permission of Wiley Blackwell.

Preoperative management

The general principles of preoperative management can be found in the principles of surgical nursing chapter, but preoperative management specific to patients with a digestive disorder will be outlined here.

The patient will need to fast in preparation for gastrointestinal surgery. In theory, this means that the patient may have light food for up to six hours and water and clear fluids for up to two hours preoperatively (ACI 2016). However, depending on the digestive disorder and the surgery's nature and site, the surgeons' preference or hospital policy, the patient may have to fast for longer. The patient's hydration and nutritional status must be monitored closely, and appropriate measures taken to prevent dehydration and malnutrition. This may include administering intravenous fluids or even total parenteral nutrition.

In addition to preoperative fasting, the patient undergoing intestinal surgery will sometimes require bowel clearance, depending on the surgeon's preference. This may involve a low-residue diet or clear fluid intake and the oral ingestion of a purgative preparation such as sodium picosulphate over the 24–48 hours prior to surgery to cleanse the bowel of faecal matter (Lichtenstein 2009). Local guidelines could be consulted for details of the policy and procedure involved. The patient should be supported during this preparation as it can be unpleasant and uncomfortable, and care should be taken to ensure that the patient's dignity is maintained.

Along with the usual risks associated with surgery, such as infection and haemorrhage, gastrointestinal surgery carries the additional risk of peritonitis and negative outcomes, such as **stoma** formation or a poor prognosis in the case of a malignancy. It is vital to provide patients with clear, comprehensive explanations of the condition, its treatment and its prognosis and ensure they fully understand what they will be asked to consent to. The stoma care specialist will need to be consulted over the stoma location and the patient's physical and psychological preparation. Setting up a meeting with a person who already has a stoma may also be helpful. Spend time with the patient listening to their concerns and answering their questions where possible.

Post-operative management

The patient may return from theatre with an intravenous infusion line, nasogastric tube, urinary catheter, wound drain and/or stoma in place. The purpose of these should be explained clearly to the patient, along with an indication of how long they may be in place and any specific care that will be required. Monitoring and documentation of vital signs and fluid balance are of the utmost priority after gastrointestinal surgery. Such complications as shock, infection, haemorrhage, dehydration and peritonitis can then be detected early. If the patient experiences nausea and vomiting post-operatively, they may require an antiemetic — the effect of which should be monitored.

Pain management is crucial in the post-operative period. Assess the patient's pain level using a pain assessment tool and note any physiological signs of pain or body cues indicating pain. The patient's reports of pain must be responded to promptly. Analgesia should be administered as prescribed, and the patient's response should be observed for any side effects and documented. Make sure that patients on patient-controlled analgesia know how to use it safely and effectively. This should be explained to the patient preoperatively. Trying to explain it to a patient immediately post anaesthesia is unlikely to be effective and may result in the patient not accessing adequate pain relief appropriately. Ensure the patient is comfortable, the wound is not under strain, and any drain or catheter tubing is not compressed or kinked.

Gastrointestinal surgery often results in a temporary cessation of peristalsis, leading to paralytic ileus. The patient may not eat or drink anything while this condition persists as doing so may result in profuse vomiting and unnecessary discomfort or pain. Monitoring for the return of bowel sounds by auscultation will signal the return of peristalsis. Once the bowel sounds have returned and the patient is no longer vomiting, they are usually commenced on sips of clear fluids followed by a light diet as tolerated, depending on the type of surgery and the surgeon's post-operative instructions. The post-operative instructions may vary greatly depending on the surgeon and the procedure. Traditionally patients following abdominal surgery have been kept on clear fluids until they pass flatus, then introduced to a light diet. Following a return of bowel sounds and having passed a bowel motion, they will proceed to a full diet. In 2001, a group of European surgeon academics developed the enhanced recovery after surgery (ERAS) protocols. These demonstrated that '**perioperative** care rather than the actual operation dictated the outcomes' (Ljundquist, Scott & Fearon 2017). The ERAS protocols have been widely recognised; however, it has taken some time for change to happen in the clinical setting. Evidence suggests that it takes 15 years after clear evidence is available to effect clinical change.

The ERAS protocols cover four areas of the patient journey from preadmission through to discharge and are multimodal and multidisciplinary.

During preadmission, the patient is encouraged to give up smoking and limit alcohol intake. There should be preoperative nutritional screening attended and, when necessary, changes made to the patient's diet. Any current chronic conditions are noted, and the patient is medically optimised in relation to these chronic conditions (Ljundquist, Scott & Fearon 2017). All these actions are taken to reduce complications and ensure that the patient is as fit for surgery as possible.

Preoperatively the patient is given structured information about the procedure, and relatives and caregivers are involved when appropriate, helping to reduce anxiety. Carbohydrate treatment to reduce insulin resistance and enhance recovery is utilised, prophylaxis against thrombolysis is implemented, and prophylaxis against nausea and vomiting are utilised (Ljundquist, Scott & Fearon 2017).

Intraoperatively minimally invasive techniques are recommended where applicable to reduce complications. Anaesthesia is standardised, avoiding long-acting opioids, and epidural anaesthesia is used where applicable to reduce the stress response. Vasopressors are recommended to support blood pressure control, and the use of surgical drains is restricted to promote mobilisation and reduce pain (Ljundquist, Scott & Fearon 2017). Body temperature is controlled using warm air flow blankets and warmed IV infusions which helps reduce complications. Fluid balance is noted carefully, ensuring the patient does not become over or under-hydrated.

Post-operatively, patients are mobilised early rather than remaining on bed rest for several days (Ljundquist, Scott & Fearon 2017). Early oral intake is advised to support energy and protein supply, and chewing gum and laxatives are offered to support the return of gut function. Urinary catheters and IV fluids should be removed the morning after surgery when possible. A multimodal approach to opioid-sparing pain control and nausea and vomiting is used.

In Australia, the ERAS protocols are being much more widely now, with guidelines available from the Clinical Excellence Commission (NSW), Queensland Department of Health and The Royal Australasian College of Surgeons.

15.5 Diagnostic investigations

LEARNING OBJECTIVE 15.5 Identify the investigations that may be necessary to aid diagnosis.

A wide variety of tests can contribute to the diagnosis of digestive disorders. These include **radiological**, ultrasound, endoscopic, laparoscopic and serum investigations (figure 15.3). In addition to these investigation results, a physical examination of the patient, description of their symptoms and their history will lead to a definitive diagnosis in most cases.

FIGURE 15.3 Radiology and imaging

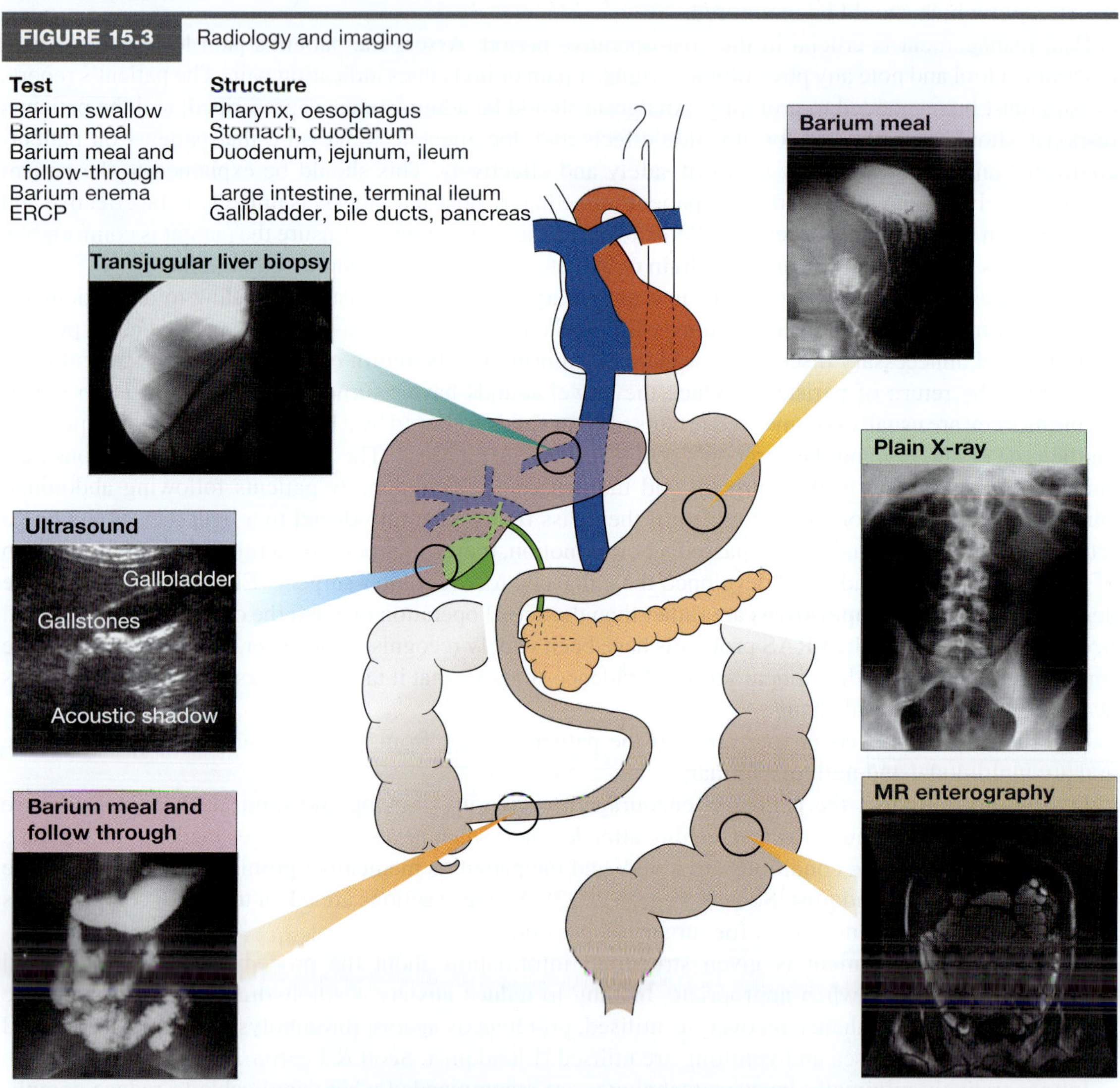

Nuclear medicine scans

Scan name	Principle and uses
Gastric emptying scan	The rate of passage of a labelled meal measures gastric motility
Meckel's scan	Labelled pertechnetate taken up by parietal cells localises ectopic gastric tissue
Red cell scan	Labelled red cells reinjected into the patient localise rapidly bleeding lesions
White cell scan	Labelled white cells reinjected into the patient accumulate at sites of inflammation
Octreotide scan	Labelled octreotide binds to somatostatin receptors, localising neuroendocrine tumours that strongly express these receptors
SeHCAT scan	Measures retention of exogenous labelled bile acid (homocholic acid taurine) to diagnose bile acid malabsorption

Source: Keshav & Baily (2012) *Gastrointestinal System at a Glance*, with kind permission of Wiley Blackwell.

Radiological investigations

A plain film (without radiopaque contrast) of the abdomen, also referred to as an abdominal X-ray, as well as contrast studies, are common investigations. The plain film allows the identification of gas and fluid levels that may indicate bowel disease or obstruction. No specific preparation or aftercare is required. Always ask if there is a chance that the patient may be pregnant. This can cause abdominal pain, and X-rays should only be done after pregnancy has been ruled out.

Imaging studies of the gastrointestinal tract commonly use the contrast medium barium sulphate and include the barium swallow, barium meal, barium follow-through and barium enema. The barium is administered orally or rectally, depending on the part of the gastrointestinal tract being investigated. Barium is radio-opaque and therefore visible on an X-ray. This enables abnormalities of the oesophagus, stomach and intestinal tract to be visualised. Air can also be used as a contract medium for gastrointestinal investigations, but this is less common. However, these procedures are contraindicated in cases of suspected obstruction or perforation of any part of the digestive tract.

The preparation for these investigations varies. In the case of a barium swallow, meal or follow-through, the patient will need to fast for 8–12 hours in advance. Medications should be withheld eight hours prior to the exam. In the case of the barium enema, however, the patient will require a low-residue diet and high fluid intake for one to three days prior to the test, in addition to bowel clearance (Knox 2017). In all cases, the barium should pass from the patient's system unaided, but occasionally a mild laxative may be required to assist its evacuation. Patients should also be encouraged to increase their oral fluid intake, where appropriate, to prevent constipation.

Abdominal ultrasound

Abdominal ultrasound is a non-invasive investigation that involves imaging the abdominal cavity using sound wave technology to produce two-dimensional images. It allows the abdominal organs and structures to be examined for inflammation and abnormalities. It aids in diagnosing several conditions, including cholecystitis, irritable bowel disease, abdominal masses and hepatomegaly. It is particularly useful for the detection of gallstones (Venables 2011).

Endoscopy

Endoscopic investigations allow direct visualisation of the mucosal lining and organs of the gastrointestinal tract using rigid or flexible scopes equipped with a light source and camera (figure 15.4). Such investigations include:

- esophagogastroduodenoscopy (visualising the oesophagus, stomach and duodenum)
- endoscopic retrograde cholangiopancreatography (ERCP; for the gallbladder and biliary and pancreatic ducts)
- proctoscopy (the rectum)
- sigmoidoscopy (the distal colon)
- colonoscopy (the entire large bowel).

In addition to directly visualising and capturing images of the gastrointestinal tract and organs, endoscopies also allow biopsies and fluid samples to be obtained to help diagnosis. Endoscopy can also be used to remove polyps (abnormal tissue growth in the intestinal mucosa) and treat certain conditions such as bleeding ulcers, oesophageal varices, bleeding intestinal lesions and some gastro-oesophageal obstructions caused by tumours, strictures or foreign bodies.

Patients are usually sedated for endoscopic investigations, and these can, if necessary, be performed under anaesthetic. The preparation of the patient varies depending on the endoscopic investigation being undertaken. Informed consent must be obtained from the patient before undergoing any endoscopic procedure. Bowel prep will be individualised to the patient. They may be on a low-residue diet for two to three days preoperatively with an aperient, or they may only be given an aperient/bowel purgative. Check carefully which regime the surgeon has requested for the patient. All patients should be on a clear fluid diet on the day of surgery (Lichtenstein 2009; ACSQHC 2018). As a general rule, patients should fast for two hours preoperatively (ACI 2016). It is important to consult local policy for their fasting guidelines and any additional preparation that may be warranted. The patient's condition and vital signs should be monitored closely during and after all endoscopic investigations to detect signs of haemorrhage, perforation or aspiration.

FIGURE 15.4 Endoscopic procedures

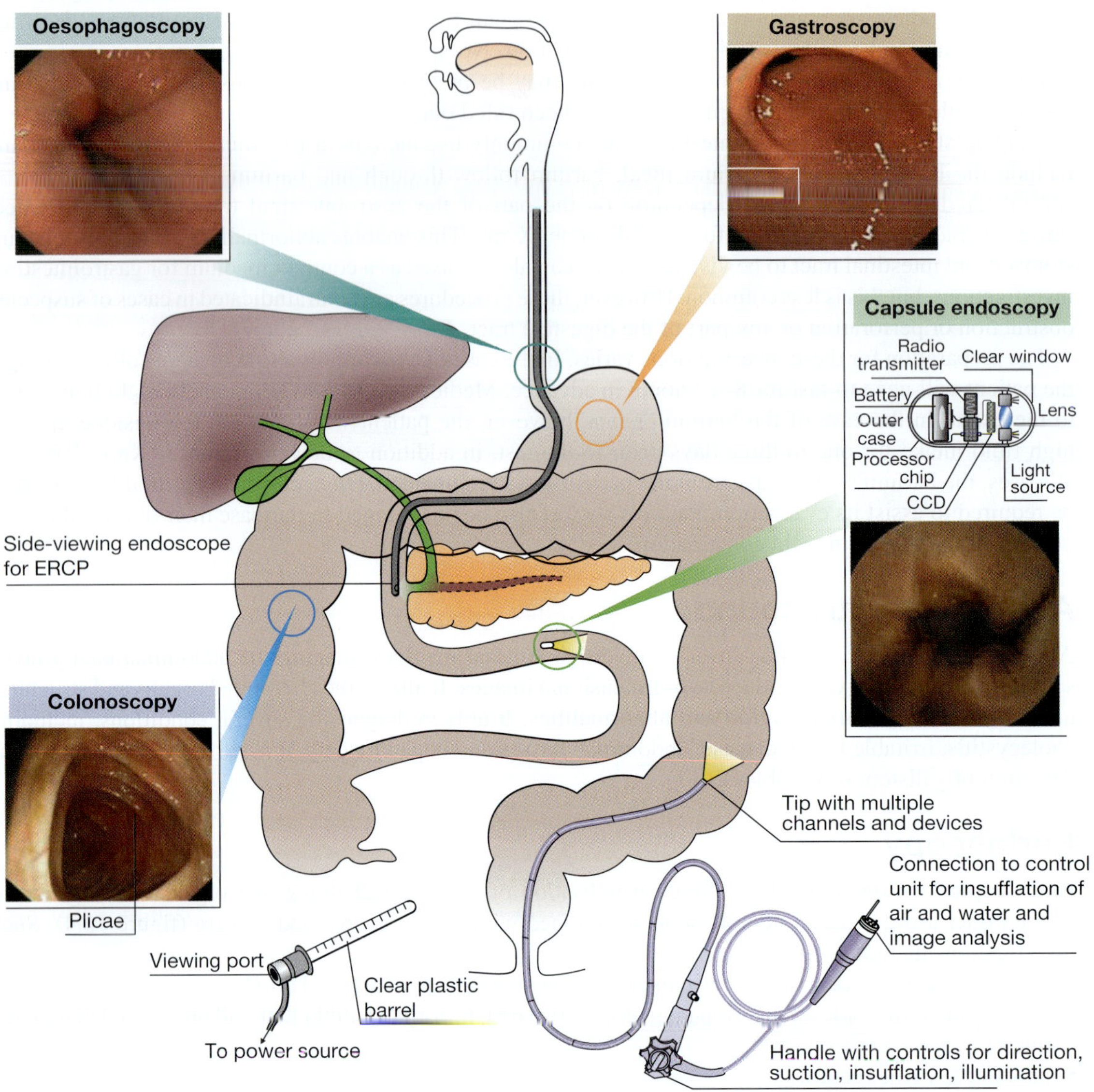

Source: Keshav & Baily (2012) *Gastrointestinal System at a Glance,* 2nd ed. with kind permission of Wiley Blackwell.

Computed tomography scanning

Computed tomography scanning produces cross-sectional images of the organs of the gastrointestinal tract. It is usually performed if the ultrasound scan has been unsuccessful or inconclusive. A contrast medium may be used to enhance the images of the abdominal organs, but this can impair renal function and cause anaphylaxis. Where these risks may prove too high, alternative means of investigation and diagnosis should be considered.

Laparoscopy

Laparoscopy is very useful in the diagnosis of digestive disorders. It is performed under anaesthetic, involving a small incision ('keyhole') through the abdominal wall to allow the injection (insufflation) of carbon dioxide into the peritoneal cavity. This moves organs and structures away from each other so they can be better visualised (Teitelbaum & Soper 2019). This technique helps in obtaining tissue and fluid samples from the abdominal structures and organs, as well as detecting inflammation, masses, gallbladder and liver disease and other abnormalities. It may be necessary to proceed to therapeutic measures such as laparoscopic excision in certain circumstances, for example, of the gallbladder, or to open abdominal surgery if needed. This possibility must be clearly stated and explained to the patient preoperatively when seeking informed consent.

Stool analysis

Stool samples can be examined for their volume, consistency, odour and colour. This initial assessment should be performed in the ward by the attending nurse each time the patient opens their bowels. Laboratory tests include checking for the presence of blood, bacteria, viruses, parasites, cysts, ova, toxins, pus cells and white cells, all of which can produce symptoms of diarrhoea and intestinal inflammation.

Blood tests

A variety of blood tests may be ordered, depending on the patient's presenting clinical features, and may include:

- full blood count
- urea, creatinine and electrolytes (E.U.C.)
- clotting factors
- liver function tests.

15.6 Common presenting symptoms of the gastrointestinal tract

LEARNING OBJECTIVE 15.6 Recognise the common presenting symptoms of gastrointestinal tract disorders

Despite the range of different disease processes that may occur throughout the **gastrointestinal tract**, many of the symptoms a patient presents with are similar.

Constipation

Constipation can be defined as passing less than two stools per week or difficulty passing stools, the incomplete or infrequent passage of hard stools, or a reduced volume of stools. It occurs more often in older adults and may result in straining and/or pain on defaecation, frequent flatus, abdominal discomfort and anorexia (Hillman 2017). The normal pattern of defaecation varies from person to person and ranges from three times a day to once every three days. It is important to establish with the patient what their normal bowel pattern is and document this in the nursing assessment. Remember to ask the patient each day if they have opened their bowels and document on the relevant chart.

Constipation may be acute or **chronic**. It may be a primary problem or a result of a disease or condition. Changes in bowel patterns that become persistent and more severe may result from a tumour or bowel obstruction. Chronic constipation may be due to functional causes that impair storage, transport or the normal passage of faeces. The causes of constipation can be differentiated into two broad categories: mechanical and functional. Mechanical causes of constipation include obstruction due to inflammatory bowel disease, postponing defaecation, lesions and scar tissue after previous surgery. Functional causes of constipation include reduced gut motility due to immobility and paralytic ileus after surgery, poor dietary fibre or fluid intake and long-term use of laxatives. Certain drugs such as iron preparations and codeine phosphate have a constipating effect. Other symptoms associated with constipation include abdominal distension and discomfort, reduced appetite, headache and indigestion (Hillman 2017).

Constipation is diagnosed by collating the patient's history and symptoms, coupled with a physical examination and investigations such as an abdominal X-ray. Particular attention is paid to the patient's normal bowel pattern and whether the constipation is a deviation from that pattern. Any recent changes to the patient's lifestyle or dietary intake or medications that may have led to constipation are also of particular interest. Treatment of constipation involves administering oral laxatives in the first instance. However, they should not be given if the patient has contraindications such as bowel obstruction, faecal impaction, undiagnosed abdominal pain or possible appendicitis. The patient should be educated on a nutritious diet high in fibre and fluid intake, if appropriate, and regular exercise and lifestyle modifications to prevent a recurrence. Prolonged constipation can lead to various complications, including haemorrhoids, impaction, hypertension and bowel perforation in extreme cases (Hillman 2017).

Diarrhoea

Diarrhoea can be described as an increase in frequency, volume and fluid content of the stool. (Hillman 2017). Some individuals may also experience abdominal and/or rectal pain.

Numerous factors can cause diarrhoea, so a comprehensive patient history should be taken. Diarrhoea can be acute or chronic, depending on the cause and/or condition. For example, diarrhoea caused by infective agents (in the case of food poisoning) is acute and usually self-limiting. In contrast, diarrhoea secondary to an underlying condition such as ulcerative colitis may be more chronic. Acute diarrhoea should be treated initially as a high transmission risk, and appropriate personal protective equipment (PPE) and isolation should be considered until the cause is confirmed. Clostridium difficile (C-diff) is recognised as a significant cause of treatment-related diarrhoea. Interestingly C-diff may be able to proliferate following antibiotic therapy (Hillman 2017).

Chronic diarrhoea may be exacerbated by milk, yoghurt and soft cheeses, fruit and juices high in fructose such as apple juice, pear juice, grapes and dates. Sugarless gums and mints that contain sorbitol or mannitol as the sugar substitute and coffee and tea can also cause or exacerbate diarrhoea (Hillman 2017).

Complications of diarrhoea can include fluid and electrolyte imbalance, which can, in extreme cases, lead to cardiac arrhythmias and other cardiac complications. If diarrhoea is extreme or prolonged, intravenous fluid and electrolyte replacement may be required.

Priorities of nursing management focus on maintaining the patient's dignity, facilitating good personal hygiene, ensuring and encouraging adequate fluid replacement and offering reassurance and support as necessary. Education about the importance of handwashing is a priority measure, especially in the case of infectious diarrhoea. Where possible, it is prudent to identify the underlying cause of the diarrhoea by sending a stool sample to the laboratory for analysis, among other diagnostic tests. Diarrhoea treatments may include fluid and electrolyte replacement, antidiarrhoeal agents, such as loperamide or codeine preparations to reduce intestinal motility, and antimicrobial agents if an infective organism has been identified. For the very young and elderly, diarrhoea may impact their skin integrity swiftly and keeping the perineal area and buttocks clean and dry is imperative. Barrier creams should be used to assist in maintaining skin integrity. All patients should have easy access to a toilet, commode or bedpan (Hillman 2017).

Nausea and vomiting

Nausea is the feeling or sensation of sickness and the desire to vomit, which may or may not result. Vomiting is the forceful expulsion of the gastric contents, which is usually preceded by nausea. It is important to note that vomiting can be a significant presenting feature of several conditions and can provide a useful indication of potential underlying conditions or the end diagnosis. Other symptoms that often accompany nausea and vomiting include sweating, increased salivation and tachycardia.

The causes of nausea and vomiting are numerous and may include pregnancy, ingested infective organisms or irritants, reduced gastric emptying and intestinal motility, peritoneal irritation, hepatobiliary or pancreatic disorders, bowel obstruction, reduced intestinal motility secondary to anaesthesia, disorders of the vestibulocochlear (VIIIth cranial) nerve, neurological conditions involving raised intracranial pressure or infections of the central nervous system, and cancer treatments such as chemotherapy or radiotherapy (Talley & O'Connor 2014). If nausea and/or vomiting are prolonged or severe, several potential outcomes can result, such as dehydration, electrolyte imbalance, weight loss, acid erosion of the teeth and oesophageal tears leading to haematemesis (vomiting blood).

Priorities of nursing care are directed towards identifying the underlying cause so that specific treatment can be initiated, in addition to correcting fluid and electrolyte imbalance and reassuring and supporting the patient. Antiemetic medications such as ondansetron, metoclopramide prochlorperazine or droperidol may be prescribed in an attempt to alleviate nausea and vomiting.

15.7 Disorders of the gastrointestinal system

LEARNING OBJECTIVE 15.7 Detail common disorders of the gastrointestinal tract.

The gastrointestinal system is a complex system involving several different organs, each with very different physiology and function. It includes hollow organs: the mouth, oesophagus, stomach, duodenum, small intestine, large intestine and anus, and solid organs: the liver, pancreas and gallbladder. Therefore a wide range of disease processes may occur.

Cancers of the gastrointestinal system

Cancer can affect any part of the digestive system, with varying disease manifestations, progression and consequences.

Colorectal cancer is the second most common cancer in men and women in Australia and is more common in those over 50. It is the second most common cause of cancer death and is responsible for nine per cent of all cancer deaths (Australian Institute of Health and Welfare 2014). In Australia, approximately 14 000 cases of colorectal cancer are diagnosed each year. Early detection is key to optimising the management and patient outcome. A National Bowel Cancer Screening Program (NBCSP) was introduced in Australia in 2006. Australians between the age of 50–74 are mailed screening kits, which they perform at home and then post back for testing. This is done every two years, with the aim to reduce the mortality of bowel cancer (Cancer Council Australia n.d.).

Diagnosis

The number and nature of investigations undertaken to reach a diagnosis will be determined by the patient's presenting features and the location of the presenting complaint. Investigations additional to those already outlined include magnetic resonance imaging (MRI) and positron emission tomography (PET) scans, both of which offer a more detailed visualisation of the relevant tissues and structures.

The signs and symptoms of gastrointestinal cancers will vary depending on the part or area affected. Commonly presenting signs and symptoms include weight loss, loss of appetite, altered eating pattern, tiredness, nausea and vomiting, and anaemia.

More specific signs and symptoms related to the specific part or area affected may include:

- dysphagia
- dyspnoea dyspepsia
- a feeling of fullness
- haematemesis
- abdominal pain and/or distension
- altered bowel pattern
- altered stools, including melaena
- rectal bleeding
- tenesmus (the feeling of a need to pass stool even when the rectum is empty)
- a palpable mass in the affected region.

In addition to reaching a cancer diagnosis, it is also standard practice to ascertain the extent of the cancer, termed staging. Stages of cancer progression generally range from stage 1, in which the tumour is confined to its primary site, through to stage 5, involving an extensive spread of the cancer to tissues and organs in other parts of the body. The earlier the stage of the cancer at the time of diagnosis, the better the prognosis will be for the patient.

Treatment

Treatment of cancer will be determined by several factors, including the site, type and stage of cancer, the impact it has had on the patient, the anticipated efficacy of interventions, their effects on the patient and any comorbidity. Standard cancer treatments usually employed include surgery, where appropriate, chemotherapy, radiotherapy, photodynamic therapy, or any combination of these. A holistic and multidisciplinary approach to patient care is essential when caring for a patient undergoing treatment for cancer of the digestive system. The nursing care plan depends on the individual patient's specific diagnosis, the particular treatment regimen prescribed, and the patient's response to that treatment. Priorities of nursing care focus on:

- psychological care
- reassurance and promotion of the patient's dignity
- observing and documenting the vital signs and the patient's condition
- preventing infections
- maintaining a high level of personal hygiene
- managing symptoms such as pain, nausea, vomiting, diarrhoea, poor appetite and dehydration
- maintaining skin integrity
- encouraging sleep and rest.

It is essential to involve members of the multidisciplinary team such as the dietitian, stoma care specialist, chaplain, social worker, counsellor, and, where necessary, palliative care team. It is also essential to support and care for the patient before, during and after any prescribed treatments, respecting their wishes at all times.

Peptic ulcer disease

A peptic ulcer is a break or ulceration in the mucosal lining of the lower oesophagus, stomach or duodenum. Peptic ulcer disease (PUD) damages the lining, usually by increased acid secretion, leading to inflammation and ulceration (figure 15.5 shows the most common sites for peptic ulcer development). PUD can range from mild, causing few symptoms, to severe and even life-threatening, as in the perforation of the gastrointestinal wall. Helicobacter pylori infection and the use of non-steroidal anti-inflammatory drugs (NSAIDs) are the primary causes of both gastric and duodenal ulcers. Helicobacter pylori infection is found in 70 per cent of people with PUD (Parrish, 2017a). Duodenal ulcers are four times more common than gastric ulcers. The onset of gastric ulcers occurs most commonly in the 50–70 year age group, while duodenal ulcers most commonly affect the 20–50 year age group (Nurgali & Wildbore 2017).

FIGURE 15.5 Common sites for peptic ulcer development

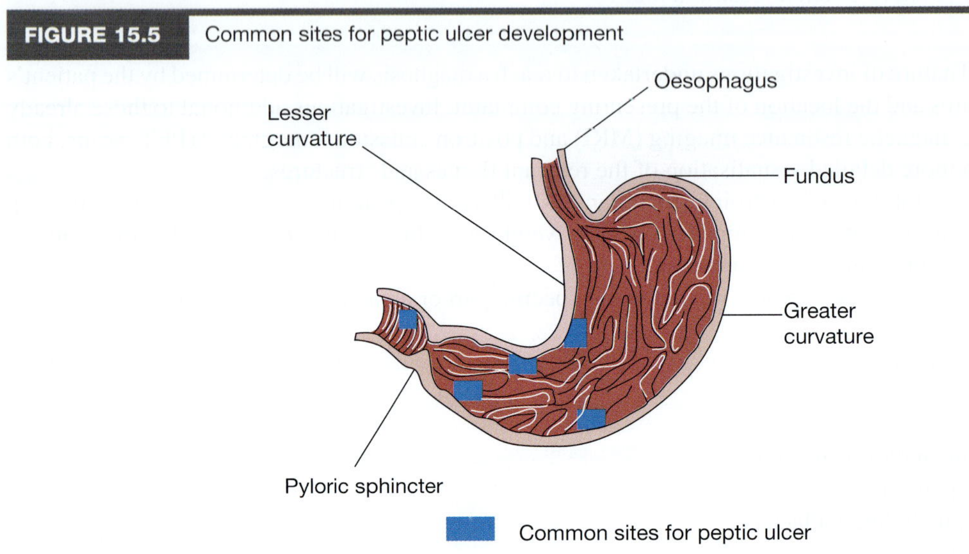

Source: Reproduced from Nair, M. & Peate, I. (2013) *Fundamentals of Applied Pathophysiology*, with kind permission from Wiley Blackwell.

Other factors that are thought to lead to PUD include smoking, alcohol, stress and genetic predisposition (Parrish 2017a; Nurgali & Wildbore 2017).

Clinical features and complications

Symptoms may vary from mild to severe, depending on the location and degree of ulceration, and can occur intermittently. **Epigastric** pain is the classic symptom of PUD. Patients with duodenal ulcers tend to have pain that occurs when the stomach is empty and is usually relieved by food, milk or antacids. This pain is typically described as gnawing or burning hunger like pain in the epigastric region. Patients with gastric ulcers are likely to have post-prandial (after eating) pain (Lanas & Chan 2017). It is often less clear in older adults and may present with vague and poorly localised pain — it may present as chest pain or dysphagia. Weight loss or anaemia may also be signs of PUD in the older population as bleeding is a frequent complication (Parrish 2017a).

Other common symptoms include:

- dyspepsia (indigestion)
- loss of appetite
- heartburn due to reflux of gastric acid and belching
- nausea and vomiting
- melaena

Hospital admission for PUD has decreased steadily over the past 20–30 years. Bleeding, perforation and gastric obstruction are the major complications of PUD with five to ten per cent mortality. Perforation is the erosion of the ulcer through the gastric or duodenal wall into the peritoneal cavity, leading to the stomach contents' movement into the peritoneal cavity causing chemical and bacterial peritonitis (Nurgali & Wildbore 2017). These complications are potentially life-threatening and require emergency treatment. Another complication of PUD is pyloric stenosis, in which the pyloric sphincter becomes obstructed due to scarring or stenosis, inhibiting the flow of the stomach contents into the duodenum.

Diagnosis

Assessment of the patient with PUD includes:

- patient history
- presenting symptoms
- physical observation and examination
- investigations to aid diagnosis, which include:
  - CT scan (often the first diagnostic procedure as it is less costly and less invasive than endoscopy)
  - gastroscopy (considered the gold standard for diagnosis)
  - biopsies
  - barium studies
  - a full blood count (a low haemoglobin level and haematocrit suggest anaemia)
  - an examination of stool samples for occult blood
  - a urease breath test and the colourimetric (CLO) test performed to detect *Helicobacter pylori* in a mucosal specimen obtained by endoscopy (Parrish 2017a).

Treatment

The cause of PUD will determine the treatment. In the case of ulcers secondary to *Helicobacter pylori* infection, antibiotic therapy using two or three antibiotics (amoxicillin, clarithromycin and metronidazole, for example) along with a proton pump inhibitor, such as omeprazole will be prescribed for 10–14 days in an attempt to eradicate the bacteria. This affects a permanent cure in 90 per cent of cases (Parrish 2017a; Nurgali & Wildbore 2017). Proton pump inhibitors and H_2 receptor antagonists such as ranitidine are used to treat ulcers that are not associated with *Helicobacter pylori*. Antacids such as calcium carbonate or magnesium salts can be used to treat symptoms such as heartburn and dyspepsia but often provide temporary relief only. Antacids may also interfere with the absorption of other drugs, including iron and antibiotics, both of which may be prescribed for these patients (Parrish 2017a). Long-term maintenance with medication may be required to prevent recurrence. The management of PUD should also incorporate advice and guidance on relevant lifestyle changes.

Nursing management

Nausea and vomiting can be treated with an antiemetic, such as prochlorperazine (Stemetil), ondansetron or metoclopramide (Maxolon). The mode of action of each of these antiemetics is different, so if one does not work, another may. The patient's response to the medication administered and the effects and side effects must be observed, documented and reported to the medical team when necessary.

Complications associated with PUD include haemorrhage, perforation and pyloric stenosis. If any of these complications occur, intravenous access will need to be established and fluid replacement initiated to correct hypovolaemia. In addition, the insertion of a nasogastric tube will allow aspiration to decompress and empty the stomach. There should be continual monitoring of vital signs and ongoing reassurance and support. Remember to document the fluid lost via nasogastric tube on the fluid balance chart. Oxygen therapy and monitoring of oxygen saturation levels will be required if there is haemorrhage, and replacement of blood components may become necessary if the haemorrhage is severe. The patient's full blood count and urea and electrolyte levels should be checked. A urinary catheter may be inserted, and the urinary output closely observed. Intravenous antibiotic therapy may be required to prevent septic shock where a perforation has occurred. Depending on the type and severity of the complication, the patient may also need to be prepared for endoscopy, for pyloric stenosis (to dilate the pylorus) or surgery, for perforation.

In order to reduce the risk of recurrence of PUD, the patient should be advised to stop smoking, reduce their caffeine and alcohol intake and modify their diet to include small regular meals and avoid foods that trigger gastrointestinal symptoms. Medications such as aspirin and NSAIDs should be avoided where possible. The patient should endeavour to reduce their stress levels if this is a contributing factor. Stress-relieving activities such as regular exercise, yoga and meditation should be encouraged.

Inflammatory bowel disease

Inflammatory bowel disease (IBD) describes inflammatory conditions of the bowel, including Crohn's disease, ulcerative colitis and diverticulitis. IBD is a chronic disorder characterised by an altered bowel pattern, abdominal pain and discomfort associated with defaecation (Hillman 2017). Other signs and symptoms may include severe diarrhoea, the presence of blood, pus or mucus in the bowel movements, nausea, vomiting, poor appetite and weight loss. IBD is typically episodic in nature, with the individual experiencing exacerbations and remissions of the disorder. Potential contributing factors that have been suggested include food intolerance or hypersensitivity, gastrointestinal infection, autoimmune, genetic and environmental factors, and stress. Almost 75 000 Australians have IBD, and this number is expected to increase. It affects approximately one in 250 people between the ages of 5–40. It tends to run in families and affects some ethnic groups more than others (Hillman 2017).

Diagnosis

IBD diagnosis is made by considering:

- patient history
- presenting symptoms
- physical observation and examination
- investigations, which can include:
  - endoscopic (sigmoidoscopy or colonoscopy)
  - barium studies
  - full blood count
  - vitamin B_{12} level
  - C-reactive protein level
  - stool samples for occult blood.

Treatment

Treatment of IBD may include the following.

- Drug therapies typically include corticosteroids, immunosuppressants (for autoimmune causes), local and systemic anti-inflammatories, antibiotic therapy and probiotic therapy.
- Depending on the symptoms, laxatives or antidiarrhoeal agents can be used.
- Antispasmodics and pain relief are used to promote comfort (Hillman 2017).

In severe cases, surgical intervention may be required, which may, in some cases, result in the formation of a stoma to rest the bowel. Some patients may need a partial or total colectomy (Hillman 2017). Dietary and lifestyle advice and psychological support are imperative in the care of individuals with IBD.

Nursing management

One of the key priorities of nursing management of the individual with IBD is psychological support and education. Given the debilitating and enduring nature of IBD, it can impact many aspects of an individual's lifestyle, including family, work and social activities. This can, in turn, result in the onset of depression. Therefore, it is essential to establish a trusting rapport with the individual and provide sufficient opportunity to voice any fears or concerns in relation to these areas. In addition, providing the individual with details of appropriate organisations that can offer ongoing support and help may prove useful in the long-term management of the condition. IBD Support Australia and IBIS (Irritable Bowel Information and Support) are two such organisations for IBD, while Beyond Blue is an organisation available 24 hours a day to offer telephone support for those concerned with anxiety and depression.

A key priority of nursing management is close monitoring of bowel pattern, fluid balance to detect any dehydration, particularly in the presence of diarrhoea, urea and electrolyte levels, nutritional intake, weight and vital signs. A low residue diet may be indicated during exacerbations. However, it is important to encourage the individual to include sufficient fibre, protein and calories in their diet during remissions. In cases of extreme diarrhoea, parenteral nutrition may be required until the diarrhoea subsides. Vitamin and mineral supplements may also be indicated.

In an acute phase of the condition, the individual should be encouraged to rest, and assistance with daily activities such as personal hygiene needs may be needed. The individual with severe diarrhoea should ideally be nursed in a single ensuite room or close to the bathroom to preserve dignity.

Close observation of the individual's condition to detect signs of potential complications is imperative. Complications that can arise include perforation and peritonitis, fistula development, bowel obstruction and toxic megacolon. The association between IBD and colorectal cancer has been recognised since 1925 and accounts for 10–15 per cent of deaths related to IBD. This increased risk of colorectal cancer is thought to be related to genetic and acquired factors. Inflammation and its link to cancer is well recognised (Dyson & Rutter 2012).

Appendicitis

The appendix is a rudimentary, blind-ending tube located at the caecum with no function in the evolved human digestive system. Its walls contain lymphatic tissue, and its inner lining secretes mucus that flows into the caecum. Appendicitis (inflammation of the appendix) occurs when the lumen becomes obstructed with materials such as faecaliths (small, hardened lumps of faeces), undigested food particles (e.g. seeds or nuts) or lymphoid tissue. This inflammation results in the presenting symptoms associated with appendicitis.

Commonly presenting appendicitis symptoms include pyrexia, nausea and vomiting, general abdominal discomfort localised to the right iliac fossa as the condition progresses, and rebound abdominal tenderness, particularly at the junction known as McBurney's point (located at the right iliac fossa). Less common symptoms such as constipation, diarrhoea or urinary symptoms may also be present. It is important to note that in elderly patients, these signs may be reduced or absent (Talley & O'Connor 2014).

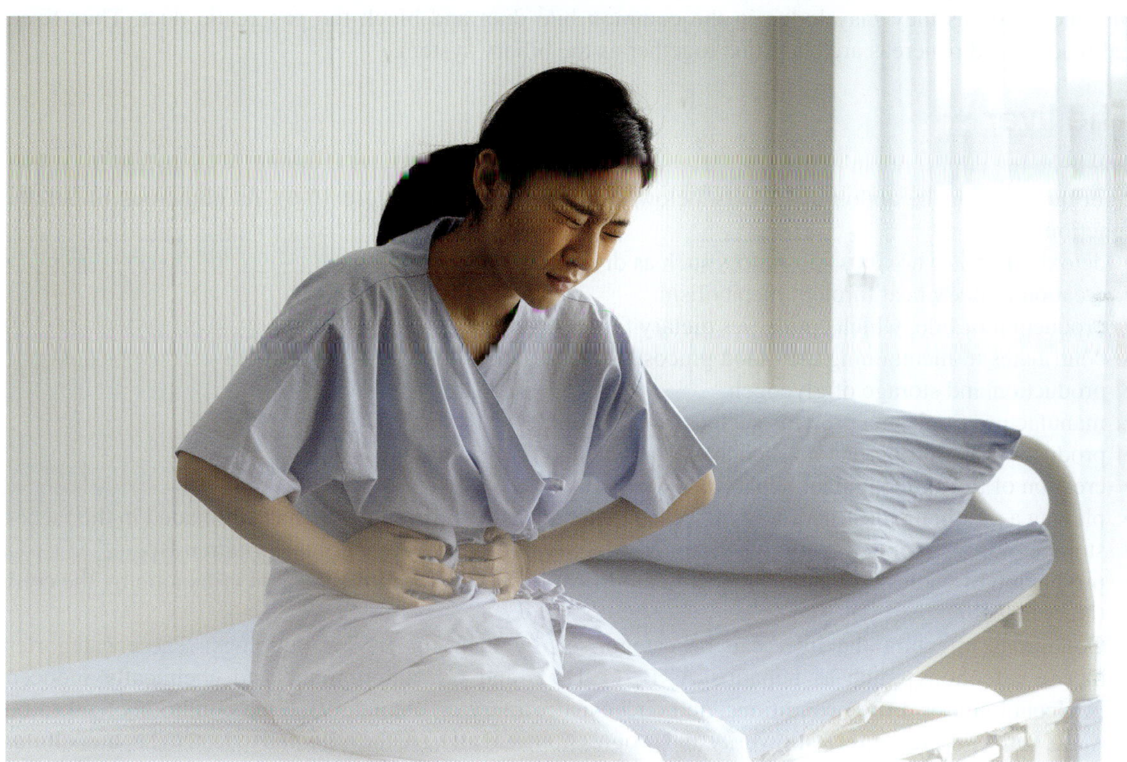

Diagnosis

Diagnosis of appendicitis involves:

- patient history
- presenting symptoms
- physical observation and examination
- investigations, including:
  - full blood count (to detect an elevated white cell count indicating the presence of infection)
  - urinalysis (to detect urinary tract infection and/or pregnancy in the case of women of child-bearing age)
  - an abdominal X-ray
  - an abdominal ultrasound.

Treatment

The treatment of appendicitis is surgical removal of the appendix (appendectomy) and antibiotic treatment. There are two surgical approaches: conventional 'open' surgery and laparoscopic surgery. If left untreated, the inflamed appendix may rupture, spilling infection into the peritoneal cavity and resulting in peritonitis and possible septic shock. Peritonitis signs and symptoms include abdominal distension and board-like rigidity, paralytic ileus, nausea and vomiting, pyrexia, tachycardia and hypotension. This is a life-threatening condition that warrants early detection and prompt intervention.

Nursing management

The nursing care principles for appendicitis include identifying potential problems, physical and psychological preparation of the patient for surgery, post-operative recovery, and early detection and prompt management of post-operative complications. The specific pre and post-operative care of a patient with a digestive disorder were addressed earlier in the chapter.

15.8 The biliary system

LEARNING OBJECTIVE 15.8 Identify the components of the biliary system and their function.

The word **biliary** relates to bile. The liver produces bile, the gall bladder stores the bile, and the pancreas produces lipase, an enzyme that works with bile to break down fats. The pancreatic duct joins the common bile duct at the sphincter of Oddi, where both flow into the duodenum. Gallstones are a common cause of pancreatitis as they may lodge in the common bile duct and block the pancreatic duct. Thus liver, gallbladder and pancreas are classified together as the biliary system.

The liver

The liver, the largest organ in the body weighing approximately 1200–1600 grams, is located in the upper right quadrant of the abdominal cavity below the diaphragm (see figure 15.6). Its numerous important functions are:

- detoxification of noxious substances such as drugs and alcohol
- creation of body heat through metabolism
- production of bile, which emulsifies dietary fat for absorption
- contributes to maintaining the blood glucose level
- production and storage of glycogen
- manufacture of plasma proteins such as albumin and globulins
- production of clotting factors such as fibrinogen and prothrombin
- creation of the anticoagulant heparin
- playing a part in the destruction of red blood cells, releasing bilirubin, which is eliminated in the faeces
- storage of iron, copper, fat-soluble vitamins A, D, E and K, and water-soluble vitamin B_{12}
- production of cholesterol and storage and modification of fats for more efficient utilisation by the cells (Nurgali 2017).

Conditions affecting the liver can be categorised by their underlying aetiology. These categories comprise infections (such as hepatitis A, B, C, D, E and G), autoimmune and chemically induced (e.g. alcohol and/or drugs) conditions, and cirrhosis (primary or secondary). Such conditions tend to be chronic, with varying degrees of severity and progression, and all have the potential to lead to hepatocellular carcinoma and liver failure with resulting portal hypertension. (Knox 2017).

Hepatitis C affects more than 230 000 Australians and is a common cause of chronic liver disease leading, in many cases, to liver cirrhosis and cancer. In March 2016, new oral direct-acting antivirals (DAA) became available on the PBS for patients over 18. These DAA medications can be administered by a primary care physician and have a 90 per cent cure rate (Khoo & Tse 2016).

The main type of injury that affects the liver is damage to the hepatocytes by cirrhosis and is strongly linked to high-fat diets and alcohol consumption. The most prevalent in Australia and New Zealand is non-alcoholic liver disease, which is the accumulation of fat in the liver cells (Nurgali & Wildbore 2017). Where possible, preventive measures should be employed to avoid contracting or developing liver disease in the first instance. However, early detection is key to optimising management and long-term outcomes for individuals who develop a liver condition.

Manifestations of liver disease can vary according to the underlying condition, and some patients may be asymptomatic for a while.

Some of the common presenting features include:

- a dull ache in the right upper quadrant
- jaundice (discolouration of the skin and sclerae due to an accumulation of bilirubin in the skin)
- fatigue
- weight loss, anorexia
- anaemia
- oedema, ascites (a collection of fluid in the peritoneal cavity)

- hepatosplenomegaly (an enlarged liver and spleen)
- clotting disorders
- dyspepsia
- altered bowel function
- gastric or oesophageal varices
- vitamin deficiency
- **portal hypertension** (increased pressure in the portal vein).

FIGURE 15.6 The liver

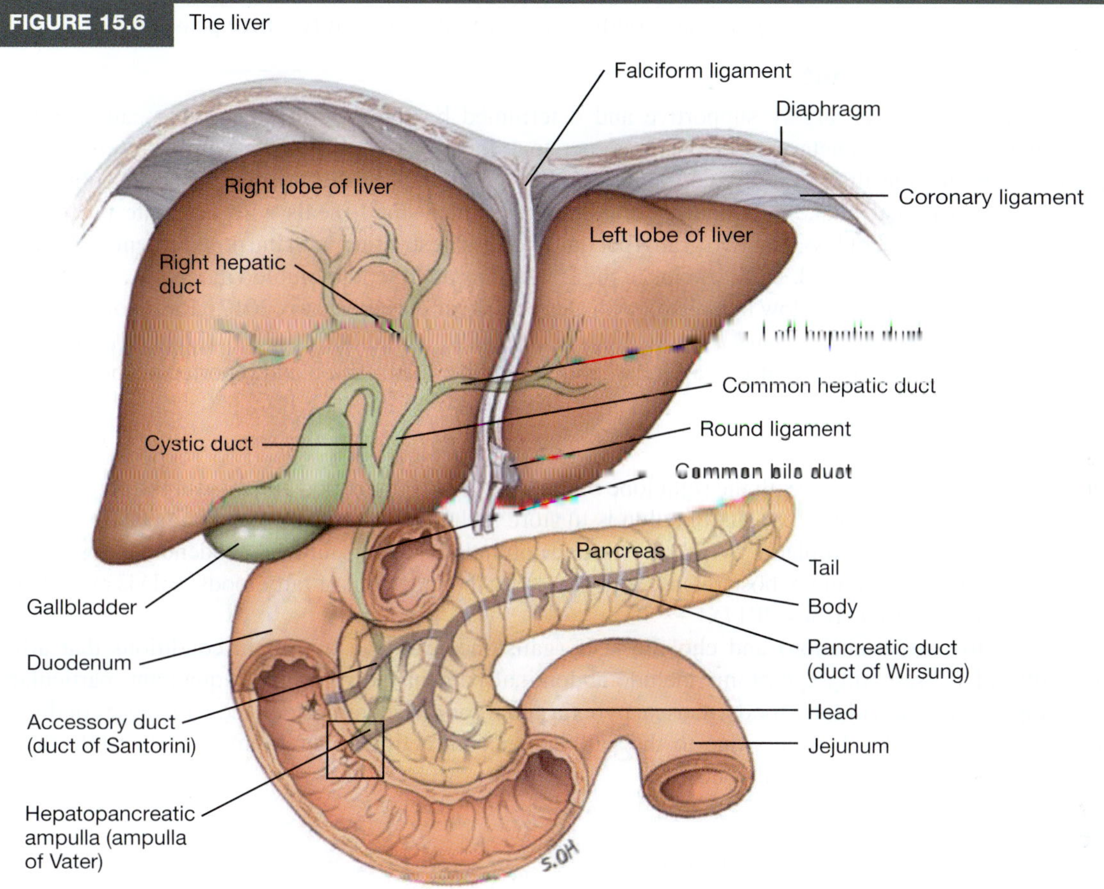

Source: Nair & Peate (2009) *Fundamentals of Applied Pathophysiology*, with kind permission from Wiley Blackwell

Diagnosis

The following are used in the diagnosis of conditions of the liver.

- patient history
- physical observation and examination
- signs and symptoms
- investigations, including:
  - full blood count
  - urea and electrolyte levels
  - liver enzymes (which may be elevated)
  - prothrombin time (which may be abnormal)
  - serum albumin (which may be low)
  - possibly, specific screening for infectious and/or autoimmune sources of hepatitis
  - stool examination
  - abdominal ultrasound
  - CT scan
  - MRI scan
  - liver biopsy (used to confirm the diagnosis and the nature and extent of the disease process).

Treatment

Therapies used to treat the diseases of the liver may include:

- antiviral treatment, as in the case of infective hepatitis (Khoo & Tse 2016) and corticosteroids
- prednisone in the case of autoimmune causes (Trivedi & Hirschfield 2013), and the pharmacological management of alcohol or drug misuse in addition to advice on abstaining from alcohol in the case of chemically induced disease and nutritional therapy (Frazier et al. 2011)
- a liver transplant in advanced disease
- in the case of irreversible liver disease, largely palliative treatment focusing on symptomatic relief, maintaining the individual's dignity and comfort and involving the family where possible.

Nursing management

Nursing management is largely supportive and determined by the specific underlying cause and the individual's symptoms. Dietary support is a cornerstone therapy for any patient with liver impairment. It is important to consult with a dietitian to develop an individualised dietary plan that will optimise an individual's nutritional intake and status. For example, regular small meals with adequate protein and calories, sodium intake of less than two grams per day and fluid restriction with the replacement of deficient vitamins should be prescribed. Deficiencies in the B vitamins and the fat-soluble vitamins A, D and E are common. Magnesium may be low in patients with alcoholic liver disease (Knox 2017). Relief of symptoms such as pain, pruritis (itching), nausea and oedema is integral to maintaining the individual's comfort. The individual's condition and response to all treatments should be documented and reported accordingly.

The gallbladder

The gallbladder is located beneath the right lobe of the liver. It is pear-shaped and measures approximately 7.5–10 cm in length (figure 15.6). Its function is to store and concentrate bile manufactured by the liver. Bile is released from the gallbladder via the cystic and common bile ducts into the duodenum in response to the hormone cholecystokinin, whose release is triggered by the ingestion of fatty foods. Bile is responsible for the breakdown of fat (Knox 2017).

Cholecystitis (inflammation) and cholelithiasis (gallstones) are the two main conditions that affect the gallbladder. Presenting symptoms include abdominal pain in the right upper quadrant, particularly following the ingestion of fatty foods, nausea, pyrexia and rigors. The pain associated with these conditions is described as colicky. It occurs due to the gallbladder contracting in an attempt to eject bile that is obstructed by the presence of gallstones.

Diagnosis

Diagnosis of gallbladder disease will involve:

- patient history
- presenting symptoms
- physical observation and examination
- investigations, including:
  - full blood count (which may reveal an elevated white cell count, indicating inflammation)
  - liver function tests (which may reveal elevated levels of biliary enzymes and bilirubin)
  - abdominal ultrasound
  - CT and/or MRI scan.

Treatment

Treatment of cholecystitis or cholelithiasis typically involves antibiotic therapy and surgical removal of the gallbladder. Cholecystectomy, conventionally an 'open' surgical procedure, is now typically performed using a laparoscopic ('keyhole') technique. The removal of gallstones only (rather than the entire gall bladder) when a patient has cholangitis is carried out using a procedure known as endoscopic retrograde cholangiopancreatography (ERCP). This involves passing an endoscope through the mouth, oesophagus and stomach into the duodenum.

Nursing management

The nursing care principles of gall bladder disease include identifying potential problems, physical and psychological preparation of the patient for surgery and post-operative recovery, and the early detection and prompt management of post-operative complications. The specific pre- and post operative care of a patient with a digestive disorder were addressed earlier in the chapter.

The pancreas

The pancreas is located behind the stomach and extends from the loop of the duodenum towards the spleen (figure 15.6). It is approximately 12–15 cm long and 2.5 cm thick. The pancreas has both endocrine and exocrine functions. Its primary function in the digestive system is to aid the digestion of carbohydrates, proteins and fats by secreting digestive enzymes into the duodenum via the pancreatic duct (an exocrine function). The endocrine cells produce the hormones glucagon and insulin necessary for normal carbohydrate, fat and protein metabolism (Parrish 2017b).

Pancreatic conditions related to digestion tend to occur primarily due to damage to the pancreatic duct by stones, tumours or trauma, releasing pancreatic enzymes that autodigest the duct tissue. In addition to possible bacterial infection, these escaping enzymes can also leak into the bloodstream. This has the potential to become a multisystem condition affecting other sites. Intravascular volume depletion leading to renal failure is a complication we must be alert to and is due to decreased intravascular volume. It will develop approximately 24 hours after onset. Acute respiratory distress syndrome (ARDS) may be another systemic complication we need to be aware of and will occur three to seven days after onset. This may be fatal. Pancreatitis can be acute or chronic in nature. Presenting symptoms include epigastric pain radiating to the back, nausea, vomiting and abdominal distension and rigidity. In addition to these symptoms, individuals with chronic pancreatitis may also present with weight loss, pain on eating and steatorrhoea (Knox 2017).

Diagnosis

The diagnosis of pancreatitis is made by considering:

- patient observation and history
- physical examination
- presenting symptoms
- investigations, which may include:
  - full blood count
  - C-reactive protein level
  - abdominal and chest X-rays
  - abdominal ultrasound scan
  - CT scan
  - MRI scan
  - an ERCP.

Treatment

Treatment of pancreatitis may include:

- oral food and fluid should be withheld in acute pancreatitis to reduce the pancreatic secretions and rest the pancreas
- intravenous fluid management in the initial phase to maintain intravascular volume and avert renal failure and ARDS
- nasogastric aspiration to relieve nausea, vomiting, abdominal distension and paralytic ileus
- pain relief as a priority
- antibiotic therapy if there is infection
- oral hypoglycaemic drugs
- palliative measures.

Nursing management

It is imperative to note that individuals with pancreatitis can deteriorate very quickly. Frequent monitoring of the patient's condition and prompt management of any complications that may arise are paramount. Key priorities of nursing care should include management of fluid and electrolyte balance, relief of pain and discomfort, optimising respiratory function, improving nutritional status, and psychological support (Knox 2017).

15.9 Obesity

LEARNING OBJECTIVE 15.9 Discuss the epidemiology of obesity and available operative treatments.

The World Health Organization (WHO) (2020) defines overweight and obesity as 'abnormal or excessive fat accumulation that present a risk to health'. Overweight refers to increased body weight when measured against the individual's height and when the body mass index (BMI) — a calculation of an individual's body fat based on their weight and height measurements — is between 25 and 29.9 kg/m^2. Obesity is said to exist when the BMI exceeds 30 kg/m^2 (WHO 2020). A BMI of 40 kg/m^2 indicates extreme obesity. These conditions predispose individuals to an increased risk of various health issues, including hypertension, heart disease, respiratory disease, type 2 diabetes mellitus, vascular disease, varicose veins, cerebrovascular accidents and bowel cancer, increasing morbidity, mortality and healthcare costs. Obesity levels have tripled worldwide since 1975 and continue to rise globally, particularly in urban settings. (WHO 2020). In Australia, 60 per cent of adults are overweight or obese, and 25 per cent of children (Department of Health, Australian Government. 2020).

Bariatric surgery

Bariatric surgery is one approach to managing obesity. It is used in cases where professionally advised weight-reducing diets and exercise programs have not proven successful. Bariatric surgery generally falls into three categories: restrictive surgery such as gastric banding; primary restrictive techniques with a malabsorptive component such as gastric bypass; and malabsorptive approaches involving various anatomical diversions of the gastrointestinal tract. Surgical approaches such as gastric banding and gastric bypass help weight loss by reducing the size of the individual's stomach, therefore, the amount of food the individual can ingest. These are known as restrictive procedures. The other type of procedure is known as malabsorptive surgery. The most common method is a Roux-en-Y procedure where the stomach is made smaller, and the duodenum is bypassed to reduce absorptive capacity. These procedures are commonly done laparoscopically (Campbell-Crofts 2017). Although this type of surgery is available, it is important to emphasise that conservative measures such as lifestyle modifications and pharmacological approaches are available and should, where possible, be considered first.

In conjunction with psychological support, all of these surgical techniques help with significant weight loss, but all bariatric procedures alter the gastrointestinal system's anatomy and physiology. Following bariatric surgery, the patient will be more susceptible to nutritional deficiencies, such as vitamin D, iron and protein being the most common (Lupoli et al. 2017), leading to anaemia, osteoporosis and muscle wasting.

Nursing management

Nursing care principles include identifying potential problems, physical and psychological preparation of the patient for surgery and post-operative recovery, and early detection and prompt management of post-operative complications. The specific pre and post-operative care of a patient with a digestive condition were addressed earlier in this chapter. It is important to ensure that the appropriate healthcare personnel, such as the dietitian, are involved in all stages of patient care delivery.

CASE STUDY 15.1

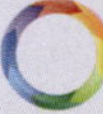

Nursing care of a patient with vomiting and diarrhoea

A 21-year-old male presents to the emergency department with a history of 4 days of vomiting and diarrhoea. He has no regular medications and is otherwise fit and healthy. On arrival, he looks pale and states he has pain of 8/10. He says he feels very nauseated and is clutching a bowl as he feels as though he is constantly about to throw up. States he has not passed urine for the last 8 hours.

His vital signs are:

- heart rate: 102 beats per minute
- blood pressure: 100/65 mmHg
- respiratory rate: 18 breaths per minute
- oxygen saturation: 99%
- pain scale: 8/10

- temperature: 37°C
- blood glucose: 3.9.

On inspection, there are no signs of blood in his vomit. He has had no diarrhoea for the last two days, but did two days previously. He hasn't tolerated any food for the past three days, and today is not tolerating fluids either. Denies illicit drug use, is a non smoker and only drinks alcohol socially. He has not travelled overseas recently.

Question

Using the information above, describe what action you would take as the nurse caring for this patient. Use the clinical reasoning cycle to guide you through the process and devise a care plan for your patient.

Answer

- *Step 1: Consider the patient.* 21-year-old male.
- *Step 2: Collect cues/information*. Include subjective and objective data here, including the patient's appearance and past medical history. Objective data will include measurable information such as his vital signs.
- *Step 3: Process information*. Separate the relevant and irrelevant data — cluster the clues together to formulate an inference about the patient.

  Patient has been vomiting for 4 days and is likely to be dehydrated. Vomiting in a younger person is most likely to be viral gastroenteritis, so he should be isolated until we confirm this. HR slightly elevated—likely linked to a combination of dehydration and pain.

  Pain 8/10 noted to be in the central abdominal region — needs analgesia.

  BGL low — related to lack of nutrition. Feels weak, likely exhausted from extended vomiting and lack of sleep due to vomiting as well as low BGL.

  Lips and tongue dry — probably dehydrated
- *Step 4: Identify problems/issues*. Nursing problems or diagnosis should be listed here.
  - Likely gastroenteritis (potentially infectious to other patients)
  - May be appendicitis; parasitic infection; new onset of IBD
  - Pain 8/10 from continual vomiting
  - Low BGL, which if it progresses, may cause a decrease in GCS
  - Dehydration.
- *Step 5: Establish goals.* Goals for this patient include decreasing pain to less than 3/10 and supplement either oral or IV to increase BGL. As they cannot tolerate oral fluids, rehydration needs IV access. Isolate patient ensuring correct use of PPE to stop the chance of spread of potential gastroenteritis to other patients.
- *Step 6: Take action.*
  - Liaise with doctor.
  - Chart and administer analgesia, antiemetics.
  - Organise IV cannula insertion and chart and commence IV fluids (always double-check with two RNs).
  - Isolate patient — ensure an adequate supply of PPE. Make sure others are aware by verbal and written communication and use of signage.
  - Collect stool sample when the patient is able to provide one and send to pathology for culture and sensitivity.
  - Continue regular obs (in ED, all patients will be on hourly obs for the first four hours).

  The patient has been given a litre of 4% dextrose N/5 saline over one hour. A second litre of fluids is now running over two hours N/S 0.9%. He has been given 2.5 mg of IV morphine and sublingual ondansetron 8 mg with good effect. Pain level now 2/10. Stool sample unable to be collected at this time.

  A single room was available and the patient has been isolated.

  Vital signs are now: HR 106; RR 18; SpO_2 100%; BP 105/70; BGL 5.2; Pain 2/10; T 37.4.
- *Step 7: Evaluate outcomes.* Two hours later, the patient now complaining of pain 7/10. Pain is now localised in the right iliac fossa. Rebound tenderness noted. Nil further vomiting.

  Vital signs: HR 110; RR 18; SpO_2 99%; BP 110/70; BGL 5.0; Pain 7/10; T 38.2

  Process new information: Pain is localised to the right iliac fossa and shows rebound tenderness. This is typical for appendicitis. Pain has increased despite a good initial response to analgesia. It seems likely that this patient has appendicitis.

  Temp and heart rate have risen, indicating an infective process. This patient may be developing sepsis, although, at this stage, BP is still within acceptable limits.

  Patient is getting teary and says he feels worse than before. He says he can't say exactly how, but he just feels really bad. You ask if he would like you to contact anyone for him, and he says he wants his Mum.

  Identify new problem: Patient is now showing signs that indicate appendicitis, which may first present with generalised abdominal pain and nausea. With the elevation of temperature, this patient may be developing sepsis. The patient is feeling alone and scared and needs support.

Establish new goal:

- Have the patient assessed by the doctor in the next 10 minutes.
- Reduce pain levels.
- Contact mother to see if she is available to come to comfort and support her son.

Take new action: Doctor notified of the deteriorating condition of the patient and organises a surgical review. IV antibiotics are ordered, and further analgesia given.

Mother was contacted and says she will be there shortly.

The surgical team confirm appendicitis diagnosis and organise emergency theatre. The patient made aware of the need for surgery and is given psychological support and education.

Prepare patient for theatre. Use preop checklist.

Evaluate new outcomes:

Vital signs: Pain now 3/10; HR 110; RR 18; SpO2 100%; BP 115/70; BGL 5.0; T 38.4

Voided 300 mL amber coloured urine. SG 1020, indicating that dehydration is slowly resolving

Mother arrives and has a calming and stabilising effect. The patient is relieved to know what is wrong and is happy to be going to theatre to be treated. He no longer needs to be isolated as deemed to be non-infectious to others as per the revised diagnosis. Patient stable pro tem.

- *Step 8: Reflect on the process and new learning.* This patient did not present with classic symptoms of appendicitis. Remember that many patients will not present with typical symptoms.

  The patient was on hourly obs as they were not stable, which is good as we could pick up on their shift in pain site and increase in temperature and realise this was not merely gastroenteritis. If they had been on four-hourly obs, we may have missed this until the appendix ruptured, which would have led to much more severe consequences, possibly peritonitis and septic shock.

  The patient is an adult, so we could not call a parent without their permission. Perhaps he should have been asked earlier if they wanted someone with them.

CASE STUDY 15.2

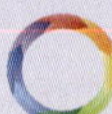

Nursing care of a patient with vaginal bleeding

Mrs Bates is a 60-year-old female who presented to emergency with a 6-week history of vaginal bleeding. She is awaiting a consult with the gynaecological team.

Her vital signs are:

- heart rate: 110 regular
- respiratory rate: 26 breaths per minute
- oxygen saturation: 89% on room air
- blood pressure: 110/70 mmHg
- pain: 0/10
- temperature: 36.5°C
- BGL: 6.8 mmol/L.

As the emergency department is extremely busy, she has been transferred to the medical acute care ward adjacent to the ED to await a consult from the gynaecological team.

Question

Using the information above and the track and trigger chart, describe what action you would take as the nurse caring for this patient. Use the clinical reasoning cycle to guide you through the process and devise a care plan for your patient.

Answer

- *Step 1: Consider the patient.* 60-year-old female presents to ED complaining of 6 weeks of vaginal bleeding. She says she went through menopause eight years ago and does not know why she has got her periods again. She is now feeling weak and breathless — past history of COPD, and congestive heart failure, ex-smoker.

  Patient is a poor historian. On questioning, she is very vague about her medical history and unsure which medications she is on or what they are for. However, she is certain she has vaginal bleeding.
- *Step 2: Collect cues/information.* Include subjective and objective data here, including the patient's appearance and past medical history. Objective data will include measurable information such as her vital signs.

  On examination, she has a pad on that has dark red blood. Full blood count shows low haemoglobin levels 11 gm/DL. She is very thin BMI 16 (underweight) and says she has lost weight over the past three months. The gynaecology team have been contacted, and the patient is awaiting review.

- *Step 3: Process information*. Separate the relevant and irrelevant data — cluster the clues together to formulate an inference about the patient
Heart and respiratory rate are high and SpO_2 low. This is likely related to her COPD and a low Hb will increase heart and respiratory rate as the blood's oxygen carrying capacity is reduced. SpO_2 may also be linked to either history of COPD or anaemia. Anaemia may be caused by vaginal bleeding.
We don't have enough information to make a definitive diagnosis and needs further data collection/examination.
Collect more cues: On examination of her perineal area, you note that the blood seems to be coming from her anus and the inner aspects of her vagina seem to be free of blood. You suspect that the patient may be losing blood from the gastrointestinal tract (GIT) and not per vagina.
Process new information: If this patient has blood loss from the gut, this will account for the low Hb. If she has rectal bleeding and we know she has had weight loss over the past three months this seems more likely to be bowel cancer.
- *Step 4: Identify the problem*. The patient remains undiagnosed, and we cannot treat her until she has a confirmed diagnosis. This no longer seems to be a likely gynaecological problem and seems more likely to be related to the GIT.
- *Step 5: Establish goals*. Patient needs a diagnosis to ensure appropriate treatment.
- *Step 6: Take action*. Inform the doctor of your new findings
- *Step 7: Evaluate outcomes*. The doctor thanks you for your focused assessment and communication. They now decide to investigate the possibility of her problem being gastrointestinal. They review the patient and ask for diagnostic tests related to GIT. The patient is sent for a CT scan which confirms a mass in the descending colon.
She is admitted under the gastroenterology team, who also book her for a colonoscopy and biopsy to confirm the diagnosis prior to deciding on surgery.
- *Step 8: Reflect on the process and new learning*. Clinical reasoning is not a linear process. It is a reiterative process that means we need to keep going back and forth collecting and analysing data until we have definitive conclusions about any potential or actual problem, allowing us to treat the patient most correctly and effectively.

SUMMARY

In this chapter, we looked at the common disorders of the digestive system. Careful assessment is essential for aiding accurate diagnosis, providing appropriate nursing care, ensuring a safe recovery and preventing complications. Key factors in the nursing assessment include observing the patient's general appearance, taking a medical and surgical history, noting symptoms, recording vital signs and the results of investigations. When caring for patients with digestive disorders, the main factors to address are communication, vital signs, nutrition, hydration, elimination, pain relief, preparation for investigations, mobility and psychosocial support.

KEY TERMS

biliary Relating to bile and the transportation of bile.

chronic A condition that is persistent or long-lasting. The term chronic is often applied when the disease process lasts longer than three months.

dysphagia Difficulty swallowing.

endoscopic Examination of the inside of the body using a flexible, lighted instrument.

epigastric The upper middle region of the abdomen.

gastrointestinal tract The tract from the mouth to the anus and includes all the organs of the digestive system (also known as the alimentary canal).

haematemesis The presence of blood in vomitus.

mastication The act of chewing.

melaena A black tarry stool resulting from bleeding in the upper gastrointestinal tract.

perioperative Before, during and after an operation. This may include a time frame of several days pre- and post-operatively.

portal hypertension Elevated pressures in the portal vein, a large vein, which carries blood from the digestive organs to the liver.

radiological A branch of medicine that uses radioactive materials or radiant energy (e.g. X-rays) in the diagnosis and treatment of disease.

stoma A Greek word meaning 'mouth' or 'opening'. The mouth, nose and anus are natural stomata. Surgical procedures that involve the creation of a stoma typically use the suffix 'ostomy' and will be referenced to the area that the stoma was created from, e.g. colostomy (from the colon), ileostomy (from the ileum).

REFERENCES

ACI. (2016) Enhanced recovery after surgery. Surgical services taskforce & anaesthesia and perioperative care network. Case study report.

Australian Commission on Safety and Quality in Health Care (ACSQHC). (2018) Colonoscopy clinical care standard.

Australian Institute of Health and Welfare. (2014) Cancer in Australia: an overview. [Version updated 16 April 2015] *Cancer series No 90. Cat. no. CAN 88.* Canberra. www.safetyandquality.gov.au/standards/clinical-care-standards/colonoscopy-clinical-care-standard

Bryant, B., Knights, K., Darroch, S. & Rowland, A. (2019) *Pharmacology for health professionals*, 5th ed. Elsevier.

Campbell-Crofts, S. (2017) 'Nursing care of people with nutritional disorders'. In Lemone & Burke (eds). *Medical-Surgical nursing. Critical thinking for person-centered care.* Pearson.

Cancer Council Australia. (n.d.) Bowel cancer screening. www.cancer.org.au/cancer-information/causes-and-prevention/early-detection-and-screening/bowel-cancer-screening

Department of Health, Australian Govt. (2020) *Overweight and obesity.* www1.health.gov.au/internet/main/publishing.nsf/Content/Overweight-and-Obesity

Dyson, J. & Rutter, M. (2012) Colorectal cancer in inflammatory bowel disease: what is the real magnitude of the risk? *World Journal of Gastroenterology.* 18(29): 3839–3848

Frazier, T., Stocker, A., Kershner, N., Marsano, L. & McClain, C. (2011) Treatment of alcoholic liver disease. *Therapeutic Advances in Gastroenterology.* 14(1): 63–81

Hillman, E. (2017) 'Nursing care of people with bowel disorders'. In Lemone & Burke (eds). *Medical-Surgical nursing. Critical thinking for person-centered care.* Pearson.

Keshav, S. & Bally, A. (2012) *Gastrointestinal System at a Glance*, 2nd ed. Wiley-Blackwell.

Khoo, A. & Tse, E. (2016) A practical overview of the treatment of chronic hepatitis C virus. *Australian Family Physician.* 45: 718–720

Knox, N. (2017) 'Nursing care of people with gallbladder, liver and pancreatic disorders'. In Lemone & Burke (eds). *Medical-Surgical nursing. Critical thinking for person centered care.* Pearson.

Lanas, A. & Chan, F. (2017) Peptic ulcer disease. *The Lancet.* 3(90): 613–624. https://doi.org/10.1016/S0140-6736(16)32404-7

Lichtenstein, G. (2009) Bowel preparations for colonoscopy: A review. *American Journal of Health System Pharmacology.* 66(1): 27–37

Ljungqvist, O., Scott, M. & Fearon, M. (2017) Enhanced recovery after surgery: A review. *Journal of the American Medical Association.* 152(3): 292–298

Lupoli, R., Lembo, E., Saldamacchia, G., Avola, C., Angrisani, L. & Capaldo, B. (2017) Bariatric surgery and long term nutritional issues. *World Journal of Diabetes.* 5(11): 464–474.

Nair, M. (2009a) 'The gastrointestinal system and associated disorders'. In Nair, M. & Peate, I. (eds). Fundament*als of Applied Pathophysiology: An Essential Guide for Nursing Students* (pp. 272–97). Chichester: Wiley Blackwell.

Nair, M. (2009b) 'Nutrition and Associated Disorders'. In Nair, M. & Peate, I. (eds). *Fundamentals of Applied Pathophysiology: An Essential Guide for Nursing Students* (pp. 298–317). Chichester: Wiley Blackwell.

Nurgali, K. (2017) 'The structure and function of the digestive system'. In Craft and Gordon (eds). *Understanding pathophysiology,* 3rd ed. Elsevier.

Nurgali, K. & Wildbore, C. (2017) Alterations of digestive function across the lifespan. In Craft and Gordon (eds). *Understanding pathophysiology,* 3rd ed. Elsevier.

O'Shea, R. S., Dasarathy, S. & McCullough, A. J. (2010) Alcoholic liver disease. *Hepatology.* 51(1): 307–328.

Parrish, T. (2017a) 'Nursing care of people with upper gastrointestinal disorders'. In Lemone & Burke (eds). *Medical-Surgical nursing. Critical thinking for person-centered care.* Pearson.

Parrish, T. (2017b) 'Nursing care of people with diabetes mellitus'. In Lemone & Burke (eds). *Medical-Surgical nursing. Critical thinking for person-centered care.* Pearson.

Talley, N. & O'Connor, S. (2014) *Clinical examination: A systematic guide to physical diagnosis*, 7th ed. Elsevier.

Teitelbaum, E. & Soper, N. (2019) 'Cholelithiasis and cholecystitis'. In Zinner, M., Ashley, S. & Hines, O. (eds). *Maingot's abdominal operations,* 13th ed. McGraw-Hill.

Tortora, G. J. & Derrickson, B. (2011) *Principles of Anatomy and Physiology.* Hoboken, NJ: Wiley.

Trivedi, P. & Hirschfield, G. (2013) Treatment of autoimmune liver disease: current and future therapeutic options. *Journal of Advanced Chronic Disease.* 4(3): 119–141.

Venables, H. (2011) How does ultrasound work? *Ultrasound.* 19(1): 44-49.

World Health Organization (WHO). (2020) *Obesity.* www.who.int/westernpacific/health-topics/obesity

ACKNOWLEDGEMENTS

Photo 15A: © Monkey Business Images / Shutterstock.com
Photo 15B: © ImagingStocker / Shutterstock.com

CHAPTER 16

Nursing care of conditions related to the urinary system

LEARNING OBJECTIVES

After studying this chapter, you should be able to:

16.1 discuss the anatomy and physiology of the urinary system

16.2 discuss the pathophysiology of the urinary system

16.3 discuss the oncological conditions of the urinary system

16.4 identify and discuss the different types of renal replacement therapy

16.5 reflect on the incidence of kidney disorders in Australia

16.6 apply patient-centred care and the clinical reasoning cycle to the management of the renal patient.

Introduction

The urinary (or renal) system's function is to filter blood and create urine as a waste by-product (Johns Hopkins Medicine 2021). The organs of the urinary system include the kidneys, renal pelvis, ureters, bladder and urethra. The urinary system plays a vital role in homeostasis (Kanpp 2020). The kidney's primary functions are regulating the amount of water and salts in the blood, filtering waste products and producing a hormone that helps control blood pressure (State Government of Victoria 2020). The urinary system is susceptible to infections, blockages and injuries that affect the system's function and harm the whole body. The assessment and management of fluid and electrolyte balance are essential to providing safe and effective care. Hence, as nurses, we need to understand the functions of the urinary system and how these functions promote wellness or loss of these functions can lead to illness.

This chapter will address the nursing management of nephrological and urological conditions and the application of the clinical reasoning cycle and patient-centred care as applied to conditions related to the urinary system.

16.1 Anatomy and physiology of the urinary system

LEARNING OBJECTIVE 16.1 Discuss the anatomy and physiology of the urinary system.

The urinary system's main role is to produce, store and excrete urine through filtration (Johns Hopkins Medicine 2021). This allows for the disposal of waste products produced within the body. The urinary system also plays a crucial role in homeostasis through the electrolyte and acid–base balance and the production of red blood cells. The human urinary tract is comprised of:

- two kidneys
- two ureters
- one bladder
- two sphincter muscles
- nerves in the bladder
- one urethra.

The kidneys

The kidneys are bean-shaped organs approximately three centimetres thick, six centimetres wide and 12 centimetres long. These organs lie in the retroperitoneal space between the 12th thoracic and third lumbar vertebrae. The left kidney sits slightly behind the spleen. The right kidney sits slightly lower than the left, behind the liver (see figure 16.1). The bean-shaped kidneys have an indentation, called the hilum, towards the middle. The hilum leads to a large cavity within the kidney called the renal sinus. The ureter and renal vein leave the kidney, and the renal artery enters the kidney at the hilum. The arterial blood supply enters via the renal artery. Each kidney is enclosed in a tough fibrous capsule and is supported and protected by fatty tissue. The parts of the kidney are illustrated in figure 16.2.

There are three major regions of the kidney:

1. the renal cortex
2. the renal medulla
3. the renal pelvis.

The renal cortex

The tissue layer surrounding the kidneys is the renal cortex. This is then covered by renal fascia (connective tissue) and the renal capsule (Jewell 2018). The renal cortex is granular tissue due to the presence of nephrons — the functional unit of the kidney — that are located deeper within the renal pyramids of the medulla. The cortex provides a space for arterioles and venules from the renal artery and vein and the glomerular capillaries to perfuse the nephrons of the kidney. Erythropoietin, a hormone necessary for the synthesis of new red blood cells, is also produced in the renal cortex.

The renal medulla

The renal medulla is the smooth inner tissue of the kidney and contains the loop of Henle and the renal pyramids (Jewell 2018). The main function of the medulla is to regulate the concentration of urine. Urine flows from the collecting ducts into the renal calyces and pelvis, undergoing unidirectional peristaltic movements to drain into the downstream ureter and bladder.

FIGURE 16.1 The renal system of a female

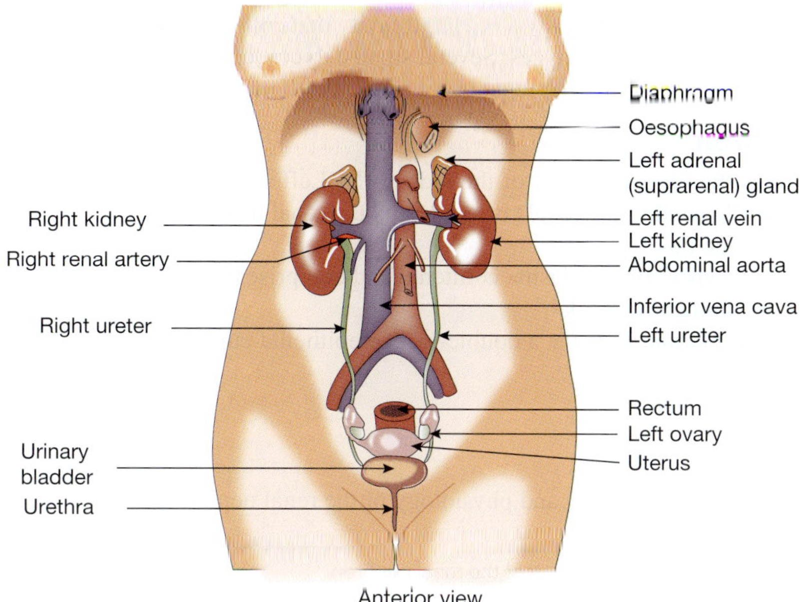

Source: Nair & Peate (2009) *Fundamentals of Applied Pathophysiology*, with kind permission from Wiley Blackwell

FIGURE 16.2 Longitudinal section of the kidney

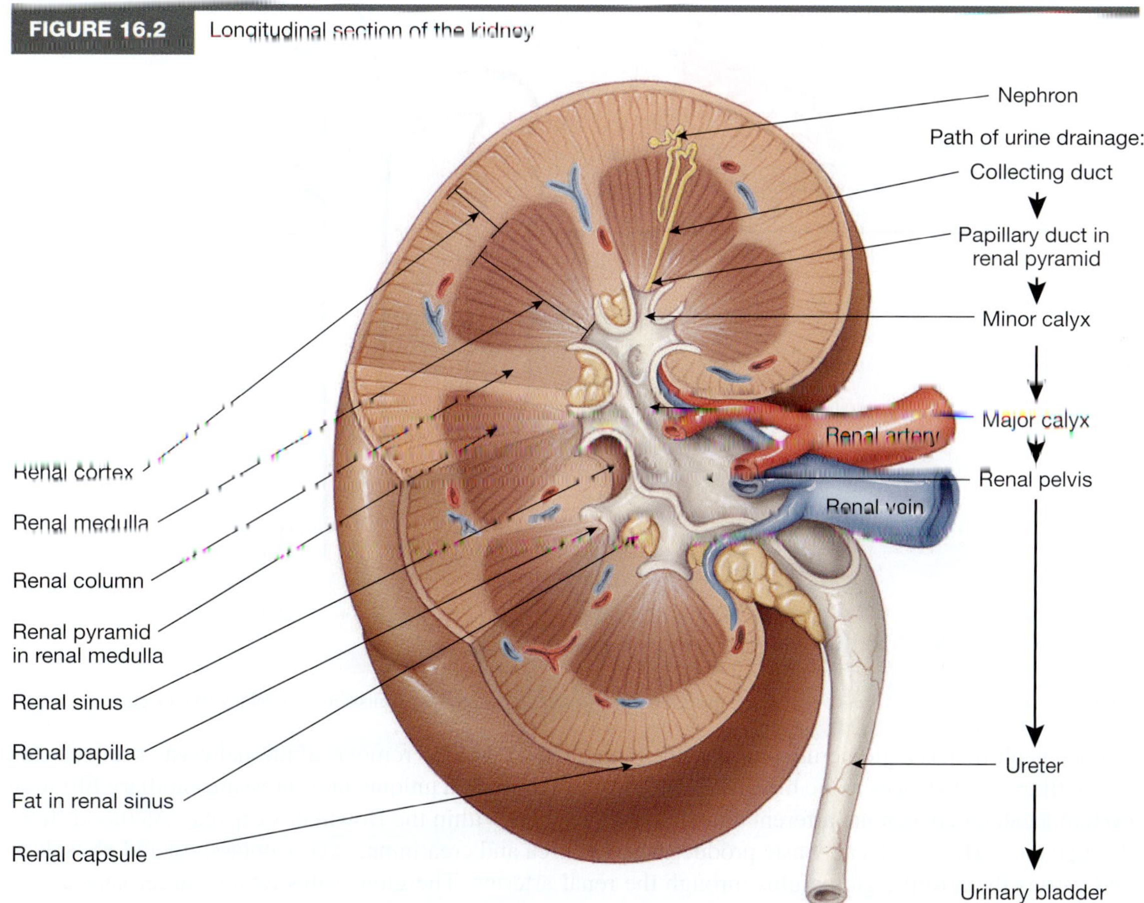

Source: Nair & Peate (2009) *Fundamentals of Applied Pathophysiology*, with kind permission from Wiley Blackwell.

The renal pelvis

The renal pelvis is the central region of the kidney (Seer Training Modules 2021) located in the renal sinus and continues to the ureter. The renal pelvis is a large cavity that collects urine. The edge of the renal pelvis has small cup-shaped spaces called calyces. Several small calyces join to form a large or main calyx. From these main calyces, urine flows into the renal pelvis and on into the ureter.

The renal nephron

The renal nephron is the functional unit of the kidney (McLafferty 2014). Each kidney has more than a million of these units located in the renal corpuscle and the renal tubule.

Each nephron is made up of:

- the renal corpuscle, where blood plasma is filtered and comprises:
  - glomerulus or capillary network
  - Bowman's or glomerular capsule, a double-walled epithelial cup
- the renal tubule
- proximal convoluted tubule
- loop of Henle
- distal convoluted tubule.

Figure 16.3 illustrates the anatomy and physiology of the renal nephron.

FIGURE 16.3 Anatomy and physiology of the renal nephron

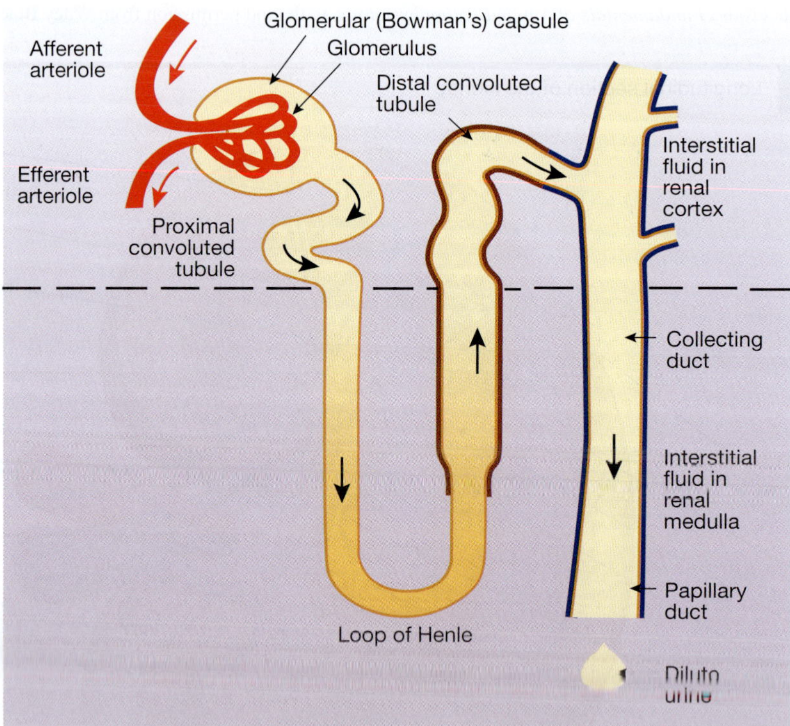

Source: Nair & Peate (2009) *Fundamentals of Applied Pathophysiology*, with kind permission from Wiley Blackwell.

Each nephron has a glomerulus to filter the blood and a tubule to remove additional waste products and return filtered substances to the bloodstream. The glomerulus is a unique, high-pressure capillary filtration system located between the afferent and efferent arterioles within the Bowman's capsule. As blood flows through the body, it picks up waste products such as urea and creatinine, excess potassium and phosphate and carries them to the glomerulus through the renal arteries. The glomerulus retains larger substances, blood cells and protein molecules that the body needs for homeostasis and growth and allows smaller molecules to pass through its membrane to eliminate waste products. Filtration produces a plasma-like fluid called the filtrate. The filtrate leaves the glomerulus and enters the tubules and collecting ducts allowing for **reabsorption** of useful substances (see figure 16.4). The reabsorption system of the peritubular capillary network surrounds the tubular parts of the nephron and starts from the efferent arteriole. The clean filtered blood then flows back to the body via the renal veins.

FIGURE 16.4 Secretion and reabsorption in the nephron

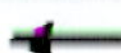

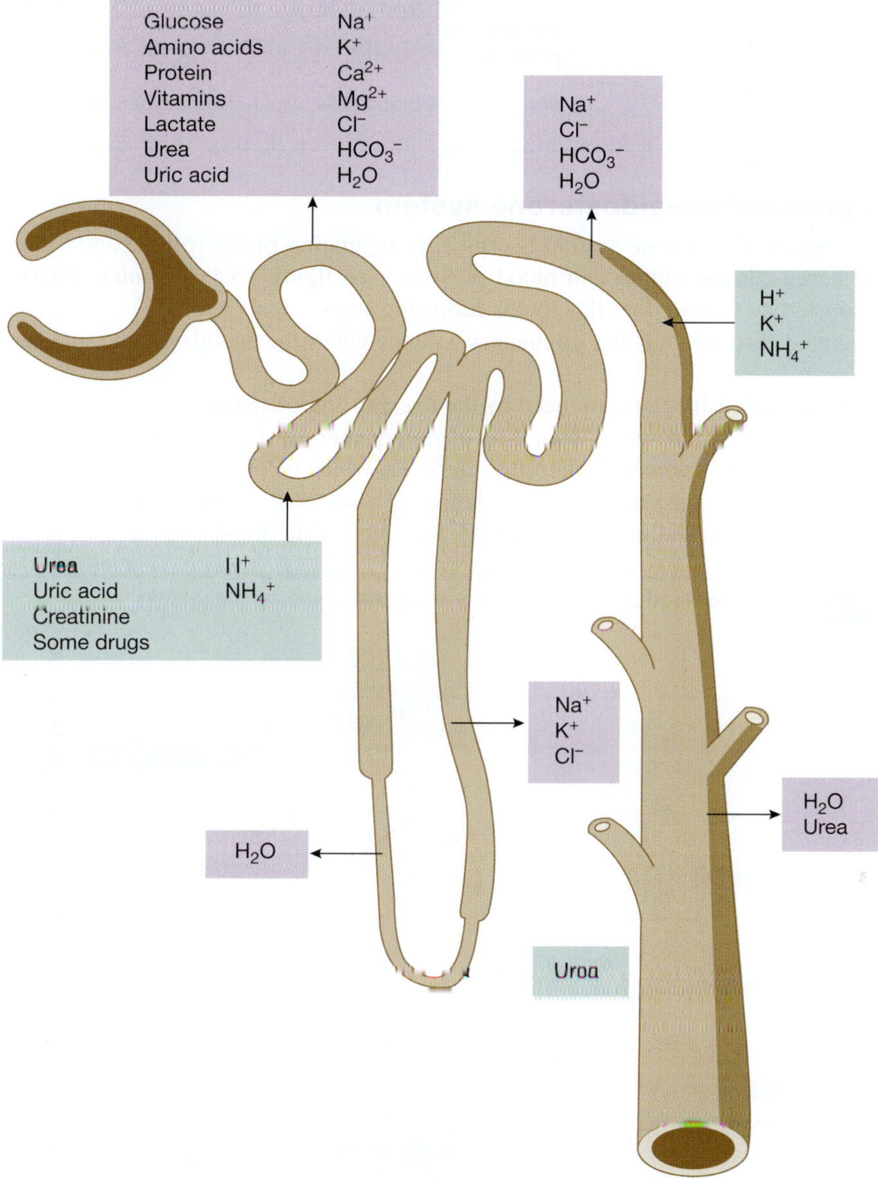

Source: Lumen Learning (n.d.).

The functions of the kidney

The kidneys are vital to homeostasis and hence, wellbeing. Table 16.1 summarises the functions of the kidneys.

TABLE 16.1 The function of the kidneys

Produce urine to remove waste products through:	• glomerular filtration tubular reabsorption • tubular secretion.
Regulate:	• blood volume by conserving or eliminating water • electrolyte balance • acid–base balance • blood pressure through the renin–angiotensin–aldosterone system.

(continued)

TABLE 16.1 *(continued)*

Produce the hormone renin:	• which regulates blood pressure and water balance.
Maintain healthy bones by:	• producing and secreting calcitriol (the active form of vitamin D), which increases the amount of dietary calcium absorbed from the digestive tract • produces erythropoietin, secreted in response to hypoxia.
Stimulates bone marrow:	• producing red blood cells, which carry oxygen to cells in the body.

The renin–angiotensin–aldosterone system

The renin–angiotensin–aldosterone system is critical in regulating blood volume and systemic vascular resistance and hence cardiac output and blood pressure (see figure 16.5) (Fountain 2020). The renin–angiotensin–aldosterone system does this by the following steps.

1. Renin is secreted directly into the circulatory system when the blood volume and blood pressure decrease.
2. Renin converts angiotensinogen (produced by the liver) to angiotensin I.
3. Angiotensin I is converted to angiotensin II by angiotensin-converting enzyme.
4. Angiotensin II causes vasoconstriction of the arterioles, which helps to increase blood pressure.
5. Angiotensin II stimulates the **secretion** of the hormone aldosterone from the adrenal cortex, increasing reabsorption of water and sodium by the tubules, thus increasing blood volume.

FIGURE 16.5 Regulating blood pressure: the renin–angiotensin–aldosterone system

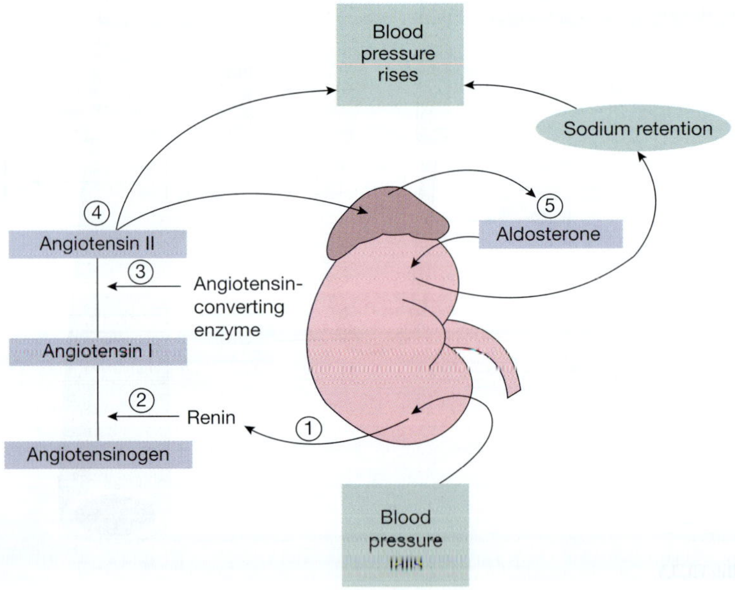

Source: MSD Manual (n.d.).

Micturition (urination)

Micturition is the process of urine excretion from the urinary bladder (LibreTexts 2020). Urine is released from the bladder and passes through the urethra to the outside of the body. The physiology of micturition is complex. It requires coordination of the central, autonomic and somatic nervous systems.

Micturition has two phases.

1. *The storage phase.* The bladder is relaxed and slowly fills with urine.
2. *The voiding phase.* The bladder contracts, forcing the external sphincter to open and discharge urine through the urethra (LibreTexts 2020).

During the storage phase, the internal urethral sphincter is tense, and the **detrusor muscle** is relaxed due to sympathetic stimulation. In the voiding phase, the autonomic and somatic nervous systems open the two sphincters to allow for micturition. During micturition, parasympathetic stimulation causes the internal urethral sphincter to relax. The external urethral sphincter is under somatic control and is consciously relaxed and opened. The micturition reflex system requires a conscious signal and an unconscious message called afferent firing from the brain to the sensory stretch fibres of the bladder and urethra. Low bladder volumes have a low afferent firing of the stretch receptors resulting in relaxation of the bladder. As bladder volume increases, so does the afferent firing of the stretch receptors. This creates a conscious urinary urge.

The colour of urine can indicate levels of hydration and the presence of blood:

- normal, healthy urine is a pale straw or transparent yellow colour
- very pale urine can indicate over hydration
- darker yellow or honey-coloured urine can indicate dehydration
- dark brownish colour may indicate a liver problem or severe dehydration
- pinkish or red urine may indicate the presence of blood (Johns Hopkins Medicine 2021).

A dipstick urine test is done on the ward or by the patient in their home (figure 16.6). The test does not require a physician's order and should be undertaken by an RN if there is any question about an infection. It will provide baseline information that could then be followed with a urine sample sent to the lab.

FIGURE 16.6 Dipstick urine test

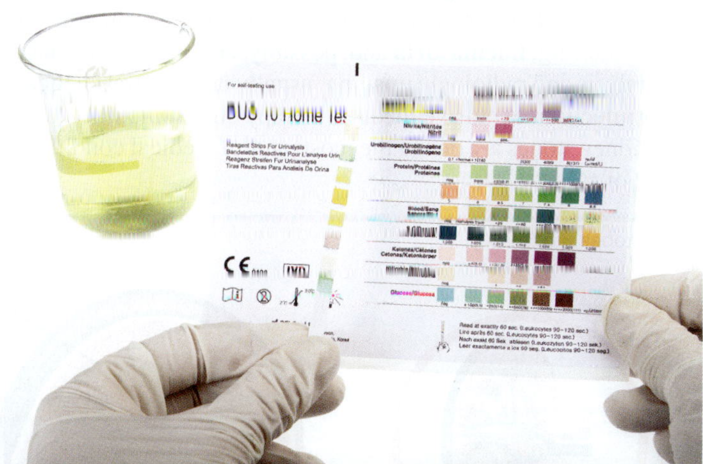

The prostate

The prostate is a walnut-sized **gland** that sits between the bladder and the penis, in front of the rectum (Hoffman 2021) The urethra runs through the centre of the prostate from the bladder to the penis providing the pathway for urine to be released. The role of the prostate is to secrete an alkaline fluid that nourishes and protects sperm. During ejaculation, the prostate squeezes this fluid into the urethra, which is expelled with sperm as semen. The **vasa deferentia** muscular tubes bring sperm from the testes to the seminal vesicles. The seminal vesicles contribute fluid to the semen during ejaculation.

The prostate is divided into three zones.

1. The peripheral zone can be felt by a finger inserted into the rectum (digital rectal examination [DRE] as seen in figure 16.7) and is the area where most prostate cancers originate.
2. The transitional zone surrounds the proximal urethra and is the area that enlarges as men get older (in benign prostatic hyperplasia [BPH]), which can lead to urinary problems.
3. The central zone surrounds the seminal vesicles and ejaculatory ducts.

FIGURE 16.7 Palpation of the prostate during DRE

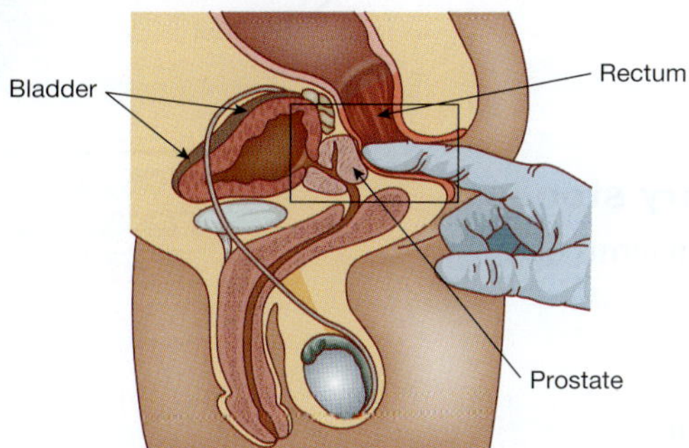

16.2 Diseases and disorders of the urinary system

LEARNING OBJECTIVE 16.2 Discuss the pathophysiology of the urinary system.

Urinary system calculi

Urinary calculi or urinary stones are solid masses of crystals made from the salts in urine. While these stones usually originate in the kidneys, they can develop anywhere in the urinary system, such as the ureters, bladder or urethra.

Urinary stones begin to form in the kidney and then enlarge in a ureter or bladder. Depending on the stone's location, it may be called a kidney stone, ureteral stone or bladder stone. The process of stone formation is called urolithiasis, renal lithiasis or nephrolithiasis (Preminger 2020). The development of stones is a common disorder of the urinary tract. It is estimated that four to eight per cent of Australians experience them in their lifetime (Kidney Health Australia 2020). While small stones may cause no symptoms, larger stones can cause agonising pain in the back between the hips and ribs (Preminger 2020). These larger stones can obstruct the urinary tract and block the flow of urine (see figure 16.8). This can cause infection as bacteria can be trapped in the urine that collects above the blockage. If stones block the urinary tract for a lengthy period, they can create excessive pressure, causing the kidney to swell. Urinary stones cause pain, nausea, vomiting, **haematuria** and, possibly, chills and fever due to secondary infection. Diagnosis is based on urinalysis and radiologic imaging, usually non-contrast helical CT. Treatment is with analgesics, antibiotics for infection, expulsive medical therapy and, sometimes, shock-wave lithotripsy or endoscopic procedures. Kidney stones are one of the most painful medical conditions. The causes of stones vary according to the type of stone.

FIGURE 16.8 Kidney stones

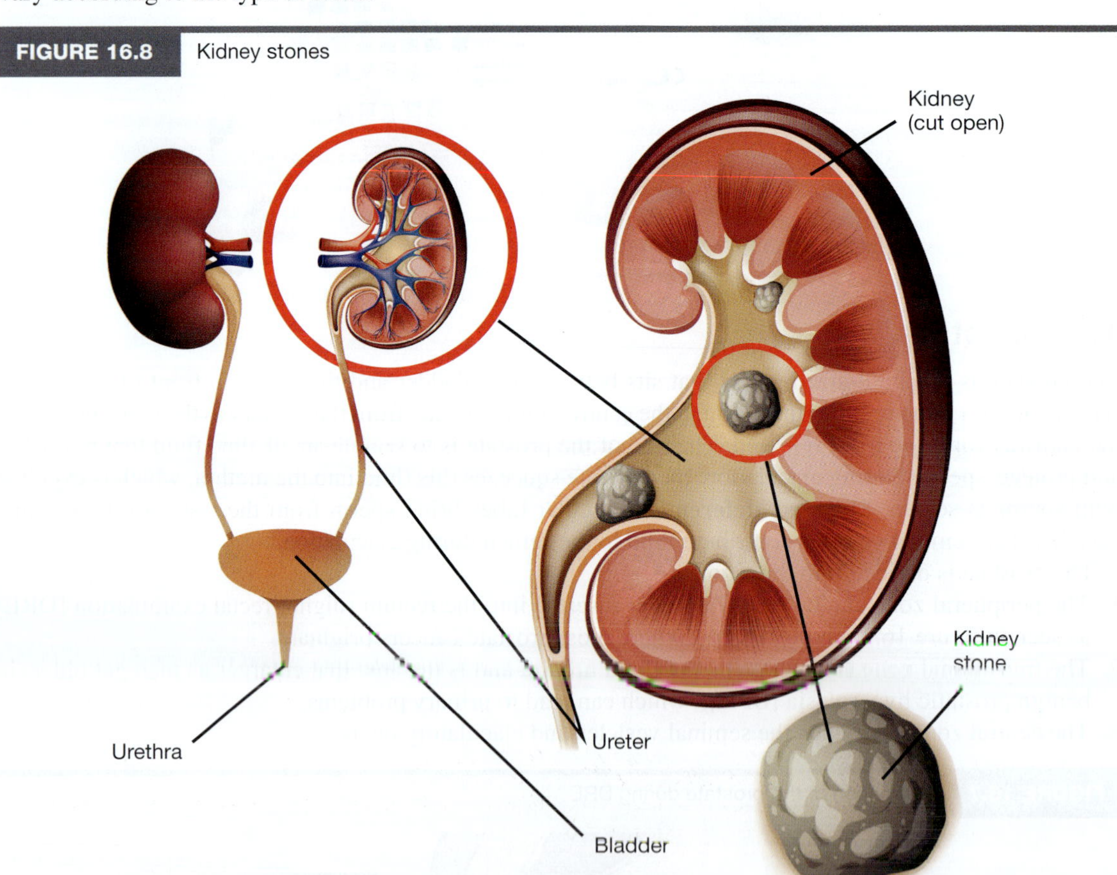

Classification of urinary stones

Urinary stones are classified in terms of:

- size
- location
- X-ray characteristics
- aetiology of stone formation

- chemical composition
- the risk group for recurrent stone formation (European Association of Urology 2021).

There are four main types of urinary system stones.

1. Stones formed from calcium that has not been utilised by the bones and muscles and has combined with oxalate or phosphate. These are the most common kidney stones.
2. Stones containing magnesium and the waste product ammonia. These stones are called struvite stones and form after urinary tract infections.
3. Uric acid stones, which are often caused by eating substantial amounts of high-protein foods.
4. Cystine stones, which are both rare and hereditary (Department of Health & Human Services 2020b).

Risk factors for urinary system stones include:

- family or personal history
- dehydration
- diets high in protein, sodium and sugar
- obesity
- digestive diseases
- digestive surgery such as gastric bypass surgery
- digestive system disorder such as inflammatory bowel disease or chronic diarrhoea
- other medical conditions such as renal tubular acidosis, cystinuria, hyperparathyroidism and repeated urinary tract infections
- supplements and medications, such as vitamin C, excessive laxatives use, calcium-based antacids and some medications used to treat migraines or depression (Mayo Clinic 2021d).

Signs and symptoms of urinary stones

While some people with kidney stones have no symptoms (Department of Health & Human Services 2020b), patients may present with signs and symptoms that are linked to the location and size of the stone (Preminger 2020). These symptoms include:

- renal colic, acute pain usually located just below the ribs on one side. This pain will radiate around to the front and sometimes towards the groin. It is often severe enough to cause nausea and vomiting
- haematuria
- cloudy or foul-smelling urine
- urinary tract infection, causing shivers, sweating and fever
- reports of small gravel-like stones in their urine
- a feeling of urgency to urinate.

Diagnosis of urinary stones

The diagnosis of urinary system stones will be based on the following criteria.

- presenting signs and symptoms
- patient history
- physical examination
- laboratory analysis including:
  - urinalysis for signs of blood, bacteria or crystallised minerals
  - serum blood samples for creatine, uric acid, calcium, sodium and potassium
- imaging including:
  - high-resolution CT scan from the kidneys down to the bladder or an X-ray of kidney, ureter and bladder (KUB)
  - ultrasonography and X-ray can be used as an alternative to a CT; however, these procedures are not considered to be as accurate as a CT scan (National Kidney Foundation 2021; Preminger 2020; European Association of Urology 2021).

Therapies to support passing urinary stones

Non-surgical treatment is preferred in cases where the patient can pass the stone spontaneously. The type of stone determines treatment and prevention (National Kidney Foundation 2019a).

Lifestyle changes that are recommended for the patient include:

- drinking two to three litres of fluid per day (preferably water)
- limiting foods with high oxalate content such and spinach, berries, chocolate, wheat bran, nuts, beets, tea and rhubarb
- avoiding calcium supplements; however, including three serves of dairy in the daily diet

- limiting protein intake
- reducing salt intake
- avoiding high doses of vitamin C.

Procedures to support the removal of the urinary stone

If the stone does not pass and prevents urination or leads to bleeding or infection, a medical decision will be made to remove the stone (Department of Health & Human Services 2020b; Lecturi 2020). Advances in surgical treatments have reduced hospital stays to as little as 48 hours. Treatments include extracorporeal shock-wave lithotripsy (ESWL), percutaneous nephrolithotomy, endoscopic removal and surgery.

Extracorporeal shock-wave lithotripsy (ESWL)

ESWL is a non-invasive therapy performed under a general anaesthetic. EWSL uses ultrasound waves to break the stone into smaller pieces, which will then be passed in urination. ESWL is used for stones less than two centimetres in size.

Percutaneous nephrolithotomy/nephrolithotripsy

Percutaneous nephrolithotomy/nephrolithotripsy is a minimally invasive surgery (National Kidney Foundation 2021) used for stones larger than two centimetres. The procedure is performed under a general anaesthetic. The stones are removed by entering the kidney through a small incision in the back. Then, a nephroscope — a miniature fibreoptic camera — is used to remove the stone. If the stone is removed whole, it is called percutaneous nephrolithotomy. If the stone is broken into pieces, it is called nephrolithotripsy. A temporary stent may be placed to help with drainage and prevent bleeding. The procedure takes around 20 to 30 minutes, and the patient remains in hospital for two to three days post-operatively.

Ureteroscopic removal

For ureteroscopic removal, an endoscope is inserted into the urethra, passed into the bladder and to where the stone is located (National Kidney Foundation 2019b). The stone is removed or broken up so that the patient can pass it more easily. This is usually an outpatient procedure, and the patient will return to have the stent removed after four to ten days (WebMD 2021).

Surgery

Advances in the treatment of urinary stones have significantly reduced the need for open surgery (European Association of Urology, 2021). However, if none of these methods is suitable due to the size of the stone or an abnormality in the urinary system, the stone may need to be removed using traditional surgery. The surgeon makes an incision (or multiple, small keyhole incisions) in the patient's side, and the kidney or ureter is opened to allow the stone to be removed (The Hospitals Contribution Fund of Australia Limited 2021). The incision is closed, and a drain is placed to allow for urine drainage. A temporary stent may also be placed to keep the urinary tract open while healing takes place. The length of stay in hospital will vary from two to nine days. The drain will be removed prior to discharge or in the initial post-op appointment.

Nursing management of urinary stones

Initial management for newly diagnosed patients with ureteral stones that are smaller than 10 millimetres diameter and whose symptoms are controlled is usually observation and ongoing assessment (RegisteredNurseRN.com 2021). In most cases, the patient will pass the stone without the need for surgical or other intervention. The nurse's role is to monitor the patient for deterioration, manage the pain, provide medications as ordered, complete and document ongoing assessments, support fluids, strain urine, monitor for complications and escalate care as needed.

Nursing management of urinary stones should include:

- providing patient and family education to support patient-centred care
- completing a full assessment and documentation
- continuing with ongoing assessments and documentation
- assessing, monitoring and managing pain by:
  - assessing the severity, location and radiation
  - administering pain relief as charted (non-steroidal anti-inflammatory [NSAIDs], opioids)
  - escalating care
- administering **antiemetics** as needed
- administering medication to support the passing of the stones as ordered — this would include alpha-blockers and calcium antagonists relax the smooth muscles of the ureters, increasing the chance of passing stone spontaneously (European Association of Urology 2021)

- maintaining and documenting fluid intake to facilitate the passing of stone fragments
- monitoring for signs and symptoms of infection
- monitoring renal function, including:
  - urine for culture and sensitivity
  - 24-hour urine collection for calculi
  - output (decreased output could indicate urinary obstruction or dehydration)
  - serum urea and creatinine levels
  - the position of the stone
  - hydronephrosis (distension and dilatation of the renal pelvis and calyces due to obstruction to urine flow from the kidney).

Nursing priorities for post-procedure care for urinary stones are outlined in figure 16.9.

FIGURE 16.9

- Assess for pain and discomfort, including what makes the pain worse or decreases pain, the quality, location and radiation of pain, severity and how long the pain has been for.
- Administer opioid analgesia and NSAID as prescribed.
- Encourage and assist the patient in assuming a position of comfort.
- Assist patient to ambulate to obtain some pain relief
- Monitor pain closely and report promptly increases in severity.
- Alleviate pain with pharmacological and non-pharmacological methods, including position change reassurance and relaxation techniques.
- Monitor for deterioration. Assess for signs of urinary tract infection such as chills or fever.
- Maintain adequate renal functioning. Assess for frequency, hesitancy or obstruction. Frequent urination of small amounts, oliguria or anuria may indicate obstruction.
- Observe urine for blood, strain for stones or gravel.
- Provide education to the patient and their families about the disease process, prognosis and treatment needs.

Source: Adapted from Vera (2014).

Urinary tract infections

Urinary tract infections are infections that occur in the bladder, urethra, ureters or kidneys. They are one of the most common infections encountered in the community. Kidney Health Australia (2018) stated that approximately one out of two women and one in 20 men would experience a UTI in their lifetime. People with diabetes and older adults are at higher risk for a UTI. The female urinary tract has a short urethra, and this increases the frequency of infections.

Common symptoms of a UTI include:

- burning sensation when passing urine
- wanting to urinate more often, if only to pass a few drops
- cloudy, bloody or odorous urine
- pain above the pubic bone
- if the UTI has moved to the kidney, the patient will experience a high-grade fever, vomiting and/or back pain (Kidney Health Australia 2018).

Signs of UTIs in children also include:

- low-grade fever
- irritability
- bedwetting in a child who has been toilet trained
- feeding difficulties in babies.

The symptoms of a UTI are dependent on the area of the urinary tract that is affected. Table 16.2 outlines the signs and symptoms of the areas affected.

TABLE 16.2 UTI signs and symptoms

Part of urinary tract affected	Signs and symptoms
Kidneys (acute pyelonephritis)	Upper back and side (flank) pain High fever Shaking and chills Nausea Vomiting
Bladder (cystitis)	Pelvic pressure Lower abdomen discomfort Frequent, painful urination Blood in urine
Urethra (urethritis)	Burning with urination Discharge

Source: Mayo Clinic (2021e).

Causes of UTI

UTIs can be caused by:

- urinary tract abnormalities from birth
- blockages in the urinary tract such as kidney stones or an enlarged prostate
- a suppressed or impaired immune system from disorders such as diabetes and other diseases that impair the immune system
- indwelling or in and out catheterisation for patients who are in hospital, people with neurological problems or paralysed people
- a recent urinary procedure such as urinary surgery or an exam of the urinary tract.

Diagnosis

Diagnosis of a UTI will be made by:

- patient history and physical assessment
- urine specimen to look for:
  - white blood cells
  - red blood cells
  - bacteria
- ultrasound, CT, MRI
- **cystoscopy**.

Prevention

Patients should be advised of the following to support the prevention of UTIs.

- Increase fluid intake to dilute urine and allow bacteria to be flushed from the urinary tract.
- Wipe from front to back to prevent bacteria in the anal region from spreading to the vagina and urethra.
- Empty the bladder soon after intercourse.
- Avoid potentially irritating feminine products such as deodorant sprays or other feminine douches or powders that can irritate the urethra.
- Consider changing birth control methods as diaphragms or spermicide-treated condoms can contribute to bacterial growth (Mayo Clinic 2021e).

Nursing management of patients with complicated UTIs

Most urinary tract infections are due to the colonisation of rectal and perineal flora in the urogenital tract (Sabih 2020). UTIs can be classified as simple or complex (Mayo Clinic 2021e). Simple UTIs, or simple cystitis, are UTIs that occur due to appropriate susceptible bacteria. Simple UTIs include cystitis and single episodes of ascending **pyelonephritis** and are treated with antibiotics and patient education on avoiding UTIs.

Complex UTIs require hospitalisation and medical treatment (Sabih 2020). Examples of complicated UTIs are:

- UTIs in males
- infections occurring due to an obstruction such as a urinary stone

- infections occurring due to an immune-compromised state
- atypical organisms
- recurrent infections despite treatment
- infections in pregnant women
- infections after surgery
- infections due to the insertion of an indwelling (Foley) catheter
- infections in patients who have undergone a renal transplant
- infections in patients with impaired renal function
- infections following prostatectomies or radiotherapy.

Nursing management for UTIs include:

- patient health history
- initial and ongoing assessment to include vital signs and pain assessment
- monitoring for signs and symptoms of deterioration and escalate concerns as needed
- measurement and documentation of urine output
- monitoring of fluid balance
- administering prescribed analgesia and antispasmodic agents
- patient and family education
- encouraging oral fluids
- reviewing for support at home with ADLs and medication management
- discharge advice on prevention, lifestyle changes and follow-up care.

Acute kidney injury

Acute kidney injury (AKI), previously known as acute renal failure (ARF), is defined as a sudden severe reduction in normal renal function. AKI requires urgent to emergent care as it results in a failure to maintain fluid, electrolyte and acid–base homeostasis. AKI develops rapidly, usually in less than a few days (Mayo Clinic 2021a). Acute kidney failure is common in people who are critically ill and hospitalised in intensive care. AKI can be fatal if not diagnosed and treated early. However, it is treatable and may be reversible unless there are underlying renal problems.

Signs and symptoms of AKI include:

- decreased urine output
- fluid retention, causing swelling in the peripheries (legs, ankles or feet)
- shortness of breath
- fatigue and weakness
- confusion and disorientation
- nausea
- irregular heartbeat
- chest pain or pressure
- seizures or coma in severe cases (Kidney Health Australia 2021; Makris & Spanou 2016; Mayo Clinic 2021a).

Causes of AKI

AKI can be caused by:

- reduced blood supply to the kidneys due to blood loss after major surgery or dehydration
- damage to kidney tissue caused by a medication, severe infection or radioactive dye
- physical trauma to the kidney in a road traffic accident or a sports injury
- an obstruction such as kidney stones or BPH.

Classification and staging of AKI

AKI is an often overlooked presentation in hospitalised patients (Ricci, Cruz & Ronco 2011). AKI is strongly associated with mortality, morbidity, cardiovascular failure and infections. To support early diagnosis, the Acute Dialysis Quality Initiative (ADQI) undertook research and developed the RIFLE criteria (risk, injury, failure, loss of function, and end-stage renal disease) designed to standardise and classify renal dysfunction (see figure 16.10).

In conjunction with the RIFLE criteria, AKI will be diagnosed with the following tests:

- 24-hour urine collection
- urine tests for abnormalities
- blood tests for urea and creatinine

- imaging tests including:
  - ultrasound
  - CT Scan
- surgery (biopsy).

FIGURE 16.10 The RIFLE criteria for AKI diagnosis

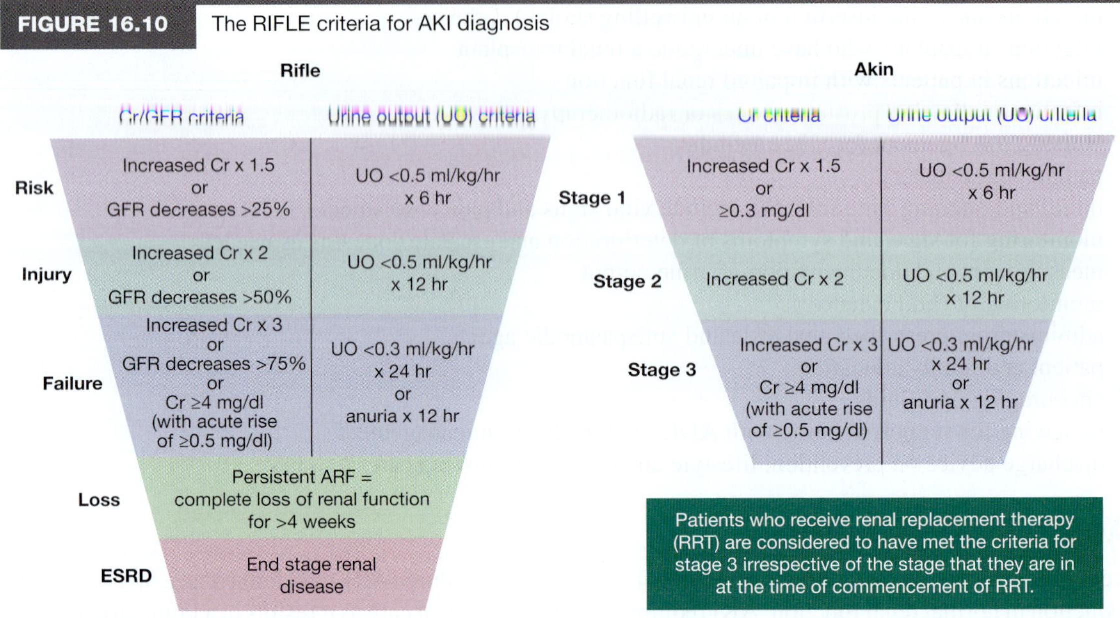

Source: Cruz, Ricci & Ronco (2009).

Treatment of AKI

The goal of treatment is to restore homeostasis and prevent the progression of injury by treating the underlying cause (Workeneh 2020). Treatment of AKI is based on:

- correction of fluid overload with furosemide
- correction of severe acidosis with bicarbonate administration, which can be important as a bridge to dialysis
- correction of **hyperkalaemia**
- correction of haematologic abnormalities such as anaemia, uremic platelet dysfunction with transfusions and administration of medications.

Nursing management of patients with AKI

Nurses caring for AKI patients must:

- obtain a patient health history
- complete assessment and documentation
- record vital signs, including pain score
- monitor fluid balance
- monitor for deterioration and escalate care
- administer prescribed oxygen therapy
- fluid management as prescribed
- provide dietary advice as prescribed
- collect urine specimens
- provide support of ADLs
- administer medications as ordered.

Chronic kidney disease

Chronic kidney disease is a progressive and irreversible condition. An estimated 1.7 million (10 per cent) Australian adults aged 18 years or more were diagnosed with chronic kidney disease (CKD) in 2011–12 (Australian Institute of Health and Welfare 2020). An estimated one in five or 18 per cent of Indigenous adults showed CKD signs in the federal government reports of 2012–13. These statistics demonstrate the severity of the problem in Australia.

Patients with CKD can remain asymptomatic and only present with the signs and symptoms of renal dysfunction in more advanced stages (Ruiz-Ortega, Rayego-Mateos, Lamas, Ortiz & Rodrigues-Diez 2020). Quality of life is lower for people with CKD than for the general population. Research has shown that patients with CKD are five to ten times more likely to die before progressing to end stage kidney disease (Webster, Nagler, Morton & Masson 2017). Its treatment can be conservative (patients without indication for dialysis, usually those with glomerular filtration rate above 15 ml/minute) or require replacement therapy (haemodialysis, peritoneal dialysis and kidney transplantation). The conservative treatment objectives for CKD are to slow down the progression of kidney dysfunction, treat complications (anaemia, bone diseases, cardiovascular diseases), vaccination for hepatitis B and preparation for kidney replacement therapy.

Risk factors for CKD include:

- diabetes mellitus
- hypertension
- cardiac disease
- family history of kidney disease
- chronic pyelonephritis
- abnormal kidney structure
- Aboriginal, Torres Strait Islander, African American, Hispanic, Native American, Asian descent
- ageing
- chronic use of NSAIDs or acetylsalicylic acid (aspirin) (Ammirati 2020; Cleveland Clinic 2021a).

Symptoms of CKD

CKD does not have notable symptoms in the early stages. As the disease worsens, symptoms will include:

- frequency of urination
- tiredness, weakness, low energy levels
- anorexia
- **peripheral oedema**
- shortness of breath
- blood in the urine
- foamy urine
- puffy eyes
- dry and itchy skin
- trouble concentrating
- trouble sleeping
- numbness
- nausea or vomiting
- muscle cramps
- hypertension
- darkening of skin (Cleveland Clinic 2021a).

Diagnosis and staging of CKD

CKD is categorised into five stages, according to the glomerular filtration rate (GFR), and in three stages, according to the albumin levels in the urine (see figure 16.11 and tables 16.3 and 16.4) (Ammirati 2020). The staging system helps physicians determine the level of monitoring and potential treatments for CKD patients.

FIGURE 16.11 Five stages of CKD

Stage 1	Stage 2	Stage 3A	Stage 3B	Stage 4	Stage 5
GFR≥90	89≥GFR≥60	59≥GFR≥40	44≥GFR≥30	29≥GFR≥15	GFR<15
Normal or high function	Mildly decreased function	Mild to moderately decreased function		Severely decreased function	Kidney failure

TABLE 16.3 CKD stages

Stages	GFR value ml/min/1.73m^2	Classification
I	>90	Normal or high
II	60–89	Slightly decreased
III A	45–59	Mild to moderately decreased
III B	30–44	Moderately to severely decreased
IV	15–29	Severely decreased
V	<15	Kidney failure

TABLE 16.4 Categories of albuminuria

Category	24-hour albuminuria mg/24 hr	Albumin/creatine ratio mg/g (in isolated urine samples)	Classification
A1	<30	<30	Normal to discrete
A2	30–300	30–300	Moderate
A3	>300	>300	Severe

In conjunction with blood tests for GFR and albumin/creatine ratio, the diagnosis of CKD will also involve:

- a patient's health history
- physical assessment
- urine tests for protein
- imaging including:
  - ultrasound
  - CT
- surgery (biopsy).

Management and treatment of CKD

Chronic renal disease has a major impact on the morbidity and mortality of patients. Appropriate management can decrease complications, with a positive impact on the prognosis of the affected population. Another important aspect is the preparation for renal replacement treatment, which significantly facilitates patients' adaptation to the chosen therapy (Physiopedia contributors 2020). Management of patients with CKD includes treatment of the underlying cause to slow the progression of the disease. Kidney failure requires an interprofessional team of healthcare professionals to support the development of a therapeutic management plan. Only open communication between the team members, patients and their families can reduce renal failure morbidity and mortality.

Nursing management of CKD patients includes:

- patient health history
- physical assessment
- ongoing urine, blood and imaging tests
- dietary referral to adjust fluid and food intake, including:
  - avoiding proteins high in essential amino acids
  - reducing foods that are high in potassium
  - managing fluids
- medication administration, including:
  - an angiotensin-converting enzyme (ACE) inhibitor or an angiotensin receptor blocker (ARB) diuretic
  - medications to lower cholesterol
  - erythropoietin, to build red blood cells
  - vitamin D and calcitriol to prevent bone loss
  - phosphate binder.

Benign prostatic hyperplasia (BPH)

BPH is an enlarged prostate (Urology Care Foundation 2019). During the male life cycle, the prostate goes through two primary growth cycles. The first growth cycle takes place in puberty when the prostate doubles in size. The second phase starts around 25 years old and continues throughout the rest of a man's life. BPH usually occurs during this second growth phase. As the prostate enlarges, it presses against the urethra (figure 16.12), and the bladder wall becomes thick. The bladder may weaken and lose the ability to empty completely leaving urine sitting in the bladder called urinary retention with aging. The narrowing of the urethra and urinary retention are the cause of many of the problems of BPH. It must be noted that BPH is benign. It is not cancer, nor does it cause or act as a risk factor for cancer. According to the Australian Journal of General Practice (Jiwrajka et al. 2018), between 2009 and 2011, some 228 000 per annum were managed by general practitioners. Management of BPH depends on the severity of symptoms (Jiwrajka et al. 2018).

FIGURE 16.12 Benign prostatic hyperplasia

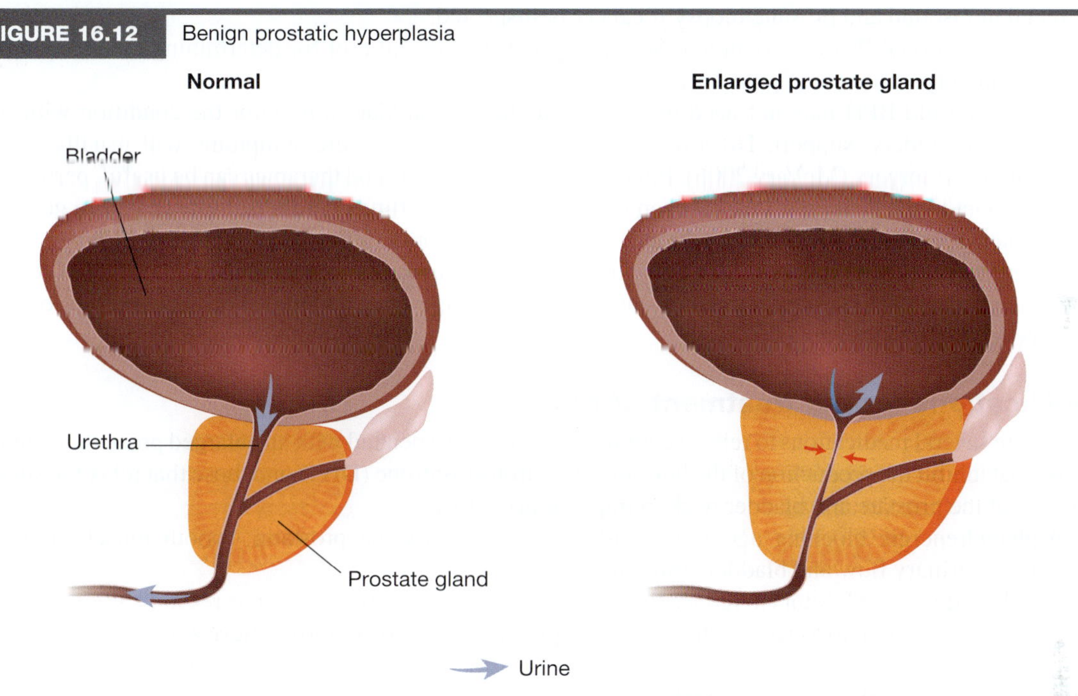

Risk factors for prostate gland enlargement include the following.

- *Age*. Prostate gland enlargement is rare in men younger than age 40. Approximately one-third of men experience moderate to severe symptoms by age 60, and about 50 per cent of men experience symptoms by the age of 80.
- *Familial history*. Particularly a close blood relative.
- *Comorbidities*. Studies show that diabetes and heart disease, and the use of beta-blockers, might increase the risk of BPH.
- *Obesity*. Obesity increases the risk of BPH, and exercise lowers the risk (Mayo Clinic 2021b).

Signs and symptoms of BPH include:

- frequency or urgency of urinate
- increased frequency of urination at night (nocturia)
- difficulty beginning urination
- a weak urine stream or a stream that stops and starts
- dribbling at the end of urination
- inability to empty the bladder completely (Jiwrajka et al. 2018; Mayo Clinic 2021b).

Less common signs and symptoms include:

- urinary tract infection
- inability to urinate
- blood in the urine.

Diagnosis and management of BPH

Assessment of the suspected BPH patient includes:

- a health history from the patient for signs and symptoms and risk factors
- **digital rectal examination (DRE)** to:
  - assesses the size of the prostate
  - palpate for malignant features
- assessment of renal function, including:
  - urinalysis
  - serum urea and creatinine levels
  - flow rate
  - post-void residual volume
- blood test for prostate-specific antigen (PSA) to rule out cancer, infection, inflammation or enlargement of the prostate
- rectal ultrasound and prostate biopsy if cancer is suspected.

The International Prostate Symptom Scoring system is a useful tool for determining the effect on the patient's quality of life (see figure 16.13).

Men with mild BPH may not need treatment but should continue to monitor the condition with their healthcare providers' support. However, men with moderate to severe symptoms will usually require medications or surgery (McVary 2006). Behavioural modifications and therapies can be useful, particularly as an adjunct to medication. Lifestyle changes include avoiding fluids before bedtime or before going out and reducing caffeine and alcohol intake as these are mild diuretics. Pelvic floor muscle training, including the use of biofeedback, may help patients with urgency with urination. Men with BPH are advised to avoid over the counter medicines such as antihistamines and decongestants that may worsen symptoms or cause urinary retention (McVary 2006).

Medications for the treatment of BPH

There are several medications to relieve common symptoms associated with an enlarged prostate, including those that inhibit the production of the hormone dihydrotestosterone (DHT) and those that relax the smooth muscle of the prostate and bladder neck to improve urine flow.

- Alpha-adrenergic blocking agents (alpha-blockers) to relax the prostatic smooth muscle and help improve urinary flow and bladder emptying.
- 5-alpha reductase inhibitors to reduce the level of dihydrotestosterone, which is responsible for prostatic growth. This will help to reduce the size of the prostate and may, in turn, relieve symptoms.

Surgical procedures for BPH

When symptoms are severe and cannot be alleviated with medications, then surgery is the preferred option The goal of surgery is to widen where the urethra passes through the prostate.

There are several surgeries aimed at relieving the physical obstruction to the urethra. In most cases, surgery is performed endoscopically via the penis. The most common endoscopic procedures are transurethral resection of the prostate (TURP) and holmium laser enucleation of the prostate (HoLEP) (Woo et al. 2017). A thin tube containing a light and a camera is introduced into the urethra, and the prostatic tissue is removed using a heated loop (TURP) or a laser (HoLEP).

Holmium laser enucleation of the prostate (HoLEP) has some advantages over the TURP. The HoLEP is a minimally invasive surgery and requires a shorter period of hospitalisation. Studies have been shown that the HoLEP reduces intraoperative haemorrhage and perioperative morbidity compared to the TURP (Woo et al. 2017).

Transurethral resection of the prostate (TURP)

TURP remains the gold standard surgical treatment for BPH (RadiologyInfo.org 2021). A TURP involves inserting a resectoscope through the urethra to remove the obstructing tissue, almost like removing the core from an apple, thus widening the channel. The nursing care for a TURP is outlined in table 16.5.

FIGURE 10.10 The International Prostate Symptom Score Sheet

INTERNATIONAL PROSTATE SYMPTOM SCORE SHEET

Docter name: ______________ Address: ______________

Patient name: ______________ Address: ______________

Date: ______________

Age group: 40–49 ☐ 50–59 ☐ 60–69 ☐ 70+ ☐

	Not at all	Less than 1 time in 5	Less than half the time	About half the time	More than half the time	Almost always	Your score
1. INCOMPLETE EMPTYING Over the past month, how often have you had a sensation of not emptying your bladder completely after you finished urinating?	0	1	2	3	4	5	
2. FREQUENCY Over the past month, how often have you had to urinate again less than two hours after you finished urinating?	0	1	2	3	4	5	
3. INTERMITTENCY Over the past month, how often have you found you stopped and started several times when you urinated?	0	1	2	3	4	5	
4. URGENCY Over the past month, how often have you found it difficult to postpone urination?	0	1	2	3	4	5	
5. WEAK STREAM Over the past month, how often have you had a weak urinary stream?	0	1	2	3	4	5	
6. STRAINING Over the past month, how often have you had to push or strain to begin urination?	0	1	2	3	4	5	
	None	**1 time**	**2 times**	**3 times**	**4 times**	**5 or more times**	
7. NOCTURIA Over the past month, how many times did you most typically get up to urinate from the time you went to bed at night until the time you got up in the morning?	0	1	2	3	4	5	

Which of the above do you regard as most troublesome (1–7) ______

TOTAL PROSTATE SYMPTOM SCORE

	Delighted	Pleased	Mostly satisfied	Mixed satisfied and dissatisfied	Mostly dissatisfied	Unhappy	Terrible
QUALITY OF LIFE DUE TO URINARY SYMPTOMS If you were to spend the rest of your life with your urinary condition just the way it is now, how would you feel about that? (pick one)	0	1	2	3	4	5	6

Source: Lawrentschuk & Perera (2016).

TABLE 16.5 Nursing management of patients undergoing TURP

Preoperative care	Post-operative care	Discharge advice for the patient

Educate patients on:
• the procedure and what they can expect
• potential complications, e.g., risk of retrograde ejaculation, bleeding and UTI.
	Monitor for and document:
	• pain, and administer analgesia
	• transurethral resection syndrome (rare; occurs when irrigating fluid is absorbed during surgery and causes low serum sodium levels, resulting in breathing problems, confusion and seizures
	• signs of excess bleeding (degree of haematuria)
	• signs of urinary retention due to clot formation:
	  • decreased urinary output
	    – abdominal distension
	    – palpable bladder
	    – increased pain.
		It takes up to 8 weeks to see a symptomatic improvement.
		Urine may be bloodstained, particularly for two weeks post-operatively.
		Drink 1.5–2 L of fluid daily (with minimal caffeine-based drinks).
		Avoid heavy lifting for two weeks.
		Resume gentle exercise and increase this as able.
		Sex can be resumed whenever the patient feels comfortable.

Stop anticoagulants as per hospital protocol Commence venous thromboprophylaxis Nil by mouth and preoperative dietary requirements	Administer intravenous fluids until the patient is drinking freely. Catheter care is part of routine personal hygiene. Continuous bladder irrigation until the urine is clear of clots. Bladder washout when urinary retention occurs. Remove catheter and observe and document urinary output. Avoid constipation and straining during defecation.	Patient may experience erectile dysfunction post-operatively; this should be reported to the surgical team at the follow-up visit. Many men will experience retrograde ejaculation following surgery. Teach the patient pelvic floor exercises. Encourage the patient to express their fears related to sexual dysfunctions and to discuss with partner.

Source: Adapted from Antipuesto (2010).

Continuous bladder irrigation post TURP

Continuous bladder irrigation is used to flush out small blood clots that can lead to urinary tract obstruction after prostate or bladder surgery (Nursekey 2016). The procedure requires the placement of a three-way or three-lumen bladder catheter. One lumen controls balloon inflation; one allows inflow, and one allows outflow. A continuous flow of irrigating solution through the bladder creates a mild tamponade that may prevent venous haemorrhage. Usually, the catheter is inserted in the operating room during surgery; however, it may be inserted at bedside (see figure 16.14).

Holmium laser enucleation of the prostate (HoLEP)

When a TURP procedure is done with a laser instead of traditional scraping, the procedures are similar although differently named, depending on the type of laser used. They include holmium laser ablation (HoLAP), PVP or greenlight laser. The physician passes the laser fibre through the urethra into the prostate and then delivers bursts of energy to vaporise obstructing prostate tissue.

Other surgical options for BPH

Other surgical options for BPH include the following.

- Transurethral incision of the prostate (TUIP) is a procedure in which the urethra is widened by making a few small incisions in the prostate gland and the neck of the bladder.
- Transurethral microwave thermotherapy (TUMT): A TUMT does not cure BPH, the aim is to reduce urinary problems. Computer-regulated microwaves are sent by way of a catheter to heat and destroy excess prostate tissue.
- Transurethral needle ablation (TUNA) is a minimally invasive approach that delivers low-level radiofrequency energy to destroy prostate tissue and widen the urinary channel, improving urine flow.
- UroLift system treatment is minimally invasive. The urethra is widened by placing tiny implants to hold the enlarged prostate tissue out of the way and improve urine flow.

- High-intensity focused ultrasound uses ultrasound waves to destroy prostate tissue. This is a new treatment area that is still undergoing clinical trials in the USA.
- Open surgery: For very large prostates, the traditional TURP and laser surgery may be ineffective and open surgery is required. An external incision allows for the removal of enlarged tissue from inside the gland. The entire prostate is not removed. The outer shell or capsule of the prostate remains intact.
- Holimum laser enucleation of the prostate (HoLEP) is another minimally invasive treatment that does not require an incision and is used for large prostates. Currently this procedure is only performed in select centres.
- Prostate artery embolisation requires an interventional radiologist to insert a hollow wire into the artery in the leg and manoeuvres it to the arteries that supply only the prostate. A material designed to slow or stop blood flow to the prostate and causing it to shrink or soften is injected through the wire. Again, this is a relatively new procedure and may require enrolling in a clinical trial to be eligible (RadiologyInfo.org 2021).

FIGURE 16.14 Continuous bladder irrigation

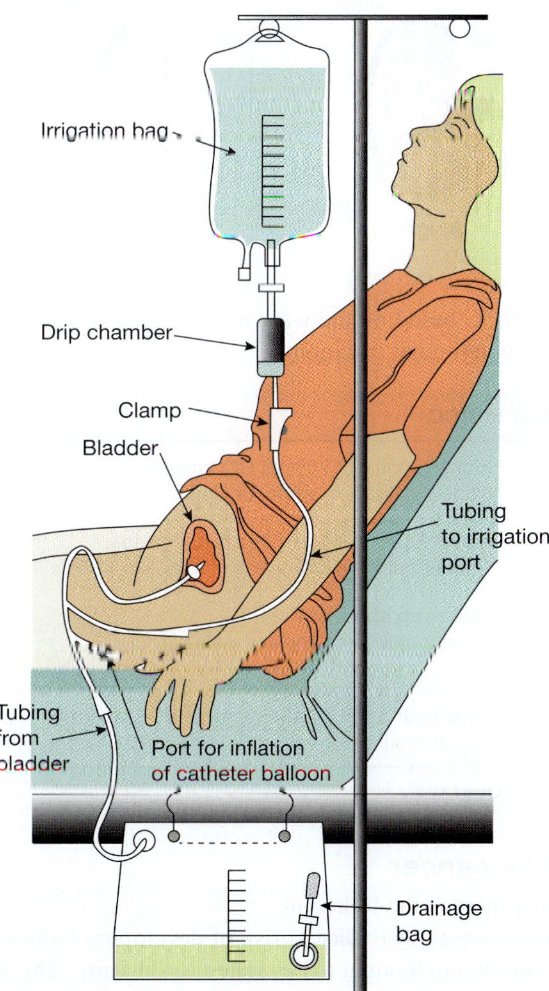

Source: Taylor et al. (2005) *Fundamentals of Nursing: The Art and Science of Nursing Care*, with kind permission of Lippincott Williams & Wilkins.

16.3 The oncological conditions of the urinary system

LEARNING OBJECTIVE 16.3 Discuss the oncological conditions of the urinary system.

Kidney cancer

Kidney cancer was the seventh most diagnosed cancer in Australia in 2016, and it is estimated that when statistics are available, this will remain unchanged in 2020 (Australian Government 2021).

In Australia, more than 3000 people are diagnosed with kidney cancer per annum. Kidney cancer makes up about 2.5 per cent of all cancers. Twice the number of men to women get kidney cancer — it is the ninth most diagnosed cancer for Australian men. Age increases the risk of kidney cancer, with the highest cancer rate being in men over 50 years old.

Renal cell carcinoma

Approximately nine out of ten kidney cancers are renal cell carcinoma (RCC), also called renal cell adenocarcinoma (Cancer Council NSW 2020). RCC starts in the cells lining the tubes in the kidney's nephrons. In the early stages, the tumour is in one kidney only. However, in rare cases, RCC affects both kidneys. As the cancer grows, it spreads to the surrounding fatty tissue, veins, adrenal glands, lymph nodes, ureters, or the liver (see figure 16.15). It may also spread to other parts of the body, such as the lungs or bones.

FIGURE 16.15 The stages of kidney cancer

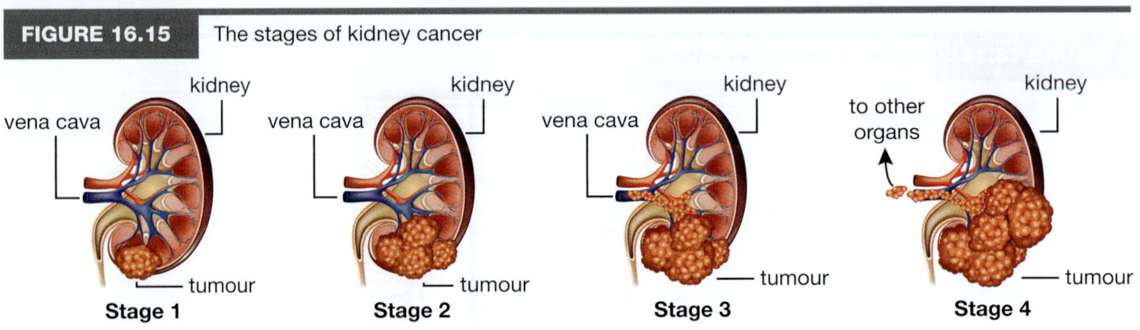

There are several types of RCC based on the way the cells look under a microscope (see table 16.6). The most common type is clear cell renal carcinoma.

TABLE 16.6 Different types of RCC

Clear cell RCC	Makes up about 75% of RCC cases Cancer cells look empty or clear
Papillary RCC	Makes up about 10–15% of RCC cases Cancer cells are arranged in finger-like fronds
Chromophobe RCC	Makes up about 5% of RCC Cancer cells are large and pale
Other types of RCC	Include renal medullary carcinoma, collecting duct carcinoma, MiT family translocation RCC, sarcomatoid RCC and other very rare types Together make up about 5–10% of RCC cases

Source: Adapted from Cancer Council NSW (n.d.).

Risk factors for kidney cancer

Risk factors for kidney cancer include the following.

- *Smoking.* People who smoke are almost twice at risk of developing kidney cancer. Approximately one in three cases of kidney cancers are thought to be related to smoking. This risk increases with the years the person smokes and the packets per day they smoke.
- *Obesity.* Excessive body fat can cause changes to some hormones that can lead to kidney cancer.
- *High blood pressure.* Whatever the cause, high blood pressure increases the risk of kidney cancer.
- *Kidney failure.* People with end-stage kidney disease have a higher risk of developing kidney cancer.
- *Family history.* People with a close relative with kidney cancer are at increased risk.
- *Inherited conditions.* About 2–3 per cent of kidney cancers develop in people who have an inherited syndrome such as von Hippel–Lindau disease, hereditary papillary RCC, Birt-Hogg-Dubé syndrome and Lynch syndrome.
- *Exposure to toxic substances at work.* The risk is thought to increase with regular exposure to chemicals including metal degreasers, arsenic or cadmium, which are used in mining, farming, welding and painting.

Tests and procedures to diagnose kidney cancer include:
- blood and urine tests
- imaging tests such as ultrasound, X-ray, CT or MRI (Cancer Council NSW 2020).

Classification and staging of kidney cancer

Kidney cancers can grow without causing any pain or other problems (American Cancer Society 2021a). Because of the kidneys' location, small kidney tumours cannot be seen or felt during a physical exam. There are no recommended early screening tests as none have demonstrated to lower the overall risk of mortality from kidney cancer. Kidney cancer will likely be first identified due to presenting signs and symptoms. Therefore, it is crucial to keep the public well informed about kidney health. The staging system most often used for kidney cancer in Australia is the American Joint Committee on Cancer (AJCC) tumour, nodes and metastases (TNM) system (table 16.7) (Cancer Council NSW 2020).

TABLE 16.7 TNM staging system

Stage 1	The cancer is found in the kidney only and measures less than 7 cm.	early
Stage 2	The cancer is larger than 7 cm, may have spread to the renal vein or the kidney's outer tissue, but no further and has not spread to any lymph nodes.	early
Stage 3	The cancer is any size and has spread to nearby lymph nodes or the adrenal gland.	locally advanced
Stage 4	The cancer has spread beyond the kidney, adrenal gland and nearby lymph nodes and is found in more distant parts of the body, such as the abdomen, distant lymph nodes or organs such as the liver, lungs, bone or brain.	advanced (metastatic)

Source: Adapted from Cancer Council NSW (n.d.).

Signs and symptoms of kidney cancer

Signs and symptoms of kidney cancer usually appear after the tumour has grown or the cancer has spread (American Cancer Society 2021b). These include:
- haematuria
- a mass in the side or lower back area
- persistent fever of unknown origin
- unexplained pain in the flank or lower back
- persistent fatigue
- oedema of the legs and ankles
- unexplained weight loss.

Investigations for kidney cancer diagnosis

The following exams and tests will be carried out to support treatment decisions to diagnose and stage kidney cancer:
- physical examination
- urinalysis for haematuria
- a full blood count for anaemia
- liver function tests
- imaging studies, including:
  - abdominal ultrasound
  - CT scan
  - MRI
- renal biopsy.

Treatment of kidney cancer

Treatment and care of patients with kidney cancer, like all other cancers, require a multidisciplinary team approach (Australian Government 2021). Treatment choices will be made in consultation with the patients and their families and will depend on:
- the stage of the disease

- the location of the cancer
- the severity of symptoms
- the patient's informed choice.

Surgery

Treatment for kidney cancer often involves surgery (Australian Government 2021). Surgery options include:

- partial nephrectomy, which involves removal of some of the kidney tissue
- simple nephrectomy, where the whole kidney is removed
- radical nephrectomy, where the kidney, adrenal gland located on top of the kidney, fatty tissue around the kidney and sometimes some of the nearby lymph nodes are removed.

Figure 16.16 illustrates a partial and radical nephrectomy.

FIGURE 16.16 Partial and radical nephrectomy

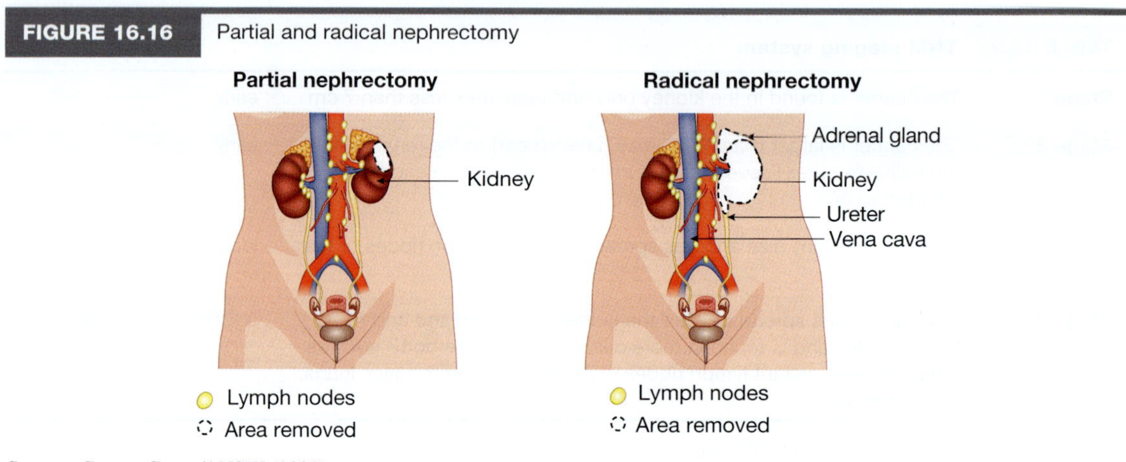

Source: Cancer Council NSW (2020).

Nursing management of renal surgery patients

Nursing management plays an important role in pre- and post-operative renal surgery, applying patient-centred care that educates and supports the patient and their family on expectations, possible outcomes and self-care. Perioperative nursing care is detailed in table 16.8.

TABLE 16.8 Nursing management of patients undergoing renal surgery care

Preoperative care	Post-operative care
Take and document full health history and physical assessment, including vital signs of cardiovascular, respiratory and renal assessment. Renal risk assessment to include a baseline assessment of renal function, urinalysis and the pattern and characteristics of the urinary output.	Ongoing monitoring, escalating any concerns to the surgeon. Vital signs including: • respirations • colour • level of consciousness and appearance • administer prescribed oxygen • place in a **semi-Fowler's position** • pulse oximetry for oxygen saturation levels.
Patient education for the early detection of deterioration. Use of patient-controlled analgesia (PCA) and the importance of treating pain and reporting pain that is not treated with the current dose of analgesia so that the surgeon can review this. Deep breathing and coughing exercises while protecting the wound.	Monitor for signs of respiratory complications such as spontaneous pneumothorax or atelectasis, such as changes in respiration, decreased oxygen saturation levels. Ensure regular use of the incentive spirometer. Use pillows to protect the wound when conducting breathing and coughing exercises. Monitor for signs of hypovolemic shock due to haemorrhage with vital signs, colour, **skin turgor**.

Use of the incentive spirometer.

Leg exercises and use of antiembolism stockings.

Care of the urinary catheter.

Care of the wound incision line.

Fasting, intravenous therapy, oral fluids and then a light diet.

Health lifestyle pursuits: exercise, diet, smoking cessation.

Wound care, including:
- monitoring for signs and symptoms of infection
- documenting wound drainage
- remove the wound drain (if present), usually 48–72 hours post-operatively as per surgeon's or physician's orders
- remove sutures/staples (if present) at 7–10 days. The patient can return to outpatients or attend a community healthcare provider for this procedure.

Monitor, assess and treat pain. If the PCA is not managing the pain, escalate the concern to the surgeon and or pain care team. Pain relief is an important factor in optimising recovery.

Monitor urinary output and record on the fluid balance chart:
- colour and odour of the urine
- post-operative voiding pattern
- renal function, e.g., serum creatinine level.
- Prevent constipation by monitoring for:
- bowel sounds
- signs and symptoms of paralytic ileus.

Early mobilisation.

Commence oral fluids followed by a light diet.

Assess for needs of support with activities of daily living on discharge.

Advise patient on follow-up treatment and care and cancer support groups.

Non-surgical treatments

Patients may undergo 'watchful waiting', which involves regular appointments to review symptoms, but they do not have routine diagnostic testing (Cancer Net 2019b).

Active surveillance or close monitoring of the cancer is used in older adults or patients who have a small renal tumour and comorbidities such as heart disease, CKD or severe lung disease that make surgery high risk (Cancer Net 2019b). It can also be used for patients who are otherwise well and have few or no symptoms.

Ablation involves removing tissue using means other than surgery and is sometimes used to attempt to destroy kidney tumours (Australian Government 2021). Types of ablation include:
- cryotherapy, which uses extreme cold delivered through a needle probe
- radiofrequency ablation using high-energy radio waves to heat the tumour delivered via a needle probe
- arterial embolisation, which involves blocking the artery that feeds the affected kidney starving it of oxygen and nutrients and causing it to shrink.

Chemotherapy is helpful in treating numerous types of cancer; however, kidney cancer is often resistant to current chemotherapy regimens (Australian Government 2021; Cancer Net 2019b). Researchers continue to study new drugs and new combinations of drugs. Immunotherapy is used in its management, with interferon-alpha being the gold standard of treatment, although interleukin-2 can also be used.

Radiotherapy can be used if it is suspected that some cancer cells are left behind after surgery (Australian Government 2021). Radiotherapy without surgery can also be used in people who are at high risk for surgery. Radiotherapy can also help ease the symptoms of kidney cancer. Research is ongoing for new and useful radiotherapy that can lead to better outcomes.

Targeted therapy is treatment with medications designed to specifically attack cancer cells without harming normal cells (Australian Government 2021). Targeted therapy can be used to treat advanced kidney cancers. The aim is to shrink or slow the growth of the cancer. To date, targeted therapies have not been shown to cause kidney cancer.

Bladder cancer

Bladder cancer is common cancer. According to Cancer Australia (2021), 2790 new cases of bladder cancer diagnosed in Australia in 2016. The more significant portion of these were males, with 2128 males to 662 females. Bladder cancer is more common in older adults than young people, especially after age 60. Cancer Australia estimates that in 2020, 3098 new bladder cancer cases will be diagnosed in Australia (2389 males and 710 females).

Bladder cancers can be classified as:

- urothelial carcinoma, previously known as transitional cell carcinoma, is the most common form of bladder cancer (80–90 per cent). It begins in the urothelial cells that line the inside of the bladder
- squamous cell carcinoma (one to two per cent) begins in the thin, flat cells that line the bladder
- adenocarcinoma is a rare form (one per cent) and begins in the mucus-producing cells in the bladder. It is the most invasive form of bladder cancer (Cancer Australia 2021).

Bladder cancer can be described based on its location (Department of Health & Human Services 2020a). Non-muscle-invasive bladder cancer has not spread to other layers of the bladder or the muscle. Muscle-invasive cancer has spread to other layers of the bladder, muscle, and other parts of the body (figure 16.17). Bladder cancer spreads by direct invasion through the bladder wall into adjacent organs such as the prostate, vagina and rectum. The lymphatic system is another route for tumours to spread, initially to the local pelvic nodes and then to the para-aortic nodes and circulatory system, giving rise to metastases in the liver, lungs and bones. The cancer can also involve the ureteric orifices, leading to unilateral or bilateral hydronephrosis and renal failure.

FIGURE 16.17 Bladder cancer

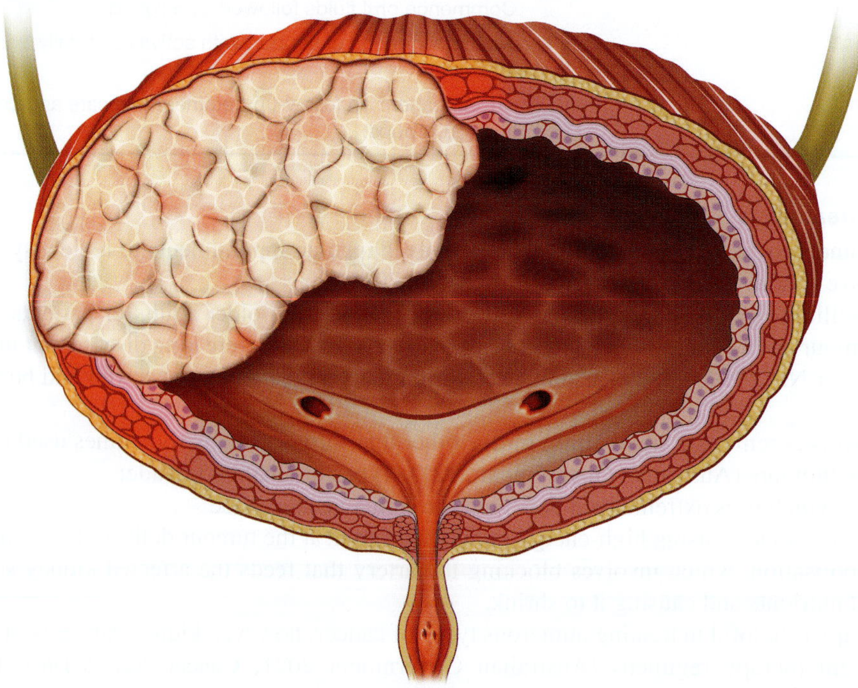

Characteristics and risk factors of bladder cancer

Bladder cancer signs and symptoms may include

- haematuria
- frequency of urination
- pain or burning sensation when passing urine
- not being able to pass urine
- back pain or lower abdominal pain (Mayo Clinic 2021c).

Risk factors for bladder cancer are:

- smoking
- ageing
- male gender
- family history
- environmental factors such as lengthy contact with aromatic amines, benzene products and aniline dyes, have been linked to bladder cancer
- chronic bladder inflammation
- radiation or chemotherapy.

Investigations for bladder cancer diagnosis

Bladder cancer is graded and staged by how far it has spread and how quickly it is growing (Mayo Clinic 2021c).

Investigations for bladder cancer will include the following.

- Examinations such as palpating for any thickening or lumps in the rectum in men and the rectum and vagina in women.
- Urine tests:
  - urine samples for cytology to detect the presence of abnormal cells. It must be noted that this is controversial in the diagnosis of bladder cancer due to the lack of sensitivity
  - midstream urine sample for culture for sensitivity.
- Blood tests:
  - a full blood count to rule out anaemia
  - a full biochemistry screen to review for renal function
  - liver function tests.
- Imaging:
  - **KUB X-ray**
  - **intravenous urogram/pyelogram**
  - CT scan
  - MRI scan
  - pelvic ultrasound
  - bone scan.
- Procedures such as cystoscopy and examination under anaesthetic.

Treatment of bladder cancer

Treatment is determined by the type, stage and grade of the cancer. Currently, the treatments that are available for bladder cancer are:

- surgery
- chemotherapy
- immunotherapy (local and systemic)
- targeted therapy
- radiation therapy.

Surgery involves the removal of the tumour and some of the surrounding tissue (Cancer Net 2019a). The choice of surgery will be made by the multidisciplinary care team and the patient and their family. Current surgical options include transurethral bladder tumour resection (TURBT). This is used for diagnosis, staging and treatment of bladder cancer and is done under procedural sedation.

A radical cystectomy entails removing the whole bladder and other tissues and organs (Cancer Net 2019a). In males, the prostate and urethra may also be removed. In females, the uterus, fallopian tubes, ovaries and part of the vagina may be removed. For all patients, lymph nodes in the pelvis will be removed. A radical cystectomy requires a surgeon who is very experienced in minimally invasive surgery. There are currently ongoing studies to determine the safety of this procedure.

Urinary diversion is a surgical procedure that creates a new way pathway for the urine to exit the body. Usually, a section of the small intestine or colon is used to divert urine to a **stoma** or **ostomy**. The stoma care nurse will be assigned to support the patient and their family in caring and providing practical advice on managing the stoma to avoid infection, skin breakdown, blockages or other problems. They will be able to reassure the patient and their family before and after the surgery and provide them with information on community support. Pre and post-operative nursing care is detailed in table 16.9.

TABLE 16.9 **Nursing management of patients with bladder cancer**

Preoperative care	Post-operative care
Identify psychological concerns and support these concerns with the appropriate members of the care team.	Ongoing monitoring and escalation of any concerns to the surgeon of vital signs including respiration, colour, level of consciousness and appearance.

(continued)

TABLE 16.9 *(continued)*

Educate the patient on the following issues: • the surgical procedure what to expect before and after the surgery • preparations for surgery • the stoma — describe the physical appearance using diagrams, videos and written information • stents inserted into the stoma to protect the anastomosis between the ureter and intestine • ostomy and related equipment • wearing of a urostomy bag • daily activities — there is no need to alter clothing, and the patient can continue to bathe or shower.	Administer prescribed oxygen. Place in a semi-Fowler's position. Pulse oximetry for oxygen saturation levels. Monitor for signs of respiratory complications such as spontaneous pneumothorax or atelectasis, such as respiration changes and decreased oxygen saturation levels. Ensure regular use of the incentive spirometer. Use pillows to protect the wound when conducting breathing and coughing exercises. Monitor for signs of hypovolemic shock due to haemorrhage with vital signs, colour and skin turgor. Wound and stoma care — coordinate with the stoma/ostomy care nurse. Monitor wound for signs and symptoms of infection. Document wound condition. Dress wounds as per protocols. Monitor, assess and treat pain level. If pain is not managed, escalate the concern to the surgeon and or pain care team. Pain relief is an important factor in optimising recovery. Monitor urinary output and record on the fluid balance chart: • colour and odour • post-operative voiding pattern • renal function, e.g., serum creatinine level. Prevent constipation by monitoring for: • bowel sounds • signs and symptoms of paralytic ileus. Early mobilisation. Diet as ordered by the surgical team. Assess for needs of support with ADLs on discharge. Advise patient on: • follow-up treatment and care with physician, stoma care nurse and dietician • lifestyle changes • cancer/ostomy support groups available.

Source: Chiba (1985).

Systemic therapy

Systemic therapy is a treatment that uses medications to destroy cancer cells and includes the following.

- Chemotherapy, given over a specific number of does or cycles over a set period. The patient and their family can plan around the treatment.
- Immunotherapy, designed to boost the body's natural defences to fight the cancer and improve, target or restore immune system function.
- Targeted therapy targets the specific genes, proteins or tissue environment that contributes to cancer growth and survival. Targeted therapy blocks the growth and spread of cancer cells while limiting damage to healthy cells (Cancer Net 2019a).

Prostate cancer

Prostate cancer is the most common cancer in Australian men aside from the common skin cancers. There are about 19 000 new cases in Australia yearly. One in six Australian men are at risk of developing prostate cancer by the age of 85. In 2018, there were 3264 deaths caused by prostate cancer, the five-year survival rate for prostate cancer is 95 per cent (Cancer Australia 2021b). The Prostate Cancer Foundation of Australia is a broad-based community organisation dedicated to reducing the impact of prostate cancer on Australian men and their families in a culturally and linguistically diverse society (Prostate Cancer Foundation of Australia 2020a).

There are two stages of advanced prostate cancer.

1. *Locally advanced prostate cancer.* In this stage, the cancer has spread outside the prostate to nearby parts of the body or glands.
2. *Metastatic prostate cancer.* In this stage, the cancer has spread to distant parts of the body.

Risk factors for prostate cancer include:

- ageing
- familial history of prostate cancer
- ethnicity or race — research has shown that Aboriginal men in NSW are nearly 50 per cent more likely to die from their prostate cancer than non-Aboriginal men (Rodger et al. 2014)
- genetic changes.

Prostate cancer symptoms

The early stages of prostate cancer are often symptom-free. Advanced prostate cancer signs and symptoms include:

- frequency of urination
- painful urinating
- blood in the urine or semen
- a weak stream during urination
- pain in the back or pelvis area
- weakness in the legs or feet
- pain or unexplained weight loss, indicative of widespread disease.

Diagnosis and staging of prostate cancer

The following tests can be used for confirming and staging a diagnosis of prostate cancer:

- a PSA — this is not a definitive test and will be used to inform the diagnosis in conjunction with other tests
- biopsy of the prostate
- DRE
- MRI, CT or bone scan.

Management of prostate cancer

The management of prostate cancer is dependent on the stage. Table 16.10 outlines the treatment options for each stage.

TABLE 16.10 Management of treatment options for each stage of prostate cancer

Stage	Management of treatment options
Localised or early	Active surveillance Surgery or radiation therapy, or both Watchful waiting
Locally advanced	Surgery of radiation therapy, or both Androgen deprivation therapy (ADT) may also be suggested
Advanced or metastatic	Usually ADT Sometimes chemotherapy or radiation therapy Watchful waiting may be an option Newer treatments as part of a clinical trial

Source: Adapted from Cancer Council Victoria (2021).

Active surveillance involves monitoring the asymptomatic or symptom-free prostate cancer to avoid or delay invasive treatment if the cancer is unlikely to spread or cause symptoms. This would include regular PSA testing, DRE and annual MRI scan and biopsies (Cancer Council Victoria 2021).

Watchful waiting is another method of monitoring prostate cancer to avoid active treatment if the patient is not experiencing symptoms. It involves less testing, and a biopsy is not usually required. Watchful waiting is often used for older patients who are not likely to experience problems during their lifetime (Cancer Council Victoria 2021).

A radical prostatectomy is used for localised prostate cancer (Prostate Cancer Foundation of Australia 2020b). A radical prostatectomy involves removing the prostate, the seminal vesicles and part of the urethra. The aim is to remove all of the cancer. The surgical approaches to a radical prostatectomy include:

- open radical prostatectomy
- laparoscopic radical prostatectomy
- robotic-assisted radical prostatectomy.

Recovery time with an open radical prostatectomy may be slower than with a laparoscopic or robotic prostate surgery but all three methods have similar side effects. The surgery is done under a general anaesthetic and will take from two to four hours. The approach used is largely dependent on the surgeon's choice in discussion with the patient and their family.

Radiotherapy is also used to treat prostate cancer. This can be done using external beam radiation therapy where the radiation is directed externally towards the prostate gland or internal radiation therapy called brachytherapy. Radioactive 'seeds' are placed inside the prostate. Some of these seeds give off low doses of radiation and are not removed after the radiation has been used up. Other seeds that give off higher doses of radiation are held in place with catheters and removed after the radiation is finished.

Cryosurgery is a less used treatment for prostate cancer. It is used after radiotherapy or if the cancer has returned after other treatments.

For prostate cancers that rely on androgen hormones, hormonotherapy can be used to reduce or slow the growth of the cancer. Hormone therapy for prostate cancer is called ADT.

Chemotherapy and immunotherapy are also used to treat prostate cancers.

Each treatment option for prostate cancer comes with its own side effects. Table 16.11 outlines each treatment option and its related side effects.

TABLE 16.11 **Prostate cancer treatment options and related side effects**

Prostate cancer treatment	Potential side effects
Surgery (prostatectomy)	Erection problems Loss of libido Dry orgasm Urine leakage during sex Infertility Urinary problems Fatigue
External beam radiation therapy (EBRT)	Erection problems Loss of libido Dry orgasm Infertility Urinary problems Bowel problems Fatigue Skin irritation Brachytherapy Erection problems Loss of libido Dry orgasm Infertility Urinary problems
Androgen deprivation therapy (ADT)	Erection problems Loss of libido Dry orgasm Infertility Bowel problems Fatigue Hot flushes Osteoporosis Heart problems Breast growth Mood swings

Source: Adapted from Cancer Council Victoria (2021).

Most treatments affect continence and potency, and adaptation to such radical body image changes may need expert practical and emotional support. Erectile dysfunction can be managed with medication or a vacuum constriction device. Continence issues can be resolved with pelvic floor exercises, medication or surgery depending on the cause.

The most common site for the spread of prostate cancer is bone (American Cancer Society 2021c). Bone metastases can cause pain, fractures and spinal cord compression if the spine is involved. This is a medical emergency, and men with bone metastases should be counselled on the signs, symptoms and action to take. Prescribing hormone deprivation therapy can impact a man's sexuality, mood and body image significantly. Men must be counselled about the side effects of hormone deprivation therapy, along with lifestyle advice to prevent longer-term complications, including metabolic syndrome and osteoporosis.

The Australian Government, through Cancer Australia, provides significant funding to the Prostate Cancer Foundation of Australia (PCFA) in support of providing national, evidence-based information, resources and psychosocial support for men and their families affected by prostate cancer. Nursing management will focus on the needs of the patient and their family, taking a person-centred care approach and using the clinical reasoning cycle to support the patient's assessment and care.

16.4 Renal replacement therapy

LEARNING OBJECTIVE 16.4 Identify and discuss the different types of renal replacement therapy.

Currently, there is no cure for CKD (Cleveland Clinic 2021a). Untreated CKD will progress to complete kidney failure, resulting in death. Options for end stages of CKD include dialysis and kidney transplantation.

Dialysis uses machines to remove waste products from your body and help maintain homeostasis. There are three primary forms of dialysis (Tandukar & Palevsky 2019):

1. haemodialysis (IHD)
2. peritoneal dialysis (PD)
3. continuous renal replacement therapies (CRRT).

Haemodialysis

Haemodialysis is the most common type of dialysis (Medical News Today 2021). A Haemodialysis machine removes the waste products and extra fluid from the blood that the healthy kidney would normally do. Blood is removed from the body and filtered by the artificial kidney and returned to the bloodstream. Toxins and excess water are removed from the blood using the principles of diffusion, osmosis and ultrafiltration. Patients are treated three times a week for three to four hours in a dialysis centre.

Vascular access for dialysis is provided by one of the following methods.

- Arteriovenous (AV) fistula connects an artery and a vein (figure 16.18) and is the preferred option for dialysis. AV fistulas have several advantages over other access methods as they provide good blood flow for dialysis, last longer than other types of access and are less likely to get infected or cause blood clots.

FIGURE 16.18 Arteriovenous (AV) fistula

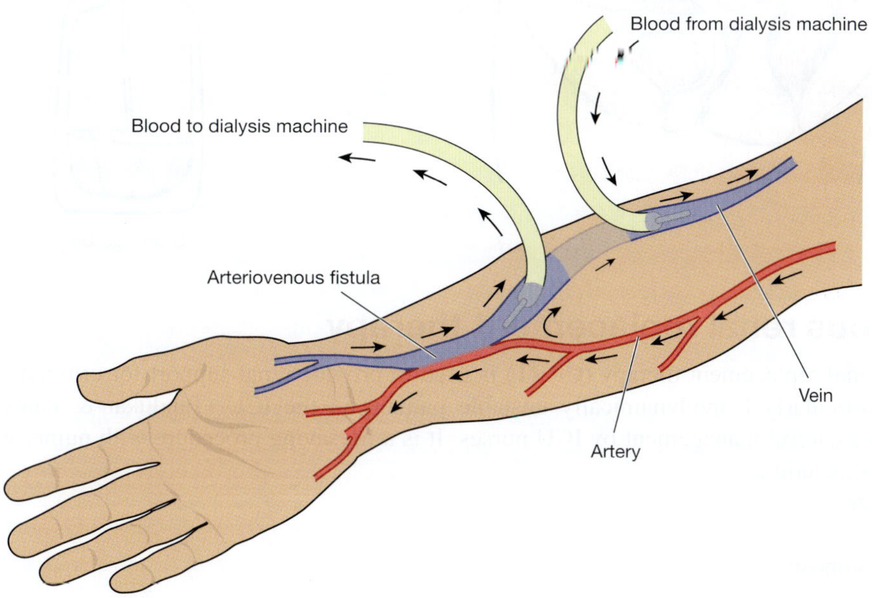

- An AV graft is a looped, plastic tube connecting an artery to a vein (The Regents of the University of California 2021). A vascular surgeon performs AV graft surgery. The surgery can be performed under procedural sedation and the patient in most cases is discharged home after the procedure.
- A vascular access catheter is inserted through either the internal jugular (neck), femoral vein (groin) or subclavian vein (upper chest) (The Regents of the University of California 2021). If fistula or graft surgery is unsuccessful and the patient needs a venous catheter for more than three weeks, the surgeon will 'tunnel' the catheter under the skin. The tunnelled catheter is more comfortable and has fewer problems.

Peritoneal dialysis

Peritoneal dialysis (PD) has an advantage over haemodialysis because it can be performed by the patient at home (Cleveland Clinic 2021b). With PD, a dialysis solution is run directly into the patient's abdomen through an access port. The solution absorbs waste, and the catheter removes this waste. Fresh solution is added to continue the process of cleaning. There are two types of PD.

1. *Continuous ambulatory PD (CAPD).* Dialysis solution is changed four times a day (see figure 16.19).
2. *Continuous cycling PD (CCPD).* Uses a machine to fill, remove wastes and refill the fluid automatically. This can be done overnight, freeing the patient up for everyday activities.

FIGURE 16.19 Peritoneal dialysis

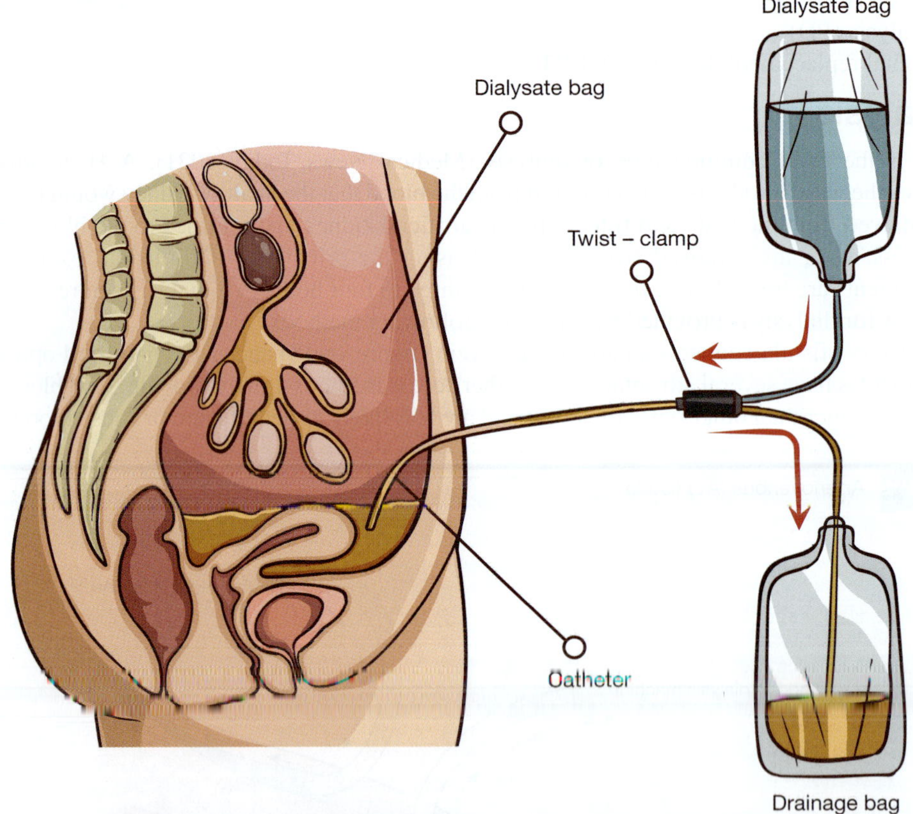

Continuous renal replacement therapy

Continuous renal replacement therapy (CRRT) is used to provide renal support for critically ill patients with AKI, particularly hemodynamically unstable patients in the ICU (Tandukar & Palevsky 2019). CRRT requires careful management by ICU nurses. It is a lifesaving procedure with numerous potential complications including:

- haemorrhage
- infection
- venous thrombosis

- venous stenosis
- traumatic arteriovenous fistula
- pneumothorax
- hemothorax
- air embolism
- visceral injury
- extracorporeal circuit-related complications
- allergic reaction to hemodialyser/hemofilter or tubing
- circuit thrombosis
- homolysis
- air embolism
- hypothermia
- hypotension
- electrolyte disturbances
- hypophosphatemia
- hypokalaemia
- hypocalcaemia
- hypomagnesaemia
- incorrect medication dosing (Tandukar & Palevsky 2019).

Kidney transplant

A kidney transplant is a surgical procedure in which a healthy kidney from a living or deceased donor into a patient with kidney failure. Kidneys come from either living donors or deceased donors. Living donors are usually family members. Donors are carefully screened for a suitable match and to prevent any transmissible diseases or complications. Deceased donors have usually willed their kidneys before their death, or their family donates the kidney after the person's death. In Australia, in 2019, there were 857 kidney transplants (Transplant.org.au 2019).

A kidney that is being transplanted is placed on the lower right or left side of the abdomen and surgically connected to nearby blood vessels. Placing the kidney in this position allows for ease of connection to blood vessels and the bladder. The vein and artery of the transplanted kidney are attached to the patient's vein and artery, and the transplanted kidney's ureter is attached to the bladder to allow for normal urination. The risks versus the benefits of a kidney transplant are outlined in table 16.12.

TABLE 16.12 Risk versus benefits of a kidney transplant

Risks of kidney transplantation	Benefits of kidney transplantation
Same as those of any surgery, including the risk of bleeding, infection or breathing problems	Increased strength, stamina and energy
Potential for side effects from the medications	Return to a more normal lifestyle
More prone to infections due to the anti-rejection medication	Greater control over ADLS
Risk of rejection	More freedom, as the patient will no longer need to attend dialysis schedules
	Return to a regular diet and more normal fluid intake
	Anaemia may be corrected after the transplant
	Fewer medications

Source: Cleveland Clinic (2019).

Post-operative nursing management

Nurses must monitor post-kidney transplantation patients for signs of deterioration and escalate care when needed.

Ongoing nursing assessment and documentation should include:

- vital signs
- airway management
- pain management
- fluid balance
- administration of IV medications, including fluids.

Prior to discharge:

- educate patient and family on:
  - follow-up care
  - medication and need for compliance
  - infection control
  - signs and symptoms of rejection
- review for referral to:
  - dietitian
  - in-home self-care assessment.

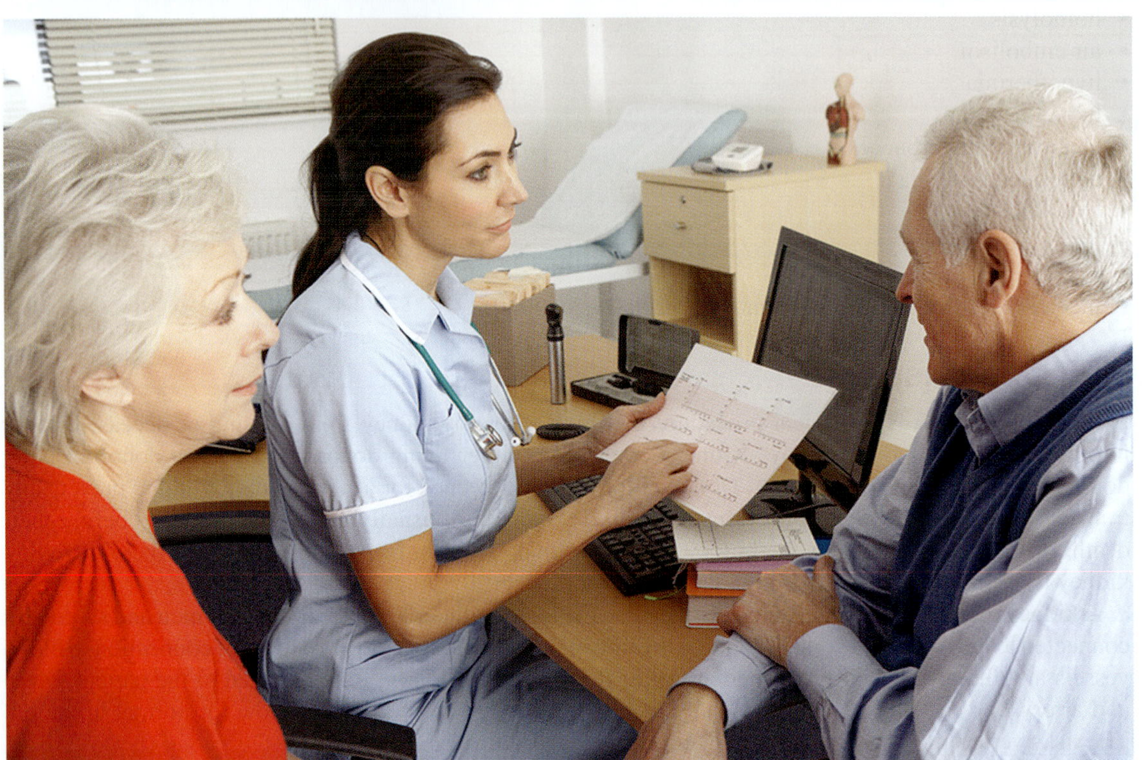

16.5 The incidence of kidney disorders in Australia

LEARNING OBJECTIVE 16.5 Reflect on the incidence of kidney disorders in Australia and the importance of understanding the function of the urinary system for a healthy community.

According to approximately one out of ten Australian adults, or about 1.7 million people in 2011–12, had biomedical signs of CKD. In 2017–18, Aboriginal and Torres Strait Islander regular dialysis rates were 11 times higher than non-Indigenous Australians. In 2018, there were 16 800 CKD-related deaths (79 per cent of deaths). Key figures from the Australian Bureau of Statistics demonstrated that in 2018:

- 237 800 Australians had kidney disease
- males and females had similar rates of kidney disease (both one per cent), with the prevalence increasing with age
- 20 851 deaths had kidney disease as a contributory factor.

The situation is much worse for at-risk groups. Kidney disease is a significant health problem for Australia. Severe kidney disease is more prevalent among Aboriginal and Torres Strait Islander peoples, and the rates of end-stage kidney disease are significantly higher than among other Australians. Kidney Health Australia (2019) has developed Australia's first *National Strategic Action Plan for Kidney Disease* (figure 16.20) due to the significant impact on Australia's health, wellbeing and economy. The focus is on the partnership between government, private and community groups to reduce kidney disease incidence through education, early detection, optimised care of patients and their families. Healthcare providers are an integral part of this action plan. Evidence-based health care to educate for prevention and optimal care is what we do.

FIGURE 16.26 Concept map for National Strategic Action Plan for Kidney Disease

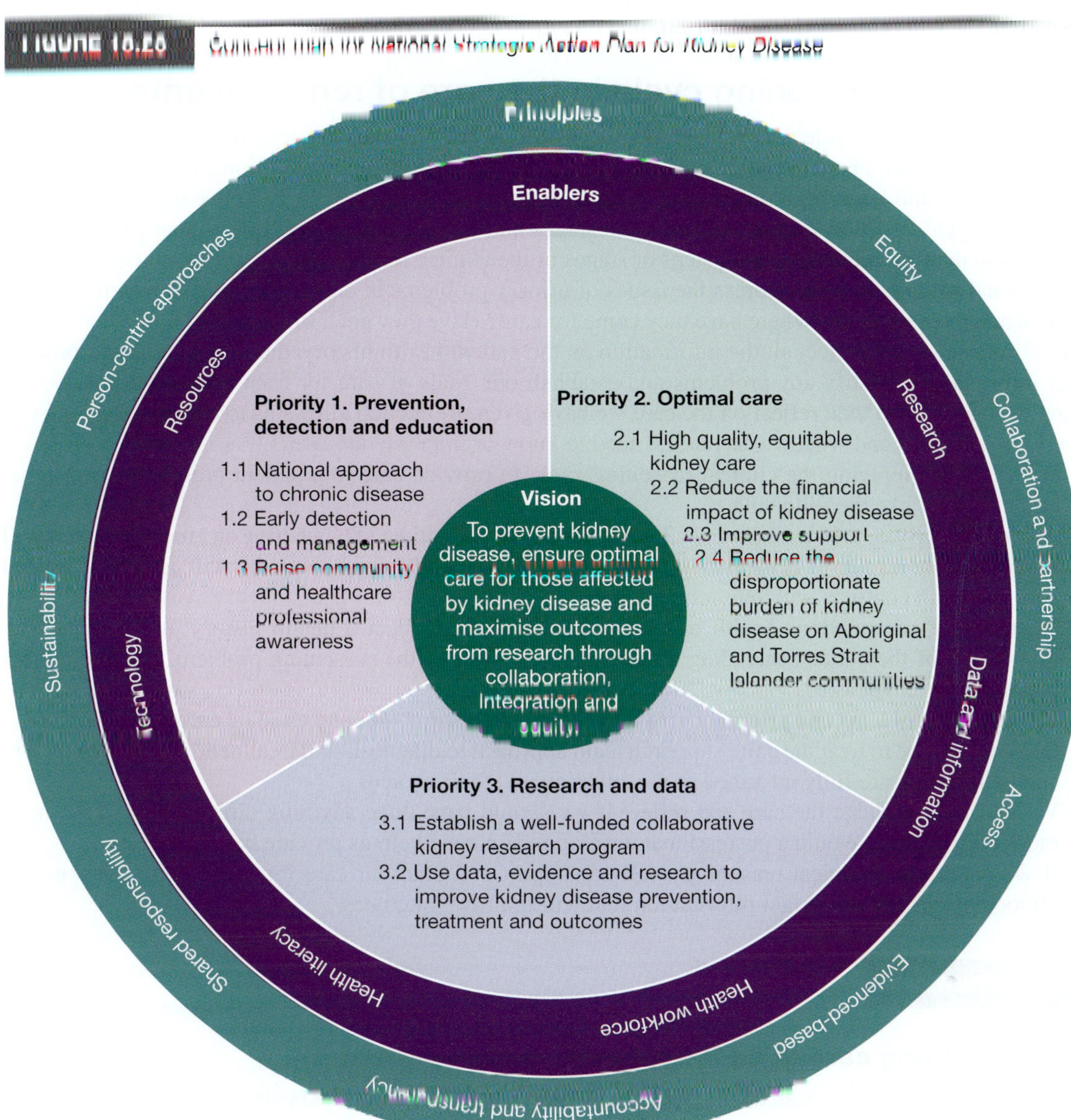

Source: Kidney Health Australia (2019).

16.6 Nursing management of the renal patient

LEARNING OBJECTIVE 16.6 Apply patient-centred care and the clinical reasoning cycle to the management of the renal patient.

Patient-centred care

Patient-centred care respects and responds to the preferences, needs and values of patients and their family. Traditionally, teaching, research and practice were organised around diseases and body systems rather than patients (O'Hare 2018). However, this is changing, and today, nurses are aware that care provided is more than performing skills. Patient-centred care promotes better outcomes through shared decision-making empowers the patient to make decisions based on knowledge and evidence-based research. Nurses need to demonstrate a willingness to listen, make time to support the patient, go beyond our job description, and understand the value in building therapeutic relationships with our patients. As nurses, we can support and educate patients and their families on options for care and treatment of kidney disease and ensure they have contact with members of the multidisciplinary team that can best support them. Renal problems often affect sexuality, and this can be particularly distressing for the patient and their families. Nurses need to be prepared to discuss such issues with patients and their partners or refer them to someone who can support them and answer their questions. Nurses play a vital role in supporting the patient and their family and providing the conduit with the multidisciplinary team.

The clinical reasoning cycle in the care of renal patients

The clinical reasoning cycle is a cyclic process by which we 'collect cues, process the information, come to an understanding of a patient problem or situation, plan and implement interventions, evaluate outcomes, and reflect on, and learn from the process' (Levett-Jones et al. 2009. p. 516). Effective use of the clinical reasoning cycle is dependent on following the stages and linking them to provide a clear picture of the patient and their problem. The eight steps or stages of the clinical reasoning cycle are essential in the care of the renal patient. To fully address the issues of urinary problems in our patients, we must consider the patient and their situation. Where have they come for care? Have they got a support person or persons with them? As nurses, we collect all the information on the patient health history, their vital signs and process that information, identify any problems and establish our goals of care for each event. We provide the care, evaluate it, and then reflect on the care we have given. Reflection allows us to consider how we can improve outcomes and what we, as nurses, need to know or improve our care.

For example, applying the clinical reasoning cycle to provide care to a patient presenting with renal stones may look like the following.

- Are we in a private area to discuss the health issue with the patient? Do we have an emergency that will require a rapid response? Is the patient demonstrating signs and symptoms as this will need to be treated before we can continue with our assessment?
- Do we have any previous health history on this patient? Collect a health history and complete an assessment of the patient, including a focused assessment of the presenting problem. Has the patient had this problem before?
- Identify the problems and prioritise care. Document the information and escalate care as needed.
- Our goal will be to treat the pain, support a team approach to diagnosis and treatment. Ensure the patient and their family are fully informed of the situation and their choices.
- We will then evaluate the care and reflect if we should have done anything differently. Did we need more information? Would a professional development course help us provide better care?

If we employ the clinical reasoning cycle to support and plan our care for the patient, there is less likelihood of missing important information that will improve outcomes.

CASE STUDY 16.1

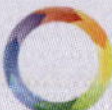

Nursing care of an 82-year-old female patient

Mrs Antoinette Parsons is an 82-year-old female who transferred to the emergency department from her residential care home. The nursing staff at the care home had documented that Mrs Parson has altered mental status, confusion and weakness that they just noted this morning. Two large-bore peripheral intravenous catheters (PIVs) are inserted, and blood is drawn for electrolytes (sodium, potassium and chloride), fats, proteins, glucose and enzymes and a complete blood count. The physician is concerned that Mrs Parson has had a stroke.

On assessment Mrs Parson's vitals are:

- heart rate: 122 beats per minute
- respiratory rate: 24 breaths per minute
- blood pressure: 92/58 mmHg
- oxygen saturation: 92% on room air
- temperature: 39.7°C
- pain score: unable to give a pain score.

Mrs Parsons has been seen by a neurologist who has ruled out stroke. The Recognition of Stroke in the Emergency Room (ROSIER) Scale (Australian Commission on Safety and Quality in Health Care 2019) is −1, and the CT scan is negative for an intracranial bleed. The nurse checks on Mrs Parsons and finds that she has been incontinent of urine. The nurse notes that the urine has a foul, sour odour. Mrs Phillips' blood pressure is now 88/52 mmHg. The nurse notifies the physician. The following order is given:

- maintain SpO_2 >92%
- blood cultures x 2
- urinalysis
- urine culture
- 500 ml NS IV bolus STAT

- 100 ml/hr NS IV continuous infusion
- Vancomycin 1000 mg IV x 1 dose NOW

The nurse obtains two sets of blood cultures and obtains a sterile urine sample using an in and out Foley catheter. The UAP reports cloudy, foul-smelling urine. The nurse initiates the IV fluid bolus and requests the vancomycin from the Pharmacy. Mrs Parsons' son has arrived and asks why she is so confused?

Question

Using the information above, describe what action you would take as the nurse caring for this patient. Which care would be prioritised? Use the clinical reasoning cycle to guide you through the process and devise a care plan for your patient.

Questions you might ask are as follows.

- Why is Mrs Phillips presenting with altered mental status?
- What may be going on with Mrs Phillips physiologically?
- What orders do you anticipate from the provider?
- What discharge education should be provided to Mrs Phillips and the caregivers at her nursing home?

Answer

- *Step 1: Consider the patient.* What is the current situation? Does the patient need additional support? Is she at risk for falls or other potential problems?
- *Step 2: Collect cues/information.* Include subjective and objective data here. The subjective will include what the patient tells you, the patient's appearance, and their past medical history. Objective data will include objective or measurable information such as vital signs, blood tests, etc.
- *Step 3: Process Information.* Separate the relevant and irrelevant data — cluster the clues together to formulate an inference about the patient. Mrs. Parsons is presenting with a Urinary tract infection. She is demonstrating signs of sepsis. She will need antibiotics, oxygen and fluids.
- *Step 4: Identify problems/issues.* Nursing problems or diagnosis should be listed here. Nursing issues include risk of falls and pressure injuries, pain, fluid imbalance and infection.
- *Step 5: Establish goals.* Goals of care for Mrs Parsons, such as improve and maintain BP as per physician orders and hypoxia management.

  Immediate and ongoing care will include management of risks, including falls risk, pressure injury risks, support ADL by cleaning Mrs Parsons, and reassuring her. Maintain fluid balance.

  Educate and reassure Mrs Parsons and her son.
- *Step 6: Take action*. Provide the required care to meet the established goals, for example? Place an IV catheter for fluids and if resuscitation is needed.

  Place the patient on a monitor to support ongoing assessment. Provide fluids as ordered, commence a fluid balance chart.

  Reassure patient.
- *Step 7: Evaluate outcomes.* Were the best outcomes achieved?
- *Step 8: Reflect on the process and new learning.* Reflect on any aspects of care that could have been done better. What went well, what did not go as well as hoped?

CASE STUDY 16.2

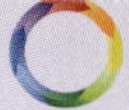

Nursing care of a male patient with urinary concerns

Andrew Ferguson, a 49-year-old Caucasian male, presented to the emergency room with confusion, disorientation, hypothermia, tachycardia, tachypnoea and hypotension. His brother has brought him in. Andrew has presented three times over the last month with complaints of being unable to pass urine.

Andrew has a history of hypertension and erectile dysfunction. Andrew is single and has no children. He is currently unemployed, having lost his job three months ago. He has advised that he has been self-catheterising at home.

Andrew is currently prescribed:

- Aspirin 81 mg QD
- Clopidogrel 75 mg QD
- Metoprolol 50 mg BID
- Viagra PRN.

His vital signs on presentation are:

- pulse: 210 beats per minute
- blood pressure: 80/40 mmHg
- temperature: 37.5°C
- oxygen saturation: 94 per cent and have dropped to 92 per cent

- pain score: states 5/10; however, clenched fists and his knees pulled are noted
- his urinalysis revealed positive white blood cells (WBC) and trace of red blood cells (RBC)
- potassium level: 5.8
- blood cultures revealed gram-negative septicaemia.

Question

Using the information above, describe what action you would take as the nurse caring for this patient. Which care would be prioritised? Use the clinical reasoning cycle to guide you through the process and devise a plan of care for your patient.

Answer

- *Step 1: Consider the patient*. What is the current situation? Does the patient need additional respiratory support? What are your concerns with the presentation? Are there any emergency actions that need to be taken?
- *Step 2: Collect cues/information*. Include subjective and objective data here. The subjective will include what the patient tells you, the appearance of the patient, and their past medical history. Objective data will include objective or measurable information such as the vital signs, blood tests etc.
- *Step 3: Process information*. Separate the relevant and irrelevant data — cluster the clues together to formulate an inference about the patient. Initially, Andrew's vital signs are of concern and he needs urgent medical treatment. This is an emergency situation and he needs to be treated for pain, rehydrated and his oxygen saturations improved. He will need to be started on antibiotics and his medications need to be reviewed in light of his presenting symptoms. Longer term, Andrew will need to be provided with support form the psychology team and be given education on infection control regarding his self catherterisation.
- *Step 4: Identify problems/issues.* Nursing problems or diagnosis should be listed here. Nursing issues include pain, anxiety, infection, fluid volume deficit/dehydration, hyperkalemia and knowledge deficit.
- *Step 5: Establish goals.* Goals of care for Andrew include stabilising Andrew and improving BP.
- *Step 6: Take action.* Provide the care that is required to meet the established goals, for example, notify the physician, rapid response of MET call.

  Provide Oxygen 6 L/min via a simple face mask to increase SpO_2 to 95 per cent or greater.

  Receive an order for and pass an indwelling urinary catheter. Commence fluid balance chart.

  Place an IV catheter for fluids and if resuscitation is needed. Place Andrew on a monitor for ongoing assessment. Arrange for admission.

  Orientate Andrew to person, time and place as necessary. Reassure Andrew and his brother.
- *Step 7: Evaluate outcomes.* Were the best outcomes achieved?
- *Step 8: Reflect on the process and new learning.* Reflect on any aspects of care that could have been done better. What went well, what did not go as well as hoped?

SUMMARY

In this chapter, we have reviewed the urinary (or renal) function in maintaining homeostasis in the human body. We have discussed the role of the urinary system's organs, including the kidneys, renal pelvis, ureters, bladder and urethra. We have discussed nursing management of patients with diseases and injuries that affect the urinary system and harm the whole body. This chapter aims to provide the nurses with the information required to provide safe, effective care of patients and promote wellness in our population.

KEY TERMS

antiemetics Medications prescribed to help with nausea and vomiting.

cystoscopy A procedure that lets the healthcare provider view the urinary tract, particularly the bladder, the urethra and the openings to the ureters.

digital rectal examination (DRE) Examines a person's lower rectum, pelvis and lower belly.

detrusor muscle A muscle that forms the wall of the bladder. The main function to contract during urination to push the urine out of the bladder and into the urethra. The detrusor muscle will relax to allow the storage of urine in the urinary bladder.

gland Organ which produces and releases substances that perform a specific function in the body.

haematuria Blood in the urine.

hyperkalaemia High potassium levels in the blood.

intravenous urogram/pyelogram X-ray exam of the urinary tract.

KUB X-ray Examines kidney, ureter and bladder. Used to assess the abdominal area for causes of pain or to assess the organs and structures of the urinary and/or gastrointestinal systems.

ostomy Refers to the surgically created opening in the body for the discharge of body wastes.

peripheral oedema Swelling of the lower legs or hands.

pyelonephritis A urinary tract infection (UTI) that begins in your urethra or bladder and travels to both kidneys. It requires prompt medical attention.

reabsorption The kidney selectively reabsorbs substances it has already secreted into the renal tubules, such as glucose, protein and sodium and returns them to the blood.

secretion Process of segregating, elaborating and releasing some material either functionally specialised such as saliva or isolated for excretion such as urine.

semi-Fowler's position Patient is positioned on their back with the head and trunk raised to between 15 and 45 degrees, although 30 degrees is the most frequently used bed angle.

skin turgor Used to determine the extent of dehydration, or fluid loss, in the body. The measurement is done by pinching up a portion of skin (often on the back of the hand) between two fingers to raise it for a few seconds.

stoma The end of the ureter or small or large bowel that can be seen protruding through the abdominal wall.

vasa deferentia The duct that conveys sperm from the testicle to the urethra.

REFERENCES

American Cancer Society. (2021a) Can kidney cancer be found early? www.cancer.org/cancer/kidney-cancer/detection-diagnosis-staging/detection.html

American Cancer Society. (2021b) Kidney cancer signs and symptoms. www.cancer.org/cancer/kidney-cancer/detection-diagnosis-staging/signs-and-symptoms.html

American Cancer Society. (2021c) Treatments for prostate cancer spread to bones. www.cancer.org/cancer/prostate-cancer/treating/treating-pain.html

Ammirati, A. L. (2020) Chronic kidny disease. *Revista da Associação Médica Brasileira.* doi: https://doi.org/10.1590/1806-9282.66.s1.3

Antipuesto, D. J. (2010) TURP (Transurethral resection of the prostate). https://nursingcrib.com/nursing-notes-reviewer/medical-surgical-nursing/turp-transurethral-resection-of-the-prostate

Australian Commission on Safety and Quality in Health Care. (2019) Acute stroke clinical care standard. www.safetyandquality.gov.au/sites/default/files/2019-12/acute_stroke_clinical_care_standard_-_october_2019.pdf

Australian Government. (2021) Kidney cancer. www.canceraustralia.gov.au/affected-cancer/cancer-types/kidney-cancer/kidney-cancer-australia-statistics

Australian Institute of Health and Welfare. (2020) Chronic kidney disease. www.aihw.gov.au/reports/chronic-kidney-disease/chronic-kidney-disease-compendium/contents/how-many-australians-have-chronic-kidney-disease

Cancer Australia. (2021) Bladder cancer. www.cancer.org.au/cancer-information/types-of-cancer/bladder-cancer

Cancer Australia. (2021b) Prostate cancer. www.cancer.org.au/cancer-information/types-of-cancer/prostate-cancer

Cancer Council NSW. (2020) Kidney cancer. www.cancercouncil.com.au/kidney-cancer

Cancer Council NSW. (n.d.) Staging and prognosis for kidney cancer. www.cancercouncil.com.au/kidney-cancer/diagnosis/staging-prognosis/#Staging

Cancer Council Victoria. (2021) Prostate cancer. www.cancervic.org.au/cancer-information/types-of-cancer/prostate_cancer/treatment_for_prostate_cancer.html

Cancer Net. (2019a) Bladder cancer: Types of treatment. www.cancer.net/cancer-types/bladder-cancer/types-treatment

Cancer Net. (2019b) Kidney cancer: Types of treatment. www.cancer.net/cancer-types/kidney-cancer/types-treatment

Chiba, M. (1985) Pre and postoperative nursing of patients with bladder cancer. Postoperative care of patients having ureterostomy—assistance given at our hospital toward patients' self care. *Kango Gijutsu.* 31(11): 1465–1470. Japanese. PMID: 3851015.

Cleveland Clinic. (2019) Kidney transplant. https://my.clevelandclinic.org/health/treatments/4350-kidney-transplant-procedure/procedure-details

Cleveland Clinic. (2021a) Chronic kidney disease. https://my.clevelandclinic.org/health/diseases/15096-kidney-disease-chronic-kidney-disease

Cleveland Clinic. (2021b) Dialysis. https://my.clevelandclinic.org/health/treatments/14618-dialysis

Department of Health & Human Services, S. G. o. V., Australia. (2020a) Bladder cancer. *Better Health Channel.* www.betterhealth.vic.gov.au/health/ConditionsAndTreatments/bladder-cancer

Department of Health & Human Services, S. G. o. V., Australia. (2020b) Kidney stones. *Better Health Channel.* www.betterhealth.vic.gov.au/health/conditionsandtreatments/kidney-stones

European Association of Urology. (2021) Urolithiasis. https://uroweb.org/guideline/urolithiasis

Fountain, J. H. & Lappin, S.L. (2020) Physiology, renin angiotensin system. *StatPearls [Internet].* Treasure Island (FL): StatPearls Publishing; *2020 Jan.* www.ncbi.nlm.nih.gov/books/NBK470410

Hoffman, M. (2021) Picture of the prostate. *Human Anatomy.* www.webmd.com/men/picture-of-the-prostate#1

Jewell, T. (2018) Kidney overview. *Healthline.* www.healthline.com/health/human-body-maps/kidney

Jiwrajka, M., Yaxley, W., Perera, M., Roberts, M., Dunglison, N., Yaxley, J. & Esler, R. (2018) Benign prostatic hyperplasia. *Australian Journal for General Practitioners.* 47: 471–475. www1.racgp.org.au/ajgp/2018/july/benign-prostatic-hyperplasia

Johns Hopkins Medicine. (2021) Anatomy of the urinary system. www.hopkinsmedicine.org/health/wellness-and-prevention/anatomy-of-the-urinary-system

Kanpp, S. (2020) Urinary system. https://biologydictionary.net/urinary-system

Kidney Health Australia. (2018, December) Fact sheet: Urinary Tract Infections. http://kidney.org.au/uploads/resources/urinary-tract-infections-fact-sheet.pdf

Kidney Health Australia. (2019) National strategic action plan for kidney disease. www.health.gov.au/sites/default/files/documents/2020/03/national-strategic-action-plan-for-kidney-disease_0.pdf

Kidney Health Australia. (2020) Kidney stones. https://kidney.org.au/your-kidneys/what-is-kidney-disease/types-of-kidney-disease/kidney-stones

Kidney Health Australia. (2021) Acute kidney injury. https://kidney.org.au/your-kidneys/what-is-kidney-disease/types-of-kidney-disease/acute-kidney-injury

Lawrentschuk, N. & Perera, M. (2016) 'Benign prostate disorders'. In Feingold, K. R., Anawalt, B., Boyce, A., et al. (eds). *Endotext [Internet].* South Dartmouth (MA): MDText.com, Inc. www.ncbi.nlm.nih.gov/books/NBK279008

Lecturi. (2020, June 9) Kidney Stones (Nephrolithiasis): Classification, Symptoms, and Treatment. https://www.lecturio.com/magazine/nephrolithiasis/#pathophysiology-and-risk-factors

Levett-Jones, T., Hoffman, K., Dempsey, J., Jeong, S., Noble, D., Norton, C., Roche, J. & Hickey, N. (2009) The 'five rights' of clinical reasoning: An educational model to enhance nursing students' ability to identify and manage clinically 'at risk' patients. *Nurse Education Today.* 30: 516. 10.1016/j.nedt.2009.10.020.

LibreTexts. (2020) 24.5E: Micturition and the micturition reflex. https://med.libretexts.org/Bookshelves/Anatomy_and_Physiology/Book%3A_Anatomy_and_Physiology_(Boundless)/24%3A__Urinary_System/24.5%3A__Urine_Transport_Storage_and_Elimination/24.5E%3A Micturition and the Micturition_Reflex

Makris, K. & Spanou, L. (2016) Acute kidney injury: definition, pathophysiology and clinical phenotypes. *The Clinical Biochemist. Reviews.* 37(2): 85–98. www.ncbi.nlm.nih.gov/pmc/articles/PMC5198510

Mayo Clinic. (2021a) Acute kidney injury. www.mayoclinic.org/diseases-conditions/kidney-failure/symptoms-causes/syc-20369048

Mayo Clinic. (2021b) Benign prostatic hyperplasia (BPH). www.mayoclinic.org/diseases-conditions/benign-prostatic-hyperplasia/symptoms-causes/syc-20370087#:~:text=Benign%20prostatic%20hyperplasia%20(BPH)%20%E2%80%94,urinary%20tract%20or%20kidney%20problems

Mayo Clinic. (2021c) Bladder cancer. www.mayoclinic.org/diseases-conditions/bladder-cancer/symptoms-causes/syc-20356104

Mayo Clinic. (2021d) Kidney stones. www.mayoclinic.org/diseases-conditions/kidney-stones/symptoms-causes/syc-20355755

Mayo Clinic. (2021e) Urinary tract infection (UTI). www.mayoclinic.org/diseases-conditions/urinary-tract-infection/symptoms-causes/syc-20353447

McLafferty, E. (2014) The urinary system. *Nursing Standard.* (27). 42–49.

McVary, K. T. (2006) BPH: epidemiology and comorbidities. *American Journal Managed Care.* 12(5 Suppl): S122–128.

Medical News Today. (2021) What is dialysis, and how can it help? www.medicalnewstoday.com/articles/genital-rash

Nair, M. & Peate, I. (2009) *Fundamentals of Applied Pathophysiology.* John Wiley and Sons Ltd.

National Kidney Foundation. (2019a) Kidney stone diet plan and prevention. www.kidney.org/atoz/content/diet
National Kidney Foundation. (2019b) Ureteroscopy. www.kidney.org/atoz/content/kidneystones_ureteroscopy
National Kidney Foundation. (2021) Percutaneous nephrolithotomy/nephrolithotripsy. www.kidney.org/atoz/content/kidneystones PNN
Nursekey. ([illegible]) Continuous bladder irrigation. https://nursekey.com/continuous-bladder-irrigation
O'Hare, A. (2018) Patient-centered care in renal medicine: five strategies to meet the challenge. *American Journal of Kidney Diseases*. (5): 732–736. www.ajkd.org/article/S0272-6386(18)30001-5/fulltext
Physiopedia contributors. (2020) Chronic kidney failure. www.physio-pedia.com/index.php?title=Chronic_Kidney_Disease&oldid=257798
Preminger, G. M. (2020) Urinary calculi. www.msdmanuals.com/en-au/professional/genitourinary-disorders/urinary-calculi/urinary-calculi
Prostate Cancer Foundation of Australia. (2020a) Prostate Cancer Foundation of Australia: About us. https://pcfa.org.au/about-us
Prostate Cancer Foundation of Australia. (2020b) Prostate cancer surgery. www.prostate.org.au/awareness/further-detailed-information/understanding-prostate-cancer-treatments-and-side-effects/understanding-surgery-for-prostate-cancer/prostate-cancer-surgery
RadiologyInfo.org. (2021) Benign Prostatic Hyperplasia (BPH) (Enlargement of the prostate). www.radiologyinfo.org/en/info.cfm?pg=bph
RegisteredNurseRN.com. (2021) Renal calculi (Kidney stones) NCLEX Review. www.registerednursern.com/renal-calculi-kidney-stones-nclex-review
Ricci, Z., Cruz, D. N. & Ronco, C. (2011) Classification and staging of acute kidney injury: beyond the RIFLE and AKIN criteria. *Nature Reviews Nephrology.* 7(4): 201–208. doi:10.1038/nrneph.2011.14
Rodger, J. C., Supramaniam, R., Gibberd, A. J., Smith, D. P., Armstrong, B. K., Dillon, A. & O'Connell, D. L. (2014) Prostate cancer mortality outcomes and patterns of primary treatment for Aboriginal men in New South Wales, Australia. *BJUI International.* 115: 16–23. https://bjui-journals.onlinelibrary.wiley.com/doi/pdf/10.1111/bju.12899
Ruiz-Ortega, M., Rayego-Mateos, S., Lamas, S., Ortiz, A. & Rodrigues-Diez, R. R. (2020) Targeting the progression of chronic kidney disease. *Nature Reviews Nephrology.* 16(5): 269–288. doi: 10.1038/s41581-019-0248-y
Sabih, A. & Leslie, S. W. (2020) Complicated urinary tract infections. www.ncbi.nlm.nih.gov/books/NBK436013
Seer Training Modules. (2021) Components of the urinary system. *Cancer Registration & Surveillance Modules.* https://training.seer.cancer.gov
State Government of Victoria. (2020) Urinary system.Department of Health & Human Services, Australia. www.betterhealth.vic.gov.au/health/ConditionsAndTreatments/urinary-system
Tandukar, S. & Palevsky, P. M. (2019) Continuous renal replacement therapy: who, when, why, and how. *CHEST.* 155(3): 626–638. doi: 10.1016/j.chest.2018.09.004
Taylor, C., Lillis, C. & LeMone, P. (2005) *Fundamentals of Nursing: The Art and Science of Nursing Care.* Philadelphia, PA : Lippincott-Raven.
The Hospitals Contribution Fund of Australia Limited. (2021) Types of kidney stone surgery. www.hcf.com.au/preparing-for-hospital/kidney-stone-surgery/types-of-kidney-stone-surgery
The Regents of the University of California, U. D. o. S. (2021) Vascular access for dialysis. https://surgery.ucsf.edu/conditions--procedures/vascular-access-for-hemodialysis.aspx
Transplant.org.au. (2019) Statistics. https://transplant.org.au/statistics
Urology Care Foundation. (2019) What is benign prostatic hyperplasia (BPH)? American Urology Association. www.urologyhealth.org/urology-a-z/b/benign-prostatic-hyperplasia-(bph)
U.S. Department of Health and Human Services, N. I. o. H., National Cancer Institute. (2021) Understanding prostate changes: a health guide for men. www.cancer.gov/types/prostate/understanding-prostate-changes
Vera, M. (2014) Urolithiasis (renal calculi). *Medical Surgical Nursing.* https://nurseslabs.com/urolithiasis-nursing-management
WebMD. (2021) When do I need surgery for a kidney stone? www.webmd.com/kidney-stones/surgery-for-kidney-stone#1
Webster, A. C., Nagler, E. V., Morton, R. L. & Masson, P. (2017) Chronic kidney disease. *The Lancet.* 389(10075): 1238–1252. https://doi.org/10.1016/S0140-6736(16)32064-5
Woo, M. J., Ha, Y.-S., Lee, J. N., Kim, B. S., Kim, H. T., Kim, T.-H. & Yoo, E. S. (2017) Comparison of surgical outcomes between holmium laser enucleation and transurethral resection of the prostate in patients with detrusor underactivity. *International Neurourology Journal.* 21(1): 46–52. doi: 10.5213/inj.1732640.320
Workeneh, B. T. (2020) Acute kidney injury treatment & management. https://emedicine.medscape.com/article/243492-treatment

ACKNOWLEDGEMENTS

Extract 16.1: © Understanding Kidney Cancer — A guide for people with cancer, their families and friends. © Cancer Council Australia 2020. Reproduced with permission of Cancer Council Victoria.
Figure 16.4: © Tubular Reabsorption. Retrieved from: https://courses.lumenlearning.com/cuny-kbcc-ap2/chapter/tubular-reabsorption-no-content/. Licensed under CCBY 4.0.
Figure 16.5: © Regulating Blood Pressure: The Renin-Angiotensin-Aldosterone System. © Merck and Co., Inc. Reproduced with permission of Merck and Co., Inc. https://www.msdmanuals.com/home/multimedia/figure/cvs_regulating_blood_pressure_renin
Figure 16.6: © Science Photo Library / Alamy Stock Photo

Figure 16.8: © BlueRingMedia / Shutterstock.com
Figure 16.10: © Cruz, D.N., Ricci, Z. & Ronco, C. Clinical review: RIFLE and AKIN – time for reappraisal. *Crit Care* 13, 211 (2009). Reproduced with permission of Springer Nature.
Figure 16.12: © Alila Medical Media / Shutterstock.com
Figure 16.13: © Nathan Lawrentschuk, Benign Prostate Disorders. © 2000–2021, MDText.com, Inc. Reproduced with permission of MDText.com, Inc. https://www.ncbi.nlm.nih.gov/books/NBK279008/.
Figure 16.15: © BlueRingMedia / Shutterstock.com
Figure 16.17: © ilusmedical / Shutterstock.com
Figure 16.18: © Blamb / Shutterstock.com
Figure 16.19: © Drp8 / Shutterstock.com
Figure 16.20: © Kidney Health Australia 2019. National Strategic Action Plan for Kidney Disease. Licensed under CCBY 4.0.
Table 16.2: © Staging and prognosis for kidney cancer. © Cancer Council Australia 2020. Reproduced with permission of Cancer Council Victoria. https://www.cancercouncil.com.au/kidney-cancer/diagnosis/staging-prognosis/#Staging.
Table 16.6: © Kidney cancer. © Cancer Council Australia 2020. Reproduced with permission of Cancer Council Victoria. https://www.cancercouncil.com.au/kidney-cancer.
Table 16.10: © Cancer Council Australia 2020. Reproduced with permission of Cancer Council Victoria. https://www.cancervic.org.au/cancer-information/types-of-cancer/prostate_cancer/treatment_for_prostate_cancer.html.

CHAPTER 17

Nursing care of conditions related to the endocrine system

LEARNING OBJECTIVES

After studying this chapter, you should be able to:

17.1 identify the main components and discuss the function of the endocrine system

17.2 discuss the pathophysiology and management of common disorders of the endocrine system

17.3 discuss the pathophysiology and management of diabetes mellitus

17.4 describe and discuss common nursing assessment and management of patients with endocrine disorders

17.5 apply patient centred care and the clinical reasoning cycle to the care of a patient with an endocrine disorder.

Introduction

The endocrine system is responsible for the regulation of hormones secreted by various glands located throughout the body. The secretion of these hormones plays a vital role in the function of cells and organs that regulate growth, metabolism, reproduction and fluid and electrolyte balance. This chapter will discuss the different parts of the endocrine system and the conditions that can occur when the **endocrine glands** do not function or function inappropriately. The chapter focuses on the most common endocrine conditions that patients experience and is designed to introduce endocrine disorders. It should be supported by further exploration of the current literature.

17.1 Anatomy and physiology of the endocrine system

LEARNING OBJECTIVE 17.1 Identify the main components and discuss the function of the endocrine system.

The endocrine and nervous systems together coordinate the functions of all the body systems. The nervous system controls homeostasis via nerve impulses, while the endocrine system releases messenger molecules, which bring about changes in metabolic activities. The science underlying the structure and function of the endocrine glands and the diagnosis and treatment of disorders of the endocrine system is called endocrinology.

The glands in the body are of two types: **exocrine** and endocrine. Exocrine glands secrete their products directly through ducts into body cavities, into the lumen of an organ or onto the outer surface of the body, as when sebaceous glands in the skin secrete oil onto the skin surface. Endocrine glands secrete hormones into the extracellular space; these then diffuse into the circulatory system and are carried to the target organ, as with gonadotrophs that are produced in the pituitary gland and stimulate the secretion of sex hormones from the testes in males and ovaries in females. Hormones have powerful effects but only affect targeted cells, which may be in multiple organs. For instance, **insulin** produced in the pancreas stimulates the transport of sugar from the blood into the cells and glycogen synthesis in the liver and triglycerides (triacylglycerols) in adipose tissue. Figure 17.1 displays the location of the endocrine organs within the body.

FIGURE 17.1 The location of the endocrine organs

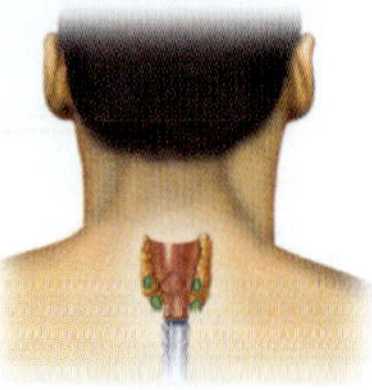

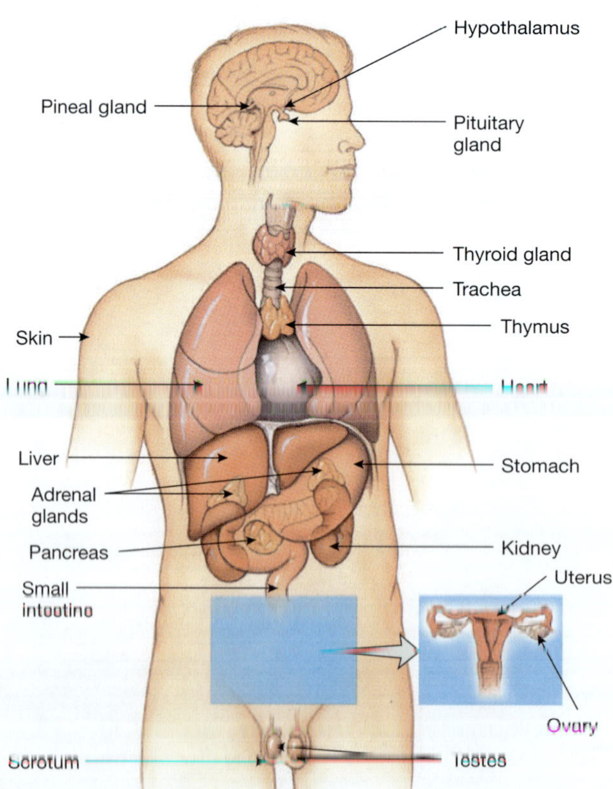

Source: Tortora & Derrickson (2011) *Principles of Anatomy and Physiology*, with kind permission of Wiley Blackwell.

The hypothalamus and pituitary gland

The hypothalamus, situated inferior to the thalamus, is the integrating link between the nervous and endocrine systems and its main role is to maintain homeostasis. It receives inputs from all parts of the brain and sensory signals from all body organs and responds by releasing appropriate hormones to [illegible] the imbalance. Cells in the hypothalamus synthesise nine different hormones, which act on either the anterior or posterior pituitary gland located just beneath it (table 17.1). The function of these hormones is to either inhibit or stimulate the release of hormones from the pituitary gland (figure 17.2).

TABLE 17.1 Function of the hormones released by the hypothalamus

Anterior pituitary	
Releasing hormones	**Inhibiting hormones**
Corticotropin-releasing hormone (CRH)	Somatostatin (inhibits growth hormone release)
Thyrotropin-releasing hormone (TRH)	Dopamine (inhibits prolactin release)
Somatotropin-releasing hormone (GHRH)	
Prolactin-releasing hormone (PRH)	
Gonadotropin-releasing hormone (GnRH)	

FIGURE 17.2 The pituitary and its target organs

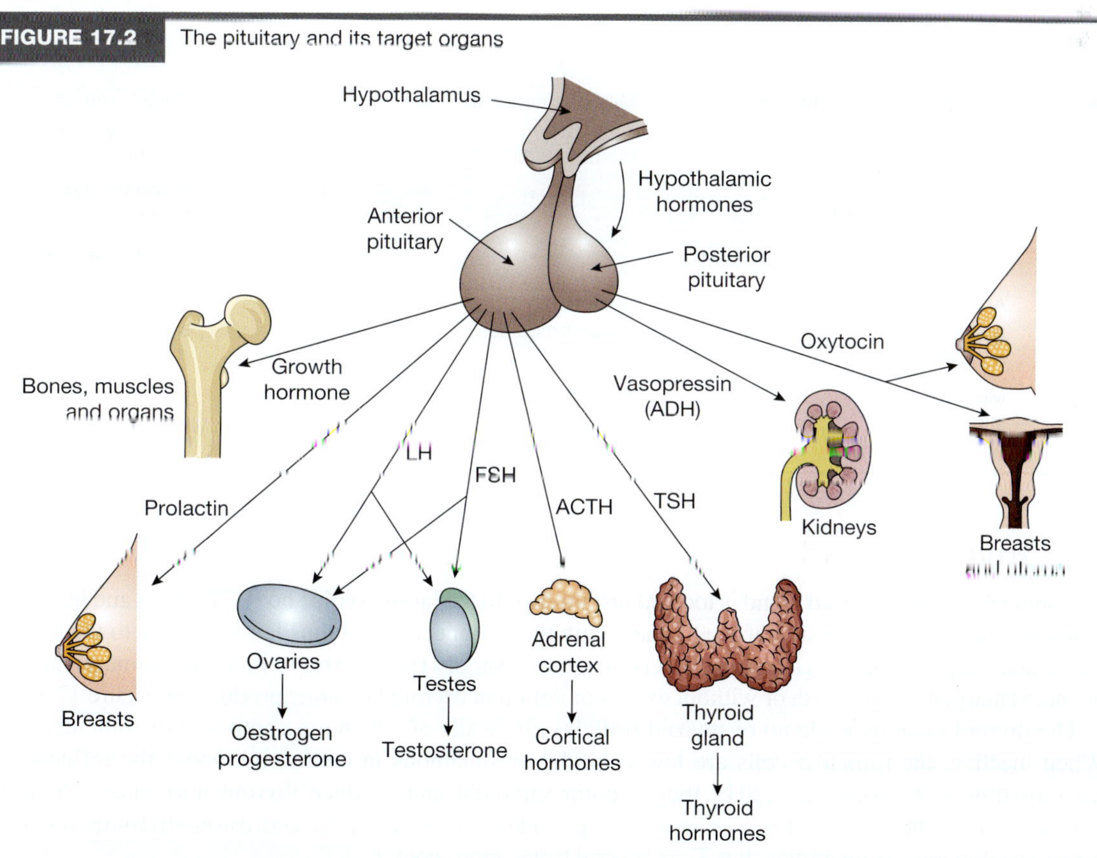

Source: Carmichael in *MSD Manual* (2020).

The posterior lobe of the pituitary does not synthesise hormones; it stores and releases oxytocin and antidiuretic hormone (ADH). During the birth of a baby, oxytocin enhances the contraction of the smooth muscles of the uterus. After delivery, it stimulates milk ejection from the mammary glands in response to the stimulus provided by a sucking infant. ADH regulates fluid volume and increases blood pressure by reducing water loss in the urine and reducing sweating. It is stimulated by plasma osmolality and hypovolemia.

The pituitary gland is pea-shaped and lies in the sella turcica of the sphenoid bone. It is subdivided into anterior and posterior lobes, an intermediate lobe between the two secretes melanocyte-stimulating hormone (MSH) responsible for skin pigmentation. Five principal types of anterior pituitary cell (secretory cells) produce seven major hormones (table 17.2).

TABLE 17.2 Anterior pituitary secretory cells

Secretory cell	Hormone produced	Target gland	Effect	Hyposecretion	Hypersecretion
Somatotrophs	Human growth hormone (HGH)	All body cells	Promote body growth Regulate aspects of metabolism	Dwarfism: • During the growth years • Occurs unless diagnosed early and treated with growth hormone	Gigantism, during the growth years Acromegaly, i.e. thickening of the bones of the face, hands and feet, which occurs during adulthood
Thyrotrophs	Thyroid-stimulating hormone (TSH)	Thyroid gland	Promote activity of the thyroid gland		Graves' disease
Gonadotrophs	Follicle-stimulating hormone (FSH) Luteinising hormone (LH)	Gonads	Growth of the reproductive system	Sterility	
Lactotrophs	Prolactin	Mammary glands	Milk production in suitably prepared mammary glands		Galactorrhoea (inappropriate lactation) Amenorrhoea (females) Impotence (males)
Corticotrophs	Adrenocorticotropic hormone (ACTH)	Adrenal gland	Secretion of glucocorticoids		Cushing's syndrome
	Melanocyte-stimulating hormone (MSH)	Skin	Promote skin pigmentation		

The thyroid gland

The butterfly-shaped thyroid gland is located just inferior to the larynx (voice box). The right and left lateral lobes are situated on either side of the trachea, with their connecting isthmus lying anterior to the trachea. The gland weighs about 30 grams, has a very rich blood supply (80–120 ml of blood per minute), and can become enlarged (goitre) with or without excess or deficient thyroid hormone production (figure 17.3).

The thyroid gland is made up of thyroid follicles, the walls of which are composed of follicular cells. When inactive, the follicular cells are low cuboidal or squamous in nature, but under the influence of thyroid-stimulating hormone (TSH), they become cuboidal and produce thyroid hormones. These are named after the number of atoms of iodine they contain: thyroxine (T_4) and triiodothyronine (T_3). T_4 is produced in greater quantities, but T_3 is several times more potent.

Their production is controlled by negative feedback and the amount of circulating iodine. Hyposecretion during foetal life or infancy results in cretinism, a failure of the body and the brain to grow. Testing of newborns ensures that thyroid dysfunction is diagnosed early and treated with replacement therapy for life. Screening occurs typically 5–7 days after birth through a simple heel prick test, with blood being analysed for both T_4 and TSH.

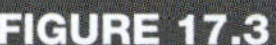

FIGURE 17.3 The position of the thyroid and parathyroid glands

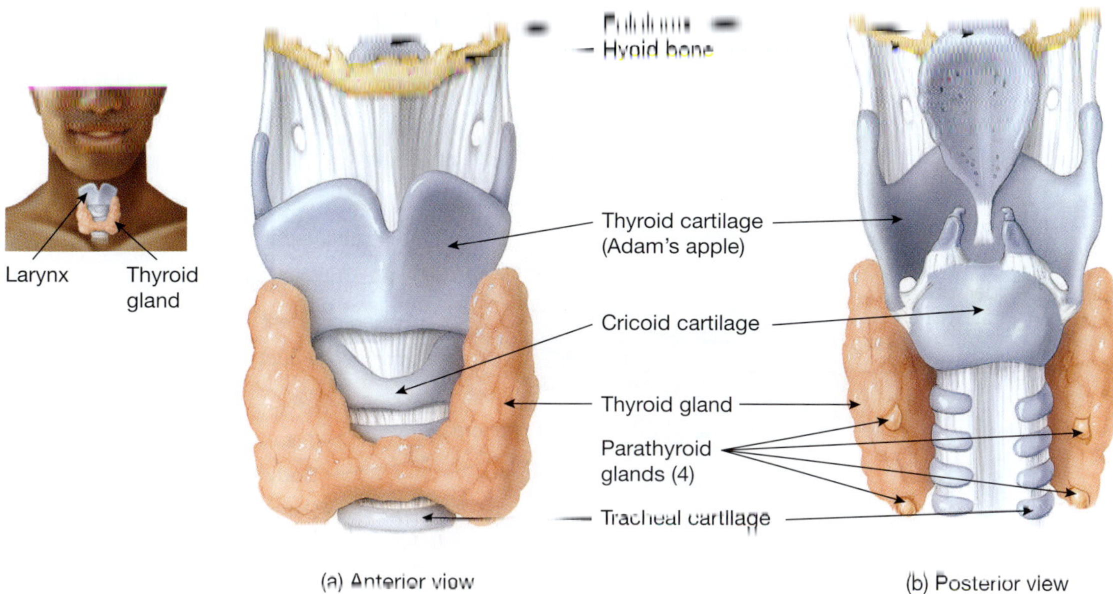

Source: Tortora & Derrickson (2011) *Principles of Anatomy and Physiology*, with kind permission of Wiley Blackwell.

The adrenal glands

There are two adrenal glands, one lying superior to each kidney; the right is triangular in shape, the left semilunar (figure 17.4a). Each gland has two distinct structures: the adrenal cortex and the adrenal medulla (figure 17.4b). The adrenal cortex is subdivided into three zones.

FIGURE 17.4 The position (a) and structure (b) of the adrenal glands

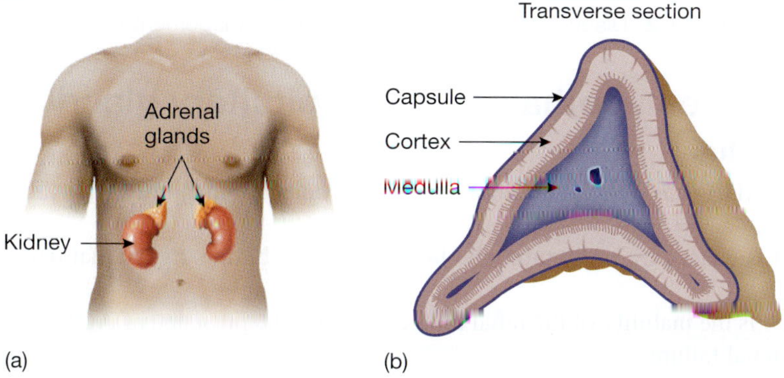

Source: Tortora & Derrickson (2011) *Principles of Anatomy and Physiology*, with kind permission of Wiley Blackwell.

The pancreas

The pancreas is composed of both endocrine and exocrine tissue. Figure 17.5 depicts the location of the pancreas in relation to the liver and gallbladder. These hormones are directly related to the maintenance of blood sugar levels, with hyposecretion or hypersecretion resulting in a group of disorders known as diabetes mellitus.

Scattered around the pancreas are one to two million tiny islets of Langerhans, which consist of four types of hormone-secreting cell:

1. Alpha or A cells secrete glucagon to raise the blood sugar level
2. Beta cells secrete insulin to lower the blood sugar level
3. Delta or D cells secrete somatostatin to slow the absorption of nutrients from the gut and inhibit insulin release
4. F cells secrete pancreatic polypeptide to control the secretion of digestive enzymes and contraction of the gallbladder.

FIGURE 17.5 View of the liver, gallbladder and pancreas

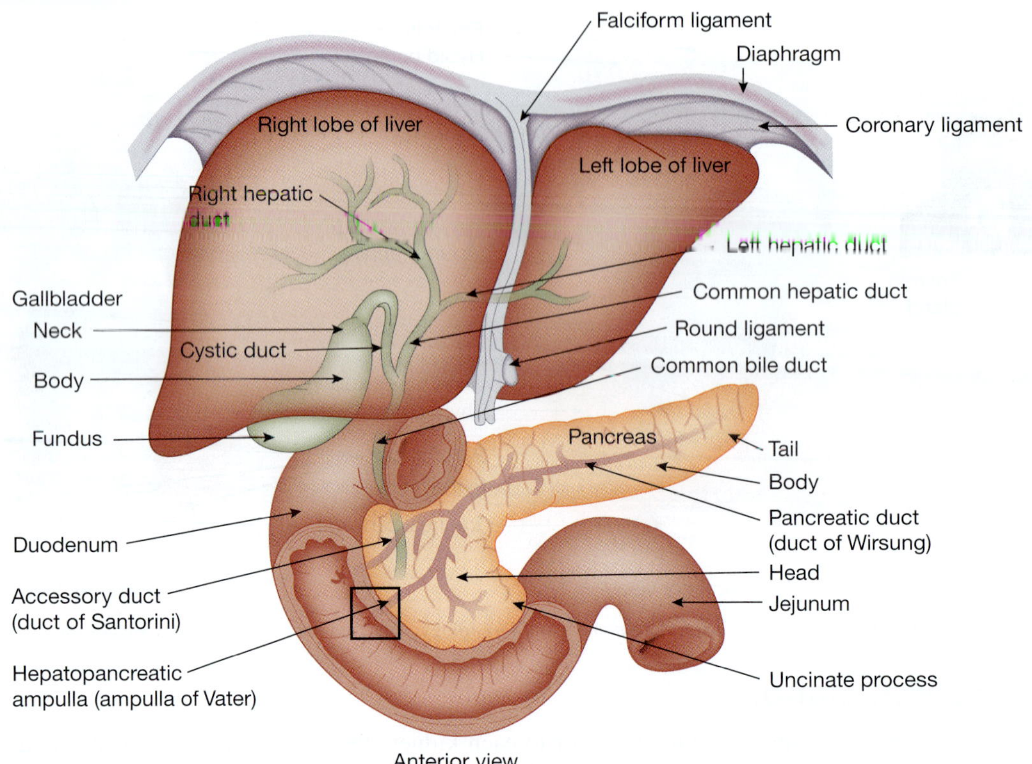

Source: Tortora & Derrickson (2011) *Principles of Anatomy and Physiology*, with kind permission of Wiley Blackwell.

17.2 Common conditions of the endocrine system

LEARNING OBJECTIVE 17.2 Discuss the pathophysiology and management of disorders of the endocrine system.

Disorders of the hypothalamus and pituitary gland

Diabetes insipidus

Hyposecretion of ADH leads to a condition known as diabetes insipidus (DI). There are two main types of DI.

1. Neurogenic DI is caused by brain tumours, head trauma or brain surgery that damages the posterior pituitary gland.
2. Nephrogenic DI is the inability of the renal tubules to sense the presence of ADH and can be hereditary or result from renal failure.

DI results in:

- increased urinary output, to as much as 20 L per day
- increased thirst (polydipsia) and dehydration
- hypernatraemia and hyperosmolality, evidenced by a low specific gravity on urinalysis.

If it has been caused by trauma, symptoms of DI generally appear within three to six days. This condition may be short-lived if the cause (e.g. raised intracranial pressure) is resolved; however, the condition may also be chronic and is then generally treated with a nasal spray such as desmopressin acetate.

Syndrome of inappropriate ADH hypersecretion

The syndrome of inappropriate ADH hypersecretion (SIADH) is a condition in which the pituitary gland produces too much **arginine vasopressin (ADH)**. SIADH causes aldosterone to be suppressed, increasing renal excretion of sodium and leading to the retention of fluid within the cells. Patients present with:

- water retention
- hyponatraemia
- decreased urinary output with concentrated urine

- hypo-osmolality
- neurological manifestations such as headaches or confusion
- generally a normal serum creatinine level, acid–base balance, adrenal function and thyroid function.

Treatment and management of SIADH

SIADH has four main causes: a malignant tumour (e.g. carcinoma of the lung or pancreas), pituitary surgery, head injury or medications (Hong 2014). SIADH is diagnosed by excluding other causes of hyponatraemia, often resulting in a delay of treatment (Hong 2014). Therefore, thorough patient history and physical examination of signs of hypovolaemia (decreased skin turgor, dry mucous membranes, tachycardia) or hypervolaemia (ascites or oedema), urine output and osmolality are essential.

Treatment of SIADH is dependent on the symptoms, the cause and speed of onset of hyponatraemia. Where possible, treating the underlying condition is the first priority. For example, if the cause is due to medication, discontinuing the medication will often resolve hyponatraemia. Further treatment of the hyponatraemia is dependent on whether it is acute or chronic in nature.

- Fluid restriction is considered the first and safest treatment. Fluid restriction is based on urine output plus insensible losses or alternatively is restricted (to 800 to 1200 ml per day) to increase serum sodium levels. This should be continued until the cause of SIADH has been identified and, where possible, eradicated. Patient compliance is often poor due to the length of time that it may take to correct the sodium level (Hong 2014).
- If symptoms are severe, furosemide and intravenous hypertonic (3 per cent) saline can be used to decrease the circulatory volume and prevent sodium excretion.
- Demeclocycline, a tetracycline antibiotic with the side effect of inducing excessive urination and inhibiting vasopressin action, may be beneficial in chronic situations and helps to maintain an adequate fluid balance.
- Vasopressin antagonists may also be prescribed and are the most beneficial medications for patients with SIADH and cardiac failure.
- Monitoring of sodium levels and correction of hyponatraemia must be undertaken with caution in order to prevent cerebral osmotic demyelination.

Disorders of the thyroid

Hyperthyroidism

Hypersecretion of T_3 and T_4 may be referred to as thyrotoxicosis or, more commonly, as hyperthyroidism. Table 17.3 outlines the effects that hypothyroidism and hyperthyroidism have on different systems of the body.

TABLE 17.3 Effects of hypothyroidism and hyperthyroidism on the body

Body system	Hyposecretion of T_3 and T_4	Hypersecretion of T_3 and T_4
Cardiovascular	Reduced cardiac output Bradycardia	Increased cardiac output Tachycardia
Metabolic	Decreased metabolism Weight gain	Increased metabolism Weight loss
Neuromuscular	Weakness Sluggish reflexes	Tremor Hyperactive reflexes
Mental/emotional	Sluggish mental processes Apathetic personality	Restlessness Irritability and emotional instability
Gastrointestinal	Constipation	Diarrhoea
General	Cold, dry skin	Warm, moist skin

The thyroid gland can produce too much T_3 and T_4; several conditions may cause this, such as:

- Graves' disease
- toxic multinodular goitre
- thyroid neoplasm.

Graves' disease

Graves' disease occurs between 20 and 40 years of age and is seven times more likely to present in women than in men. This condition may result from an autoimmune process and is characterised by a triad of thyrotoxicosis, exophthalmos (protruding eyeballs; see figure 17.6) and infiltrative dermopathy (thick, scaly skin lesions, which may appear like an orange-peel texture).

FIGURE 17.6 Exophthalmos

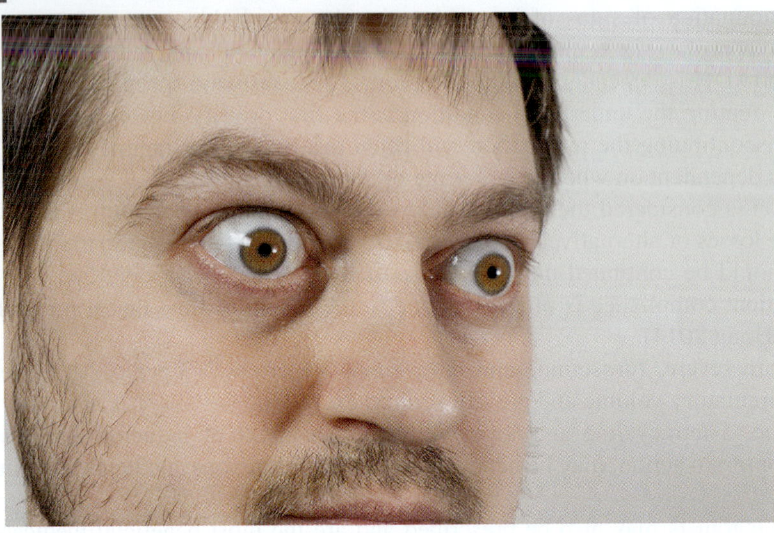

The symptoms are those listed for hyperthyroidism in table 17.3, including the distinctive triad described above. The diagnosis is normally established by a thyroid function test, with results demonstrating elevated T_3 and T_4 levels and low levels of TSH.

Toxic multinodular goitre

This form of hyperthyroidism is caused by a tumour and is characterised by several small nodules that are discrete and function independently. These nodules secrete excessive amounts of thyroid hormones, resulting in symptoms associated with hyperthyroidism. The aetiology is not fully understood; however, genetic mutation of the follicle cells has been suggested as one possible cause. This condition is not associated with the eye or skin pathology as seen in Graves' disease.

Thyroid neoplasm

Thyroid neoplasms, such as follicular adenomas, may cause hypersecretion from the thyroid gland. Thyroid neoplasms take on a wide variety of morphological patterns, although follicular adenoma tends to present as a benign encapsulated mass of follicles. The most common malignant neoplasm found within the thyroid gland is papillary carcinoma. This slow-growing neoplasm is typically found in countries where the dietary intake of iodine is either sufficient or excessive. The prognosis following treatment for papillary carcinoma is very good.

Thyroid crisis

Thyroid crisis (or thyroid storm) occurs as the result of a rapid increase in metabolic rate resulting in excessive thyroid hormone production; it is a medical emergency and is considered life-threatening. Thyroid crisis is associated with undiagnosed hyperthyroidism but is rare due to effective diagnosis and treatment. Signs and symptoms include:

- hyperthermia (39–41°C)
- tachycardia
- hypertension
- abdominal pain
- gastrointestinal disturbances
- restlessness
- agitation
- seizures.

Patients must be treated urgently as any delay may result in increased mortality. Treatment for thyroid crisis comprises fluid replacement, management of electrolyte imbalance, cooling, avoidance of aspirin (it may increase free thyroid hormone levels), stabilisation of cardiovascular function and reduction of the synthesis and production of thyroid hormones

Treatment and management of hyperthyroidism

Hyperthyroidism is confirmed by the presence of elevated levels of T_3 and T_4. Patients suspected of having thyroid nodules or neoplasms may undergo a thyroid scan or magnetic resonance imaging scan for a full evaluation. There are three main treatment options (figure 17.7). A number of potential complications are associated with thyroid surgery (table 17.4).

FIGURE 17.7 Treatment and management for hyperthyroidism

Medication

- Anti-thyroid medications, e.g. carbimazole or methimazole
- Reduces the synthesis of new T_3 and T_4
- Symptoms may take a number of weeks to reduce due to existing stores of thyroid hormone within the gland

Radioactive iodine therapy

- Radioactive iodine (^{131}I) is given
- The thyroid absorbs the radioactive iodine
- This destroys thyroid tissue, resulting in the production of lower levels of thyroid hormones
- It is administered orally
- This is an outpatient procedure
- The treatment effect may take as long as 6–8 weeks
- It is not suitable for pregnant women as radioactive iodine crosses the placenta, affecting the development of the foetal thyroid gland
- It is not always possible to control how much of the thyroid gland is destroyed, so patients may go on to develop hypothyroidism as a result of treatment

Surgery

One of six procedures may be undertaken.

- Partial thyroid lobectomy — removal of the upper or lower portion of one lobe
- Thyroid lobectomy — removal of one entire lobe
- Thyroid lobectomy with isthmusectomy — removal of one lobe and the isthmus
- Subtotal thyroidectomy — removal of one lobe, the isthmus and most of the other lobe
- Total thyroidectomy — removal of the entire gland
- Radical total thyroidectomy — removal of the entire gland and cervical lymphatic nodes

TABLE 17.4 Complications and nursing care of patients after thyroid surgery

Complications	Nursing interventions
Haemorrhage	The thyroid gland is situated within an abundant supply of blood vessels Surgical intervention for haemorrhage occurs in approximately 0.1–1.5% of patients Normal post-operative observations are required Monitor for signs of haemorrhage in the post-operative period Haemorrhage is likely to occur between 6 and 12 hours post-surgery Assess anterior and posterior dressings as this is where blood tends to accumulate If there is evidence of haemorrhage, surgical intervention should be sought immediately
Respiratory distress	Occurs as a result of: • haemorrhage • oedema, causing compression of the trachea • laryngeal spasms due to hormone imbalance Assess: • respiratory rate, depth and rhythm • patient's colour • oxygen saturation level Any signs of distress should be acted upon immediately

(continued)

TABLE 17.4	(continued)
Complications	**Nursing interventions**
Laryngeal nerve injury	Is due to: • incision clamping • stretching of the nerve • local compression due to oedema, haematoma or electrocoagulation during surgery Assess quality of voice and the swallow reflex, and report any concerns to the medical team Some weakness of the vocal cords may occur, but these should resolve within 6 weeks
Tetany	The parathyroid gland is located in close proximity to the thyroid There is a risk of injury or accidental removal of the parathyroid gland This results in calcium deficiency after surgery, with signs and symptoms of: • tingling of the toes, fingers and lips • muscular twitches • positive Chvostek's and Trousseau's signs. Calcium gluconate should always be available locally and administered immediately intravenously, if necessary
Wound infection	There is potential for wound infection The most likely causative organisms are staphylococcal or streptococcal bacteria Wound infection is rare after thyroid surgery (0.3–0.8%) Monitor: • temperature • wound site for signs of infection, such as the presence of an odorous discharge

Hypothyroidism

Hypothyroidism affects one per cent of the adult population and is six times more common in women than men (one in 50 women and one in 300 men). Hypothyroidism may be classified as primary or secondary (table 17.5). Primary hypothyroidism accounts for up to 95 per cent of cases in adults.

TABLE 17.5 Causes of primary and secondary hypothyroidism

Primary hypothyroidism	Secondary hypothyroidism
Autoimmune destruction of the thyroid gland	Pituitary failure
Other autoimmune conditions, e.g.: • type 1 diabetes • Addison's disease • pernicious anaemia	Hypothalamic failure After pituitary surgery
Following treatment for hyperthyroidism Congenital hypothyroidism — the absence of a thyroid gland after birth, which occurs at a rate of approximately one in 3000 live births Iodine deficiency	

The thyroid gland produces insufficient quantities of T_4 in hypothyroidism; low levels of T_4 are also associated with high levels of TSH. The onset of the symptoms is generally slow, and often tiredness and lethargy are mistaken for the effects of normal ageing, resulting in a prolonged period before seeking medical assistance. The patient may present with:

- myxoedema (non-pitting oedema) affecting the hands, feet and eyelids, with facial swelling and puffiness
- an inability to think quickly
- constant tiredness
- weight gain
- sensitivity to the cold
- constipation, which may give rise to faecal impaction

- coarse, brittle hair
- a decreased glomerular filtration rate
- anovulatory cycles or severe menorrhagia.

Treatment and management of hypothyroidism

Diagnosis of hypothyroidism is through a thyroid function test. A low plasma level of T_4 confirms hypothyroidism (<5 pmol/L) and a raised TSH level (>20 mU/L). The measurement of T_3 as a diagnostic tool for hypothyroidism is not recommended as it is considered unreliable and may lead to a missed diagnosis

Treatment is through oral replacement therapy of thyroid hormones. Low-dose T_4 (25–50 µg daily) is initially commenced, gradually increasing in increments of 25–50 µg on a monthly basis until the serum TSH level is normal. Patients education on the management of hypothyroidism must be on:

- their condition
- the reason why replacement therapy must be life-long
- the need to take the medication in the morning, as a single dose on an empty stomach
- the importance of not missing a dose
- the fact that symptomatic relief is achieved in about 2–4 weeks
- that it may take six weeks before normal TSH levels are achieved
- the potential for overreplacement
- the signs of hyperthyroidism, including anxiety, restlessness, palpitations and diarrhoea.

Failure to ensure patients' adequate understanding may result in poor adherence to medication or increased anxiety levels.

Nurses should be aware that T_4 interacts with several other medications, such as anticoagulants, oral hypoglycaemic agents and insulin, with a possible need to adjust the medications in these situations. In addition, approximately 40 per cent of patients with angina are unable to tolerate full T_4 replacement therapy even with the addition of beta-blockers or vasodilators. Such patients may need to be referred for coronary angioplasty or coronary bypass grafting before tolerating full T_4 replacement. Patients taking T_4 replacement therapy are reviewed annually in order to assess the effectiveness of their treatment and provide them with the opportunity to express any concerns they may have.

Disorders of the adrenal gland

Cushing's syndrome

Cushing's syndrome is a chronic disorder characterised by excessive production of cortical hormones. It is more common in women than men and is usually diagnosed between 30 and 50 years, although it can occur at any age. Cushing's syndrome has a number of causes (figure 17.8). Signs and symptoms include:

- rapid weight gain, particularly of the trunk and face
- hirsutism (facial hair growth), especially in women
- an irregular or absent menstrual cycle
- fat pads along the collar bone
- hyperhidrosis (excessive sweating)
- thinning of the skin
- mood swings, irritability, anxiety, depression
- the appearance of purple lines over the abdomen, thighs or buttocks (as a result of weakening and rupture of the deeper layers of skin).

FIGURE 17.8 Causes of Cushing's syndrome

- Iatrogenic (the most common) — from long-term use of pharmacological glucocorticoid preparations. Glucocorticoids are commonly used in inflammatory conditions such as asthma, rheumatoid arthritis and lupus erythematosus
- Pituitary adenoma — hypersecretion of adrenocorticotropic hormone occurs, referred to as Cushing's disease
- Ectopic tumours — adrenocorticotropic hormone (ACTH)-secreting tumours, e.g. small cell lung cancer
- Adrenal causes:
  - Excessive production of cortisol
  - Benign or malignant tumour

Treatment and management of Cushing's syndrome

The treatment for Cushing's syndrome is dependent on the cause. In the case of a tumour, the treatment will usually require surgery to remove the adrenal gland. Usually, only one adrenal gland is removed; however, in the presence of an adrenocorticotropic hormone-producing tumour, bilateral adrenalectomy may be performed. Follow up care may include radiation therapy or chemotherapy. In these cases, there is often a need for ongoing hormone replacement therapy.

Specific aspects of nursing care that need to be considered for patients undergoing an adrenalectomy are outlined in figure 17.9.

FIGURE 17.9 Specific preoperative and post-operative care following an adrenalectomy

Preoperative care
- Dietary consultation — stress the importance of a diet high in vitamins and proteins, which are necessary for tissue repair and wound healing
- If hypokalaemia exists, include foods high in potassium
- Glucocorticoid excess increases catabolism
- Ensure medical and surgical asepsis when providing care and treatments (as cortisol excess increases the risk of infection)
- Monitor electrolyte and glucose levels — any imbalances should be corrected before surgery
- Educate patients on:
  - coughing techniques
  - deep-breathing exercises
  - changing positions in bed.
  - These activities are particularly important for patients at risk of infection

Post-operative care
- Results in adrenal insufficiency
- Addison's crisis and hypovolaemic shock may occur
- Cortisol is given on the day of surgery and in the post-operative period to replace inadequate hormone levels
- Assess:
  - body temperature
  - white blood cell levels
  - wound drainage
  - use **aseptic technique** as impaired wound healing increases the risk of infection.

Where the cause is induced iatrogenic Cushing's syndrome, the reduction or ceasing of medication will resolve the symptoms. The reduction of glucocorticoid medication should only be under the doctor's care as the sudden withdrawal of medication may cause adrenal suppression leading to a life-threatening Addisonian crisis (State Government of Victoria Department of Health & Human Services 2020).

Addison's disease

Addison's disease (primary adrenal insufficiency) is a chronic endocrine disorder resulting from complete destruction or dysfunction of the adrenal cortex. The adrenal cortex no longer produces aldosterone, glucocorticoids or adrenal androgens. The condition affects around 2500 Australians and is generally found in adults under 60 years of age (Hormones Australia 2019). Causes include:
- autoimmune processes
- adrenal haemorrhage
- bacterial or fungal infections, e.g. tuberculosis
- removal of both adrenal glands
- cancers or tumours affecting both adrenals.

The onset of the disease is slow, symptoms often remaining absent until 90 per cent of cortical function has been lost. Symptoms include:
- lethargy
- muscle weakness
- weight loss
- hypotension
- hypoglycaemia
- hyponatraemia

- hyperkalaemia
- hyperpigmentation, which is most obvious on exposed areas of skin.

Treatment and management of adrenal insufficiency

Treatment of adrenal insufficiency will vary from person to person and is dependent on whether it is primary or secondary insufficiency and the hormones involved. Treatment will usually require the use of long-term medications (see table 17.6).

TABLE 17.6 Medications used in the treatment and management of adrenal insufficiency

Medication class and name	Dosage	Indication	Action	Precautions
Glucocorticoid replacement therapy — hydrocortisone	15–25 mg daily	Primary and secondary adrenal insufficiency	Replacement of cortisol	Should not be ceased abruptly Needs to be adjusted during illness, surgery, trauma and stress
Cortisone acetate	20–30 mg daily			
Prednisolone	3–6 mg daily			More side effects than other medications
Mineralocorticoid replacement therapy — fludrocortisone	0/05–0.3 mg daily	For primary adrenal insufficiency where aldosterone levels are low		

Source: Information from Hormones Australia (2019).

During times of illness, surgery, trauma or stress, cortisol levels rise; however, in people with adrenal insufficiency, this does not happen, so glucocorticoid therapy is increased to avoid an adrenal crisis (Hormones Australia 2019). A sick day management plan (figure 17.10) allows patients to self-manage their medication when they are unwell. Many people also carry injectable hydrocortisone for emergencies.

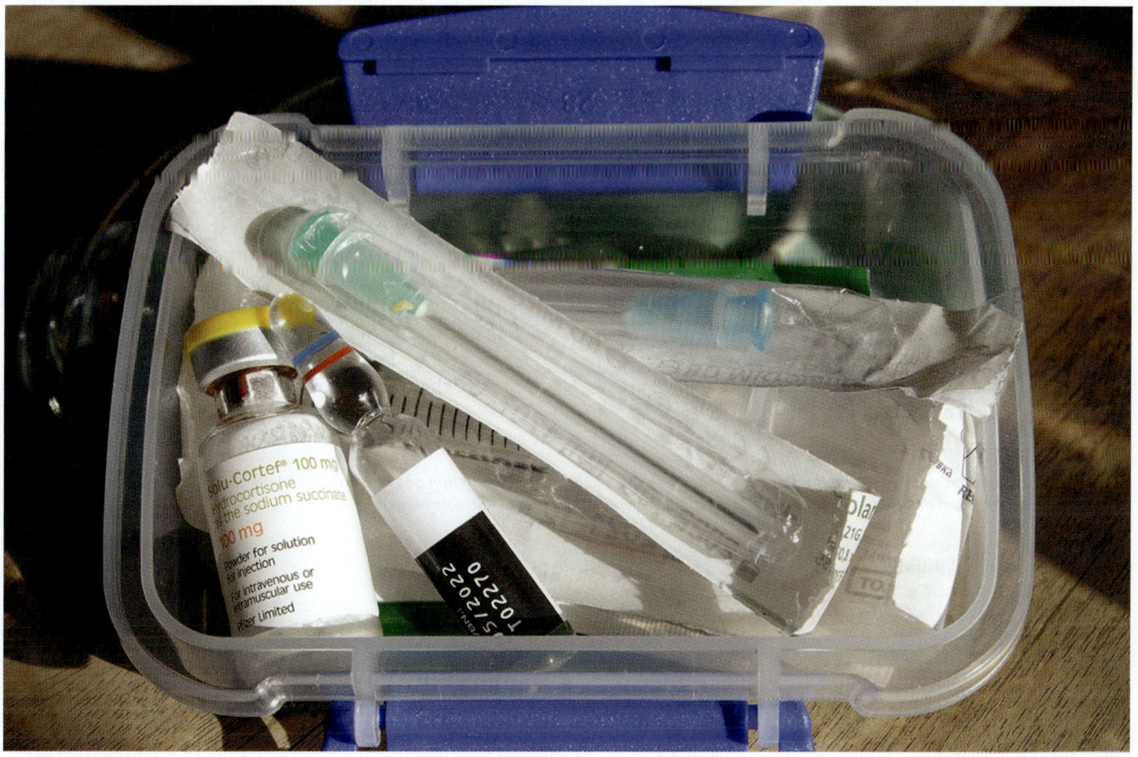

FIGURE 17.10 Sick day management plan

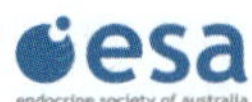

Adrenal Insufficiency Advice for Patients & Doctors

Sick Day Management for Patients on Glucocorticoid Therapy

ESA recommends two (2) copies of this form be provided to the patient: one for them to keep and the other to give to their partner/next of kin. A copy should also be sent to the patient's GP.

Name...**DOB**....................................

Diagnosis...

Contact details of usual public hospital OR private endocrinologist

....

....has a form of **adrenal insufficiency.**

Replacement medications will keep them well, but at times of **illness or other stress to the body**, they are at risk of **adrenal crisis**. Unless additional glucocorticoids are given at these times, they could become very unwell. This is a simple guide about what to do in such situations. If there is any doubt or concern about their health, their endocrinologist or their usual hospital's Endocrinology Department should be contacted for further specific advice.

	Usual Dose		
	AM	Mid	PM
Tablet Name:	mg	mg	mg

Issue	Examples	Temperature	Dose Change[1]	Adjusted Dose		
				AM	**Mid**	**PM**
Trivial illness or emotional stress	Mild cold, Exam stress, Bereavement	No temperature, able to complete usual daily activities and physically well	Usually **NO** change (advice may be varied at the discretion of the endocrinologist)	mg	mg	mg
Mildly unwell	A fever, Urine infection	37.5 – 38.5° C	2 x normal dose for at least 2 days	mg	mg	mg
More unwell	High fever, Diarrhoea	Above 38.5° C	3 x normal dose for at least 3 days	mg	mg	mg
Vomiting or persistent diarrhoea		Normal or raised	***Hydrocortisone Injection*** is required either by self-injection (e.g. 100 mg Solu-Cortef Act-o-Vial™)[2], a GP or an Emergency Department as soon as possible. After receiving the injection, the person should then proceed to the nearest Emergency Department for further treatment. If unable to access this treatment, call 000 and request an urgent ambulance.			

[1] If the person is still unwell despite following the suggested dose changes, they should seek immediate medical attention.

[2] Ensure the self-injected Solu-Cortef Acto-o-Vial has not expired.

Acknowledgement: Modified from material initially developed by Julie Hetherington and Prof Kate Steinbeck (Royal Prince Alfred Hospital), and material from Prof David Torpy and Carmen Bischoff (Royal Adelaide Hospital).

Source: Hormones Australia (2018)

Addison's crisis

This is a life-threatening condition that results from acute destruction of the adrenal cortex (by surgery or trauma) or an abrupt withdrawal of long-term corticosteroid therapy. The condition may manifest with:

- any of the symptoms of Addison's disease
- severe vomiting, dehydration and diarrhoea leading to circulatory collapse

- abdominal pain
- high fever
- hypotension
- tachycardia.

Treatment and management of Addison's crisis

This is a medical emergency and treatment must commence immediately, requiring skilful management of fluid replacement in conjunction with the administration of glucocorticoids until an appropriate fluid balance has been restored and the symptoms have been negated.

17.3 Diabetes mellitus

LEARNING OBJECTIVE 17.3 Discuss the pathophysiology and management of diabetes mellitus.

Diabetes mellitus (DM) refers to the group of disorders that have one common sign — an elevation in blood glucose level (hyperglycaemia) caused by deficient production of insulin and/or resistance to its action. It is estimated that 1.2 million Australians (approximately 5 per cent of the population) had diabetes in 2017–18 (Australian Institute of Health and Welfare [AIHW] 2020), increasing in prevalence for both males and females from 2014 to 2015. Diabetes is a chronic condition that places a significant burden on the individual and the healthcare system; it is the 10th leading cause of death in Australia. Socioeconomic advantage plays a significant role in the prevalence, with diabetes being twice as high in the lowest socioeconomic areas. Indigenous Australians are almost three times more likely to have diabetes than non-Indigenous Australians (12.6 per cent compared to 4.3 per cent) (AIHW 2020).

As hyperglycaemia increases:

- glucose spills out into the urine (glucosuria), causing
- osmotic diuresis (not correctable in the loop of Henle), which leads to
- excessive urine production (polyuria) and
- excessive thirst (polydipsia).

There are four clinical classes of diabetes (see figure 17.11). The most common form of diabetes is type 2, which is normally associated with diagnosis above the age of 40 years. Type 1 diabetes accounts for approximately 10 per cent of diagnosed diabetes and is normally associated with individuals diagnosed below the age of 30 years (National Institute for Health and Clinical Excellence [NICE] 2009). Although type 1 and type 2 diabetes are both associated with a relative or absolute lack of insulin, the two conditions have very different disease patterns and are therefore managed differently.

FIGURE 17.11 Clinical classes of diabetes

- *Type 1 diabetes.* Results from β-cell destruction due to an autoimmune process usually leading to insulin deficiency.
- *Type 2 diabetes.* Results from a progressive insulin secretory defect on the background of insulin resistance.
- *Gestational diabetes mellitus (GDM).* Defined as glucose intolerance with onset or first recognition during pregnancy.
- *Other specific types of diabetes (impaired fasting glucose or impaired glucose tolerance).* Due to other causes such as genetic defects in beta-cell function, genetic defects in insulin action, diseases of the exocrine pancreas (e.g. cystic fibrosis), and drug-induced or chemical-induced causes (e.g. treatment of human immunodeficiency virus/acquired immune deficiency syndrome [HIV/AIDS] or after organ transplantation).

Type 1 diabetes

Type 1 diabetes is an autoimmune disorder resulting from T cell-mediated destruction of the beta-cells in over 90 per cent of cases. The remaining 10 per cent of cases are referred to as idiopathic diabetes, often classified as type 1B diabetes mellitus. The exact aetiology of this autoimmune process is not completely understood, with environmental, toxic, nutritional, viral and infective factors all being implicated. Genetic susceptibility to type 1 diabetes is associated in particular with human leucocyte antigen genes.

Beta-cell destruction leads to a near-total insulin deficiency, resulting in the development of hyperglycaemia. In the absence of insulin, the body is unable to utilise the glucose present within the bloodstream prompting the following.

- The liver releases further stores of glucose to maintain normal cell function and homeostasis.
- This results in a further increase in hyperglycaemia.
- To sustain energy levels and maintain normal function, the body utilises both muscle and fat stores.
- This results in lethargy and weight loss.
- High levels of circulating glucose lead to osmotic diuresis.
- This, in turn, leads to polyuria, polydipsia, dehydration, severe electrolyte imbalance and coma (if untreated).
- Increased circulating levels of fatty acids lead to hyperlipidaemia (a risk factor for atherosclerosis).
- Fat metabolism results in the production of ketones, an acidic by-product, which are toxic to the body at high levels.
- If left untreated, this leads to diabetic ketoacidosis (DKA), a life-threatening condition that is the leading cause of mortality and morbidity in children and young people with type 1 diabetes. Approximately 25 per cent of children and young people with new-onset diabetes present in DKA (NICE 2009).

Type 2 diabetes

Type 2 diabetes develops as a consequence of insulin resistance, reduced insulin production and utilisation, and has been associated with poor lifestyle choices and obesity. Type 2 diabetes tends not to be associated with autoimmunity; however, recent evidence suggests that type 2 diabetes in the young may result from both insulin resistance and autoimmunity.

Type 2 diabetes develops over years and progresses from normal glucose tolerance to abnormal glucose tolerance (postprandial blood glucose levels increasing first) and eventual fasting hyperglycaemia. The aim of treatment is to control:

- hyperglycaemia, thought to be the determinant of microvascular complications, such as renal and retinal complications
- hyperlipidaemia, related to insulin resistance, which results in raised low-density lipoprotein (LDL) cholesterol, reduced high-density lipoprotein (HDL) cholesterol, and raised levels of triglycerides and fibrinogen (a thrombotic agent)
- hypertension, more common in people with diabetes and varies between different ethnic, racial and social groups.

The care of patients with type 2 diabetes has been shaped by findings from the UK Prospective Diabetes Study (UK Prospective Diabetes Study Group 1998). This landmark 20-year study remains important today. The study of 5102 people newly diagnosed with type 2 diabetes showed that the complications of type 2 diabetes, previously regarded as inevitable, could be reduced by improving blood glucose and/or blood pressure control. As all people with type 2 diabetes are at high risk of cardiovascular events, the control of cholesterol attains equal importance. Table 17.7 presents the differing nature of type 1 and type 2 diabetes mellitus.

TABLE 17.7 Characteristics of type 1 and type 2 diabetes mellitus

Characteristic	Type 1	Type 2
Risk factors	Genetic + Exposure to environmental factors + Exposure to trigger factors	Poor diet Overweight Sedentary lifestyle Genetics ≥40 years of age High-risk ethnic group Previous altered blood glucose metabolism, e.g. gestational diabetes Certain medications
Nature of the illness	An autoimmune condition — beta-cells are destroyed, resulting in an absolute deficiency of insulin	Both insulin inefficiency and insulin deficiency must be present, i.e.: • Inadequate beta-cell insulin production • Peripheral body cells resisting insulin

Symptoms — some overlapping	Fast onset of: • extremely high blood sugar levels • weight loss • hunger • fatigue • thirst • frequent urination	Medium to long onset of: • dry mouth • thirst • nocturia • fatigue, especially after a meal • recurrent, difficult to treat infections The patient may have no symptoms The condition is diagnosed on presentation: • In a routine health check • With symptoms of a complication of diabetes
Onset	Quick onset — within a few weeks or months	Slow onset over years
Treatment	Daily self-management of insulin — balancing the effects of food intake and/or exercise on blood sugar levels Multiple injections of insulin or infusion through an insulin pump	Daily self-management of food in take Exercise Medication to enhance insulin usage or/and insulin production May need to use insulin injections
Age of onset	Early childhood or teenage years Can occur at any age	Adults, but can occur at any age
Complications	Short-term complications give rise to acute emergencies such as: • DKA • hypoglycaemia (as a side effect of medical management) Long-term exposure to low blood sugar levels can cause hypoglycaemic unawareness Long-term exposure to high blood sugar levels causes micro- and macrovascular changes	May have following complications at diagnosis from damage to the large and small blood vessels, resulting in: • retinopathy/blindness • cardiac disease • kidney disease • amputation • gastroparesis • earlier mortality
Preventable	No	Yes, by as much as 58%, by: • a healthy diet • keeping the weight under control
Reversible	No	No But easily managed by losing excessive weight and with a healthy diet

Diabetes risk assessment

It is recommended that all people be screened for diabetes risk from age 40 using the **AUSDRISK** (Australian Type 2 Risk Assessment Tool [figure 17.12]) (RACGP 2016; Colagiuri et al. 2009a). Due to the increased prevalence of diabetes in the Indigenous Australian population, it is recommended that this group be screened from 18 years of age. A risk score of ≥12 indicates the need for further laboratory testing.

In asymptomatic patients, a positive laboratory result is confirmed with a repeated result within a day or two before a diagnosis of diabetes. Those patients with elevated glucose not high enough to diagnose type 2 diabetes are considered to have either impaired fasting glucose (IFG) or impaired glucose tolerance (IGT), which indicates a future risk of diabetes development.

Diagnosis of diabetes

Diagnosis of diabetes is by means of biochemical analysis considering the presence or absence of symptoms and presenting the patient's risk factors. The diagnostic criteria for type 2 diabetes are outlined in the figure 17.13. In symptomatic patients with hyperglycaemia or a single elevated laboratory test value, this is considered definitive of diabetes. Where a patient presents asymptomatic, a second laboratory result is required for confirmation.

FIGURE 17.12 AUSDRISK Assessment Tool

The Australian Type 2 Diabetes Risk Assessment Tool (AUSDRISK)

1. Your age group

Under 35 years	☐	0 points
35 – 44 years	☐	2 points
45 – 54 years	☐	4 points
55 – 64 years	☐	6 points
65 years or over	☐	8 points

2. Your gender

Female	☐	0 points
Male	☐	3 points

3. Your ethnicity/country of birth:

3a. Are you of Aboriginal, Torres Strait Islander, Pacific Islander or Maori descent?

No	☐	0 points
Yes	☐	2 points

3b. Where were you born?

Australia	☐	0 points
Asia (including the Indian sub-continent), Middle East, North Africa, Southern Europe	☐	2 points
Other	☐	0 points

4. Have either of your parents, or any of your brothers or sisters been diagnosed with diabetes (type 1 or type 2)?

No	☐	0 points
Yes	☐	3 points

5. Have you ever been found to have high blood glucose (sugar) (for example, in a health examination, during an illness, during pregnancy)?

No	☐	0 points
Yes	☐	6 points

6. Are you currently taking medication for high blood pressure?

No	☐	0 points
Yes	☐	2 points

7. Do you currently smoke cigarettes or any other tobacco products on a daily basis?

No	☐	0 points
Yes	☐	2 points

If you scored 6-11 points in the AUSDRISK you may be at increased risk of type 2 diabetes. Discuss your score and your individual risk with your doctor. Improving your lifestyle may help reduce your risk of developing type 2 diabetes.

8. How often do you eat vegetables or fruit?

Every day	☐	0 points
Not every day	☐	1 point

9. On average, would you say you do at least 2.5 hours of physical activity per week (for example, 30 minutes a day on 5 or more days a week)?

Yes	☐	0 points
No	☐	2 points

10. Your waist measurement taken below the ribs (usually at the level of the navel, and while standing)

Waist measurement (cm) ☐

For those of Asian or Aboriginal or Torres Strait Islander descent:

Men	Women		
Less than 90 cm	Less than 80 cm	☐	0 points
90 – 100 cm	80 – 90 cm	☐	4 points
More than 100 cm	More than 90 cm	☐	7 points

For all others:

Men	Women		
Less than 102 cm	Less than 88 cm	☐	0 points
102 – 110 cm	88 – 100 cm	☐	4 points
More than 110 cm	More than 100 cm	☐	7 points

Add up your points ☐

Your risk of developing type 2 diabetes within 5 years*:

☐ *5 or less: Low risk*
Approximately one person in every 100 will develop diabetes.

☐ *6-11: Intermediate risk*
For scores of 6-8, approximately one person in every 50 will develop diabetes. For scores of 9-11, approximately one person in every 30 will develop diabetes.

☐ *12 or more: High risk*
For scores of 12-15, approximately one person in every 14 will develop diabetes. For scores of 16-19, approximately one person in every 7 will develop diabetes. For scores of 20 and above, approximately one person in every 3 will develop diabetes.

**The overall score may overestimate the risk of diabetes in those aged less than 25 years.*

If you scored 12 points or more in the AUSDRISK you may have undiagnosed type 2 diabetes or be at high risk of developing the disease. See your doctor about having a fasting blood glucose test. Act now to prevent type 2 diabetes.

Source: RACGP (2016).

FIGURE 17.13 Diagnostic criteria for type 2 diabetes

- Fasting blood glucose (FBG) $\geq$7.0 mmol/L or random blood glucose $\geq$11.1 mmol/L confirmed by a second abnormal FBG on a separate day
- Oral glucose tolerance test (OGTT) before (fasting) and two hours after an oral 75 gm glucose load is taken. Blood glucose is measured. Diabetes is diagnosed as FBG $\geq$7.0 mmol/L or two-hour blood glucose is $\geq$11.1 mmol/L
- Glycated haemoglobin (HbA1c) $\geq$48 mmol/mol (6.5 per cent; on two separate occasions). These are via venous sampling under laboratory methodology

Source: RACGP (2016).

Complications of diabetes

The complications of diabetes may be described as either emergency or chronic.

The emergency complications of diabetes are classified as:

- hypoglycaemia
- diabetic ketoacidosis (DKA)
- hyperosmolar hyperglycaemic syndrome (HHS).

Long-term complications include:

- diabetic retinopathy
- neuropathy
- nephropathy
- cardiovascular disease, including myocardial infarction and stroke.

Hypoglycaemia

Hypoglycaemia is considered to be any blood glucose level below 4 mmol/L and may be:

- mild — patients experience symptoms and self-treat their low blood glucose levels
- moderate — patients need help to treat their low blood glucose
- severe — patients are unconscious or unable to treat their low blood glucose and require a third party to do this for them.

The blood glucose targets for both type 1 and 2 diabetes are as follows.

- Type 1 diabetes.
  - Fasting/before meals: 4–8 mmol/L.
  - Two hours after starting meals: <10 mmol/L.
- Type 2 diabetes.
  - Fasting/before meals: 6–8 mmol/L.
  - Two hours after starting meals: 6–10 mmol/L (National Diabetes Services Scheme (2020).

Tables 17.8 and 17.9 detail the symptoms and treatment of hypoglycaemia.

TABLE 17.8 Symptoms of hypoglycaemia

Autonomic signs/symptoms	Neuroglycopenic symptoms
Pallor	Loss of concentration
A sense of anxiety	Blurred vision
Sweating	Aggressive behaviour
Tremor	Lack of cooperation or confusion
Palpitations (tachycardia)	Seizures
Numbness around the lips and fingers	Transient neurological deficits Reduced level of consciousness Headache

TABLE 17.9 Treatment for hypoglycaemia

Mild hypoglycaemia (adults who are conscious, orientated and able to swallow)

Step 1

- Immediate action:
- Give 15 g fast-acting carbohydrate using one of the following:
  - 100 mL of Lucozade
  - 150 mL of any non diet drink
  - 150 mL of pure fruit juice
  - 3–5 glucose tablets
  - 3–4 regular sweets, e.g. jelly babies
- Wait 15 minutes for the sugar to be absorbed into the bloodstream
- If, after 15 minutes, the blood sugar is:
  - still <4 mmol/L, a sugary option from the above list should be given again
  - >4 mmol/L, proceed with Step 2

Step 2

- The actions outlined in Step 1 must be followed by a slow-acting carbohydrate snack, which may be any one of the following if the person's next meal is more than 15 minutes away:
  - A roll/sandwich
  - A portion of fruit
  - A cereal bar
  - Two plain biscuits
  - One tub of natural low-fat yoghurt
  - One glass of milk
- Test glucose every one to two hours for the next four hours

Moderate hypoglycaemia (adults who are conscious but confused, disorientated, unable to cooperate or aggressive, or have an unsteady gait, but can swallow)

- If the patient is capable and cooperative, follow the treatment outlined for mild hypoglycaemia
- If the patient is not capable and/or is uncooperative but is able to swallow, give either:
  - 1.5–2 tubes of Glucogel or Dextrogel squeezed into the mouth between the teeth and gums. If this is ineffective give:
  - Glucagon 1 mg intramuscularly or subcutaneously into the thigh, buttock or upper arm (although this may be less effective in patients who are prescribed sulphonylurea therapy)
  - Monitor the blood glucose level after 15 minutes — if it is still <4.0 mmol/L, repeat the treatment (up to three times)
  - If the blood glucose level remains <4.0 mmol/L after 45 minutes (or three cycles of initial treatment), consider intravenous 10% glucose infusion at 100 ml per hour
  - Once the blood glucose is >4.0 mmol/L and the patient has recovered, follow Step 2 for mild hypoglycaemia

DO NOT omit an insulin injection if it is due (although a dose review may be required)

- NB: Patients given glucagon require a larger portion of long-acting carbohydrate to replenish their glycogen stores (double the amount suggested above)
- Ensure regular capillary blood glucose level monitoring is continued for 24–48 hours, whether at home or in hospital. Give hypoglycaemia education or refer the patient to a diabetes specialist nurse

Severe hypoglycaemia (adults who are unconscious and/or having seizures and/or are very aggressive)

- Check the:
  - Airway
  - Breathing
  - Circulation
- Call an ambulance, or if in hospital seek medical help immediately
- If in hospital, the following three options are all appropriate (adhering to local hospital policy):
  - Glucagon 1 mg intramuscularly (although it may be less effective in patients prescribed sulphonylurea therapy). Glucagon may take up to 15 minutes to take effect. It mobilises glycogen from the liver and will not work if given repeatedly or in starved patients with no glycogen stores, or those with severe liver disease. If this is the situation or if prolonged treatment is required, intravenous glucose is better
  - If intravenous access is available, give 75 ml of 20% glucose (over 12 minutes):
- Repeat the capillary blood glucose measurement 10 minutes later
- If the blood glucose is <4.0 mmol/L, repeat the treatment
- If intravenous access is available, give 150 ml of 10% glucose (over 12 minutes):
- Repeat the capillary blood glucose measurement 10 minutes later;
- If the blood glucose is <4.0 mmol/L, repeat the treatment
- Once the blood glucose is >4.0 mmol/L and the patient has recovered, follow Step 2 for mild hypoglycaemia
- Ensure regular capillary blood glucose level monitoring is continued for 24–48 hours, whether at home or in hospital
- Give hypoglycaemia education or refer the patient to a diabetes specialist nurse

Source: Adapted from Diabetes Australia (2020).

Diabetic ketoacidosis (DKA)

DKA is a complex disordered metabolic state characterised by hyperglycaemia, acidosis and ketonaemia. It usually occurs as a consequence of absolute or relative insulin deficiency that is accompanied by an increase in counterregulatory hormones (i.e. glucagon, cortisol, growth hormone and epinephrine). This type of hormonal imbalance enhances hepatic gluconeogenesis and glycogenolysis, resulting in severe hyperglycaemia.

Enhanced lipolysis increases serum free fatty acids that are then metabolised as an alternative energy source in the process of ketogenesis, which results in the accumulation of large quantities of ketone bodies and subsequent metabolic acidosis. Ketones include acetone, 3-beta-hydroxybutyrate and acetoacetate. The predominant ketone in DKA is 3-beta-hydroxybutyrate (NHS Diabetes 2010a).

Signs and symptoms of DKA include:

- vomiting
- dehydration
- fruity smell on the breath
- deep laboured breathing (Kussmaul breathing) or hyperventilation
- tachycardia
- confusion and disorientation
- coma
- BGL <16 mmol/L
- ketones present

Management of DKA is a medical emergency and carries a significant risk of mortality for the patient as their condition may change rapidly. The management of DKA requires a multi-disciplinary team to:

- establish IV access and begin fluid and electrolyte replacement therapy
- administer 0.9% saline at a rate to restore urine output to 30 to 60 ml/hr
- administer intravenous insulin infusion — titrated to BGL
- monitor BGL regularly
- assess vital signs — cardiovascular and respiratory status
- assess venous blood gasses
- assess precipitating factors, i.e. missed insulin dose, infection, myocardial infarction.

Hyperosmolar hyperglycaemic syndrome (HHS)

HHS is one of the most serious acute metabolic complications of type 2 diabetes. The main difference between HHS and DKA is the absence of a build-up of keto acids in the bloodstream, with a more severe fluid loss in HHS, many patients showing a fluid deficit of up to nine litres. As HHS is associated with type 2 diabetes, it is suggested that the presence of small amounts of endogenous insulin inhibits the breakdown of fats, preventing ketosis.

Diabetic retinopathy

Diabetic retinopathy is a complication of diabetes that affects the blood vessels in the retina. Diabetes causes the retinal capillaries to become blocked, resulting in an inhibition of sight. If retinopathy is identified early by retinal screening and treated appropriately, blindness can be prevented in 90 per cent of those at risk. According to the Center for Eye Research Australia (2020), of Australians who have diabetes, one in three of these people have some level of diabetic retinopathy.

Neuropathy

Neuropathy is nerve damage. There are three different types of neuropathy: sensory, autonomic and motor. Each type will affect the body in different ways, for example, loss of feeling, erectile dysfunction or disrupted movement.

Nephropathy

Nephropathy is kidney damage and is a microvascular complication associated with diabetes mellitus. This condition mainly affects the glomerulus of the kidney, leading to basement membrane thickening and expansion of the mesangium, which results in a declining glomerular filtration rate and, ultimately, renal failure. No protein can usually leak through the renal glomeruli; however, long-term high blood sugar and/or high blood pressure causes stresses in the walls of the glomeruli, allowing progressively larger protein molecules to pass through. All people with diabetes are routinely prescribed renoprotective antihypertensive agents from puberty. Nurses have a responsibility to help patients understand the importance of taking this medication, even when they are not hypertensive.

Angiopathy

Angiopathy is a disease of the blood vessels (arteries, veins and capillaries). Long-term exposure to high blood sugar causes inflammation of the blood vessels and contributes to the build-up of fatty plaques within them. Microangiopathy occurs when smaller blood vessel walls become weak and thick, for example, in retinopathy. Macroangiopathy occurs when fat and blood clots build-up in larger blood vessels, adhere to the walls and impede the blood flow; this is seen in, for example, cardiovascular disease.

Gestational diabetes

Gestational diabetes is diagnosed in pregnant females during pregnancy and disappears immediately after delivery. It is due to changes in glucose metabolism during pregnancy as a direct result of the antagonistic effect of pregnancy hormones.

Diagnosis of gestational diabetes

All women not previously known to have pre-pregnancy diabetes or gestational diabetes should have a pregnancy oral glucose tolerance test (POGTT) at 24–28 weeks gestation. In POGTT, an extra plasma glucose at one hour is performed. The diagnostic glucose levels are also lower in pregnant women (Nankervis et al. 2014).

According to the Australasian Diabetes in Pregnancy Society (ADIPS) recommendations for a diagnosis of gestational diabetes could be made on one or more of these values:

- fasting — >5.1 mmol/L
- 1 hour — >10.0 mmol/L
- 2 hour — ≥8.5 mmol/L.

Previous ADIPS guidelines (Hoffman et al. 1998) for the testing and diagnosis of gestational diabetes in Australia are still in use among some clinicians:

- fasting — ≥5.5 mmol/L
- 2 hour glucose — ≥8.0 mmol/L.

Ongoing monitoring of diabetes

Ongoing management of diabetes is assessed largely through blood glucose control, though other diagnostic tests may also indicate the progression of the disease or the presence of any other complications (table 17.10). Self blood glucose monitoring as a useful practice to promote self-management of the disease will be discussed in nursing management.

TABLE 17.10 **Laboratory testing for ongoing management of type 2 diabetes**

Test	Indication	Reference Range	Consideration
Urine albumin/creatinine ratio (UACR)	Assess and monitor changes to renal function due to diabetes	Normal: <30 mg/day Moderate: 3.4 to 34 mg/mmol of creatinine	Baseline test at diagnosis of diabetes and then annually. First urine of day to be tested.
Lipid profile Triglycerides Cholesterol HDL LDL	Assess and monitor for indicators of atherosclerosis and cardiovascular disease	Normal: ≤2.5 mmol/L Normal: ≤5.2 mmol/L 1.00–2.50 mmol/L ≤3.5 mmol/L	Patient is required to fast for 9–12 hours prior.
Glycated haemoglobin (HbA1c)	Ongoing maintenance of type 2 diabetes	≤53 mmol/L (7.0%)	Non-fasting — no preparation required. Interpret with care for haemoglobinopathies or abnormal red cell lifespan

Source: Adapted from Mayo Clinic (2021).

Diabetes goals of management include improving the quality of life for the individual, reducing symptoms and preventing both acute and long-term complications associated with the disease. Improved glycaemic management has been shown to reduce the complications of retinopathy, renal disease and neuropathy in people with type 2 diabetes (Colagiuri et al. 2009b).

Management of diabetes involves a multi-disciplinary team using a patient-centred care approach. A multi-disciplinary care team will ensure that the patient benefits from a broad perspective to their health and wellbeing (RACGP 2016). The exact make-up of the team will be dependent on the individual needs of the patient and access to services (see figure 17.14), though the approach should be consistent with components of the chronic care model (CCM).

FIGURE 17.14 Potential members of the multi-disciplinary diabetes care team

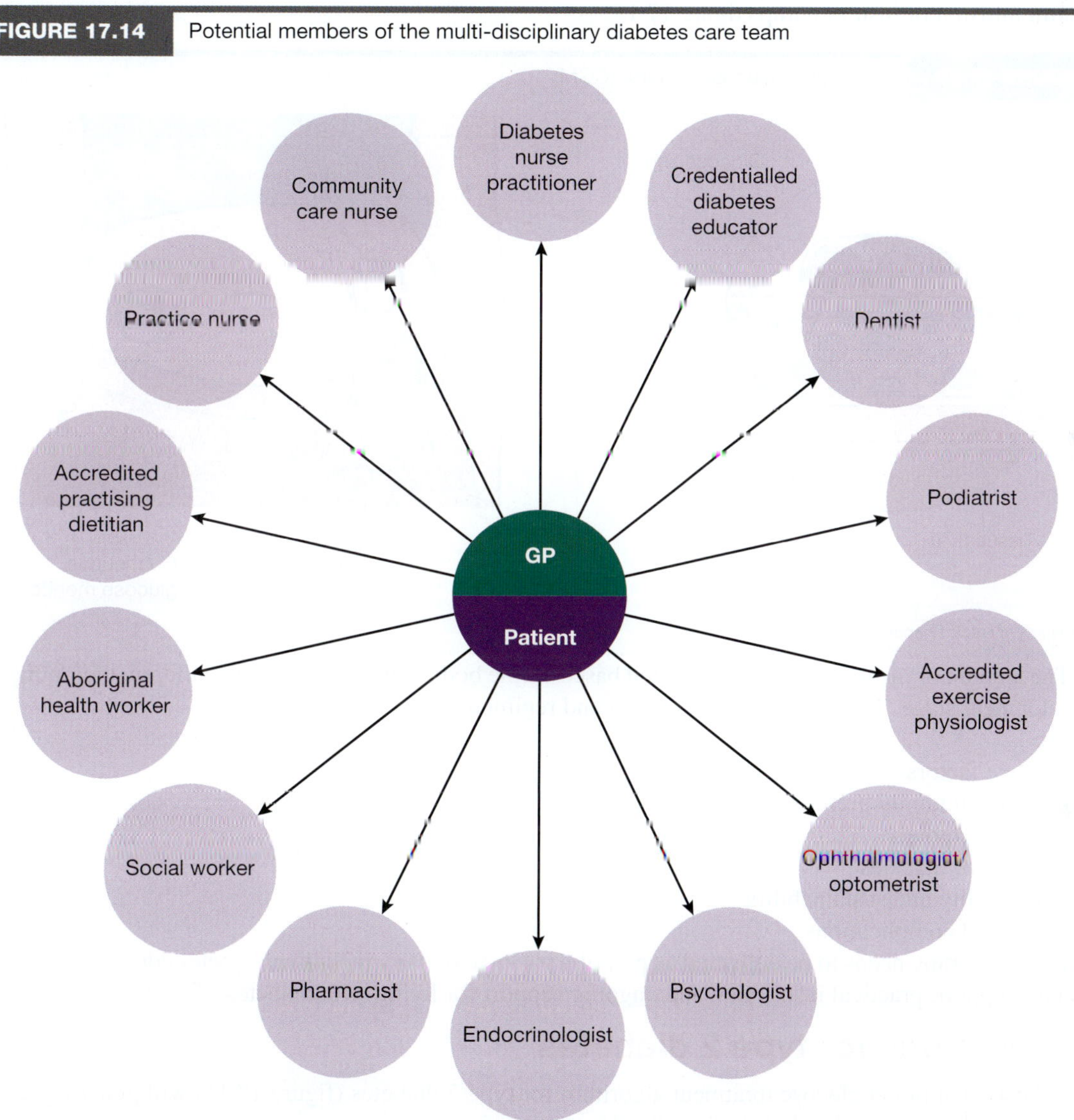

Source: RACGP & Diabetes Australia (2016).

The CCM ensures that patients are provided with the education and support needed to take responsibility for the day to day management of their condition. Patient education is at the centre of a structured management plan for diabetes and integral in enabling self-management of the disease (RACGP 2016).

When caring for Indigenous Australians with a chronic illness such as diabetes, the addition of an Aboriginal liaison officer, Indigenous healthcare worker or care co-ordinator to the multi-disciplinary care team is essential to ensure cultural sensitivity.

Medications for type 1 diabetes

The aim of insulin therapy regimes in type 1 diabetes is:

- to provide sufficient basal insulin for a 24-hour period
- to deliver boluses of rapid-acting insulin matched to the carbohydrate content of meals or snacks throughout the day
- to minimise blood glucose fluctuation and risk of hypo and hyperglycaemia.

Insulin therapy has dramatically changed since it was first used in 1922, with many insulin products and insulin regimens now being used throughout the world. Insulin regimes can be delivered via multiple daily injections as a part of a basal-bolus approach or rapid-acting therapy insulin via a continuous subcutaneous insulin infusion or insulin pump (figure 17.15).

FIGURE 17.15 Continuous glucose monitor (CGM)

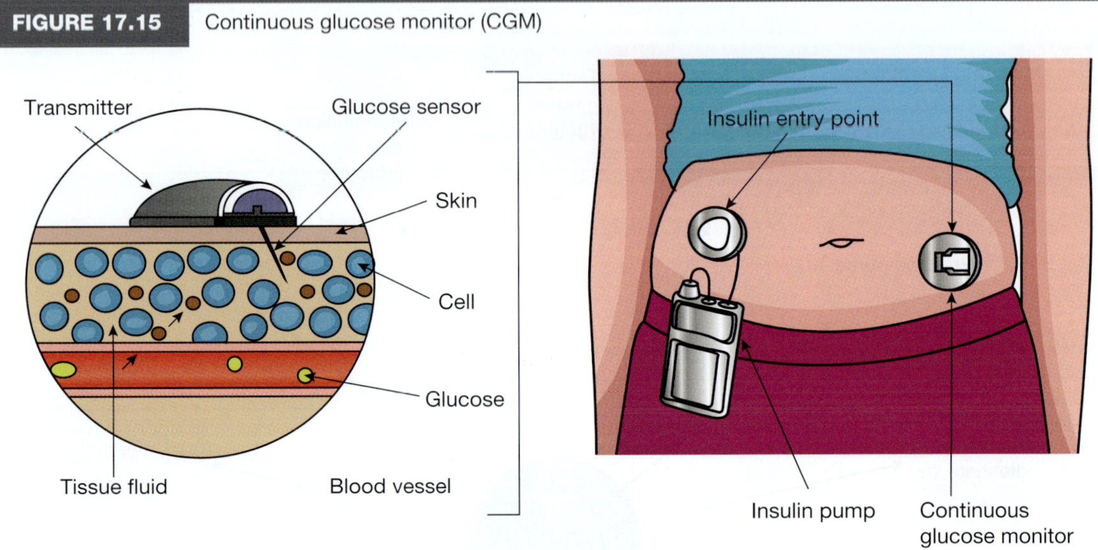

Source: OnTrack Diabetes (2016).

The amount of insulin required is adjusted based on the body weight, age, and in children, their pubertal development stage. The choice of insulin type and regimen will be guided by:

- age
- lifestyle factors
- patient and family preference
- metabolic targets
- duration of diabetes
- affordability and sustainability
- associated complications.

Insulin therapy needs to be delivered as part of a package of care, including diabetes education, specific dietary support, practical instruction and ongoing support for living with diabetes.

Medications for type 2 diabetes

The Australian blood glucose treatment algorithm for type 2 diabetes (figure 17.16) will generally guide decision making about the choice of medications and regimen.

People with type 2 diabetes will generally be taking medication to control hypertension and hyperlipidaemia and may also be on oral hypoglycaemic agents. The first-line oral hypoglycaemic agents are biguanides, which increase the effectiveness of insulin (e.g. metformin [Glucophage]), and are introduced when dietary and exercise modifications are unable to achieve appropriate glycaemic control.

Second-line (dual) therapy may then be introduced.

- Failure to achieve glycaemic control using biguanides and lifestyle modifications necessitates the addition of a second drug class.
- Glitazones and dipeptidyl peptidase-4 (DPP-4) inhibitors are the choice for second-line therapy.
- Older sulphonylureas (e.g. gliclazide [Diamicron MR]) are less commonly used; they encourage the pancreas to produce more insulin and are used in non-obese people or when metformin is not well tolerated. Alternative options for these patients or patients with irregular daily blood glucose patterns are the second-generation sulphonylureas known as insulin secretagogues (e.g. nateglinide [Starlix]).

FIGURE 17.16 The Australian blood glucose treatment algorithm for type 2 diabetes

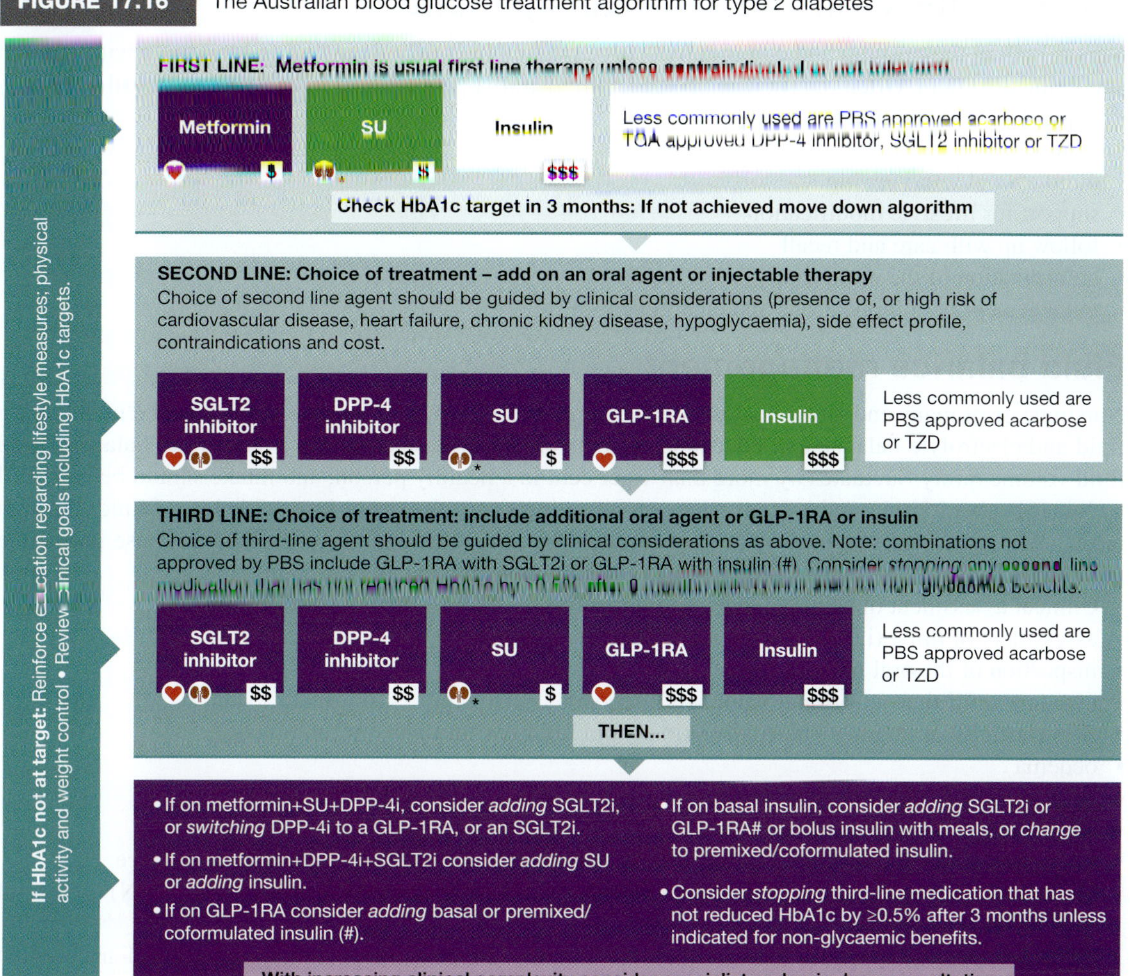

Source: Australian Diabetes Society (2016).

There are several alternative medical options.

- Glitazones makes available insulin work more effectively (e.g. rosiglitazone [Avandia]).
- Glucagon like peptide 1 (GLP-1) receptor agonists delay the breakdown of insulin; they are only available as injectables (e.g. exenatide [Byetta]).
- DPP-4 inhibitors delay the breakdown of insulin and are given orally (e.g. sitagliptin [Januvia]).
- Prandial glucose regulators stimulate extra insulin production when sugar is taken; however, the effects do not last very long and it is only taken with meals (e.g. repaglinide [NovoNorm]).
- Alpha-glucosidase inhibitors help to slow the break-up of food in the digestive system; side effects can include stomach upsets and problems with wind (e.g. acarbose [Glucobay]).

Insulin therapy becomes necessary when other medications fail to achieve adequate control or when the presence of liver or renal dysfunction contraindicates their usage.

17.4 Nursing management of endocrine disorders

LEARNING OBJECTIVE 17.4 Describe and discuss nursing assessment and management of patients with endocrine disorders.

Endocrine disorders are complex and chronic conditions that will require ongoing management both from the patient and the multi-disciplinary care team. Nursing care of the person with an endocrine disorder will consider physical, psychological and social needs. The person's age, culture, socioeconomic status and health literacy may all impact the person's ability to engage in self-management of the disease or disorder. Assessment, interventions and planning require adjustment as the person progresses from diagnosis to maintenance, with acute complications also presenting challenges to care.

Patient education and self-management

Nurses both in the hospital and community setting play an integral role in caring for people with chronic endocrine disorders. Often nurses take on both administrative and clinical roles being responsible for:

- clinical assessment of the patient
- education
- motivational interviewing
- support for lifestyle modification
- follow up with care and recall
- co-ordination of the multi-disciplinary team
- management of complications and emergencies.

Fluid balance management

Nursing care of many endocrine disorders and their associated complications revolves around maintaining fluid and electrolyte balance and educating patients on the need to maintain a strict fluid balance. Total fluid volume rarely fluctuates by more than 1 per cent in a healthy person, and intake should be balanced by loss (Shepherd 2011). Aside from urine output, patients can experience insensible loss of fluids through faces, skin, sweat and evaporation of fluid through the lungs that cannot be measured. These insensible losses are influenced by dietary intake, illness, medications and the environment.

Clinical assessment of fluid balance should involve:

- assessment of thirst (i.e. ask the patient if they are thirsty)
- inspection of the oral mucosa
- capillary refill time — normal value is ≤2 seconds
- skin elasticity or turgor — normally skin should fall back into place when pinched
- oedema
- body weight — should be measured at the same time each day using the same scales
- urine output — should be 0.5 ml/kg/hour
- vital signs — respiratory rate, blood pressure and heart rate are all affected by fluid balance
- blood chemistry — sodium, potassium, chloride, bicarbonate and blood urea nitrate (BUN) are useful in assessing hydration.

Patients should be taught to monitor their fluid intake independently where possible. A diary is often recommended when first diagnosed to assist in recognising times of the day, volumes and types of fluid consumed.

Nursing care of patients on long-term corticosteroid therapy

Corticosteroids are used extensively for:

- adrenal insufficiency
- suppressing inflammation
- suppressing autoimmune reactions
- controlling allergic reactions
- reducing the rejection process in transplantation.

The anti-inflammatory and anti-allergy actions of corticosteroids make them an effective treatment method for conditions such as rheumatoid arthritis and systemic lupus erythematosus. Corticosteroids may also be used to manage other chronic conditions, such as asthma and multiple sclerosis. As with all medications, the use of corticosteroids is not without consequence as they have numerous side effects and drug interactions that need to be considered (table 17.11).

Nursing care of the patient with diabetes

Several nursing interventions can be made for a patient with diabetes:

- instruct patients on basic food types and their effect on blood sugar levels.
- assist in:
  - meal planning to normalise blood sugar levels and meet weight loss targets, if appropriate
  - designing a personalised physical activity plan
  - helping patients to achieve mastery in glucose testing and insulin administration, if appropriate
  - advising on the need for diabetes reviews, and stress the importance of regular medical follow-ups
  - instructing patients on good foot care and hygiene to minimise complications.

TABLE 17.11 Nursing care of patients on long-term corticosteroid therapy

Potential complication	Nursing action
Cardiovascular Hypertension Thrombophlebitis Thromboembolism Accelerated atherosclerosis	Monitor blood pressure for signs of hypertension Assess for a positive Homans' sign (indicating a deep vein thrombosis) Educate patients on: • Avoiding positions and situations that restrict blood flow (e.g. crossing the legs or prolonged sitting in the same position) • Foot and leg exercises • Low-sodium intake • A low saturated fat diet
Immunological Increased risk of infection	Assess for signs of infection (bacterial and fungal) and inflammation Encourage: • Patients to avoid exposure to others with known infections or colds • Hand-washing and good hygiene practices
Eye changes Glaucoma Corneal lesions	Encourage yearly eye examinations Refer patients to an ophthalmologist if changes in visual acuity are detected
Musculoskeletal Muscle wasting Poor wound healing Osteoporosis: • Vertebral compression fractures • Pathological fractures of the long bones • Aseptic necrosis of head of the femur	Refer to a dietitian Encourage a diet high in protein, calcium and vitamin D Calcium and vitamin D supplementation, if indicated Take measures to avoid falls and other trauma Use caution when moving and turning patients Encourage postmenopausal women on corticosteroids to consider bone mineral density testing and treatment, if indicated Instruct the patient to rise slowly from the bed or chair in cases of postural hypotension Promote regular physical activity
Metabolic Alterations in glucose metabolism Steroid withdrawal syndrome	Monitor blood glucose levels In the event of steroid-induced diabetes, refer to the diabetes nurse for education and management Report signs of adrenal insufficiency Monitor fluid and electrolyte balance Administer fluids and electrolytes as prescribed Educate patients on: • The importance of taking corticosteroids as prescribed without abruptly stopping therapy • Obtaining and wearing a medical identification bracelet • Notifying all healthcare providers (e.g. the dentist) about the need for corticosteroid therapy
Changes in appearance Moon face Weight gain Acne Thinning of the skin Tendency to bruise easily	Encourage a low-calorie, low-sodium diet Assure patients that most changes in appearance are temporary and will disappear if and when corticosteroid therapy is no longer necessary Monitor skin changes Instruct on active bruising avoidance, e.g. the use of stockings to prevent injury to the shins in affected individuals

Blood glucose monitoring

Self-monitoring of blood glucose (SMBG) is a good educational tool for people with diabetes and is usually indicated:

- for patients on insulin and glucose-lowering agents that can cause hypoglycaemia
- when monitoring hyperglycaemia arising from illness
- with pregnancy and pre-pregnancy planning
- when changes in treatment, lifestyle or other conditions require data on glycaemic patterns
- when **HbA1c** estimations are unreliable (e.g. haemoglobinopathies).

Not all people with type 2 diabetes will benefit from SMBG, so consideration must be given to the daily stress and inconvenience for the individual compared with the potential benefits. Routine SMBG for people with type 2 diabetes who are considered low risk and using oral glucose-lowering medications is not recommended (RACGP 2016). When a person is undertaking SMBG, they should be aware of their target values and what to do when these are not achieved. Targets for SMBG levels are 6–8 mmol/L for fasting and pre-prandial and 6–10 mmol/L for 2 hours postprandial (Colagiuri et al. 2009b; Harkins 2008).

Dietary modifications

Eighty per cent of people diagnosed with type 2 diabetes are overweight, so the inclusion of a practising dietician is highly recommended in assisting patients in making successful dietary modifications. Three themes exist when guiding people with diabetes to make dietary modifications:

1. emphasising nutrient-dense foods in appropriate proportions
2. eating for cardiovascular protection
3. glycaemic management and meal planning.

Dietary advice should always be given in consideration of the patient's individual circumstances with respect to current health, comorbidities and personal preferences regarding cultural, religious and economic preferences. Some general guidelines include:

- consume a wide variety of foods from the core food groups everyday
- drink plenty of water.
- consider the amount and quality of carbohydrates eaten within a meal. Eating low GI load foods (i.e. wholegrain breads and low-fat dairy products) may improve glycaemic control.
- limit intake of foods such as:
  - those high in saturated fats, e.g.: biscuits, pastries, pies and fast food
  - food and drink containing added salt
  - avoiding food and drink containing added sugar, e.g. soft drink and confectionary (RACGP 2016).

Diabetes and alcohol

Current Australian guidelines for people with and without diabetes recommend no more than two standard drinks (150 ml) for both men and women per day. Alcohol can have many effects, including:

- weight gain
- damage to the pancreas, nerves, brain and liver
- difficulty in managing diabetes, causing both high and low blood glucose levels.

Patients taking insulin or oral hypoglycaemics are at particular risk of alcohol-related hypoglycaemia. This may occur while drinking or for several hours after, because typically when glucose levels decline, the liver will release glucose to correct the derangement. However, the liver will always process alcohol first instead of the stored glucose, increasing hypoglycaemia. Patients taking insulin or oral hypoglycaemic medication that may cause low blood sugar levels should be advised to alternate their drinks so that some sugar is consumed to prevent hypoglycaemia.

Exercise modification

The benefits of regular exercise for those diagnosed with diabetes include:

- increased insulin sensitivity
- reduced weight gain
- improved psychological health
- a reduced risk of cardiovascular disease (Michaliszyn et al. 2009).

Aerobic exercise has been shown to achieve a similar reduction in HbA1c as some oral hypoglycaemics (RACGP 2016). Recommendations for patients with type 1 diabetes are the same as for the general population. The universal recommendations with regard to physical activity are as follows.

- Accumulate at least 30 minutes of moderate-intensity physical activity on most days of the week.

- A total of 30 minutes spread over the entire day is equally beneficial to one 30-minute walk.
- Activities of daily living such as housework and using the stairs are valuable in increasing physical activity

FIGURE 17.17 The Australian Guide to Healthy Eating

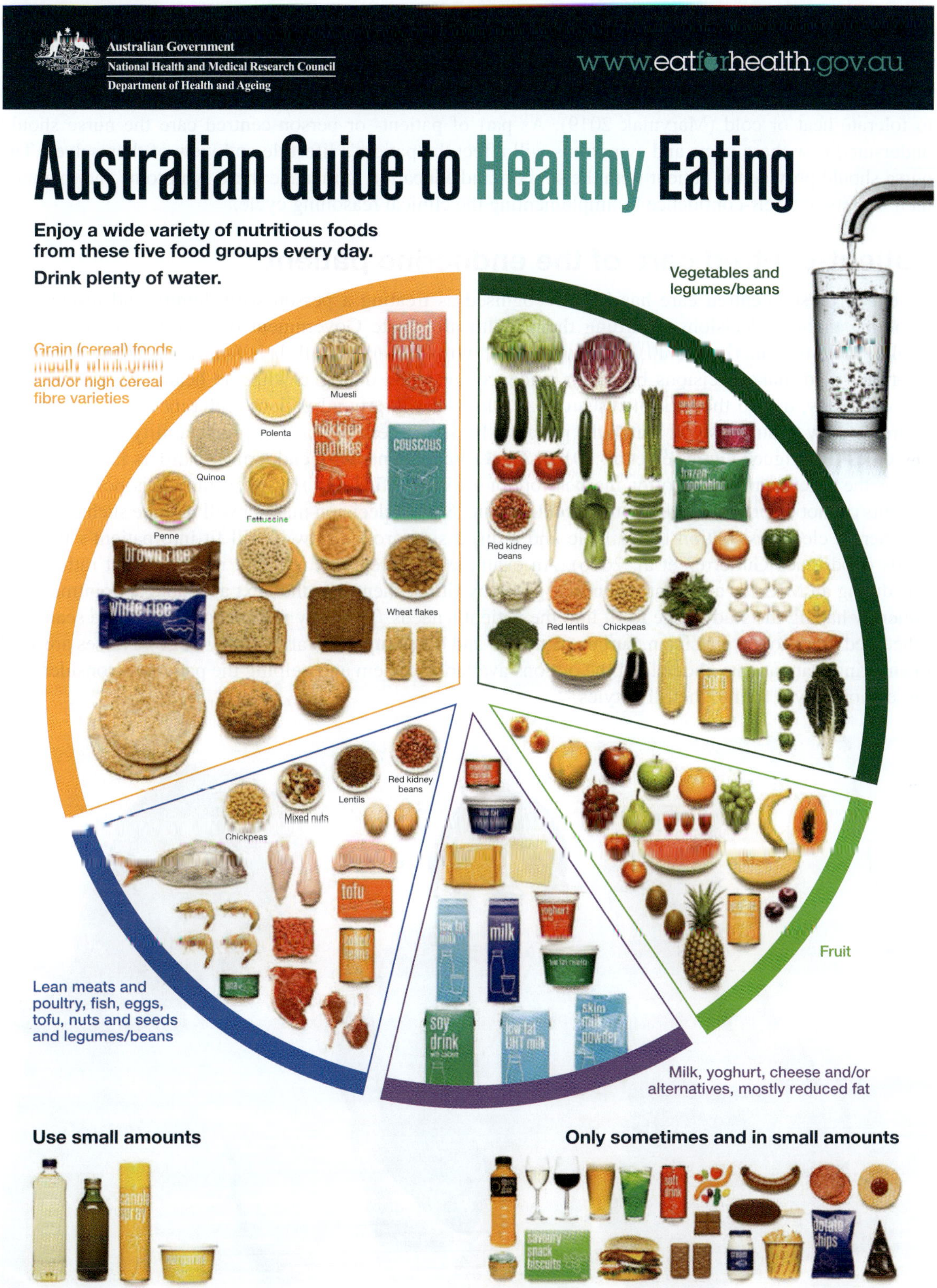

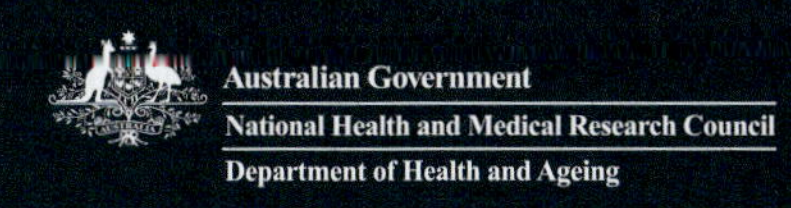

Use small amounts

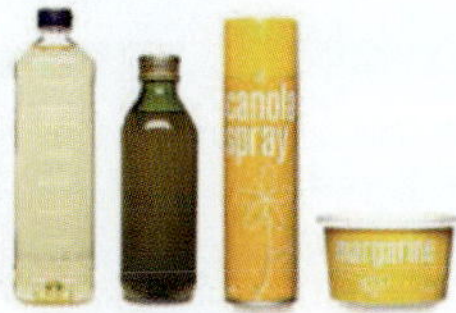

Only sometimes and in small amounts

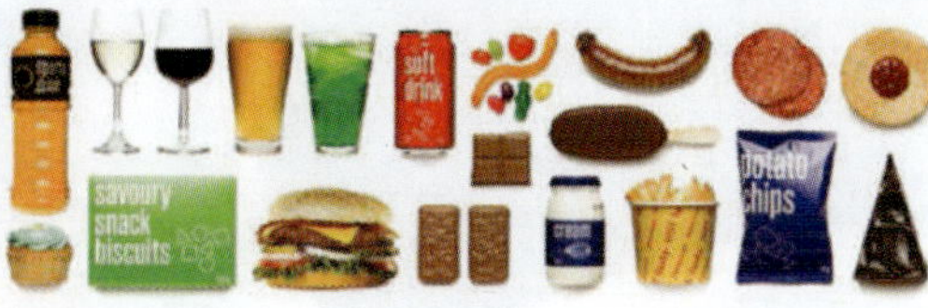

Source: NHMRC (2017).

17.5 Patient-centred care and the clinical reasoning cycle for patients with endocrine disorders

LEARNING OBJECTIVE 17.5 Apply patient-centred care and the clinical reasoning cycle to the care of a patient with an endocrine disorder.

The nurse has a significant role to play in helping the patient understand their disease process and changes that may need to be made in their lifestyle. Signs and symptoms of endocrine diseases can include fatigue, lethargy, change in appetite and weight changes, dizziness, depression, irritability, anxiety, pain, decreased libido, nausea, vomiting, changes in urinary or bowel habits, vision changes and changes in the ability to tolerate heat or cold (Maryniak 2019). As part of patient- or person-centred care the nurse should understand how these signs and symptoms will affect the patient's lifestyle and view of themselves. The nurse should provide the patient with the support and education to manage these symptoms and maintain their dignity and self-confidence by implementing the clinical reasoning cycle.

Patient-centred care of the endocrine patient

Patient or person-centred care has been recognised as treating a person with dignity and respect and involving them in decisions regarding their healthcare (State Government of Victoria Department of Health & Human Services 2020). It includes providing the patient and their families with the necessary information to make decisions based on evidence and open dialogue with the healthcare provider. In endocrinology, due to the lack of research, a lack of clarity around patient preferences, or an inability to predict how treatments will match the patients' lifestyle, there is a lack of predictability around patient outcomes (Rodriguez-Gutierrez et al. 2016). Therefore, patients with endocrine disorders face situations where the care team cannot offer the best options with confidence. However, this does not mean that patients cannot be provided with patient-centred care. Shared decision making will include such decisions as where a clear best option is available and a discussion around how it will fit into patient's lifestyle needs (Rodriguez-Gutierrez et al. 2016). An example of patient-centred care might be that rather than scheduling an MRI for a patient's pituitary gland by fitting them into the next available appointment but rather by having the study done to fit into the patient's needs. This may mean coordinating the scan with scheduled visits to the physician, surgeons, nurses and other support staff (Bagley 2017). Nurses are vital to ensuring that patients understand the options available to them and helping the patient to consider how these choices will fit into their lifestyles.

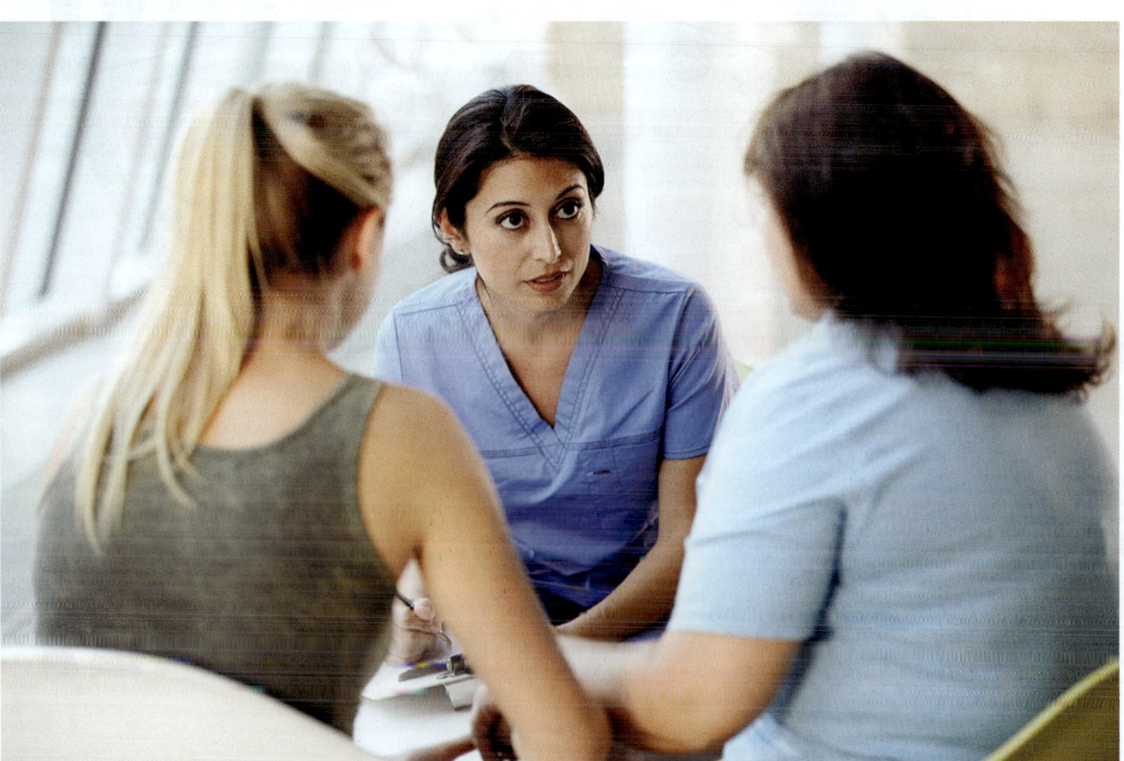

The clinical reasoning cycle and the endocrine patient

Clinical reasoning is essential for the provision of safe and effective nursing care. In nursing, the thought process that supports clinical reasoning involves cognitive, behavioural and mental habits. In cognitive skills, the health care provider seeks information, analyses the information and interprets it based on knowledge, policies, procedures and standards of practice. Behavioural skills require self-confidence, open-mindedness and a systemised approach. Mental habits require reflection, intellectual perspective and intellectual integrity (Carvalho et al. 2017). The clinical reasoning cycle (Levett-Jones 2017) organises the clinical reasoning process into a set of steps that support a systematic process of assessing and planning care for the patient. Endocrine diseases can be challenging to diagnose, treat and care for. Familiarity with the endocrine glands and the hormones they secrete, and the signs and symptoms of abnormalities in these hormones' production will help healthcare providers identify endocrine disorders. Understanding the endocrine system and the functions of that system is necessary to assess, treat and care for patients with endocrine abnormalities. This knowledge of how the system works and then a focused endocrine assessment begins with a history of chief complaints followed by a focused physical assessment. Using the clinical reasoning cycle as a supportive structure will help the healthcare providers provide the best care for patients and their families.

CASE STUDY 17.1

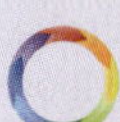

Nursing care of a male patient with an endocrine disorder

Francis Johns is a 19-year-old recruit to the Army who was brought into the Army base healthcare facility after collapsing during his basic training.

Two weeks ago, Francis experienced an episode of weakness, general malaise and drowsiness. He reported to the hospital, was seen by the medics and a diagnosis of dehydration was given. He received 1 litre of normal saline via IV and was returned to duty.

Upon this presentation, Francis reports ongoing thirst and the repeated need to urinate. He has recently lost 8 kilograms without intending to. His baseline body weight is 69 kilograms and his height is 153 centimetres. He looks flushed and breathless. He complained of vague abdominal pain, and he had vomited once prior to his collapse. On examination, he appears pale and dehydrated with dry mucous membranes and poor skin turgor.

Vital signs on presentation are:

- respiratory rate: 36/minute with deep, laboured breathing
- heart rate: 138 beats per minute regular
- blood pressure: 90/60 mmHg
- temperature: 37°C
- Glasgow Coma Scale: 10/15
- pain score: 3/10
- chest clear; heart sounds normal
- urine dipstick was positive for glucose and acetone
- blood glucose: 25 mmol/L.

Question

Using the information above, describe what action you would take as the nurse caring for this patient. Which care would be prioritised? Use the clinical reasoning cycle to guide you through the process and devise a plan of care for your patient.

Questions you might ask are as follows.

- Why was he given IV saline on his initial visit?
- Why is he presenting with dyspnoea?
- What are you considering the underlying problem to be?
- What needs to be done urgently?

Answer

- *Step 1: Consider the patient.* Francis Johns is a 19-year-old recruit to the Army
- *Step 2: Collect cues/information*. Include subjective and objective data here. The subjective will include what the patient tells you, the appearance of the patient, and their past medical history. Objective data will include objective or measurable information such as the vital signs, blood tests etc.
- *Step 3: Process information.* Separate the relevant and irrelevant data — cluster the clues together to formulate an inference about the patient. What is the current situation? Does the patient need additional support? What are the risks for this patient?

- *Step 4: Identify problems/issues.* Nursing problems or diagnosis should be listed here. Nursing problems will be identified during the assessment of your patient and then will require focused assessments. Nursing problems for this case would include pain and blood sugar management, fluid volume deficit, fatigue, knowledge deficit and the potential for a feeling of powerless and concern about his career.
- *Step 5: Establish goals*. The goals of care for Francis would include pain relief, managed glucose levels, maintaining fluid balance, education and reassurance.
- *Step 6: Take action*. Provide the care that is required to meet the established goals. In the initial stages, the focus will be to treat the pain and discomfort, BSL and lab testing, fluids IV or orally as ordered, maintain a strict fluid balance chart, and provide reassure and education to Francis.
- *Step 7: Evaluate outcomes*. Were the best outcomes achieved?
- *Step 8: Reflect on the process and new learning*. Reflect on any aspects of care that could have been done better. What went well, what did not go as well as hoped. What continuing professional development could you do to better support cases like this in the future?

CASE STUDY 17.2

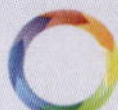 Nursing care of a patient with type 2 diabetes

Mrs Priti Patel is an 89-year-old woman who is currently residing in an aged care facility. She has been a widow for five years. She has been living in the aged care facility since she suffered a left-sided stroke two years ago. The stroke affected her right side and her speech. She is unable to perform her activities of daily living without support. Mrs Patel's son and his wife both work and have been unable to support her care. Her son and his wife visit Mrs Patel weekly and are very attentive to her needs. Mrs Patel was diagnosed with type 2 diabetes twenty years ago. Until her stroke and the death of her husband, Mrs Patel took an active role in managing her diabetes. She is becoming increasingly frustrated because she is unable to communicate her needs or how she is feeling. You notice that Mrs Patel has had very little to eat today and says she does not want anything to eat. She had her usual medications and her gliclazide 80 mg and metformin 1 gm at 1000 hours. At 1400 hours, you note that Mrs Patel is sweating profusely, is pale and drowsy but looks up at you when you call her name.

Question

Using the information above, describe what action you would take as the nurse caring for this patient. Which care would be prioritised? Use the clinical reasoning cycle to guide you through the process and devise a plan of care for your patient.

Questions you might ask are as follows.

- What are Mrs Patel's vital signs?
- What is Mrs Patel's glucose level?
- Do you need to escalate her care immediately?

Answer

- *Step 1: Consider the patient*. Mrs Priti Patel is an 89-year-old woman with type 2 diabetes and residing in a residential care home.
- *Step 2: Collect cues/information.* Include subjective and objective data here. The subjective will include what the patient tells you, the appearance of the patient, and their past medical history. Objective data will include objective or measurable information such as the vital signs, blood tests etc.
- *Step 3: Process information*. Separate the relevant and irrelevant data — cluster the clues together to formulate an inference about the patient. What is the current situation? Does the patient need additional support? What are the risks for this patient? Blood glucose levels can drop too low after taking diabetes medication if the patient is eating less than usual.
- *Step 4: Identify problems/issues*. Nursing problems or diagnosis should be listed here. Possible issues include diabetic hypoglyceamia, seizures or unconsciousness.
- *Step 5: Establish goals*. Our immediate goals of care for Mrs Patel are to stabilise her condition. She will also need transfer to a hospital for emergency care.
- *Step 6: Take action*. Provide the care that is required to meet the established goals. Take a blood glucose level urgently and consider the results of the test. Notify her physician and arrange transfer to the local hospital for urgent care. Reassure Mrs Patel, provide a drink of juice or glucose sweets.
- *Step 7: Evaluate outcomes*. Were the best outcomes achieved?
- *Step 8: Reflect on the process and new learning*. Reflect on any aspects of care that could have been done better. What went well, what did not go as well as hoped. What continuing professional development could you do to better support cases like this in the future.

SUMMARY

This chapter provides readers with a basic knowledge of the endocrine system's anatomy and physiology and the common endocrine disorders. It includes valuable information on the challenges nurses encounter when caring for patients with complex endocrine disorders and provides an overview of relevant nursing management. An understanding of the major endocrine glands, the hormones they secrete, and the symptoms of hormone imbalances support nurses to provide holistic patient-centred care. Endocrinology is a challenging nursing discipline. It offers the nurse the opportunity to experience both acute interventions and ongoing management of chronic diseases. Endocrine nursing is a specialist role that is evolving and growing as new information and treatments become available. Endocrine nurses can make a difference for their patients and the families by providing support, reassurance and education and applying their specialist knowledge to clinical practice. This chapter should not be considered sufficient and should be used in conjunction with other published material to ensure further development of knowledge and keep up to date in this ever-changing field.

KEY TERMS

arginine vasopressin (ADH) A hormone made by the hypothalamus in the brain and stored in the posterior pituitary gland. ADH regulates and balances the amount of water in the bloodstream.

aseptic technique Strict practices and procedures to prevent contamination from pathogens.

AUSDRISK The Australian type 2 diabetes risk assessment tool consists of a short list of questions designed to assess the risk of developing type 2 diabetes over the next five years.

diabetes mellitus (DM) A group of diseases that result in too much sugar in the blood stream (high blood glucose levels).

endocrine glands The glands of the endocrine system that secrete hormones directly into the bloodstream. The major glands of the endocrine system are the pineal gland, pituitary gland, pancreas, ovaries, testes, thyroid gland, parathyroid gland, hypothalamus and adrenal glands.

exocrine Refers to the secretion of a substance out through a duct. The exocrine glands include the salivary glands, sweat glands and glands within the gastrointestinal tract.

gestational diabetes High blood sugar affecting pregnant women.

HbA1c A blood test that measures how well-controlled a patient's blood sugar has been over approximately three months.

insulin A hormone created by the pancreas that controls the amount of glucose in the bloodstream and helps to store glucose in the liver, fat cells and muscles, and regulates the metabolism of carbohydrates, fats and proteins.

type 1 diabetes A chronic condition in which the pancreas produces little or no insulin.

type 2 diabetes A chronic condition that affects the way the body processes blood sugar (glucose).

REFERENCES

Australian Diabetes Society. (2016) Type 2 diabetes treatment. http://t2d.diabetessociety.com.au

Australian Government Department of Health. (2010) The Australian type 2 diabetes risk assessment tool (AUSDRISK). www.health.gov.au/resources/apps-and-tools/the-australian-type-2-diabetes-risk-assessment-tool-ausdrisk

Australian Institute of Health and Wefare. (2020) Diabetes. Australian Government. www.aihw.gov.au/reports/diabetes/diabetes/contents/how-many-australians-have-diabetes

Bagley, D. (2017) Handle with care (Part 2). *Endocrine News*. https://endocrinenews.endocrine.org/handle-care-part-2

Carmichael, J. D. (2020) Overview of the Pituitary Gland. *MSD Manual*. www.msdmanuals.com/en-au/home/hormonal-and-metabolic-disorders/pituitary-gland-disorders/overview-of-the-pituitary-gland

Carvalho, E. C., Souza Oliveira-Kumakura, A. R. & Coelho Ramalho Vasconcelos Morais, S. (2017) Clinical reasoning in nursing: teaching strategies and assessment tools. *Revista Brasileira de Enfermage*. 70(3): 662–668. doi:https://doi.org/10.1590/0034-7167-2016-0509

Center for Eye Research Australia. (2020) Diabetic eye disease. www.cera.org.au/conditions/diabetic-eye-disease

Colagiuri, S., Davies, D., Girgis, S. & Colagiuri, R. (2009a) National Evidence Based Guideline for case detection and diagnosis of type 2 diabetes. Diabetes Australia and the NHMRC, Canberra.

Colagiuri, S., Dickinson, S., Girgis, S. & Colagiuri, R. (2009b) National Evidence Based Guideline for blood glucose control in type 2 diabetes. Diabetes Australia and the NHMRC, Canberra.

Diabetes Australia. (2020) *Living with Diabetes*. www.diabetesaustralia.com.au/living-with-diabetes/managing-your-diabetes/hypoglycaemia

Harkins, V. (2008) *A Practical Guide to Integrated Type 2 Diabetes Care.* Kildare: Health Service Executive.

Hoffman, L., Nolan, C., Wilson, J. D., Oats, J. J. N. & Simmons, D. (1998) Gestational diabetes mellitus — management guidelines. The Australasian Diabetes in Pregnancy Society. *The Medical Journal of Australia.* 169: 93–97.

Hong, L. (2014) Management of hyponatremia associated with syndrome of inappropriate antidiuretic hormone secretion. *Topics in Clinical Nutrition.* 29(2): 187–196. doi: 10.1097/01.TIN.0000445902.90393.82

Hormones Australia. (2018) *Sick day management for patients on glucocorticoid therapy.* www.hormones-australia.org.au/wp-content/uploads/2020/11/Sick-Day-Management-Plan-FINAL-fillable.pdf

Hormones Australia. (2019) Adrenal insufficiency. Endocrine Society of Australia. www.hormones-australia.org.au/endocrine-diseases/adrenal-insufficiency

Levett-Jones, T. (2017) *Clinical Reasoning, Learning to Think Like a Nurse*, 2nd ed. Melbourne, Australia: Pearson.

[illegible] (2010) The endocrine system. www.[illegible].com/clinical-insights/endocrine-system

Mayo Clinic. (2021) *Type 2 diabetes.* Mayo Foundation for Medical Education and Research (MFMER). www.mayoclinic.org/diseases-conditions/type-2-diabetes/diagnosis-treatment/drc-20351199

Michaliszyn, F. S., Shaibi, G. Q., Quinn, L. et al. (2009) Physical fitness, dietary intake and metabolic control in adolescents with type 1 diabetes. *Pediatric Diabetes.* 10: 389–394.

Nankervis, A., McIntyre, H. D., Moses, R., Ross, G. P., Callaway, L., Porter, C., Jeffries, W., Boorman, C., De Vries, B. & McElduff, A. (2014) *ADIPS Consensus Guidelines for the Testing and Diagnosis of Hyperglycaemia in Pregnancy in Australia and New Zealand, The Australasian Diabetes in Pregnancy Society.*

National Diabetes Services Scheme. (2020) *Blood glucose monitoring fact sheet.* www.ndss.com.au/about-diabetes/resources/find-a-resource/blood-glucose-monitoring-fact-sheet

National Health and Medical Research Council. (2017) Australian guide to healthy eating. Australian Government. www.eatforhealth.gov.au/guidelines/australian-guide-healthy-eating

National Institute for Health and Clinical Excellence (NICE). (2009) Diabetes update. London: NICE.

NHS Diabetes. (2010a) *Joint British Diabetes Societies Inpatient Care Group Guidance on the Management of Diabetic Ketoacidosis.* London: NHS Diabetes.

OnTrack Diabetes. (2016) What is a continuous glucose monitoring (CGM)? www.ontrackdiabetes.com/type-1-diabetes/what-continuous-glucose-monitor-cgm

Rodriguez-Gutierrez, R., Gionfriddo, M. R., Ospina, N. S., Maraka, S., Tamhane, S., Montori, V. M. & Brito, J. P. (2016) Shared decision-making in endocrinology: present and future directions. *The Lancet Diabetes & Endocrinology.* 4(8): 706–716. doi:https://doi.org/10.1016/S2213-8587(15)00468-4

Royal Australian College of General Practitioners (RACGP). (2016) *General practice management of type 2 diabetes: 2016–18.* East Melbourne, Vic.

Shepherd, A. (2011) Measuring and managing fluid balance. *Nursing Times.* 107(28): 12–16.

State Government of Victoria Department of Health & Human Services. (2020) *Patient-centred care explained. Better Health.* www.betterhealth.vic.gov.au/health/ServicesAndSupport/patient-centred-care-explained#bhc-content

Tortora, G. J. & Derrickson, B. (2011) *Principles of Anatomy and Physiology.* Wiley Blackwell.

UK Prospective Diabetes Study Group. (1998) Tight blood pressure control and risk of macrovascular and microvascular complications in type 2 diabetes: UKPDS 38. *British Medical Journal.* 317: 703–713.

ACKNOWLEDGEMENTS

Figure 17.2: © John D. Carmichael, Overview of the Pituitary Gland.

Figure 17.6: © Garna Zarina / Shutterstock.com

Figure 17.10: © Sick Day Management for Patients on Glucocorticoid Therapy, Adrenal Insufficiency Advice for Patients & Doctors. Endocrine Society of Australia. https://www.hormones-australia.org.au/wp-content/uploads/2020/11/Sick-Day-Management-Plan-FINAL-fillable.pdf

Figure 17.12: © The Australian Type 2 Diabetes Risk Assessment Tool (AUSDRISK), Department of Health, Commonwealth of Australia.

Figure 17.13: © General practice management of type 2 diabetes 2016–18, RACGP.

Figure 17.14: © Management of type 2 diabetes: A handbook for general practice, RACGP.

Figure 17.15: © Amy Hess Fischl, "What Is a Continuous Glucose Monitor (CGM)?". © Remedy Health Media, LLC. Reproduced with permission of Remedy Health Media, LLC.

Figure 17.16: © Australian Type 2 Diabetes Management Algorithm, © Australian Diabetes Society. Reproduced with permission of Australian Diabetes Society.

Figure 17.17: © National Health and Medical Research Council, https://www.eatforhealth.gov.au/guidelines/australian-guide-healthy-eating. Reproduced with permission.

Photo 17A: © Kathy deWitt / Alamy Stock Photo

CHAPTER 18

Nursing care of conditions related to the neurological system

LEARNING OBJECTIVES

After studying this chapter, you should be able to:

18.1 describe the anatomy and physiology of the neurological system

18.2 discuss the components of a neurological assessment

18.3 list important investigations required to diagnose neurological conditions

18.4 discuss the pathophysiology, treatment and management of neurological conditions.

Introduction

The nervous system is one of the most complex body systems, controlling and integrating all other body systems. An understanding of this complex system underpins many aspects of patient care. This chapter includes an overview of the central and peripheral nervous systems' anatomy and physiology and appropriate management plans for key neurological disorders.

18.1 The anatomy and physiology of the neurological system

LEARNING OBJECTIVE 18.1 Describe the anatomy and physiology of the neurological system.

This system receives and processes information and initiates actions through an intricate network of specialised cells called neurons (nerves). It regulates, controls and coordinates the actions and activities of all body systems, thereby maintaining homeostasis. The nervous system has two parts:

- the central nervous system (CNS) — the brain and spinal cord
- the peripheral nervous system (PNS) — the cranial and spinal neurons.

The PNS refers to neurons outside the CNS and consists of the somatic and autonomic nervous systems, which can be subdivided into sympathetic and parasympathetic (figure 18.1).

FIGURE 18.1 Divisions of the human nervous system

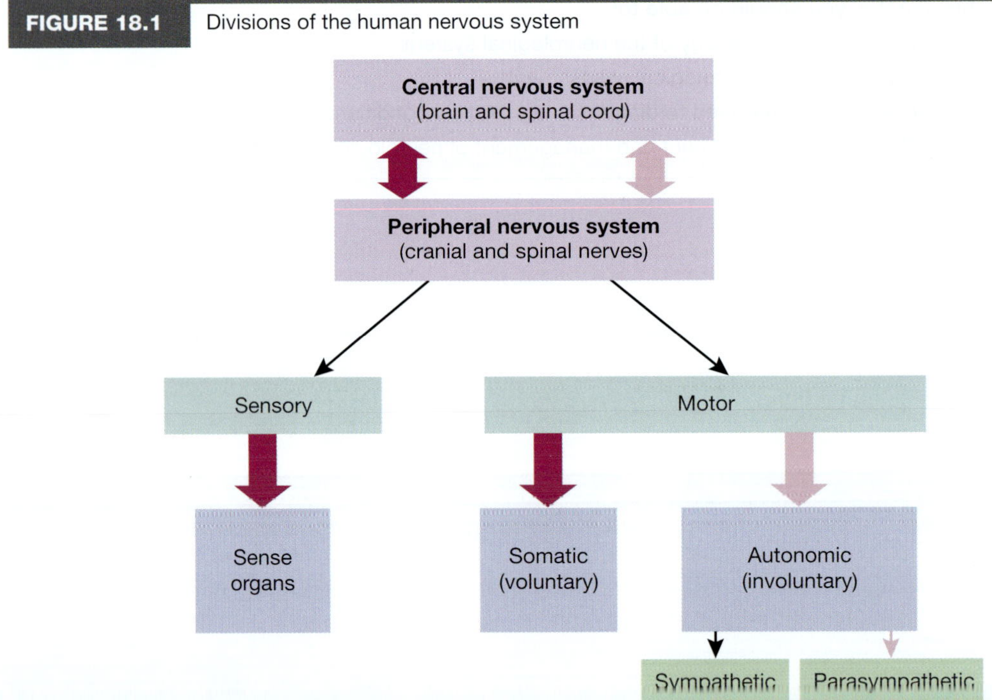

Source: Nair & Peate (2009) *Fundamentals of Applied Pathophysiology*, with kind permission from Wiley Blackwell.

The cells

The cells of the neurological system are:

- the neuroglia (glia), which support, nourish and protect the neurons (table 18.1)
- the neurons (nerves) communicate with and are connected to other neurons and cells in the body (table 18.2 and figure 18.2).

Impulses or action potentials are received by the dendrites and cell bodies of one neuron and transmitted in a firing pattern, via the axon, to the next neuron. Action potentials are responsible for the release of neurotransmitters at the synapse. Axons can be myelinated or unmyelinated.

The different types, locations and functions of neurons are outlined in table 18.3. Neuronal cell bodies, found in groups in the CNS called nuclei, make up the grey matter. Elsewhere in the body, these groups are called ganglia. The axons of the cell groups form the white matter.

TABLE 18.1	Neuroglia		
Neuroglia	**Description**	**Function**	**Location**
Polydendrocytes	Recently discovered	Are the stem cells of the CNS Generate both glia and neurons	CNS
Macroglia	Astrocytes: • Are star-shaped • Have many processes • Are the biggest, most numerous glia • Can be reactive • Are known as astroglia when clumped together	Fill the spaces between the neurons (supportive role) Regulate extracellular chemicals and ions Transport glucose and other substances from the blood Reactive astrocytes together with microglia respond to injury	CNS
	Oligodendroglia: • The cytoplasm and nucleus are denser than in astrocytes • Have smaller and fewer processes than astrocytes	Provide support to axons Produce myelin/myelin sheath to insulate the axons	CNS and PNS
	Schwann cells — the equivalent of oligodendrocytes in the PNS	As above Also facilitate neuronal regeneration after injury	PNS
Microglia	Are small round cells Have many processes and little cytoplasm Are resting or active/reactive	Have a phagocytic macrophage function in response to injury or invasion of pathogens	CNS
Ependymal cells	Line the ventricles and central canal of the spinal cord	Are involved with the directional flow of cerebrospinal fluid, which facilitates the transport of nutrients and removal of waste	CNS

TABLE 18.2	Neuronal components	
Component of neuron	**Description**	**Function**
Cell body (perikaryon)	The enlarged portion of the nerve cell from which the dendrites and axon extend Is greyish in colour	The nucleus produces all neurotransmitters, hormones and proteins
Dendrites	Are hair-like structures or processes Extend from the cell body The ends have synaptic knobs	Conduct incoming signals Synaptic knobs form connections with adjacent neurons
Axon (nerve fibre)	Extends from the cell body The length varies (millimetre to metre) Has processes or branches at its end	Conducts outgoing signals
Schwann cell	See table 18.1	
Myelin sheath	A fat-like sheath Composed of a complex mix of protein and phospholipids (fat)Is white in colour	Surrounds and protects the axon Acts as an insulator Increases the rate of impulse transmission
Nodes of Ranvier	Gaps occurring at regular intervals in the myelin sheath that surrounds the axon	Assist impulse transmission through repolarisation and depolarisation of the nerve membrane Allow entry of nutrients Allow exit of waste
Synapse	The small gap between the axon of one cell and the dendrite of another	Releases neurotransmitters, such as acetylcholine or dopamine

FIGURE 18.2 (a) Parts of a neuron. (b) Motor neuron. LM, light microscope

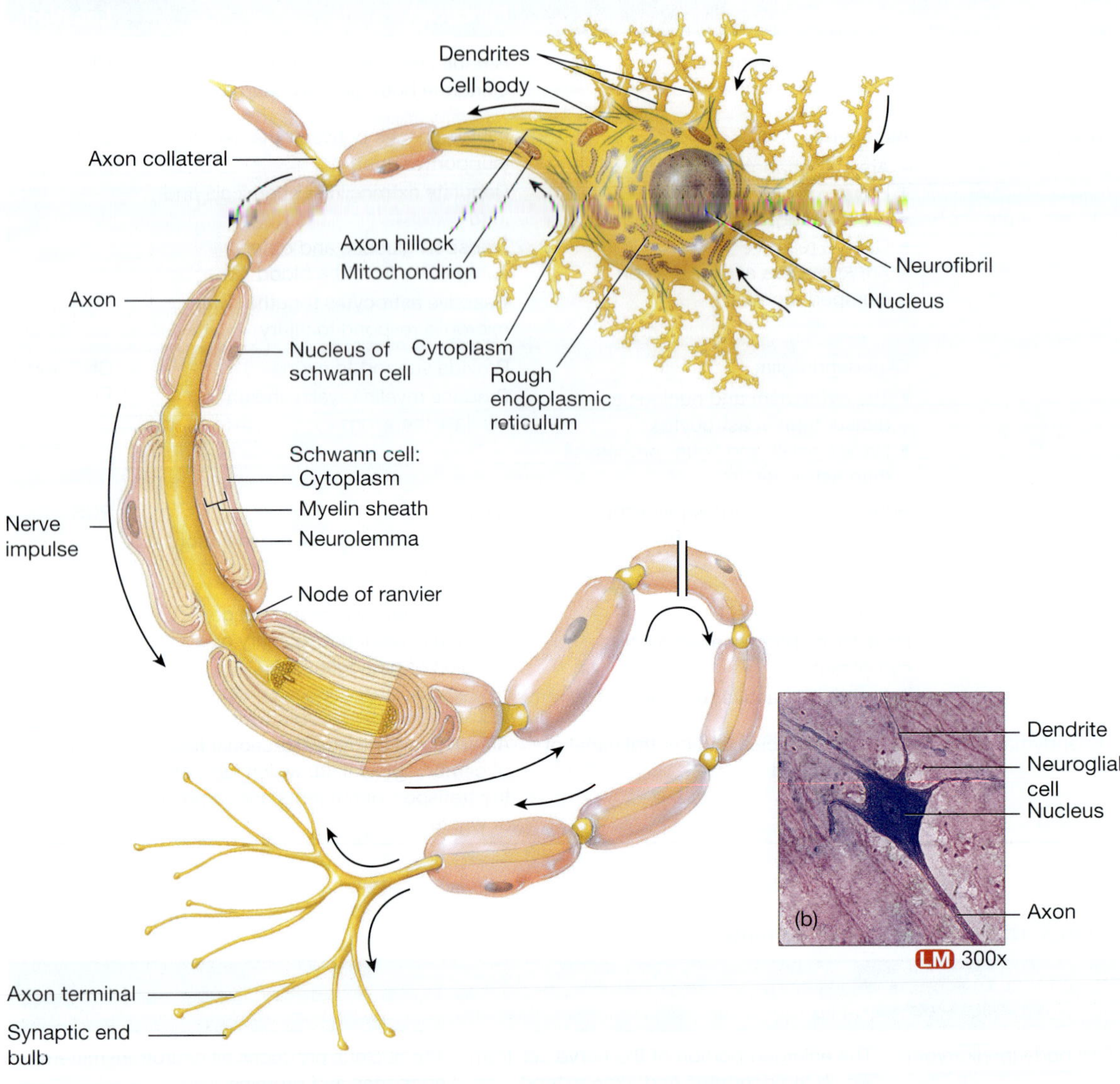

Source: Tortora & Derrickson (2011) *Principles of Anatomy and Physiology*, with kind permission of Wiley Blackwell.

TABLE 18.3 Types of neuron

Type	Location	Function
Motor (efferent)	CNS and PNS Originate in the brainstem and spinal cord	Controlled by the motor areas of the brainstem and the cerebral cortex, and influenced by the basal ganglia and cerebellum Transmit impulses from the CNS to muscles and glands within the body
Sensory (afferent)	PNS and CNS Originate in the sensory organs	Transmit impulses from the sensory organs and other parts to the CNS These are processed by relay nuclei, including the thalamus, before being analysed by the cortex
Mixed	PNS and CNS Include most large nerves, e.g. the brachial and spinal nerves	Consist of both sensory and motor nerves
Relay	CNS	Transmit impulses generated by stimuli to other neurons within the CNS

The brain

The brain consists of over 100 billion neurons, accounts for 2 per cent of body mass and in adults, weighs approximately 1.3–1.5 kilograms. The main divisions of the brain are outlined in figure 18.3 and table 18.4.

FIGURE 18.3 The four main parts of the human brain

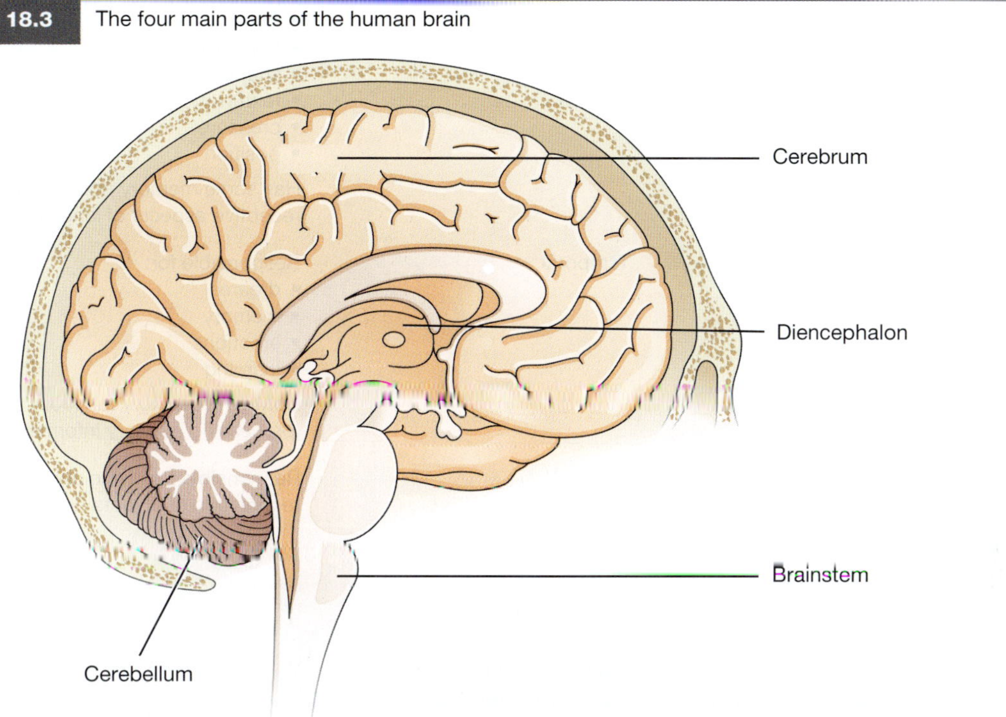

Source: Nair & Peate (2009) *Fundamentals of Applied Pathophysiology*, with kind permission from Wiley Blackwell.

TABLE 18.4 The brain

Main division	Lobe	Function
Cerebrum The largest division Is divided into the right and left cerebral hemispheres The two hemispheres: • are 'twins' • are connected by the corpus callosum • receive sensory (afferent) impulses • initiate motor (efferent) impulses • are made up of grey matter (outside) and white matter (inside) • are subdivided into four further lobes The left lobe of the cerebrum sends and receives information from the right side of the body The right lobe sends and receives information from the left side of the body Contains the basal ganglia	Frontal	Controls fine movements and smell Is the centre for abstract thinking and judgement In the left hemisphere, incorporates the language centre for expressive and motor speech

(continued)

TABLE 18.4 *(continued)*

Main division	Lobe	Function
	Parietal	Coordinates sensory information (spatial orientation and perception) Deals with: • pain • form • temperature • shape • texture • pressure • position Has some memory function (in the receptive aspects of language)
	Temporal	Responsible for: • dreams • memory • emotions • learning Centre for auditory function (processing auditory information)
	Occipital	Responsible for vision and the recognition of objects
Cerebellum The second largest division Is found below the cerebrum Is composed of two hemispheres Has an outer cortex of grey matter Receives and sends impulses via the brainstem Incoming information is received from the cortex via the pons Outgoing information goes to the cortex via the thalamus	Balance Muscle tension Fine motor control Eye movement Equilibrium of the trunk Spinal nerve reflexes Posture and balance of the limbs	
Main division	**Structure**	**Function**
Diencephalon Located between the cerebrum and the midbrain Contains two important structures: • Thalamus • Hypothalamus	Thalamus: • An egg-shaped mass of grey matter • Divided into right and left parts	Is the main synaptic relay centre and processes motor information; acts as the 'gatekeeper' to the cerebral cortex Receives and relays sensory information to and from the cerebral cortex
	Hypothalamus: • A collection of ganglia • Is located below the thalamus • Is closely associated with the pituitary gland	Senses change in body temperature Regulates sympathetic and parasympathetic nervous systems Controls the pituitary gland Regulates appetite Is part of the arousal/alerting mechanism
Brainstem Consists of: • Medulla oblongata • Pons • Midbrain (mesencephalon or cerebral peduncles) The medulla is the most important All functions of the brainstem are associated with cranial nerves III–XII	Medulla and pons Medulla Midbrain and pons	Breathing, respiration Heart rate, blood pressure, vomiting coughing, swallowing, hiccupping, sneezing Reflex centres for the pupils and eye movements

Blood supply

The main arteries supplying the brain (figure 18.4) are:

- two internal carotid arteries
- two vertebral arteries, which join to become the basilar artery.

  Both sets of arteries give rise to the arteries that form the circle of Willis (figure 18.5).

FIGURE 18.4 The arteries supplying the brain

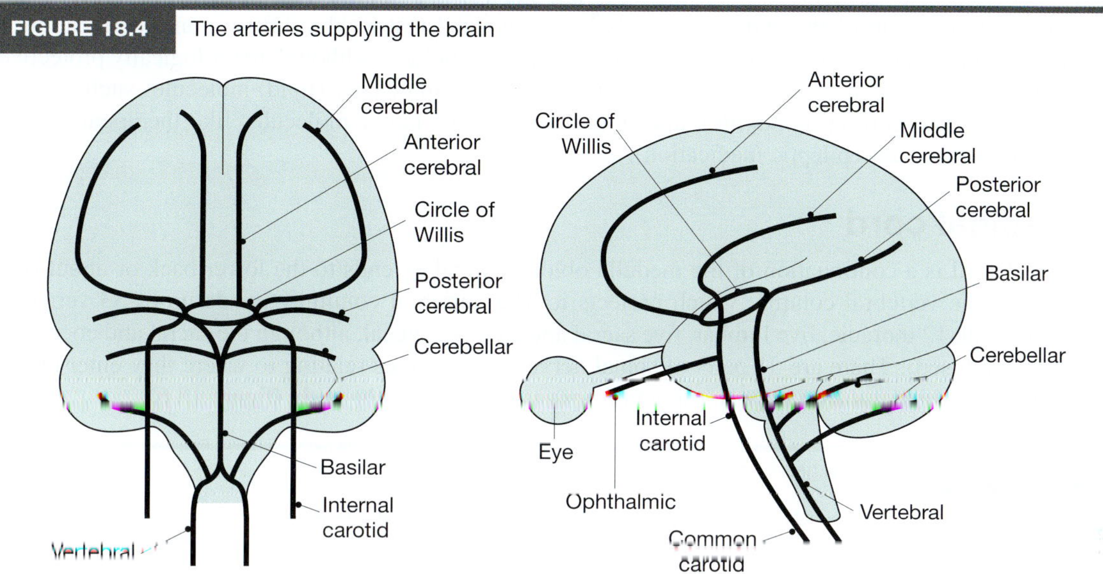

Source: Wilkinson & Lennox (2005) *Essential Neurology*, with kind permission of Wiley Blackwell.

FIGURE 18.5 The circle of Willis

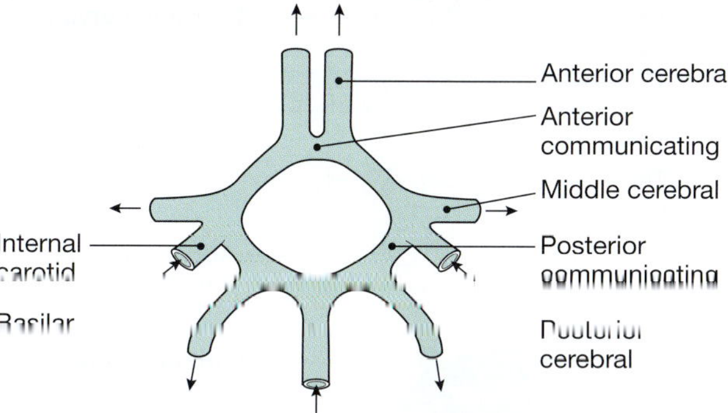

Source: Wilkinson & Lennox (2005) *Essential Neurology*, with kind permission of Wiley Blackwell.

The coverings of the brain and spinal cord

The brain and spinal cord are covered by three membranes (the meninges):

1. *the dura mater* — the thick outer fibrous membrane, which has two layers and contains large venous sinuses
2. *the arachnoid mater* — the middle thin avascular membrane, which is covered with mesothelial cells and has arachnoid villi or granulations that project into the venous sinuses and veins
3. *the pia mater* — the thin inner fibrous membrane, which is attached to the surface of the brain and the spinal cord. It is connected to the arachnoid mater by delicate fibrous trabeculae.

Cerebrospinal fluid

About 400–500 millilitres of cerebrospinal fluid (CSF) is produced each day by specialised ependymal cells in the choroid plexus of the brain. The CSF is clear and colourless and flows in the subarachnoid space (between the arachnoid and the pia) in a unidirectional flow. Its functions are to:

- remove waste and potentially noxious substances such as drugs

- lubricate the meninges and provide frictionless movement of the brain
- cushion and protect against impact injury.

The blood–brain/CSF barrier

The blood–brain barrier (BBB) and the CSF barrier act to regulate the exchange of substances entering the brain to maintain optimum levels of, for example, glucose, proteins and electrolytes for normal brain activities. The function of the endothelial cells is to filter and restrict the diffusion and permeation of molecules to protect the brain against harmful toxins and metabolites. Although neurologically protective, it can be a hindrance as it allows, for example, the entry of small or fatty (lipid) molecules such as some viruses and toxins (carbon monoxide), and limits the entry of larger molecules like therapeutic drugs (e.g. antibiotics and antiepileptic medication).

The spinal cord

The spinal cord is a continuation of the medulla oblongata and extends to the lower back or about two-thirds down the vertebral column, which protects it. The vertebral column is made up of 33 vertebrae (seven cervical, 12 thoracic, five lumbar, five sacral and four coccygeal, although the sacral and coccygeal vertebrae are fused). There are 31 pairs of spinal nerves (their names relating to where they enter or exit the vertebrae), which transmit impulses to and from various parts of the body (figure 18.6).

FIGURE 18.6 The spinal nerves and their areas of innervations

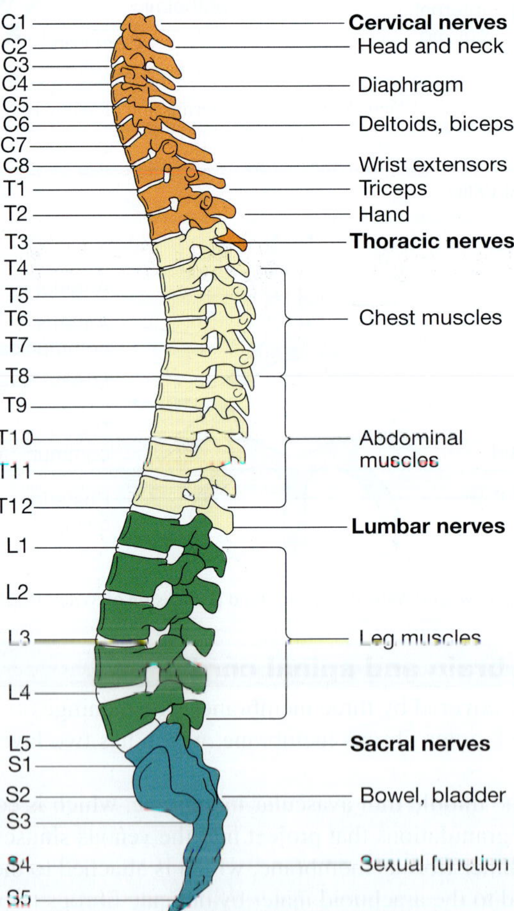

Source: Woodward & Mestecky (2011) *Neuroscience Nursing: Evidence Based Practice*, with kind permission of Wiley Blackwell.

The cranial neurons

There are 12 pairs of cranial nerves (I–XII), the majority of their functions relating to structures within the head and neck; however, the functions of three cranial nerves extend beyond these areas (table 18.5).

TABLE 18.5 Cranial nerves (type and function)

Number	Name	Motor (M) or sensory (S)	Function
I	Olfactory	S	Sense of smell
II	Optic	S	Sensory function of the retina
*III	Oculomotor		Most eye movements Pupillary constriction
*IV	Trochlear	Mainly M with some S	Downward and inward eye movements
*VI	**Abducen**		Lateral eye movements
V	Trigeminal (has three branches): • Ophthalmic • Maxillary • Mandibular	M, S	Cornea Face Mouth Jaw
VII	Facial	M, S	Facial muscles Lacrimal glands Salivary glands Taste
VIII	Known as: • Acoustic • Auditory, or • Vestibulocochlear	M, S	Hearing Equilibrium Balance Body position Orientation to space
IX	Glossopharyngeal	M, S	Coordination of swallowing Sensation in the pharynx Taste Salivation
X	Vagus	M, S	Controls swallowing, phonation and movement of the soft palate and uvula Sensation of the mucosa of the pharynx, soft palate, tonsils, viscera of the thorax and abdomen Smooth muscles of the thorax and abdomen
XI	Spinal accessory	M, S	Sternocleidomastoid muscles Upper trapezius Palate and pharyngeal muscles
XII	Hypoglossal	M, S	Tongue movement in swallowing and speech

*These three neurons are usually grouped together because they are concerned with eye movement.

18.2 Nursing assessment of the neurological system

LEARNING OBJECTIVE 18.2 Discuss the components of a neurological assessment.

Neurological assessment evaluates the mental status, cranial nerve function, motor system, sensory system, reflexes, etc. This should start by collecting detailed history from the patients. Sometimes it would be necessary to collect history from the family members as the clients may be confused or unconscious. Ask the client about medications (anti-depressants, sedatives), drug (cocaine, heroin) and alcohol use, toxin exposure, past neurological symptoms (syncope, seizures, tremors, dizziness, vertigo), numbness or tingling, difficulty swallowing, difficulty speaking, head injury and falls as part of history collection. Subtle observations during history collection could provide a general impression about anxiety, depression, hypochondriasis, memory, language comprehension and behaviour (Lowenstein, Martin & Hauser 2018).

For a conscious client, neurological assessment begins as soon as the client enters the room. Level of consciousness is the most important parameter to detect neurological deterioration. Arousal and awareness are the fundamental constituents of consciousness. Arousal is by evaluating the patient's ability to respond to a variety of stimuli, and AVPU is a common acronym used for this assessment. A stands for alert, where the patient is alert without the need for any stimuli. V, if the patient responds to voice or light touch. P, if the patient responds only to painful stimuli (sternal rub, trapezius pinch, suborbital pressure). U iss for unresponsive.

If arousable, then a detailed assessment of awareness using the Glasgow Coma Scale is conducted. Awareness means the patient can interact with and interpret their environment.

Glasgow Coma Scale

The **Glasgow Coma Scale (GCS)** is an assessment instrument extensively used to assess the depth and duration of impaired consciousness and **coma**, awareness and arousability (Teasdale & Jennett 1974).

Damage to or a lesion in the cerebral hemisphere impairs its function so that it is unable to respond to afferent stimuli. Damage in the brainstem affects the structures there and limits or stops the access of afferent neurons to the cerebral hemispheres. Impaired pupillary reactions to light and pupillary dilatation may indicate damage or a lesion in the midbrain. The GCS assessment (figure 18.7) provides a framework for eliciting information on the following.

FIGURE 18.7 Documentation of the GCS

Neurological observation chart																			
Glasgow Coma Scale	Eye opening	Open spontaneously (4)	•																(C) = Eyes closed due to swelling
		Open to speech (3)		•	•														
		Open to pain (2)				•	•												
		Closed (1)						•	•	•									
	Verbal response	Orientated (5)																	(T) = intubated
		Confused (4)	•	•	•														
		Inappropriate words (3)				•	•												
		Incomprehensible sounds (2)						•	•										
		No verbal response (1)								•									
	Motor response	Obeys commands (6)	•	•															Record best arm response
		Localises to pain (5)			•														
		Flexion withdrawal (4)				•	•												
		Abnormal flexion (3)						•											
		Extension to pain (2)							•										
		No movement (1)								•									
		Total (out of 15)	14	13	12	9	9	6	5	3									

Source: Woodward & Mestecky (2011) *Neuroscience Nursing: Evidence Based Practice*, with kind permission of Wiley Blackwell.

The GCS score

The score is used as an indication of neurological status and to monitor any changes effectively. The maximum score of 15 indicates that patients are fully conscious, alert and responsive. The minimum score of 3 indicates comatose and unresponsive patients. Scores may also be affected for other reasons.

The first part is to check the patient's eye-opening (E). This parameter assesses arousal ability or wakefulness. Points range from 1 to 4. If the patient's eyes are already open, or the patient opens their eyes without stimulation, then the score is 4. The lowest score of 1 is given if there is no eye-opening, even with painful stimuli. If the patient opens their eyes to verbal stimuli, a score of 3 is given, and 2 is given for opening eyes to painful stimuli. Patients may sometimes be unable to open their eyes due to peri-orbital oedema. The letter C is sometimes used in such situations against the lowest score.

The second part is to check verbal response (V). This measures the appropriateness of speech and awareness. It has a score ranging from 1 to 5. A maximum score of 5 is given when the patient responds appropriately and is orientated to person, place and time. If the patient is confused and disorientated to person, place and/or time, a score of 4 is given. A score of 3 is given when the patient uses words or phrases but makes little or no sense. If the patient can only make unintelligible sounds, moaning or groaning, a score of 2 is allocated. If the patient does not make any sound or speech, the lowest score of 1 is given.

The third parameter in GCS is to assess the patient's motor response. This parameter is used for overall awareness and ability to respond to external stimuli. A score of 6 is given if the patient obeys commands. The patient receives a score of 5 if the patient can bring their hand (above the nipple line) when painful stimuli are applied to the trapezius muscle (localising to pain). If the patient moves the body away from the source of pain, a score of 4 is given. If there is flexion of the elbow with painful stimuli, 3 is given. A score of 2 is given when there is an extension to pain. This is assessed by observing for extension of the elbow and internal rotation of the wrist in response to pain. The verbal and motor responses may be absent or reduced due to intubation, muscle relaxants or sedation.

Frequent GCS assessment (every 30 minutes) is needed for head injury patients depending on hospital policy. A similar or modified version of this approach could be used for other neurological conditions, after anaesthesia or neurosurgery, as well as with paediatric patients (see figure 18.8 for a modified version of the GCS used in paediatric patients). Staff using the GCS should be adequately trained and have the necessary skills and experience to recognise changes. Individual components of the assessment should be adequately described and communicated, both verbally and in writing. For example, patients with a total score of 13 (4 for eye-opening, 4 for verbal response and 5 for motor response) should be reported as E4, V4 and M5.

A limb strength assessment commonly follows the GCS. The strength of each limb should be assessed separately, moving from upper to lower limbs.

FIGURE 18.8 Paediatric Glasgow Coma Scale

	Response	Score
Eyes opening	Spontaneously	4
	To verbal stimuli	3
	To pain	2
	No response to pain	1
Motor response	Obeys verbal commands or performs normal spontaneous movements	6
	Localises to pain or withdraws to touch	5
	Withdraws from pain	4
	Abnormal flexion to pain (decorticate)	3
	Abnormal extension to pain (decerebrate)	2
	No response to pain	1
Verbal response	Alert, babbles, coos, words or sentences to usual ability	5
	Less than usual words and or spontaneous irritable cry	4
	Cries inappropriately to pain	3
	Occasionally whimpers and or moans	2
	No vocal response	1

Source: Aitken, Marshall & Chaboyer (2013).

Pupillary response assessment

This is done by shining fine light using a penlight torch from the side of each eye and noting the pupil's response. This must be done in a dark or dimly lit room. The eyes are assessed for size, equality, reaction to light and consensuality of pupil reaction (pupil reaction on the right eye when shining light on the left eye and vice versa). Document the size of the pupil before the penlight is directed into the eye. Pupils normally constrict and return to their original size in response to the light. PERRLA (pupils, equal, round, react to light and accommodation) or PEARL (pupils, equal and reacting to light) are some of the common acronyms used for documentation. Pupillary reaction is recorded as + or – or SL next to the size. + is recorded when there is a reaction, – is recorded when there is no reaction. SL is recorded if the pupil has constricted but took slightly longer. No reaction to light must be reported to a physician immediately.

Vital signs

Abnormal vital signs indicate problems in the pons and/or medulla. An increase in temperature, pulse, respiration and blood pressure denotes autonomic dysregulation. The initial measurements of respiration, blood pressure, temperature and pulse will form the baseline for monitoring and assessing deterioration or improvement.

The rate, depth and pattern of respiration should be closely observed. Shallow, rapid respirations, low blood pressure and tachycardia may result from a reduced circulating volume following surgery or injury. If patients require oxygen, their oxygen saturation should be maintained to avoid hypoxia, which leads to reduced cerebral blood flow (CBF). If blood flow to any part of the brain is reduced, the following can occur:

- ischaemia
- a reversible loss of function
- if it is prolonged and/or severe, infarction and irreversible cell death.

Ischaemic brain damage with swelling results from a combination of hypotension and hypoxia. A one degree increase in temperature increases the cerebral metabolic rate by 10 per cent, which can affect neurological recovery. Hence, pyrexia should be treated, and temperature should be kept within normal range.

Mini-mental state examination (MMSE)

A mini-mental state examination (MMSE) is a standardised screening examination of cognitive function and is widely used in healthcare settings. An MMSE is a 30-point test of cognitive function, with each correct point being scored as 1 point. It includes tests in the areas of orientation, memory, speech, language, insight, judgement, calculation and ability.

The ABCDE assessment

The mnemonic ABCDE is used to prioritise the initial treatment of neurological disorders.

- **A**irway — intubation may be required for patients with severe traumatic brain injury and those with a Glasgow Coma Score of <8.
- **B**reathing — maintain oxygenation and normocapnia.
- **C**irculation:
  - measure the heart rate and blood pressure
  - treat hypotension, aiming for a target mean arterial pressure (MAP) of over 80 mmHg.
- **D**isability — GCS assessment to detect changes in level of consciousness and assess the severity of the impairment.
- **E**xposure and environment — look for signs of injury, e.g. scalp wounds.

18.3 Investigations for the neurological system

LEARNING OBJECTIVE 18.3 List important investigations required to diagnose neurological conditions.

Following physical and neurological examinations, a number of diagnostic tests may be ordered to investigate any abnormal findings. The least invasive procedures are normally carried out first, proceeding to more invasive investigations. These investigations can be anxiety provoking for both patients and their families. Nurses need to provide emotional support to patients by educating them on the procedure and appropriate nursing care before, during and after the procedure.

Radiological examinations

Radiological examinations include:

- skull and spine X-rays, used to identify:
  - fractures
  - displacement of the vertebrae
  - spinal curves
  - tissue displacement
- CT scans (may require an injection of contrast medium prior to the scan to provide anatomical clarity, however, no additional nursing preparation is needed; close observation is not required unless patients' consciousness is impaired)
- MRI.

Cerebral blood flow tests

These can be non-invasive or invasive procedures and are used to visualise blood vessels in the brain and neck, and include:

- magnetic resonance angiography (MRA) — performed with or without the injection of **contrast medium**
- CT angiography (CTA) — involves the injection of contrast medium via a peripheral cannula followed by a series of images of the cerebral vessels being taken.

Cerebral angiography is an invasive procedure, undertaken with or without sedation, that involves the injection of contrast medium, usually via catheterisation of the femoral artery. Patients may need to be nil by mouth for a period before the procedure. Specific nursing considerations include:

- regular neurological observations including vital signs, both before and after the procedure
- assessment of the puncture site for haemorrhage and haematoma
- bed rest, usually for four hours after the procedure.

Neurophysiology tests

Clinical neurophysiologists usually perform neurophysiology tests, such as nerve conduction studies, electromyograms (EMGs), evoked potentials (EPs) and **electroencephalograms (EEGs)**.

- EMG and nerve conduction studies test the integrity and functioning of the skeletal muscles and large myelinated nerve fibres in the arms and legs.
- EPs measure the brain's response to particular stimuli; for example, visually evoked potentials measure the visual pathway from the retina to the occipital cortex.
- EEGs are used to measure the electrical activity of the brain.
- Lumbar puncture:
  - used to measure CSF pressure and obtain a sample of CSF by inserting a spinal needle into the subarachnoid space of the spinal canal, usually between the L3–L4 or L4–L5 vertebrae, once a local anaesthetic has taken effect
  - is normally performed at the patient's bed, with the patient lying on their left side with their knees drawn up to their chest
  - involves observations being recorded after the procedure
  - involves patients being encouraged to rest and drink plenty of fluids.
- A muscle biopsy is indicated if the integrity of the muscle unit is disrupted.

18.4 The pathophysiology of neurological conditions

LEARNING OBJECTIVE 18.4 Discuss the pathophysiology of neurological conditions.

Traumatic brain injury

Traumatic brain injury (TBI) or head injury refers to any injury to the scalp, skull (cranium or facial bones) or brain that disrupts the brain's function. The leading causes of TBI are falls, road traffic accidents and assaults. TBI in young people is a major ethical and social burden with regard to long-term disability and socioeconomic costs. The magnitude, duration and orientation of the force applied to the cranium significantly impact the nature of the resulting lesion (Mesfin, Gupta, Hays Shapshak & Taylor 2020). TBI can be classified according to the mechanism of injury, the morphology of the injury or clinical severity. Investigations to establish the morphology and severity of TBI include MRI and CT scans.

- An open (penetrating) head injury occurs when the outer layer of the meninges is breached (e.g. by a knife or bullet).
- A closed head injury is one that occurs without the integrity of the skull being compromised (Temporary alteration in consciousness related to a closed head injury in the presence of a normal head CT scan is commonly called concussion) (Mesfin, Gupta, Hays Shapshak & Taylor 2020).

When TBI occurs at the site of impact, it is referred as a coup injury. Contre coup occurs opposite the initial impact site and is often referred to as a contrecoup injury (Mesfin, Gupta, Hays Shapshak & Taylor 2020). TBI can also be divided into primary and secondary injuries. Primary injury occurs at the time of impact whereas secondary injury develops later in response to the primary injury. Primary injuries mainly include:

- acceleration injury — the head is struck by a moving object
- deceleration injury — the head hits a stationary object

- acceleration–deceleration injury — the head hits an object, and the brain 'rebounds' within the skull
- injuries to the brain including concussion, contusion and diffuse axonal injury
- intracranial haemorrhage, including haematomas; this can be extradural, subdural or intracerebral
- injuries to the skull (including fractures).

Secondary injuries include:

- occurring after the initial injury as a result of progression events, which affect the perfusion and oxygenation of the brain cells
- most commonly occurs due to brain swelling, with an increase in intracranial pressure (ICP).

Symptoms of raised ICP include:

- altered mental status
- a progressive deterioration in consciousness
- nausea and vomiting, usually in the morning, with an accompanying headache
- headache that is often worse on waking in the morning (due to lying flat and the ICP typically increasing at night), and worse on coughing or moving the head
- restlessness, weakness and incoordination
- pupillary changes, including irregularity, i.e. changes in pupil size or dilatation in one eye with impaired reactivity to light, a sluggish pupillary reaction to direct light or no response.

Other late signs of increased ICP include 'Cushing's response' (hypertension, a widening pulse pressure, bradycardia and irregular respiration), papilloedema (optic disc swelling) and fundal haemorrhage.

If the raised ICP is left untreated, a decrease in cerebral perfusion leads to ischaemia. The ability to cope with an increase in ICP differs from person to person and ultimately depends on the compliance of the brain tissue.

Monro-Kellie doctrine is frequently used to describe the volume and pressure relationship when discussing ICP management. According to Monro-Kellie doctrine, the skull is rigid, and the brain, cerebrospinal fluid and blood are the incompressible structures within it. Careful equilibrium exists between the structures so that the ICP is maintained within normal range. So, managing ICP requires manipulating the volume of these contents in the intracranial space (in the absence of pathologic mass within the cranium).

Classification of TBI

The classification of TBIs is important in determining treatment and rehabilitation plans and for patient outcomes, including prognosis and long-term disability. TBIs are graded according to their severity (table 18.6), based on several parameters, including:

- duration of loss of consciousness (LOC)
- level of consciousness, as per the GCS, at the time of the injury
- the length of time (after the injury) that the patient remains in a post-traumatic amnesic state, which is a period of confusion and disorientation after emergence from coma.

TABLE 18.6 TBI grading

Grade of TBI	Length of LOC	GCS	Post-traumatic amnesia duration
Mild	<30 minutes	13–15	Less than 24 hours or none
Moderate	1–24 hours	9–12	More than 24 hours — less than seven days
Severe	>24 hours	3–8	1–4 weeks or more

Source: Adapted from Bullock & Hales (2019).

Individualised multidisciplinary care initiated early and continued throughout the patient's journey is critical in maximising recovery and reducing long-term disability. Physical disabilities are varied and depend on the severity and area of injury. Patients may experience:

- language and swallowing problems
- impaired mobility and coordination
- visual and sleep disturbances
- a number of cognitive, behavioural and emotional difficulties.

Care for patients after a TBI should start as early as possible and include:

- individualised rehabilitation interventions aimed at promoting functional recovery
- the prevention and treatment of secondary complications
- control of CBF which is the focus of care strategies and forms the basis of patient management.

Patients who sustain a moderate or severe TBI require close monitoring and medical management strategies aimed at minimising secondary injury. This may require patients to be cared for in intensive care units where they can be closely observed and systematically monitored. Table 18.7 provides detailed information on the nursing management of patients with a TBI and raised ICP.

TABLE 18.7 Nursing management of patients with a TBI and raised ICP

Nursing intervention	Rationale
GCS Monitor neurological status using the GCS. A score of ≤8/15: • is indicative of coma • requires patients to be intubated and ventilated immediately Observe and control any seizure activity	The GCS is the gold standard tool for assessing LOC In sedated, ventilated patients with no ICP monitor, regular pupil checks are crucial as pupillary changes may be the only sign of further neurological deterioration Seizure activity will increase cerebral metabolic rate for oxygen and exacerbate cerebral hypoxia
Respiratory status Observe and monitor respiratory gases and status May be mechanically ventilated to control the partial pressure of oxygen (PO_2) and carbon dioxide (PCO_2) to within set parameters, avoiding hypoxia and hypercapnia Monitor and record pulse oximetry Administer prescribed oxygen The brain accounts for 20% of total body oxygen consumption, and hence it is extremely susceptible to injury from lack of oxygen	Blood oxygen levels regulate CBF Hypoxia — an arterial partial pressure of oxygen (PaO_2) ≤60 mmHg (8 kPa) — will impair autoregulation and increase CBF Hypercapnia ($PaCO_2$ >45 mmHg, or approximately 6 kPa), a potent cerebral vasodilator, can increase CBF and ICP and impair cerebral perfusion Administer prescribed oxygen
Cardiovascular status Maintain MAP sufficiently to maintain a CPP 50–70 mmHg Aim to achieve a target MAP of 90 mmHg until ICP monitoring has been established	Hypotension is associated with decreased CPP
Fluid status Maintain fluid levels to ensure hydration Avoid overhydration and dextrose solutions Monitor and maintain normal blood glucose levels	Overhydration and dextrose solutions can exacerbate cerebral oedema and increase ICP The brain uses glucose for energy; hypoglycaemia will cause neurons to die A high blood glucose level increases cerebral metabolism and oedema, increasing ICP
Nutritional status Maintain nutritional support May require an enteral feeding regimen (nasogastric or percutaneous endoscopic gastrostomy)	Cerebral trauma induces a state of hypermetabolism and hypercatabolism A high-energy, high-protein diet avoids the effects of protein catabolism and loss of lean body mass
Temperature Monitor core temperature Maintain normothermia (36–36.5°C)	Hyperthermia increases brain oxygen and glucose demand, increasing CBF and CPP With each 1°C increase in temperature, cerebral metabolic rate for oxygen increases by 6–9%, and ICP subsequently rises
Mobility Nurse in a head-up position of 30° Maintain the head and neck in a neutral position Minimise physical activity and cluster care activities	A 30° head-up position promotes cerebral venous drainage, optimises CPP and can reduce ICP Positioning patients at more than 90° at the hip when in bed can increase intraabdominal pressure Minimising movement will prevent increased metabolic demand

(continued)

TABLE 18.7 *(continued)*

Nursing intervention	Rationale
Elimination Maintain a normal urine output (0.5 ml/kg per hour) Monitor bowel movements Avoid constipation	Neuroendocrine disturbances can result in diabetes insipidus, leading to severe dehydration and increasing the risk of ischaemia Constipation increases intraabdominal pressure, increasing intrathoracic pressure and increasing ICP
General Minimise sensory stimulation like bright light, loud noise etc. (applicable to critically unwell sedated patients admitted in ICU)	
Families/carers Assess families and carers for coping strategies Involve them in care, as appropriate Prepare them for the potential outcomes of the injury Collaborate with other support services, e.g. a chaplain or support organisations	

Cerebral perfusion pressure (CPP) is another common measurement used in the management of TBI. The pressure gradient drives blood flow to the brain tissue or pressure gradient, which maintains perfusion to the brain. CPP depends on MAP and ICP. This mathematical equation is given below:

$$CPP = MAP - ICP$$

In severe TBI cases, disorders of consciousness can arise and present one of the most challenging conditions of the human brain (table 18.8). Table 18.9 lists non-physical problems associated with TBI.

TABLE 18.8 Disorders of consciousness

Coma (absent wakefulness and absent awareness)	A state of unrousable unresponsiveness, lasting more than six hours in which a person: • is unconscious and unresponsive to the world around them • won't respond to pain, light or sound • lacks a normal sleep-wake cycle • does not initiate voluntary actions (such as coughing or swallowing).
Post-coma unresponsiveness (wakefulness with absent awareness)	A state of wakefulness without awareness in which there is preserved capacity for spontaneous or stimulus-induced arousal, evidenced by sleep-wake cycles and a range of reflexive and spontaneous behaviours. Characterised by an absence of behavioural evidence for self or environmental awareness.
Minimally conscious state (wakefulness with minimal awareness)	A state of severely altered consciousness in which minimal but clearly discernible evidence of self or environmental awareness is demonstrated. Characterised by inconsistent but reproducible responses above the level of spontaneous or reflexive behaviour, which indicate some degree of interaction with their surroundings.

Source: Adapted from Royal College of Physicians (2020).

TABLE 18.9 Non-physical problems associated with TBI

Cognitive	Emotional	Behavioural
Memory	Emotionally labile	Disinhibition
Poor attention and concentration	Depression	Impulsivity
Lack of insight and awareness	Manic features	Apathy

Impaired problem-solving	Anxiety	Restlessness
Poor initiation		Agitation
		Aggression and anger outbursts on a 'short fuse'
		Personality changes — 'not the same person'

Source: Adapted from Agency for Clinical Innovation (2015).

Treatment of TBI

Patients with TBI require constant monitoring of ICP using special devices, and hence they are typically managed in intensive care units. Management focuses on the three main structures within the cranium — CSF, blood and brain. Ventriculostomy may be performed to drain CSF. The next treatment strategy is the manipulation of CBF to bring the ICP to normal range. Removing or loosening devices that may compress the jugular veins, elevating the head of the bed and optimising analgesia and sedation to prevent elevation in intrathoracic or intraabdominal pressures are some of the strategies to promote venous outflow (Mesfin, Gupta, Hays Shapshak & Taylor 2020).

Osmotherapy is a strategy used to minimise cerebral oedema. The plasma's osmolarity in the brain is increased by administering substances such as mannitol and hypertonic saline solution intravenously. This increased osmolarity helps to draw water from the brain tissue. Inducing a pharmacological coma using sedatives to reduce brain metabolism and induce cerebral vasoconstriction is another option to reduce ICP. Cerebral vasoconstriction can also be achieved by inducing systemic respiratory alkalosis using hyperventilation strategies (increasing respiratory rate in mechanical ventilator). Hyperventilation should be used only as a temporary short-term measure to bring down ICP when all the other measures have failed. Prophylactic treatment using antiepileptic is necessary as seizures can exacerbate intracranial hypertension. Most patients require lengthy rehabilitation to return to normal function following TBI.

Intracranial tumours

Intracranial tumours are tumours arising within the cranium; their causes are mostly unknown. Their origin can be primary or secondary (spreading from the lung, breast, kidney, colon or skin [melanoma]).

Brain tumours are usually named after the area where they grow; for example, a tumour of the meninges is called a meningioma. Table 18.10 outlines other examples. Intracranial tumours are classified in terms of their growth rate and are graded accordingly (the more rapidly the tumour grows, the higher the grade), and whether they are benign or malignant (low-grade tumours tending to be benign and high-grade tumours tending to be malignant). Tumours can also be referred to as:

- space-occupying lesions
- localised or focal — a clear distinction between the brain tissue and the tumour can be seen on a scan or during surgery
- diffuse — with no clarity between the tumour and the tissue.

TABLE 18.10 Examples of CNS tumours

Tumour name	Where it develops from	Rate of growth	Benign (B) or malignant (M)	Spread	Who is affected
Gliomas Astrocytomas including glioblastoma multiforme (GBM) • The most common type • Graded 1 to 4, e.g. GBM grade 4, anaplastic **astrocytoma** grade 3	Astrocytes	Slower fast Higher low grade	M	To other parts of the brain	Adults Children

(continued)

TABLE 18.10 *(continued)*

Tumour name	Where it develops from	Rate of growth	Benign (B) or malignant (M)	Spread	Who is affected
Oligodendrogliomas • Often found in the frontal and temporal lobes	Oligodendrocytes	Slower fast	M	Within the CNS via the CSF	Mostly adults Can occur in children
Acoustic neuromas May grow for a long time before being diagnosed Associated with the genetic condition neurofibromatosis type 2If genetic, is more likely to occur in younger people Can be bilateral May develop menin-giomas	Acoustic nerve	Slow growing	B	Do not spread	Mainly older people
Hemangioblastomas Can grow in the brainstem Difficult to treat Can be part of another syndrome called von Hippel–Lindau syndrome (which runs in families)	Grow from blood vessel cells	Slow growing	Behave differently in different people	Do not spread	Can affect any age, but mainly occur in middle-aged adults
Pituitary tumours Or pituitary adenomas	Pituitary gland tissue	Slow growing	B	Do not spread	Mainly adults
Primitive neuroectodermal tumours The most common type is the medulloblastoma Grow in the cerebellum	Develop from cells left over from early development in the womb that become cancerous	Fast growing	M	Within the CNS via the CSF	Children and young adults
Primary cerebral lymphomas Can originate elsewhere Most are a type called diffuse large B cell non-Hodgkin's lymphoma	Lymphocytes	Fast growing	M	One or more tumours may occur in the CNS	Affect anyone with poor immunity due to AIDS or medications after organ transplant
Meningiomas Atypical meningiomas: • Grow more aggres-sively than normal meningiomas • Grow into the brain tissue • Recur after surgery	Meninges	Slow growing	Usually benign		More common in older people and in women
Germ cell tumours Commonly occur in the pineal and suprasellar areas	Primitive developing cells in the embryo that develop into the reproductive system	Slow or fast growing	B or M	Dependent on cell type	Young adults

Spinal cord

Meningiomas and neurofibromas:

- Are most common in adults
- Grow outside the spinal cord

Astrocytomas and ependymomas:

- Astrocytomas are most common in children; ependymomas are most common in adults
- Grow in the spinal cord tissue

There are often exceptions to brain tumours' general rules; for example, benign tumours are sometimes treated with radiotherapy and chemotherapy. Irrespective of whether a tumour is benign or malignant, it can be life-threatening or cause severe deficits depending on its location. One such area is the brainstem, which controls the vital signs, so any pressure from a tumour, for example, on the respiratory centre, could result in a respiratory arrest. It is often not possible to remove tumours from delicate areas as this may cause more disability or even death. High doses of radiotherapy are also not recommended if these will cause more damage to the surrounding area.

Investigations for the diagnosis of intracranial tumours include:

- blood tests; for example, germ cell tumours produce chemicals that can be detected in the blood
- CT and MRI scans of the brain
- biopsy
- laboratory tests, including:
  - haematoxylin and eosin staining
  - immunohistochemical staining (to determine the type and proliferation of the tumour cells)
- radiotherapy
- chemotherapy
- surgical resection.

Treatment of intracranial tumours

Treatment of intracranial tumours will be dependent on the location of the tumour.

Tumour treating fields (used in the treatment of **glioblastoma**) are battery-powered, insulated electromagnetic transducers placed on the scalp and deliver alternating, low-intensity, intermediate-frequency electric fields that aim to disrupt cell division and inhibit tumour growth (Hottinger, Pacheco & Stupp 2016).

Some very slow growing benign tumours are less likely to recur or spread after complete removal and may not need chemotherapy or radiotherapy post-surgery. Malignant tumours tend to recur and may spread to other parts of the brain or spinal cord even if, macroscopically, they seem to have been completely removed. Therefore, they may require radiotherapy and/or chemotherapy to slow their growth to prevent a recurrence.

A brain tumour diagnosis could signal the start of a long period of uncertainty, anger, guilt and fear for those involved. Patients may have neurological and cognitive deterioration, which they and their families and carers have to cope with before and/or after surgery. In addition, disorders of consciousness (see table 18.8) can arise, especially after surgery. Patients may also experience side effects from chemotherapy and following radiotherapy, including:

- loss of pituitary function
- diminished intellectual function
- hydrocephalus
- cerebral necrosis.

The key elements of nursing management are the same as for patients with a TBI and/or raised ICP (see table 18.7). In addition:

- physical and cognitive abilities need to be assessed
- an individualised rehabilitation program should be started as early as possible.

Cerebrovascular disorders

A **stroke** is a sudden decrease in blood flow to a localised area of the brain, characterised by a gradual or rapid onset of neurological deficits due to compromised CBF. It is a medical emergency requiring rapid treatment in order to prevent avoidable death and long-term disability. It is the third most common cause of death worldwide. An estimated 20–30 per cent of people who have had a stroke will die within one month. Few stroke victims will make a full recovery as most are left with some form of disability.

Risk factors include:

- certain diseases, such as diabetes mellitus or heart disease
- lifestyle habits, for example, smoking and a sedentary lifestyle
- dietary factors, such as saturated fats and high alcohol consumption
- race, higher incidences being seen in Asian and African-Caribbean individuals
- gender, strokes being more common in men than women
- age, as the incidence of stroke increases dramatically over the age of 55 years.

The main types of stroke are ischaemic and haemorrhagic.

Ischaemic stroke

An ischaemic stroke is a sudden vascular occlusion resulting in reduced blood oxygen supply to the brain cells and occurs in 85 per cent of all strokes. This occlusion leads to irreversible brain damage and the death of brain cells, known as infarction. Ischaemic stroke is most commonly caused by atherosclerosis, which leads to stenosis of the blood vessels.

Primary pathophysiologic mechanisms responsible for ischaemic stroke can be divided into thrombosis, embolism and hypoperfusion. Other less common ischaemic stroke mechanisms include hypercoagulable states and genetic conditions.

Investigations for ischæmic stroke include:

- CT angiography
- MRI angiography
- catheter cerebral angiography
- ECG
- echocardiogram
- serum glucose level
- serum electrolytes
- cardiac enzymes
- blood cell count
- coagulation profile.

Treatment

Acute reperfusion therapy should be commenced at the earliest once the initial evaluation is completed. Tissue plasminogen activators such as alteplase is given via intravenous route. Major contraindications for tissue plasminogen activator include coagulopathy, recent surgery or trauma, uncontrolled blood pressure, active bleeding, thrombocytopenia, elevated prothrombin time or international normalised ratio (INR). Endovascular thrombectomy can be beneficial in acute ischaemic stroke patients with large vessel occlusion.

Long-term treatment to prevent recurrent ischaemic stroke consists of antithrombotic agents (aspirin, clopidogrel) and statin therapy.

Haemorrhagic stroke

Haemorrhagic stroke is seen in 20 per cent of strokes and may be due to intracerebral haemorrhage or subarachnoid haemorrhage. Both of these are caused by a rupturing of cerebral blood vessels producing haemorrhage (bleeding) into the brain. Chronic hypertension, coagulopathies that arise endogenously or because of anticoagulant medications, vascular malformations of the brain, cranial trauma, and haemorrhage that occurs within the area of an ischaemic stroke are some of the major causes for intracerebral haemorrhage (Ropper, Samuels, Klein & Prasad 2019a).

Subarachnoid haemorrhage can be caused by rupture of a developmental aneurysm arising from the vessels of the Circle of Willis, cerebral trauma and arteriovenous malformations (Ropper, Samuels, Klein & Prasad 2019a).

Transient ischaemic attacks (TIAs), also known as minor or mini-strokes, occur when stroke symptoms resolve within 24 hours and are a warning that a further stroke may occur.

The neurological deficits vary according to the cerebral artery involved, the size and area of the brain affected, and the length of time the blood flow decreases or stops.

Signs and symptoms of haemorrhagic stroke include:

- a sudden onset
- a focal nature
- usually a one-sided deficit
- **hemiplegia** (paralysis on one side of the body); as the motor pathways cross (decussate) at the junction of the medulla and spinal cord, loss or impairment of sensorimotor functions occurs on the side of the body opposite to the side of the brain that is damaged
- a stroke in the right hemisphere of the brain manifested by deficits in the left side of the body, and vice versa.

Management of cerebrovascular disorders

Early assessment and diagnosis are critical if early and effective management decisions are to be implemented. This is especially important for those patients with thrombotic strokes as a small window of opportunity exists in which thrombolytic treatment (to break up the thrombosis or emboli) can be administered. The earlier thrombolysis is started, the greater the benefits. CT scans of the brain play a crucial role in the diagnosis of acute stroke.

Diagnosis begins with a complete history and careful physical assessment, including a thorough neurological examination. One way of identifying suspected acute stroke patients is the FAST stroke identification tool (figure 18.9), a quick score based on three specific symptoms of stroke; if any one of the three symptoms is positive, patients should seek urgent medical attention.

FIGURE 18.9 FAST assessment

Facial weakness
- Can the person smile?

Arm weakness
- Can the person raise both arms?

Speech problems
- Can the person speak clearly and understand what you say?

Time
- Time is critical. It is important to bring the person to a medical facility if any of these signs are present.

An important component in TIA and ischaemic stroke management is minimising the high risk of recurrent stroke. Therefore, treatment will include antithrombotic regimens such as antiplatelet therapy (e.g. aspirin) and anticoagulants (e.g. warfarin). The nursing management of a stroke is outlined in table 18.11.

TABLE 18.11 Nursing management of patients following stroke

Nursing interventions	Rationale
Neurological status Use the GCS and/or National Institutes of Health Stroke Scale (NIHSSS)	The NIHSS, a systematic assessment tool, provides a quantitative measure of stroke-related neurological deficit Neurological examination serves as a baseline for assessment of neurological improvement or worsening
Physiological monitoring Monitor vital signs — maintain blood pressure within specified limits observing for severe hypertension (systolic blood pressure >200 mmHg) or relative hypotension (systolic blood pressure <110 mmHg) Maintain a normal blood sugar level (4–11 mmol/L)	Vital signs and neurological status may fluctuate rapidly immediately after a stroke 78% of acute stroke patients are hyperglycaemic on admission. High blood sugars can cause further damage to the neurons in the brain; this is associated with an increased risk of death and more severe disability

(continued)

TABLE 18.11 *(continued)*

Nursing interventions	Rationale
Respiratory status Assess respiratory status Monitor and record pulse oximetry, and maintain oxygen saturations levels above 95% Administered prescribed oxygen	Oxygen saturation <95% should be treated with oxygen therapy) Blood oxygen levels regulate CBF
Temperature Monitor core temperature	Hyperthermia increases brain oxygen and glucose demand, thus increasing CBF and CP
Mobility Mobilise the patient as soon as possible (their condition permitting) Maintain correct and careful handling and positioning of the limbs Refer early to physiotherapy Administer antispasmodics Splinting and passive range of movement exercises	Prevents potential complications arising from reduced mobility, e.g. deep vein thrombosis Prevents complications associated with incorrect positioning: • Spasticity • Shoulder (glenohumeral) subluxation • Pressure sores • Contractures Optimises muscle function and recovery Helps patients to learn to deal with their disabilities Ensures correct and appropriate use of devices, e.g. walking aids and sticks Prevents spasticity, which may interfere with the patient's rehabilitation and recovery
Communication Early identification of communication difficulties Referral to speech and language therapist Patients are screened for visual problems Expression of pain management Assessment and management of post-stroke pain	Ensures an appropriate communication strategy is identified and implemented Stroke patients with visual deficits have an increased risk of falling Post-stroke neuropathic pain is common; this is caused by central or peripheral nerve damage Hemiplegic shoulder pain occurs in approximately 24% of stroke patients and is associated with poor upper limb recovery
Nutritional status Patient will remain nil by mouth until after a swallow assessment by an appropriately trained healthcare professional, e.g. a speech and language therapist An enteral feeding regimen is used if the patient is unable to swallow safely (nasogastric or percutaneous endoscopic gastrostomy) Assess nutritional status using a recognised assessment tool, e.g. the Malnutrition Universal Screening Tool	Assesses appropriateness of oral feeding and minimises complications associated with dysphagia, e.g. aspiration pneumonia Dysphagia is common Maximises nutritional intake; enables early nutritional management to be identified and implemented
Elimination Assess for incontinence Monitor fluid intake and output volumes and frequency Monitor bowel movements	Incontinence is common Assesses: • Minimal and maximal bladder volumes • The length of time between voidings of urine Enables appropriate bladder training programs to be instigated
Psychological support Observe for signs of anxiety and depression Refer to an appropriately trained professional for assessment Assess for post-stroke fatigue Help patients and their families adjust to their disability Provide patient education, advice and support	Anxiety may be associated with post-traumatic stress disorder Depression is common and can inhibit engagement with the rehabilitation process Fatigue is common, adversely impacting on quality of life and recovery

Families/carers Provide advice and support about being a carer Include caregivers in the discussions Provide information about benefits, stroke support groups, family support workers and specialist services	Care giving can be both stressful and distressful, resulting in emotional, physical and social disruption

The National Institutes of Health Stroke Scale (NIHSS) score is also used globally to assess the clinical severity of a stroke. It measures several aspects of brain functions such as consciousness, vision, sensation, movement, speech and language. The scale can be accessed here: www.ninds.nih.gov/sites/default/files/nih_stroke_scale_booklet_508c.pdf.

Stroke is among the top ten causes of death in children. Please refer to the clinical guidelines provided by The Stroke Foundation to find information on childhood stroke management (Stroke Foundation 2020): www.informme.org.au/en/Guidelines/Childhood-stroke-guidelines

Epilepsy

Epilepsy affects up to 50 million people of all ages, races, and ethnic backgrounds worldwide. It is not one condition but a diverse group of disorders, all having in common the presence of at least one seizure. It is a chronic disorder characterised by an abnormal recurring, excessive and self-terminating electrical discharge from the neurons in the brain. It is this electrical discharge that can be recorded with EEG scalp electrodes. This abnormal neuronal activity may involve all or part of the brain and disturbs skeletal motor function, sensation, autonomic function of the viscera, behaviour and/or consciousness.

Epilepsy may be:

- idiopathic (no identifiable cause), with multiple episodes diagnosed as a seizure disorder
- secondary to conditions affecting the brain or other organs, for example, drug and alcohol overdose and withdrawal, **meningitis** and cerebral bleeding.

Signs of seizures are dependent on the brain location of the epileptogenic focus and the extent and pattern of the epileptic discharge. Typical signs include:

- temporary changes in mental status and LOC
- abnormal sensory changes
- abnormal movements.

There are currently over 30 different types of epilepsy, with no agreed definitive classification system. Most systems rely heavily on descriptions of the seizures. Three main categories can be identified: focal or partial seizures, generalised seizures and unclassified seizures (figure 18.10).

FIGURE 18.10 Classification of epilepsy

Partial or focal seizures

- The hyperactive activity of the epileptogenic focus remains localised, causing partial or focal seizures.
- They involve an area in one of the cerebral hemispheres at the onset.
- All types of partial seizures can spread, resulting in secondarily generalised tonic-clonic seizures.
- Typically, a portion of the motor cortex is affected, causing recurrent muscle contractions.
- Partial seizures can be further subdivided into:
  - simple partial seizures, without impaired consciousness
  - complex partial seizures, with impaired consciousness
  - partial seizures evolving into secondary generalised seizures.

Generalised seizures

- Abnormal activity begins simultaneously in both hemispheres of the brain, resulting in impaired consciousness.
- They can be further subdivided into six major categories:
  1. generalised tonic-clonic seizures, also known as 'grand mal' seizures
  2. tonic seizures
  3. clonic seizures
  4. myoclonic seizures
  5. atonic seizures
  6. absence seizures, also known as 'petit mal':

- sudden brief cessations of all motor activity accompanied by a blank stare and unresponsiveness
  - last only 5–10 seconds
  - vary from occasional episodes to several hundred per day
  - are more common in children than adults.

Unclassified epilepsies

- Seizures that cannot be clearly classified into one of the existing categories until further information permits diagnosis.

Tonic-clonic and absence seizures are the most common forms of generalised seizure activity, with tonic-clonic seizures following a typical pattern (table 18.12). Status epilepticus occurs when patients' seizure activity is continuous, and they do not regain consciousness between seizures. Prompt treatment is required to prevent irreversible neurological damage and preserve life.

TABLE 18.12 Tonic-clonic seizure pattern

Phase	Description
Aura (a warning)	A vague sense of uneasiness or an abnormal gustatory, visual, auditory or visceral sensation (e.g. a metallic taste in the mouth or a smell of burning rubber) Seizures can occur without warning
Tonic phase	Sudden LOC Tonic muscle contractions Loss of postural control, so if standing, patients will fall to the floor Rigid muscles, with the arms and legs extended Clamping down of the jaw; the tongue may get caught between the teeth and be bitten Incontinence may occur Respiration may stop and cyanosis develop The phase lasts 10–20 seconds and may persist for up to a minute
Clonic phase	Alternating contraction and relaxation of the muscles Phase varies in duration
Postictal period or phase	Patients remain unconscious and unresponsive to stimuli Gradually regain consciousness May be confused and disorientated Often amnesic of the seizure and the events just prior to the seizure activity

Psychogenic non-epileptic seizures (PNES) or psychogenic syncopes:

- are events that resemble epileptic seizures and are relatively common
- are not associated with abnormal EEG discharges
- are presumed to be caused by a psychological disorder
- are often mistaken for epileptic seizures
- if misdiagnosed, they can lead to inappropriate treatment with antiepileptic drugs (AEDs) and can be life-threatening.

Diagnosis is based on several sources and should only be confirmed by an epilepsy specialist. The distinction between epilepsy and non-epileptic seizures is complex, so patients should be referred for a neurological assessment if either PNES or psychogenic syncope is suspected. Typical investigations that are conducted to support a diagnosis are:

- a clinical history from the patient or an eye-witness to the attack, along with a physical examination
- diagnostic testing to determine any treatable causes and precipitating factors, e.g. a skull X-ray, MRI or CT scan
- an electroencephalogram to help localise the epileptogenic focus and confirm the diagnosis.

Other tests may include:

- a lumbar puncture to assess spinal fluid for CNS infections
- blood tests, e.g. for plasma electrolytes, glucose and calcium, to rule out other causes.

Treatment of epilepsy

Treatment of all types of epilepsy focuses mainly on four aspects; antiepileptic drugs, surgical intervention, removal of causative or precipitating factors and regulation of physical and mental activity (Ropper, Samuels, Klein, & Prasad 2019b). Some of the commonly used antiepileptic medications include valproic acid, phenytoin, carbamazepine, phenobarbital, levetiracetam, clonazepam, diazepam and pregabalin. Many of these medications can cause toxicity. Hence it is essential to measure serum concentration of the drugs regularly to make dose adjustments. Most of these medications are metabolised by liver, and serum concentration must be checked more frequently in patients with liver failure. Antiepileptic drugs interact with many other commonly used medications. Chloramphenicol causes an accumulation of phenytoin and phenobarbital whereas erythromycin causes the accumulation of carbamazepine. Antacids reduce the concentration of phenytoin in blood. Phenobarbital or carbamazepine decrease warfarin level.

Antiepileptic drugs (AEDs), also known as anticonvulsant medications, aim to:

- reduce or control the seizure activity
- prevent irreversible complications (e.g. cerebral and cardiovascular changes) as a result of seizures.

The choice of AEDs is dependent upon the type of seizure and any side effects that patients may experience. In some cases, brain surgery is an option and aims to remove the epileptogenic focus. Other treatment options include:

- stereotactic radiotherapy (gamma knife surgery), aimed at destroying the abnormal brain cells;
- neurostimulation therapy — for example, deep brain stimulation and **vagus nerve** stimulation, is designed to prevent seizures by sending regular small pulses of electrical energy to the brain via the vagus nerve.

Patients with epilepsy may require hospitalisation for seizure monitoring, for management or to confirm a diagnosis. Immediate care during a seizure will depend upon the type of seizure but generally involves:

- providing a safe environment, aiming to protect patients from any injury
- securing the airway by inserting an oropharyngeal airway to prevent the patient from biting their tongue; also provide access to the back of the mouth to remove secretions using a suction cannula
- loosening clothing around the neck
- positioning patients in the recovery position (after the clonic phase)
- assessing cardiac and respiratory function
- suction if excessive salivation has occurred
- administration of oxygen therapy
- intravenous access for AEDs to be administered (especially in status epilepticus)
- documenting an account of the seizure, including:
  - any aura
  - behavioural/motor activity
  - LOC
  - incontinence
  - the time the seizure commenced
  - the length of time of the entire seizure
  - the period elapsed since the last seizure.

Timely information, training and support to assist patients and their families in accepting, understanding and psychosocially adjusting to their diagnosis are important nursing interventions. Monitor serum concentration, drug interaction and toxic signs of AEDs and stress the importance of compliance with the prescribed medication regimen.

Neurological infections

The brain and spinal cord are extremely well protected by the skull, the vertebral column, the BBB and the CSF barrier; however, infections of the CNS ranging from mild to fatal do occur. These include the following.

- Meningitis (infection of the meninges), primarily caused by viruses. Life-threatening if bacterial in nature (although it is less common). Rarely caused by spirochaetes and fungi.
- **Encephalitis** (infection of the brain substance), mainly caused by viruses such as herpes simplex virus (the most common).
- Human immunodeficiency virus (HIV), which causes mild meningitis. In full-blown acquired immune deficiency syndrome (AIDS) may cause subacute encephalitis.

- Brain abscesses, usually defined, localised lesions. Occur singularly or in multiples after surgery, trauma, extending osteomyelitis or ear infections.
- Rabies, a fatal infection. Enters the PNS following a bite from an infected animal and migrates to the CNS.
- Rubella and measles are linked to a rare complication called subacute sclerosing panencephalitis, which is fatal and may only manifest 10 years after uncomplicated measles.
- Spongiform encephalopathies such as Creutzfeldt–Jakob disease (CJD) and variant CJD are progressive neurodegenerative diseases resulting in death.
- *Clostridium tetani* (which causes tetanus) blocks inhibitory mediators at the nerve synapses, resulting in intense muscle spasm and causing injury to the tissues and eventually death.
- *Clostridium botulinum* blocks the release of acetylcholine, resulting in flaccid paralysis and death from respiratory or cardiac failure.

Management of neurological infections

For most neurological infections, biochemical and microbiological tests, especially on the CSF and blood, can yield important information to assist diagnosis. CSF is obtained via a lumbar puncture, and its colour may also indicate the diagnosis (table 18.13). Difficulties may be experienced in culturing pathogens such as bacteria if patients have received antibiotics prior to the lumbar puncture. A lumbar puncture is not without risk to patients; if the ICP is significantly raised, as may be the case with an abscess, a lumbar puncture may result in fatal cerebellar coning. CT scans and brain biopsies may be undertaken in, for example, brain abscesses, encephalitis and rabies. For some infections, antibiotics and immunisation have markedly reduced the risk of contracting infections such as meningitis and tetanus. Other drugs, such as acyclovir for viral encephalitis, have similar effects.

TABLE 18.13 Diagnosing infections of CNS: the colour of the CSF

Possible diagnosis	CSF colour
Viral meningitis Chronic meningitis	Slight opalescence
Acute bacterial meningitis	Markedly turbid or cloudy
Traumatic lumbar puncture Subarachnoid haemorrhage	Bloodstained
Tuberculosis meningitis	A spider's web clot appearance due to the high-protein content of the CSF

Patients may be extremely ill, requiring basic nursing care in addition to constant monitoring. The early detection and prevention of neurological deterioration and life-threatening complications is a priority. Nursing management includes the following:

- monitoring neurological function, vital signs and GCS
- using isolation or barrier nursing (if required)
- seeking advice from the infection prevention and control team
- following local policy
- addressing patients' emotional wellbeing (mental health, safety)
- identifying the mode of transmission (airborne, faecal/oral route)
- assessing the risk of spread (to other patients and health workers)
- providing information and prophylaxis (treatment and screening) to close family and carers, for example, to eliminate the nasopharyngeal carriage of organisms.

Meningitis is one of the most common infections of the neurological system. It refers to an inflammatory reaction in the subarachnoid space. Headache, fever and neck stiffness are the main symptoms of meningitis. The causative pathogen can be bacterial or viral. Some viruses may cause encephalitis, myelitis or encephalomyelitis in addition to meningitis. An altered level of consciousness is commonly seen in bacterial meningitis, which is not present in viral meningitis. Seizures can occur in bacterial meningitis. Antibiotics, depending on the bacteria cultured, should be initiated, and corticosteroids are sometimes given in addition to antibiotics (Agnihotri 2020). Headache is severe with nausea and vomiting in viral meningitis. Acyclovir is used to treat viral meningitis caused by the herpes zoster virus, and antiretroviral therapy should be commenced on HIV patients. Eosinophilic meningoencephalitis is seen with parasitic infection. Eosinophils are detected in CSF for this type of meningoencephalitis. Meningitis seen in autoimmune disorders following medications use (Intravenous immunoglobulin) or as part of neoplastic disorders is referred to as aseptic meningitis.

Multiple sclerosis

Multiple sclerosis (MS) is an autoimmune disease that attacks the CNS, resulting in damage to the myelin sheath and the formation of localised areas of inflammation called 'plaques'. Damage to the CNS primarily occurs through the demyelination of axons within the brain, optic nerves and spinal cord (Meador 2020). It is thought that there is damage to the blood–brain barrier, resulting in cells entering the CNS and triggering an immune response. This immune response is thought to be triggered by prior viral infection or environmental exposure in childhood in a genetically susceptible person. The onset is usually between 20 and 40 years of age, peaking around the age of 25. MS is more common in women than men.

There are four main types of MS:

1. relapsing-remitting, the most common type of MS, which accounts for approximately 80 per cent of cases of MS
2. primary progressive
3. secondary progressive
4. progressive relapsing.

The signs and symptoms are determined by where in the CNS the demyelination plaques occur and can vary in character, number and duration. Common signs and symptoms include:

- sensory impairment
- transient muscle weakness
- fatigue, which is the most disabling symptom
- sleep disorders
- visual changes (diplopia and visual loss)
- cognitive impairment.

MS is characterised by:

- periods of exacerbation or 'relapse':
  - signs and symptoms that are highly pronounced
  - lasting for days, weeks, or months
- periods of remission:
  - a period of relapse followed by a period when the damaged myelin sheath undergoes remyelination
  - the symptoms thus improving.

In the early stages, MS is commonly a relapsing and remitting disease. Over time, however, the myelin sheath becomes unable to repair itself completely during the remission period, and patients are left with residual deficits. Repeated healing and inflammation can lead to scarring (gliosis) and loss of axons. Axonal and neuronal degeneration is evident on MRI scanning as black holes. As the disease progresses, remissions become shorter and fewer, and patients become more physically disabled.

Diagnosis of MS is based on the following.

- A clinical history and examination are necessary. A common feature of MS is blurred vision due to optic neuritis, caused by demyelination of the nerve fibres.
- MRI scans may reveal white areas within the white matter.
- Lumbar puncture may reveal the presence of oligoclonal bands in the CSF, reflecting proteins synthesised within the CNS during the immune response (which is found in 95 per cent of patients with established MS).
- Evoked response testing (visual, auditory and somatosensory) may show delayed conduction (slowing of the nerve messages).

Management of MS

The management of MS varies according to the acuity of exacerbations (relapses) and the presenting signs and symptoms. It involves the treatment of acute relapses, disease modification and symptom management, all of which require an interdisciplinary individualistic approach. Although there is no cure for MS, many medical therapies are available, which may slow the progression of the disease and help manage some of its symptoms (table 18.14).

Please visit the MS Australia website to find further information about medications and treatment (www.msaustralia.org.au/about-ms/medications-treatments).

TABLE 18.14 **Medical therapies used in MS**

Therapies	Examples
Disease-modifying therapies • Reduce the number of exacerbations (relapses) by reducing the production of interferon gamma, thought to be involved in the formation of demyelination plaques • Reduce antibody/lymphocyte activity • Prevent specific inflammatory events leading to the development of lesions	Interferon beta-1a and interferon beta-1b are the drugs of choice in relapsing-remitting MS, and are given intramuscularly Glatiramer acetate (Copaxone), given subcutaneously Natalizumab (Tysabri), given intravenously
Disease-suppressing therapies • Are given in the early inflammatory phase (in relapses) • Suppress the immune response	Immunosuppressant drugs, e.g. methotrexate
Corticosteroids — hastens recovery from a relapse	Methylprednisolone — a high dose given intravenously or orally
Medications for the treatment of signs and symptoms	Muscle relaxants (e.g. baclofen and dantrolene) to relieve muscle spasms and spasticity; in severe cases, botulinum toxin may be injected into specific sites Antidepressant drugs for depression Urinary frequency and urgency may be treated with anticholinergic drugs Amantadine for fatigue

The goal and focus of nursing care are to retain as much independence and function as possible, control symptoms, and reduce potential complications. Supportive and symptomatic care may help minimise patients' disability and help achieve optimal physical and psychological adjustment levels. As the disease often affects young adults, the psychosocial and economic effect can be devastating. Many nursing care interventions relate to the inability to perform activities of daily living and to problems arising from musculoskeletal changes or altered nerve conduction.

Encourage the patient to maintain a healthy lifestyle, such as maintaining a healthy weight, being active, avoiding smoking and control alcohol consumption, engaging in reading, education and artistic or creative pastimes to keep their mind active.

Additional advice for MS patients includes:

- educating the patient about the benefits of early intervention with disease-modifying therapy
- empowering the patient by providing relevant information about local support
- monitoring treatment adherence and developing individualised treatment plans
- encouraging the patient to self-monitor their disease by keeping a diary or mobile app.

Please visit the website MS Brain Health (www.msbrainhealth.org/article/brain-health-in-multiple-sclerosis-a-nursing-resource) to find additional information about nursing care.

Motor neuron disease

Motor neuron disease (MND) is a devastating and progressive life-limiting disease leading to advancing paralysis and eventual death, with the intellect remaining intact throughout. Sensory neurons, bladder and bowel function, emotional feelings, and sexual desire generally remain intact. The upper motor neurons (in the brain) and/or the lower motor neurons (in the brainstem, spinal cord, arms, legs and torso) may be affected. The neurons become damaged and eventually stop working, resulting in weakness, wasting and atrophying of the muscles supplied by these neurons. The average life expectancy is two to three years. MND can affect adults of any age, but is more common in people over 50.

There are different types of MND (table 18.15). The disease initially affects the hands, feet or mouth and throat, depending on the type of MND. Although the signs and symptoms of the different types may differ initially, they tend to overlap as the disease progresses, so in the final stages, there is very little or no differentiation between all types of MND.

TABLE 18.15 Types of MND

Type	Description
Amyotrophic lateral sclerosis (ALS)	The most common form Referred to as classic MND Patient may experience: • muscle wasting • fasciculation • speech and swallowing problems • muscle spasms
Progressive muscular atrophy (PMA)	Less common and tends to progress more slowly than ALS Patients may go on to develop ALS
Isolated bulbar palsy	Mainly affects the muscles in the tongue, throat and face Causes difficulties with speech, swallowing, coughing and clearing the throat Emotional lability — individuals laugh or cry for no apparent reason
Primary lateral sclerosis	Very rare Patients experience spasticity, but no muscle wasting or fasciculations, slower disease progression and in some cases a normal life expectancy

Management of motor neuron disease

There is no definitive test to diagnose MND, the diagnosis being based on:

- a full and thorough history and neurological examination
- interpretation of the clinical signs and symptoms
- investigations to exclude other causes.

There are no distinct laboratory tests to diagnose various forms of MND. Laboratory and radiologic studies should be considered as an extension of neurologic evaluations. They should not be interpreted alone to make MND diagnosis. Studies used in the diagnosis of MND may include:

- blood tests (to exclude problems such as kidney, liver, thyroid and inflammatory conditions)
- lumbar puncture
- EMG
- nerve conduction studies
- transcranial magnetic stimulation, which measures the activity of the neurons from the brain to the spinal cord
- MRI
- muscle biopsy.

The only medication found to be beneficial in MND is riluzole. Liver function test should be checked before commencing and every three months while the patient is on riluzole (Kazamel, 2020). Edaravone is another medication used in the treatment of ALS. Drug therapy should aim to treat symptoms such as muscle cramps, spasticity (quinine, gabapentin, baclofen), drooling (**glycopyrrolate**, carbocisteine), depression, insomnia, etc.

Nursing care involves implementing measures to ensure the best quality of life for patients and using measures to compensate for the progressive loss of bodily functions such as mobility, speech, swallowing, breathing, cognition and behaviour. Among other approaches, treatment should include:

- collaboration and close working with the multidisciplinary team; physical therapy, occupational therapy, speech therapy, nutritionist, counsellor and a social worker should be involved in care
- respiratory care — cough augmentation techniques are used to help with secretion clearance. Invasive and non-invasive ventilation is used to support the patient during critical phase
- a high-calorie diet that is easy to swallow for the patient with dysphagia. Regular monitoring of weight is also important. Gastric feeding tubes may be required to maintain nutrition in severe cases
- implementation of the patient's wishes, i.e. information on healthcare advocates and advanced directives being made available
- hospice care for later stages of the disease, which can be introduced gradually in the form of respite care for the family and carers.

Additional resources for the management of MND can be found at the following websites:

- www.mndaust.asn.au
- www.alsa.org
- www.mdausa.org
- www.neuro.wustl.edu.

Parkinson's disease

Parkinson's disease is a common, slowly progressive neurodegenerative disorder that affects older adults. It usually develops after the age of 60 and is more common in men than in women. Parkinson's disease involves:

- the death of dopamine-releasing neurons
- the formation of 'Lewy bodies' (small spherical protein deposits that are found in neurons).

There is progressive development of motor and non-motor symptoms. There is no cure, and in most cases, the cause is unknown, although there is evidence that both genetics and environmental factors play a role.

Parkinson's disease is characterised by:

- motor impairment
- **bradykinesia**
- rigidity
- repetitive tremor
- disorders of gait, balance and posture.

Non-motor symptoms include:

- anxiety
- depression
- hallucinations
- sensory changes
- sleep disturbances
- autonomic and gastrointestinal dysfunction
- fatigue
- apathy
- cognitive decline
- dementia (Hoogland et al. 2019).

Symptoms may present at any stage but tend to occur in the later stages. The severity of symptoms fluctuates, making them difficult to predict and control. Patients subsequently experience a reduction in motor function. These fluctuations in symptoms can be accompanied by high rates of depression, reduced psychological wellbeing and caregiver distress. Table 18.16 presents some of the common terminology used in describing the signs and symptoms of Parkinson's disease.

TABLE 18.16 Terminology to describe the signs and symptoms of Parkinson's disease

Terminology	Description
Bradykinesia	Slowness of movement or difficulty in starting to move
Dyskinesia	Abnormal involuntary movements of the limbs, trunk or face occurring with: • Peak plasma **levodopa** levels • Fluctuating plasma levodopa levels • Low plasma levodopa levels
Dystonia	Sustained and painful muscle contractions Often affect the neck, trunk and limbs, and result in abnormal postures
'On–off' phenomenon	Severe fluctuations in motor function during levodopa treatment 'On' — states of good mobility or the patient is asymptomatic when the medication is effective 'Off' — states of poor mobility or the patient is symptomatic, e.g. bradykinesia, rigidity and/or tremor, as the medication wears off
Freezing	States in which patients suddenly stop and become 'stuck' when walking, talking or performing any movement

Management of Parkinson's disease

The mainstay of treatment for Parkinson's disease is medication, which aims to increase dopamine or mimics its effect by stimulating the area of the brain where dopamine works. Patients are often prescribed a combination of medications to control and manage their symptoms (figure 18.11).

FIGURE 18.11 Medications used for the treatment of Parkinson's disease

Levodopa therapies
- Are highly effective
- Are commonly prescribed drugs that are converted to dopamine in the brain

Dopamine agonists
- Stimulate the dopamine receptors in the brain, in particular, the dopamine D2-receptors
- An example is bromocriptine, an ergot-derived dopamine agonist

Non-ergot dopamine agonist (NEDAs)
- Stimulate the dopamine receptors in the brain, in particular the D2- and D3-receptors
- Examples of NEDAs are ropinirole, pramipexole and apomorphine (which cannot be given orally)

Monoamine oxidase type B (MAO-B) inhibitors
- Block the enzyme MAO-B, which breaks down dopamine in the brain
- An example is selegiline

Catechol-O-methyl transferase inhibitors
- Block the enzyme that breaks down levodopa, prolonging its effect
- Are used in combination with levodopa; examples are entacapone and tolcapone

Nurses' assessment needs to include the many symptoms that can accompany Parkinson's disease. Therefore, the following should be assessed:
- the intensity, frequency and duration of symptoms
- the distress associated with the symptoms as this enables nurses to understand patients' complete symptom experiences.

This assessment will identify symptoms that need to be targeted and the necessary interventions to address those symptoms. Nurses can then evaluate the effectiveness of these interventions on the targeted symptoms.

Nurses should administer medications at the prescribed time and consider supporting self-medication (in which patients control their own medication) if they are able to ensure a constant therapeutic level of symptom control.

As Parkinson's disease is a chronic, progressive disease, intervention is unlikely to eliminate a symptom completely. However, some symptoms are associated with potential complications, such as **freezing**, and postural instability is associated with a high risk of falls. Nurses should assess patients for risks such as falling and implement strategies to improve their posture and balance (see the chapter on geriatric nursing for more detailed information on falls and risk assessment).

Alzheimer's disease

Alzheimer's disease is a progressive disease during which protein (senile) plaques and neurofibrillary tangles develop in the brain's structure, resulting in the death of cells and synapses. This loss occurs mainly in the cerebral cortex and leads to atrophy of the brain. There is a shortage of acetylcholine, which, apart from functioning as a neurotransmitter, has a role in memory and learning. Alzheimer's disease is characterised by a gradual decline in:
- mental abilities
- cognition
- reasoning
- exercising judgement
- spatial and language abilities
- planning and executing familiar tasks
- personality and mood.

Alzheimer's disease is the most common cause of dementia (table 18.17). The progress of Alzheimer's disease and its associated signs and symptoms are individual to the person and may not manifest in everyone. It is important to remember that:

- each stage of Alzheimer's disease is more devastating not only to the individual, but also to their family and carers
- an individual with mild cognitive impairment (difficulty remembering or thinking clearly) may not have Alzheimer's disease.

TABLE 18.17 Stages, signs, symptoms and medication in Alzheimer's disease

Stage of disease	Some common signs and symptoms	Medication/drug treatments
Early/initial	Lapses of memory Problems finding the right words or names Work performance affected Loss of interest Reluctant or hesitant to use own initiative, make decisions or act Difficulties with planning and organising	Donepezil (Aricept) Rivastigmine (Exelon)
Mild/moderate	Obvious memory loss Difficulties with simple tasks and/or instructions Decreased ability to perform mental challenges, e.g. counting backwards from 100 Confusion or agitation — this is called sundowning or sundown syndrome when it is more noticeable in the late afternoon or early evening Verbal outbursts and threatening and/or violent behaviour Purposeless and inappropriate activities (fidgeting, pacing, moving things around) May have periods of irritability, paranoia and anxiety Wandering, getting lost	Galantamine (Reminyl) All of the above for mild and moderate stages
Late/severe	Inability to manage independently Becomes bedridden Loss of intelligible speech Urinary incontinence Faecal incontinence Motor problems such as inability to smile, grimacing instead Requires support to sit up without falling Difficulty holding head up Physical and neurological changes (rigidity, re-emergence of the grasp and sucking reflexes, contractures)	Memantine (Ebixa) Only for moderate to severe stages

Non-pharmacological interventions include:

- psychological support
- behavioural management
- environmental therapies.

Diagnostic investigations

There is no specific test for Alzheimer's disease, and diagnosis is made based on the exclusion of other conditions with similar signs and symptoms. Diagnostic investigations will include:

- a detailed medical history
- thorough physical and neurological examination
- blood tests — to exclude infections, nutritional deficiencies, thyroid problems and side effects of medication
- X-rays — to exclude chest infection
- assessment of memory — to assess both recent and past memory recall
- lumbar puncture for CSF tests
- MRI, Positron Emission Tomography (PET) scan.

Families and carers should be involved in the history-taking as they may be extremely useful in providing information patients may have forgotten. Furthermore, a detailed assessment is undertaken by a clinical psychologist. The patient is assessed for impaired ability to learn or recall information, impaired language skills, impaired visuospatial abilities, executive dysfunction and changes in behaviour or personality.

Nursing management of Alzheimer's disease is profoundly life-changing, and the approach to nursing care should be centred on the individual. Patient needs vary depending on the stage of the disease. It is important to remember that nurses need to care for Alzheimer's patients in various settings, and hence an individualised plan may be needed for patients.

The nurse should:

- ensure the care plan is tailored to patients' needs
- regularly assess, evaluate and identify patients' and carers' needs
- engage and work in partnership with patients and their families and carers
- be sufficiently knowledgeable to recognise the progression of the disease
- have the knowledge, skills and time to deal with problems as they occur
- refer patients and/or families to the relevant agencies that can offer assistance and support.

Some of the specific interventions are as follows.

- Encourage the patient to participate in hobbies, community activities, etc.
- Identify stressors that cause agitation and confusion and eliminate or minimise them.
- Avoid corrections, criticism and conflicts with the patient.
- Reduce overstimulation. Some strategies are to turn off the TV, provide a quiet environment and set up a calm atmosphere such as relaxing music. These measures will help to manage agitation exhibited by some Alzheimer's patient.
- Establish regular sleep and wake times, increasing day time activities and starting calming night-time rituals could help with sleep disturbance associated with Alzheimer's disease.
- Provide reassurance.
- Write down the answer to repeatedly asked questions and visual reminders such as a calendar to orientate the patient to date and day.
- Educate the family and patient about medications and their side effects.

There is currently no cure for Alzheimer's disease, but if the disease is diagnosed early, medication may help to improve or stabilise symptoms. The condition's progression varies, with some individuals progressing rapidly and others more slowly, but care becomes more challenging and intensive as the condition worsens. Families and carers should be viewed as equal partners. Where possible, the initial care should be in the individual's home, with respite care periods offered. As the disease progresses, there may be occasions when a stay in hospital is beneficial, and palliative care should be available if and when required. Additional information on the nursing care of older people with dementia can be found in the chapter on geriatric nursing.

Additional resources for Alzheimer's disease can be found at the Dementia Australia website: www.dementia.org.au.

CASE STUDY 18.1

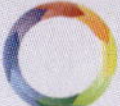

Nursing care of a patient with ischaemic stroke

John, a 72-year-old man, was brought in by ambulance with right-sided weakness. The patient was eating breakfast when he suddenly lost strength on the right side of his body such that he was unable to move his right arm or leg. He also noted a loss of sensation in the right arm and leg and difficulty speaking. His medical history includes hypertension, hypercholesteraemia and recently diagnosed coronary artery disease. On physical examination, his blood pressure is 190/90 mmHg. Right facial droop present on examination. No movement to right upper and lower limbs. CT angio scan of the brain showed mid cerebral artery occlusion. The patient is admitted to neurologic ICU and commenced acute reperfusion therapy using intravenous alteplase. John lives with his wife, Delma, 65.

His vital signs are:

- temperature: 37.6°C
- blood pressure: 190/90 mmHg
- heart rate: 96 beats per minute
- respiratory rate: 20 breaths per minute
- oxygen saturation: 97% on room air

- blood glucose level: 7.2 mmol/L
- height: 172 cms
- weight: 72 kg
- Glasgow Coma Scale: E4 V5M6
- pupils are equal and reacting light.

Question

Using the information above, describe what action you would take as the nurse caring for this patient. Use the clinical reasoning cycle to guide you through the process and devise a care plan for your patient.

Answer

- *Step 1: Consider the patient*. John, 72 years old.
- *Step 2: Collect cues/information*. Include subjective and objective data here, including the appearance of the patient, investigation results and their past medical history — CT angio shows mid cerebral artery occlusion, hypertension, hypercholesteraemia and recently diagnosed coronary artery disease. Right-sided weakness, right facial droop. Objective data will include measurable information such as vital signs. Subjective data — no movement to right upper and lower limbs.
- *Step 3: Process information*. Separate the relevant and irrelevant data — cluster the clues together to formulate an inference about the patient. Right-sided weakness, blood pressure 190/90 mmHg, CT angio mid cerebral artery occlusion.
- *Step 4: Identify problems/issues*. Nursing problems or diagnosis should be listed here: inadequate cerebral tissue perfusion as evidenced by CT angio result, high blood pressure, impaired mobility to right-sided weakness, altered body image due to facial droop.
- *Step 5: Establish goals*. Goals of care for John focus on reducing blood pressure and restoring cerebral perfusion to minimise permanent damage to brain damage due to ischaemia.
- *Step 6: Take action*. Nursing priority is to commence reperfusion therapy at the earliest. However, the baseline coagulation profile should be established before commencing therapy. Antihypertensive medications should be administered to bring blood pressure down, and frequent neurological observations to detect changes early. The patient should remain in bed during the acute phase. Later on, John may need mobility aids for movement.
- *Step 7: Evaluate outcomes*. Blood pressure returned to a range that is normal to the client. Decreased weakness to the right side and gradual return to normal functional status.
- *Step 8: Reflect on the process and new learning*. Reflect on any aspects of care that could have been performed in a way to achieve an improved outcome.

CASE STUDY 18.2

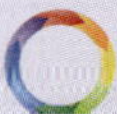

Nursing care of a patient with traumatic brain injury

Chelsey is a 22-year-old female transferred to ICU following a motor vehicle accident. The car she was driving hit a tree at high speed. The patient lost consciousness at the scene. On arrival to emergency, Chelsey's GCS was low (E2 V2 M2), and she has obtained multiple lacerations over the forehead and both arms. A CT scan revealed subdural haematoma. Chelsey had surgery to evacuate a haematoma. She was transferred to ICU post-surgery with ICP device in situ for monitoring. Chelsey is sedated and on ventilator support. Past medical history of Juvenile diabetes diagnosed at the age of 10 years. Chelsey works as a retail assistant in a local store and lives with friends Jemma and Erin in a shared apartment. Chelsey is a social drinker. Her blood alcohol reading was 0 on arrival in ED.

Her vital signs are:

- temperature: 38.2°C
- blood pressure: 90/50 mmHg (MAP: 63 mmHg)
- heart rate: 102 beats per minute
- respiratory rate: (frequency on the ventilator) 18
- oxygen saturation: 94% with 50% FiO_2 on the ventilator
- ICP: 22
- CPP: MAP–ICP = 41
- GCS: not applicable. Sedated
- height: 155 cm
- weight: 60 kg.

Question

Using the information above, describe what action you would take as the nurse caring for this patient. Use the clinical reasoning cycle to guide you through the process and devise a care plan for your patient.

Answer

- *Step 1: Consider the patient.* Chelsey, 22 years, female.
- *Step 2: Collect cues/information.* Include subjective and objective data here, including the patient's appearance, investigation results and past medical history. Juvenile diabetes objective data will include measurable information such as her vital signs. Investigations: CT shows subdural haematoma.
- *Step 3: Process information*. Separate the relevant and irrelevant data — cluster the clues together to formulate an inference about the patient. Chelsey's temperature is elevated, CPP is low; MAP is low, ICP is high, SpO_2 is low.
- *Step 4: Identify problems/issues*. Nursing problems or diagnosis should be listed here. Maintaining normal CPP and ICP is urgent.
- *Step 5: Establish goals*. Goals of care include reducing ICP, reducing temperature, improving BP, improving SpO_2.
- *Step 6: Take action.* The nurse should take immediate intervention to bring down ICP. High temperature and low oxygen saturation can be responsible for elevated ICP. Administer antipyretics and apply a cooling blanket to bring down temperature to normal. Adjust FiO_2 on the ventilator to improve saturation. It is also vital to maintain CPP. Chelsey may need intravenous fluids or inotropic support to bring blood pressure to normal range.
- *Step 7: Evaluate outcomes.* ICP within normal range, CPP above 70, temperature around 36.7°C, SpO_2 above 96%.
- *Step 8: Reflect on the process and new learning*. Reflect on any aspects of care that could have been performed in a way to achieve an improved outcome.

SUMMARY

To ensure good practice, staff caring for neurological patients should have the necessary skills and experience, especially in utilising tools such as the GCS. The nursing care of conditions related to the neurological system lends itself to acquiring valuable, diverse skills and knowledge, which are transferable to other disciplines. Nurses have to collaborate with patients and/or their families and carers and the multidisciplinary team according to patients' holistic needs, goals and care requirements.

KEY TERMS

abducen One of the cranial nerves.
Alzheimer's disease Type of neurodegenerative disease with memory loss as one of the main characteristics.
astrocytoma Type of central nervous system tumour.
axon Part of neuron which conducts outgoing signals.
bradykinesia Slowness of movement or difficulty in starting to move.
cerebral perfusion pressure (CPP) Pressure gradient to maintain perfusion to brain tissues.
coma Stage of unconsciousness where the person is unrousable and unresponsive.
dendrite Part of neuron which conducts incoming signals.
dystonia Sustained and painful muscle contractions.
electroencephalograms (EEGs) Test to assess electrical activity of the brain.
encephalitis Infection of the brain substance.
epilepsy Seizure disorder resulting from abnormal recurring, excessive and self-terminating electrical discharge from the neurons in the brain.
freezing States in which patients suddenly stop and become 'stuck' when walking, talking or performing any movement.
Glasgow Coma Scale (GCS) Tool to assess awareness and arousability.
glioblastoma Type of central nervous system tumour.
glycopyrrolate Medication to decrease secretions.
hemiplegia Paralysis to one side of the body.
levodopa Medication used to treat Parkinson's disease.
meningitis Infection of the meninges or brain covering.
multiple sclerosis (MS) Autoimmune disease that attacks the central nervous system.
osmotherapy Treatment strategy to decrease brain swelling using hypertonic solutions.
stroke Decreased perfusion to the brain, either due to a blocked blood vessel or a ruptured blood vessel.
vagus nerve One of the cranial nerves, which controls smooth muscles of the thorax and abdomen.

REFERENCES

Aitken, L., Marshall, A. & Chaboyer, W. (2015) *ACCCN's Critical Care Nursing*. Elsevier Health Sciences.

Agency for Clinical Innovation. (2015) *NSW Brain injury rehabilitation program: Case management.* https://aci.health.nsw.gov.au/__data/assets/pdf_file/0006/289392/DIRP-Case-Management-MOC2.pdf

Agnihotri, S. P. (2020) 'Neurologic infections'. In F. R. Amthor, A. B. Theibert, D. G. Standaert & E. D. Roberson (Eds.). *Essentials of Modern Neuroscience.* New York, NY: McGraw Hill.

Bullock, S. & Hales, M. (2019) *Principles of Pathophysiology*, 2nd ed. Melbourne: Pearson Education Australia.

Douglas, V. C. & Aminoff, M. J. (2021) 'Multiple sclerosis'. In Papadakis, M.A.,McPhee S.J. & Rabow M.W. (Eds.). *Current Medical Diagnosis & Treatment.* McGraw-Hill.

Hoogland, J., Boel, J. A., de Bie, R. M. A., et al. & MDS Study Group. (2019) Validation of mild cognitive impairment in Parkinson disease. Risk of Parkinson's disease dementia related to level I MDS PD-MCI. *Mov Disord.* Mar, 34(3): 430–435. doi. 10.1002/mds.27617

Hottinger, A. F., Pacheco, P. & Stupp, R. (2016) Tumor treating fields: a novel treatment modality and its use in brain tumors. *Neuro-oncology.* 18(10). 1338–1349. https://doi.org/10.1093/neuonc/now182

Jankovic, J. (2021). 'Parkinson disease and other movement disorders'. In J. M. D. Jankovic, J. C. M. D. P. Mazziotta, S. L., M. D. P. Pomeroy & N. J. M. D. Newman (Eds.). *Bradley and Daroff's Neurology in Clinical Practice*, 8th ed. (pp. 1498–1534.e1495).

Jennett, J. & Teasdale, G. (1981) *Management of Head Injuries.* Philadelphia: FA Davies.

Kazamel, M. (2020) 'Neuromuscular disorders'. In F. R. Amthor, A. B. Theibert, D. G. Standaert & E. D. Roberson (Eds.). *Essentials of Modern Neuroscience.* New York, NY: McGraw Hill.

Lowenstein, D. H., Martin, J. B. & Hauser, S. L. (2018) 'Approach to the patient with neurologic disease'. In Jameson, J., Fauci, A. S., Kasper, D. L., Hauser, S. L., Longo, D.L, & Loscalzo, J. (Eds.). *Harrison's Principles of Internal Medicine*, 20th ed. McGraw-Hill

Meador, W. (2020) 'Neuroimmunology & neuroinflammatory disorders'. In F. R. Amthor, A. B. Theibert, D. G. Standaert & E. D. Roberson (Eds.) *Essentials of Modern Neuroscience*. New York, NY: McGraw Hill

Mesfin, F. B., Gupta, N., Hays Shapshak, A., & Taylor, R. S. (2020) 'Diffuse axonal injury'. In StatPearls [Internet]. Treasure Island (FL): StatPearls Publishing. PMID: 28846342.

Nair, M, & Peate, I. (2009) *Fundamentals of Applied Pathophysiology*. Wiley Blackwell.

National Institute for Health and Clinical Excellence. (2007) *Head injury: Triage, assessment, investigation and early management of head injury in infants, children and adults.* NICE Clinical Guideline No. 56 (Partial update of NICE Clinical Guideline No. 4). London: NICE.

Parkinson's Disease Society. (2008) *Life with Parkinson's today – Room for improvement.* London: Parkinson's Disease Society.

Prince, M., Bryce, R. & Ferri, C. (2011) *The benefits of early diagnosis and intervention.* World Alzheimer Report 2011. www.alz.co.uk/research/WorldAlzheimerReport2011.pdf

Ropper, A. H., Samuels, M. A., Klein, J. P. & Prasad, S. (2019a) 'Stroke and cerebrovascular diseases'. In *Adams and Victor's Principles of Neurology,* 11th ed. New York, NY: McGraw-Hill Education.

Ropper, A. H., Samuels, M. A., Klein, J. P., & Prasad, S. (2019b) 'Epilepsy and other seizure disorders'. In *Adams and Victor's Principles of Neurology,* 11th ed. New York, NY: McGraw-Hill Education

Royal College of Physicians. (2020) *Prolonged disorders of consciousness following sudden onset brain injury.* National Clinical Guidelines. London: RCP.

Royal College of Physicians. (2008) *Stroke. National Clinical Guidelines for Diagnosis and Initial Management of Acute Stroke and Transient Ischaemic Attack (TIA).* London: RCP.

Saxena, M. K. (2019) 'Neuromuscular disorders'. In A. D, Bersten & J. M. Handy (Eds.), *Oh's Intensive Care Manual* (pp. 721–730.e722).

Stroke Foundation. (2020) Childhood stroke clinical guidelines. https://informme.org.au/en/Guidelines/Childhood-stroke-guidelines

Woodward, S. & Mestecky, A. (2011) *Neuroscience Nursing: Evidence Based Practice.* Wiley Blackwell.

Teasdale, G. & Jennett, B. (1974) Assessment of coma and impaired consciousness. A practical scale. *Lancet.* 13;2(7872): 81–84. doi: 10.1016/s0140-6736(74)91639-0

Tortora, G. J. & Derrickson, B. (2011) *Principles of anatomy and physiology.* Wiley Blackwell.

Waxman, S. G. (Ed.). (2020) Fundamentals of the nervous system. *Clinical Neuroanatomy*, 29th ed. McGraw-Hill.

Wilkinson, I. & Lennox, G. (2005) *Essential Neurology*. Wiley Blackwell.

ACKNOWLEDGEMENTS

Figure 18.8: © Aitken, Marshall, Chaboyer (2015), *ACCCN's Critical care nursing*, page 531, Elsevier. Reproduced with permission.

CHAPTER 19

Nursing care of conditions related to the immune system

LEARNING OBJECTIVES

After studying this chapter, you should be able to:

- **19.1** discuss the role of key cells and organs of the immune system in protecting individuals from infection
- **19.2** outline the immune defences that protect against invading foreign organisms
- **19.3** identify the inflammatory immune response
- **19.4** explain the lymphatic system's role in the immune system function
- **19.5** outline the conditions and diseases that can result from altered immune response
- **19.6** outline key nursing considerations for patients with immunodeficiency or altered immune response.

Introduction

The human body is an ideal host for many pathological organisms that live in the environment around us. On invading the body, these organisms can cause disease and ultimately death. The human body has developed an immune response to invading organisms to keep us healthy and free from infection. This chapter will explore the organs, cells and responses of the immune system. When alterations of the immune response occur, people can develop a range of conditions such as allergy, anaphylaxis, immunodeficiency disorders or autoimmune conditions. General nursing care for patients with immune-related conditions will be also be explored.

19.1 The immune system

LEARNING OBJECTIVE 19.1 Discuss the role of key cells and organs of the immune system in protecting individuals from infection.

The immune system is a unique body system that is spread throughout the entire body. Its role is to recognise cells that belong in the body and differentiate them from **pathogens** (foreign substances) that may cause damage, and remove them from the body.

Foreign substances include anything that comes from outside of the body (external factors), such as bacteria, viruses, fungi, parasites and environmental factors, such as the sun, chemicals, pollutants and trauma. Internal factors that are considered foreign include cancer and transplanted or grafted organs.

The immune system organs include the thymus, liver, blood, bone marrow, tonsils, lymph nodes and spleen. Their locations in the body are identified in figure 19.1.

19.2 Immune defence mechanisms

LEARNING OBJECTIVE 19.2 Outline the immune defences that protect against invading foreign organisms.

The human body has two types of defence mechanisms, innate and adaptive, that work together to protect us from foreign substances.

Innate immunity

The innate defences are those we are born with and include:

- skin and mucous membranes to provide physical barriers
- immune cells and proteins
- inflammation and fever.

These defences combine to provide a generalised response to injury/infection (Garvan Institute of Medical Research 2020b; Hendrick 2019b).

Intact skin

Our body is defended first by skin, acting as a physical barrier. High levels of keratin in the epidermis prevent many foreign substances from entering the body. Secretions in the skin form an acid mantle (acid layer) that prevents bacteria from growing on the skin, and normal skin flora helps to protect against invading foreign bodies.

Intact mucous membranes

Mucous membranes continue the physical barrier to prevent foreign substances from entering the body where there is an opening from inside the body to the outside, such as the respiratory, gastrointestinal and genitourinary tracts. The lining of the lungs has the largest surface area of the entire body that connects to the outside (Kikkert 2020). Mucous is a physical barrier that traps substances in the respiratory and digestive tracts.

Other physical barriers of the innate immune system include:

- nasal hair and cilia that trap foreign substances in the nasal passages and move them away from the respiratory tract
- gastric fluids containing acids and enzymes that destroy foreign substances in the stomach
- the acid mantle in the vagina prevents bacteria and fungi from growing
- enzymes in saliva, respiratory mucous (mucin), ear wax (cerumen) and eye fluid (lacrima) destroy bacteria
- acidic urine flushes the urinary tract and prevents bacteria from growing (Hendrick 2019b; Maricb & Hoen 2016).

FIGURE 19.1 Organs of the immune system

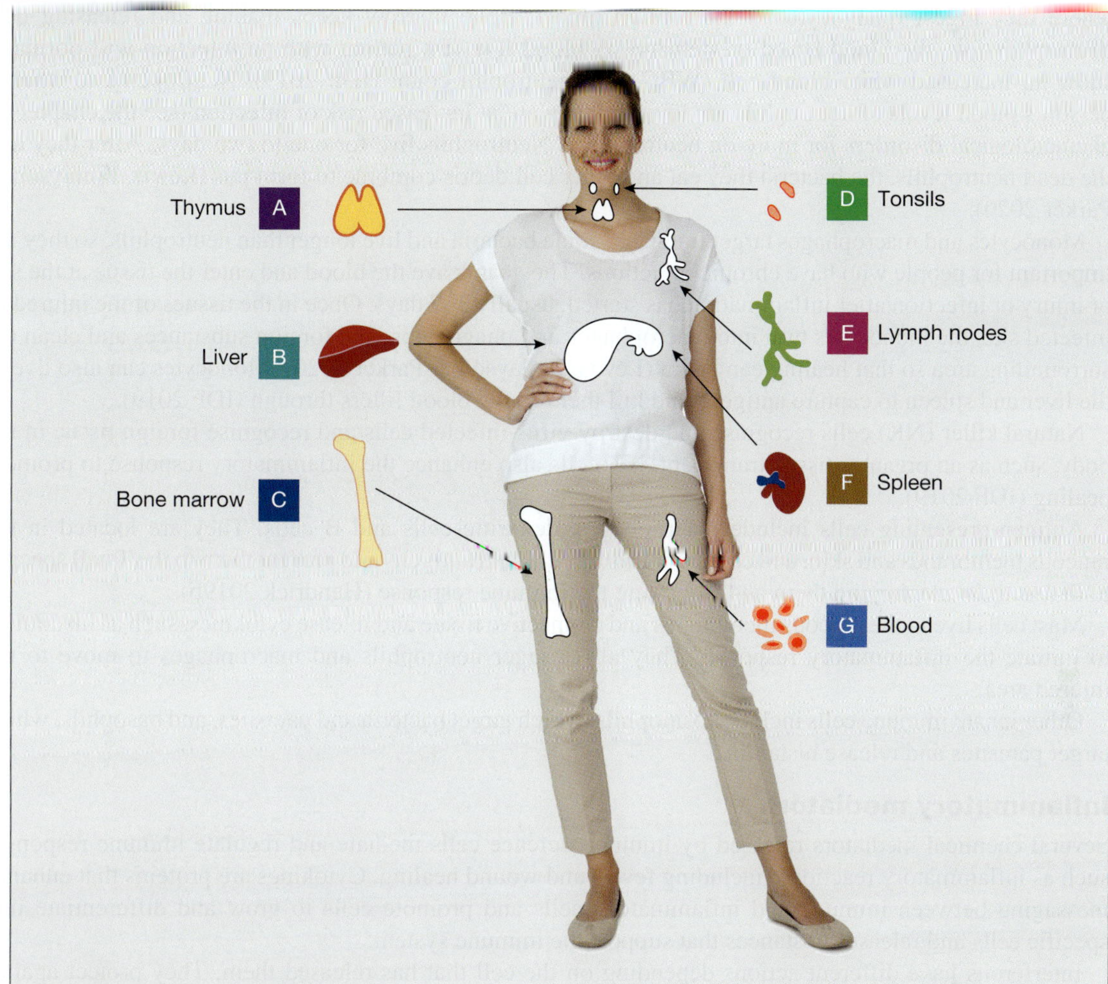

A: The thymus is where T lymphocytes go to mature when they leave the bone marrow. When they have matured, they learn to differentiate between normal, healthy cells that they should not attack and infected cells that they must respond to.
B: Phagocytic cells of the liver clean bacteria from our blood as it moves through the liver. The liver also produces enzymes that support the complement system. Complement is the process of opsonisation coating pathogens in a substance that helps the neutrophils and monocytes to break down their protective outer layer.
C: Our immune cells are made in our bone marrow and begin as stem cells, which can develop into any type of blood cell.
D: Tonsils in our throat contain lymphocytes, and adenoids that trap antigens (bacteria and viruses).
E: Lymph nodes are throughout the body, in our throat, armpits, groin and GIT system (Peyers Patches) and contain B and T lymphocytes.
F: The spleen filters our blood and contains B lymphocytes and monocytes that kill pathogens that pass through it.
G: Blood carries immune cells and proteins around the body.

Source: Adapted from Immune Deficiency Foundation (IDF) (2019).

Cells of the innate immune system

The cells of the innate immune system include **phagocytes**, natural killer cells, antigen-presenting cells and cytokines. Phagocytes are made in the bone marrow and circulate in the blood. These cells eat the cells of invading foreign substances, damaged or dead cells. They include neutrophils and **monocytes**.

When an infection is detected, large numbers of neutrophils (also called **granulocytes** because they contain granules) leave the bloodstream and enter the tissue at the site of injury or infection (chemotaxis), where they ingest (phagocytosis) the foreign object. Bone marrow keeps making and releasing new neutrophils into the blood based on demand. A blood test of a patient with an infection will normally show an increased white blood cell (WBC) and neutrophil count (IDF 2019). Neutropenia is when a person's blood levels of neutrophils are low, and they are at increased risk of infection (see the chapter on haematological disorders for more on neutropenia). Neutrophils live for one to two days. After they die, the dead neutrophils, the bacteria they eat and other cell debris combine to form pus (Lewis, Finlayson & Parker 2020).

Monocytes and macrophages target fungi and some bacteria and live longer than neutrophils, so they are important for people who have chronic infections. They can leave the blood and enter the tissue at the site of injury or infection after inflammation has started, usually 3–7 days. Once in the tissues of the injured or infected site, the monocytes turn into macrophages and phagocytose the foreign substances and clean the surrounding area so that healing can begin (Lewis, Finlayson & Parker 2020). Monocytes can also live in the liver and spleen to capture antigens and kill them as the blood filters through (IDF 2019).

Natural killer (NK) cells recognise and destroy virus-infected cells and recognise foreign tissue in the body, such as an organ or tissue transplant. NK cells also enhance the inflammatory response to promote healing (IDF 2019).

Antigen-presenting cells include macrophages, dendritic cells and B cells. They are located in the mucous membranes and skin, and capture invading cells and antigens and present them to the T cell specific to that antigen, destroying them and triggering the immune response (Hendrick 2019b).

Mast cells live in the mucous membranes and connective tissue and release cytokines, such as histamine, to initiate the inflammatory response. They also trigger neutrophils and macrophages to move to the injured area.

Other innate immune cells include eosinophils, which target bacteria and parasites, and basophils, which target parasites and release histamine.

Inflammatory mediators

Several chemical mediators released by immune defence cells mediate and regulate immune responses such as inflammatory reactions (including fever) and wound healing. Cytokines are proteins that enhance messaging between immune and inflammatory cells and promote cells to grow and differentiate into specific cells and release substances that support the immune system.

Interferons have different actions depending on the cell that has released them. They protect against viral infections and work to protect uninfected cells or increase macrophage activity (Lewis, Finlayson & Parker 2020).

Complement is an enzyme produced in the liver. When the complement system is activated, antigens are coated in chemicals that help the phagocytes to identify and ingest the foreign substance and enhance the inflammatory response to promote healing (Lewis, Finlayson & Parker 2020).

Adaptive immunity

Adaptive immunity is acquired after the body has been exposed to a specific foreign substance, and it can provide us with long-term immunity. Exposure to the substance allows specific antibodies and lymphocytes to develop, which speeds up the immune response the next time that same substance is detected. For example, vaccines are made of weakened viruses or an inactive part of a virus that cannot make a person sick. When a person is administered a vaccine, it mimics the active virus, which causes the immune system to produce an **antibody** specific to that virus; however, the person does not become sick (Hendrick 2019b).

There are two types of adaptive immune responses, humoral immunity and cell-mediated immunity.

Humoral immunity is when plasma cells create specific antibodies (immunoglobulin [Ig]) in response to a foreign substance circulating in the blood or lymph and produce memory cells to make the immune response faster in the subsequent exposure to that same **antigen** (Hendrick 2019b).

Cell-mediated immunity is when T cells also undergo differentiation and develop into several types of cells in response to the presence of an antigen. For example, helper T cells help active both cell-mediated and humoral immune responses. Memory cells induce the secondary immune response, cytotoxic cells attack and remove pathogens and infected cells, and macrophages secrete cytokines that activate or signal other cells (Hendrick 2019b).

Cells and proteins of the adaptive immune system

Cells of the adaptive immune system include antibodies and lymphocytes.

Antibodies prevent infection by bind to the surface of viruses, preventing the virus from attaching to healthy tissue of the body. Other antibodies activate the complement system (Lewis, Finlayson & Parker 2020). Antibodies live for a long time and protect us from infections that may have happened a long time ago. For example, we may have been exposed to an antigen (or been immunised) during childhood; however, we still have antibodies that protect us and prevent us from becoming ill from that specific antigen (IDF 2019).

Lymphocytes are cells that travel in the lymph fluid. Lymphocytes turn into B and T cells as part of the adaptive immune response.

B lymphocyte cells are WBCs that originate in the bone marrow but are found in lymph fluid. Their job is to produce plasma cells (which produce specific immunoglobulins (antibodies) to an antigen/infection). For example, when an antigen is detected, some of the B lymphocytes turn into memory cells to allow a rapid response to future infections. Other B lymphocytes turn into plasma cells, which are responsible for making antibodies (immunoglobulins). There are a number of classes of immunoglobulins.

- IgM (immunoglobulin M), which moves through the body in the blood and is the first responder to infection and the first to reach the antigen.
- IgA (Immunoglobulin A) found in the mucous membranes (mouth, nose, lungs and GIT). These antibodies move into the bloodstream, tissue, tears and secretions in the GIT and respiratory system to recognise and attack specific antigens.
- IgG (Immunoglobulin G) travel in the blood and move easily into the tissues. This antibody is able to cross the placenta and provide the foetus with some immune protection.
- IgE are responsible for allergic reactions.
- IgD are thought to help maintain haemostasis of the GIT system (IDF 2019).

T lymphocytes respond to specific antigens, and as B cells, they are also WBCs that develop from stem cells made in the bone marrow and mature in the thymus. Once mature, they leave the thymus and move to other organs in the immune system (spleen, lymph nodes and bone marrow), where they can directly attack the antigen. T cells in the blood become memory T cells after exposure to a specific antigen (IDF 2019).

Types of T cells include:

- helper T cells help killer T cells by producing antibodies and binding to target cells
- regulatory T cells tell the immune system when the infection is under control or when more lymphocytes are needed. Without these cells, the immune system would keep working and attacking cells (IDF 2019).

Table 19.1 provides a comparison of the key differences between the innate and adaptive immune responses.

TABLE 19.1 Comparison of the innate and adaptive immune responses

Feature	Innate immune response	Adaptive immune response
Activation time	Begins quickly, within minutes to hours.	Slow to respond, can take a number of days.
Response time and duration	Responds to general pathogens or foreign substances. Short-term protection.	Specific response; can differentiate between pathogens. Long-term protection.
Cells	Macrophages, neutrophils, NK cells, dendritic cells, basophils, eosinophils.	Lymphocytes (T cells, B cells) and antigen-presenting cells.
Chemicals	Cytokines, interferons, complement.	Antibodies, cytokines, interferons, complement.
Self-cell differentiation	Yes, can differentiate between self-cells and invading cells.	Yes, can differentiate between self-cells and foreign cells but not as well as innate immunity. Problems differentiating cause autoimmune diseases.
Memory	No	Yes, provides long-term protection and a faster response on next exposure.

Source: Adapted from Hendrick (2019b).

Table 19.2 summarises the immune system's response to bacterial and viral infection.

TABLE 19.2 Summary of the response of the immune system to invading bacteria and viruses

Invading bacteria	Invading viruses
If bacteria are able to penetrate into the tissues of the body: 1. Complement 2. Antibodies (immunoglobulin). These allow the neutrophils to differentiate the foreign substance from normal body cells and respond by 3. Phagocytosing (engulfing) and granulocytosis occurs to kill the bacteria. All three stages must be working together to kill the invading bacteria. Invading bacteria can overwhelm the immune response if there are large numbers of if there are deficits in complement, antibody production or neutrophils.	If a virus enters a cell, the cell releases cytokines to prevent other cells from becoming infected. If this is not effective and other cells become infected, T cells and NK cells go to the site of infection to kill the infected cells (which also kills other uninfected cells). While the T cells are destroying the virus, B cells make specific antibodies to prevent infection, and memory T cells are made so that if the same infection occurs a second time, it will be minor or not as severe.

Source: Adapted from Immune Deficiency Foundation (IDF) (2019).

Organ transplants and the immune system

Transplanted body organs, tissues and fluids can be recognised as foreign substances because the acquired immune system recognises the antigens on the transplanted organ's surface and begins to attack it. Immunosuppressant drugs help to reduce the risk of rejection by reducing the immune response; however, they are not always successful (Lewis, Finlayson & Parker 2020).

The human **leukocyte** antigen (HLA) genes are responsible for rejecting foreign tissue; therefore, patients receiving an organ transplant require a good HLA match. The poorer the HLA match, the greater likelihood that rejection will occur. Typing of donors and recipients is done to identify a potential donor match.

In Australia in 2019, 1444 people received a lifesaving organ donation from 548 deceased organ donors and 239 living organ transplants. There are currently 1600 people on the organ transplant waiting list (DonateLife 2020).

19.3 The inflammatory response

LEARNING OBJECTIVE 19.3 Identify the inflammatory immune response.

When pathogenic organisms gain access to the body, the next line of defence is the inflammatory response. Inflammation is important because it limits the spread of the infective agents to other cells, gets rid of cell debris and pathogens, alerts the adaptive immune system and prepares the injured site for healing to commence. Inflammation can be a therapeutic response to injury or disease; however, if it becomes chronic, it can worsen the condition by damaging cells and tissue, which delays wound healing (Marieb & Hoen 2016).

The inflammatory response begins with:

1. vasodilation to slow blood flow and increase blood volume at the injured area
2. plasma escapes out of the vessels (exudation), which causes further swelling and pain and increases blood viscosity (thickening), further slowing the blood flow and increasing the RBC concentration, bringing oxygen and nutrients to the area
3. granulocytes and monocytes then commence phagocytosis.

On assessment of your patient with an infection, heat/fever, swelling, redness and/or pain are the primary findings.

Fever is when body temperature is greater than 37 degrees Celsius and is how the body increases the defences against invading organisms. It is caused when pyrogens are released by leukocytes and macrophages when they are exposed to foreign substances. Pyrogens produce prostaglandins that trigger the thermoregulatory centre in the hypothalamus to increase the body's temperature (set point) and enhance the immune response. Shivering, decreased perspiration and peripheral blood flow result, causing the patient to feel cold until a higher temperature is reached (Lewis, Finlayson & Parker 2020; van de Mortel 2017).

Nursing care of fever

Nursing management of fever begins by:

- obtaining and documenting the patient's vital signs
- encouraging oral fluids to replace the fluid lost from the increased body temperature and metabolism
- administration of prescribed antipyretic medications, salicylates (aspirin), acetaminophen or non-steroidal anti-inflammatories (NSAIDs), which lower temperature by acting on the thermoregulatory centre or interfere with the prostaglandins. Remember to assess your patient's response to the medication.

Despite a fever, any intervention to cool the patient that may cause shivering (such as a fan directly blowing on the patient or tepid sponge) is not recommended. Shivering is the body's response to increased body temperature (Lewis, Finlayson & Parker 2020).

Extremely high fevers of over 40 degrees can be harmful, causing seizures and damaging cells and the bodies temperature control centre in the hypothalamus. Fever in patients who have altered immune response is a potentially serious complication because severe infections can develop quickly (Lewis, Finlayson & Parker 2020).

19.4 The lymphatic system's role in immunity

LEARNING OBJECTIVE 19.4 Explain the lymphatic system's role in the immune response.

The lymphatic system is complex, and its role is to support the cardiovascular and immune systems. The role of the lymph system in immunity is to filter lymph, trap and destroy specific pathogens and trigger the immune response (Knight & Nigam 2020).

Interstitial fluid containing vital gases and nutrients moves from the vascular system and bathes cells in oxygen and other substances that help the body to function normally. The interstitial fluid that is not absorbed by the cells is absorbed by the lymphatic system and is returned to the vascular system, providing an avenue for cellular waste products and excess fluid to be returned to the circulating blood (Al-Kofahi et al. 2017).

Lymphoedema

If interstitial fluid accumulates in the tissues, it can cause swelling. Swelling may damage tissue by compressing tiny blood vessels with the accumulated fluid (Knight & Nigam 2020). This is a chronic (long lasting) condition called lymphoedema (Marieb & Hoen 2016).

Lymphoedema occurs because the normal flow of lymph is decreased. A primary cause is when a person is born with a malformation of the lymph vessels.

Secondary causes of lymphoedema are because of:

- a tumour
- lymph nodes have been removed or radiated because of cancer treatment
- damage during trauma or surgery
- obesity
- immobility
- filariasis — parasitic worm infestation transmitted via mosquito bites that lodge in the lymph glands and nodes (ALA 2021).

Lymphoedema can affect a person of any age and develop in a person's head, neck, arms and legs, trunk, breast or genitals/groin.

Lymphoedema can cause:

- physical discomfort and interference with normal limb movement, which may cause problems for the person in managing their normal activities of daily living such as dressing and mobility
- psychological distress, anxiety and depression due to altered body image and function. This may be particularly challenging for children and teenagers to learn to adapt to and manage as part of their life
- impaired wound healing, cellulitis (infections) and ulcers from decreased cellular oxygen delivery to swollen areas (ALA 2021).

Nursing care of lymphoedema

Management of lymphoedema should include:

- avoiding anything that may slow the flow of lymph through the limb, such as applying a blood pressure cuff, tourniquet or administering injections
- encouraging limb mobility
- keeping skin in good condition to help minimise the risk of infection
- compression garments, undergoing lymphatic drainage massage or physiotherapy to promote lymph drainage (CCN 2018).

19.5 Conditions resulting from an altered immune response

LEARNING OBJECTIVE 19.5 Outline the conditions and diseases that can result from altered immune responses.

The inflammatory and immune response is integral for tissue growth and repair following injury and protection against disease. These usually protective mechanisms can sometimes produce reactions in the body, such as allergy or anaphylaxis. Alternatively, people may have altered immune responses to injury or infection, such as immunodeficiency and autoimmune conditions.

Allergy

When the body's immune system overreacts to an otherwise harmless substance, it is called an allergy. An allergen is a specific substance that triggers the immune system to overreact.

In Australia, 4 million people have an allergy, which can result from exposure to dust mites, medications, insect stings/bites/venom, ticks, pollen, grasses, moulds, domestic animals or proteins that are in food (Asthma & Anaphylaxis Australia 2020).

When the immune system has its first exposure to an allergen, it responds by producing antibodies that adhere to mast cells and basophils. The mast cell releases histamine when they come into contact with the allergen, which causes redness, swelling and discomfort. Other symptoms can include irritated eyes (conjunctivitis), nose (hay fever/allergic rhinitis) and skin (eczema or hives), allergic asthma and anaphylaxis (Asthma & Anaphylaxis Australia 2020).

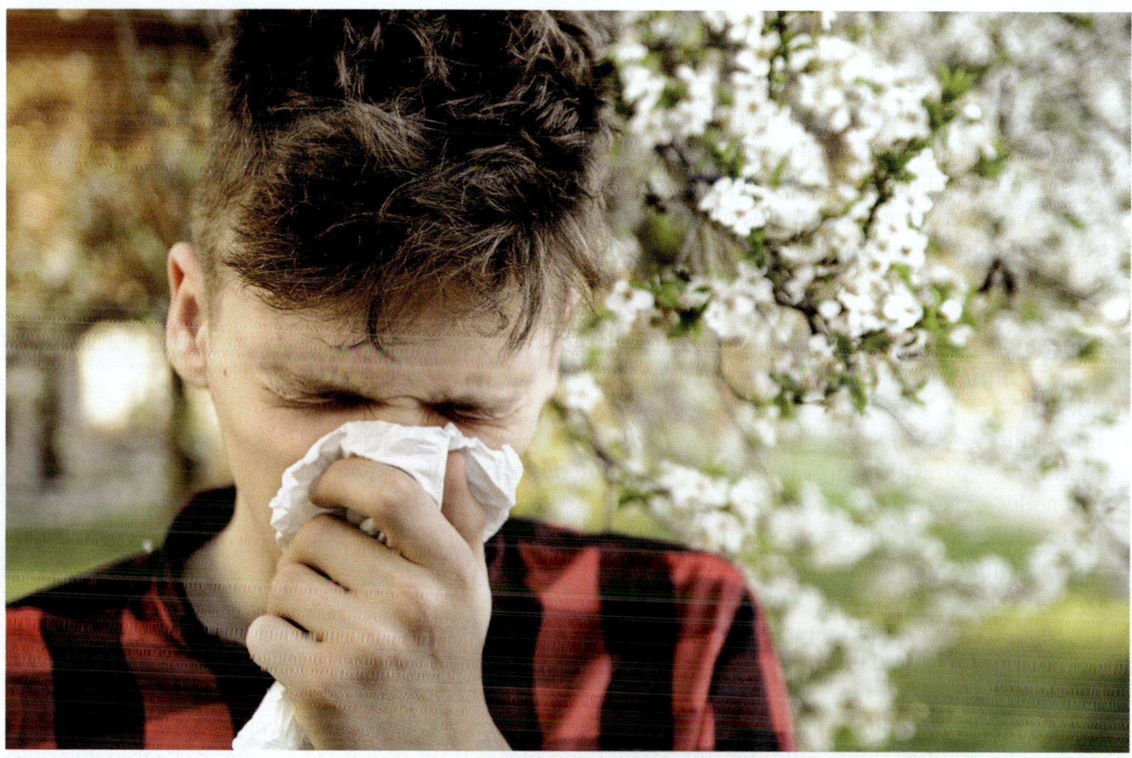

Atopy is used to identify a person who has a genetic predisposition to develop an allergy, and allergy is 60 per cent more likely to develop in a person if they have a biological parent who has an allergy (National Asthma Council Australia 2021).

There are strong links between asthma and allergies that may trigger an asthma attack, for example, allergic rhinitis. If exposure to known allergens can be limited, episodes of asthma may be reduced. Triggers can include dust mites, pollen, food, mould, pets and latex (see figure 19.2). Careful management of known allergies will help to limit exacerbations of asthma (National Asthma Council Australia 2021).

To identify asthma allergens, a person may undergo skin prick tests and blood tests to identify the presence of specific IgE antibodies in the blood (National Asthma Council Australia 2021).

For more information on living with asthma, visit The National Asthma Council: www.nationalasthma.org.au/living-with-asthma.

In Australia and New Zealand, food allergies are more common in children, with up to 10 per cent of infants, 8 per cent of children and 2 per cent of adults experiencing allergy. Food allergy signs and symptoms can include excessive crying in young babies (colic), eczema, asthma, and anaphylaxis (Australasian Society of Clinical Immunology and Allergy 2019). You can watch a summary of food allergy and the immune system here: www.allergyfacts.org.au/allergy-anaphylaxis/what-is-allergy.

Adults and children who have a food allergy can undergo a food challenge in a controlled setting that determines if the person has an allergy or if the allergy has resolved.

Almost any substance can be an allergen for some individuals. These allergens can enter the body through various routes such as inhalation, injection, ingestion or direct contact with the skin (Asthma & Anaphylaxis Australia 2020). Allergy usually appears on repeated contact with the allergen.

Allergic reactions can be:

- localised, affecting one body part or a limited area, for example, hives, sneezing, abdominal cramps or swelling of the lips
- systemic, affecting several parts or the entire body, for example, acute anaphylaxis or bronchoconstriction.

FIGURE 19.2 Examples of allergens

- Plant pollens
- Dust mites
- Latex
- Certain foods, e.g. milk, peanuts, shellfish, wheat, soy and eggs
- Antibiotics, e.g. penicillin and tetracycline
- Insect bites and venom, e.g. wasp, honeybee, ant and snake.

Anaphylaxis

A severe allergic reaction to an allergen causes a person to develop allergy symptoms in more than one body system suddenly. Anaphylaxis can be life-threatening and must be treated immediately (Burchum & Rosenthal 2019b).

Warning signs of anaphylaxis can include:

- swelling of lips, face or eyes (angio-oedema)
- hives or welts
- tingling mouth
- abdominal pain, vomiting (if the allergic reaction is from insect bites or stings).

Signs that a person is having an anaphylactic reaction include:

- difficulty or noisy breathing (bronchospasm)
- swelling of the tongue
- swelling/tightness in the throat
- wheeze or persistent cough
- difficulty talking and/or hoarse voice
- persistent dizziness or collapse
- pale and floppy (in young children).

People known to suffer anaphylaxis will have an anaphylaxis action plan and carry an epinephrine injection (EpiPen) (Asthma & Anaphylaxis Australia 2020; ASCIA 2020b).

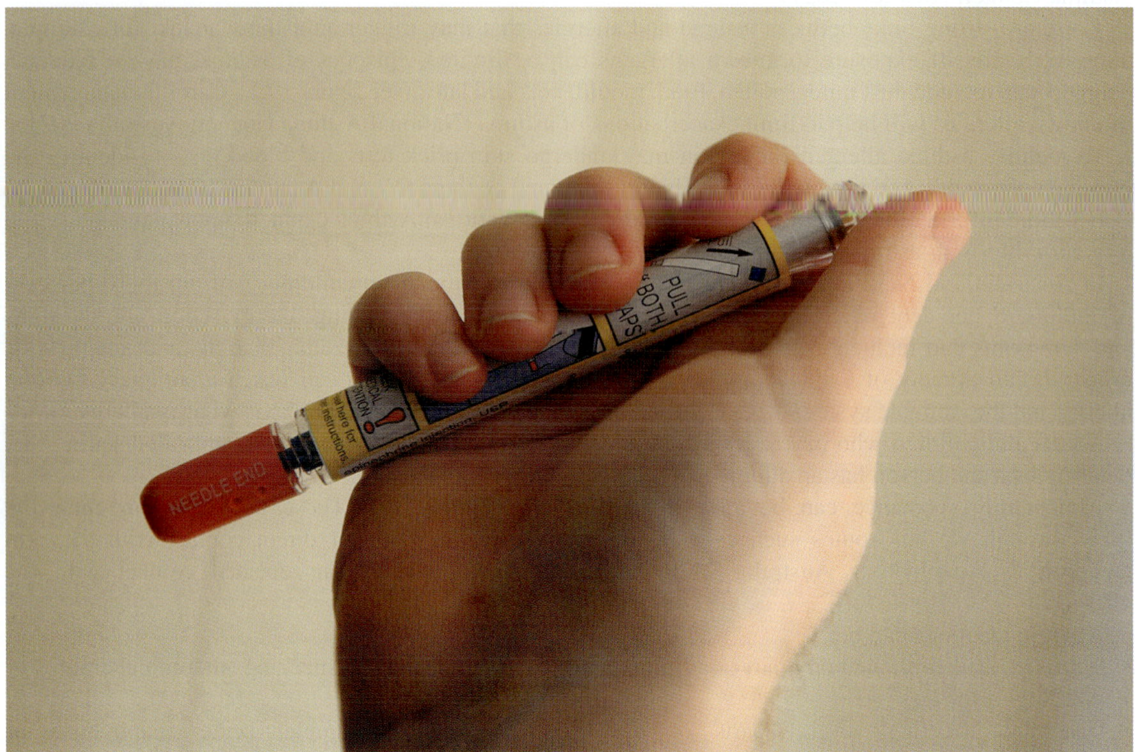

In Australia, the NSQHS Medication Safety Standard addresses the obligations of health services to patients with known drug allergies or who experience an adverse reaction while in hospital. In healthcare facilities, patients with allergies or adverse drug reactions wear a red wrist band and have the allergy documented in their patient history and on their medication chart. They also have an alert sticker on their hard-copy healthcare record or electronic allergy/ADR alerts in a digital healthcare record (Australian Commission on Safety and Quality in Health Care 2019).

The NSQHS Medication Safety Standard can be viewed at the following link: www.safetyandquality.gov.au/standards/nsqhs-standards/medication-safety-standard.

The two videos in this link explain the signs and symptoms of anaphylaxis and demonstrate how to administer an EpiPen to a person experiencing anaphylaxis: www.allergyfacts.org.au/resources/videos-from-a-aa.

Adrenaline and anaphylaxis

Epinephrine is a catecholamine — a hormone naturally produced by the body and contributes to our fight or flight response. Epinephrine is administered during anaphylaxis because it triggers the fight or flight response to increase blood flow to muscles, the heart and lungs.

Epinephrine acts on the:

- alpha 1 receptors in smooth muscles to cause vasoconstriction and elevate blood pressure
- beta 1 receptors in the heart to increase heart rate and the strength of the heart's contractions
- beta 2 receptors in the lungs to relax the bronchioles (bronchodilation) and improve gas exchange (Burchum & Rosenthal 2019a).

Anaphylaxis is a severe allergic reaction that is of rapid onset and can have a potentially fatal outcome, even with immediate medical intervention. It affects many organs within seconds or minutes of exposure to the allergen, so prevention is critical (Asthma & Anaphylaxis Australia 2020).

More anaphylaxis resources can be accessed here: www.allergy.org.au/hp/anaphylaxis.

Allergy treatment involves removing or discontinuing the causative agent and administering drugs such as adrenaline, corticosteroids and antihistamines. Nurses have a responsibility to recognise the signs and symptoms of anaphylaxis and respond promptly and efficiently. Table 19.3 outlines the medications and treatments for allergy and anaphylaxis.

TABLE 19.3 **Medications and treatment for allergy and anaphylaxis**

Medication	Pharmacology
Antihistamines	Available to buy over the counter (OTC) in pharmacies. They are used to block the release of histamine from mast cells, reducing allergic symptoms There are two types of antihistamines: H1 receptor blockers, which cause drowsiness, and H2 receptor blockers, which do not cause drowsiness.
Corticosteroids	Corticosteroids are used suppress the immune response (in the case of organ or tissue transplant) or when the body is under stress (such as allergic reaction) to reduce swelling that develops. They increase the number of RBCs, leukocytes and decrease the number of lymphocytes, eosinophils, basophils and monocytes.
Epinephrine (Adrenaline)	Epinephrine is administered during anaphylaxis because it triggers the fight or flight response to increase blood flow to our muscles, heart and lungs.

Source: Adapted from Burchum & Rosenthal (2019b & c).

Immunodeficiency

Sometimes the body does not respond properly to an infection. This can be from a primary or secondary cause.

Primary immunodeficiency (PID) is thought to be genetically inherited and can be diagnosed in people of any age. PID occurs because there is a problem with the immune cells, such as complement or phagocytic deficiencies or combined immunodeficiencies, which alter the body's immune response (ASICA 2021, IDF 2019).

People who have PID have an increased risk of developing infections, may have several infections simultaneously, or have an infection that is difficult to treat because of the type of infection or location in the body (IDF 2019). Delayed treatment may result in severe or life-threatening complications, and treatments may include antibiotics, immunoglobulin replacement therapy (IRT), immunomodulation (to increase or suppress immune function) or stem cell transplant (ASCIA 2020a).

Some people with PID may develop '**autoimmunity**' and is when the immune response is triggered when there is no infection, and the immune system attacks itself (ASCIA 2021).

Secondary immunodeficiencies are an antibody deficiency resulting from medical treatment that suppresses the immune system, such as when a person has:

- chemotherapy
- haematological malignancies
- renal or gastrointestinal immunoglobulin loss
- organ transplantation
- infectious diseases
- corticosteroid, anticonvulsant or immunosuppressive medications (ASICA 2019, IDF 2019).

HIV and AIDS

In 1981, the first reports of deaths from acquired immune deficiency syndrome (AIDS) were reported. By the year 2000, AIDS was the eighth leading cause of death worldwide. Between the start of the human immune deficiency virus (HIV) epidemic in the early 1980s and 2019, 33 million people died from AIDS-related illnesses globally. Testing, diagnosis and treatment (pre-exposure prophylaxis [PReP], antiviral medications and post-exposure prophylaxis [PREP]) has reduced death from AIDS from the eighth leading cause of death globally in 2000, to the 19th leading cause of death in 2019 (WHO 2020a). Of all people living with HIV globally, two-thirds live in sub-Saharan Africa (WHO 2020b). Currently in Australia, 0.14 per cent of the population live with HIV (Australian Federation of AIDS Organisations 2021).

AIDS is a blood-borne infection transmitted through blood or blood products, the sharing of intravenous needles, unprotected anal and vaginal intercourse or from mother-foetus transmission. Healthcare workers can come into contact with the virus through needle-stick injuries and open wounds (Hendrick 2019a) HIV is the most severe secondary immunodeficiency. It destroys helper T cells, which control the humoral immunity response to create specific antibodies (Ig) in response to a previously detected foreign substance, and cell-mediated immunity, when T cells also undergo differentiation and develop into several types of cells that react directly with the antigen on the surface of foreign substances or infectious agents.

HIV is a retrovirus, which means that it is able to change the DNA of a cell and remain dormant inside the cell until it is activated. If activated, the virus replicates, and the person develops AIDS, causing multiple infections, cancers and chronic conditions because of their severely diminished immune response, and the person is unlikely to survive (Hendrick 2019a). The effects of HIV/AIDS on the body is outlined in figure 19.3.

FIGURE 19.3 Alterations in immune function

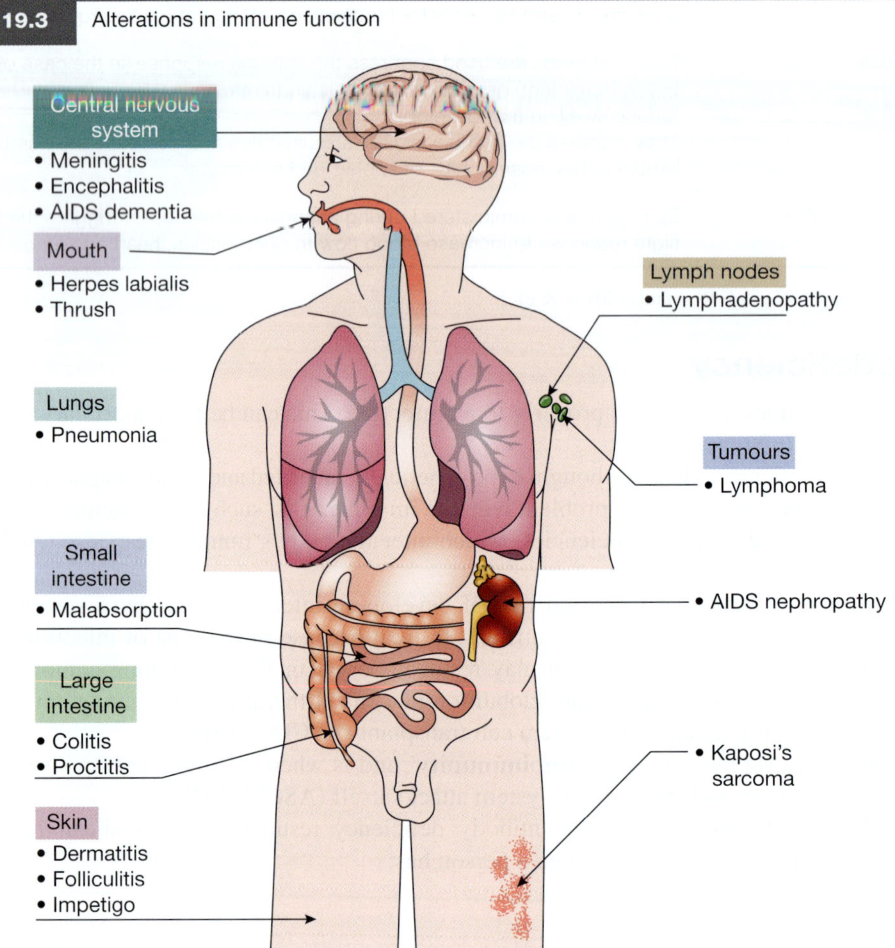

Source: Hendrick (2019a).

Autoimmune disorders

Autoimmune conditions occur when a person's immune system is overactive and does not recognise its own 'self' cells. The immune system produces antibodies that attack cells, tissues and organs as if they were foreign substances, which causes injury, inflammation and impaired function. There are more than 100 autoimmune disorders, and in Australia and New Zealand, approximately five per cent of people have an autoimmune disease. More than 12 per cent of people will be affected by one autoimmune disease during their lifetime (Garvan Institute of Medical Research 2020a).

Some people develop an autoimmune disease secondary to an infection, while some medications may trigger disease in others. Autoimmune diseases can be genetic, passed from parent to child, and females more likely to be affected than males (ASICA 2020a).

There is no cure for autoimmune diseases, and treatment and management of the condition are by clinical specialists who aim to:

- manage the specific symptoms
- reduce further tissue/organ damage
- maintain the existing tissue/organ function.

The symptoms will depend on the type of disease and how far it has progressed. Some people may require medications that replace hormones their body is no longer able to produce (insulin, thyroid hormone and corticosteroids), and other people may need anti-inflammatories, immunosuppressants or antibody replacement (immunoglobulin therapy) (ASCIA 2020b).

Some people may undergo a treatment called apheresis, wherein the person's blood is collected and separated with a specific component removed before the blood is returned to the patient. For example, leukocytapheresis removes WBCs from patients with some leukemias who have high levels of abnormal WBCs. In comparison, plasmapheresis (sometimes called plasma exchange) is used to remove inflammatory mediators and autoantibodies from patients with autoimmune diseases, including systemic lupus erythematosus (SLE), glomerulonephritis, Goodpasture's syndrome, myasthenia gravis, thrombocytopenic purpura, rheumatoid arthritis and Guillain-Barré syndrome (van de Mortel 2017).

Myasthenia gravis

Myasthenia gravis (MG) is an autoimmune neuromuscular disease characterised by weakness and easy fatigability of the voluntary muscles during activity but improves with rest. Voluntary muscles are used for eyelid and eye movement, facial expression, talking, chewing and swallowing, breathing and limb movement. Symptoms may develop over days or weeks, and the muscles involved and degree of weakness is widely variable (Brain Foundation 2020). Weakness occurs due to an antibody attack on the acetylcholine receptors, which interferes with impulse conduction at the neuromuscular junction, reducing the muscles' ability to contract.

Women have a higher incidence than men in developing MG, and the disease can be diagnosed at any age, although it typically occurs between the ages of 20 and 30 years. MG is diagnosed based on clinical presentation and by testing the person's response to anticholinesterase medication. As MG is a rare disorder, the diagnosis is often delayed or missed. People who have MG may experience a relapse of symptoms triggered by infection, fever, emotional stress or adverse medication reaction.

The signs and symptoms of a mild form of MG include disturbances of the ocular muscles presenting as weakness, double vision and a droopy or sleepy appearance of the face.

Severe symptoms include:

- difficulties with swallowing and chewing
- generalised muscle weakness
- fatigue
- altered bladder and bowel function
- respiratory difficulties.

Treatment involves the use of anticholinesterases and immunosuppressants, which reduce the symptoms and increase the periods between remissions and relapses. Removal of the thymus gland (thymectomy) may also improve the symptoms. Some patients may have plasmapheresis to temporarily removes specific antibodies from the blood and replaces them with donated antibodies (Brain Foundation 2020).

Nursing care priorities include:

- assessing and managing symptoms associated with reduced muscle function and fatigue
- promoting mobility and self-care (which improves muscle strength)
- encouraging rest during times of weakness and fatigue
- close observation of respiratory function (as there is a potential for a weakening of the diaphragm and intercostal muscles); check for:
  - difficulty breathing
  - coughing
  - increased secretions
- assistance with communication, eye care and nutritional support if patients have difficulty swallowing or have weakness in their eyes or facial muscles
- close monitoring of patients' responses to drug therapy, enabling an early recognition of myasthenic or cholinergic crises.

Systemic lupus erythematosus (SLE)

Lupus affects one in 600 people in Australia, with 90 per cent of those affected being females between 15 and 45 years of age (Garvan Institute of Medical Research 2020c). Lupus occurs when the immune system produces antibodies that affect connective tissue, causing joint pain, inflammation and tissue damage to any body system or organ. The most commonly affected areas are the skin and joints; however, the heart, lungs, kidneys and blood cells can also be affected. People with lupus can develop skin rashes, experience hair loss, fatigue and lethargy, fever and weight loss. Nursing care is focused on minimising or relieving the symptoms that individual patients develop.

The course and severity of SLE vary, so early signs and symptoms, such as fever, fatigue and weight loss, may be non-specific and mimic those of other disorders. Clinical manifestations of the disease are included in table 19.4.

TABLE 19.4 Signs and symptoms of SLE

System affected	Signs and symptoms
Musculoskeletal	Morning stiffness Joint pain and swelling Muscle weakness Arthritis
Dermatological	Photosensitivity Malar rash (butterfly rash) on the cheeks and bridge of the nose Alopecia
Renal	Proteinuria Haematuria Nephritis
Cardiovascular	Pericarditis Myocarditis Endocarditis Atherosclerosis
Gastrointestinal	Anorexia Nausea Vomiting Abdominal pain Peritonitis
Pulmonary	Pleuritis Pleural effusion Pneumonitis Pulmonary hypertension
Haematological	Anaemia Thrombocytopenia
Neurological	Headaches Seizures Psychosis Depression

There are several medications used in the treatment of lupus to prevent flare-ups of symptoms and reduce their severity and duration. These include NSAIDs, corticosteroids, disease-modifying antirheumatic drugs (DMARD) and immunosuppressants. More information on the medications used to treat SLE can be access from this link: www.msk.org.au/lupus.

Patients may be very well when in remission and have no limitations on their daily activities. However, during periods of relapse, symptoms may be so severe that patients may have to be admitted to a critical care unit. Nursing interventions are directed towards assessing and managing individual patient symptoms, including fatigue and confusion, preventing infection, maintaining skin integrity, managing joint pain, preventing seizures, and monitoring renal and respiratory function.

The Australian Society of Clinical Immunology and Allergy (ASCIA) is the peak body for allergy and immunology in Australia and New Zealand and provide further information about lupus on their web page: www.allergy.org.au/patients/autoimmunity/systemic-lupus-erythematosus-sle.

Common autoimmune conditions

Type 1 diabetes, Hashimoto's thyroiditis and rheumatoid arthritis (RA) are three common autoimmune conditions in Australia.

In Australia, ten per cent of people with diabetes have type 1. In this type of diabetes, the immune system begins to destroy the beta cells in the islets of Langerhans in the pancreas, causing an insulin, amylin and glucagon hormone imbalance. Initially, beta cells can compensate, and insulin and amylin are still produced; however, as more cells are destroyed, production decreases until insufficient insulin and amylin are being released (List 2019).

Patients with type 1 diabetes may have blood glucose levels that are difficult to control when they are unwell, have an infection or experience stress as blood glucose levels increase as part of the body's response. Patients with diabetes will require regular checks of their blood glucose levels and insulin injections. The checks may need to be between four and six times each day, depending on how stable their diabetes is. The blood glucose checks are taken before the person eats to see if the blood glucose is in the target range (between 4 and 6 mmol/L) (Diabetes Australia 2020). Stable blood glucose levels help reduce the risk of the patient developing complications, such as ketoacidosis, stroke, kidney failure and amputations from poor wound healing (Diabetes Australia 2020).

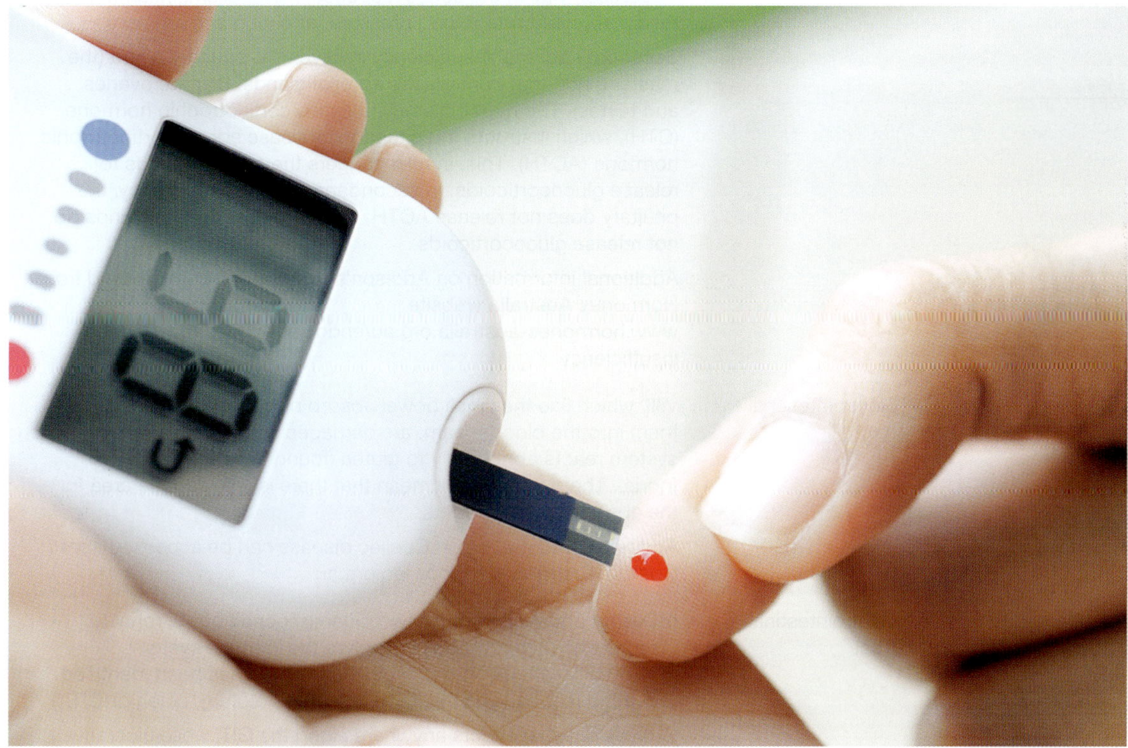

Insulin is used to treat patients with type 1 diabetes. More on the pharmacokinetics of insulin can be accessed from this link: www.diabetesaustralia.com.au/living-with-diabetes/medicine/insulin.

Diabetes Australia is Australia's national body for diabetes support and education. You can learn more about all types of diabetes from their website: www.diabetesaustralia.com.au

Hashimoto's thyroiditis is caused when the immune system produces antibodies that attack the cells of the thyroid gland. As a result, the levels of thyroid hormones released fluctuate as the cells die. Thyroid hormones control the rate of body metabolism, which influences all body functions, including energy levels, heart rate, digestion, sleep and menstruation (Endocrine Society of Australia 2019). Patients with Hashimoto's thyroiditis may experience a wide range of symptoms because of all the affected body systems.

The Australian Thyroid Foundation provides further information on thyroid diseases, and their website can be accessed via this link: www.thyroidfoundation.org.au/Hypothyroidism-&-Hashimotos-Disease.

In rheumatoid arthritis (RA), the immune system makes antibodies that symmetrically attack the synovium (lining) of small joints in the hands, feet, and sometimes in larger joints like the hips and knees. The joints become swollen, painful and stiff (Arthritis Australia 2017; Endocrine Society of Australia 2019).

There are several medications used to treat RA. More information on these medications and their pharmacokinetics can be access here: www.nps.org.au/australian-prescriber/articles/disease-modifying-drugs-in-adult-rheumatoid-arthritis.

Arthritis Australia is Australia's peak body for arthritis and musculoskeletal conditions. Further information about all types of arthritis, including RA, can be accessed from their website here: www.arthritisaustralia.com.au.

Autoimmune diseases can be localised (affecting one specific organ/tissue) or systemic (affecting more than one organ/tissue at the same time).

Localised autoimmune diseases

There are many types of localised autoimmune diseases, some of which can be reviewed in table 19.5.

TABLE 19.5 Localised autoimmune disorders

Disorder	Organ affected	Description and resources
Addison's disease	Adrenal glands	Addison's disease (primary adrenal insufficiency) develops when the adrenal glands do not produce enough corticosteroid hormone — cortisol, vital in the stress response, metabolism, inflammatory response, heart rate, blood pressure, attention and memory. Secondary adrenal insufficiency involves the pituitary gland (the master gland that controls the adrenal glands, thyroid, ovaries and testes). The hypothalamus releases corticotrophin hormone (CTH), which instructs the pituitary to release adrenocorticotrophic hormone (ACTH). This, in turn, triggers the adrenal glands to release glucocorticoids. In secondary adrenal insufficiency, the pituitary does not release ACTH; therefore, the adrenal glands do not release glucocorticoids. Additional information on Addison's disease can be accessed from Hormones Australia website: www.hormones-australia.org.au/endocrine-diseases/adrenal-insufficiency
Coeliac disease	Gastrointestinal tract	Villi, which line the small bowel absorb nutrients and transfer them into the bloodstream, are damaged because the immune system reacts abnormally to gluten (found in wheat and many foods). The damaged villi mean that there is less surface area for the absorption of nutrients. Additional information on Coeliac disease can be accessed from Coeliac Australia: www.coeliac.org.au
Inflammatory bowel disease (IBD)	Gastrointestinal tract	IBD is an umbrella term for two different conditions (Crohn's disease and ulcerative colitis), where the immune system continues to attack after a foreign substance has been identified and removed, causing inflammation of the rectum, colon or GIT. Crohn's disease affects anywhere along the GIT, while ulcerative colitis occurs in the large bowel (transverse and descending colon). Additional information on Crohn's disease can be accessed from Crohn's & Colitis website via this link: www.crohnsandcolitis.com.au/about-crohns-colitis
Autoimmune hepatitis type 2	Liver	This condition predominantly affects females between 2 and 14 years of age and occurs when the immune system attacks the liver cells, causing inflammation. Additional information on autoimmune hepatitis can be accessed from Melbourne's Royal Children's Hospital website: www.rch.org.au/kidsinfo/fact sheets/Autoimmune_hepatitis
Primary biliary cholangitis (cirrhosis)	Liver	Chronic inflammation of the bile ducts in the liver means the ducts are gradually destroyed over a long period. Additional information on cholangitis can be accessed from the PBC website: www.pbcaustralia.org/pbc-australia
Sclerosing cholangitis	Liver	The flow of bile to and from the liver is altered because of scarring, thickening and inflammation of the bile ducts. Eventually, the build-up of bile in the liver can lead to liver cirrhosis and liver failure. Additional information on sclerosing cholangitis can be accessed from the PSC Australia website: www.psc-australia.com.au/what-is-psc.html

Grave's disease (hyperthyroidism)	Thyroid	Antibodies target the thyroid gland to increase in size and produce excessive amounts of thyroid hormone, which increases the activity of every bodily function. Additional information on Graves' disease can be accessed from the Australian Thyroid Foundation: www.thyroidfoundation.org.au/hyperthyroidism-Graves-Disease-&-Thyroid-Eye-Disease
Guillain-Barré syndrome	Nervous system	The peripheral nerves are attacked by antibodies and lymphocytes, which causes weakness/paralysis, abnormal sensations and pain. Additional information on Guillain-Barré syndrome can be accessed from the Brain Foundation: www.brainfoundation.org.au/disorders/guillain-barre-syndrome
Multiple sclerosis (MS)	Nervous system	Scars occur in the CNS that interfere with nerve impulses in the brain, spinal cord and optic nerves, which causes fatigue, vertigo, pins and needles, neuralgia and visual disturbances, urinary incontinence and constipation, depression, cognitive difficulties and memory loss. Additional information on multiple sclerosis can be accessed from the MS Australia website: www.msaustralia.org.au/what-ms
Myasthenia gravis	Nerves and muscles	Antibodies block, alter or destroy the acetylcholine receptors at the neuromuscular junction, preventing signals between nerve impulses and muscles from being transmitted. This causes weakness in the skeletal muscles involved with breathing and movement that worsens with activity but improves with rest. Additional information on MG can be accessed from the Brain Foundation: www.brainfoundation.org.au/disorders/myasthenia-gravis

Systemic autoimmune diseases

Systemic diseases affect more than one body system. Connective tissue provides support and holds together joints, muscles, internal organs, skin and other body tissues. There are a number of systemic autoimmune diseases, some of which can be reviewed in this table 19.6.

TABLE 19.6 **Systemic autoimmune disorders**

Disease	Body system affected	Description and resources
Antiphospholipid antibody syndromes	Blood cells	This condition causes an increased risk of blood clotting and is linked to miscarriage and pregnancy complications. www.melbournehaematology.com.au/fact-sheets/antiphospholipid-syndrome.html
Dermatomyositis	Skin and muscles	Affects more women than men and is more likely to develop if the person has a diagnosis of diabetes melilites. Weakness in muscles starts closest to the trunk of the body and then progresses to distal limbs and neck. www.mda.org.au/disorders/inflammatory-myopathies/dermato
Mixed connective tissue disease	Connective tissue	This disease overlaps with other connective tissue diseases (lupus, scleroderma and polymyositis and RA) and affects mostly young women. www.arthritis.org/diseases/mixed-connective-tissue-disease

(continued)

TABLE 19.6 *(continued)*

Disease	Body system affected	Description and resources
Polymyalgia rheumatica	Large muscles	A type of arthritis caused by inflammation of the joints and tissues around the joints causing widespread muscle pain. www.arthritisaustralia.com.au/types-of-arthritis/polymyalgia-rheumatica
Polymyositis	Skin and muscles	It is thought that the immune system attacks muscle fibres that have been infected with a virus. The resulting inflammation causes muscle weakness. Other connective tissue disorders may also be present. www.myositis.org.au/polymyositis-info
Scleroderma	Skin, intestine; less commonly lungs and kidneys	This condition is a connective tissue disorder that results in thickening and hardening of tissues. www.msk.org.au/scleroderma
Sjögren's syndrome	Salivary glands, tear glands and joints	This disease causes abnormally dry eyes, mouth, throat, nose, skin, and vagina. Most people can live a normal life but may be at higher risk of developing eye and mouth infections. www.arthritisaustralia.com.au/types-of-arthritis/sjogrens-syndrome

Other autoimmune conditions

Table 19.7 identifies other autoimmune system diseases. Use the links to support your independent research to develop your knowledge of the conditions further.

TABLE 19.7 Other autoimmune system diseases

Disease	Australian web resources
Ankylosing spondylitis	www.arthritisaustralia.com.au/types-of-arthritis/ankylosing-spondylitis
Autoimmune haemolytic anaemia and pernicious anaemia	www.gastrohealthaustralia.com.au/about-your-health/digestive-health/anaemia
Autoimmune vitiligo	www.healthdirect.gov.au/vitiligo
Chronic inflammatory demyelinating neuropathy	www.brainfoundation.org.au/disorders/chronic-inflammatory-demyelinating-polyneuropathy
Dermatomyositis	www.mda.org.au/disorders/inflammatory-myopathies/dermato
Goodpasture's syndrome (anti-GBM disease)	www.kidney.org/atoz/content/goodpasture
Giant cell arteritis	www.arthritisaustralia.com.au/types-of-arthritis/giant-cell arteritis
Henoch-Schönlein purpura	www.rch.org.au/clinicalguide/guideline_index/HenochSchonlein_Purpura
Immune thrombocytopenia	www.itpaustralia.org.au/about-itp
Membranous nephropathy	www.kidney.org.au/uploads/resources/iga-nephritis-fact-sheet-%E2%80%93-kidney-health-australia.pdf
Motor neurone disease	www.mndaust.asn.au/Get-informed/What-is-MND.aspx
Primary antiphospholipid syndrome	www.melbournehaematology.com.au/fact-sheets/antiphospholipid-syndrome.html

19.6 Nursing management of patients with immunodeficiency or altered immune response

LEARNING OBJECTIVE 19.6 Outline the nursing considerations for patients with immunodeficiency or altered immune response.

Nursing care for patients with immunodeficiency is specific to the condition they have. General nursing considerations for patients with conditions of altered immunity include the following.

- Employ the five moments of hand hygiene.
- Ensure patient and bed hygiene, as one of the greatest sources of infection is the patient's own body flora.
- Educate patients on hand hygiene after using the toilet and before meals.
- Monitor the vital signs for indications of infection.
- Ensure regular mouth care and oral hygiene.
- Aseptic techniques must be used when managing wound dressings or any break in the skin's integrity.
  - Monitor intravenous (IV) cannulas for signs of inflammation and infection.
  - Monitor blood tests for signs of an increased white cell count as this may indicate the presence of infection.
  - Use of PPE and standard precautions for all patients

Following the diagnosis and stabilisation of symptoms, most people with conditions related to altered immunity will manage their conditions at home, which requires patient education and psychosocial support to support coping and self-esteem. Nurses help patients, their carers and families living with a chronic condition by providing support and education on:

1. their condition
2. their medications and medication regimen (including side effects)
3. how to identify potential complications and what to do if they occur
4. prevention — lifestyle modifications to reduce risk of exacerbating the condition
5. relaying of information to primary health services that are in place.

Person-centred care for conditions of altered immunity

Conditions of altered immunity or immune response have no cure and are chronic lifelong conditions that affect a person's quality of life. In Australia, chronic health conditions are a major cause of illness, premature mortality and are linked to nine of every ten deaths (Australian Health Ministers Advisory Council 2017; Department of Health and Human Services 2019). In Australia, 50 per cent of people have a chronic health condition, and 60 per cent of people over the age of 65 have more than one chronic condition (Department of Health 2020).

Regardless of the setting, nurses will provide care based on Australia's National Strategic Framework for management of chronic conditions, which can be accessed from this link: www.health.gov.au/resources/publications/national-strategic-framework-for-chronic-conditions. When caring for patients with immunodeficiency and autoimmune-related conditions, awareness of the patient's symptoms and management means that the care planned and delivered is specific to the patients' needs and their condition, regardless of the setting.

CASE STUDY 19.1

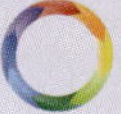

Nursing care of a patient with lupus

Jedda McCormack is 26-year-old female and has been admitted to the medical ward with a flare-up of her lupus. Yesterday Jedda attended her GP clinic because her symptoms have become worse. Jedda's symptoms include fever, extreme fatigue, weight loss, painful hips, knees and shoulder joints and unexplained headaches.

Jedda's vital sign are:

- temperature: 38.1°C
- pulse: 85 beats per minute
- blood pressure: 109/72 mmHg
- respiratory rate: 19 breaths per minute
- oxygen saturation: 98% on room air.

Jedda is very worried about being in hospital. She has a 2-year-old child who is at home with her partner, and she has expressed a number of times that she wants to go home and be with her family as soon as she can.

Question

Using the information above, describe what action you would take as the nurse caring for Jedda. Use the clinical reasoning cycle to guide you through the process and devise a plan of care for Jedda.

Answer

- *Step 1: Consider the patient*. Jedda 26-year-old mother of a young child and has been admitted with a diagnosis of lupus.
- *Step 2: Collect cues/information*. Include subjective and objective data here, including the patient's appearance and their past medical history.
  Jedda reports extreme fatigue, nausea and weight loss, painful hips, knees and shoulder joints, and unexplained headaches. Vital signs indicate Jedda currently has a fever of 38.1; all other vital signs are within normal parameters. Jedda has NKA and no previous medical or surgical history. Regular medication includes the contraceptive pill. There are no tests or investigations planned for Jedda today. Jedda tells you that she feels exhausted because she didn't sleep well again. She feels nauseous, has another headache, and her body is aching all over.
- *Step 3: Process information*. Separate the relevant and irrelevant data — cluster the clues together to formulate an inference about the patient.
  The information you have about Jedda is that she has a fever, has pain and nausea, and is extremely fatigued. You conclude that Jedda's general condition means she will need your help over the day to complete several normal daily activities. Jedda's medication chart has a number of PRN medications that may be administered to help improve how Jedda feels.
- *Step 4: Identify problems/issues*. Nursing problems or diagnosis should be listed here. Jedda's nursing problems include decreased oral intake secondary to nausea, joint pain causing difficulty mobilising, decreased activity tolerance due to extreme fatigue, potential fluid imbalance due to fever and nausea and anxiety due to separation from her young child and partner.
- *Step 5: Establish goals.* Goals of care for Jedda should focus on improving her pain so she can ambulate safely and easily, treating her temperature so she feels more comfortable, resolving her nausea so her oral food and fluid intake can return to normal and maintaining personal hygiene.
- *Step 6: Take action*. The nurse should administer the prescribed medications when they are needed to treat Jedda's fever, nausea and pain and check their effectiveness after 30 minutes. Assist Jedda with ADLS (showering, dressing and toileting) to maintain her personal hygiene. Position her call bell, over bed table and other items within easy reach. Ask Jedda if there is anything, in particular, she would like you to do for her, or if there is anything she is worried about.
- *Step 7: Evaluate outcomes*. How effective have your nursing interventions been?
  Jedda will have improved pain allowing her to have increased ambulation without any problems. Nausea will be improved, allowing an increased oral food and fluid intake. Fever will be improved or resolved and Jedda will feel more comfortable.
- *Step 8: Reflect on the process and new learning*. What important new pieces of knowledge about lupus that you have learned by completing this case study. Reflect on any aspects of Jedda's nursing care that could have been managed differently.

CASE STUDY 19.2

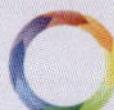

Nursing care of a patient with anaphalaxis

Nick Nguyen is a 19-year-old male patient admitted to the surgical ward to treat a severely infected pilonidal sinus he has had for the last 8 days.

Nick has severe pain at the site of the abscess that he rates at 8/10. Nick's vital signs indicate that he has a fever:

- temperature: 38.2°C
- pulse: 95 beats per minute
- blood pressure: 135/80 mmHg
- respiratory rate: 22 breaths per minute
- oxygen saturation: 98% on room air.

Nick has a medical history of well-controlled asthma and takes both reliever and preventer medications as per his asthma management plan. Nick has no surgical history, has no known allergies, and is otherwise well.

Nick has been commenced on a multimodal pain relief regimen and is currently receiving an intravenous (IV) antibiotic called metronidazole.

Shortly after the antibiotic infusion commenced, Nick tells his nurse that he thinks he is experiencing asthma and would like to use his puffer. Nick complains of feeling nauseous and says his shortness of breath is becoming worse. The nurse notices that Nick's face is beginning to swell very quickly, his skin is pale, and his breathing is very noisy, and he is using all his accessory muscles.

Question

Using the information above, describe what action you would take as the nurse caring for this patient. Use the clinical reasoning cycle to guide you through the process and devise a plan of care for your patient.

Answer

- *Step 1: Consider the patient*. Nick Nguyen is a 19-year-old male patient.
- *Step 2: Collect cues/information.* Include subjective and objective data here, including the patient's appearance and their past medical history.

  Nick is very anxious and distressed, telling the nurse he feels light-headed, his mouth tingling and a tight feeling in his throat. Nick has a history of well-controlled asthma and no known allergies.

  Objective data will include measurable information such as his vital signs. Nick is febrile at 38.3 degrees.
- *Step 3: Process information.* Separate the relevant and irrelevant data — cluster the clues together to formulate an inference about the patient.

  Nick has rapidly developing symptoms of respiratory distress, swelling of his face, lips and eyes, and is suddenly hypotensive. Given the sudden onset of the symptoms across several body symptoms and knowledge that penicillin antibiotics are a known cause of anaphylaxis in some people, it is reasonable to conclude that Nick is experiencing a life-threatening anaphylactic reaction to the antibiotic that has been administered. Nick does have a history of asthma; however, the respiratory symptoms that Nick is experiencing are far more severe than his usual asthma symptoms and are not consistent with an allergy to the medication.
- *Step 4: Identify problems/issues*. Nursing problems or diagnosis should be listed here. Nick is experiencing life-threatening symptoms, and the nurse must respond quickly.

  Nick's priority nursing problems are respiratory distress, compromised airway, decreased oxygenation and impaired gas exchange.
- *Step 5: Establish goals*. Goals of care for Nick should focus on immediately restoring a clear airway, improving oxygenation and supporting circulatory function to restore blood pressure.
- *Step 6: Take action.* The nurse should immediately recognise that Nick's respiratory distress and facial swelling mean he is experiencing a life-threatening condition. Nick meets the criteria for a medical emergency call to be initiated. The nurse should stay with Nick and let him know that they have organised help and that they are aware he is having difficulty breathing. This should reassure Nick that the nurse is aware of his symptoms and that help is on the way. Administer O_2 via Hudson mask at 15 L/m and prepare the Ambu bag in case Nick stops breathing. Check Nick's IV access and make sure it is secure. Stop any IV infusions.

  Once the Met team arrives, medications to treat Nick's anaphylaxis will be administered. Epinephrine (adrenaline) IV and/or via nebuliser may be administered as first-line treatment of anaphylaxis. Other medications may include hydrocortisone and glucagon, depending on Nick's response to treatment. Obtain new vital sign readings.
- *Step 7: Evaluate outcomes*. Once the medical emergency team has attended and Nick has been stabilised he may be transferred to ICU or a high dependency ward where he can be closely observed and monitored.
- *Step 8: Reflect on the process and new learning*. Consider what important new knowledge about anaphylaxis you have learned by completing this case study. Reflect on one aspect of Nick's nursing care that could have been managed differently.

SUMMARY

The human immune system plays a significant role in ensuring that individuals live a healthy, disease-free life. This chapter has discussed the role of the key immune cells, chemicals and organs in the immune response. Sometimes, however, the system whose role it is to protect the body falls victim to disease or responds in a way that damages health and can cause illness. Conditions resulting from altered immune responses are chronic conditions, including allergy, anaphylaxis, immunodeficiency and autoimmune diseases, have been outlined. Considerations for people living with chronic conditions have also been explored.

KEY TERMS

antibody Also known as an immunoglobulin, is a large protein used by the immune system to identify and neutralise foreign objects such as bacteria and viruses.

antigen A substance on a pathogen that can trigger the immune response.

autoimmunity The innate immune response is triggered when there is no infection.

granulocytes White blood cells that contains granules, released in response to invading foreign substances.

leukocyte White blood cells that help fight infection; include granulocytes (neutrophils, basophils and eosinophils), monocytes and lymphocytes.

lymphocytes Immune cells in the blood and lymph tissue (NK cells, B and T cells).

monocytes White blood cell that can change into macrophage and live longer than leukocytes.

pathogens Foreign substances that can cause disease.

phagocytes Cells that ingests invading foreign cells.

REFERENCES

Al-Kofahi, M., Yun, W., Minigar, A. & Alexandar, S. (2017) Anatomy and roles of lymphatics in inflammatory diseases. *Clinical and Experimental Neuroimmunology.* 8(8): 199–214.

Arthritis Australia. (2017) Rheumatoid Arthritis. https://arthritisaustralia.com.au/types-of-arthritis/rheumatoid-arthritis

Asthma & Anaphylaxis Australia. (2020) Allergy & anaphylaxis. https://allergyfacts.org.au/allergy-anaphylaxis

Australian Commission on Safety and Quality in Health Care(ACSQHC). (2019) Medication Safety Standard. The National Safety and Quality Health Service (NSQHS). www.safetyandquality.gov.au/standards/nsqhs-standards/medication-safety-standard/documentation-patient-information/action-47

Australasian Society of Clinical Immunology and Allergy (ASCIA). (2019) Food allergy. www.allergy.org.au/patients/food-allergy/food-allergy

Australasian Society of Clinical Immunology and Allergy (ASCIA). (2020a) Autoimmune diseases. www.allergy.org.au/patients/autoimmunity/autoimmune-diseases#:~:text=Autoimmune%20diseases%20are%20a%20broad,thyroiditis%2C%20rheumatoid%20arthritis%20and%20diabetes

Australasian Society of Clinical Immunology and Allergy (ASCIA). (2020b) What is allergy? www.allergy.org.au/patients/about-allergy/what-is-allergy

Australian Federation of AIDS Organisations. (2021) HIV in Australia 2021. www.afao.org.au/about-hiv/hiv-statistics/

Australian Health Ministers Advisory Council. (2017) *National Strategic Framework for Chronic Conditions.* Canberra: Australian Government. www.health.gov.au/resources/publications/national-strategic-framework-for-chronic-conditions

Australian Lymphology Association. (2021) About lymphoedema. www.lymphoedema.org.au/about-lymphoedema/what-is-lymphoedema

Brain Foundation. (2020) Myasthenia gravis. https://brainfoundation.org.au/disorders

Burchum, J. & Rosenthal, L. (2019a) 'Adrenergic agonists'. In *Lehne's Pharmacology for Nursing Care*, 10th ed. (pp. 147a–158). Canada: Elsevier.

Burchum, J. & Rosenthal, L. (2019b) 'Anaphylaxis'. In *Lehne's Pharmacology for Nursing Care*, 10th ed. (pp. 844–846). Canada: Elsevier.

Burchum, J. & Rosenthal, L. (2019c) 'Glucocorticoids in nonendocrine disorders'. In *Lehne's Pharmacology for Nursing Care*, 10th ed. (pp. 871–880). Canada. Elsevier.

Chronic Care Network. (2018) *Lymphoedema: A guide for clinical services.* Chatswood: NSW Government. www.aci.health.nsw.gov.au/__data/assets/pdf_file/0008/417998/lymphoedema-guide.pdf

Department of Health. (2020) Chronic conditions in Australia. www.health.gov.au/health-topics/chronic-conditions/chronic-conditions-in-australia

Department of Health and Human Services. (2019) Care for people with chronic conditions. Victoria: Victorian Government. www2.health.vic.gov.au/primary-and-community-health/community-health/community-health-program/chip-guidelines

Diabetes Australia. (2020) Managing type 1 diabetes. www.diabetesaustralia.com.au/living-with-diabetes/managing-your-diabetes/managing-type-1

[illegible]

Endocrine Society of Australia. (2019) Thyroid gland. www.hormones-australia.org.au/the-endocrine-system/thyroid

Garvan Institute of Medical Research. (2020a) Autoimmune diseases explained. www.garvan.org.au/research/collaborative-programs/hope/autoimmune-disease

Garvan Institute of Medical Research. (2020b) 'Immunity and inflammation research'. www.garvan.org.au/research/immunology

Garvan Institute of Medical Research. (2020c) Lupus. www.garvan.org.au/research/diseases/lupus

Hendrick, L. (2019a) 'Alterations of immune function across the life span'. In J. Craft, C. Gordon, S. Heuther, V. Brashers & N. Rote (Eds.). *Understanding Pathophysiology. Australia and New Zealand edition,* 6th ed. (pp. 357–382). Chatswood NSW: Elsevier.

Hendrick, L. (2019b) 'The structure and function of the immune system'. In J. Craft, C. Gordon, S. Heuther, V. Brashers & N. Rote (Eds.). *Understanding Pathophysiology. Australia and New Zealand edition*, 6th ed. (pp. 281–303). Chatswood Australia: Elsevier.

Immune Deficiency Foundation (IDF). (2019) *IDF Patient & Family Handbook for Primary. Immunodeficiency Diseases*, 6th ed. USA. www.idfa.org.au/wp-content/uploads/2020/09/IDF_Patient_Family_Handbook_-6th_Edition.pdf

Kikkert, M. (2020) Innate immune evasion by human respiratory DNA viruses. *Journal of Innate Immunology.* 12: 4–20. doi: https://doi.org/10.1159/000503030

Knight, J. & Nigam, Y. (2020) The lymphatic system 1: structure, function and oedema. *Nursing Times* [online]. 116(10): 39–43. www.nursingtimes.net/clinical-archive/immunology/the-lymphatic-system-1-structure-function-and-oedema-21-09-2020

Lewis, S., Finlayson, K. & Parker, C. (2020) 'Nursing management. Inflammation and wound healing'. In R. Aitken, T. Buckley, H. Edwards & D. Brown (Eds.). *Lewis's Medical-Surgical Nursing*, 5th ed. (pp. 188–209). Elsevier.

List, S. (2019) 'Alterations of endocrine function across the life span'. In J. Craft, C. Gordon, S. Heuther, K. McCance, V. Brahshers & N. Rote (Eds.). *Understanding Pathophysiology*, 3rd ed. (pp. 255–277). Chatswood NSW: Elsevier.

Marieb, E. & Hoen, K. (2016) 'The immune system: Innate and adaptive body defences'. In E. Marieb & K. Hoen (Eds.). *Human Anatomy & Physiology*, 10th ed. (pp. 791–826). Essex, England: Pearson.

National Asthma Council Australia. (2021) What role does allergy play in your Asthma? www.nationalasthma.org.au/living-with-asthma/resources/patients carers/brochures/asthma allergy#all

van de Mortel, T. (2017) 'Inflammation and fever'. In T. B. R. Aitken, H. Edwards & D. Brown (Eds.). *Lewis's Medical-Surgical Nursing*, 5th ed. (pp. 305–332). Elsevier.

World Health Organization (WHO). (2020a) HIV/AIDS key facts. www.who.int/news-room/fact-sheets/detail/hiv-aids

World Health Organization (WHO). (2020b) WHO top 10 causes of death [Press release]. www.who.int/news-room/fact-sheets/detail/the-top-10-causes-of-death

ACKNOWLEDGEMENTS

Figure 19.1: © Patient & Family Handbook, Immune Deficiency Foundation. © Immune Deficiency Foundation of America. Reproduced with permission of Immune Deficiency Foundation of America.

Figure 19.1 (Photo): © wavebreakmedia/Shutterstock.com

Figure 19.3: © Hendrick, Alterations of immune function across the life span in Understanding Pathophysiology, p. 375, Elsevier. © Elsevier. Reproduced with permission of Elsevier.

Photo 19A: © Leonard Zhukovsky/Shutterstock.com

Photo 19B: © Leonard Zhukovsky/Shutterstock.com

Photo 19C: © Seasontime/Shutterstock.com

CHAPTER 20

Nursing care of conditions related to haematological disorders

LEARNING OBJECTIVES

After studying this chapter, you should be able to:

20.1 differentiate the functions and components of the haematology system
20.2 describe the phases and components contributing to haemostasis
20.3 describe the considerations and indications for the safe transfusion of blood and blood products
20.4 outline the conditions that may develop with abnormal function of the haematology system
20.5 describe the oncological conditions of the haematology system and the nursing care for these patients.

Introduction

Nursing knowledge and skills related to the haematological system are applicable to all areas of medical and surgical nursing. Sound knowledge and understanding of the haematological system underpin patient assessment and nursing care planning for haematological conditions. This chapter provides an introduction to the components of blood and commonly ordered blood tests, haemostasis and the clotting cascade, blood types and blood transfusions. It also covers the basic pathophysiology of common conditions, and the nursing care and treatment of patients with haematological conditions, including anaemia, bleeding disorders and blood cancers — leukaemia, lymphoma and myeloma.

20.1 The haematological system

LEARNING OBJECTIVE 20.1 Differentiate the functions and components of the haematology system.

The haematological system comprises blood, bone marrow and lymph nodes. Blood is considered to be a connective tissue that:

- works as a transport system to cells and organs, carrying oxygen, nutrients, blood cells, hormones, enzymes, chemicals and minerals
- removes waste products of cellular metabolism, e.g. carbon dioxide from the lungs and excretory waste from the kidneys
- regulates body heat by distributing the temperature
- provides haemostasis (control of bleeding) and regulates water and electrolyte balance
- protects from infection by circulating antibodies, providing a protective immune function (Rome & Hargreaves 2020).

Overview of blood

The pH of the blood should be between 7.35 and 7.45 for normal function to be maintained. The total blood volume is estimated to be 4 to 5 litres in females and 5 to 6 litres in males, accounting for approximately 8 per cent of body weight.

All blood cells originate from a specific stem cell (pluripotent) in the bone marrow (see figure 20.1). Bone marrow is in the centre of long flat or irregular shaped bones, such as the iliac crest of the pelvis, the humerus, vertebrae, skull, ribs, sacrum, scapula and sternum. **Erythropoietin** is a hormone released by the kidneys, which stimulates the bone marrow to make **red blood cells (RBCs)** (Rome & Hargreaves 2020).

Cellular components

The key components of blood (identified in table 20.1) are erythrocytes (red blood cells [RBCs]), leukocytes (**white blood cells [WBCs]**) and **thrombocytes** (platelets), which are transported around the body in **plasma**.

Erythrocytes

Erythrocytes or RBCs transport oxygen and nutrients in the blood. Normal RBCs are discs that can pass through capillary walls, facilitate gaseous exchange and the carriage of essential oxygen around the body.

Haemoglobin

Haemoglobin (Hb) is a protein within RBCs that enables them to carry oxygen molecules. Iron is needed to help the body make haemoglobin, and we consume iron in our diet. The amount of Hb in the blood indicates the oxygen-carrying capacity of blood and is measured as Hb level. A normal Hb level for men is 130–170 g/L and for women is 120–160 g/L (Leukaemia Foundation 2020b).

Haemoglobin gives arterial blood its red colour — oxygenated blood is a brighter red colour than deoxygenated blood. When haemoglobin binds with oxygen, it produces oxyhaemoglobin, which makes up the oxygen-carrying capacity of blood. As the RBCs move through the body, the oxygen molecule jumps off the haemoglobin and moves into the tissue. Carbon dioxide moves in the reverse, from the cells tissue to the haemoglobin molecule, which carries it to the lungs to be released from the body (Rome & Hargreaves 2020). RBCs use anaerobic respiration to produce energy, thus conserving the oxygen they are carrying.

In addition to iron, B vitamins (B12, B9 and B6) and other factors are required for the healthy synthesis of red blood cells. Where there is a deficiency during **erythropoiesis** (making of RBCs), a decreased number of erythrocytes are produced, and anaemia occurs.

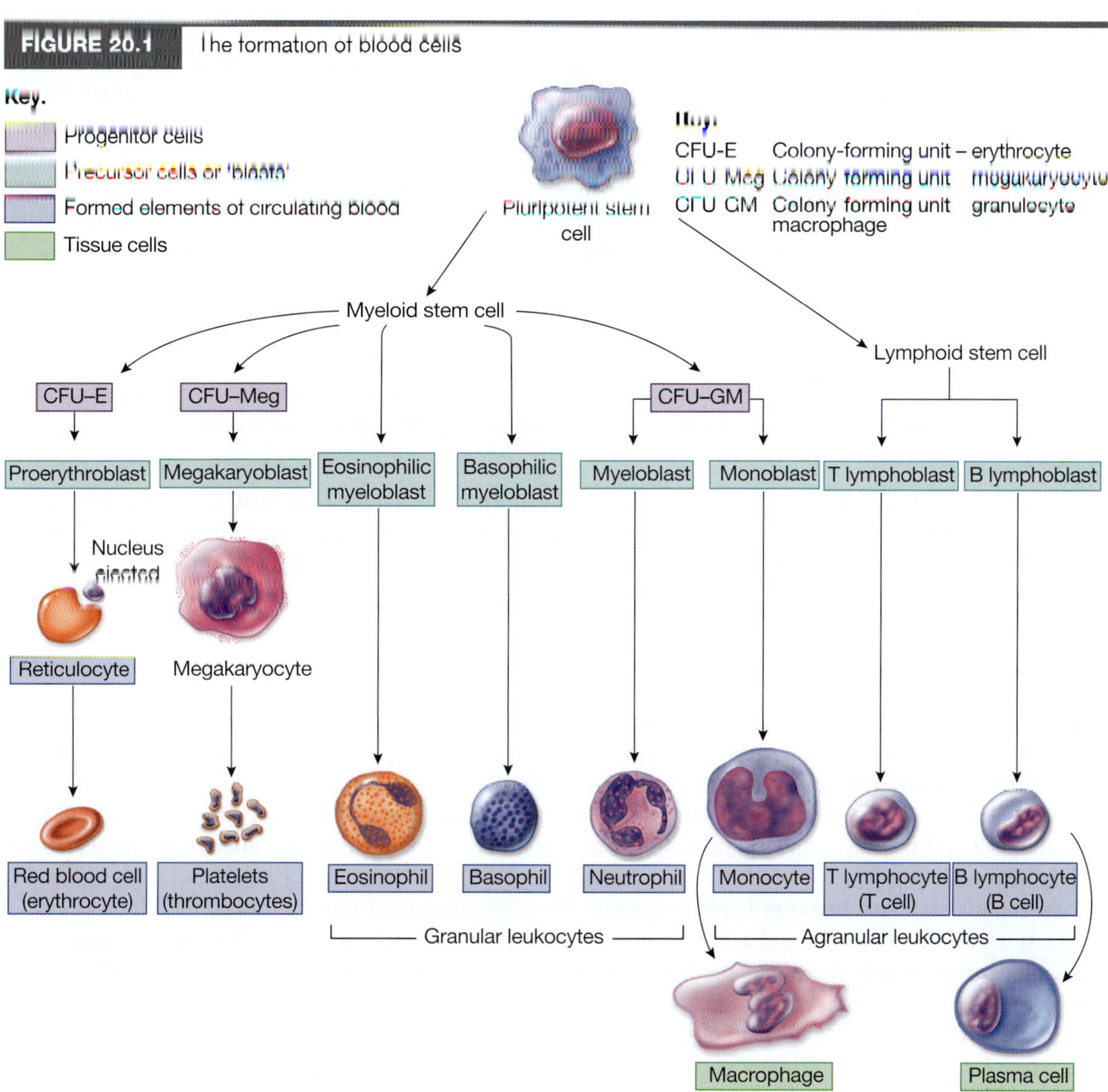

FIGURE 20.1 The formation of blood cells

Source: Nair and Peate (2009) *Fundamentals of Applied Pathophysiology*, with kind permission from Wiley Blackwell.

TABLE 20.1 The components of blood

Component	Description
Plasma	Transports nutrients, hormones, and proteins. It is a yellow liquid that makes up about 55% of the body's blood volume. Provide energy to cells and signal for growth and tissue repair.
Platelets	Form clots to stop bleeding. Platelets make up less than 1% of blood and are constantly being produced because they have an average lifespan of eight to 10 days within the body.
Red blood cells	Carry fresh oxygen through the body and remove carbon dioxide. Red blood cells make up about 40 to 45% of blood. Contain a protein called haemoglobin, which contains iron and binds to oxygen, giving blood its red colour.
White blood cells	Part of the body's immune system, they detect and fight viruses and bacteria. There are five major types of white blood cells, and they make up less than 1% of blood. Work with plasma, platelets and red blood cells to enable normal body function.

Source: Adapted from The Conversation (2017).

Erythropoiesis

Erythropoiesis is the production of RBCs and is triggered by tissue hypoxia, causing the kidneys to produce erythropoietin, which stimulates the bone marrow to produce RBCs. As a result, the number of RBCs and the amount of oxygen uptake increases, reducing the hypoxic state.

When RBCs become old (average life of 120 days), damaged or defective, they are destroyed by a process known as haemolysis, which occurs in the liver, spleen and bone marrow. When RBCs are haemolysed (broken down), bilirubin (a yellowish-orange pigment) is produced. The liver conjugates the bilirubin and excretes it into bile (a digestive fluid) so that it can be released from the body (Rome & Hargreaves 2020). Iron released from haemoglobin during bilirubin formation is carried in the plasma to the bone marrow on a protein called transferrin and used to produce new haemoglobin.

Leukocytes

Leukocytes or WBCs, are immune cells that protect the body from infection. WBCs are divided into two groups: granulocytes (60 per cent) and agranulocytes (mononuclear cells; 40 per cent).

Granulocytes

Granulocytes have granules inside the cell (cytoplasm). They are larger than RBCs, and the number of circulating granulocytes remains constant except in the presence of infection, during which numbers increase (leukocytosis). A decrease from normal values is called leukopenia. Granulocytes are further divided into three groups:

1. basophils
2. eosinophils
3. neutrophils.

Basophils react to harmful substances. They contain granules of heparin, histamine and other substances, which cause inflammation. Allergens — antigens that cause an allergy — stimulate the basophils to release the contents of their granules (Rome & Hargreaves 2020).

Eosinophils have a specific phagocytic mode of action. They contain enzymes and peroxidase in their granules, which function against parasites. Eosinophil numbers increase during allergic reactions (Rome & Hargreaves 2020).

Neutrophils' primary function is phagocytosis. They are capable of moving out of the blood vessel in response to foreign material and are present at the site of inflammation within an hour. The number of neutrophils increases in the presence of infection or injury to tissue in the body (Rome & Hargreaves 2020).

Agranulocytes (mononuclear leukocytes) are WBCs that do not have granules inside them. There are two types: lymphocytes and monocytes.

Lymphocytes are suspended in lymphatic fluid, which is found in the lymphatic tissues and spleen. Their lifespan is between a few hours and years, and they differ from other WBCs in their mode of action as they are not phagocytic.

There are two types of lymphocytes: T and B lymphocytes. T cells are formed in the thymus gland, while B cells originate in the bone marrow.

T lymphocytes are involved in graft reactions and in fighting cancer and viruses by direct cellular destruction.

B lymphocytes make antibodies in response to antigens in the body. Once this occurs, assisted by T lymphocytes, B lymphocytes enlarge and divide into either **plasma cells** or **memory B cells**.

Plasma cells release antibodies (immunoglobulins). Once antibodies have bound to antigens, they are prime targets for helper T lymphocytes, cytotoxic T lymphocytes and macrophages. Antibodies bind to the toxin and activate the complement system, which in turn accelerates the phagocytic response. This process of the combination of B and T lymphocyte production leads to the release of cytokines and is more specifically referred to below in relation to macrophage activity. The cytokines produced are chemical messengers released by specific cells of the immune system used by immune cells to communicate with one another. Examples of cytokines include interleukins and interferons.

Memory B cells hold within them the memory of the interaction that has occurred for a variably long period afterwards, providing immunity against the same antigens.

Monocytes are the largest of the WBCs and have two modes of action: phagocytosis (eating bacteria, dead or old blood cells and debris from tissues). The other function is to become macrophages and relocate permanently to specific locations around the body. For example, macrophages that live in the liver are called Kupffer cells, and macrophages that live in the bone are called osteoclasts, alveolar macrophages in the lungs, and some organs of the lymph system (Rome & Hargreaves 2020). Both types of monocytes assist the immune response by releasing interleukin 1, which signals the hypothalamus to increase temperature (fever response) and also stimulates the development of some globulins in the liver and enhances the activation of T lymphocytes.

Thrombocytes (platelets)

Platelets are disc-shaped particles lacking a nucleus and arise from the bone marrow. Platelets usually circulate for approximately 1 week before being destroyed and have a crucial role in haemostasis (the control of bleeding).

Platelets assist with vasoconstriction at the site of injury to slow blood flow and promote healing, as well as sticking to damaged blood vessels and the formation of a platelet plug (platelets sticking together) to stop bleeding. This provides the foundation for the coagulated blood to form a stable fibrin clot and begin the tissue repair process (Hendrick 2019).

Plasma

Plasma is the water component of blood that carries the components of blood around the body. Plasma contains albumin, plasma cells, clotting factors and electrolytes.

Albumin carries normal components of blood and drugs and helps to maintain colloid osmotic pressure, which stops fluid from passing out of the blood and into the surrounding tissue. A low albumin level means that large amounts of fluid move from the vascular space into the surrounding tissue, causing swelling (oedema) and decreased blood volume (Hendrick 2019).

Plasma cells release antibodies (immunoglobulins). Antibodies bind to antigens and activate the complement system, which in turn accelerates the phagocytic response. The cytokines produced are chemical messengers released by specific cells of the immune system that communicate with one another. Examples of cytokines include interleukins and interferons.

More information about antibody products can be accessed from the National Blood Authority Australia via this link: www.blood.gov.au/plasma-and-recombinant-products.

Clotting factors such as fibrinogen work to stop bleeding by helping the platelets stick together (coagulation).

Electrolytes such as sodium, potassium, calcium and chloride and phosphate, are essential for maintaining normal cell function, osmotic pressure and the pH level of the blood (Hendrick 2019; National Blood Authority n.d.).

20.2 Haemostasis (blood clotting)

LEARNING OBJECTIVE 20.2 Describe the phases and components contributing to haemostasis.

When a vessel or tissue has been injured, bleeding is the result. Haemostasis has been achieved when bleeding has stopped. There are four phases to achieving haemostasis:

1. vasoconstriction of the injured blood vessel
2. formation of a platelet plug
3. formation of a fibrinogen clot
4. fibrinolysis (the breakdown of the clot).

Phase 1: Vasoconstriction

Blood vessel injury initiates the first phase of clotting, and the vessel goes into spasm and constricts. The decreased size of the vessel reduces the amount of blood loss and brings the surfaces of the vessel together (Rome & Hargreaves 2020). Thrombocytes produce serotonin, causing the muscles of the vessel wall to constrict and decrease the blood flow. Constriction also results from stimulation of pain receptors and the release of thromboxanes by the damaged cell wall.

Phase 2: Platelet plug formation

Collagen from the injured tissue causes the platelets to become adhesive (stick together) and aggregate (form clumps). Platelets release thromboxanes and ADP (adenosine diphosphate), which further promote platelet aggregation and the formation of a primary platelet plug. Factors released into the blood help an adhesive bridge to form between the platelets and the subendothelial tissue. The platelets also assist the clotting factors to work (Rome & Hargreaves 2020).

Phase 3: Fibrinogen clot formation

Fibrin forms a mesh across the damaged vessel, which pulls the edges together and seals the site, trapping blood cells. Trapped platelets retract, which pulls the fibrin closer together, making the clot stable and secure.

There are two pathways by which the fibrin clot forms to achieve coagulation — the extrinsic and the intrinsic pathway (figure 20.2) — in collaboration with the various clotting factors listed in table 20.2.

FIGURE 20.2 Blood clotting process

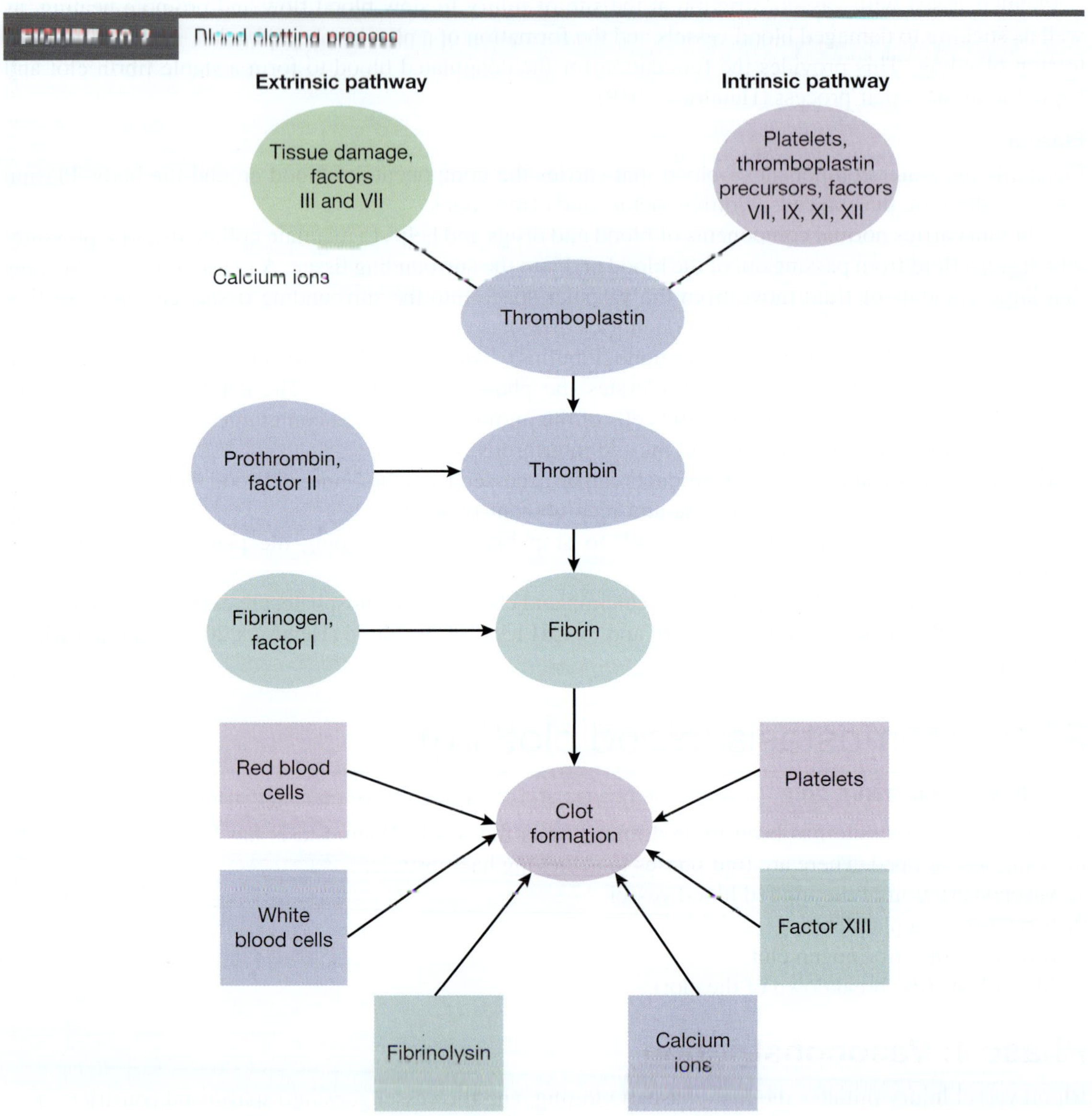

The intrinsic, extrinsic and common clotting pathways work together to achieve haemostasis.

The intrinsic clotting pathway is triggered when clotting factor XII in the blood comes into contact with subendothelial substances (collagen) exposed as a result of vascular injury. This triggers factor X in the common clotting pathway. Therefore, the intrinsic pathway occurs inside the vessel.

The external clotting pathway occurs outside the vessel in the tissue. When clotting factors from the vascular damage react with other clotting factors, the pathway is triggered, activating factor X in the common clotting pathway.

In the common clotting pathway, factor X activates prothrombin, which becomes thrombin. Thrombin converts fibrinogen to fibrin, which is the foundation of the fibrin mesh (clot).

TABLE 20.2 **Clotting factors**

I	Fibrinogen
II	Prothrombin
III	Thromboplastin
IV	Calcium
V	Proaccelerin, labile factor
VII	Serum prothrombin conversion accelerator
VIII	Antihaemophillic factor
IX	Christmas factor, plasma thrombin component
X	Stuart–Power factor
XI	Plasma thromboplastin antecedent
XII	Hageman factor
XII	Fibrin-stabilising factor

Source: Nair & Peate (2009) *Fundamentals of applied pathophysiology*, with kind permission from Wiley Blackwell.

Phase 4: Fibrinolysis

The enzyme plasmin dissolves the fibrin clot. This occurs when the vessel is undergoing repair. The clots are removed from the tissue and blood vessel by the fibrinolytic system, and normal blood flow is returned (Hendrick 2019).

20.3 The transfusion of blood and blood products

LEARNING OBJECTIVE 20.3 Describe the considerations that govern and indications for the safe transfusion of blood and blood products.

Blood types

Blood types are inherited from a mix of both parent's genes. It identifies what antigen the blood cell is carrying, which will be either A antigen, B antigen, AB (both antigens) or O (no antigen) (Australian Red Cross Lifeblood 2017).

The Rhesus (Rh) factor further classifies the blood type (see figure 20.3). People who also have an Rh antigen on their blood cell are Rh-positive, and people who do not have an Rh antigen are Rh-negative (Healthdirect 2017). Administering blood can cause life-threatening complications if the blood types do not match, as the immune system will recognise the blood as foreign and attack it (Healthdirect 2017).

FIGURE 20.3 Rhesus disease

Rhesus disease can be a complication of pregnancy. If a Rh-negative mother is carrying an Rh-positive baby, there is a chance that blood from the baby can pass to the mother's circulation during pregnancy or childbirth. The mother's immune system becomes sensitised and produces antibodies against the Rh-positive cells (Rh-positive mothers and Rh-negative babies do not experience problems as there are no antibodies from the baby to trigger the mother's immune system). If the mother has a Rh-positive baby in subsequent pregnancies, her immune system will send antibodies through the placenta to destroy the baby's RBCs. The baby will develop haemolytic disease of the newborn, which can cause anaemia, jaundice, blindness, brain damage, miscarriage, stillbirth or infant death (Pregnancy Birth & Baby 2020).

Rhesus disease is detected in pregnant women through a screening blood test early in the pregnancy. If the woman is Rh-negative, and has a Rh-positive partner, she is given an anti-D immunoglobulin injection later in the pregnancy. Australian scientists pioneered the Rh program, developing this treatment in the 1960s, and was the first country in the world to offer immunisation to pregnant women who were Rh D negative, making the condition uncommon in Australia today (Australian Red Cross Lifeblood 2017).

More on the efforts of Australian scientists can be accessed from the Australian Red Cross via this link: www.transfusion.com.au/bsib_july2017_2.

When people need a blood transfusion, knowing the donor's blood type and the recipient is critical to ensure that transfusion is safe. The universal blood type is O negative and can be given to anyone; useful in emergency circumstances. Use figure 20.4 below to match safe options for transfused blood from donor to recipient.

FIGURE 20.4 Compatible blood types

Patient's blood type	Donor's blood type: O–	O+	B–	B+	A–	A+	AB–	AB+
AB+	✓	✓	✓	✓	✓	✓	✓	✓
AB–	✓		✓		✓		✓	
A+	✓	✓			✓	✓		
A–	✓				✓			
B+	✓	✓	✓	✓				
B–	✓		✓					
O+	✓	✓						
O–	✓							

Source: Australian Red Cross Lifeblood (n.d.).

Use the link to this video to learn more about blood types ABO and Rh (with doughnuts and sprinkles): www.dailymotion.com/video/x2l5r9w.

Table 20.3 shows the percentages of blood types in Australia.

TABLE 20.3 **Blood types, percentages in Australia**

Blood type	How many Australians have it	About this blood type
O+	40%	This is the most common blood type.
O–	9%	O– can be safely given to any patient, regardless of their blood type.
A+	31%	Type A platelets (a component of blood that is important for clotting) can be safely given to any patient.
A–	7%	
B+	8%	Type B is more common in South Asian and black communities.
B–	2%	
AB+	2%	
AB–	1%	This is the rarest blood type.

Source: Healthdirect (2017).

The following resources are available to help you further explore concepts related to safe blood and blood products management.

- For detailed guidelines on the administration of blood, go to https://anzsbt.org.au/wp-content/uploads/2018/06/ANZSBT_Guidelines_Administration_Blood_Products_3rdEd_Jan_2018.pdf
- Blood safe E-learning Australia. https://bloodsafelearning.org.au
- NSQHS Standards. Blood management: www.safetyandquality.gov.au/sites/default/files/migrated/National-Safety-and-Quality-Health-Service-Standards-second-edition.pdf

Figure 20.5 shows an example of a label on RBC for transfusion. Note the approximate cost of one bag of blood.

FIGURE 20.5 Example of a red cell component label with cost indicator for 2013–14

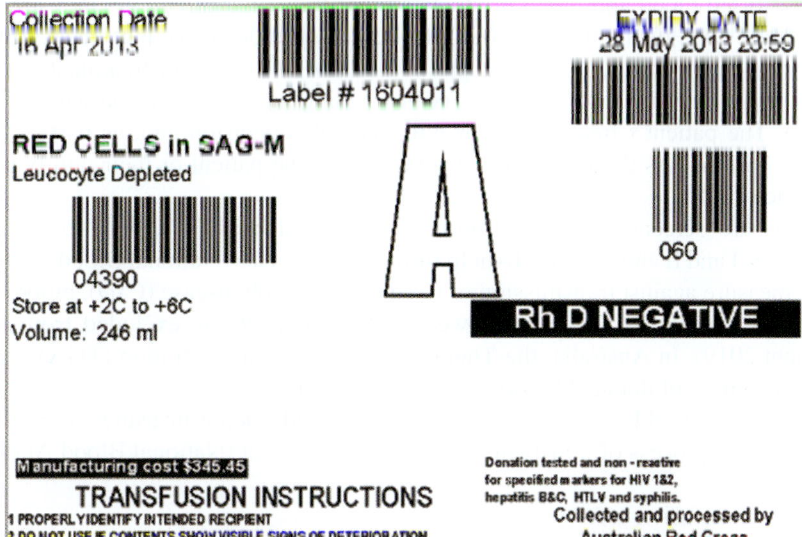

Source: National Blood Authority Australia (n.d.c).

In Australia, patients are not charged for blood or blood products they receive, and blood donors are not paid for the blood donations they make. To find a blood donation centre near you, use this link: www.abmdr.org.au.

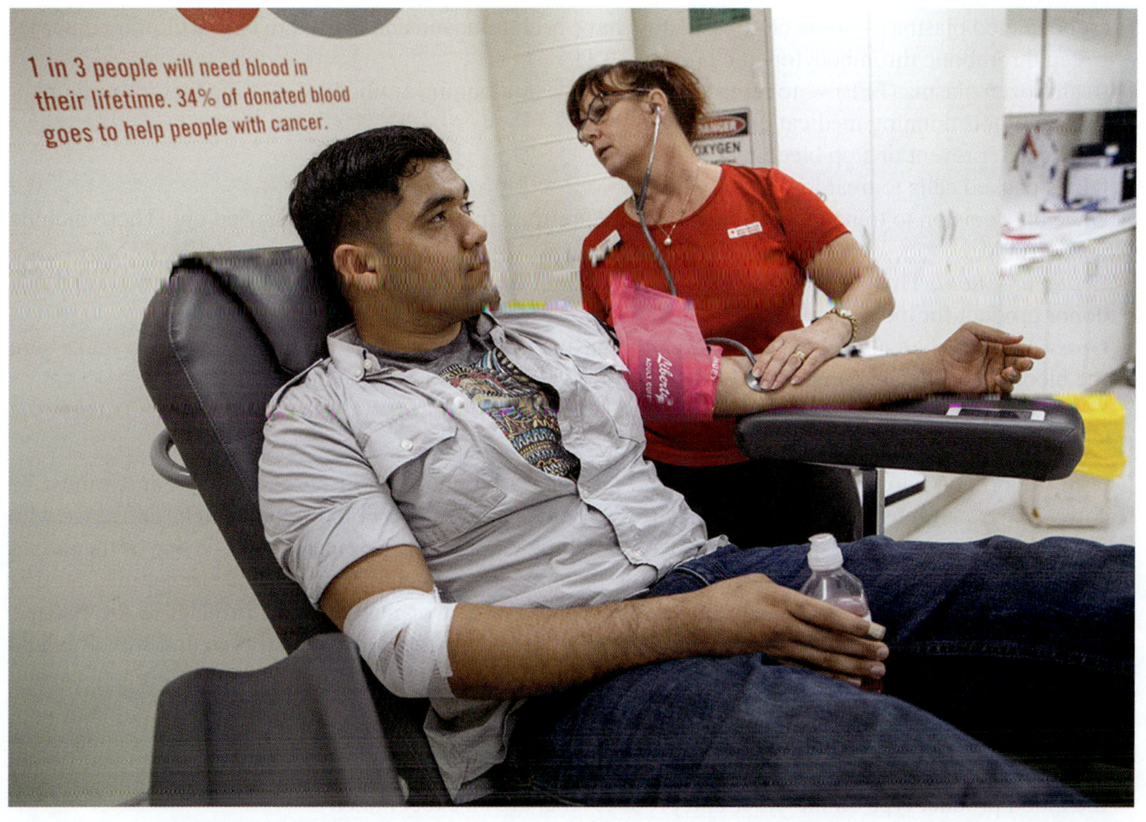

The rationale for blood transfusion

The effects of transfused blood and blood products are not fully understood, yet they are known to have the potential to cause side effects ranging from mild reactions to death. To help reduce the risk of harm to patients, the decision to proceed with a transfusion comes after all other treatment options have been explored, and the conclusion is that the benefits of proceeding with a transfusion will outweigh the risks (ACSQHC 2017). The patient's treating doctor will make this decision and, as part of obtaining valid informed consent, will discuss the risks and advantages with the patient or their family (Australian Red Cross Blood Service 2018).

Blood donations are screened for blood borne diseases, such as HIV, hepatitis B and C, human T-lymphotropic types I and II and syphilis To help further reduce risks (National Blood Authority Australia n.d). As a safety measure against transmission of Creutzfeldt–Jakob disease (CJD), blood donations from people who lived in the United Kingdom between 1980 and 1996 are excluded from donating blood (NSW Government 2019). In Australia, the Therapeutic Goods Administration (TGA) is responsible for coordinating the screening of donated blood and blood products.

All blood that is transfused has strict checking, tracking and tracing measures to ensure the blood is safe to transfuse and the process of transfusion is safe for the patient (National Blood Authority Australia n.d.c).

The reasons for a transfusion are:

- critical bleeding and patients requiring a massive blood transfusion
- perioperative — blood loss is anticipated during or after surgery
- medical reasons — such as acute or chronic conditions, e.g. anaemia, haemophilia or sickle cell disease
- patients requiring critical care
- obstetrics and maternity care
- neonates and paediatrics (National Blood Authority Australia n.d.b).

Types of blood products that can be transfused include:

- cryoprecipitate — contains fibrin and other clotting factors and is used for people who do not have enough fibrin or have defective fibrin, or when a massive blood transfusion is required (National Blood Authority Australia n.d.b)
- cryodepleted plasma — some clotting factors have been removed and is used to treat a clotting disorder called thrombotic thrombocytopenic purpura (TTP)
- fresh frozen plasma (FFP) — to replace proteins such as albumin, antibodies, clotting factors, or quickly reverse blood-thinning medications
- platelets to prevent or stop bleeding
- RBCs packed cells to treat low haemoglobin.

Once the decision to transfuse has been made, a pre-transfusion blood test is carried out. These include the following.

- *Group and hold.* This test identifies the patient's blood group and antibodies to provide a compatible donor product for the transfusion.
- *Cross match.* When a sample of the patient's plasma is mixed with potential donor cells to make sure the blood and cells are compatible (Australian Red Cross Blood Service 2018).

Checking blood and blood products

Due to the critical nature of transfusing blood and blood products, strict checking procedures must be followed. Two staff must complete the check to verify the patient and blood product match. The nurse who hangs the blood product is responsible for overseeing the whole transfusion and must be one of the nurses who has completed the check and confirmed the patient and product are correct and compatible. During the checking process, if there is any concern about the product or match of the product to the patient, the product should not be used and instead returned to the service provider (Australian and New Zealand Society of Blood Transfusion & Australian College of Nursing 2018).

The check is comprehensive and includes:

- patient's full name, date of birth and medical record number are an exact match to the label attached to the blood product and the blood product order
- the blood product type on the order and product label are an exact match
- the blood group, donation or batch code/number on the compatibility label are an exact match the information on the product from the blood service
- any special requirements on the order are identified

- the blood group on the blood component is compatible with the blood group of the patient as indicated on the compatibility label attached to the pack; if the blood group of the blood component and the patient are not identical, the transfusion service provider must make a specific comment to indicate that it is compatible (or is the most suitable available)
- the blood component or product is not out of date/time
- the integrity of the blood product and packaging is checked for leaks, unusual discolouration and clots.

Administering the transfusion

Transfusion of the blood product should commence immediately, but if there has been a delay and it has not started within 30 minutes, the product should be returned to the blood fridge.

Once a transfusion of RBCs has commenced, it must be completed within four hours and only approved IV lines that have a standard filter to remove clots, and other debris that may have formed can be used. Importantly, platelets cannot be transfused through a blood administration set that has been used for red cells, because the platelets and RBCs may not be compatible. Medications must not be added to the blood bag or IV line because they may interact with the blood or other additives such as anticoagulants in the blood product.

Vital signs, including the patient's temperature, pulse, respiration rate and blood pressure, must be measured and recorded (and the patient skin checked for a rash) before the transfusion is commenced, and again within 15 minutes of commencing the transfusion (some facilities may also require constant visual observation of the patient for the first 15 minutes), and when the infusion is completed. Measuring and documenting the patient's vital signs throughout the transfusion is determined by the health service.

Transfusion reactions

Blood reactions can occur when transfusing blood products. During the transfusion, the nurse must be alert for signs of transfusion reactions that can range from mild to life-threatening. General signs and symptoms of transfusion reaction are outlined in table 20.4.

TABLE 20.4 Nursing management of a transfusion reaction

Reaction type	Signs and symptoms	Management
Mild reaction	Temperature increase of 1°C to 1.5°C above the baseline Localised rash or pruritus (itchy skin)	Stop the transfusion Ensure the IV access is secured Monitor and record the patient's temperature, pulse, respirations and blood pressure Repeat all documentation and identity checks of the patient and blood pack Contact medical staff immediately for further management and investigation
Moderate and severe reactions	Temperature of 1.5°C or more above baseline Skin rash Hypotension, shock or hypertension Tachycardia Severe anxiety or 'feeling of impending doom' Respiratory symptoms (dyspnoea, stridor, wheeze and hypoxia tachypnoea, wheeze or stridor) Rigors or chills Nausea or vomiting Pain (localised, chest, flank or discomfort at infusion site)	Stop the transfusion immediately Seek urgent medical advice Remove the blood bag and IV line (do not throw away) and replace with a new IV line and bag of normal saline. Repeat all documentation and identity checks of the patient and blood pack Monitor and record the patient's temperature, pulse, respirations and blood pressure Immediately report the event to the transfusion service provider, who will advise on return of the implicated product and administration set, and any further blood or urine samples needed from the patient

Source: Adapted from Australian and New Zealand Society of Blood Transfusion & Australian College of Nursing (2018).

Investigations

Since the collection of specimens requires an invasive procedure, consent must be sought from patients, who are informed about:

- the purpose of the test
- the time frame in which they will know the result
- how the result will be communicated.

Care of the venepuncture site and specimen collection should adhere to good clinical practice guidelines.

Blood tests

Full blood count (FBC) is one of the most common blood tests ordered and is a window into the general health status of a patient. An FBC can also be used to check the severity of blood loss, diagnose the presence of infection or diseases and ascertain the patient's response to treatments.

A blood film may be requested if there is a suspected disease or disorder affecting blood cell production and examines the appearance, quantity and maturity of all the blood cells (RBCs, WBCs and platelets) (Lab Tests Online 2020e). More on blood film tests can be accessed via this link: www.labtestsonline.org.au/learning/test-index/blood-film. Table 20.5 outlines the implications of altered cell counts in blood test results.

TABLE 20.5 Altered cell counts in blood tests results

Test	Name	Increased/decreased
WBC	White blood cell	May be increased with infections, inflammation, allergies, cancer, myeloproliferative neoplasm, leukaemia; decreased with some medications (such as methotrexate), some autoimmune conditions, some viral or severe infections, bone marrow failure, lymphoma, enlarged spleen, liver disease, alcohol excess and congenital marrow aplasia (marrow doesn't develop normally), diseases of the immune system (e.g. HIV/AIDS).
Neutrophils	Neutrophil/PMNs/Neuts	This is a dynamic population that varies somewhat from day to day depending on what is going on in the body. Significant increases are associated with different temporary/acute and/or chronic conditions. See Blood film examination and WBC.
Lymphocytes	Lymphocyte	An increase in the number of lymphocytes may be seen in a variety of conditions including viral illness (e.g. cytomegalovirus, Epstein-Barr virus, certain drug treatments and chronic lymphocytic leukaemia). Decreases in lymphocytes may be seen in autoimmune disorders (e.g. lupus and rheumatoid arthritis), infections (e.g. HIV, viral hepatitis), bone marrow damage.
Eosinophils	Eosinophil	The number of eosinophils may be increased in allergies such as hay fever, asthma and parasitic infections.
RBC	Red blood cell	Decreased with anaemia; due to acute or chronic bleeding, RBC destruction, bone marrow disorders. Increased when too many made (polycythaemia) and with fluid loss due to diarrhoea, dehydration, burns, living at high altitude.
Hb	Haemoglobin	Mirrors RBC results.
PCV/Hct	Haematocrit	Mirrors RBC results.
MCV	Mean cell volume	Increased (larger than normal RBCs — macrocytic) with vitamin B12 and folate deficiency. Decreased (smaller than normal RBCs — microcytic) with iron deficiency and thalassaemia.
MCH	Mean cell haemoglobin	Mirrors MCV results.

MCHC	Mean cell haemoglobin concentration	May be decreased when MCV is decreased. Increases limited to amount of Hb that will fit inside a RBC
RDW	RBC distribution width	Increased RDW indicates mixed population of RBCs. This may be due to an increase in the numbers of immature RBCs, which tend to be larger. It can also be seen following a blood transfusion or iron therapy.
Platelet	Platelet	Increased number of platelets occur after bleeding, inflammation and surgery. Decreased numbers are associated with some inherited disorders (such as Wiskott-Aldrich, Bernard-Soulier), with Systemic lupus erythematosus, pernicious anaemia, hypersplenism (spleen takes too many out of circulation), leukaemia and chemotherapy.
MPV	Mean platelet volume	Vary with platelet production; younger platelets are larger than older ones. A low MPV indicates that a condition is affecting the production of platelets by the bone marrow. A high MPV indicates that a condition is causing an overproduction and rapid release of platelets into circulation

Source: Lab Tests Online (2015).

Erythrocyte sedimentation rate

Erythrocyte sedimentation rate (ESR) is requested to measure and monitor the degree of inflammation in the body. A raised ESR is indicative of an infection, inflammatory disorder and/or malignancy, while a decreasing ESR may be indicating a satisfactory response to treatment (Lab Tests Online 2020b).

Coagulation screen

This test may be requested for patients who have altered coagulation factors, to identify the patients clotting times before a procedure, when a patient has a condition that is associated with bleeding, when there is a concern that the patient may bruise easily, or if the patient is on mediations that affect clotting times or if the patient has had an envenomation (some snake bites interfere with normal clotting mechanisms) (Lab Tests Online 2020f).

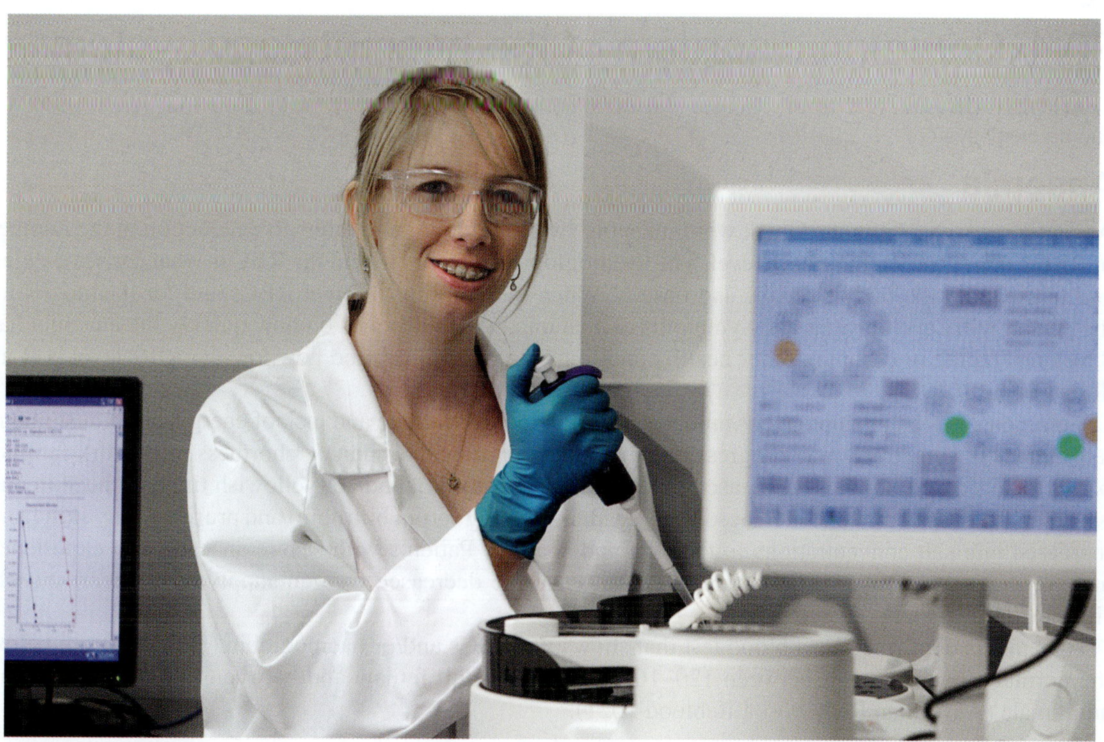

This test measures various bleeding times by measuring the activity of certain components of the intrinsic and extrinsic clotting pathway.

- *Prothrombin time (PT) — assesses the extrinsic clotting pathway.* It is prolonged in patients who are on warfarin therapy and in patients with liver disorders and disseminated intravascular coagulation (DIC).
- *Activated partial thromboplastin time (APTT) — assesses the intrinsic clotting pathway.* It is prolonged in patients receiving heparin and those who have liver disease and DIC.
- *International normalised ratio (INR) — assesses the extrinsic pathway.* This will be increased in patients receiving warfarin or who have liver dysfunction of DIC (Lab Tests Online 2020f).

Sickling test

This is the diagnostic test for sickle cell anaemia. In this condition, the patient has a genetically inherited variation of the shape of their haemoglobin molecule, which affects its ability to carry oxygen (Lab Tests Online 2020d).

Direct antiglobulin test (Coomb's test)

This test is requested if there is suspicion a patient's immune system is destroying their RBCs. The test screens or monitors patients who already have conditions that destroy RBCs, such as haemolytic anaemia, transfusion reactions or haemolytic disease of the newborn (Lab Tests Online 2020a).

Human leukocyte antigen (HLA) typing

This test is requested to identify a patient's inherited HLA genes and antigens and to match organ and bone marrow donors with recipients.

The HLA genes and antigens work as part of the immune response to recognise the body's 'self' cells and attack foreign cells. The HLA genes in the donor and recipient need to be the same or match as closely as possible for a transplant to be successful and for the tissue not be attacked or rejected by the recipient's immune system.

The degree of likeness between the recipient and donor must be matched as closely as possible or else the recipient's immune system will attack and reject the donor organ or bone marrow (Lab Tests Online 2020c).

Bone marrow aspiration/biopsy

This test is requested for patients with anaemia from an unknown cause, who have cancer that affects RBC production or are immunocompromised. This test assesses the blood cells or other substances and diagnoses cancers of the blood and bone marrow (Lab Tests Online 2020g).

20.4 Common disorders of the haematology system

LEARNING OBJECTIVE 20.4 Outline the conditions that may develop with abnormal function of the haematology system.

Anaemia

Anaemia is derived from the Greek word meaning 'without blood' and refers to a reduction in the number of RBCs and/or the haemoglobin level. The haemoglobin molecule within the RBC is what carries oxygen and nutrients to the body's organs and tissues. When there are insufficient RBCs and /or haemoglobin, the person will develop signs and symptoms of anaemia, which depends on how quickly the anaemia has developed (acute or chronic), other health conditions the person has, and how low the RBC level is (Lab Tests Online 2019).

Common signs and symptoms of mild anaemia can include fatigue and lack of energy, but if anaemia is left untreated, symptoms may progress and include palpitations, dyspnoea (shortness of breath), fatigue, pallor (pale skin colour from decreased blood flow to the skin), jaundice (yellowish tinge to the skin and whites of the eyes because of increased RBC death increasing serum bilirubin) and pruritis (itchy skin from increased bile salt concentrations in the skin and **serum**). Patients with severe anaemia can experience angina pectoris and myocardial infarction because of the decreased oxygen supply to the heart muscle (Rome 2020).

Anaemia is confirmed by a blood test that shows the RBCs and/or haemoglobin (Hb) levels are below the normal range, which is between 120–160 g/L for an adult female and between 130–180 g/L for an adult male (Australian Red Cross Lifeblood 2021).

Table 20.6 outlines the different types of anaemia and their causes.

TABLE 20.6 Types of anaemia

Type of anaemia	Description	Examples of causes
Iron deficiency	Lack of iron leads to decreased amount of haemoglobin; low levels of haemoglobin, in turn, leads to decreased production of normal RBCs	Blood loss; diet low in iron; poor absorption of iron
Pernicious anaemia and B vitamin deficiency	Lack of B vitamins does not allow RBCs to grow and then divide as they normally would during development; leads to decreased production of normal RBCs	Lack of intrinsic factor (pernicious anaemia, atrophic gastritis); diet low in B vitamins; decreased absorption of B vitamins
Aplastic	Decreased production of all cells produced by the bone marrow of which RBCs are one type	Cancer therapy; exposure to toxins; autoimmune disorders; viral infections
Haemolytic	RBCs survive less than the normal 110–120 days in the circulation; leads to overall decreased numbers of RBCs	Inherited causes include sickle cell and thalassaemia; other causes include transfusion reaction, autoimmune disease, certain drugs (e.g. penicillin)
Anaemia of chronic diseases	Various conditions over the long term can cause decreased production of RBCs	Kidney disease, diabetes, tuberculosis or HIV

Source: Lab Tests Online (2019).

Use this link to access more information on each of the types of anaemia in the table above www.labtestsonline.org.au/learning/index-of-conditions/anemia.

Nursing care of patients with anaemia

When planning the care of anaemic patients (table 20.7), it is useful to plan according to the basic needs assessment, putting the first priority on symptoms that can be life-threatening, such as blood loss and hypoxia.

TABLE 20.7 General nursing management of anaemic patients

	Management
Care of life threatening complications	Cardiac failure can occur in acute blood loss or where anaemia is experienced in conjunction with other conditions such as chronic obstructive pulmonary disease, cardiogenic shock or chronic pre-existing blood loss Dyspnoea in extreme cases causes collapse and respiratory failure Shock can occur where the condition is acute or untreated
Diagnosis and monitoring	Recognise signs and symptoms Take routine blood tests and correctly interpret them Assist with investigations Prevention of infection
Administration of medication	Administer prescribed medications when dietary supplementation is insufficient Administer blood transfusion as per local policy Oral iron sulphate 200 mg, three times a day with food for up to six months as required As constipation is a side effect, stool softeners may need to be given Intramuscular iron supplements are given in malabsorption disorders or when there is poor compliance; these need to be given in a 'Z-track' manner to prevent tracking and discolouration of the skin For patients on corticosteroids: • monitor blood sugars • daily urinalysis — if glucose is detected, check the blood glucose for secondary diabetes mellitus; insulin may be required if the result is positive

(continued)

TABLE 20.7 *(continued)*

	Management
	Mild to moderate pain — anti-inflammatory drugs Severe pain — opiates Oxygen therapy
Dyspnoea	Nurse the patient in the upright position to maximise lung expansion Use an integrated approach that concurrently manages both anxiety and breathlessness Physical demands will be great due to this symptom; care must be taken to assist patients with activities of daily living while promoting independence
Blood transfusions	Caution is required with elderly patients to ensure against overload of the circulatory system; blood may need to be given more slowly or spaced over a longer period of time Monitor fluid balance Administer erythropoietin if prescribed; this may improve quality of life as hospitalisation for blood transfusions will no longer be necessary
Tiredness	Patients can experience tiredness with the slightest exertion Educate patients that tiredness should lessen as the treatment takes effect Assistance should be given as required; periods of rest are encouraged Patients may be debilitated and may need to be on bed rest; and attend to pressure sore prevention and risk of deep vein thrombosis
Anxiety and depression	Patients may experience light-headedness and confusion due to hypoxia Anaemia may cause altered body image and loss of normal personal body state, which is replaced by a more dependent life-limiting persona This can increase anxiety and bring about feelings of depression Patients need: • assistance to restore functioning • reassurance • monitoring • understanding of the condition. Specific management is required in severe cases
Maintaining a safe environment	Patients are susceptible to falls due to symptoms of anaemia Skin integrity is impaired — skin is easily damaged so must be monitored carefully Educate patients on the maintenance of body heat and mobilisation Mental attention span is lessened; time off work and assistance in the home may be required A social services referral may be required following assessment
Mouth care	Assist patient to maintain oral hygiene (cleaning teeth/dentures) Monitor and record any injuries to lips, gums and mucous membranes Patients may experience soreness at the corners of the mouth; instruction on mouth care and maintenance of nutrition is necessary
Nutritional assessment and guidance	Dietary support and maintenance of good supplies of essential nutrients for blood cell regeneration Patient education to support recommendations from dietitian reinforce the essential foods
Discharge planning	Ensure patients are safe to go home Educate patients on self-care, recognition of anaemia and medications Where required, dietetic support is ongoing Arrange an outpatient appointment Alternatively, a follow-up appointment can be made with the GP Elderly people or those who struggle with family responsibilities may need community support services

Polycythaemia

Polycythaemia is a very rare condition characterised by an abnormally higher than normal haemoglobin level (and sometimes RBCs and platelets) that accumulate in the bone marrow and blood stream, which causes the blood to become thick (hyperviscosity).

Patients may have headaches, visual disturbances, fatigue, weakness and itchy skin. Some patients will develop splenomegaly (enlarged spleen), hepatomegaly (enlarged liver) and a feeling of fullness because of the enlarged organs pressing on the stomach.

Venesection of 450–500 ml of blood (removal of blood from the circulation) is the treatment of choice. The frequency of venesection depends on (Haemophilia Foundation Australia 2020) the patient's haematocrit and may be needed as frequently as every month to as infrequently as every year (Leukaemia Foundation 2019).

Von Willebrand disease (VWD)

This condition is the most common inherited bleeding disorder globally and affects both males and females. Von Willebrand is a factor found in blood. When there is not enough of this factor, or the factor does not work the way it should, it takes longer for the blood to clot; therefore, the person bleeds for longer (Haemophilia Foundation Australia 2018).

This condition may cause people to bleed more easily from the delicate mucous membranes that line the nose, mouth, stomach and intestines, vagina and uterus. This means the person may bruise easily, bleed for longer from minor injury or cuts, have heavy menstrual periods or heavy bleeding after childbirth. In most people, the condition is only problematic if they experience severe trauma or surgery (Haemophilia Foundation Australia 2018).

If treatment is required, hormones and the von Willebrand clotting factor are administered to the patient (Haemophilia Foundation Australia 2018).

Haemophilia

In Australia, almost 3000 people have haemophilia, with more males being affected than females. Haemophilia is an inherited disorder that results from a life-long deficiency of clotting factors (factor VIII; haemophilia A) or Christmas factor (factor IX; haemophilia B). Haemophilia is diagnosed when a person has less than 40 per cent of the normal level of clotting factors in their blood (Haemophilia Foundation Australia 2020).

Over a period, internal bleeding into joints and muscle can cause chronic pain, joint damage and arthritis.

In Australia, people with haemophilia have their care coordinated at the Haemophilia Treatment Centre (HTC) located within a public hospital in their state or territory. Treatment involves the replacement of the clotting factors, either prophylactically to prevent bleeding/injury or on-demand (when they are bleeding) (Haemophilia Foundation Australia 2020).

Thrombocytopenia

Thrombocytopenia is a reduced platelet count resulting from excessive bleeding or an inability of the bone marrow to produce a normal number of platelets.

Thrombocytopenia is an autoimmune disease where there is a low number of platelets resulting in spontaneous bleeding or prolonged bleeding after trauma or injury. There are three types of this condition. Thrombocytopenia can occur during pregnancy, because of medications, cancers or infections, or an enlarged spleen. Children are more likely than adults to develop acquired thrombocytopenia (Healthdirect 2019). There are three types of thrombocytopenia.

1. Immune thrombocytopenia (ITT) occurs when the immune system coats the platelets in an antibody that causes the spleen to destroy the platelets when they pass through.
2. Thrombotic thrombocytopenia (TTP) is when there is bleeding and clotting at the same time, with tiny micro thrombi developing in arterioles and capillaries. This condition is a medical emergency.
3. Heparin-induced thrombocytopenia (HIT) is when the commonly used medication heparin releases particles that activate thrombin (from the clotting cascade) to form clots.

Thrombocytopenia will often resolve on its own or if the cause is treated (e.g. cancer, stopping medications). Some patients may require a platelet or immunoglobulin transfusion, or steroid therapy to increase the number of platelets, or splenectomy (removal of the spleen) (Healthdirect 2019).

Disseminated intravascular coagulation (DIC)

DIC is a serious life-threatening condition that results from simultaneous overactivation of the coagulation system and fibrinolytic pathways, which decreases the number of platelets and clotting factors. The causative factors include transfusion reactions, leukaemia and cytotoxic treatment, which trigger the clotting cascade. It requires intensive monitoring and specialist haematological input. A balance needs to be achieved between replacing clotting factors by means of infusing cryoprecipitate and FFP and anticoagulating patients with heparin (Rome 2020).

Neutropenia

Neutropenia is a low number of circulating WBCs called neutrophils, which provide immune defence against bacterial infections. Neutropenia can result from treatments for conditions such as cancer, immune system dysfunction, autoimmune disease, infection or genetics.

Neutropenic patients are very vulnerable to developing severe infections. Neutropenia may resolve if the underlying cause can be treated or stopped (Rome 2020).

20.5 Oncological disorders of the haematology system

LEARNING OBJECTIVE 20.5 Describe the oncological conditions of the haematology system and the nursing care for these patients.

Blood cancers can affect the blood cells, bone marrow or the lymphatic system. Three common blood cancers in Australia include myeloma, leukaemia and lymphoma.

Myeloma

Myeloma is cancer of the plasma cells. When the plasma cells become malignant and change, they are called myeloma cells. They multiply and take over the bone marrow, which leaves no space for other cells, causing pancytopenia (decreased levels of RBC, WBCs and platelets). This means the person can develop anaemia (from decreased RBCs), infections (from decreased WBCs) and bleeding (from decreased platelets). Myeloma cells in bone marrow (located in the long and flat bones) become tumours that grow on the surface of bones throughout the body (multiple myeloma), releasing chemicals that trigger osteoclasts in the bone to remove calcium, causing brittle bones that break easily (osteoporosis) (Leukaemia Foundation 2020). The incidence is higher in those over the age of 60 years, and the condition is common in men. The cause of multiple myeloma is unknown (Cancer Council Victoria n.d.). However, there is increased risk:

- in patients who have relatives with *BRCA1* and *BRCA2* gene mutations
- with previous exposure to radiation, rubber, wood, chemicals and textiles.

There is evidence of high levels of abnormal proteins in the blood and urine, which can cause renal failure. Increased blood viscosity can cause clotting, while abnormal proteins surrounding the organs and blood vessels can cause proteins to build up and accumulate (amyloidosis). There is also a reduction in immunoglobulins, increasing the risk of infection. Other signs and symptoms include:

- bone pain and/or fractures is a common symptom and can develop due to thinning of the bones (osteoporosis) or holes in the bones, causing an increased risk of injury and calcium from the damaged bones entering the bloodstream (hypercalcaemia)
- tiredness
- spinal cord compression
- bleeding and bruising.

Medical management and nursing care for patients with myeloma

Multiple myeloma is not curable, but many effective treatments are available that can delay the progression of the disease for a number of years and provide supportive therapy and improved quality of life. The medical and nursing management are outlined in figures 20.6 and 20.7.

FIGURE 20.6 Medical management of myeloma

- Chemotherapy
- Autologous stem cell transplantation
- Radiotherapy is given as a supportive therapy to treat bone lesions; it can be a palliative measure
- Bisphosphonates (to treat bone destruction), corticosteroids
- Surgical intervention, may be required to treat pathological fractures or stabilise bones

Other treatments include the following.

- Erythropoietin
- Management of:
  - pancytopenia
  - infection
  - renal failure.

FIGURE 20.7 Nursing priorities for patients with myeloma

Spinal cord compression

- This is an oncological emergency; patients can either collapse or have severe sensorimotor impairment and require prompt medical management.

Pain management

- Initiate pain assessment and ongoing management of pain.
- The patient may require:
  - drug therapy
  - supportive approaches through the use of mobilisation aids
  - referral to the palliative care team early in the illness journey for management of pain and control of symptoms.

Maintenance of a safe environment

- The patient is often elderly with impaired mobility, which requires referral to the physiotherapy and occupational therapy departments for suitable equipment.
- Bone fractures and lesions put these patients in a high-risk category for falls and pressure sores.

Prevention and management of renal failure

- The patient may present with renal failure, which must be treated.
- Ongoing disease and its management can cause renal failure.
- Fluid balance monitoring and electrolyte assessment is important.
- Education on the need for adequate fluid intake is required prior to discharge.

Pancytopenia

- Low RBC and platelet counts are usually treated with transfusions; administration is as per local hospital guidelines.

Infection

- Ascertain the microbiology results.
- Administer antibiotic therapy.
- Educate patients on how to protect themselves from contracting infections and adhere to a good nutritional diet.

Hypercalcaemia

- This results from bone destruction and the release of excessive amounts of calcium into the blood.
- Observe the patient for confusion.
- Gentle mobilisation reduces the release of calcium.

Physiological and psychological support

- Ongoing support from a specialist centre is needed due to the range of problems that patients experience.
- Refer the patient to social services, financial support and patient support groups, all of which can assist patients to deal with the longevity of the disease.

Discharge planning

- Involve the palliative care team and community specialists.
- The level of mobility will be assessed and suitable aids provided.
- Organise appropriate home care.
- Family support is important to support patients at home and assist with transport to hospital for monitoring.

Leukaemia

Leukaemia is a cancer in the bone marrow, where all blood cells are made. Leukaemia causes the stem cells in the bone marrow to develop abnormally, which then multiply, but leaves them unable to fulfil their normal function. Leukaemia can affect either myeloid cells (which turn into RBCs, WBCs and platelets) or lymphoid cells (which affects the B and T lymphocyte cells). Leukaemia is classified as either acute or chronic (Leukaemia Foundation 2020). Leukaemia is diagnosed with blood tests and bone marrow biopsy (Rome 2020).

Acute leukaemia is characterised by a rapid increase in the number of immature blood cells, leaving the bone marrow unable to produce healthy blood cells. Immediate treatment is required due to the rapid progression and accumulation of the malignant cells, which spill over into the bloodstream and spread to other organs of the body.

Chronic leukaemia is characterised by the excessive build-up of relatively mature, but still abnormal, WBCs. Cells are produced at a higher rate than normal cells, resulting in many abnormal WBCs being seen in the blood. Chronic leukaemia may be monitored for some time before there is any need for treatment; it can take months or years to progress and mostly occurs in older people but can theoretically occur in any age group.

The classification of leukaemia is outlined in table 20.8.

TABLE 20.8 Classification of leukaemia

Cell line	Acute	Chronic
Lymphoid	Acute lymphoblastic leukaemia (ALL)	Chronic lymphocytic leukaemia (CLL)
Myeloid	Acute myeloid leukaemia (AML)	Chronic myeloid leukaemia (CML)

Acute lymphoblastic leukaemia (ALL)

In ALL, abnormal WBCs (lymphoblasts) grow too quickly and outnumber the RBCs, normal WBCs and platelets. The bone marrow becomes crowded, and the blood cannot develop properly. Excess cells are forced out of the bone marrow and into the circulation, accumulating in the lymph glands, spleen, liver, brain and spinal cord (Leukaemia Foundation 2020). ALL diminishes the body's ability to fight infection.

Acute myeloid leukaemia (AML)

In AML, the immature myeloid cells are cancerous and the proliferation of abnormal WBCs is uncontrollable, causing an abundance of blast cells to be present. These crowd out the bone marrow and prevent the normal growth of WBCs, RBCs and platelets, causing anaemia and increased risk of bleeding/bruising (Leukaemia Foundation 2020).

Chronic lymphocytic leukaemia (CLL)

This is a slow growing cancer of the lymphoid B cells (B lymphocytes), whose normal function is to produce antibodies to fight infection. Lymphocytes usually die off naturally at the end of their lifespan. In CLL, these cells live on even when they are no longer useful in fighting infection. They build up in the bone marrow until there is no space for normal blood cells to develop. CLL is the most common form of leukaemia diagnosed in Australia (Leukaemia Foundation 2020).

Chronic myeloid leukaemia (CML)

CML is a cancer of the WBC called granulocytes, leading to a hyperproliferation of immature abnormal granulocytes in the bloodstream. Because the cells are immature and not working properly, they are not able to protect against infection, and like in other leukaemias, they can cause anaemia and increased bleeding or bruising (Leukaemia Foundation 2020).

Causes and signs of leukaemia

The exact causes of leukaemia are unknown, but risk factors include:

- increasing age
- smoking
- exposure to high doses of radiation
- radon gas
- benzene

- previous treatment for cancer
- Down's syndrome
- blood disorders such as Fanconi anaemia.

Symptoms are vague and vary depending on the type of leukaemia and how advanced it is. There may be no symptoms in the early stages, especially with chronic leukaemia, or they may be mild at first and then worsen (figure 20.8). Chronic leukaemia usually presents with enlarged lymph glands (in the neck, underarms and groins).

FIGURE 20.8 Signs and symptoms of leukaemia

- Tiredness, breathlessness and pale skin (due to anaemia)
- Fever (pyrexia)
- Infections that do not clear
- Abnormal bruising or bleeding
- A petechial rash
- Bone and joint pain (due to overcrowding of the bone marrow)
- Swollen lymph nodes
- Abdominal discomfort (due to an enlarged spleen)
- Loss of appetite and weight loss
- Swollen gums
- Swollen testicles
- Headaches and vision problems
- Itchy skin
- Night sweats and fevers

Diagnosis of leukaemia

The following investigations are performed for the diagnosis of leukaemia:

- physical examination
- FBC
- blood film
- bone marrow aspirate and biopsy
- analysis of abnormal cells found in the blood and bone marrow (cytogenetics and immunophenotyping)
- computed tomography (CT)
- magnetic resonance imaging (MRI)
- ultrasound scans
- lumbar puncture (in ALL).

Treatment of leukaemia

The type of leukaemia determines treatment. Combinations of chemotherapy, corticosteroids, radiation therapy and stem cell transplant can be used to achieve remission for the different types of leukaemia. Ultimately, the treatment regimen depends on the type of leukaemia the patient has, their comorbidities and patient preferences.

Nursing care of the patient with leukaemia incorporates those identified in table 20.9, outlining care of the patient with anaemia and figure 20.9.

TABLE 20.9 **Diagnostic tests**

Blood tests	FBC
	ESR
	Liver and kidney function
	Lactate dehydrogenase level
	Uric acid

(continued)

TABLE 20.9 *(continued)*

Imaging	Chest X-ray CT scan Ultrasound MRI scan Positron emission tomography
Biopsy/cytology	Biopsy of any suspicious lesions (the most important diagnostic test), usually lymph nodes (surgical biopsy being the preferred method) Fine-needle aspiration Bone marrow aspiration and/or biopsy Lumbar puncture (spinal tap)
Molecular analysis	Immunophenotyping Genotyping

FIGURE 20.9 Nursing management of leukaemia and lymphoma

Prevention of infection
- Hand-washing
- Protective isolation while neutropenic
- Prophylactic antibiotics and antifungal agents
- 4-hourly vital signs while neutropenic
- Blood cultures when pyrexial
- Antipyretics (e.g. paracetamol)
- Monitoring for signs of infection
- Granulocyte colony-stimulating factor therapy to reduce the length of neutropenia
- Dietary restrictions, e.g. no unpasteurised foods
- Patient education:
  - Avoid unnecessary crowds and people who may have an infection
  - Contact the healthcare team if symptoms of infection develop
  - Wear loose cotton clothing
  - Layer clothing and bedding for easy temperature adjustment
  - Use sprays and moist wipes to cool the skin

Fatigue/anaemia
- If anaemic, use:
  - Blood transfusions
  - Drug therapy (e.g. erythropoietin)
- Patient education:
  - Eat a healthy, well-balanced diet
  - Take regular gentle exercise
  - Have adequate rest
  - Avoid caffeine just before bedtime

Bleeding/thrombocytopenia
- Severe risk of bleeding if the platelet count is below 10–20 × 10^9/L
- Platelet transfusion
- Replacement of clotting factors, if required
- Patient education:
  - Avoid cuts, bruises and falls
  - Take care when:
    - blowing your nose
    - shaving
    - cleaning your teeth

Fertility
- Sperm banking
- Oocyte/embryo cryopreservation (if time allows)

Psychosocial care
- Anxiety
- Information needs
- Education on the illness and the side effects of treatment

Nausea/vomiting
- Give an antiemetic before and after chemotherapy and/or radiotherapy
- Arrange a prescription for nausea control at home
- Try serotonin receptor antagonists
- Patient education:
  - Drink plenty of fluids before, during and after therapy
  - Eat frequent small meals and snacks
  - Adapt meals and drinks according to symptoms
  - Consider complementary therapy (e.g. relaxation techniques and aromatherapy)

Hair loss
- Refer to a hospital wig services or wig supplier experienced in fitting people with cancer
- Patient education:
  - Visit a wig supplier before all hair is lost to ensure a good colour, texture and style match
  - Alternatively, use hats, hair bands, scarves and bandanas

Sore throat/mouth (mucositis)
- Monitor for signs of infection:
  - Pink or red bleeding lesions
  - Dry mucosa or tongue
  - Painful, white patches
- Adequate pain management
- Regular oral assessment and mouth care
- Patient education:
  - Use a soft toothbrush and brush the teeth (and tongue) gently after every meal
  - Avoid mouthwashes containing alcohol; saltwater or baking soda may be used instead
  - Rinse the mouth with water as often as needed
  - Avoid irritating acidic and spicy foods
  - Drink plenty of fluids

Lymphoma

Lymphoma is the sixth most common cancer in Australia. It is a disease that affects the lymphocytes, which become malignant, grow and multiply uncontrollably, and may not die off when and how they ought to. Lymphomas are divided into two major categories.

1. *Hodgkin's lymphoma.* Initiates in a lymph gland, then spreads around the body through the lymphatic system, affecting other lymph glands, lymph organs and the bone marrow. Hodgkin's lymphoma can be caused by viruses, a weakened immune system (from an autoimmune disease or medications that suppress the immune system), or it can be genetically inherited (Cancer Council NSW n.d.-a).
2. *Non-Hodgkin's lymphoma (NHL).* More common than Hodgkin's lymphoma. NHL also initiates in the lymphocytes and travels through the lymph system to other lymph glands, organs and bone marrow. The difference between the two conditions is in the appearance of the cells, and that NHL can move outside of the lymphatic system to the central nervous system, skin, bone and stomach. There are several non-Hodgkin's lymphomas that can develop, based on whether the B or T lymphocyte is affected (Cancer Council NSW n.d.-b).

The signs and symptoms of lymphoma are similar to those of leukaemia and include:
- painless swelling of the lymph glands in the neck, under the arms or in the groin
- loss of appetite and weight loss
- fever
- excessive sweating at night
- itchiness all over the body
- a feeling of weakness
- breathlessness with swelling of the face and neck.

The initial assessment includes a full physical examination, special attention being paid to all lymph node-bearing regions and Waldeyer's ring (the ring of tissues formed by the tonsils and their connecting lymphatic tissue). Nurses can help patients through the diagnosis and disease evaluation period by providing reassurance, support and information on the disease and the diagnostic tests (table 20.9).

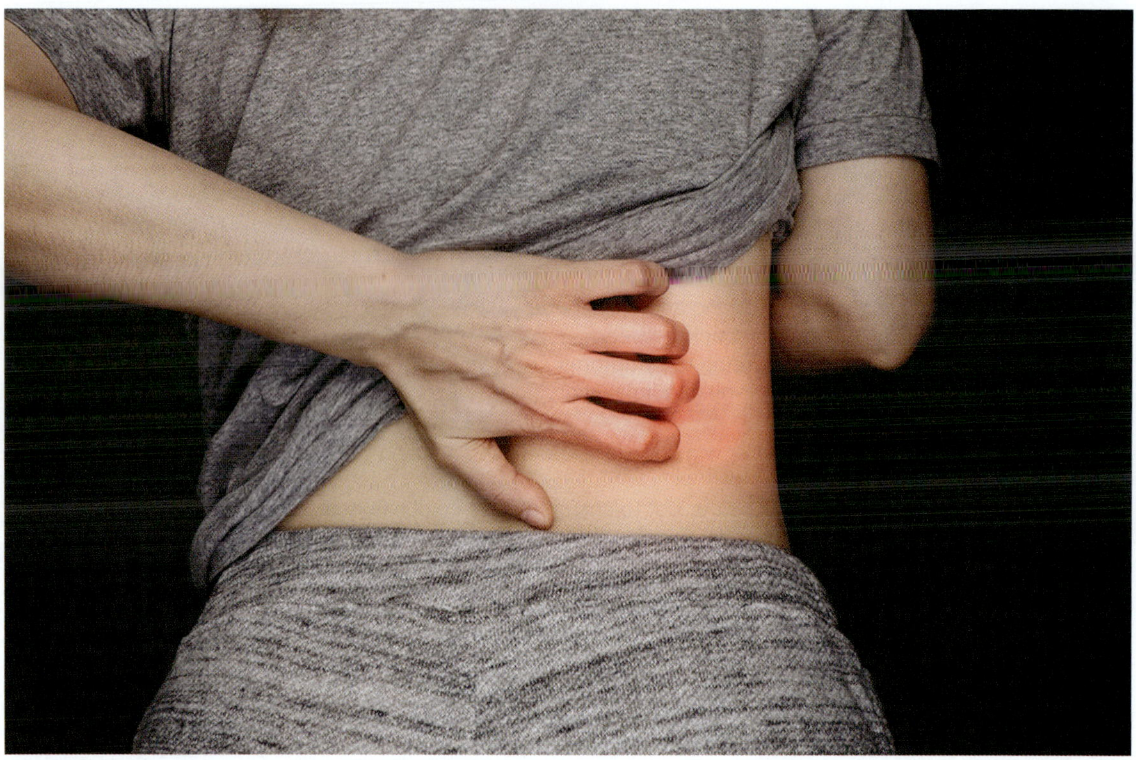

Treatment of lymphoma

Chemotherapy is commonly used and may be given as a single agent or may be combined with radiotherapy or monoclonal antibody therapy and in combination with other drugs. Treatment is tailored to patients' specific disease needs.

Lymphomas may become resistant to chemotherapy, so many different regimens, including experimental drugs, can be used.

Chemotherapy can be delivered:

- orally (as a liquid, tablet or pill)
- intravenous (IV)
- intramuscular (IM)
- intra-arterial
- intraperitoneal (injected into the abdomen)
- intrathecal (injected into the cerebrospinal fluid)
- subcutaneously (into the tissue just under the skin).

Chemotherapy is administered to kill the cancer cells, but it also kills or damages healthy cells. The remaining healthy cells can repair damage that is caused by the chemotherapy.

Access this link www.canceraustralia.gov.au/affected-cancer/treatment for more information on the types of cancer treatments and side effects.

The nursing management of leukaemia and lymphoma is outlined in figure 20.9.

Haematopoietic stem cell transplant

Stem cells are the cells inside the bone marrow, from which all cells are made. A stem cell transplant can be used to eliminate an underlying disease and restore the function of blood and immune cells for people diagnosed with leukaemia, myeloma or lymphoma, as well as for other diseases. The transplant removes all the cells in the bone marrow, including the damaged and cancerous cells, and replaces them with healthy cells that produce properly functioning blood cells.

There are two types of transplant.

- *Autologous transplantation.* Sometimes stem cells are collected from patients when they are in remission and frozen until required. Any cancerous cells are removed, and the remaining cells then reinfused after high-dose chemotherapy has been administered. There is a risk that not all cancerous cells were removed and the patient will relapse (Cancer Australia 2021).

- *Allogeneic transplantation* is when cancer-free stem cells are collected from a carefully matched donor (often a sibling) and administered to patients following high-dose chemotherapy and/or radiotherapy. The risk is that the patient's body might reject the new stem cells (called graft versus host disease), and anti-rejection medication might be required for some months after the transplant (Cancer Australia 2021).

Both procedures can be physically and emotionally difficult, so patients often require support and counselling. Patients are hospitalised for a few weeks while the bone marrow and blood cell count returns to normal. The risk of infection during this period is high, so patients may be placed under reverse isolation, and special precautions are taken to reduce infection.

Sources of cells for haematopoietic stem cell transplant are:

- bone marrow, which is aspirated from the posterior iliac crests under general anaesthesia, marrow volumes of 800–1200 ml usually being taken
- peripheral blood stem cells, obtained following the administration of granulocyte colony-stimulating factor and collected by apheresis
- umbilical cord blood cells, which are collected from the umbilical cord at birth.

For more information on bone marrow donation, use this link to access the Australian Bone Marrow Donor Registry www.abmdr.org.au.

CASE STUDY 20.1

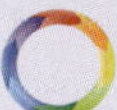

Nursing care of an elderly patient with anaemia

Indira Kaur is a 70-year-old widow who has been admitted to the medical ward with anaemia for investigation. Indira has had increasing shortness of breath, fatigue and episodes of dizzy spells over the last six weeks. Indira lives alone but has a large family and grandchildren who visit her at home most days. Indira has no known allergies, has a history of controlled atrial fibrillation, for which she is prescribed anticoagulant medication to reduce her risk of stroke. Indira is very anxious that she feels short of breath and is worried that she will not be able to return to her own home if she cannot properly care for herself.

Vital signs are:

- temperature: 36.5°C
- heart rate: 90 beats per minute
- blood pressure: 135/80 mmHg
- respiratory rate: 28 breaths per minute
- oxygen saturation: 94% on room air
- blood test: Hb level of 80 gm/L.

Question

Using the information above, describe what action you would take as the nurse caring for this patient. Use the clinical reasoning cycle to guide you through the process and devise a plan of care for your patient.

Answer

- *Step 1: Consider the patient.* Indira Kaur is a 70-year-old female who has been admitted to the medical ward.
- *Step 2: Collect cues/information.* Include subjective and objective data here, including the patient's appearance and their past medical history. Objective data will include measurable information such as their vital signs.

  Indira is very thin and pale, and is resting in bed, saying she has little energy to do anything. Vital signs indicate that Indira is afebrile.
- *Step 3: Process information.* Separate the relevant and irrelevant data — cluster the clues together to formulate an inference about the patient.

  Indira is anxious and looks tired, saying she has little energy, consistent with a diagnosis of anaemia. A Hb level of 80 gm/L is below the normal HB range for females. Without adequate oxygen being delivered to the cells, Indira's symptoms will continue and her condition will deteriorate further.
- *Step 4: Identify problems/issues.* Indira's nursing problems or diagnosis should be listed here.
  - Activity tolerance due to extreme fatigue
  - Dyspnoea causing anxiety
  - Risk of falls due to general debility
  - Potential for bruising/bleeding due to anticoagulant medications
  - Potential for confusion and tissue damage due to hypoxia
  - Low body weight

- *Step 5: Establish goals.* Goals of care for Indira include reducing anxiety related to breathlessness and improve oxygenation.

  Administering prescribed iron replacement medications and improving oral food and fluid intake to achieve satisfactory body weight and iron intake.

  Maintain personal hygiene. Eliminate falls risks.
- *Step 6: Take action.* The nurse should place Indira in the sitting position to increase lung expansion and manage symptoms of breathlessness to reduce anxiety.

  Initiate a dietitian review and recommend the necessary dietary changes.

  Administer prescribed iron replacement medications to increase Hb and restore normal RBC oxygen-carrying capacity. Assist Indira with ADLS (showering, dressing and toileting) to maintain her personal hygiene and reduce falls risks.

  Position her call bell, over bed table and other items within easy reach and ask Indira if there is anything in particular she would like you to do for her or if there is anything she is worried about.
- *Step 7: Evaluate outcomes.* How effective have your nursing interventions been?

  Indira will have improved activity tolerance allowing her to have increased ambulation without dyspnoea or risk of falls. Respiratory rate will be within normal parameters

  Lethargy will subside, appetite will be restored increased oral food and fluid intake. An understanding of dietary modifications and medications will be required to maintain normal Hb levels.
- *Step 8: Reflect on the process and new learning.* Consider what important new knowledge about anaemia you have learnt by completing this case study. Reflect on one aspect of Indira's nursing care that could have been managed differently.

CASE STUDY 20.2

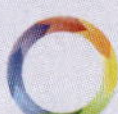

Nursing care of a patient receiving a blood transfusion.

James Bourke is a 74-year-old widower who has been admitted to the medical ward with anaemia for investigation. James blood test on admission indicates his Hb is 72 gm/L. James has had PR bleeding and increasing fatigue, and episodes of dizzy spells over the last ten weeks. James has been on anticoagulant medication since his mitral valve replacement 10 years ago. James has been prescribed a blood transfusion. James has had the necessary pre-transfusion tests to identify his blood type and a cross match to identify a suitable blood donor, and the nurse is completing the checking processes to administer the blood transfusion.

Vital signs are:

- temperature: 36.3°C
- heart rate: 100 beats per minute
- blood pressure 115/80 mmHg
- respiratory rate: 28 breaths per minutes
- oxygen Saturation: 90% on nasal prongs at 2 L pm.

Question

Using the information above, describe what action you would take as the nurse caring for this patient. Use the clinical reasoning cycle to guide you through the process and devise a care plan for your patient.

Answer

- *Step 1. Consider the patient.* James Bourke, a 74 year-old male patient.
- *Step 2. Collect cues/information.* Include subjective and objective data here, including the patient's appearance and their past medical history. Objective data will include measurable information such as his vital signs.

  Baseline assessment at the commencement of the transfusion identifies that James is very pale and extremely short of breath while sitting.

  Twenty minutes into the transfusion, James becomes very anxious and reports a feeling of nausea and begins to vomit. The nurse repeats the vital signs, which indicate: temp: 37.9; HR 120; BP: 90/55; oxygen saturation 90% on nasal prongs at 2 L pm.
- *Step 3: Process information.* Separate the relevant and irrelevant data – cluster the clues together to formulate an inference about the patient.

  Considering the sudden change in James's vital signs and presentation, the nurse recognises that James is experiencing a severe transfusion reaction.
- *Step 4: Identify problems/issues.* The immediate problem for James is that the symptoms he is experiencing are because of a reaction to the blood transfusion he is receiving.

- *Step 5: Establish goals*. Goals of care should focus on immediately removing the cause of the reaction and supporting James through the associated anxiety.
- *Step 6: Take action*. The nurse should immediately stop the transfusion and seek urgent medical advice by initiating a met call/code blue. Remove the blood bag and IV line (do not throw away) and replace them with a new IV line and bag of normal saline.

  Repeat all documentation and identity checks of the patient and blood pack and continue to monitor and record the patient's temperature, pulse, respiration and blood pressure.

  Report the event to the transfusion service provider, who will advise on the return of the product and administration set, and any further blood or urine samples needed from the patient.
- *Step 7: Evaluate outcomes*. Once the medical emergency team has attended and James has been stabilised, he may be transferred to ICU or a high dependency ward where she can be closely observed and monitored.
- *Step 8: Reflect on the process and new learning*. Consider what important new knowledge about managing a blood transfusion reaction you have learned by completing this case study. Reflect on one aspect of James's nursing care that could have been managed differently.

SUMMARY

Blood is essential for the body to function; therefore, it is imperative that nurses know the components and functions of the haematological system to understand haematological disorders and conditions that can develop. This chapter explored the functions and components of the haematology system, haemostasis, blood types and principles for safe nursing care when administering a blood transfusion. Nursing care for patients who have developed disorders and diseases secondary to abnormal function of the haematology system were also explored. Knowledge provides a sound basis for the safe nursing care of haematology patients in a haematology setting and in medical and surgical care settings.

KEY TERMS

erythropoiesis The production of red blood cells (RBCs). Erythro means 'red', and poiesis means 'to make'.

erythropoietin A hormone released by the kidneys that stimulates the bone marrow to start haematopoiesis (RBC production).

plasma A liquid that makes up more than half of our blood and contains RBCs, WBCs, clotting factors, lipids, steroid hormones and vitamins, and transports them around the body.

plasma cells A type of white blood cell (WBC) that are made in the bone marrow. Plasma cells release specific antibodies (immunoglobulins) when an antigen is detected.

red blood cells (RBCs) Cells that are made in the bone marrow. They have a haemoglobin protein that enables oxygen molecules to attach and to be transported around the body. RBCs are also called erythrocytes.

serum From the liquid component of blood. It contains protein such as albumin, which carries electrolytes, hormones and antibodies around the body but has no clotting factors.

thrombocytes Also known as platelets, they develop in the bone marrow and are released into the circulation to form blood clots to stop or prevent bleeding and maintain haemostasis.

white blood cells (WBCs) Work with the immune system to fight infection. They are categorised into granulocytes (have granules in the centre and include basophils, eosinophils and neutrophils), lymphocytes (including B cells, T cells and natural killer cells) and monocytes.

REFERENCES

ACSQHC. (2017) Blood Management Standard. NSQHS Standards. https://www.safetyandquality.gov.au/sites/default/files/migrated/National-Safety-and-Quality-Health-Service-Standards-second-edition.pdf

Australian and New Zealand Society of Blood Transfusion, & Australian College of Nursing. (2018) Guidelines for the administration of blood products. Sydney, Australia: Australian & New Zealand Society of Blood Transfusion Ltd.

Australian Red Cross Blood Service. (2018) Transfusion resource handbook — Blood matters. https://www2.health.vic.gov.au/-/media/health/files/collections/policies-and-guidelines/b/transfusion-resource-handbook-2018-pdf.pdf?la=en&hash=E3E9272CC3BE6C12379900D688DFA7E560B0E846

Australian Red Cross Lifeblood. (2017) Australia's pioneering Rh program turns 50. https://transfusion.com.au/bsib_july2017_2

Australian Red Cross Lifeblood. (2021) Anaemia. https://[illegible]transfusion/anaemia

Cancer Australia. (2021) Stem cell transplant. https://www.canceraustralia.gov.au/affected-cancer/treatment/stem-cell-transplant

Cancer Council NSW. (n.d.-a) Hodgkin lymphoma. https://www.cancercouncil.com.au/hodgkin-lymphoma

Cancer Council NSW. (n.d.-b) Non-Hodgkin's lymphoma. https://www.cancercouncil.com.au/non-hodgkin-lymphoma

Cancer Council Victoria. (n.d.) Multiple myeloma. https://www.cancervic.org.au/cancer-information/types-of-cancer/multiple_myeloma/multiple-myeloma-overview.html

Dougherty, L. & Lamb, J. (2009) *Intravenous therapy in nursing practice*, 2nd ed. Oxford: Blackwell Publishing.

Haemophilia Foundation Australia. (2018) Von Willebrand disease. https://www.haemophilia.org.au/publications/bleeding-disorders

Haemophilia Foundation Australia. (2020) Haemophilia. https://www.haemophilia.org.au/about-bleeding-disorders/haemophilia

Healthdirect. (2019) Thrombocytopenia. https://www.healthdirect.gov.au/thrombocytopenia

Healthdirect. (2017) Blood types. https://www.healthdirect.gov.au/blood-types

Hendrick, L. (2019) 'The structure and function of the haematological system'. In J. Craft, C. Gordon, S. Heuther, K. McCance, V. Brahshers & N. Rote (Eds.). *Understanding Pathophysiology*, 3rd ed. (pp. 383–406). Chatswood, NSW: Elsevier.

Lab Tests Online. (2015) Full blood count: At a glance. https://www.labtestsonline.org.au/learning/test-index/fbc#glance

Lab Tests Online. (2019) Anaemia. https://www.labtestsonline.org.au/learning/index-of-conditions/anemia

Lab Tests Online. (2020) Direct antiglobulin test. https://www.labtestsonline.org.au/learning/test-index/direct-antiglobulin

Lab Tests Online. (2020b) Erythrocyte sedimentation rate (ESR). https://www.labtestsonline.org.au/learning/test-index/esr
Lab Tests Online. (2020c) HLA testing. https://www.labtestsonline.org.au/learning/test-index/hla-testing
Lab Tests Online. (2020d) Sickle cell. https://www.labtestsonline.org.au/learning/test-index/sickle
Lab Tests Online. (2020e) Blood film examination. https://www.labtestsonline.org.au/learning/test-index/blood-film
Lab Tests Online. (2020f) Coagulation factors. https://www.labtestsonline.org.au/learning/test-index/coag-factors
Lab Tests Online. (2020g) Bone marrow biopsy. https://www.labtestsonline.org.au/learning/test-index/bone-marrow
Leukaemia Foundation. (2019) Polycythaemia (rubra) vera. https://www.leukaemia.org.au/blood-cancer-information/types-of-blood-cancer/myeloproliferative-neoplasms/polycythaemia-rubra-vera
Leukaemia Foundation. (2020) Types of blood cancer. https://www.leukaemia.org.au/blood-cancer-information/types-of-blood-cancer/
Leukaemia Foundation. (2020b) What is blood? Blood cancer information. https://www.leukaemia.org.au/blood-cancer-information/types-of-blood-cancer/understanding-your-blood/what-is-blood
Nair, M. & Peate, I. (2009) *Applied Pathophysiology. An Essential Guide for Nursing Students.* Oxford: Wiley Blackwell.
National Blood Authority Australia. (n.d.a) Overview: About blood. https://www.blood.gov.au/about-blood
National Blood Authority Australia. (n.d.b) Safety of patient blood management guidleines. hhttps://www.blood.gov.au/pbm-guidelines
National Blood Authority Australia. (n.d.c) Safety of blood products. https://www.blood.gov.au/safety-blood-products
NSW Government. (2019) Creutzfeldt-Jakob disease (CJD) factsheet. In NSW Government.
Pregnancy Birth & Baby. (2020) Rhesus D negative and pregnancy. https://www.pregnancybirthbaby.org.au/rhesus-d-negative-in-pregnancy
Rome, S. (2020) 'Nursing management. Haematological problems'. In *Lewis's Medical Surgical Nursing*, 5 ed. (pp. 702–720). Chatswood, Sydney: Elsevier.
Rome, S. & Hargreaves, M. (2020) 'Nursing assessment; The haematological system'. In R. Aitken, T. Buckley, H. Edwards & D. Brown (Eds.). *Lewis's Medical-Surgical Nursing*, 3rd ed. (pp. 616–636). Chatswood: Elsevier.
Waugh, A. & Grant, A. (2010) *Ross and Wilson's Anatomy and Physiology in Health and Illness,* 11th ed. Edinburgh: Churchill Livingstone/Elsevier.

ACKNOWLEDGEMENTS

Figure 20.5: © Best donation by blood type. ©Australian Red Cross Lifeblood. Reproduced with permission of Australian Red Cross Lifeblood.
Figure 20.6: © Manufacturing costs on all blood component labels, Commonwealth of Australia. Licensed under CC BY 3.0.
Table 20.2: © Blood types. Retrieved from: https://www.healthdirect.gov.au/blood-types.
Table 20.4: © Full blood count. © Lab Tests Online Australasia. Reproduced with permission of Lab Tests Online Australasia. https://www.labtestsonline.org.au/learning/test-index/fbc#glance.
Table 20.5: © Anaemia. © Lab Tests Online Australasia. Reproduced with permission of Lab Tests Online Australasia. https://www.labtestsonline.org.au/learning/index-of-conditions/anemia.
Photo 20A: © AB Forces News Collection / Alamy Stock Photo
Photo 20B: © PR Handout Image / AAP images
Photo 20C: © ANN PATCHANAN / Shutterstock.com

CHAPTER 21

Nursing care of conditions related to the musculoskeletal system

LEARNING OBJECTIVES

After studying this chapter, you should be able to:

21.1 identify key features and elements of the musculoskeletal system
21.2 discuss the implications of osteoarthritis on the ageing population
21.3 explain the difference between rheumatoid arthritis and osteoarthritis
21.4 discuss the implications of osteoporosis
21.5 recognise the clinical signs and symptoms of a fracture
21.6 discuss the different types of pathogenesis of osteomyelitis
21.7 outline the potential implications of hip fracture in the elderly
21.8 recognise the importance of neurovascular assessment in preventing potential complications
21.9 explain the causes and management of bony metastases.

Introduction

Orthopaedic and trauma care is a dynamic and constantly evolving area of practice. Patients are increasingly being seen in settings other than the traditional ward and clinic areas, with an increased focus on shared care, day case interventions and community-based care. This chapter outlines the musculoskeletal anatomy and provides an overview of common conditions related to the skeletal system, including **osteoarthritis**, **osteomyelitis**, **rheumatoid arthritis**, **fracture** injuries, osteoporosis, femoral neck fracture and **bone metastases**. A glossary of common orthopaedic related terms such as the one at the end of this chapter or online (available at www.bosmc.com.au/glossary-of-terms) may assist the reader in understanding this chapter.

21.1 Anatomy and physiology of the musculoskeletal system

LEARNING OBJECTIVE 21.1 Identify key features and elements of the musculoskeletal system.

The musculoskeletal system is composed of bones, joints, muscles, tendons and ligaments. The skeletal system provides a form for the body, protects the vital organs, acts as a framework for muscle attachment and permits the body's motion (figure 21.1). The skeleton consists of 206 bones that are divided into the **axial skeleton** and the **appendicular skeleton**, with the spine viewed as having cervical, thoracic, lumbar, sacral and coccygeal sections (figure 21.2).

FIGURE 21.1 The bones of the adult skeletal system

Division of the skeleton	Structure	Number of bones
Axial skeleton	**Skull**	
	Cranium	8
	Face	14
	Hyoid	1
	Auditory ossicles	6
	Vertebral column	26
	Thorax	
	Sternum	1
	Ribs	24
	Number of bones =	**80**

Division of the skeleton	Structure	Number of bones
Appendicular skeleton	**Pectoral (shoulder) girdles**	
	Clavicle	2
	Scapula	2
	Upper limbs	
	Humerus	2
	Ulna	2
	Radius	2
	Carpals	16
	Metacarpals	10
	Phalanges	28
	Pelvic (hip) girdle	
	Hip, pelvic, or coxal bone	2
	Lower limbs	
	Femur	2
	Patella	2
	Fibula	2
	Tibia	2
	Tarsals	14
	Metatarsals	10
	Phalanges	28
	Number of bones =	**126**
	Total bones in an adult skeleton =	**206**

Source: Tortora & Derrickson (2011) *Principles of Anatomy and Physiology*, with kind permission of Wiley Blackwell.

At birth, the spine is one concave primary curve, which remains in the thoracic, sacral and coccygeal bones (figure 21.3). The upper extremities include the shoulder girdle, arm, elbow, forearm, wrist and hand. The lower extremities similarly comprise the hip, thigh, knee, leg and foot.

The bones

In essence, the bones protect and shape the body; bone tissue makes up about 18 per cent of body weight. There are two types of bone tissue, compact (cortical/hard) and spongy (cancellous/soft) bone. The components of a typical long bone are depicted in figure 21.4. The bone's functions include giving the body a framework, providing attachment sites for muscle and tendons, allowing movement of the body as a whole and in parts by forming joints that are moved by muscles. Some bones, particularly flat bones, e.g. the skull and pelvic bones, bones of the hip and vertebrae, and the metaphyseal and epiphyseal ends of long bones, contain red bone marrow, responsible for the production of red and white blood cells, and platelets through a process called haemopoiesis. Yellow bone marrow consists mainly of adipose cells, and these store triglycerides. Bones also provide a storage site for minerals (calcium phosphate) and a reservoir for blood calcium.

FIGURE 21.2 Divisions of the skeletal system (with the axial skeleton indicated in blue)

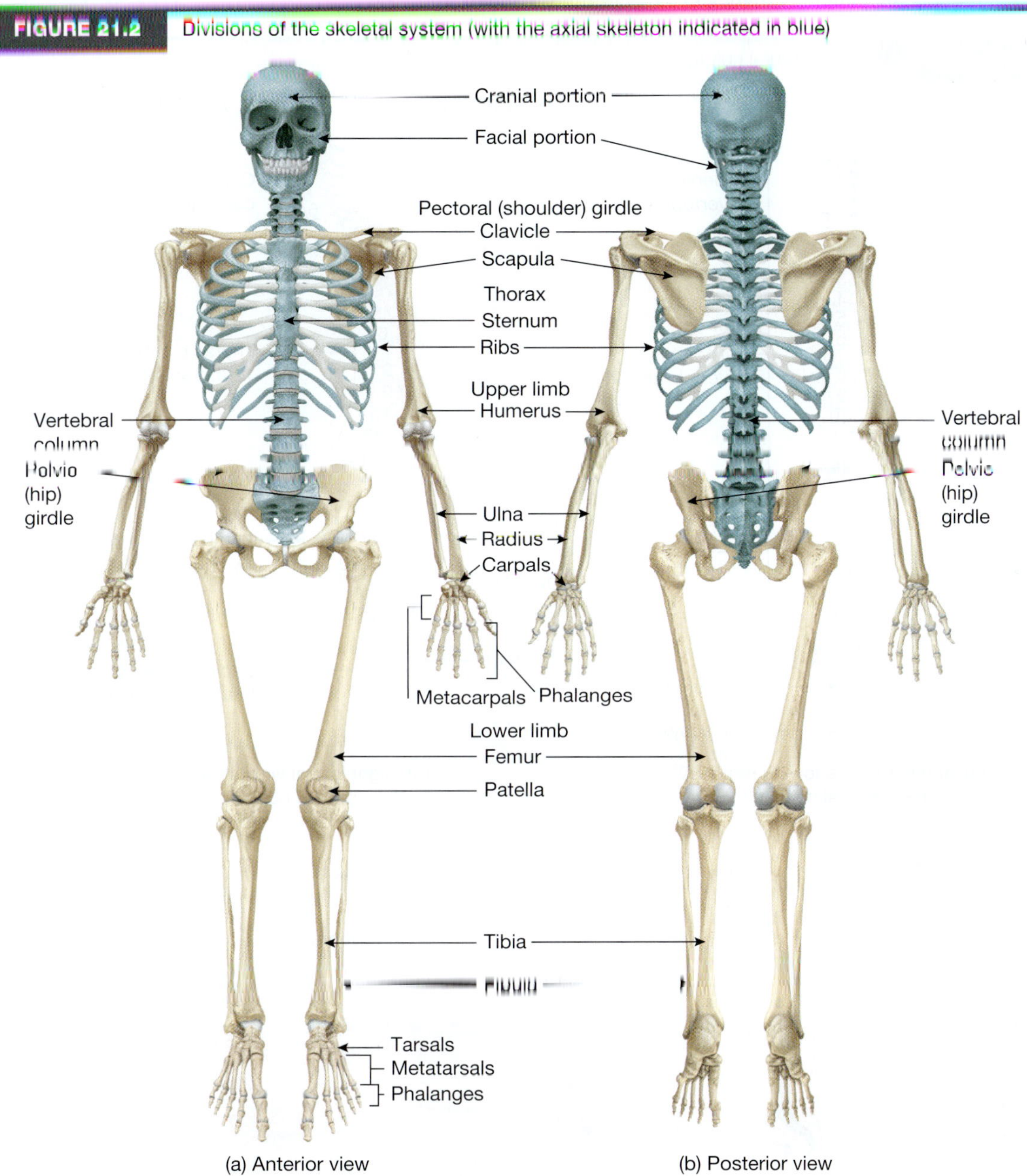

Source: Tortora & Derrickson (2011) *Principles of Anatomy and Physiology*, with kind permission of Wiley Blackwell.

Types of bones and their structure

There are five types of bones in the human body.

1. *Long bones* consist of a shaft and two extremities. Examples are the femur, tibia and fibula. The lengthwise growth of long bones occurs at the epiphyseal plate (growth plate), which is located between the diaphysis (shaft) and the epiphysis. The periosteum is a vascular membrane composed of two layers, an outer tough and fibrous layer, with an inner layer containing cells that build bone (osteoblasts) and cells that reabsorb bone (osteoclasts). Most bones of the limbs, including the fingers and toes, are long bones.
2. *Flat bones* are found in the skull, rib cage, scapula and pelvis. The function of these bones is to protect organs. They also provide large areas of attachment for muscles.
3. *Short bones* are cube-shaped. They are found in the wrist and ankle joints and provide stability and some movement.

4. *Irregular bones* have a variety of shapes and structures and thus do not fit into any other category. Examples are the vertebra, and the ilium and ischium (hip bones).
5. *Sesamoid bones* are embedded in tendons. Their function is to protect tendons from stress and wear. An example is the patella. Others can be found in the hands and feet.

FIGURE 21.3 The vertebral column

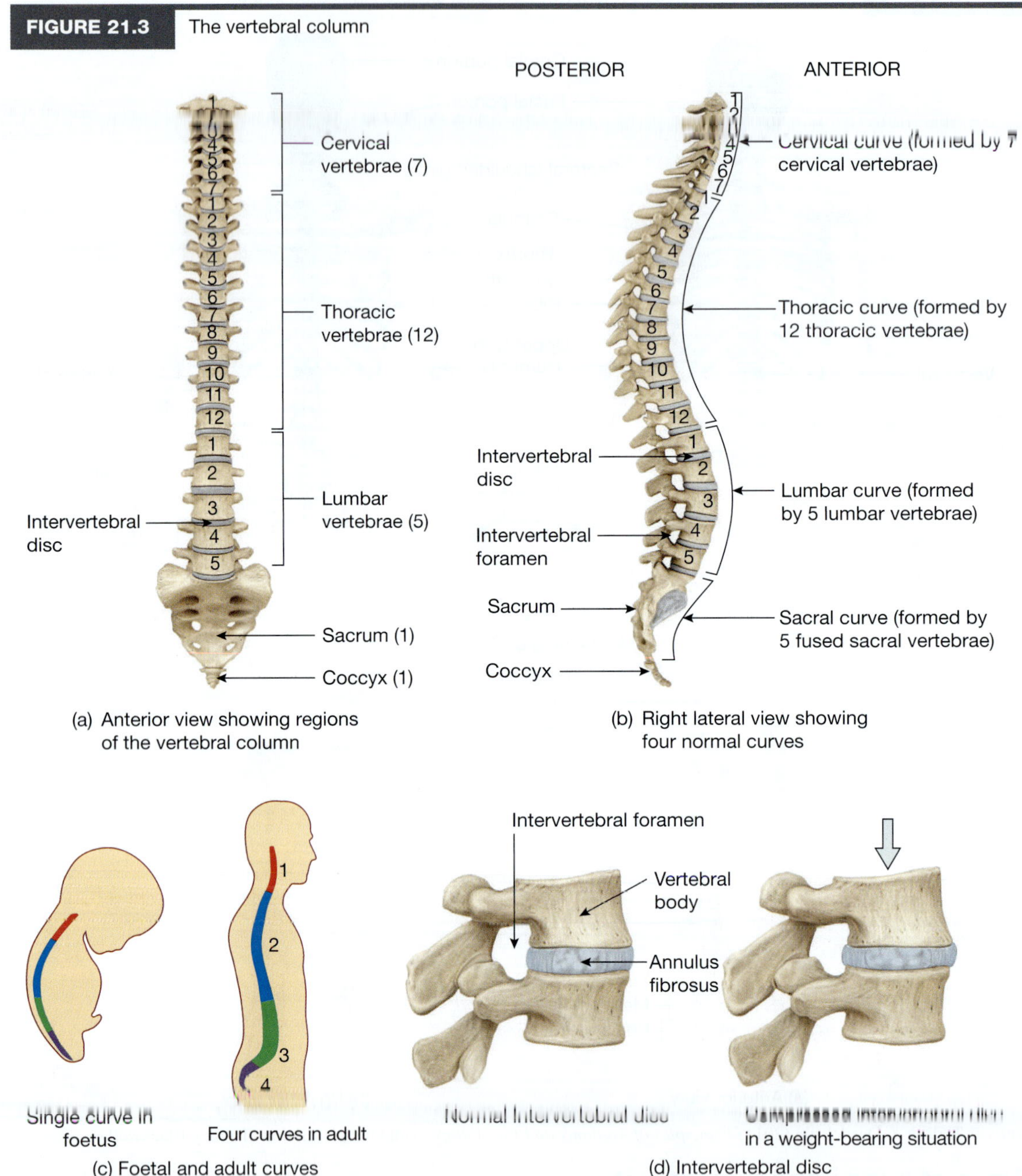

(a) Anterior view showing regions of the vertebral column

(b) Right lateral view showing four normal curves

(c) Foetal and adult curves

(d) Intervertebral disc

Source: Tortora & Derrickson (2011) *Principles of Anatomy and Physiology*, with kind permission of Wiley Blackwell.

The muscles

The bones cannot move the body on their own, so the muscles provide movement and also generate heat. The motion of the skeletal system arises from the contraction and relaxation of the skeletal muscles. Four major muscle groups of the body include the muscles of the head and neck, the trunk, and the upper and lower extremities. The principal anterior superficial skeletal muscles are depicted in figure 21.5. The muscles constitute approximately 23 per cent of body weight in females and 40 per cent in males.

There are three types of muscular tissue: smooth (located in the walls of the hollow visceral organs), cardiac (located in the walls of the heart) and skeletal, which occurs in the muscles attached to the skeleton. The skeletal muscle fibres are striated in appearance and are under voluntary control (figure 21.6).

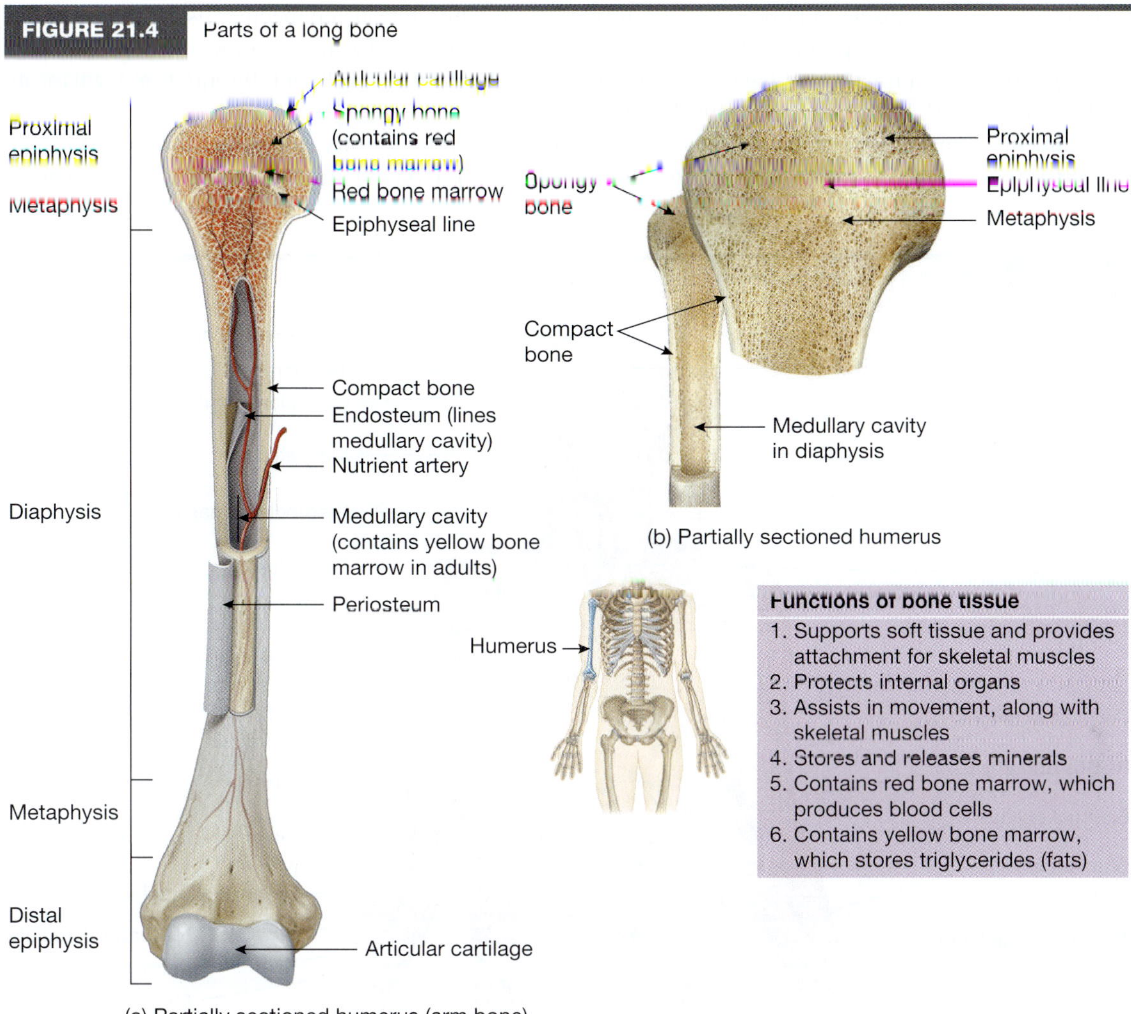

FIGURE 21.4 Parts of a long bone

Source: Tortora & Derrickson (2011) *Principles of Anatomy and Physiology*, with kind permission of Wiley Blackwell.

By sustained contraction or alternating contraction and relaxation, muscle tissue has six main functions.

1. It brings about body movement.
2. It maintains body posture.
3. It assists in stabilisation of the joints.
4. It assists in the movement of substances in the body.
5. It aids temperature control.
6. It helps regulate breathing (the diaphragm).

Tendons and ligaments

Tendons and ligaments are two types of connective tissue. Both are made of dense connective tissue that is 70 to 80 per cent collagen (Leong et al. 2020). Dense connective tissue has a relatively limited blood supply, and collagen fibres are not living. This is why they are relatively slow to heal. Intra-articular tendons and ligaments have the most limited blood supply and so may not heal at all and need surgery to repair any damage. Extra-articular tendons and ligaments have a slightly better but still limited blood supply. Injury to ligaments and tendons accounts for 50 per cent of musculoskeletal injuries (Maffulli, Wong & Almekinders 2003).

Tendons connect muscle to bone. They are formed from white fibrous connective tissue, the fibres of which are arranged as compact parallel bundles and provide support and a small degree of elasticity. These tough yet flexible fibrous tissue bands attached to the skeletal muscles essentially allow movement by acting as intermediaries between the muscles and the bones.

Ligaments connect bone to bone. They are formed from yellow fibrous connective tissue interwoven in a crisscross pattern allowing greater elasticity and providing strength and stability needed to stabilise joints.

FIGURE 21.5 The principal superficial skeletal muscles

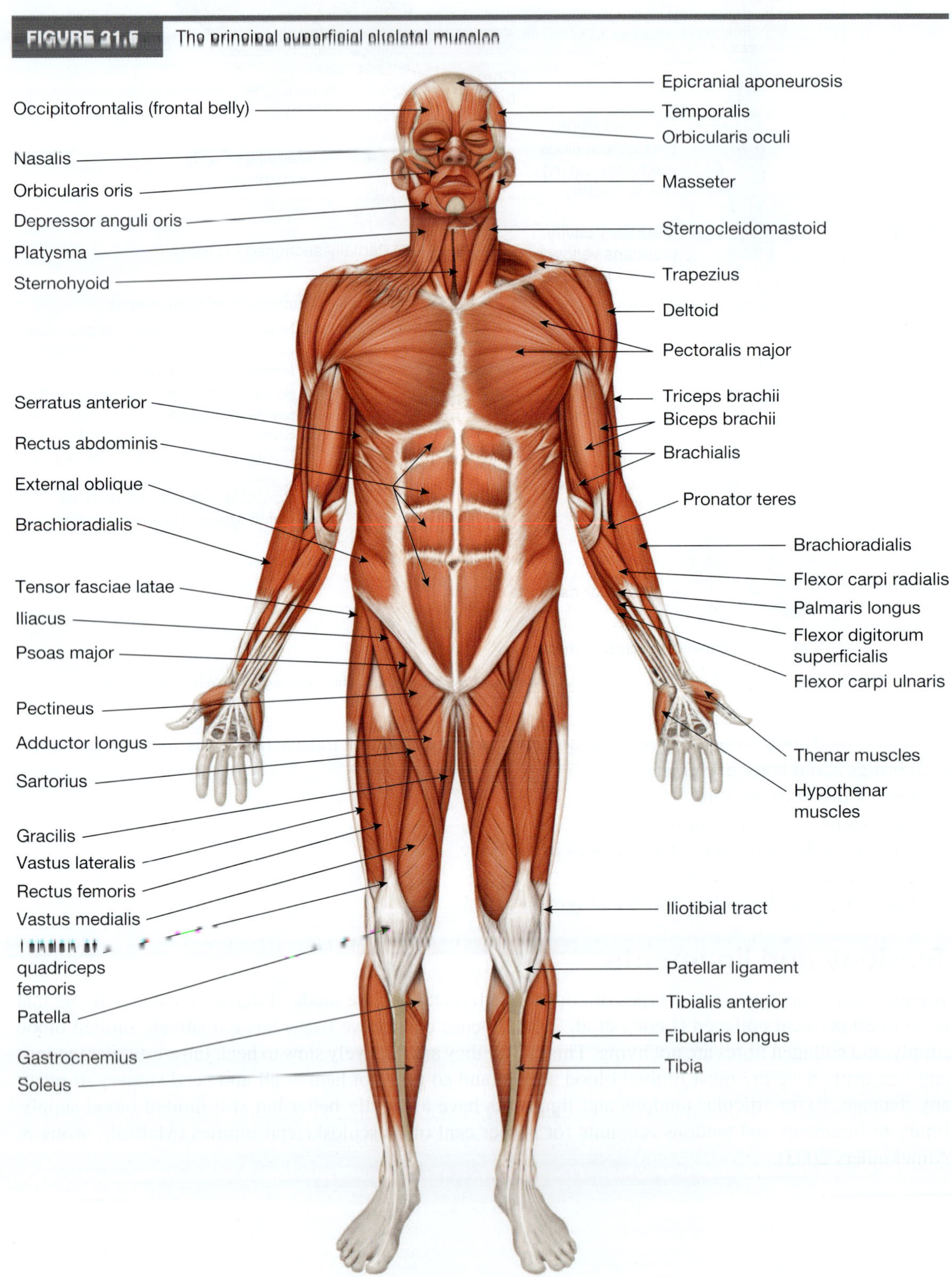

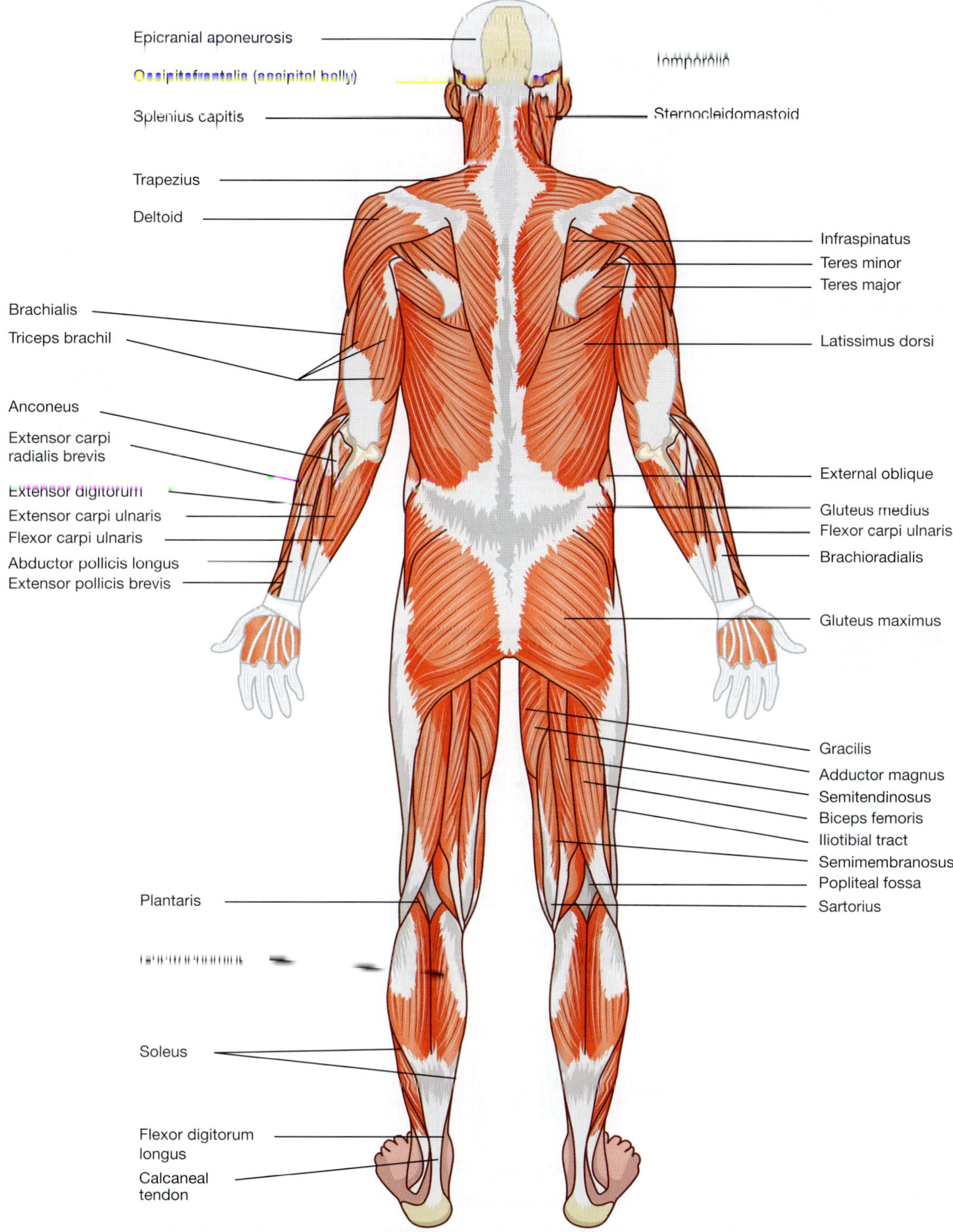

Source: Tortora & Derrickson (2011) *Principles of Anatomy and Physiology*, with kind permission of Wiley Blackwell.

Joints

A joint, or articulation, is where two bones come together, for example, the knee. In terms of the amount of movement they permit, there are three main joint types: immovable (synarthrosis) examples of which are the fibrous joints of the skull sutures, slightly movable (amphiarthrosis) such as the cartilaginous joint that unites the bodies of the vertebrae and freely movable (diarthrosis). Synovial joints (diarthroses), such as the hip or knee, are by far the most common joint classification within the human body. Additional examples of synovial joints include pivotal, ball and socket, and hinge. A key aspect of synovial joints is that they incorporate a fluid-filled capsule, which surrounds the articulating surfaces. This lubricates the joint surface, nourishes the cartilage and acts as a shock absorber (figure 21.7).

FIGURE 21.6 Skeletal muscle: light microscope (LM)

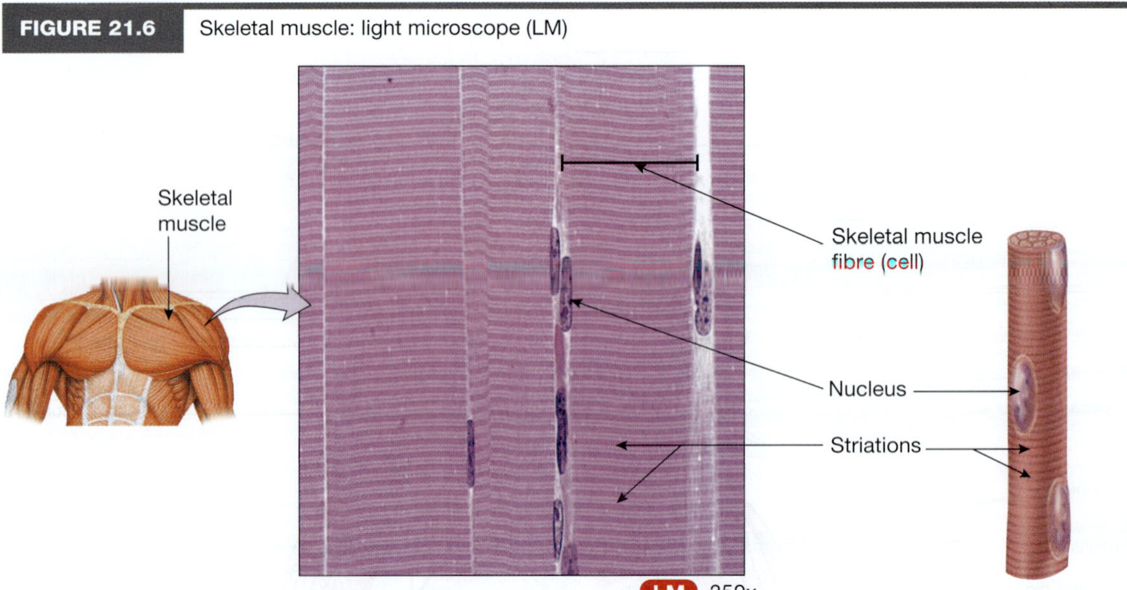

Source: Tortora & Derrickson (2011) *Principles of Anatomy and Physiology*, with kind permission of Wiley Blackwell.

FIGURE 21.7 A synovial joint

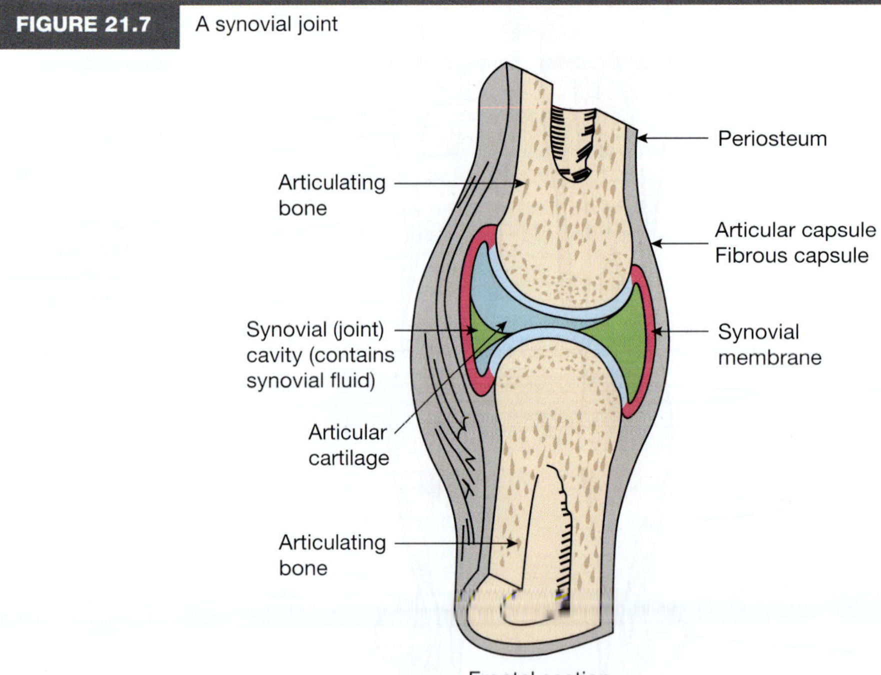

Source: Nair & Peate (2009) *Fundamentals of Applied Pathophysiology*, with kind permission from Wiley Blackwell.

Blood and nerve supply

The blood and nerve supply of the body is a vast subject. Bones receive their blood supply from several different sources, all of which have their importance. These sources include nutrient arteries, epiphyseal arteries, periosteal arteries and metaphyseal arteries. Most of the nerves supplying bones are **sympathetic and vasomotor** in function (figure 21.8). It is important to note that the bones not only have a blood supply, but they also supply blood for the body by haematopoiesis. This is covered in the chapter on haematological disorders.

FIGURE 21.8 Partially sectioned tibia (shin bone)

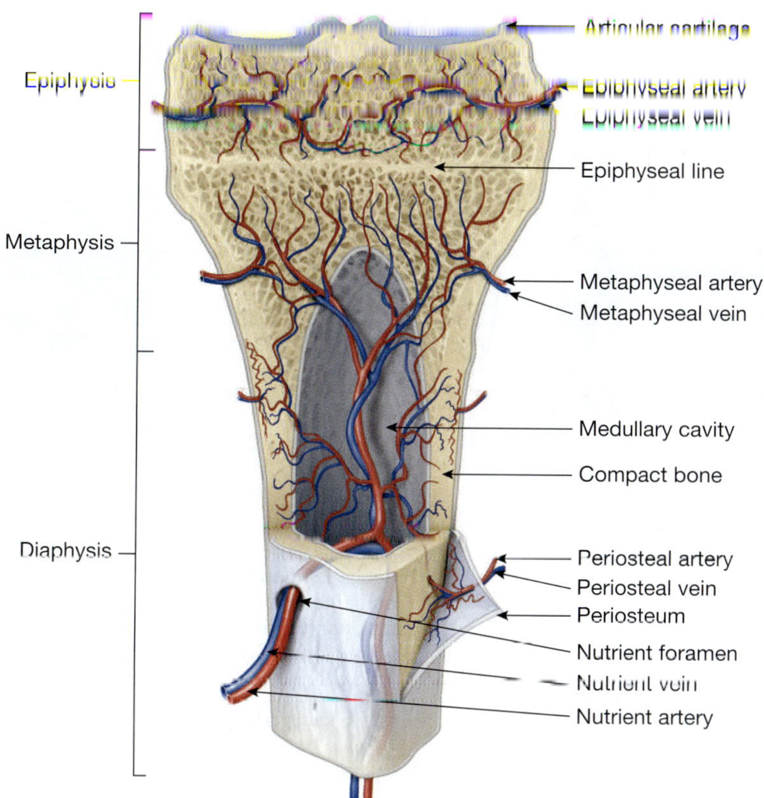

Source: Tortora & Derrickson (2011) *Principles of Anatomy and Physiology*, with kind permission of Wiley Blackwell.

21.2 Osteoarthritis

LEARNING OBJECTIVE 21.2 Discuss the implications of osteoarthritis on the ageing population.

Osteoarthritis is a degenerative disease of synovial joints. Typically, progressive deterioration and loss of articular cartilage of the joint, new bone formation of the joint margins and subchondral bone changes occur. Osteoarthritis can present in any synovial joint but commonly occurs in hips, knees, hands and spine. Figure 21.9 shows the changes in a knee with osteoarthritis. In particular, articular cartilage and mechanical damage lead to problems with mobility and daily living activities, with dependence on others occurring in severe cases. The disabling symptoms of pain, joint swelling, stiffness and restricted movement commonly cause patients to seek help. Initially, pain will be felt during and immediately after activity, but as the disease progresses, the pain worsens and may be constant even when resting. Individuals are further affected if they have to adapt or change their work or cannot carry on working, have reduced social contact or can no longer participate in physical activities such as sports. Globally osteoarthritis is the leading cause of chronic disability in the over 70 population and has been named a priority disease by the World Health Organization (WHO). In Australia, osteoarthritis affects one in 11 people (9.3 per cent of the population) and one in five Australians over 45 (22 per cent of the population). It is the leading cause of chronic pain, disability and early retirement (AIHW 2020). In Australia, osteoarthritis accounted for 19 per cent of the total burden of disease due to musculoskeletal conditions in 2015.

Notable osteoarthritic changes are seen in adults from 30 years of age onwards, with the incidence increasing in older age groups. These changes can result from a variety of causes. The cartilage's normal collagen fibres break down, causing a loss of resistance and a frayed appearance with loose bodies, exposing the underlying bone. A protective inflammatory reaction occurs, resulting in the synovium producing more synovial fluid. Eventually, both bones lose areas of cartilage. The two bone surfaces then come into contact and rub against each other due to joint space loss. This leads to further abrasion, microfractures in the subchondral bone surface, the necrosis (death) of small areas of bone, and cyst formation from increased pressure in the joint forcing synovial fluid into the bone. The production of osteophytes (new bony projections) is evident at the joint margins. This damage eventually distorts the bone surfaces with the potential for subluxation or dislocation.

FIGURE 21.9 A knee joint with osteoarthritis

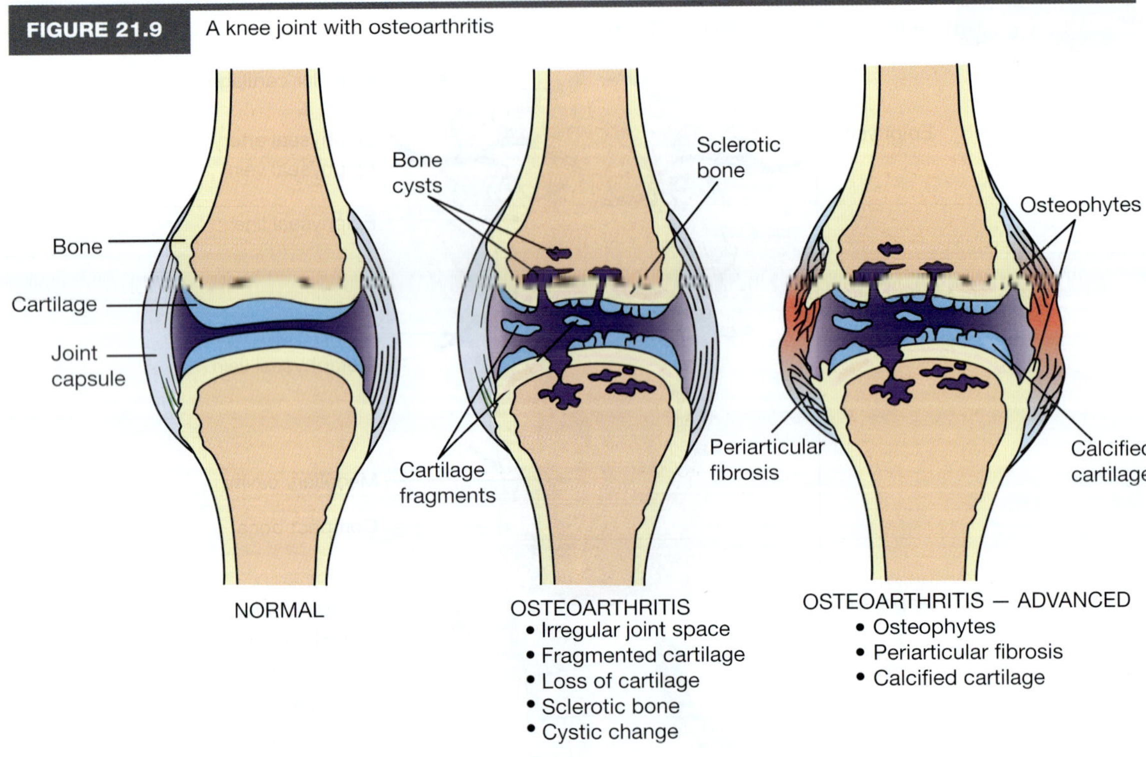

Source: Peate (2017) *Fundamentals of Applied Pathophysiology*, with kind permission from Wiley Blackwell.

Predisposing factors and diagnosis of osteoarthritis

Osteoarthritis has no specific cause; however, several factors contribute to the onset and progression:

- being female (women account for approximately 60 per cent of cases)
- excess weight (obese people are five times more likely to have osteoarthritis of the knee and twice as likely to have osteoarthritis of the hip)
- congenital joint deformities, e.g. developmental dysplasia of the hip
- genetic disease affecting a joint, e.g. haemophilia or sickle cell anaemia
- developmental changes in bone, e.g. Perthes' disease
- metabolic changes, e.g. gout
- infection of the bone or joint, e.g. osteomyelitis and septic arthritis due to tuberculosis or *Staphylococcus*
- traumatic injury to the bone or joint, e.g. a fracture damaging the articular cartilage or a ligament tear causing joint instability
- physically demanding activities, sports and repetitive joint injuries, e.g. farming and football, kneeling, squatting and heavy lifting
- avascular necrosis, e.g. following a fracture
- other skeletal changes, e.g. ankylosing spondylitis
- hereditary factors, e.g. nodal arthritis affecting women's hands
- ethnic origin (osteoarthritis is more common in the white European population).

The joint changes occur slowly over several years. In the early stages, one joint is affected, with the patient experiencing tenderness around the joint and pain that is often worse following exercise and initially relieved by rest. As the disease advances, surgery is considered when joint pain, for example, hip pain radiating down towards the knee, is experienced at rest and night.

Osteoarthritis is diagnosed by the symptom pattern, the exclusion of other conditions that can affect a joint and radiographic examination of the joint. An X-ray, magnetic resonance imaging (MRI) scan, or computed tomography (CT) scan may show a combination of changes: a reduction or loss of the joint space, osteophytes, cysts in the subchondral bone, loose bodies, angulation, subluxation or dislocation of the joint. Even though joint damage can be severe, this does not always equate to the patient's symptoms — some patients with moderate changes have severe pain and disability. In contrast, others with severe damage may only have mild discomfort.

Common radiological investigations for osteoarthritis include the following.

- X-rays use a type of high-energy ionising radiation to quickly create a two-dimensional picture. X-ray views include anteroposterior (AP) and lateral (from the side). The radiation doses used in medical X-rays are lower than those used in MRI and CT scans.
- MRI scanning uses a strong magnetic field to identify radio signals emitted by different tissues to create a three-dimensional picture of the bone and soft tissues. It is an expensive technique, and many patients find the procedure claustrophobic. A MRI of an ankle could take 20–30 minutes.
- CT scanning uses high-dose radiation beams at multiple angles to create three-dimensional images of tissue structures or cross-sectional images of the tissues. It only shows bone tissue clearly, and not soft tissues. CT scanning is much quicker than MRI.

Put the term 'orthopaedic X-rays' into an online search engine to view some examples of X-rays of the skeletal system.

Table 21.1 reflects an adapted 'at-a-glance' summary of the 2014 guidance from the National Institute for Health and Care Excellence (NICE) on the care and management of osteoarthritis in adults (see www.nice.org.uk/guidance/cg177).

TABLE 21.1 Treatment protocol*

Option	Intervention	Additional information
Pharmacological options	Paracetamol (given regularly if needed) Topical NSAIDs for OA of the knee or hand Topical capsaicin for OA of the knee or hand Intra-articular corticosteroid injections for moderate to severe pain	Identify drug allergies and check the medical history Injections can provide pain relief for several weeks but do not benefit all patients
If paracetamol and/or topical NSAIDs are ineffective	Add an opioid Prescribe an oral NSAID or COX-2 inhibitor in addition to paracetamol or instead of a topical NSAID Co-prescribe this with a proton pump inhibitor Use the lowest effective dose for the shortest possible duration Choose the agent and dose based on risk factors for gastrointestinal, liver and cardiorenal toxicity and monitor for any side effects If the patient is already taking low-dose aspirin for another condition, consider an alternative analgesic Do not prescribe etoricoxib 60 mg as first-line treatment	Review the patient's analgesic history to prevent complications such as falls Establish whether the patient is opioid-naive (i.e. does not take this type of analgesic) or has a tolerance Patients who are used to opioids may need a higher dose
Non-pharmacological options	Heat and cold packs TENS Manipulation and stretching Assessment for bracing, joint supports or insoles Assistive devices (e.g. walking sticks, tap turners) to address specific problems. Seek expert advice if needed	Seek expert advice if needed Particularly for OA Assistive devices help with biomechanical joint pain or instability Assistive devices help with biomechanical joint pain or instability
Treatments not recommended	Rubefacients Intra-articular hyaluronan injections Electroacupuncture Chondroitin or glucosamine	

(continued)

TABLE 21.1 *(continued)*

Option	Intervention	Additional information
Self-management	Exercise Weight loss (if overweight) Suitable footwear Heat and cold packs TENS	Knee pain may decrease if the patient is obese and loses weight
Referral to joint surgery	Consider referral for joint surgery if symptoms continue to substantially affect quality of life despite medical treatment Arthroscopic lavage and debridement should be used only for patients with OA of the knee and a clear history of mechanical locking in the knee Scoring tools are not advocated to prioritise patients or refuse referral on the grounds of age, gender, smoking, obesity, etc.	

*aCOX-2 = cyclooxygenase-2; NSAID = non-steroidal anti-inflammatory drug; OA = osteoarthritis; TENS = transcutaneous electrical nerve stimulation.

Common surgical interventions of osteoarthritis

An **arthrodesis** (joint fusion), for example of the first metatarsal and first phalanx, creates a pain-free joint, but there is a loss of all movement and may be an increase in the stress on adjacent joints. An **osteotomy** is where the bones are cut and realigned to stop subluxation (an incomplete or partial dislocation). This can reduce the level of pain and postpone the need for joint replacement surgery.

Arthroplasty or joint replacement is an effective way of removing damaged bone and replacing it with an artificial joint (prosthesis), reducing or removing the pain and improving joint function and mobility (Brown 2017). This is routinely done for the hip and knee joints, and 95 per cent of replacements will last for 15 years, 78.8 per cent for 20 years and 58 per cent will last for 25 years. (Evans et al. 2019). Complications include loosening of the prosthesis and infection, wear, dislocation pain and fracture (Evans et al. 2019). Arthroplastic surgery may include both components of the joint (total arthroplasty) or only one component (hemiarthroplasty).

Nursing care of the patient having joint replacement surgery

Whenever possible, a patient who is about to undergo either hemi or total arthroplasty must be prepared both physically and psychologically to ensure the best recovery. The Enhanced Recovery After Surgery (ERAS) guidelines that were initially implemented in 1997 for patients undergoing bowel surgery are being implemented into many other surgical spheres. Joint surgery is one of them. The key concepts include preoperative evaluation, assessment, education, current health optimisation and clear communication with the patient. The guidelines specify the need for the patient's preoperative preparation both through education and nutritional perspectives. Good communication between the teams involved in the patient's journey from pre-operation through the intra-operative phase and then post-operative through to discharge. Where ERAS guidelines are implemented, patients have reduced hospital stays, decreased readmissions, improved functional ability and higher patient satisfaction levels.

Preoperative care

Assessment of the patient's understanding of what surgery they are having and their degree of understanding of what this means is crucial. Patients may often be able to give the name of the surgery they are having but, on questioning, have very little understanding of what is going to happen to them. Therefore, it is important to determine the patients' level of health literacy and ensure that the communication with them has been clear. Ensure the patient understands any preoperative exercises and why they are important in their recovery. Give the patient time to ask any questions they may have. Knowledge decreases anxiety and increases the likelihood of the patient participating fully in necessary activities post-operatively (Kaye et al. 2019).

Preoperative preparation includes the following.

- Gain informed consent.
- A health and physical assessment — this allows nurses to tailor care to the individual's needs and serves as a baseline to measure progress against.

- Justify the need for the surgery and its impact on patient outcome.
- Teach respiratory techniques, such as the use of incentive spirometry, deep breathing and coughing. Explain why they are necessary post-operatively.
- Physical preparation — inform the patient of expected theatre time and fasting times to help minimise anxiety and increase collaboration from the patient. Explain the need for skin prep and the gown and cap they will be asked to wear during surgery. Both these actions help reduce the potential for post operative infections.
- Social preparation — identify any difficulties with the home environment.
- Discuss post-operative pain control, including how to use the patient controlled analgesia (PCA), epidural infusions or tap blocks or any other analgesic regimens the surgical team may use (Lucas 2008a).

If the joint surgery is elective, these actions should be attended by the preoperative clinic, but the ward nurse needs to ensure that the patient has the required information and, when necessary, give any extra education.

Patient education prior to surgery should include clear information on the operative procedure. Explain the placement of the incision, the extent of the dressings that they will see, and what lines they may be connected to when they return to the ward. Patients can be taken by surprise by a larger than anticipated wound or dressing, which may induce anxiety and fear of mobilisation.

The physiotherapy team should be contacted to provide preoperative education on post-operative activities. When moving techniques are practiced prior to surgery, patients can use them more effectively in the post-operative period (Brown 2017).

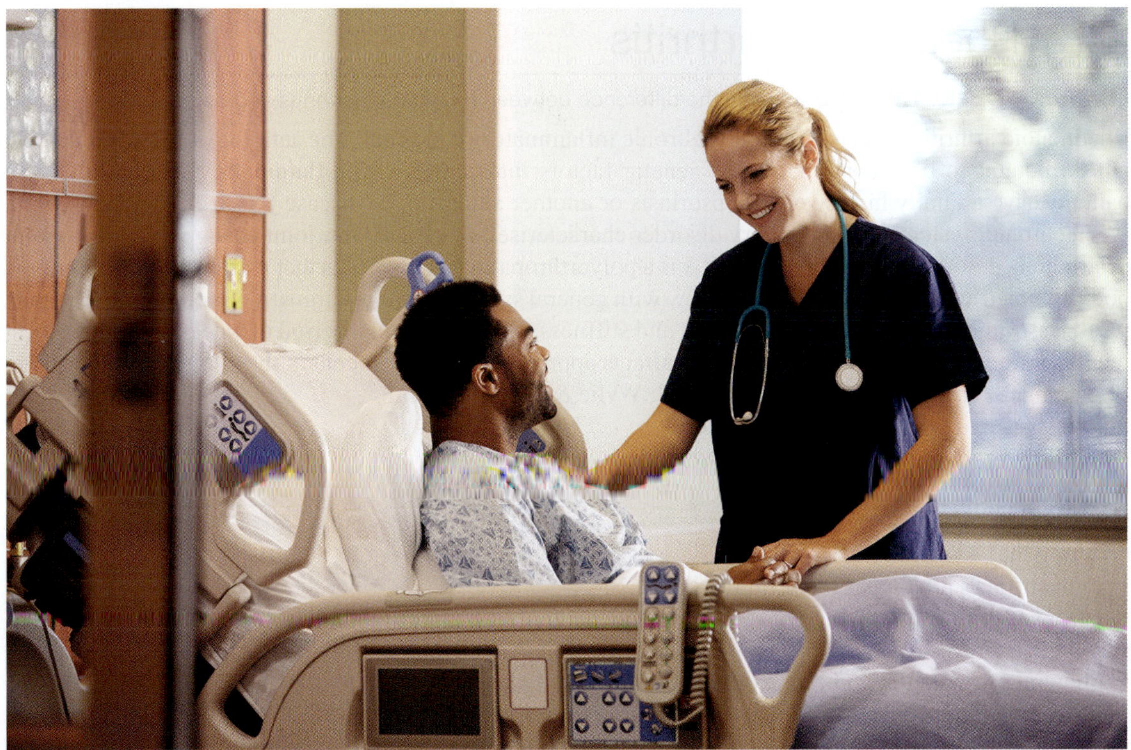

Post-operative care

The immediate recovery period (recovery from anaesthetic — general or spinal) is a specialised area of nursing. The patient remains in the recovery unit until they can maintain their airway, have a GCS of 14–15 and vital signs are stable.

On return to the ward, take a full handover from the recovery staff. Check all documentation, including orders for analgesia, antiemetics, IV fluids and regular medications. Perform an immediate primary survey (airway, breathing, circulation and neurological status) and a vital signs assessment, including pain score and neurovascular assessment. Check all wound sites, dressings, drips, drains and catheters. Check oxygen if in progress.

As a general rule, post-operative observations should be conducted immediately on return to the ward. Then twice at 15-minute intervals. If the patient is stable, do the next set after 30 minutes and then, if the patient remains stable, continue for three hours on hourly observation. If stable and depending on ward policy, the patient can be put on 4-hourly observation. The first four hours post-operation and anaesthetic are vital, and the patient must be carefully observed. Report any abnormal findings immediately.

Post-operative care of the joint replacement patient includes assessment of the following.

- *Pain.* Ensure adequate pain relief at all times (watch for constipation. Opioids, in particular, slow peristalsis of the bowel, and may cause constipation. Aperients may be needed).
- *Wound care.* Perform neurovascular obs hourly for the first 12 hours. Then if stable every two to four hours. Monitor incisional drainage by checking the dressing and drain output. Significant blood loss can occur in joint replacement, particularly total hip replacement (THR) surgery.
- *Fluid status.* Maintain accurate fluid balance documentation for the first week as these patients are at risk of fluid deficit due to potential blood loss.
- *Mobilisation.* This should be initiated early as per the surgeon's instructions. Clear communication with the physiotherapy team is vital. If the patient has had a THR, a key issue in the first six weeks is the potential for dislocation of the joint. For this reason, the patient must not abduct their operative leg (bring it across the midline). Patients may return to the ward with an adduction pillow or other device between their legs to stop this from happening. Nurses need to be very alert to this potential issue when moving the patient around in the bed or mobilising them.
- *VTE.* Prophylaxis to prevent deep venous thrombosis, such as TED stockings. A variety of anticoagulants may be prescribed (heparin and enoxaparin are commonly used).
- *Discharge preparation.* Assess home circumstances and support.
- *First six weeks after discharge.* Patient education.
- *Long-term recovery and outcomes.* Review these and provide patient education (Lucas 2008b).

21.3 Rheumatoid arthritis

LEARNING OBJECTIVE 21.3 Explain the difference between rheumatoid arthritis and osteoarthritis.

Rheumatoid arthritis (RA) is a complex, chronic inflammatory condition. The aetiology of RA is unknown but is thought to be a combination of genetic factors interacting with inflammatory mediators. Some patients have a family history of RA, psoriasis or another autoimmune disease (Nash & McLeish 2017). It is a chronic, systemic inflammatory disorder characterised by progressive joint changes leading to joint destruction, deformity and immobility. RA is a polyarthropathy which means that it affects both sides of the body symmetrically. Onset is generally slow with general symptoms of inflammation such as fever, fatigue, weakness, anorexia and generalised aching and stiffness. Gradually over a period of weeks to months, local manifestations will occur. In Australia, RA affects approximately 2.1 per cent of the population 63 per cent of whom are female (Nash & McLeish 2017; Wylie & Clarke 2014).

The signs and symptoms of RA include:

- swelling or inflammation of the affected joints
- joint pain
- erythema
- a joint that is warm to the touch
- joint stiffness after a period of immobility
- early morning stiffness
- joint deformity
- bilateral presentation with, for example, both hands or knees affected
- restriction in movement from joint changes and ligaments being stretched
- fixed flexion deformities, e.g. flexion of the proximal interphalangeal (PIP) joint and extension of the distal interphalangeal (DIP) joint causes a boutonnière deformity, whereas a fixed extension of the PIP joint and flexion of the DIP joint causes swan-neck deformity
- subluxation of the joints, e.g. the metacarpophalangeal joints with or without palmar and ulnar deviation of the fingers, and subluxation and radial deviation of the wrist with prominence of the ulnar styloid process
- instability of the cervical spine at the atlantoaxial (C1–C2) joint
- tenosynovitis, i.e. inflammation of the synovium membrane covering the tendon
- bursitis — inflammation of the fluid-filled sac (bursa) that lies between a tendon and skin, or between a tendon and bone.

These symptoms generally need to have lasted for more than six weeks to exclude post-viral changes, which are likely to resolve. Although RA can occur at any age, the peak age for onset is 40–60 years, and there is a higher incidence of RA in women.

Diagnosis is determined by physical examination, X-ray of the joint to determine joint space, bone erosion and joint deformity, along with a serum test for rheumatoid factor (RF). However, this is not an absolute indicator as it may not be positive. Ultrasound scanning is being used as standard practice to determine the degree of synovitis in joints and soft tissue. The disabling effects of joint change are exacerbated by the range of systemic effects seen in patients with more advanced disease that have an impact on the psychosocial wellbeing of patients and their families.

Systemic changes seen with advanced RA include:

- cardiac system, e.g. pericarditis
- circulatory system, e.g. Raynaud's phenomena
- eyes, e.g. scleritis
- haematological changes, e.g. anaemia
- nervous system, e.g. sensorimotor neuropathy
- respiratory system, e.g. pulmonary effusions or basal fibrosis
- skin, e.g. vasculitis (ulcers or haemorrhages) and erythema
- soft tissues, e.g. muscle wasting or nodules
- other changes, e.g. weight loss, exhaustion, pyrexia and malaise.

Paediatric rheumatoid arthritis

Childhood RA accounts for 5 per cent of all cases. It differs from adult RA in a number of ways.

- oligoarthritis (affecting four or fewer joints) is more common in paediatric RA than in adult-onset RA
- large joints are most commonly affected
- chronic uveitis is more common (inflammation of the anterior chamber of the eye)
- rheumatoid nodules and RF are usually absent.

RA that continues throughout adolescence may severely affect growth and health in adult life (Nash & McLeish 2017).

Interdisciplinary care of rheumatoid arthritis

Patients are regularly seen by other members of the healthcare team. Physiotherapists will assess the patient's general fitness, encourage exercises to maintain joint function and muscle strength, and help with pain relief. Occupational therapists can provide protective splints for joint protection and assist with hand problems and give advice on home, work, and lifestyle adaptations. Referral to a podiatrist is essential for patients with foot problems as insoles or adapted footwear may be required. Patients are referred to an orthopaedic surgeon if they have persistent pain due to joint damage, worsening joint function, progressive joint deformity, persistent, localised synovitis, tendon rupture, nerve compression or stress fracture. Surgical options can include joint replacement surgery, arthrodesis (joint fusion), nerve decompression and tendon repair (NICE 2018).

Good communication and patient education of their condition and treatment options will ensure they can make informed decisions about their care (NICE 2018). Where possible, the family or carers should be involved in this as well. Care must be patient-centred, with a full multidisciplinary team involved. Most centres have a rheumatologist and a rheumatoid specialist nurse who regularly sees each patient, assessing the progress of joint and systemic changes. Many specialist nurses provide patient education and support and amend or prescribe drug regimens within agreed protocols.

The current recommendation is for aggressive early treatment to prevent or delay the onset of severe joint deformity and disability. Drugs will not reverse the damage that has already occurred to a joint but will reduce the inflammation and pain and slow the disease progression (table 21.2).

TABLE 21.2 Drugs commonly used in RA

Drug group	Patient type	Drug type/complications
Disease-modifying antirheumatic drugs (DMARDs)	Administered to newly diagnosed patients within the first three months of symptom onset	Aim to halt the disease progression and include methotrexate and one other DMARD, e.g. hydroxychloroquine, sulphasalazine or leflunomide, plus a short-term glucocorticoid. DMARDs can have severe side effects and should be reduced to a maintenance dose when the disease is under control

(continued)

TABLE 21.2 *(continued)*

Drug group	Patient type	Drug type/complications
Oral steroid therapy Joint (intra-articular) steroid injections	Used to control symptoms when the disease is active Used for direct pain relief in an acute joint flare-up as they appear to have no long-term effect on the joint, however, drug action is short-lived	Steroids can have severe side effects, so require close monitoring
Non-steroidal anti-inflammatory drugs (NSAIDs)	Short-term pain control	Cyclo-oxygenase-2 inhibitors, e.g. celecoxib, are favoured as they have fewer gastrointestinal side effects

21.4 Osteoporosis

LEARNING OBJECTIVE 21.4 Discuss the implications of osteoporosis.

Osteoporosis literally translates as 'porous bones' and is characterised by the loss of bone mass and increased bone fragility, leading to an increased risk of fractures. Osteoporosis is diagnosed based on bone mineral density (BMD) or bone mass. It is a condition in which normal bone gradually loses mineral density. The BMD relies on the balance between osteoblast and osteoclast activity within the bone. Thus, the bone mass increases in childhood and plateaus at skeletal maturity until about 35 years of age, when it begins to decrease as part of the natural ageing process in both sexes. In females, the bone loss is most rapid in the first years after menopause. Men lose bone density with ageing also, but because they begin with higher bone density and have a slower rate of loss, they become osteoporotic at an older age than women (Nash & McLeish 2017). The whole skeleton is affected, but the condition may go unnoticed until the patient presents with one of three typical osteoporotic fractures:

1. fracture of the distal radius (a Colles' fracture)
2. fracture of the femoral neck (a hip fracture)
3. crush fracture of the vertebral body (commonly of a thoracic vertebra).

The main risk factors that accelerate the rate of bone density loss are:

- female gender, age (over 60 years), Caucasian or Asian origin
- a maternal history of a hip fracture
- oestrogen deficiency, e.g. due to early (premature) menopause, prolonged amenorrhoea or primary hypogonadism
- corticosteroid therapy, e.g. prednisolone therapy of more than 7.5 mg per day for more than 6 months
- low BMI (<19 kg/m^2), owing to a combination of reduced oestrogen levels and a reduction in impact loading
- low calcium levels and/or vitamin D deficiency
- smoking
- excess alcohol
- sedentary lifestyle, lack of weight-bearing exercise and prolonged immobilisation
- anorexia nervosa (low weight, menstrual irregularity and a low-calcium diet)
- endocrine syndromes (hyperparathyroidism, hyperthyroidism and Cushing's syndrome)
- inflammatory arthropathy
- a history of fractures in adulthood, especially a previous Colles', hip or vertebral fracture
- breast cancer, especially for postmenopausal women.

The key message is to:

- have a healthy diet high in calcium and vitamin D or take alternative supplements
- increase the level of activity, particularly weight-bearing exercise
- stop or reduce levels of smoking
- avoid excess levels of alcohol
- seek medical advice about reducing or stopping steroid drugs.

Table 21.3 outlines the drugs used in the prevention and treatment of osteoporosis.

TABLE 21.3 **Drugs used for the prevention or management of osteoporosis**

Drug	Rationale for use
Bisphosphonate group, e.g. risedronate, alendronate and etidronate	Inhibit osteoclast action and slow the rate of bone resorption to maintain the patient's current bone mass density and reduce the risk of a fracture. Known for their poor rate of absorption and potential gastrointestinal side effects.
Many patients will be advised to take with vitamin D and calcium supplementation	Guidance on taking these include swallowing them on an empty stomach with a glass of water while standing, and then remaining upright and fasting for 30 minutes. Compliance is difficult to achieve, and often poor
Selective oestrogen receptor modulators, e.g. raloxifene	Can reduce the rate of bone loss and reduce the risk of vertebral fractures. They are better tolerated but have an increased risk of deep vein thrombosis formation
Strontium	Stimulates bone formation in the natural cycle of remodelling of bone tissue. Has a beneficial effect in reducing vertebral and femoral neck fractures
Hormone replacement therapy	Currently used for management of menopause symptoms and has a role in maintaining BMD
Testosterone	Used for men if hypogonadism is present or is the main cause of osteoporosis
Teriparatide (synthetic parathyroid hormone)	Stabilises BMD. Only used for the treatment of severe osteoporosis for 18 months due to a potential increased risk of osteosarcoma (bone cancer) with prolonged use

Source: Adapted from Tu et al. (2018).

The best approach to osteoporosis is that of prevention. The multidisciplinary team need to be involved in giving timely and appropriate advice on prevention, along with diagnosing and treating osteoporosis. Such health promotion would promote peak bone mass in adulthood and decrease the rate of loss of bone density with age. This should not be confined to the orthopaedic or trauma teams but include practitioners in primary care settings — physiotherapists, dietitians and occupational therapists all have a role in this area of health promotion (Brown 2017).

21.5 Fracture injuries

LEARNING OBJECTIVE 21.5 Recognise the clinical signs and symptoms of a fracture.

A bone becomes fractured when a force exerted on it is stronger than the bone's strength, for example, when an individual is hit by a moving object such as a car. A fracture can occur when a normal force is exerted on a bone that has not developed correctly, as in osteogenesis imperfecta, or when a normal bone is weakened from changes to its structure, as with osteoporosis. A repeated force on a bone can also slowly damage the internal bone structure, leading to fatigue or spontaneous fracture, such as stress fractures of the tibia seen in runners.

Figure 21.10 demonstrates the four main fracture types of fractures, with table 21.4 providing a more detailed fracture classification.

The bone healing process follows several clearly defined stages.

- Stage 1: *The inflammatory phase.* When the bone breaks, bleeding from the bone and surrounding tissues create a fracture haematoma that seals the bone ends. An inflammatory response then occurs.
- Stage 2: *The reparative phase.* A capillary network forms within the haematoma, and granulation tissue develops. Osteoblast cells that create new bone begin to form a bridge between the bone ends and new bone (callus) is formed.
- Stage 3: *The remodelling stage.* There is a gradual spread of callus, and the creation of the compact and cancellous bone structures occurs over several months to two years, depending on the type and degree of damage to the bone. Osteoclast cells will absorb fragments of dead bone tissue and callus to reform the bone's internal and external structure.

Usually, by 6 weeks, the bone can support movement and normal function. However, in some areas where there are a compound and comminuted fracture of mainly compact bone, for example, the femoral shaft, it can take 16 weeks for the bone to unite, and possibly longer before the bone can support weight and the patient mobilise unaided (Brown 2017).

FIGURE 21.10 The four types of fracture: (a) simple, (b) incomplete (greenstick), (c) comminuted and (d) compound

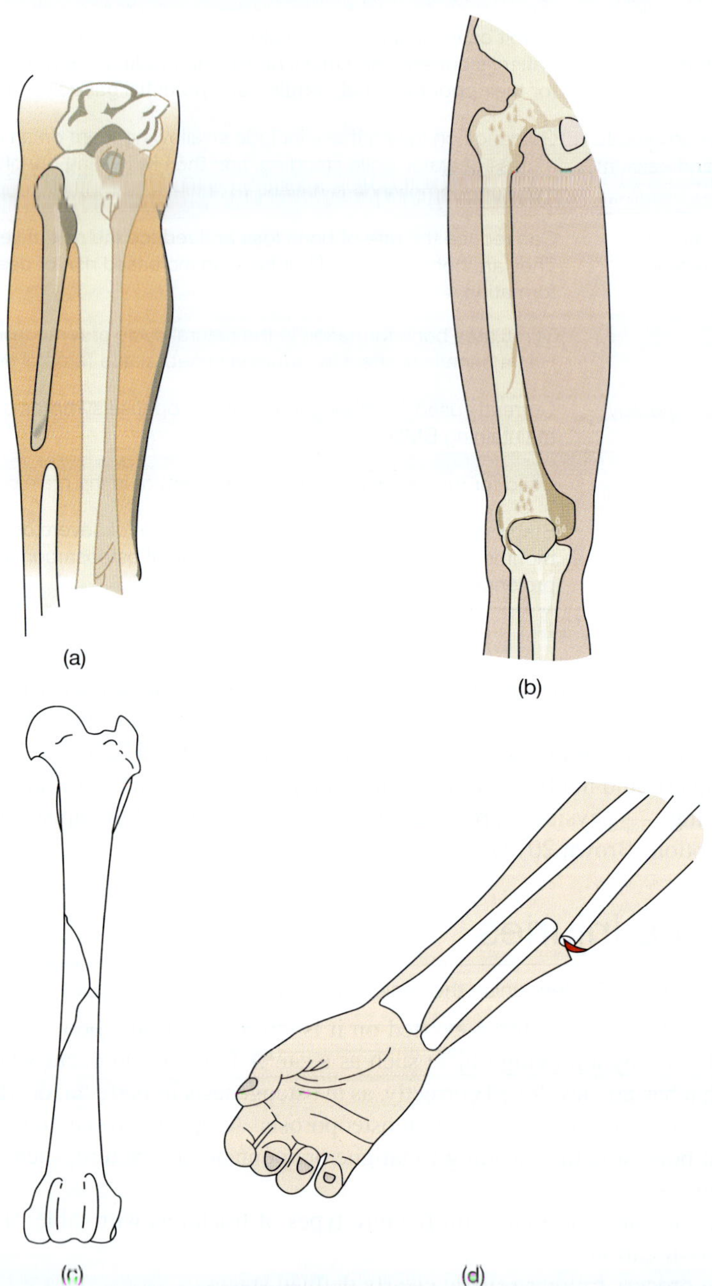

Source: Nair & Peate (2009) *Fundamentals of Applied Pathophysiology*, with kind permission from Wiley Blackwell.

When a patient with a suspected or actual joint or bone injury is admitted, the mechanism of injury that describes the incident is documented. However, immediate assessment of the patient's airway, breathing and circulation are essential, and these functions must be stabilised before other orthopaedic care is provided (see the chapter on special nursing care). Monitoring of vital signs and neurovascular observations, including the pulses distal to the site of injury, skin colour, sensory changes and movement of the limb or area distal to or around the injury is crucial. The corresponding limb is compared, with joints and muscles checked for their ligaments. X-rays are taken of potential and actual injury sites, along with an MRI or CT scan if a head or abdominal injury is suspected.

TABLE 21.4 Classification of fractures

Fracture terms	Descriptions
Closed	Where there is no wound present over or near the fracture
Open or compound	A wound near or over the fracture site makes it an open or compound fracture. All wounds are assumed to be dirty and must be cleaned to reduce the risk of a bone infection (osteomyelitis), as an infection that occurs at a fracture site will stop the bone healing. Patients with an open fracture are generally given prophylactic antibiotics to prevent this
Stable or unstable	The fracture is stable if the bone ends do move without a significant additional force being applied
Extra-articular	Fractures away from a joint
Intra-articular	Fractures within a joint, which must be reduced with a high degree of accuracy to reduce the risk of further joint problems such as osteoarthritis
Pathological fracture	These injuries occur when the bone has been damaged by disease, such as osteoporosis or bone metastases
Greenstick fracture	Seen in children; the malleable bone bends away from the direction of the force and is left at an angle but not broken
Avulsion fracture	Results from the sudden contraction of a muscle that results in a small area of bone being pulled away
Transverse fracture	The fracture occurs across the bone at 90°; these are usually stable as the surrounding muscles contract and hold the bones in place
Oblique fracture	The fracture is at 30° or more to the bone axis; these are often unstable as the bone is liable to slip when the muscles around it contract
Spiral fracture	Arises from a twisting force creating a spiral break around the bone
Impacted fracture	Caused by crushing of the bone where one part is driven into another; these are usually stable injuries
Comminuted fracture	Involves multiple bone fragments that arise from very high-impact or high-energy forces; such injuries often damage more than one bone or joint, and there will be damage to other structures, e.g. skin, blood vessels and nerves

Common intervention in the treatment of fractures

The treatment of a fracture depends on the site, type and extent of injury. Pain relief is essential and based on a regular assessment. Figure 21.11 outlines the common interventions used in treating fractures.

FIGURE 21.11 Common interventions to treat fractures

- Splinting — taping one finger or toe to its neighbour(s) (with mild analgesia).
- Reduction — manual manipulation to ensure correct positioning of the fractured bone (with or without analgesia and sedation).
- Internal fixation — (which is not usually visible to the patient) using metal screws, plates, wiring or intramedullary nails to ensure accurate reduction and allow early mobilisation (with analgesia dependent on fracture type).
- External fixation — visibly seen on the outside of the fractured limb. Hoffman and Ilizarov are two examples. External fixation is achieved by inserting pins into the bone through the skin (percutaneously). The fixation apparatus is then attached to the pins, which act as a scaffold and stabilises the fracture. Since the pins go directly from the external environment into the bone this leaves the patient vulnerable to infection, particularly osteomyelitis. There is no specific guideline in Australia for pin site care, and a Cochran review found that there was insufficient evidence to determine a best practice standard. The key consideration is scrupulous attention to asepsis and aseptic technique. Further recommendations are weekly cleaning of pin sites with alcoholic chlorhexidine, and pin sites should be

covered with a dressing that keeps excess moisture and exudate away from the wound. The frequency of dressing changes should be increased with increasing exudate. Any patient-reported symptoms of pain, decreased movement, swelling or redness should be taken very seriously.

- Traction — used to immobilise the fractured limb and reduce pain (with or without analgesia or sedation).

Source: Nash & McLeish (2017).

Following treatment, patients will need information on how to look after their injury and how to protect it from further trauma (table 21.5). Ideally, both verbal and written information will be given. Where possible, a relative or carer should be involved in the discussion if the patient does not understand any of the information.

TABLE 21.5 Patient information

Information topic	Why this is needed
Analgesia and anti-inflammatory drugs	To ensure the correct type and usage of analgesics and anti-inflammatory drugs
Elevating the limb	To reduce and prevent further swelling of the area; the area must be supported correctly. Reduction of swelling also decreases pain
Sling	A high arm sling is used to reduce swelling of the fingers or wrist. A broad arm sling is used to take the weight and support the arm. Advice is needed on when to use or to remove the sling
Using a walking aid	If the leg is in a cast, or a ligament or muscle injury is affecting mobility, the patient must be taught how to use crutches, a walking stick or other walking aids correctly to prevent further falls and injury
Care of a plaster or fibreglass cast	A cast is used for immediate care of factures that do not require surgery or is used following surgery. It is often applied and then split. Alternatively, only a back slab is used, and this is initially bandaged on to the limb to allow for swelling. This is replaced by a full plaster or fibreglass cast in the next 2–3 days once the swelling has subsided. Advice is essential to ensure it keeps the fracture stable and to protect the skin from damage

Complications of fractures

Complications can arise when a fracture occurs or later as healing takes place, and include the following.

- Hypovolaemic shock from loss of blood at the time of injury.
- Arterial and nerve trauma at the time of injury.
- Tendon and muscle trauma at the time of injury.
- Avascular necrosis, when a bone fragment does not have an adequate blood supply; the area then needs to be removed (debrided) and a new secure internal or external fixation created, possibly with bone graft materials applied to the area.
- Compartment syndrome, in which swelling into a muscle increases the pressure within that muscle, causing extreme pain when it is touched or moved. If left untreated, this leads to muscle ischaemia and a permanent contraction of the distal limb. Any cast or bandages are removed if they are preventing circulation. If no improvement is seen, the patient is taken to theatre, where the muscle fascia is split and left open to allow the swelling to reduce. Secondary closure of the wound and any skin grafting is carried out later. Peripheral neurovascular assessment is pivotal to the patient's outcome (Brown 2017; Hill et al. 2016).
- Non-union where the bone ends do not unite.
- Malunion where the bone ends have united but at an inappropriate position or angle.
- Joint or muscle stiffness or weakness, especially if the joint has been encased in a cast or the patient has not used their joints and muscles for a long time; physiotherapy can help to reduce the effect and enable full or near-full function to be restored.
- Wound infections, arising from an open injury and a contaminated wound, or in a surgical wound following surgery to stabilise the fracture.
- Osteomyelitis, an infection in the bone, which must be suspected if the patient has pain and the bone is not healing.

21.6 Osteomyelitis

LEARNING OBJECTIVE 21.6 Discuss the different types of pathogenesis of osteomyelitis.

Osteomyelitis is an infection of a bone usually caused by *Staphylococcus aureus*, Pseudomonas or *Mycobacterium tuberculosis*. This condition is considered to be an orthopaedic emergency. Patients at increased risk of osteomyelitis include those with diabetes mellitus, malnourished or immunosuppressed patients and those who have been on long-term steroid treatment.

A bone infection can occur from a direct spread of the organism due to the following.

- Exogenous infection, where infection enters the bone from outside the body (e.g. open fractures, surgical procedures, burns, human and dog bites or penetrating wounds). In people who abuse IV drugs, this tends to occur in the arms and hands.
- Endogenous infection, caused by the movement of infective organisms from a site of infection elsewhere in the body (e.g. respiratory infections). Endogenous infection occurs more commonly among infants, children and the elderly.
- An abscess at the metaphysis of a long where blood flow is slow and bacteria can collect (usually the cause of osteomyelitis in children) (Nair & McLiesh 2017).

Symptoms and diagnosis of osteomyelitis

Osteomyelitis begins with an inflammatory response, and the increased pressure within the bone causes pain and local tenderness. The increase in infected material towards the cortex of the bone causes the periosteum to lift, resulting in swelling. The affected bone tissues start to necrose and an abscess forms within the bone. If left untreated, the abscess can rupture and eventually form a sinus leading to the skin.

Local symptoms of acute osteomyelitis include:

- pain at the site of infection
- local tenderness
- heat
- swelling
- redness over the area
- later on, a sinus between bone and skin.

Diagnosis of the specific microorganism requires a needle aspiration bone biopsy at the site of infection. The infection will not be initially evident on an X-ray until changes in the bone have occurred, which can take several weeks. MRI, CT or bone scans will show the extent of the infection at an earlier stage. An elevation in the white cell count and positive blood cultures may also not be seen initially. The patient will develop systemic signs of an infection, including pyrexia, lethargy and irritability (Brown 2017).

A prompt diagnosis and early treatment are essential. Treatment requires management of the patient's symptoms, the primary cause of infection if known and the bone infection. The degree of pain can be reduced by elevation, supporting the affected limb using a cast or splint and pre-emptive analgesia (Brown 2017). Using a removable splint allows any wound to be treated and the infection area to be inspected. Paracetamol and aspirin are prescribed for their analgesic and antipyretic properties. If the pain is severe, opiate analgesia is prescribed.

A broad-spectrum antibiotic such as flucloxacillin or vancomycin is prescribed until the causative microorganism has been isolated. Antibiotics are initially given intravenously and then orally. Patient compliance is essential as antibiotics are often prescribed for four weeks to several months. Topical antibiotic therapy using antibiotic cement or removable beads in the affected area can be employed if the patient undergoes surgery (Brown 2017).

Surgical intervention is required if the pressure within the bone continues to increase, requiring the removal of necrotic tissues or the draining of an abscess. Extensive debridement may be required and the wound left open for continued irrigation and removal of the exudate. Secondary wound closure is carried out once the area is clean and granulation is evident. A persistent organism, such as *Staphylococcus aureus* or *Mycobacterium tuberculosis*, can lie dormant in the tissues for years, leading to recurrence of the infection, causing chronic osteomyelitis.

21.7 Hip fracture

LEARNING OBJECTIVE 21.7 Outline the potential implications of hip fracture in the elderly.

Hip fractures may occur in any age group; however, those sustained in the younger cohort are usually due to trauma (e.g. motor vehicle accident). A majority of hip fractures occur in the older population. In Australia and New Zealand, it is estimated that by the age of 90, 33 per cent of females and 19 per cent of males will have had a hip fracture. Indigenous Australians have a 5 per cent higher risk of hip fractures than the rest of the population (AIHW 2018). Ten to 20 per cent of patients who suffer a hip fracture will be institutionalised after the fracture. Hip fractures in the elderly are associated with a decline in mental health and cognitive impairment. A 2017 study showed that people over the age of 65 who suffered a hip fracture were 3.5 per cent more likely to die within a year of surgery than those who had surgery for a non-fracture-related procedure (AIHW 2018). Although most hip fractures result from osteoporosis, they are also caused by the increased risk of falling that is seen with age.

Once an older person has fallen and sustained a fracture, they are unable to get up and weight-bear, they experience tenderness or pain over the lateral aspect of the thigh and the leg is externally rotated and shortened due to contraction of the dominant muscles, but there is rarely any bruising evident. If the fracture is impacted, the patient may attempt to stand and walk, but the bone remains painful, and the leg is shortened.

Classification and management of hip fracture

The patient is given opiate analgesia and an intravenous infusion is commenced in emergency room. An X-ray of the hip will confirm the diagnosis of a hip fracture.

There are two main classifications of hip fracture.

1. An *intracapsular fracture* occurs within the joint capsule and presents as a subcapital fracture across the femoral neck high under the femoral head. This is the most common type of hip fracture and is four times more common in females than males. Femoral neck fractures have a 14–36 per cent associated mortality in the first year after injury.
2. An *extracapsular fracture* occurs outside the joint capsule, either at the base of the femoral neck or through the greater and/or lesser trochanter. These fractures have a better prognosis (Cusack 2020).

A full patient assessment should be completed where the patient's pre-injury health status is recorded, and any medical issues such as those related to osteoporosis or a history of repeated falls are noted. Patients are then transferred to the orthopaedic trauma unit. Surgery will ideally take place within 24 hours because a poor health status prior to surgery and a delay in surgical intervention are known to affect recovery and possibly increase mortality risk. Additional benefits from early surgery are an increased ability to return to independent living and a reduced hospital stay (Roberts et al. 2015; Koizia et al. 2019; Cusack 2020). The following points related to surgery should be remembered.

- The surgical procedure depends on the extent and type of injury.
- A subcapital fracture is liable to compromise the blood supply from the vascular ring outside the base of the femoral neck, which has several arterial entry points with vessels going up the femoral neck to the head.
- Trauma to the vessels risks avascular necrosis (AVN) of the femoral head (bone death); therefore, the femoral head is removed and replaced (a hemiarthroplasty).
- No acetabular component is required unless there are severe osteoarthritic changes in the joint. With an extracapsular fracture, the blood supply is unaffected, but this tends to be a more unstable fracture.
- An extracapsular fracture is treated with a dynamic hip screw into the femoral neck and attached to a plate that is screwed on to the lateral surface of the femur below the greater trochanter.

Potential complications of a hip fracture are detailed in table 21.6.

TABLE 21.6 **Potential complications of a hip fracture pre- and post-surgery**

Complications from the injury and the preoperative phase	Post-surgical and rehabilitation-related complications
Hypovolaemic shock	Complications of bed rest include pressure sores, chest infection, urinary tract infection
Pain	Deep vein thrombosis and pulmonary embolism

Limb deformity (the limb is externally rotated and shortened)	Joint dislocation if a hemiarthroplasty has been used
Dehydration	Loosening of fixation
Avascular necrosis of the femoral head	Non-union of the fracture
Delirium	Post-operative confusion
Electrolyte imbalances	Pressure sores
	Osteomyelitis

Special considerations in the elderly with hip fractures

A common but infrequently discussed complication of hip fractures in the elderly is delirium. A quarter of patients admitted with a proximal femoral fracture suffer an episode of delirium. For patients with co-existing dementia, this can be particularly difficult to recognise. Delirium may be due to several factors, including infection, pain and hypovolaemia, either due to dehydration, blood loss or a combination of the two. Delirium leads to increased morbidity and mortality and increased loss of independence following discharge. Recommendations to address this are the use of a multidisciplinary team involving multiple specialties. Regional anaesthesia with multi-modal pain control include minimising narcotic use, minimising surgery delays, nutritional support and intensive physical therapy. Close attention should also be paid to reversing any fluid and electrolyte abnormalities (Roberts et al. 2015; Koizia et al. 2019).

Overall, patients' length of stay is related to their comorbid conditions, where they lived before the injury, the timeliness of their transfer to rehabilitation and where they are discharged to. Unfortunately, many patients with comorbid conditions require an extensive rehabilitation period (Cusack 2020).

21.8 Neurovascular assessment and plaster care

LEARNING OBJECTIVE 21.8 Recognise the importance of neurovascular assessment in preventing potential complications.

All patients who have a musculoskeletal injury or have undergone orthopaedic surgery or cast immobilisation of a limb (figure 21.12) are at risk of developing neurovascular compromise, leading to compartment syndrome. Peripheral neurovascular assessment involves a systematic assessment of a limb's neurological and vascular integrity, intending to promptly recognise any neurovascular deficit. Damage to the tissues worsens as time passes, so prompt recognition and intervention are necessary (Hill et al. 2016).

Physiological indicators of vascular compromise are caused by a lack of oxygen within the muscles and all the tissues and neurological compromise due to an interruption of the nerve supply to the tissue (Hill et al. 2016). Dykes (1993) recognised '5Ps' approach to neurovascular assessment integrates the assessment of the patient's limb with regard to pain, pulses, pallor, paraesthesia and paralysis. Documentation on a dedicated chart noting pain intensity and type, warmth, sensation, colour, capillary refill time and the movement of the affected and unaffected limb are key to provide a baseline for comparison.

Pain is a critical early sign of compartment syndrome. Pain may not be relieved by analgesia and may be greater on passive motion and out of proportion to the injury. Paraesthesia is a subtle early sign which may need careful questioning to elicit. This may show as tingling or burning and can lead to numbness. Pallor and paralysis are later signs and must be acted on swiftly. Pulselessness is a late and ominous sign.

FIGURE 21.12 Key principles of plaster cast care

Patient education

- Keep the plastered arm or leg raised on a pillow for the first 12 hours and at rest as elevation aids the reduction of swelling. Continue to do this for another 12 hours if the cast still feels tight.
- Don't get the plaster cast wet as this will weaken the cast, and the bone will no longer be fully supported and will become a source for infection (osteomyelitis or septic arthritis).
- Baths and showers should be avoided, but in reality, a plastic bag can be used to cover the cast. Try using sticky tape or a rubber band to seal the bag at the top and bottom to make it as water-tight as possible. Alternatively, it is possible to buy special covers for plaster casts to keep them dry.

- Always remove the bag as soon as possible to avoid sweating, which could also damage the cast.
- Even if the plaster cast makes the skin feel very itchy, do not 'poke' anything down the cast to try to relieve the itch as it could cause a wound or source of infection. The itchiness should settle down after a few days (or contact your GP about taking an antihistamine).

Plaster cast tips

- Don't let any small objects fall inside the cast as they could irritate the skin.
- Don't try to alter the length or position of the cast.
- Don't lift anything heavy or drive until the cast has been removed and it has been agreed by a doctor that it is safe to lift or drive.
- Use a sling, as advised by your health professional.
- Don't write on the cast for at least 24 hours to prevent denting of the cast and skin problems; allow it to dry naturally.

Plaster cast problems

Contact A&E, the fracture clinic, the plaster unit or the ward if:

- the plaster cast still feels too tight after keeping it elevated for 24 hours
- the cast is rubbing or cutting into the skin
- the fingers on the affected limb feel swollen, tingly, burning, painful (even after taking painkillers) or numb
- the fingers turn blue or white
- the cast feels too loose or slips
- the cast is broken or cracked
- the skin underneath or around the edge of the cast feels sore
- there is an unpleasant smell, discharge or staining coming from the cast.

Document in the patient's notes when verbal and written advice has been given.

Source: Adapted from Clarke (2003).

21.9 Bone metastases

LEARNING OBJECTIVE 21.9 Explain the causes and management of bony metastases.

As bone metastases are more commonly seen in adults than primary bone tumours, the latter are not discussed here. Although many primary tumours are known to result in bone metastases, 70 per cent arise from primary breast and prostate cancers. They occur in bones with a rich blood supply, such as the vertebrae, humerus, acetabulum and femur. Patients generally present with dull, aching bone pain that increases during the day and may disturb sleep at night. Movement, especially weight-bearing, can increase the pain, leading to difficulty in weight-bearing and reduced mobility. The sudden onset of severe pain identifies a pathological fracture. If bone metastases are suspected, a bone scan will identify the extent of the metastatic spread. If a spread is shown, this should be followed by plain X-ray, CT or MRI scans to help plan patient care (Macedo et al. 2017).

A diagnosis of bone metastases often indicates that the primary cancer has advanced or that treatment has been unsuccessful, causing a raised level of anxiety and fear in patients and their families. The median survival rates following diagnosis of bony metastases are between three and 58 months; therefore, psychological and social aspects of care are essential for these patients, as is the management of their pain (Macedo et al. 2017). Conservative management is essential to reduce the level of pain experienced, reduce the risk of a fracture occurring and ensure that a patient's level of health and quality of life are maintained. Options for pain relief include analgesia, radiotherapy, chemotherapy, surgery and bisphosphonate drugs. For this reason, the oncology, orthopaedic and palliative care teams will collaborate to ensure appropriate care for the patient concerning the management of the primary cancer and any palliative care needs (Macedo et al. 2017). Patients presenting with a fracture require symptomatic treatment, including appropriate analgesia and fracture management, for example, internal fixation, bed rest on traction and a plaster cast. The decision to operate on the fracture will depend on the patient's health and life expectancy.

CASE STUDY 21.1

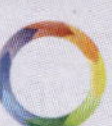

Nursing care of a patient with osteoarthritis

Madeline Vargas is a 58-year-old female who has presented with a 24-month history of increasing pain in her left knee. She says the pain initially only occurred after she had been doing a lot of bending and lifting, which she does a lot in her job as a landscape gardener. Initially, the pain was relieved by rest and paracetamol. Madeline is overweight (BMI 26) but feels she is fit and is trying to lose weight.

Over the past few months, the pain has been getting worse, and paracetamol no longer seems effective. Her knee is beginning to hurt even when at rest. She also notes that sometimes her knee seems to 'crack'.

She has mild hypertension, which is treated with 25 mg metoprolol mane.

You do a set of observations and find:

- temperature: 36.0°C
- heart rate: 88 bpm
- respiratory rate: 16 breaths per minute
- blood pressure: 115/80 mmHg
- oxygen saturation: 98% on room air
- pain scale (in left knee): 5/10.

Question

Using the information above, describe what action you would take as the nurse caring for this patient. What examinations might you expect this patient to need for diagnosis? What medications might be indicated as the paracetamol is no longer effective? What non-pharmacological interventions can be used for this patient? Use the clinical reasoning cycle to guide you through the process and devise a plan of care for your patient.

Answer

- *Step 1: Consider the patient.* Madeline Vargas is a 58-year-old female with a 24-month history of increasing pain in her left knee.
- *Step 2: Collect cues/information.* Include subjective and objective data here, including the patient's appearance and past medical history. Objective data will include measurable information such as his vital signs. Think here about what extra tests you might consider they should have.
- *Step 3: Process information.* Separate the relevant and irrelevant data — cluster the clues together to formulate an inference about the patient.

  Patient's only comorbidity is hypertension, which is well controlled on a minimal dose of metoprolol. She works as a landscape gardener, which indicates that she is likely relatively healthy and mobile and is in a role that requires the use of her knees. Her pain relief is not as effective as desired. Paracetamol is indicated in knee and hip pain. Her osteoarthritis of the knee is likely to become worse over time. Her weight will exacerbate both the pain and the rate of deterioration. If she loses weight this will help relieve the knee pain and may also have a positive effect on her hypertension.
- *Step 4: Identify problems/issues.* Nursing problems or diagnosis should be listed here. The main problems are the patient's excess weight and knee pain, which is no longer responding well to recommended analgesia.
- *Step 5: Establish goals*. Knee pain may decrease if the patient loses weight. Think about how you might communicate this to the patient in a patient-centred, compassionate and supportive way.
- *Step 6: Take action*. How might you best communicate the concept of weight loss with your patient? Remember that this can be a very emotional issue for many people.
- *Step 7: Evaluate outcomes.* Has the patient lost weight? If so how much? Has the pain diminished?
- *Step 8: Reflect on the process and new learning*. Reflect on any aspects of care that could have been performed in a way to achieve an improved outcome.

  Weight loss can be difficult. If the patient was successful ask, 'What did you find easy? What was hard? What kept you motivated?' This can be useful information for another patient that may need to lose weight. If the weight loss was not successful, try to find the reasons. Again, this is all useful information when assisting another patient on their weight loss journey. Always elicit information in a supportive and collaborative manner. People sometimes have to change the habits of a lifetime. Often people are not aware of their behaviours. Quietly and calmly going over the patient's weight loss journey with them may highlight some key problems that can be slowly modified.

CASE STUDY 21.2

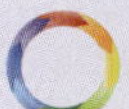

Nursing care of a deteriorating patient post-THR

Mrs Brauer is a sprightly 90-year-old female patient who has recently returned from theatre following a THR for osteoarthritis. She has a history of asthma controlled with preventer inhalers and occasional salbutamol PRN. She has no other significant comorbidities.

You are given a handover from the recovery nurse. It is brief as they are in a hurry to get back to the busy unit. You take a set of obs, all of which are within normal limits. She has a Glasgow Coma Scale of 15 and a pain score of 4/10.

She has a dressing on her left leg with nil ooze. One drain at the inferior aspect of the incision, minimal drainage noted. PCA is running with a background infusion of morphine 1 mg per hour. She has oxygen running at 2 L per minute via nasal prongs.

You settle her and make sure she has her call button and water within reach. She indicates she is aware of how to use the PCA, which is also within her grasp.

Fifteen minutes later, you do her second set of obs, and she seems drowsy. Respiratory rate is 15 breaths per minute, slightly lower than before, as is he oxygen saturation at 96 per cent. Otherwise, she seems fine, and you understand that she will still be having residual effects of the anaesthetic.

Ten minutes later, while attending to another patient, you look over, and she seems semi-conscious and barely breathing. You quickly attempt to rouse her with minimal success. You do another set of obs, and her respiratory rate is six breaths per minutes, and she cannot be roused except to pain. Her oxygen saturation is 85 per cent. You immediately call for help and lay her down while maintaining her airway.

The team arrive and assist her respiration with a bag and mask. After a quick but thorough check of wounds, drains etc. and auscultation of her heart, the team administer Narcan 0.4 mg IV. This has an immediate effect. Mrs Brauer opens her eyes and begins to breathe on her own. You feel your breathing settle down as well.

Question

Using the information above, describe what action you would take as the nurse caring for this patient. Use the clinical reasoning cycle to guide you through the process and devise a plan of care for your patient.

Answer

- *Step 1: Consider the patient*. Mrs Brauer, a 90-year-old female patient post-THR for osteoarthritis.
- *Step 2: Collect cues.* Include subjective and objective data here, including the patient's appearance and past medical history. Objective data will include measurable information such as vital signs. Patient is immediately post-op THR. She has severely decreased respirations (bradypnoea), SpO_2 is decreased. Level of consciousness has decreased.
- *Step 3: Process information*. Separate the relevant and irrelevant data — cluster the clues together to formulate an inference about the patient. Unresponsiveness and apnoea are not normal. You can't think of anything that correlates with what might be happening to help process the information.
- *Step 4: Identify problems.* Patient is semi-conscious and has severe respiratory difficulty. If this is not addressed, she will become hypoxic and may die.
- *Step 5: Establish goals*. Goals for care include getting oxygen into her system and correcting her level of consciousness.
- *Step 6: Take action*. The nurse should immediately recognise that the patient meets the criteria for a medical emergency call. Call for help and establish patent airway.
- *Step 7: Evaluate outcomes*. The patient was stabilised with oxygen delivery via a bag and mask. While this was happening, the medical team looked through her recovery notes. It noted that shortly before her return to the ward, she had become bradypnoeic, and orders were written to give Narcan 4 mg IV stat and to cease the background infusion of morphine via the PCA. Narcan lasts for 30 minutes, after which time it wears off quickly. The PCA was not adjusted.
- *Step 8: Reflect on the process and new learning.* In future, make sure that even if a staff member is in a hurry, you get a full and considered handover. Breakdown in the transfer of information or in 'communication' has been identified as one of the most important contributing factors in serious adverse events and is a major preventable cause of patient harm (AIHW 2012).

  Clinical handover is the effective 'transfer of professional responsibility and accountability for some or all aspects of care for a patient, or group of patients, to another person or professional group on a temporary or permanent basis' (AIHW 2012).

SUMMARY

This chapter has outlined some of the common conditions associated with the musculoskeletal system. The musculoskeletal system encompasses not only the bones, which give the body its core structure and protects many vulnerable and essential organs, it includes the muscles, ligaments and tendons, which enable movement as well as being the source of all blood cells. The flat bones are responsible for haematopoiesis, so many haematological disorders are also linked to a disease process having a skeletal origin. The problems that may arise due to damage or dysfunction of components of the musculoskeletal system are varied and can impact many other body systems. Any loss of integrity of the musculoskeletal system will impact multiple aspects of a persons' daily living activities, which in turn highly influences a person's perception of self. Pain is also a key aspect of any musculoskeletal injury, and pain is in itself extremely debilitating. Acute observation and focused communication with the emphasis on the individual is essential in assisting any patient with a musculoskeletal injury to achieve the best possible outcome for their ongoing health and continuing engagement in all aspects of their life.

KEY TERMS

appendicular skeleton The upper and lower extremities including the shoulder girdle and pelvis.

arthrodesis Joint fusion. The purpose is to inhibit movement between two bones.

arthroplasty Joint replacement. Includes hip, knee, shoulder, ankle, metacarpal and metatarsal joints.

axial skeleton The bones of the head and thoracic vertebrae. This includes the rib cage and vertebral column and consists of 80 bones.

bone metastases The spread of malignant cancer cells to bone.

fracture Any break in the bone from a crack to a complete break.

osteoarthritis Chronic arthritis, usually mechanical, not caused by inflammatory process.

osteomyelitis Inflammation of bone marrow, cortex, tissue and periosteum; can be caused by any organism, but usually bacteria.

osteotomy Where the bones are cut and realigned to stop subluxation (an incomplete or partial dislocation).

rheumatoid arthritis (RA) A chronic, systemic inflammatory disorder characterised by progressive joint changes leading to joint destruction, deformity and immobility.

sympathetic and vasomotor The sympathetic response relates to the sympathetic nervous system which activates what is commonly known as the 'flight or fright' response. The vasomotor response to this is the dilation or constriction of the blood vessels.

REFERENCES

Australian Institute of Health and Welfare (AIHW). (2012) NSQHS Standards (first edition) fact sheet on clinical handover. www.safetyandquality.gov.au/sites/default/files/migrated/NSQHS-Standards-Fact-Sheet-Standard-6.pdf

Australian Institute of Health and Welfare (AIHW). (2018) Hip fracture incidence and hospitalisations in Australia 2015–2016. www.aihw.gov.au/getmedia/296b5bb1-0816-44c6-bdce-b56e10fd6c0f/aihw-phe-226.pdf.aspx?inline=true

Australian Institute of Health and Welfare (AIHW). (2020) Reports and data. *Osteoarthritis*. www.aihw.gov.au/reports/arthritis-other-musculoskeletal-conditions/osteoarthritis/data

Brown, A. (2017) 'Nursing care of people with musculoskeletal disorders'. In Lemone and Burke (Eds.). *Medical surgical nursing: critical thinking for person centered care*, 3rd ed.

Clarke, S. (2003) Orthopaedic paediatric practice: an impression of pain assessment. *Journal of Orthopaedic Nursing*. 7: 132–136.

Craft, J. & Gordon, C. (2017) *Fundamentals of applied pathophysiology*, 3rd ed. Wiley.

Cusack, S. (2020) 'Hip injuries'. In Cameron, P., Little, M., Mitra, B. & Deasy, C. (Eds.). *Textbook of adult emergency medicine*, 5th ed.

Dykes, P. C. (1993) Minding the five P's of neurovascular assessment. *American Journal of Nursing*. 6: 38–39.

Evans, J. T., Evans, J. P., Walker, R., Blom, A., Whitehouse, M. & Sayers, A. (2019) How long does a hip replacement last? A systematic review and meta-analysis of case series and national registry reports with more than 15 years of follow-up. *The Lancet*. 393: 647–654.

Hill, C., Atalla, B. & Keady, J. (2016) 'Major orthopaedic and neurovascular trauma'. In Curtis, K., Ramsden, C., Shanban, R., Fry, M. & Considine, J. (Eds.). *Emergency and trauma care for nurses and paramedics*, 3rd ed.

Kaye, A., Urman, R., Cornett, E., Hart, B., Chami, A., Gayle, J. & Fox, C. (2019) Enhanced recovery pathways in orthopaedic surgery. *Journal Anaesthesiology Clinical Pharmacology*. 35(sup 1): 35–39.

Koizia, L., Wilson, F., Reilly, P. & Fertleman, M. (2019) Delerium after emergency hip surgery — common and serious but rarely consented for. *World Journal of Orthopaedics.* 10(6): 228–234.

Leong, N., Kator, J., Clemens, T., James, A., Enamoto-Iwamoto, M. & Jiang, J. (2020) Tendon and ligament healing and current approaches to tendon and ligament regeneration. *Journal of Orthopaedic Research.* 38(1): 7–12.

Lucas, B. (2008a) Total hip and total knee replacement: preoperative nursing management. *British Journal of Nursing.* 17(21): 1346–1351.

Lucas, B. (2008b) Total hip and total knee replacement: postoperative nursing management. *British Journal of Nursing.* 17(22): 1410–1414.

Macedo, F., Ladiera, K., Pinho, F., Saraiva, N., Bonito, N., Pinto, L. & Goncalves, F. (2017) Bone metastases: An overview. *Oncology Review Journal.* 11(1).

Maffulli, N., Wong, J. & Almekinders, L. C. (2003) Types and epidemiology of tendinopathy. *Clinical Sports Medicine.* 22: 675–692.

Nair, M, & Peate, I. (2009) *Fundamentals of applied pathophysiology.* Wiley.

Nash, D. & McLiesh, P. (2017) 'Alterations of musculoskeletal function across the life span'. In Craft, J., Gordon, C., Huether, S., Brashers, V. & Rote, N. (Eds.). *Understanding Pathophysiology*, 3rd ed.

National Institute for Health and Care Excellence (NICE). (2014) Osteoarthritis: care and management. Summary of Clinical Guideline 117. London: Department of Health. www.mims.co.uk/Guidelines/1087441/care-management-osteoarthritis-adults

National Institute for Health and Care Excellence (NICE). (2018) Rheumatoid arthritisin adults: management. Clinical Guideline 100. London: Department of Health.

Roberts, K., Brox, W., Jevsevar, D. & Sevarino, K. (2015) Management of hip fractures in the elderly. *Journal of the American Academy of Orthopaedic Surgeons.* 23(1): 131–137.

Tortora, G. & Derrickson, B. (2011) *Principles of anatomy and Physiology*, 13th ed. Wiley.

Tu, K., Lie, J., Wan, C., Caneron, M., Austel, A., Nguyen, J., Van, K. & Hyun, D. (2018) Osteoporosis: A review of treatment options. *Journal of Pharmacy and Therapeutics.* 43(2): 93–104.

Wylie, E. & Clarke, S. (2014) 'Key conditions and principles of orthopaedic'. In Clarke, S. & Santy-Tomlinson, J. (Eds.). *Orthopaedic and trauma nursing: an evidence-based approach to musculoskeletal care.* Wiley.

ACKNOWLEDGEMENTS

Figures 21.9 and 21.10: © Peate, I., *Fundamentals of Applied Pathophysiology: An Essential Guide for Nursing and Healthcare Students*, 4th ed., 2021. © John Wiley & Sons Inc. Reproduced with permission of John Wiley & Sons Inc.

CHAPTER 22

Nursing care of conditions related to the ear, nose, throat and eyes

LEARNING OBJECTIVES

After studying this chapter, you should be able to:

22.1 describe the anatomy and physiology of the ear, and the management of patients with ear disorders

22.2 describe the anatomy and physiology of the nose, and the management of patients with nose disorders

22.3 describe the anatomy and physiology of the throat, and the management of patients with throat disorders

22.4 describe the anatomy and physiology of the eye, and the management of patients with eye disorders

22.5 apply patient-centred care to care of the patient with conditions affecting the ear, nose, throat and eye.

Introduction

As nurses, we care for patients across the lifespan who experience a wide range of acute and chronic conditions related to their ears, nose, throat (ENT) and eyes. Disorders of the ENT and eyes affect our ability to communicate and can also affect balance. This impacts an individual's ability to perform activities of daily living. In some circumstances where the airway is affected, these conditions constitute a medical emergency. Nursing care for patients experiencing problems with their eyes, ears, nose and throat is provided in various locations, including acute inpatient, outpatient, primary care and community settings. This chapter will provide an overview of the anatomy and physiology of the ENT and eyes. It will also review the pathophysiology of these systems providing a broad overview of common conditions of the ENT and eyes and their nursing management. The chapter will also and consider the application of patient-centred care and the clinical reasoning cycle to these cases.

22.1 The ear

LEARNING OBJECTIVE 22.1 Describe the anatomy and physiology of the ear, and the management of patients with ear disorders.

The auditory system is responsible for hearing and balance and consists of the ears and nerves, which transmit electrical impulses from the ear to the brain. Hearing is the transduction of sound waves into a nerve signal (Garvan Institute of Medical Research 2021). This transduction of sound waves is made possible by the structures of the ear.

Anatomy and physiology of the ear

Hearing starts with the outer ear. When a sound is made, the sound waves travel down the external auditory canal and strike the eardrum (tympanic membrane). The tympanic membrane vibrates, and these vibrations are passed to the ossicles. The ossicles amplify the sound. They send the sound waves to the inner ear and into the fluid-filled hearing organ called the cochlea. Once these sound waves reach the inner ear, they are converted into electrical impulses and sent by the auditory nerve to the brain. The brain then translates these electrical impulses as sound.

Balance is controlled by signals to the brain from the inner ear and by vision and movement sensors in our skin, muscles and joints (Department of Health & Human Services 2020). The organs of balance in the inner ear are called the vestibular system. The vestibular system includes three semi-circular canals, which are filled with fluid and respond to the rotation of the head. Near the semi-circular canals are the utricle and saccule, which detect gravity and back-and-forth movement. As the head moves, signals from the utricle and saccule are sent through the vestibular nerve to the brain, where they are processed. The brain uses the information from the inner ear, our vision and our body's ability to sense location, movement and action to identify the body's position.

The ear is made up of the:

- outer or external ear
- the **middle ear**
- the **inner ear** (Ervin 2021).

The outer ear

The **outer ear** includes the visible structures of the ear.

- The pinna or auricle is a concave structure made of cartilage that collects and directs sound waves into the ear canal or external auditory meatus.
- The ear canal is an S shape, approximately 24 mm long and 6 mm wide and ends at the tympanic membrane (Ervin 2021).

In adults, the ear canal is curved downward and forward. In children less than three years of age, the ear canal is directed upward and backward. The role of the ear canal is to direct airborne sound waves towards the tympanic membrane. It also helps maintain the temperature and humidity of the ear and preserve the elasticity of the tympanic membrane. Glands, which produce cerumen (earwax), and the small hairs in the ear canal, protect against insects and foreign particles from entering and damaging the tympanic membrane.

The middle ear

The main function of the middle ear is to transmit vibrations from the tympanic membrane to the inner ear by way of the auditory ossicles. The middle ear is in an air-filled space that lies within the temporal bone.

It is separated from the external ear by the tympanic membrane and consists of the following.

- Three small bones called auditory ossicles (malleus, incus and stapes). These bones link the tympanic membrane to the inner ear. The auditory ossicles lay next to the tympanic membrane and transmit the vibrations from the membrane to the inner ear.
- The eustachian tube, connecting the middle ear to the throat, helping to equalise pressure in the middle ear. The eustachian tube is normally closed and opens with yawning and swallowing actions.
- The oval window, a connective tissue membrane located at the end of the middle ear and the beginning of the cochlea of the inner ear (Healthline 2021b). Sound waves cause the tympanic membrane to vibrate. The ossicles transmit the vibrations to the oval window, causing the fluid within the cochlea to vibrate, activating the receptors for hearing.

The inner ear

The inner ear contains a bony canal structure located in the temporal bone. Sound waves enter the inner ear and then the cochlea, a snail-shaped organ. The cochlea is filled with the **perilymph** fluid that moves due to the vibrations from the oval window. As the fluid moves, the 25 000 nerve endings are set into motion. These nerve endings transform the vibrations into electrical impulses that then travel along the eighth cranial nerve (auditory nerve) to the brain. The brain then interprets these signals, and this is how we hear. The inner ear also contains the vestibular organ that is responsible for balance. Figure 22.1 illustrates the anatomy of the ear.

FIGURE 22.1 Anatomy of the ear

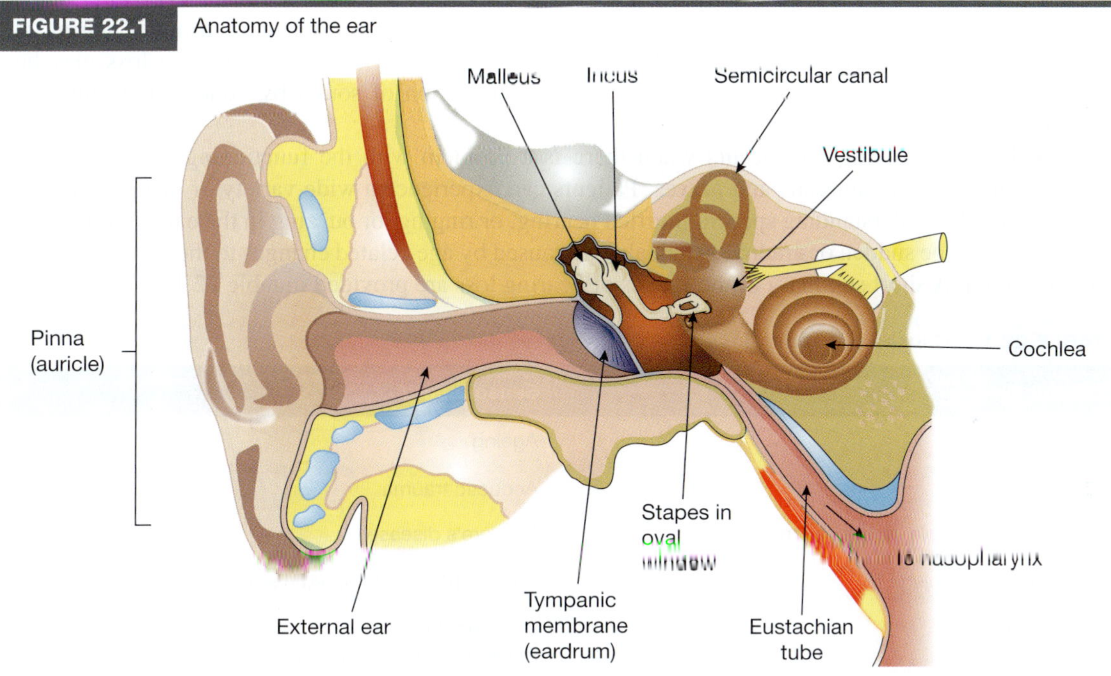

Source: Nair & Peate (2009) *Fundamentals of Applied Pathophysiology*, with kind permission from Wiley Blackwell.

Common disorders of the ear

Ear conditions may be caused by problems in the ear itself or the neck, the sinuses or the head. Babies and children are the most vulnerable to ear infections. Other common disorders include hearing loss, otitis media, tinnitus, Ménière's disease and barotrauma. All disorders of the ears can affect hearing and balance and hence create safety issues for the patient along with discomfort and concern.

Auditory dysfunction

The prevalence of hearing loss in Australia in 2019–20 was estimated to be 3.95 million people, or 15.3 per cent of the total population (Health Care Industry Association 2021). An additional 350 000 people now live with hearing loss, an increase of 9.7 per cent since 2017. By 2025, it is estimated that hearing loss will increase by more than 10 per cent to 4.4 million cases and to 7.8 million cases by 2066, which is almost double the current number.

A definition of deafness or hearing loss can include:

- decreased audibility or loss of ability to hear some sounds at all
- decreased dynamic range or less ability to hear a range of soft to loud sounds
- decreased frequency resolution or less ability to separate speech from background noise
- decreased temporal resolution (less ability to differentiate intense sounds from weaker sounds).

Impaired hearing or loss results in difficulty communicating. A person with hearing loss may experience a combination of these factors and struggle to hear and understand speech. Whether categorised as mild, moderate, severe or profound, hearing loss can impact work, general health and personal relationships (Amplifon n.d.). Individuals may experience social disengagement resulting in social isolation, loneliness, decreased self-esteem and depression. Congenital or early childhood hearing loss adversely affects speech and language development. Loss of hearing in the later years due to aging will affect the older adult's ability to be a part of their community. Individuals that miss parts of a message require repetition, leading to frustration and emotional distancing from family and friends (Preminger & Meeks 2010). There may also be safety issues, such as an inability to hear traffic or warning alarms. The degree of hearing impairment and loss, whether it is transient or permanent, and the patient's age group will have a bearing on management, treatment and the patient's response to care.

Hearing impairment can be sensorineural (nerve), conductive (mechanical) or a mixture of both and can be caused by a range of different conditions and environmental factors.

Conductive hearing loss occurs when sound conduction from outer to middle ear is impeded. The presence of cerumen (ear wax), foreign bodies, and blockages of the eustachian tube can all cause conductive hearing loss. Patients with conductive hearing loss often have trouble hearing and can have an altered perception of sound. For example, people with conductive hearing loss may hear their own voice louder than it actually is, due to the conduction of sound by bone to the middle ear (Craft & Gordon 2015).

Sensorineural hearing loss occurs when there is a problem with the functioning of the inner ear, including the cochlea, hair cells and nerves. Patients can experience a wide variety of symptoms. These include difficulty understanding speech, muffled hearing, or ringing, or buzzing in the ears. Sensorineural hearing loss can be sudden or gradual. It can also be caused by age-related changes to the auditory system, and congenital. A short summary of the causes of hearing loss are provided in table 22.1.

TABLE 22.1 Causes of hearing loss

Conductive	Sensorineural
Foreign bodies	Ageing
Wax	Acoustic trauma
Trauma, for example, to the ear, middle ear	Ménière's disease
Surgery or head injury	Presbycusis (age-related hearing loss)
Otitis media	Ototoxic drugs Platinum-based antineoplastic agents

Ear trauma

Trauma can be caused by a range of different mechanisms, including the insertion of a foreign body, for example, beads, toys or cotton buds, into the external auditory canal. Foreign bodies in the ear canal are often seen with children and can cause perforation of the tympanic membrane.

Trauma can also be caused by external blunt force trauma to the external structures of the ear in sports, motor vehicle accidents, falls and fights, etc. Trauma to the pinna can lead to swelling bruising known as a sub-perichondrial haematoma.

Otitis media

Otitis media is inflammation located in the middle ear. Otitis media can occur due to a cold, sore throat, or respiratory infection. It is common in children but can also occur with adults (Healthline 2021a). A simple guide to the symptoms of otitis media is provided in figure 22.2. Patients diagnosed with serious otitis media may require a myringotomy and the insertion of grommet or tympanostomy tubes to facilitate drainage. Patients with chronic otitis media require antibiotic eardrops. Patients should be educated on the condition, treatment and self care or care of the child.

FIGURE 22.2 Symptoms of otitis media

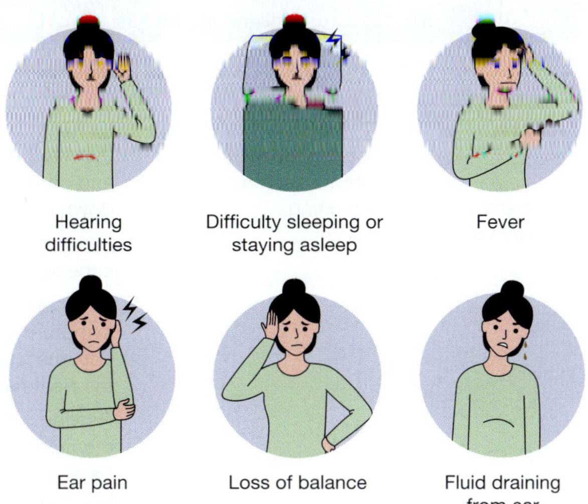

Ménière's disease

Ménière's disease is a disorder of the inner ear characterised by episodes of vertigo, ringing in the ears (tinnitus) and hearing loss. The causes of Ménière's disease is not fully understood but thought to be related to an imbalance in the production and absorption of endolymph within the inner labyrinth.

A brief summary of the symptoms, assessment and management of each of the above conditions is supplied in table 22.2.

TABLE 22.2 **Summary of common auditory dysfunction**

Condition	Signs and symptoms	Assessment	Management
Trauma	Presence of a foreign body: Pain Discharge Visible foreign body. External trauma to the ear: Redness Pain Swelling Bruising.	Patient health assessment, vital signs, examination of the external ear looking for swelling, discharge, redness or other abnormalities Assess internal ear using an otoscope, looking for wax, foreign bodies and visualising the tympanic membrane.	Foreign bodies need to be removed as to not push them in further. This may be achieved by gentle irrigation or using instruments such as alligator forceps, wax loops or right-angle hooks. Some foreign bodies may need surgical removal. Trauma: apply ice to the ears to reduce swelling and provide analgesia as needed. Ear lacerations may require suturing.
Otitis media	Pain Decreased hearing on the affected side Sensation of popping in ears In tympanic membrane rupture, possible serous discharge Fever. Indications in children include fussiness and intense crying, clutching the ear and wincing in pain or complaints of ear pain in older children.	Patient health assessment, including health history, vital signs and physical examination of the external and internal ear. The external ear is observed for signs of swelling, discharge, redness, or other abnormalities. The internal ear is assessed using an otoscope to examine the tympanic membrane for redness, bulging and decreased movement.	Most cases of acute otitis media occur in children. Guidelines indicate that most cases will resolve spontaneously — routine prescribing of antibiotics is no longer recommended. Antibiotics may be prescribed in severe cases or where signs of systemic infection are present. Decongestants, antihistamines and corticosteroids are not effective and are no longer recommended. Simple analgesics such as over-the-counter medications may be required for pain management. Provide patient education on risk factors and prevention, including avoiding secondhand smoke and bottle feeding while laying down for babies.

(continued)

TABLE 22.2 *(continued)*

Condition	Signs and symptoms	Assessment	Management
Ménière's disease	Vertigo Tinnitus Nausea Vomiting Sensorineural deafness (a feeling of fullness in the affected ear) Sweating	Patient health assessment, including vital signs and physical examination. Assess for associated symptoms such as nausea and vomiting	Management is focused on symptom control. If patient is acutely dizzy, encourage them to position themselves in a safe and comfortable position either lying down or sitting upright Monitor and maintain oral hydration, especially if vomiting is present. Medication may be prescribed for symptom management, including antiemetics and medications used in the treatment of vertigo. Provide patient education on monitoring and avoiding triggers; for example, caffeine and alcohol are known triggers in some patients.

Source: MedlinePlus (2014).

Assessment of the ears

An assessment of the ears and hearing will include a detailed medical history and physical examination. The health history will ask about the patient's general health, including comorbidities, etc. and then focus on the auditory system.

- What brought you to the clinic/ hospital today?
- What problems have you noticed? How long have you been experiencing these problems?
- Describe your hearing difficulties. Are the hearing problems in the left or the right ear or both ears?
- When did you first notice that you had hearing difficulties?
- Do you have ringing in your ears? If so, what time of the day, and does it go on for long?
- Have you had a lot of ear infections?
- Do you have pain in your ears? Please describe the pain. What makes the pain better or worse? What is the pain like? Where is the pain, and does it radiate anywhere? On a scale of one to ten, please score the pain. How long has it been going on?
- Have you noted drainage from your ears? Please describe the drainage.
- Do you ever feel dizzy?
- Do you have a family history of hearing loss?
- Do you find it harder to hear female voices, male voices or children's voices?
- Are you told you that you have the television or radio on too loud?
- Are you told you that you speak too loudly?
- Do you have to ask people to repeat what they said? If so, how often does this happen?
- Do you hear people speaking but cannot understand what they are saying?
- Have you worked in places that are very loud and noisy? Have you served in the military? Do you shoot guns or take part in other loud activities? Do you play music loudly?
- Are there times when you have more trouble hearing, such as in a car, restaurant, theatre or in large groups?

With children, the assessment will include the presence of the parents or carer and will include:

- a health history and the health history of the family
- the ability of the child to understand and respond to familiar sounds
- the child's response to loud, unexpected sounds the startle response
- a history of the child's hearing, including any prior hearing tests
- speech and language development
- motor and thinking skills.

The nurse will also conduct a physical and general health assessment for both adults and children that includes:

- vital signs including blood pressure, pulse, temperature, respiratory rate, oxygen saturations and pain assessment, and assessment of nausea and vomiting
- assessment of dizziness and balance

- physical examination of the ear. Both ears must always be examined. If the patient states that the problem is on one side only, it is recommended to examine the ear without the problems first (Chang 2005). This allows for any variation in normal anatomy to be recognised for that individual patient. It will also reduce the potential for cross-infection if one ear has noted discharge or signs or symptom of an infection. For common forms of the assessment of hearing, see table 22.3.

TABLE 22.3 Assessment of hearing and diagnostic tests

Assessment	Indication and method	Results
Weber test	The Weber test is a quick and simple test using a tuning fork to assess hearing loss. It is best used for unilateral hearing loss. The examiner holds the tuning fork by the stem between their thumb and first finger. The fork tines are tapped on a surface, such as the examiner's knee or elbow, and then placed on the patient's forehead. The patient is asked 'Is the sound louder in your right ear, your left ear or in the middle?' (Wahid 2020 Mar 28).	In hearing loss, the sound will be different in one ear depending on the type of hearing loss. Conductive hearing loss: sound will be heard louder in the deaf ear. Sensorineural hearing loss: the sound will be heard louder in the normal ear Bilateral hearing loss: the sound will be the same in both ears.
Rinne test	The Rinne test is used to assess the conduction of sound through bone and detect conductive hearing loss. The examiner holds the tuning fork by the stem between their thumb and first finger. The fork tines are tapped on a surface such as the examiner's knee or elbow, and placed on the patient's mastoid process and then close to the external auditory meatus. The patient is asked in which position is the sound the loudest?	Positive Rinne test: the tuning fork is loudest when positioned near the external auditory meatus. Negative Rinne test: the sound is loudest when the fork is placed on the mastoid process.
Otoscopic examination	An otoscope is used to examine the ear canal and tympanic membrane. The ear is gently pulled back up and out by the pinna to straighten the ear canal. The otoscope speculum is gently inserted into the ear to inspect the walls of the ear canal and the tympanic membrane.	A healthy tympanic membrane will look translucent or pearly coloured. If an infection is present, the tympanic membrane may appear pink, red or opaque. The tympanic membrane may bulge or show a perforation.
Audiometry	Audiometry tests the intensity and tone of sounds, balance issues and other issues related to the function of the inner ear. It assesses hearing levels at a range of frequencies. The patient is asked to listen to pure tones through a set of headphones at different levels of loudness and indicate when the sound is heard. The unit of measure for sound intensity is a decibel (dB).	Results are plotted on an audiogram, and degrees of hearing loss measured. Normal hearing will fall between 0–20 dB less than this indicates hearing loss and degree of loss.
Brainstem auditory evoked potential (BAEP)	A neurological test used to assess the auditory nerve to determine if changes to the auditory nerve are the cause of the hearing loss. Electrodes are connected to the patient's head or ears, and the patient will then listen to a series of clicks through a set of headphones. The neural response to the clicks are recorded on an electroencephalogram.	The amplitude of the signal is averaged and plotted against time and interpreted by a specialist.

Nursing management of patients with hearing impairment

Nursing care of patients with a hearing impairment is dependent on the type, cause, onset and duration of the loss or impairment. Effective communication is paramount in caring for individuals with a hearing impairment. Education and support include the patient and their family.

Emotional support is an essential factor in the care of these patients, especially if the hearing impairment has been newly diagnosed and will be permanent. Patients and their families may require additional support in the form of counselling to come to terms with the diagnosis and prognosis, and patient education is an essential nursing role (table 22.4).

TABLE 22.4 Hearing loss health education

Communication strategies	Prevention education
Minimise background noise; for example, turn the radio or TV off when speaking with patients	Encourage the use of earplugs in noisy situations
When talking to patients, face them at eye level to facilitate non-verbal communication utilising facial cues	Reduce exposure to excessive noise
Speak clearly but do not shout	Maintain hand hygiene and personal hygiene — keep ears clean
Take time to communicate	Advise not to use cotton tips to clean ears as this can push wax or foreign bodies further into the ear
Do not exaggerate lip and mouth movements as this causes distortion and can adversely affect lip-reading	Encourage attending regular hearing assessments
Patients may be proficient in lip-reading using sign language, writing or texting and these modes of communication are to be supported	Any changes in the patient's condition should be reported to their healthcare team
Review the condition of any hearing aids and check they are working correctly	

Approximately 39 children in every 10 000 Australians live with a degree of hearing loss. This is usually related to congenital conditions (Amplifon n.d.), including trauma during birth, childhood diseases, chronic ear infections. High-quality public healthcare and healthcare screenings have led to a lower percentage of childhood hearing loss in Australia than in much of the world (Amplifon n.d.). What is important is that people who are hearing impaired consider themselves part of a global community and do not consider themselves impaired but culturally different. Culture is concerned with our actions, beliefs and values systems. The deaf communities have distinctive characteristics. Some of these cultural characteristics are shared not only across Australia but globally. The recognition of this approach is important to healthcare providers who are caring for people in the deaf community.

Ear surgery

There are a number of surgeries that are performed on the ear. The nursing management pre and post-operatively will vary depending on the type of surgery that is performed. Many surgeries performed on the ear occur in outpatient clinics or day surgeries. See table 22.5 for more information.

TABLE 22.5 Overview of ear surgeries

Surgery	Type/indication
Acoustic neuroma surgery	Surgical procedure to remove a noncancerous tumour that develops on the vestibular nerve leading from your inner ear to the brain
Cochlear implant	A surgical procedure to implant an electronic device that helps provide sound to people with severe hearing loss

Congenital atresia ear reconstruction	A surgical procedure that is aimed are repairing parts of the ears anatomy, such as the ear canal, the tympanic membrane and the Ossicular chain
CyberKnife® radiosurgery	A surgical technique used to treat ear and hearing disorders related to brain conditions
Labyrinthootomy	A surgical procedure that removes remaining inner ear balance function causing vertigo and disequilibrium from a diseased ear
Myringotomy	A surgical procedure where an incision is made in the tympanic membrane, allowing drainage of fluid. Insertion of ear tubes helps to ventilate the ear and prevent fluid accumulation
Myringoplasty	A surgical procedure to repair tympanic membrane perforation. A graft made from tissue is used to repair the hole
Mastoidectomy	A surgical procedure used to remove air cells. Mastoid air cells may require removal due to infection or to facilitate the insertion of a cochlear implant
Osseointegrated bone conduction hearing system	A surgical procedure that anchors a bone hearing aid to the skull and allows for the transmission of sound through the bone to the inner ear
Ossiculoplasty	A surgical procedure performed to repair or reconstruct the ossicles with the intention of improving sound conduction and treat specific causes of hearing loss
Otologic laser procedures	A surgical procedure that uses lasers with micro-millimetre spot size, it is highly accurate and minimises trauma to the inner ear
Particle repositioning manoeuvre	A surgical procedure that redirects minute calcium crystals floating freely in the inner ear back into the inner ear
Stapedectomy/stapedotomy	A surgical procedure to treat a progressive hereditary condition of the temporal bone that can result in hearing loss
Tympanoplasty	A surgical procedure on the eardrum and middle ear bones to restore the mechanism for middle ear hearing

Source: University of Pittsburgh Medical Center (2021).

Nursing care for post-operative ear surgery includes:

- monitoring vital signs
- treating pain
- pressure bandages, which may be left in situ and should remain until instructed by medical staff to remove
- dissolvable foam packing, which may be used and should be left in situ — used to help protect grafts
- any ear tubes will eventually fall out of their own accord
- patient education to avoid increasing pressure to head and should avoid blowing nose or sneezing with mouth open
- avoiding swimming or getting water into ears when showering or washing.

22.2 The nose

LEARNING OBJECTIVE 22.2 Describe the anatomy and physiology of the nose, and the management of patients with nose disorders.

The human nose is part of the respiratory system and is our primary organ for smell. Air enters the body via the nose, hairs in the nose clean the air, and the air passes over the specialised cells of the olfactory system. The brain recognises and identifies the smells. The sense of smell is closely linked to memory and smell is highly emotive (Fifth Sense n.d.). The perfume industry is built around this concept. Unlike the loss of sight, the loss of smell is only apparent to the individual. One of the indicators of COVID-19 is a loss of smell. Research has shown that the loss of smell can indicate Parkinson's disease and Alzheimer's disease long before motor skill problems become apparent. It should be part of our holistic assessment of patients.

Anatomy and physiology of the nose

The nose has two main components. The external component is composed of:

- the nasal bone
- cartilage tip
- nares (nostrils).

And the internal component is composed of:

- the nasal cavity formed by the ethmoid, maxillae, lacrimal and palatine bones
- the nasal septum, which divides the nasal cavity into two
- the lateral nasal wall, which includes turbinates or fleshy protrusions from the nasal wall
- paranasal sinuses.

See figure 22.3 for an overview of the anatomy of the nose.

FIGURE 22.3 Anatomy of the nose

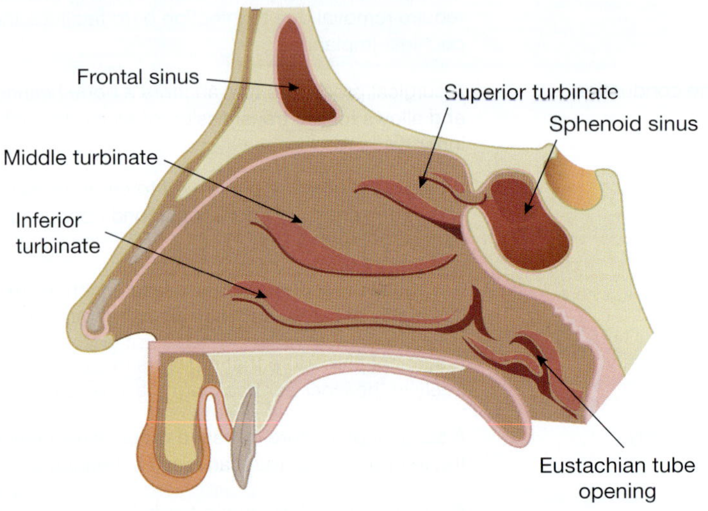

Source: Nair & Peate (2009) *Fundamentals of Applied Pathophysiology*, with kind permission from Wiley Blackwell.

The functions of the nose, which leads to the pharynx are to:

- facilitate the passage of air to and from the lungs
- warm, filter and moisten the incoming air
- be the sense organ for smell. The olfactory sense receptors are located on either side of the nasal septum in the superior part of the nasal cavity. These receptors are innervated by the olfactory nerve.
- facilitate speech sounds (nasal cavity).

Common disorders of the nose

Epistaxis

Epistaxis is bleeding from the nose and usually originates from the small blood vessels in the nose bursting. Epistaxis is classified as either an anterior or a posterior bleed, dependent on where the bleeding blood vessel is located. The most common bleed is an anterior bleed.

The causes of nose bleeds can be classified as local, systemic environmental, medication or idiopathic and can include:

- trauma
- nasal septal perforation or nasal septal abnormalities
- sinus tumours
- leukaemia
- thrombocytopenia
- anticoagulant therapy
- upper respiratory infection
- a genetic blood vessel disorder that can lead to haemorrhage such as Osler-Weber-Rendu syndrome (haemorrhagic telangiectasia) and haemophilia
- changes in the climate
- illicit drug use such as cocaine.

Epistaxis is often a simple and time-limited condition that resolves with simple interventions. In the case of severe bleeding, there is a risk of hypotension, tachycardia or hypovolaemic shock. Blood that does not flow out through the nostrils can pass into the nasopharynx and be either swallowed or expectorated. The patient can experience nausea and vomiting if large amounts of blood are swallowed.

The assessment of patients with epistaxis involves:

- a health history, including an assessment of the current nosebleed (duration, severity and what side the bleed is on), previous nose bleeds, as well as brief medical–surgical history including regular medications
- vital signs including pulse, blood pressure, respiration, oxygen saturation, temperature and pain score
- physical examination the nose is examined for appearance noting presence of swelling, bleeding, discharge.

Patients should be advised to sit up with their head forward to prevent aspirating or swallowing blood. Bleeding can be controlled by applying pressure to the cartilaginous part of the nose below the bridge. If the patient can tolerate it, an ice pack can be applied. For uncontrolled bleeding, dependent on the bleed site, the physician may insert either an anterior or a posterior nasal pack. A nasal pack may be either a gauze pack or an inflatable balloon. If the nasal pack is inserted, the patient will be instructed to mouth breathe. Nursing care following nasal pack insertion is outlined in table 22.6.

TABLE 22.6 Nursing care of patients following nasal pack insertion

Nursing care	Rationale
Provide patient and their family with complete information on the procedure	Reduces anxiety
Advise the patient to inform you of any discomfort, breathing problems or concerns	Supports early detection of deterioration
Administer sedative as prescribed	Relieves anxiety — if the patient is anxious and a sedative has not been prescribed, consult with the physician in charge of the case
Place patient in semi-fowlers position and ensure they are comfortable	Supports the pack to stay in position and helps to keep airway open
Monitor for signs of hypoxia and airway occlusion, including vital signs: pulse, blood pressure temperature, respiratory rate, oxygen saturation and pain	Supports early detection of deterioration
Pay specific attention to signs and symptoms of airway constriction, including skin colour (cyanosis), agitation, changes in level of consciousness, difficulty breathing, wheeze, stridor	
Check the position of the pack	Ensure the pack is in the optimal position to stop bleeding and is not blocking the airway
Provide cool fluids A soft or liquid diet is recommended	Hot fluids may cause local blood vessel dilatation and increase bleeding
Packing to remain until physician's instructions, usually 48–72 hours	Ensures bleeding has stopped

Further management includes:

- electrical or chemical cauterisation
- arterial ligation surgery, for example, septoplasty with ethmoidal ligation
- radiological embolisation for patients with poor medical health.

Chronic sinusitis

Sinusitis is inflammation and swelling of the sinuses, usually caused by an infection. Sinusitis can be acute or chronic and is characterised by nasal congestion, facial pain, altered hearing and nasal discharge, which can be posterior or anterior. In chronic sinusitis, symptoms are the same as those of acute sinusitis for around 12 weeks despite active treatment. Complications from chronic sinusitis are rare but can include:

- orbital cellulitis
- orbital abscesses
- visual changes
- cavernous sinus thrombosis
- systemic infection.

Assessment of chronic sinusitis involves:

- patient health history
- a detailed history of the condition, including symptoms and duration
- physical assessment
- vital signs including blood pressure, pulse, temperature, respiratory rate, oxygen saturation and pain.

The initial management is like that of acute sinusitis, including regular nasal irrigation with normal saline and topical steroids. However, an unresolved bacterial nasal infection and orbital cellulitis that is unresponsive to antibiotic treatment may indicate a need for surgery, such as functional endoscopic sinus surgery. Sinus surgery involves removing the damaged mucosal tissue and enlarging the nasal openings, enhancing drainage.

Deviated nasal septum

A deviated nasal septum occurs when the nasal septum is displaced to one side, making one nasal passage smaller than the other. This can result from developmental problems of the septum or from external trauma. The condition may be asymptomatic, or it may present with the following signs and symptoms:

- unilateral nasal obstruction of varying degrees
- sinus infection or otitis media
- hypertrophy of the unaffected side of the nose.

Assessment involves:

- a detailed health history including symptoms and duration
- physical assessment
- vital signs including blood pressure, pulse, temperature, respiratory rate, oxygen saturation and pain.

Depending on the underlying cause and severity of the deviation, surgery may be required. The main surgical procedures are septoplasty (straightening of the nasal septum) and submucosal resection. Turbinates, small structures in the nose that cleanse and humidify the air as it passes through the nostrils into the lungs, can become enlarged (Stanford Health Care 2020). This makes it difficult to breathe through the nose. Submucosal resection of turbinates reduces the size of the turbinates and opens the airway. It may be done to:

- relieve a blockage in the nasal passages
- improve breathing through the nose by increasing airflow and moisture
- reduce a postnasal drip and excess drainage.

Nasal injuries

Nasal injuries can be caused by external trauma and foreign bodies. Small children are more likely to experience nasal obstruction from the insertion of foreign bodies such as paper, toys, beads, food into their nasal cavity.

Signs and symptoms of nasal injury will vary depending on the type of injury but may include:

- visible foreign body
- lacerations and swelling
- bleeding
- pain
- discharge from the nasal cavity.

The type of injury will dictate the assessments and subsequent management. Assessments will generally involve:

- a detailed health history
- a detailed history of the current presentation to include signs and symptoms and duration of the presenting problem
- vital signs including blood pressure, pulse, temperature, respiratory rate, oxygen saturation and pain
- physical examination of the nose and assessment of airway
- X-ray (for nasal trauma).

Management will vary depending on the type of injury. Foreign bodies will need to be removed and can be done with small forceps or cerumen loop. Sometimes a small suction catheter can be used. If the patient is old enough to follow instructions, encourage patient to block one nostril and then blow out the other nostril to help dislodge the foreign body. Nasal fractures are usually conservatively treated. Analgesia and ice therapy for pain and swelling are indicated after nasal trauma.

Tumours of the nose

The primary causes of nasal and sinus cancers are chemicals and carcinogenic substances such as those used in the furniture, textiles, shoe, paint and chemical industries.

Nasal tumours include:

- juvenile nasopharyngeal angiofibromas
- inverting papillomas
- malignant tumours of the paranasal sinus cavities.

Risk factors for nasal tumours include:

- infection with human papillomavirus (HPV)
- male and older than 40 years
- smoking
- exposure to workplace chemicals or dust, such as those found in:
  - furniture-making
  - sawmill work
  - carpentry
  - shoemaking
  - metal-plating
  - flour mill or bakery work (National Cancer Institute n.d.).

The signs and symptoms of nasal and paranasal tumours can include:

- nasal congestion
- facial pain
- blockage to one side of the nose
- bleeding.

A range of tests and assessments can be used in the diagnoses of nasal tumours, including:

- a full patient history including family history
- nasal endoscopy and biopsy: a small camera is used to visualise the inside of the nose. If abnormalities are detected, a biopsy will be taken for further analysis
- medical imaging: CT and MRI scans may be used to identify any abnormalities such as a mass, bony obstruction or erosion.

The management of patients undergoing surgery for nasal tumours will vary depending on the procedure being performed (see figure 22.4). Patients may require further treatment such as chemotherapy and or radiation.

FIGURE 22.4 Nursing management of post-operative nasal surgery

Assessment

- Monitor vital signs.
- Maintain hand and personal hygiene to reduce the potential for infection.
- Review signs or symptoms of infection such as redness, irritation and fever.
- Perform a swallow test to determine the need for a liquid or soft diet.
- Document assessment and treatments.

Pain management

- Support with non-pharmacological pain management, positioning, relaxation techniques, reassurance and low lightening.
- Administer analgesia and medications as prescribed.

Wound care

- Assess for crusting of the sinus and/or nasal cavity.
- Inspect the incision site for signs of symptoms of infection and healing.
- Monitor wound drainage and document the amount, colour and presence of mucus.
- Monitor for signs of **cerebrospinal fluid (CSF)** leakage and escalate care if noted.

Sensory and/or motor deficits assessment
- Decreased vision
- Diplopia (double vision)
- Epiphora (excessive tear production)
- Trismus (jaw clenching)
- Facial paraesthesia
- Pain

Patient management
- Refer to counselling services and support groups — patients may experience anxiety due to the diagnosis and concerns about an altered body image facial incision, sinus removal or facial disfigurement.
- Administer analgesia and medications as prescribed.
- Refer to a speech therapist to determine any speech difficulties.
- Increase humidification with a bedside humidifier, steam or nasal saline spray.

Patient education
- Advise not blow nose for 10 days post-operatively — sniff the secretions in and either swallow or expectorate them.
- Reiterate the importance of attending post-operative appointments with the medical team, including the surgical team, speech therapist and general practitioner.
- Patients and their families may need to be instructed how to remove, clean and reinsert a palate obturator or how to camouflage defects with an eye patch or make-up, depending on the type of surgery.

22.3 The throat

LEARNING OBJECTIVE 22.3 Describe the anatomy and physiology of the throat, and the management of patients with throat disorders.

The throat also called the pharynx. The throat is a funnel-shaped tube that starts at the internal nares and extends partway down the neck. The throat acts as a passageway for air from the nasal cavity and mouth to the larynx, and a pathway for food. It acts as a resonating chamber for speech sounds and houses the tonsils.

Anatomy and physiology of the throat

The pharynx extends from the nose to the cricoid cartilage and is divided into three anatomical regions.

1. *The nasopharynx, which lies behind the nasal cavity, has openings to the auditory tubes and the internal nares.* The adenoids are situated in the posterior wall.
2. *The oropharynx forms the middle part of the pharynx and lies behind the oral cavity.* It extends from below the soft palate to the level of the hyoid bone and contains two pairs of tonsils: the palatine and lingual.
3. *The hypopharynx forms the lower part of the pharynx, beginning at the level of the hyoid bone.* It is the lower portion continuing anteriorly into the larynx and posteriorly into the oesophagus.

See figure 22.5 for more detail.

The larynx connects the pharynx with the trachea. The epiglottis covers the glottis during swallowing, preventing food and fluid from entering the trachea and into the lungs. The larynx, with vibrations of the vocal cords in conjunction with the pharynx, mouth, nasal cavity and paranasal sinuses, is responsible for voice production.

Common disorders of the throat

Laryngeal obstruction

Laryngeal obstruction is a narrowing or complete closure of the airway due to oedema or blockage of the airway. This is a life-threatening emergency event and must be resolved immediately. Causes include:

- acute laryngitis
- epiglottitis
- anaphylactic reaction
- oedema following endotracheal intubation
- laryngeal spasm
- urticaria
- inflammatory disease of the throat.

FIGURE 22.5 Anatomy of the throat

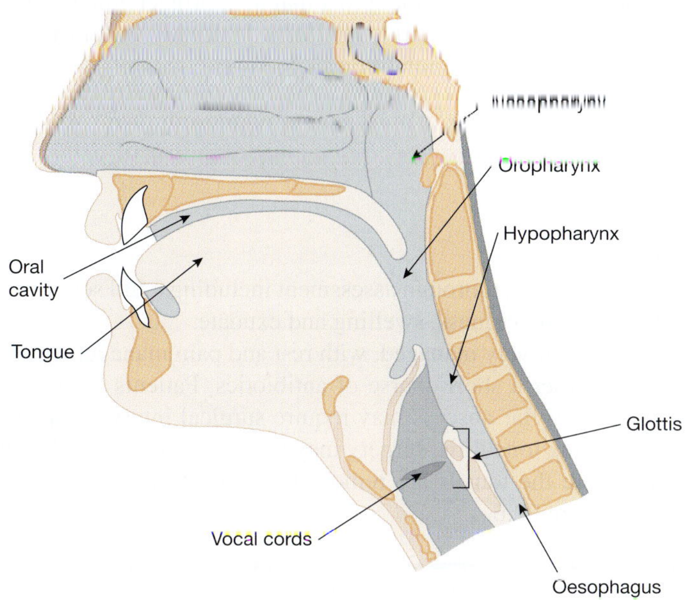

Source: Nair & Peate (2009) *Fundamentals of Applied Pathophysiology*, with kind permission from Wiley Blackwell.

Laryngeal obstruction can be mild or severe depending if the obstruction is partial or complete. It must be recognised that even a mild compromise can quickly deteriorate into a full obstruction. Signs and symptoms of laryngeal obstruction vary depending upon the cause and severity of the obstruction but can include:

- hoarse voice
- stridor
- drooling
- increased work of breathing
- cough
- agitation
- cyanosis
- tachycardia.

Laryngeal obstruction is a medical emergency. Early detection and intervention are vital to patient survival. Obstruction can occur gradually or rapidly. A rapid response or medical emergency team need to be called using facility protocol. Assessment is performed in a calm concise manner as not to distress the patient further. Assessment will involve a respiratory assessment including:

- respiratory rate
- oxygen saturation or end-tidal CO_2
- identification of respiratory difficulties such as nasal flaring
- the use of accessory muscles
- cyanosis
- decreased or absent breath sounds and chest movement
- a focused cardiovascular assessment and peripheral vascular system assessment (British Columbia Institute of Technology (BCIT) n.d.)
- collecting subjective data about diet, nutrition, exercise and stress levels
- patient's and the patient's family history of cardiovascular disease
- signs and symptoms of cardiovascular and peripheral vascular disease, such as peripheral oedema, shortness of breath (dyspnoea) and irregular pulse rate.

Management of a laryngeal obstruction will depend on the cause and severity of the obstruction. Nurses should focus on reassuring the patient and sitting them in an upright position. Patients with an airway obstruction can be very distressed, and portraying a calm manner is important to prevent the patient from panicking. Oxygen may need to be applied for acutely short of breath and hypoxic patients. Medications aimed at reducing swelling and opening the airways may be ordered depending on the cause of the obstruction. These may include adrenaline and corticosteroids. Close monitoring of the patient is required because deterioration can happen quickly, and the patient may require advanced airway management.

Tonsillitis

The tonsils are bilateral glands at the back of the throat that help protect you against infection (S. G. o. V. Department of Health & Human Services 2021a). Tonsillitis is usually caused by a virus or bacteria, and can follow a cold. Tonsillitis is a common condition in paediatric patients however can occur in adults. Symptoms include:

- sore throat
- hoarse voice
- fever
- lack of appetite
- pain with swallowing.

The patient with tonsillitis require a thorough assessment including a full set of vital signs and a focused assessment of the throat, noting any redness, swelling and exudate.

Tonsillitis is generally conservatively managed, with rest and pain management. If a bacterial infection is suspected, the doctor may order a short course of antibiotics. Patients with signs of severe infection or complications such as peritonsillar abscess may require surgical intervention such as drainage of the abscess. In patients with recurring tonsillitis, surgery may be considered. Tonsillectomy is the name given to the surgical procedure where the tonsils are removed. The post-operative care of the patient after a tonsillectomy is outlined in figure 22.6.

FIGURE 22.6 Nursing management of patients after tonsillectomy

Assessment
- Monitor vital signs
- Monitor for post-operative complication such as post-tonsillectomy bleed

Pain management
- Regular pain assessments
- Administer analgesia as ordered

Patient management
- Nutrition and hydration
- Monitor hydration and nutrition status
- Encourage soft diet and regular sips of water
- Avoid hot or spicy foods and fluids
- Support patient with a dietary referral
- Speech pathology should review the patient for the ability to swallow

Patient education
- Provide discharge education, including monitoring signs of complications such as secondary haemorrhage, which can occur 5–10 days post-operative, or infection
- Provide diet and exercise advice — patients should avoid strenuous exercise and avoid hard, crunchy or spicy foods

Throat tumours

Head and neck cancer relates to cancers that occur in the throat (pharynx and larynx), nose, sinuses and mouth. The number of head and neck cancers diagnosed in Australia is increasing due mainly to Australia's increasing and ageing population.

Throat (pharyngeal) tumours can occur in the oropharynx, nasopharynx or hypopharynx and can be benign or malignant. Tumours are staged according to the TNM (tumour, node and metastasis) system. Primary causes of throat cancer are smoking, alcohol, carcinogens, nutrition and riboflavin deficiency. Signs and symptoms include:

- painless mass
- enlarged cervical nodes
- hoarseness
- pain on swallowing (odynophagia)
- referred pain
- dysphagia
- weight loss.

Assessment for throat tumours includes a detailed health history, including risk factors and family history of cancer.

Physical assessment should include:

- vital signs, including pulse, blood pressure, temperature, oxygen saturation and pain score
- weight loss and nutritional status
- a focused assessment of the throat and airway.

Diagnostic tests include:

- laryngoscopy
- chest X-ray
- barium swallow
- endoscopy
- CT and MRI scans.

Management will depend on the type and location of the tumour and the patient's preference. Surgical interventions may be required to resect (remove) the tumour. Reconstructive surgery may also be required if more extensive surgery is required to remove metastasis. Chemotherapy and radiation may also be required.

The nursing management is outlined in figure 22.7.

FIGURE 22.7 Nursing management of throat tumours

Assessment
- Monitor the vital signs. A drop in blood pressure and an increase in pulse rate may indicate blood loss.
- Observing for haemorrhage.
- Undertake tracheostomy care if necessary — temporary or permanent tracheostomy may have been inserted.
- Monitor for signs of respiratory distress:
  - Skin and mucosal colour — look for signs of cyanosis (blue tinge to the lips, skin). This is a late sign
  - Respiration rate, depth and pattern, and use of accessory muscles
  - Oxygen saturation or end-tidal CO_2 levels
  - Level of consciousness/Glasgow Coma Scale
  - Administer oxygen as prescribed

Pain management
- Assess pain level
- Administer prescribed analgesia

Nutrition and hydration
- Monitor hydration status and keep a strict fluid balance chart
- Administer IV as ordered
- Monitor nutritional status
- Monitor and assess for swallowing deficits
- Patients may require nasal gastric (NG) feeding and should be provided as directed by the medical staff, dietician and speech pathologist

Wound management
- Assess and monitor:
  - incision site
  - skin integrity
  - wound healing
  - wound drains.
- Care of the skin flap as per facility guidelines

Education and emotional support
- Provide emotional support, especially given the diagnosis and possible altered body image
- Educate patients on:
  - treatment and self care
  - monitoring for signs and symptoms of infection
  - diet and nutrition.

Laryngeal cancer

Laryngeal cancer is a cancer of the larynx and is the most common site for head and neck cancers (Koroulakis & Agarwal 2021). Cancer can develop in the three main areas of the larynx; the glottis, supraglottic or subglottic. The signs and symptoms will depend on the location of the cancer. Signs and symptoms can include:

- a lump in the throat
- otalgia
- dysphagia
- dyspnoea
- a cough
- enlarged lymph nodes.

A range of different diagnostic test can be used in the diagnosis of laryngeal cancer and can include:

- laryngoscopy
- endoscopy and biopsy
- medical imaging including X-ray, CT or MRI scans
- a detailed health history to include risk factors and family history of cancer
- physical assessment, including vital signs
- weight loss and nutritional status
- focused assessment on the throat and airway
- psychosocial assessment.

The location and staging of the cancer will influence management strategies. Surgical intervention may be required and can range from localised extraction to a total laryngectomy. The nursing management of a patient following a laryngectomy is outlined in figure 22.8.

FIGURE 22.8 Management of laryngeal cancer

Preoperative education and support

- Educate patients on:
  - the type and extent of the laryngectomy (partial or total)
  - the possibility of neck dissection and reconstructive surgery
- Provide emotional support to patients and their families
- Refer patients to the speech and language therapist
- Provide patients with information on support groups

Post-operative care

Assessment:

- Regular vital signs
- Monitor for signs of complications such as bleeding, airway obstruction and infection
- Administer analgesia as required

Wound care:

- Monitor for signs and symptoms of infection
- Monitor surrounding skin
- Monitor drains
- Document wound care

Special considerations

- Patients may experience altered communication — with a total laryngectomy, patients will experience an initial lack of ability to talk, and this will be frustrating for the patient and their family.
- Patients may require radical neck dissection for metastases, which will require reconstructive surgery and a referral and education.
- Patients may require further treatment such as radiation and chemotherapy and will need referrals and education.
- Patient may require a temporary or permanent tracheostomy, which will require referrals and patient and family education.

Tracheostomy

A tracheostomy is the formation of an opening into the front of the trachea and may be temporary, as seen in figure 22.9, or permanent. A permanent tracheostomy is usually performed in conjunction with a total laryngectomy as seen in figure 22.10. The relevant nursing management is outlined in figure 22.11.

FIGURE 22.9 Temporary tracheostomy

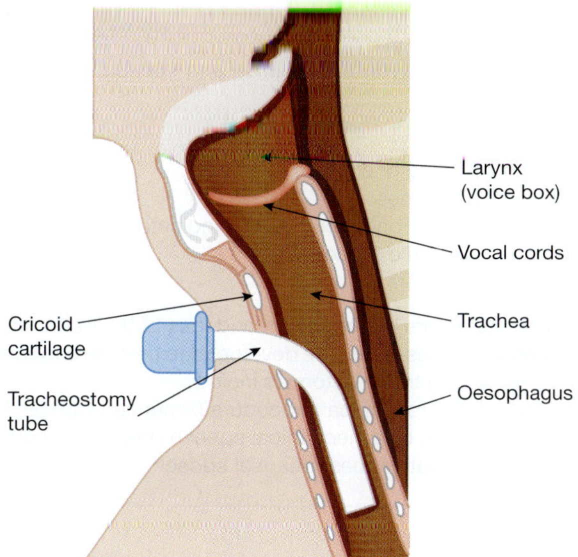

Source: Nair & Peate (2009) *Fundamentals of Applied Pathophysiology*, with kind permission from Wiley Blackwell.

FIGURE 22.10 Total laryngectomy

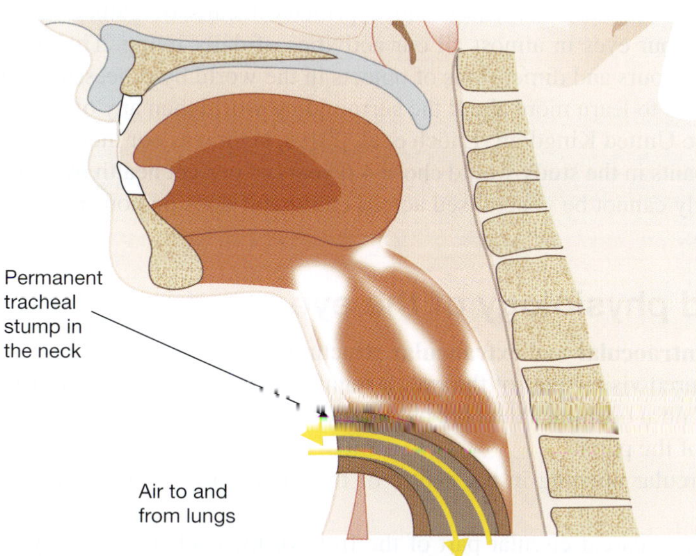

Source: Nair & Peate (2009) *Fundamentals of Applied Pathophysiology*, with kind permission from Wiley Blackwell.

FIGURE 22.11 Care of the patient with a tracheostomy

Assessment

- Assess the reason for the tracheostomy and the type of tracheostomy tube used
- Assess the availability of emergency equipment for example tracheal dilators, spare tracheostomy tubes and tracheostomy masks
- Assess vital signs
- Focused respiratory assessment
- Assess tracheostomy tube securement (Velcro straps, cotton ties, sutures)
- Assess cuff pressure (if cuff tubed in situ) as per policy usually every 8 hours
- Document assessment including tracheostomy care

Nutrition and hydration

- Assess hydration status — adequate hydration is important for secretion clearance
- Monitor input and output
- Patients may be initially nil by mouth (NBM) — dietitian and speech pathology may be required when re-introducing oral intake

Wound care

- Monitor the tracheostomy for bleeding or signs of infection
- Attend to dressing as per local guidelines
- Suctioning of a tracheostomy should only occur when indicated — signs of shortness of breath or secretion build up (suctioning is a sterile procedure)

Communication

Loss of ability to communicate as before the operation and loss of their normal voice can be distressing and alternative communication strategies should be developed to provide support to patients and families.

The current options for patients with tracheostomies include:

- tracheooesophageal puncture (TEP), a surgical procedure (American Cancer Society 2021)
- electrolarynx, which is the placement of a mechanical speech box in the mouth
- less frequently today, teaching the patient oesophageal speech.

22.4 The eye

LEARNING OBJECTIVE 22.4 Describe the anatomy and physiology of the eye, and the management of patients with eye disorders.

Sight is the most used of the five senses and a primary means of gathering information from our surroundings. We use our eyes in almost all our activities of daily living. The eye allows us to see and interpret the shapes, colours and dimensions of objects in the world by processing the light they reflect or emit. The eye allows us to learn more about the surrounding world than any of our other four senses. In a survey of adults in the United Kingdom (Enoch et al. 2019), sight was our most valued sense, followed by hearing. The participants in the study would chose 4.6 years of perfect health over 10 years of life without sight. While this study cannot be generalised across cultures it does demonstrate the importance of sight to the western culture.

Anatomy and physiology of the eye

The eye consists of **intraocular** and **extraocular** structures.

- *The iris.* The coloured visible part of the eye. It regulates the amount of light that enters the eye. Light enters through a central opening called the pupil. The iris controls the widening and narrowing (dilation and constriction) of the pupil.
- *The pupil.* The circular opening in the centre of the iris through which light passes into the lens of the eye.
- *The cornea.* The transparent circular part of the front of the eyeball. It is very sensitive to pain. The cornea does not contain blood vessels. The cornea refracts light as it enters the eye onto the lens and focuses it onto the retina.
- *The lens.* Enclosed in a thin transparent capsule and is located behind the pupil. The lens helps to refract incoming light and focus it onto the retina.
- *The choroid.* The middle layer of the eye between the retina and the sclera. It contains a pigment that absorbs excess light to prevent blurring of vision.
- *The ciliary body.* The part of the eye that connects the choroid to the iris.
- *The retina.* A light sensitive layer that lines the interior of the eye. It is made up of light-sensitive cells known as rods and cones. The human eye contains some 125 million rods and six to seven million cones. The rods and cones are necessary for seeing in dim light. However, they function best in bright light. The rods and cones are essential for receiving a sharp image and for distinguishing colours.
- *The macula.* A yellow spot on the retina at the back of the eye that surrounds the fovea.
- *The fovea.* Forms a small indentation at the centre of the macula and is the area with the greatest concentration of cone cells. When the eye is directed at an object, the part of the image that is focused on the fovea is the image most accurately registered by the brain.

- *The optic disc.* The visible (when the eye is examined) portion of the optic nerve, also found on the retina. The optic disc identifies the start of the optic nerve, where messages from cone and rod cells leave the eye via nerve fibres to the optic centre of the brain. This area is also known as the 'blind spot'. *The optic nerve.* Leaves the eye at the optic disc and transfers all the visual information to the brain.
- *The sclera.* The white part of the eye, a tough covering with which the cornea forms the external protective coat of the eye (Moorfield Public Hospital 2017).

An overview of the major anatomical features is illustrated in figure 22.12.

FIGURE 22.12 Anatomy of the eye

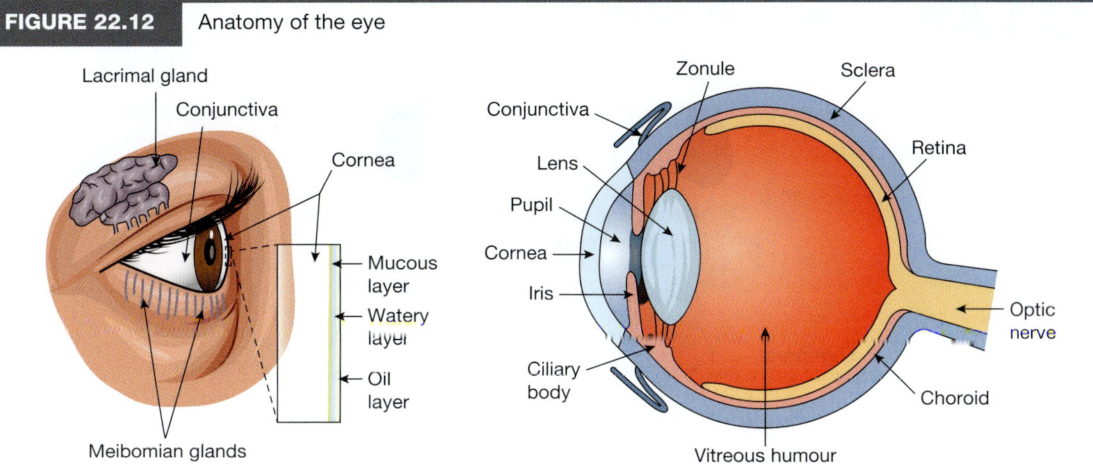

Source: American Academy of Ophthalmology (2021).

Sight

Light is reflected by an object into the eye and passes through the lens. The lens then projects an inverted image of the object on to the retina at the back of the eye by accommodation (which focuses the image). The light rays are refracted (bent) as they pass through the cornea, aqueous humour, lens and vitreous humour, converging at a point in the retina. The signals produced by the rod and cone cells in the retina, travel to the brain through the optic nerve. The two optic nerves meet at the optic chiasma, where axons from the nasal side of each retina cross to the opposite side and join axons from the temporal side of the retina of the other eye. These pairs continue as the left and right optic tracts. The crossing of the axons results in each optic tract carrying information from both eyes. The nerves continue to the thalamus, where projections extend to the visual areas in the occipital lobe of the cerebral cortex (figure 22.13). The brain interprets the image so that the person perceives it as it occurs.

Common disorders of the eye

According to the Australian Institute of Health and Welfare, in 2017, some 13 million Australians have one or more chronic eye conditions (Australian Bureau of Statistics 2018). Chronic eye conditions vary in presentation, treatment and outcomes; however, most are more common in the ageing population. In 2017–18, chronic eye conditions affected 93 per cent of people aged 65 and over. Females have a higher prevalence of chronic eye conditions than males at 59 per cent and 51 per cent, respectively.

Visual impairment

Visual impairment varies from mild to extreme and can be immediate or progressive, depending on the cause of the impairment. Visual impairment is broadly divided into:

- sudden loss (trauma, retinal detachment, vitreous haemorrhage, acute angle-closure glaucoma and retinal vein/artery occlusion)
- gradual loss (cataracts, chronic angle-closure glaucoma, age-related macular degeneration [AMD] and diabetic retinopathy).

An overview of the nursing considerations for providing care to the visually impaired is as follows.

- Orientate patients to the ward environment (the position of the bed, toilet facilities, tv, call bell, etc.).
- Describe the activities going on around patients.
- Introduce yourself as you enter the room and inform patients when you are leaving.
- Identify potential hazards.

- Replace items in same place.
- Explain loud noises to avoid unnecessary worry and concern.
- Describe the position of food on the plate in terms of a clock face (for example, your potato is at 3 p.m., etc.).
- Allow patients to hold your arm when assisting them with walking. Do not hold their arm. Describe the environment as you walk (e.g. 'there are two steps ahead').
- Ask patients if they require assistance (Vision Australia n.d.).

FIGURE 22.13 Visual pathways and visual fields

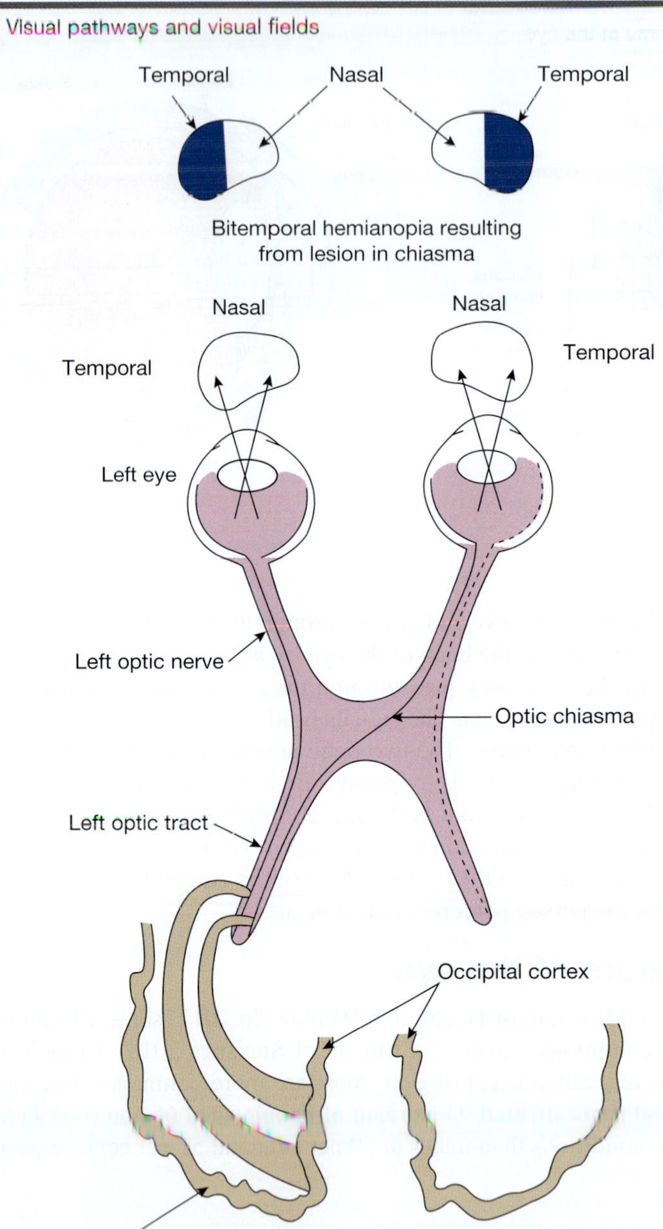

Source: Dougherty & Lister (2011), with kind permission of Wiley Blackwell.

Glaucoma

When the optic nerve is damaged, there are a number of eye diseases that can result. Because the deterioration of sight happens slowly, a diagnosis may not be made for some time. Glaucoma is defined as optic nerve disease with changes on the optic disc and defects in the visual field often associated with raised intraocular pressure (National Institute for Health and Clinical Excellence 2009; Hodge & Roberts 2003). Glaucoma is broadly divided into acute and chronic forms.

In Australia, up to 90 per cent of people diagnosed with glaucoma have primary open angle glaucoma (POAG). This condition begins with gradual loss of peripheral vision, and diagnosis is often not made until significant vision is lost.

If a person has acute angle glaucoma (ACG), it is a medical emergency. ACG is caused by angle narrowing and prolonged raised intraocular pressure, resulting in unilateral ischaemic optic nerve damage. Symptoms can include severe eye pain, blurred vision, visual disturbances (seeing a halo around a light) headache, nausea and vomiting (Glaucoma Australia 2021).

Chronic glaucoma is a progressive disease characterised by chronic raised intraocular pressure resulting in optic nerve damage.

An overview of the signs and symptoms, assessment and management of the forms of glaucoma is provided in table 22.7.

TABLE 22.7 **Overview of glaucoma**

	Signs and symptoms	Assessment and diagnostic tests	Management	Nursing management
Primary acute angle-closure glaucoma	Severe pain Redness Blurring of vision Nausea Vomiting A general feeling of being unwell	Patient assessment and history Vital signs Visual acuity testing with a Snellen chart to determine the clarity of distance vision Diagnostic tests: • Tonometry • Fundoscopy • Gonioscopy	Medical management aims to reduce intraocular pressure, thus limiting ischaemic damage. Interventions include medications or surgical interventions A peripheral iridotomy using YAG (yttrium aluminium garnet) laser therapy may be required once the inflammation has subsided; this creates an alternative drainage channel for the aqueous flow. It may also be performed prophylactically on the non-affected eye.	Ensure the patient's comfort. Provide analgesia as required. Monitor the patient, including ongoing pain assessments and intraocular pressure. Monitor the response to treatment. Alert medical staff if symptoms persist.
Chronic open-angle glaucoma	Vague symptoms with: • peripheral visual loss • mild headaches • difficulty focusing on near objects. A lack of symptoms until the disease is advanced	Patient assessment and history Assess vital signs Visual acuity testing Diagnostic tests: • Tonometry • Fundoscopy • Gonioscopy	The aim is to preserve vision and prevent deterioration. This requires life-long monitoring and treatment adherence.	Patient education and support.

Diabetic retinopathy

Diabetic retinopathy is a condition caused by chronically elevated blood glucose levels, which damage the retinal blood vessels (Bhavsar 2021). Damage to the retinal blood vessels can lead to progressive deterioration in sight. Diabetic retinopathy often presents with little to no symptoms, but when the symptoms occur, they can include blurred vison, floaters, which are small shadows that float across the eye and decreased visual acuity. Control of diabetes and maintaining the glycaemic haemoglobin (A1C HbA1c) level in the six to seven per cent range are the goals in the optimal management of diabetic retinopathy. Assessments include:

- a detailed patient health history
- vital signs, including blood pressure, pulse, temperature, respiratory rate, oxygen saturation and pain
- blood glucose level

- pathology investigations, including fasting glucose and HbA1c
- radiology investigation, including fluorescein angiography, optical coherence tomography and b-scan ultrasonography.

Corneal disorders

The cornea is the translucent surface at the front of the eye and focuses light onto the retina to form a visual image. Corneal disorders can include keratoconus, usually a bilateral eye condition that affects the cornea's shape, causing it to bulge outward, or corneal ulceration, which can be caused by trauma or infection. Signs and symptoms of corneal disorders can include:

- pain
- the sensation of a foreign body
- blurred or reduced vision
- photophobia
- watering of the eye
- corneal scarring or perforation after long-term damage.

The management of corneal disorders will depend upon the cause. Most corneal disorders will be treated in the outpatient setting and may include antibiotic eyedrops and analgesia as required. Patients may also receive relief while wearing dark glasses. The patient should be educated on not rubbing the eye or using contact lenses until the cornea has healed and advised by a doctor.

Cataracts

A cataract is a decrease in opacity or clouding of the lens leading to interference with the transmission of light to the retina and a decreased ability to perceive images clearly. Causes for cataracts can include congenital factors, trauma, ocular inflammation and some medications, such as long-term corticosteroids.

Signs and symptoms of cataracts include:

- a variable density of the cataract
- decreased visual acuity
- difficulty adjusting between light and dark environments
- a condition that may be bilateral unless related to eye trauma
- sensitivity to glare
- an inability to distinguish colour hues
- pupils that appear cloudy grey or white.

An illustration of the before and after of a cataract removal can be seen in figure 22.14.

FIGURE 22.14 Eye before and after cataract removal

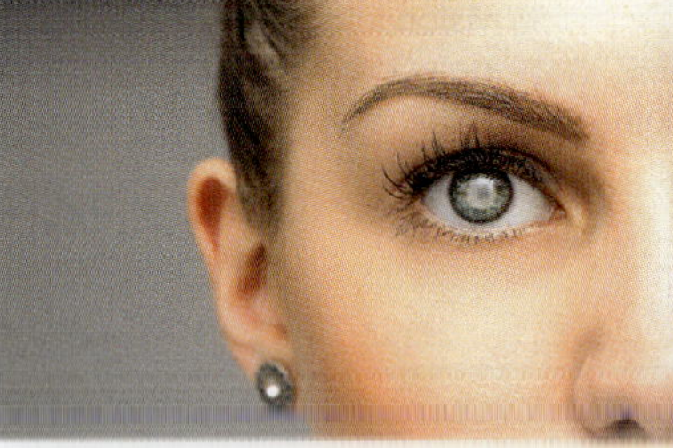

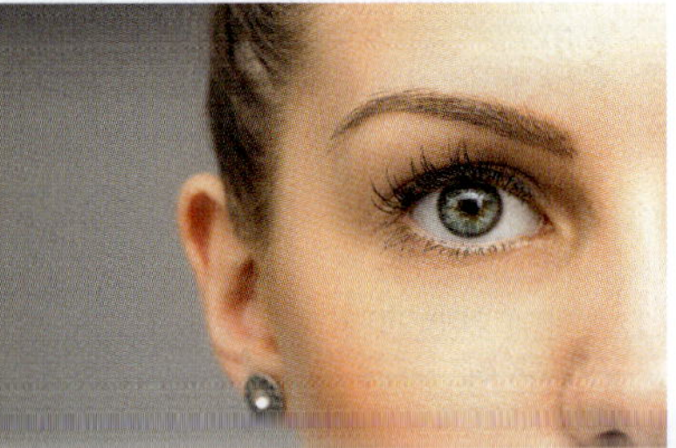

As with other types of eye conditions, the patient with cataracts or suspected cataracts will need a thorough assessment, including the current presentation and symptoms, patient history and a physical assessment of the eye itself.

Cataracts can be removed surgically. The most common form of cataract surgery is phacoemulsification. In most cases, cataract surgery is performed as a day procedure, under procedural sedation, and the patient is discharged home the same day. Patient education is important and will be dependent on the specialist's recommendations. These include:

- wearing an eye shield at night for protection
- avoiding activities that could increase ocular pressure
- monitoring for complications such as infection.

Eye trauma

Eye trauma can come in many forms, from a foreign body to a direct impact to the eye. Other forms of eye trauma include ocular burns, which can be chemical injuries (alkaline and acid) or radiant injuries caused by heat, radiation or electricity. Signs and symptoms of eye trauma will vary depending on the underlying cause but can include:

- vital signs — pulse, blood pressure, temperature, oxygen saturation and pain
- redness
- swelling
- loss of vision
- changes to the cornea
- visible foreign bodies
- bleeding and bruising.

As with other types of eye conditions, the patient with eye trauma will need a thorough assessment, including the current presentation and symptoms, patient history and a physical assessment of the eye itself. Investigations may include X-rays or CT scans in the case of trauma or when there is suspicion of an ocular penetrating foreign body. The management of eye trauma will be based on the underlying cause. Ongoing assessment of visual acuity and pain management is essential for patients experiencing eye trauma.

Foreign body

If a foreign body is lodged in the cornea, medical treatment will include the following.

- A vision test to locate the foreign body.
- Once the foreign body has been located, the eye will be numbed with anaesthetic eye drops.
- If the foreign body is central or deep, an ophthalmologist will be called to remove the object.
- The eye may be washed with saline to flush out any dust and dirt.
- X-rays may be required to find an object that has entered the eyeball or orbit.
- The eye may require an eye patch to allow it to rest and scratches to heal.
- Patient should be advised not to drive until the eye patch is removed and vision has returned to normal and to ensure they attend follow up appointments.

An example of a foreign body in the eye is illustrated in figure 22.15.

FIGURE 22.15 Foreign body in the eye

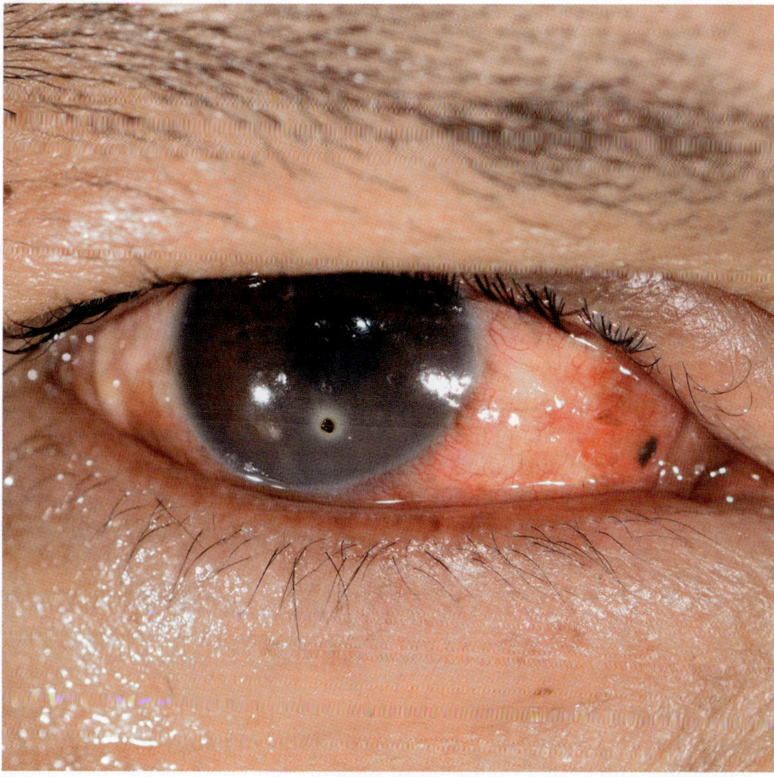

Penetrating wounds

Penetrating wounds require surgery with immediate care focused on pain management and protecting the eye from further injury. A sterile gauze or an eye pad is placed over the eye to prevent further damage. If a foreign body is embedded in or sticking out of the eye, the object is left in situ until an ophthalmologist can be seen. Patients may require analgesia, sedation, an antiemetic and prophylactic intravenous antibiotic.

Chemical burns

Chemical burns are flushed with copious amounts of normal saline. Topical anaesthetic will be applied for pain and support inspection and irrigation of the eye. During irrigation, the fluid is directed from the inner canthus of the eye to the outer canthus. The patient's head should be slightly turned to the affected side to prevent contamination of the unaffected eye. Irrigation is continued until the pH of the eye is normal (use pH paper to test this and ensure the range is 7.2–7.4). A topical antibiotic ointment is applied following irrigation.

Retinal detachment

Retinal detachment is a condition in which the retina detaches from the back of the eye. Retinal detachment can be caused by trauma; however, it can also be spontaneous. This is a time-critical emergency and requires immediate attention. Signs and symptoms can vary and patients may report:

- floaters — irregular dark lines or spots in the visual field
- flashing lights
- blurred vision with progressive deterioration
- a sensation of a curtain falling across the field of vision
- if the macula is involved, a loss of central vision

An illustration of retinal detachment can be seen in figure 22.16.

FIGURE 22.16 Retinal detachment

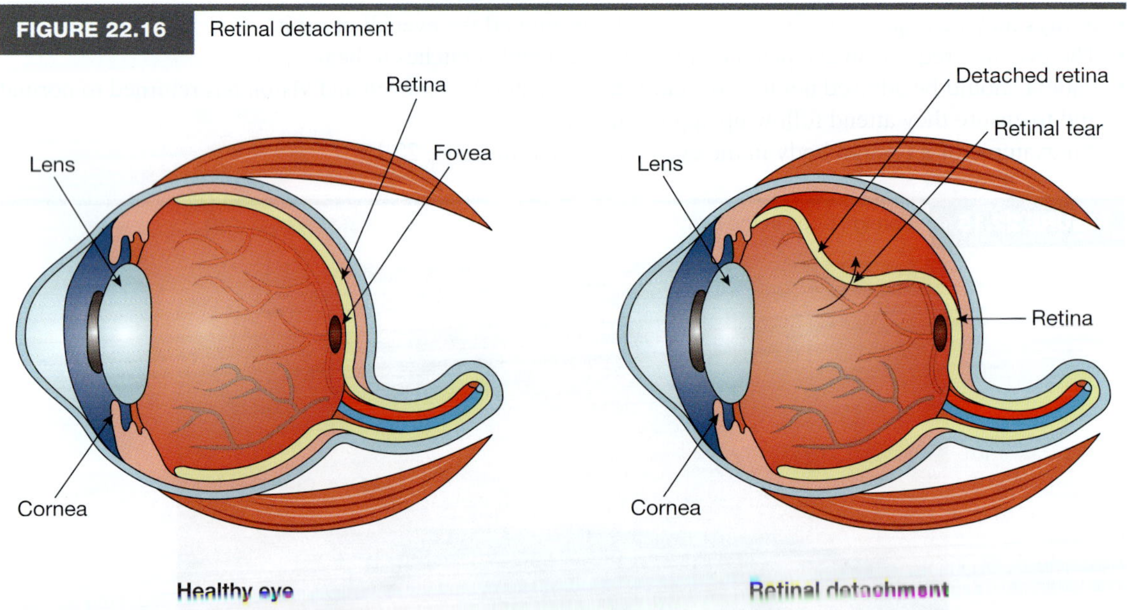

As with other types of eye conditions, the patient with retinal detachment or suspected retinal detachment will need a thorough assessment, including the presenting signs and symptoms, patient history, vital signs and a focused assessment of the eye, including visual acuity testing.

The management of retinal detachment varies depending on the cause. Providing patient comfort and ongoing monitoring is essential. Patients may require surgery to repair the detachment and could include a procedure known as 'scleral buckling' where the retina is reattached or a vitrectomy — replacement of the vitreous gel with gas, air or silicone oil, which helps to restore normal pressure in the eye.

Laser surgery

The use of lasers in ENT and eye surgery has become common place in healthcare practice (Jena Surgical 2021). With the advancement of laser sources, surgical **otolaryngology** and **ophthalmology** approach has been transformed. Approximately 75 per cent of patients with new larynx cancers and 50 per cent of patients with new mouth or pharynx cancers may be eligible for laser surgery. Laser surgery allows the specialist to perform minimally invasive, highly-precise surgery, suitable for a wide range of treatments for diseases of ENT and eye (Lexington Clinic 2021). Lasers are used to improve or correct myopia (short-sightedness), hypermetropia (long sightedness) and astigmatism (uneven curvature of the eye's surface) (S. G. o. V. Department of Health & Human Services 2021b). The first laser sculpting procedures for eyes were performed more than 30 years ago. Advantages of laser surgery include reduced post-operative pain, less scarring and fewer wound problems, all of which support a reduced hospital stay. One of the most important advantages of laser surgery is that it offers an improved quality of life. Laser surgery can help avoid trouble eating and tasting, progressive difficulty swallowing, loss of voice or speech, neck and shoulder disfigurement, and often tracheostomies.

22.5 Patient-centred care of the ENT and eye patient

LEARNING OBJECTIVE 22.5 Apply patient-centred care to care of the patient with conditions affecting the ear, nose, throat and eye.

Patient-centred care is care that values the patient and their family and considers the patient and their family as integral to planning and decision on care planning. The patient and their family are at the centre of all care and care is organised around the patient as opposed to around the schedules of the health care service. Patient-centred care will involve placing the patient in an environment where they feel safe, are provided with privacy and confidentiality, and supported with clear communication. When nursing patients who have diseases or disorders of the ENT and eye we must recognise that these organs affect how we interact with the rest of the world. The anxiety and confusion that can result from this must be understood and considered by the healthcare provider.

Levett-Jones et al. (2009, p. 5160) stated that the clinical reasoning cycle provided a framework for the nurse to use knowledge, skills and attitudes to 'collect cues, processes the information, come to an understanding of a patient issue, plan and implement interventions, evaluate outcomes, and then reflect on and learn from the process'. It is essential to realise that this is an ongoing cyclic process used with every patient every time they are met.

The eight steps or stages of the clinical reasoning cycle are as important in the care of the patient who is experiencing problems with their ear, nose, throat or eyes. Suppose we apply this to providing care to a patient presenting with a retinal detachment. We are aware that this can be a time-sensitive emergency, so we need to notify the ophthalmologist prior to taking a lengthy history. We also need to place the patient in a quiet area with low lighting and reassure them and their families.

We can collect a health history and a history of the presenting problem from a family member if present. If the patient has come on their own, we can take a brief history and a set of vital signs while we wait for the arrival of the specialist. If the patient is in pain, we need to request pain relief from the physician and treat the pain. If the patient will be treated in the operating room or need an anaesthetic we need to prepare the patient with informed consent, gowns, and check on their last meal, etc.

In this situation, we identified the problem and prioritised care. We recognised that this is an urgent situation and needs immediate care. Our goal will be to treat the pain and support a team approach to diagnosis and treatment. Ensure the patient and their family are fully informed of the situation and their choices.

We will then evaluate the care and reflect if we should have done anything differently. If we employ the clinical reasoning cycle to support and plan our care for the ENT and eye patient, there is less likelihood of missing important information to improve outcomes.

CASE STUDY 22.1

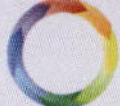

Nursing care of a patient complaining of a sore throat

Aiden Stephens, a 19-year-old male, presented to the urgent care clinic with complaints of a sore throat. Aiden had a negative COVID-19 test two days prior, but the sore throat persists. He is accompanied by his mother. Aiden is a fit and healthy male who plays soccer regularly and works out to keep his fitness levels up. He does not smoke and drinks a couple of beers with his friends on the weekend. He was unable to play soccer on the weekend and did not feel well enough to go out with his friends.

Vital signs and observations on presenting to urgent care were:

- pulse: 50 beats per minute
- blood pressure: 122/74 mmHg
- temperature: 38.9°C
- respirations: 15 breaths per minute
- pain score 8/10 (I have a sore throat. It hurts to eat and drink hot drinks. Cold drinks really help. It is almost a burning pain. It is at the back of my throat. It is not radiating anywhere. It started last night.)
- medications: Nil
- vaccinations are up to date; however, he has not yet had a COVID-19 vaccination
- previous surgeries: Nil
- allergies: Nil

Question

Use the clinical reasoning cycle to describe what action you would take as the nurse caring for this patient. Which care would be prioritised?

Answer

- *Step 1: Consider the patient.* Aiden Stephens, a fit and usually healthy 19-year-old male.
- *Step 2: Collect cues/information*. Include subjective and objective data here. The subjective will include what the patient tells you, the appearance of the patient, and their past medical history. Objective data will include objective or measurable information such as the vital signs, blood tests
- *Step 3 Process information.* Separate the relevant and irrelevant data — cluster the clues together to formulate an inference about the patient. What is the current situation? What additional vital signs or tests need to be undertaken?
- *Step 4: Identify problems/issues.* Nursing problems or diagnosis should be listed here, Pain, Discomfort, Anxiety
- *Step 5: Establish goals*. Goals of care for Aiden should be to manage the pain or discomfort and reassure the patient and their family. A medical diagnosis needs to be established by his attending physician.
- *Step 6: Take action*. Provide the care that is required to meet the established goals. For example, provide cool soothing drinks and pain relief as ordered.

  Do a top-to-toe assessment and blood tests to rule out infection — use a lighted instrument to view the throat, ears and nasal passage. Palpate the next for swollen lymph nodes and perform a respiratory assessment.

  Repeat COVID-19 test.

  Consider acid reflux or GERD and prepare patient for possible. Complete full physical examination to rule out GERD. Discuss with the health care team the need for a procedure such as a endoscopy, bariums swallow etc.
- *Step 7: Evaluate outcomes*. Were the best outcomes achieved? Was pain and discomfort alleviated? Was a diagnosis determined and was the patient prepared for any further care? In this case we will be working to alleviate the symptoms and find a definitive cause of the problem. It must be a team approach with medical, nursing and possibly dietary involved.
- *Step 8: Reflect on the process and new learning*. Reflect on any aspects of care that could have been done better. What went well, what did not go as well as hoped.

CASE STUDY 22.2

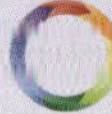

Nursing care of a patient suffering from loss of vision

Don Fredericks is a 61-year-old Caucasian male. Mr Fredricks has presented to the emergency room with a loss of vision in his left eye. He reports having had cataract surgery in his left eye 3 weeks ago. Mr Fredricks states that it started yesterday morning and has become progressively worse. He describes it as a curtain coming up over his eye, and the curtain has now affected his central vision. Mr Fredericks said he experienced flashing lights and then floaters in the same eye a week ago. The patient has no complaints of pain, diplopia or other symptoms.

Mr Fredricks teaches at the local university. He is married with one son who lives in another state. Mr Fredricks has a medical history of hypertension, which is well controlled on medication. He has been diagnosed with osteoarthritis and had a right knee replacement in 2005. He is a non-smoker, drinks socially and does not use illicit drugs. He states that there is no family history of retinal detachment, glaucoma or blindness. His mother suffered from macular degeneration.

Vital signs upon presentation were:

- pulse: 85 beats ber minute

- blood pressure: 140/90 mmHg
- respirations: 12 breaths per minute
- temperature: 36.9°C
- oxygen saturation: 98% on room air
- medications: hydrochlorothiazide 25 mg orally once daily; lisinopril 40 mg orally once daily
- allergies: Nil known.

Question

Use the clinical reasoning cycle to describe what action you would take as the nurse caring for this patient. Which care would be prioritised?

Answer

- *Step 1: Consider the patient.* Don Fredericks is a 61-year-old male post-cataract surgery with loss of vision
- *Step 2: Collect cues/information.* Include subjective and objective data here. The subjective will include what the patient tells you, the appearance of the patient, and their past medical history. Objective data will include objective or measurable information such as the vital signs, blood tests etc.
- *Step 3 Process information.* Separate the relevant and irrelevant data — cluster the clues together to formulate an inference about the patient. What is the current situation? Does this situation need immediate treatment? Who would you inform?
- *Step 4: Identify problems/issues.* Nursing problems or diagnosis should be listed here. Include recognition of a medical emergency and early notification of the ophthalmologist involved in the care of this patient, risk of falls or trauma due to loss of vision, anxiety due to loss of vision, knowledge deficit.
- *Step 5: Establish goals.* Goals of care for Mr Fredricks should focus on reducing anxiety and continue to assess for pain, notifying the medical team immediately, reduce risks of falls or trauma due to loss of sight.
- *Step 6: Act.* Provide the care that is required to meet the established goals, including full assessment including Snellen's test. Set up for ophthalmoscopy or slit-lamp biomicroscopic examination. Your role will be to support the patient and ensure that he is seen by the medical team and cause of loss of sight diagnosed. You will provide a safe and quiet environment for the patient and ongoing education of the status of the issue at hand.
- *Step 7: Evaluate outcomes.* Were the best outcomes achieved? What went well? What could have been done better?
- *Step 8: Reflect on the process and new learning.* Reflect on any aspects of care that could have been done better. What went well, what did not go as well as hoped.

SUMMARY

This chapter provided a review of the pathophysiology of the systems of the ear, nose, throat (ENT) and eyes and an overview of the common conditions that affect these organs. We considered how these health issues impact communication and an individual's ability to perform activities of daily living. An integral part of this chapter was the required nursing management for these cases and how we support our patients with evidence-based practice, patient-centred care and the clinical reasoning cycle.

KEY TERMS

cerebrospinal fluid (CSF) A clear fluid that surrounds the brain and spinal cord, cushioning the brain and spinal cord from injury and delivering nutrients and removing wastes from the brain.

conductive hearing loss Hearing loss caused primarily by a blockage impeding sound conduction from outer to middle ear.

extraocular Structures occuring or situated outsie the eyeball, e.g. the lacrimal gland, eyelids, etc.

inner ear The innermost part of the ear, mainly responsible for sound detection and balance.

intraocular Structures occuring inside the eyeball, e.g. the scleara and retina.

middle ear The small membrane-lined cavity separated from the outer ear by the tympanic membrane and transmits sound waves from the tympanic membrane to the inner ear by way of the auditory ossicles.

ophthalmology A branch of medicine and surgery which deals with the diagnosis and treatment of eye disorders.

otolaryngology A medical specialty focused on the ears, nose and throat. An otolaryngologist is often called an ear, nose and throat doctor, or an ENT for short.

outer ear The visible structures of the ear.

perilymph Extracellular fluid located within the inner ear, found within the scala tympani and scala vestibuli of the cochlea. The ionic composition of perilymph is comparable to that of plasma and cerebrospinal fluid.

sensorineural hearing loss Hearing loss that occurs when there is a problem with the functioning of the inner ear, including the cochlea, hair cells and nerves.

REFERENCES

American Cancer Society. (2021) Living as a laryngeal or hypopharyngeal cancer survivor. www.cancer.org/cancer/laryngeal-and-hypopharyngeal-cancer/after-treatment/follow-up.html

Amplifon, H. C. P. (n.d.) Hearing loss in Australia. www.amplifon.com/au/hearing-loss/how-does-the-ear-work/hearing-impairment-australia

Australian Bureau of Statistics. (2018) 2017–18 National Health Survey. www.abs.gov.au/statistics/health/health-conditions-and-risks/national-health-survey-first-results/latest-release

Bhavsar, A. R. (2021) Diabetic neuropathy. *Medscape.* https://emedicine.medscape.com/article/1225122-overview

British Columbia Institute of Technology (BCIT). (n.d.) Clinical procedures for safer patient care. Chapter 2 Patient Assessment. https://opentextbc.ca/clinicalskills/chapter/2-5-focussed-respiratory-assessment

Chang, P. & Kesley, P. (2005) Ear examination. A practical guide. www.racgp.org.au/afpbackissues/2005/200510/200510chang.pdf

Craft, J. & Gordon, C. (2015) *Understanding Pathophysiology*, 2nd ed. Chatswood, N.S.W: Elsevier Australia.

Department of Health & Human Services, S. G. o. V., Australia. (2021a). Tonsillitis. www.betterhealth.vic.gov.au/health/ConditionsAndTreatments/tonsillitis

Department of Health & Human Services, S. G. o. V., Australia. (2021b) Eyes — laser eye surgery. www.betterhealth.vic.gov.au/health/ConditionsAndTreatments/eyes-laser-eye-surgery

Department of Health & Human Services, S. G. o. V., Australia. (2020) Ears. *Better Health Channel.* www.betterhealth.vic.gov.au/health/conditionsandtreatments/ears

Enoch, J., McDonald, L., Jones, L., Jones, P. R. & Crabb, D. P. (2019) Evaluating whether sight is the most valued sense. *JAMA Ophthalmol.* 137(11): 1317–1320. doi: 10.1001/jamaophthalmol.2019.3537

Ervin, S. E. (2021) Assessment tools: Introduction to the anatomy and physiology of the auditory system. www.workplaceintegra.com/hearing-articles/Ear-anatomy.html

Fifth Sense. (n.d.) Psychology and smell. www.fifthsense.org.uk/psychology-and-smell

Garvan Institute of Medical Research. (2021) Hearing loss: About hearing loss. www.garvan.org.au/research/diseases/hearing-loss/about?

Glaucoma Australia. (2021) What is glaucoma? https://glaucoma.org.au/what-is-glaucoma?gclid=EAIaIQobChMIl7imjcm88QIVz6mWCh2KKAdcEAAYASAAEgKmPD_BwE

Hearing Care Industry Association. (2021) About hearing loss. www.hcia.com.au/about-hearing-loss/#.YC8yrXlxVPY

Healthline. (2021a) Acute otitis media: Causes, symptoms, and diagnosis. www.healthline.com/health/ear-infection-acute#symptoms

Healthline. (2021b) Oval window. www.healthline.com/human-body-maps/oval-window#1

Hodge, C. & Roberts, T. (2003) Glaucoma. Eye series 1. *Australian Family Physician*. 32(8): 643–644. PMID: 12973875.

Jena Surgical. (2021) ENT. www.jenasurgical.com/en/ent

Koroulakis, A. & Agarwal, M. (2021) 'Laryngeal cancer'. In *StatPearls* [Internet]. Treasure Island (FL): StatPearls Publishing. PMID: 30252332.

Levett-Jones, T., Hoffman, K., Dempsey, J., Jeong, S., Noble, D., Norton, C., Roche, J. & Hickey, N. (2009) The 'five rights' of clinical reasoning: An educational model to enhance nursing students' ability to identify and manage clinically 'at risk' patients. *Nurse Education Today*. 30: 515–520. 10.1016/j.nedt.2009.10.020.

Lexington Clinic. (2021) Laser surgery. www.lexingtonclinic.com/services/associate-practices/kentucky-ear-nose-and-throat/patient-resources/laser-surgery

MedlinePlus. (2014) Ear disorders. U.S. Library of medicine. https://medlineplus.gov/eardisorders.html

Moorfield Public Hospital, N. T. (2017) Anatomy of the eye. www.moorfields.nhs.uk/content/anatomy-eye

Nair, M. & Peate, I. (2009) *Fundamentals of Applied Pathophysiology*. USA: JohnWileyandSonsLtd.

National Cancer Institute. (n.d.) Paranasal sinus and nasal cavity cancer treatment (adult) (PDQ®) — Patient Version. www.cancer.gov/types/head-and-neck/patient/adult/paranasal-sinus-treatment-pdq

National Institute for Health and Clinical Excellence (NICE). (2009) Glucoma. https://pathways.nice.org.uk/pathways/glaucoma

Preminger, J. E. & Meeks, S. (2010) The influence of mood on the perception of hearing-loss related quality of life in people with hearing loss and their significant others. *International Journal of Audiology*. 49(4): 263–271. doi: 10.3109/14992020903311396

South Eastern Melbourne PHN. (2019) Tonsillitis management adults. https://melbourne.healthpathways.org.au/39262.htm?zoom_highligh(semphn.org.au)

Stanford Health Care. (2020) Turbinate reduction. https://stanfordhealthcare.org/medical-treatments/n/nasal-surgery/types/turbinate-reduction.html

University of Pittsburgh Medical Center. (2021) Surgical treatments at the ear and hearing center. www.upmc.com/services/ear-nose-throat/services/hearing-and-balance/ear-and-hearing-center/treatments/surgical-options

Vision Australia. (n.d.) Tips for assiting people who are blind or have low vision. www.visionaustralia.org/information/family-friends-carers/tips-assisting

Wahid, N. W. B., Hogan, C. J. & Attia, M. (2020) Weber test. In *StatPearls* [Internet]. Treasure Island FL. www.ncbi.nlm.nih.gov/books/NBK526135

ACKNOWLEDGEMENTS

Figure 22.12: © Eye Anatomy: Parts of the Eye and How We See. © American Academy of Ophthalmology. Reproduced with permission of American Academy of Ophthalmology.

Figure 22.13: © Dougherty & Lister, *The Royal Marsden Manual of Clinical Nursing Procedures*, 9th ed., 2011, © John Wiley & Sons Inc. Reproduced with permission of John Wiley & Sons Inc.

Figure 22.14: © sruilk / Shutterstock.com

Figure 22.15: © ARZTSAMUI / Shutterstock.com

Figure 22.16: © VectorMine / Shutterstock.com

Photo 22A: © Medicimage / UIG / Alamy Images

Photo 22B: © Andrey_Popov / Shutterstock.com

Photo 22C: © Peakstock / Shutterstock.com

Photo 22D: © BSIP / Getty Images

CHAPTER 23

Nursing care of conditions related to reproductive health

LEARNING OBJECTIVES

After studying this chapter, you should be able to:

23.1 describe the anatomy and function of the female reproductive system

23.2 describe the anatomy and function of the male reproductive system

23.3 identify common disorders of the female reproductive system and nursing management

23.4 identify the common types of female gynaecological surgery and the physical and psychological care required

23.5 summarise the methods of contraception and identify screening programs available for women's health in Australia

23.6 identify common breast disorders and discuss treatment options in breast cancer

23.7 outline common testicular disorders and their management.

Introduction

Reproductive health is defined as 'a state of physical, mental, and social well-being in all matters relating to the reproductive system at all stages of life. Reproductive health implies that people are able to have a satisfying and safe sex life and that they have the capability to reproduce and the freedom to decide if, when, and how often to do so' (United Nations 1994).

Reproductive health is a concept that encompasses much more than simply the study of biological factors. All aspects of reproduction are deeply embedded within our social and cultural values and expectations. Humans are mammals, and the three basic drives that are hardwired for survival are the need for food and shelter, which ensure that an individual can survive, and the need for sex, which links to the species' ability to survive. The inability of males or females to reproduce can be devastating and may remove their sense of self-worth, masculinity or femininity. It may affect the persons social standing, both in the family and wider social setting. This, in turn, can have a devastating effect on the person's integral sense of self and psychological health.

The male and female reproductive systems are homologous, meaning they are fundamentally similar in structure and function. The genetic sex of the **embryo** is determined at fertilisation, but until eight weeks, the developing **foetus** exhibits no differentiation. At about 8 weeks, the expression of a gene on the Y chromosome initiates testosterone production, resulting in the development of male characteristics of the foetus. At this time, the external genitals still appear similar, and it is not until approximately week 16 that visual determination of sex is possible. At 12–24 weeks, the testes descend into the inguinal canal. In simple terms, the ovaries develop into testes and move down the inguinal canal into the labia majora, which becomes the scrotum.

Reproductive health is vital for men and women and affects sexuality, fertility and body image. Care is delivered within different settings, including primary care, outpatient clinics and day surgery, with more complex conditions being managed in an inpatient hospital setting. The provision of psychological support is paramount within this specialty.

23.1 The female reproductive system

LEARNING OBJECTIVE 23.1 Describe the anatomy and function of the female reproductive system.

The main components of the female reproductive system are shown in figures 23.1 and 23.2.

FIGURE 23.1 The female external genitalia

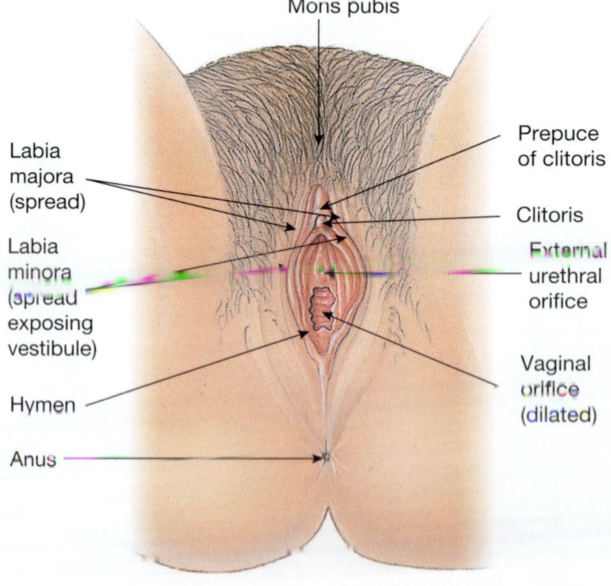

Source: Tortora & Derrickson (2011) *Principles of Anatomy and Physiology*, with kind permission of Wiley Blackwell.

FIGURE 23.2 The uterus and associated structures

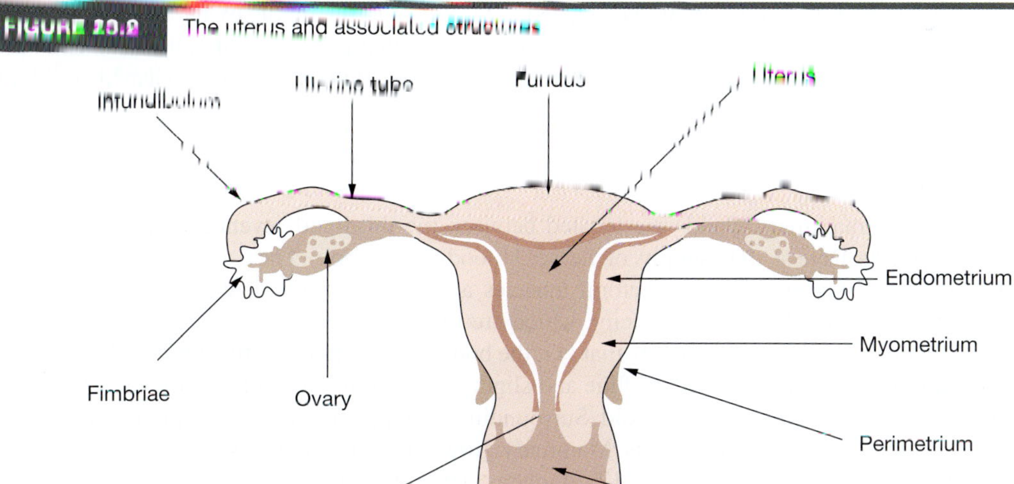

Source: Nair & Peate (2009) *Fundamentals of Applied Pathophysiology*, with kind permission from Wiley Blackwell.

The pelvic floor consists of muscles, pelvic fascia, ovarian ligaments and round ligaments. The vagina starts at the introitus (the opening to the vagina). It is a distensible muscular structure that is held in place by the levator ani muscles acting through the perineal body. The upper end of the vagina is attached to the cervix, which divides into the anterior, lateral and posterior walls. To the front of the vagina lie the urethra and bladder neck; to the back is the rectum.

The cervix (figure 23.3) is cylindrical in shape and connects to the uterus, a pear-shaped and sized organ with an inverted triangle-shaped cavity. The uterus is composed of three layers: the peritoneum — the outer serous layer; the myometrium — the middle muscular layer; and the **endometrium** — the inner functional layer. The uterus sits at right angles to the vagina and tilts forward (anteversion); in 15 per cent of women, the uterus tilts backward (retroversion).

FIGURE 23.3 The cervix

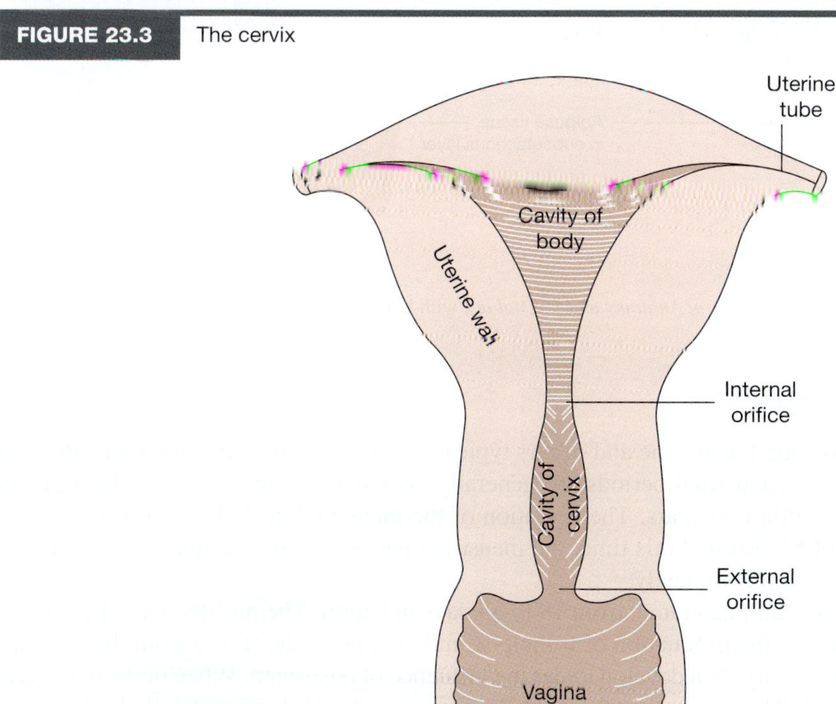

Source: Nair & Peate (2009) *Fundamentals of Applied Pathophysiology*, with kind permission from Wiley Blackwell.

Leading from the fundal portion of the uterus are the fallopian tubes attached at both corners of the uterus. They are tubular structures containing small cilia. The waves of movement produced by the cilia propel the ovum (egg) gently down the fallopian tubes to the uterus. The fallopian tubes end at the fimbriae, where the ovaries can be found. Each ovary is attached to the cornu of the uterus by the ovarian ligament. A single layer of cuboidal cells covers the surface of the ovary called the germinal epithelium and has a central vascular medulla and an outer thicker cortex. In the young adult, it is almond-shaped, solid and white in colour.

Breast structure

The female breasts or mammary glands are located between the third and seventh ribs on the anterior chest wall. The breasts have a rich supply of nerves, blood and lymph. They are made up of 15–20 pyramid-shaped lobes supported by the pectoral muscles and Cooper's ligaments. Each lobe contains lobules that contain functional units called acini, which are lined by epithelial cells capable of secreting milk. The acini empty into a network of ducts that exit the body through pores in the nipples. The nipple is a pigmented cylindrical structure located midline and slightly inferior to the centre of the breast. Nipples become erect in response to stimulation and cold. Surrounding the nipple is the areola, a pigmented circular area containing a number of sebaceous glands. Mammary growth is stimulated by the onset of puberty and is often the first overt sign of this (Hogarth 2017; Stephens 2017). The structure of the breasts can be seen in figure 23.4.

FIGURE 23.4 Structure of the breasts

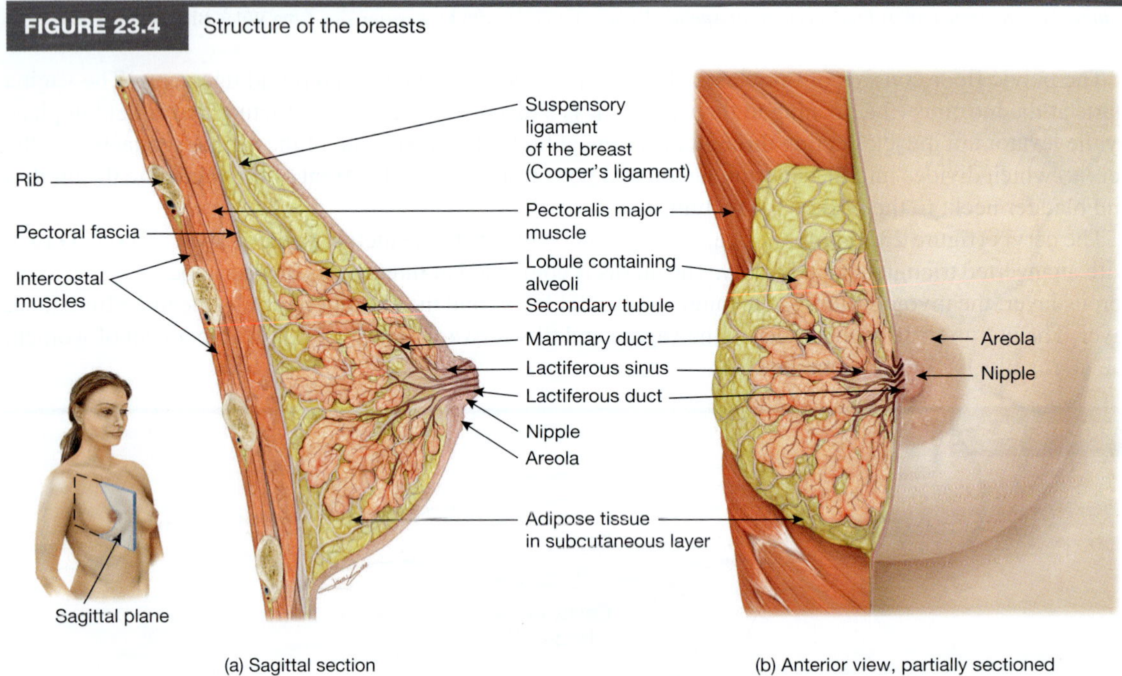

Source: Tortora & Derrickson (2011) *Principles of Anatomy and Physiology,* with kind permission of Wiley Blackwell.

The menstrual cycle

The onset of menstruation is called menarche and occurs typically at age 12–13 years, two years after the first signs of puberty. The first menstrual periods are generally anovulatory (non-ovum producing) and irregular, but usually settle within two years. The cessation of the menstrual cycle is menopause, which happens at an average age of 51. Around this time, the menstrual periods change frequency, with longer gaps between them until they stop completely.

The menstrual cycle (figure 23.5) can range from 19 to 35 days in length. The proliferative phase is the first stage, which is governed by the production of follicle-stimulating hormone (FSH) from the pituitary gland. The follicles within the ovary then develop under the influence of oestrogen. When oestrogen levels rise, there is suppression of FSH via a negative feedback system, and one dominant follicle develops. Oestrogen also acts on the endometrium, causing the endometrial glands to grow and new blood vessels to form.

FIGURE 23.5 The menstrual cycle

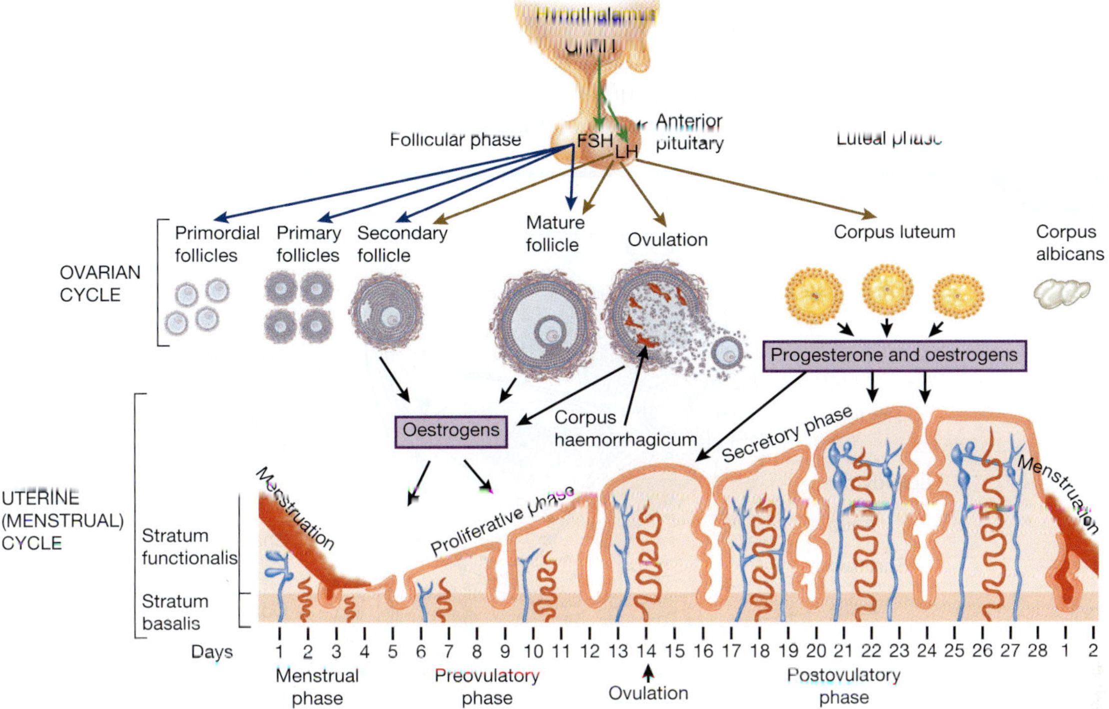

(a) Hormonal regulation of changes in the ovary and uterus

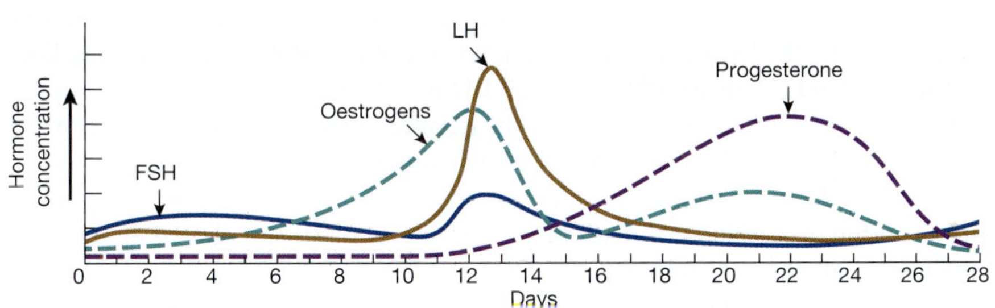

(b) Changes in concentration of anterior pituitary and ovarian hormones

Source: Tortora & Derrickson (2011) *Principles of Anatomy and Physiology,* with kind permission of Wiley Blackwell.

The second stage is the secretory phase. A surge of luteinising hormone (LH) from the anterior pituitary gland leads to maturation of the dominant follicle followed by a rise in progesterone release from the corpus luteum. A release of prostaglandins and cytokines leads to rupture of the follicle wall and ovulation, about 38 hours after the initiation of the LH surge. The empty follicle then becomes the corpus luteum. Progesterone is synthesised by the corpus luteum, its concentration rising above 25 mmol/L, suggesting that the cycle is ovulatory. The endometrium thickens to become secretory, with an increased number of glands in readiness for a pregnancy to implant. The gradual fall of oestrogen and progesterone levels finally results in menses (loss of blood).

Menstruation refers to the shedding of superficial layers of the endometrium. It is initiated by the fall in progesterone that follows the failure of the corpus luteum cyst as it starts to resolve. The amount of blood loss in a regular cycle is up to 80 ml, with menstruation starting on day one of a cycle and usually lasting up to seven days.

Along with changes within the ovary and endometrium, other changes occur under the control of hormones at this time. Cyclical changes occur in the cervical mucus, which becomes thinner at the time of ovulation to facilitate penetration of the cervix by the sperm. It then becomes thicker under the influence of progesterone.

23.2 The male reproductive system

LEARNING OBJECTIVE 23.2 Describe the anatomy and function of the male reproductive system.

The male reproductive system (figure 23.6) consists of the external organs (the penis and scrotum) and the internal organs (the testes, epididymis, vasa deferentia, ejaculatory ducts, seminal vesicles, prostate gland and bulbourethral glands). The purpose of the male reproductive system is to produce, transport and discharge sperm, and the production and secretion of male sex hormones.

FIGURE 23.6 The male reproductive tract

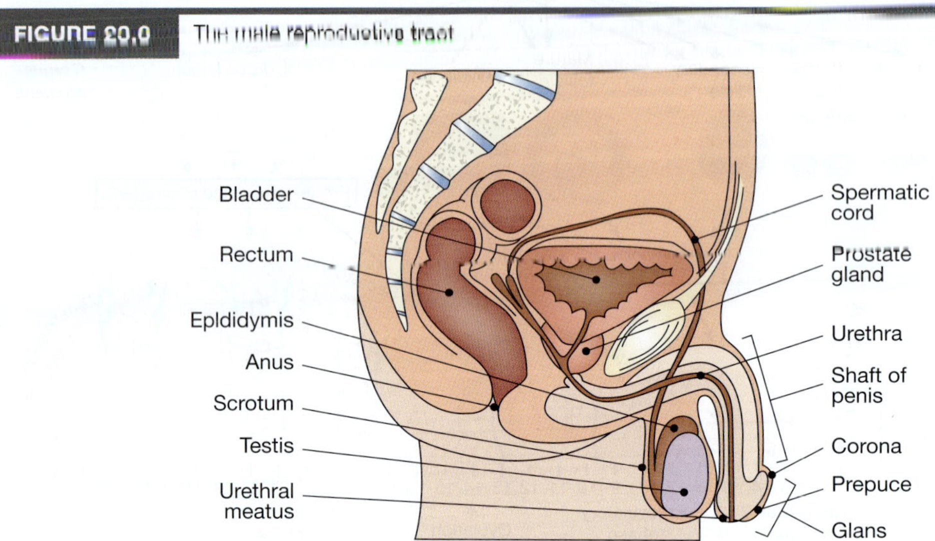

Source: Nair & Peate (2009) *Fundamentals of Applied Pathophysiology*, with kind permission from Wiley Blackwell.

The testes sit within the scrotum and are responsible for producing sperm and testosterone. Testosterone production is regulated by the hypothalamus via the release of gonadotrophin-releasing hormone (GnRH), causing the pituitary gland to release LH and FSH. LH travels to the testes and triggers the production of testosterone. Testosterone initiates and maintains the development of the male sexual characteristics (such as the development of the genitalia and pubertal changes) and governs the sex drive.

Each testis is surrounded by a fibrous capsule called the tunica albuginea, covered by the double-layered tunica vaginalis. Within each testis are small tubes (the seminiferous tubules) that lead to a coiled tube at the back of the testes called the epididymis.

FSH acts on the cells in the seminiferous tubules to stimulate the production of sperm. Specialised cells within the tubules divide many times to become the sperm; the sperm are released from the tubules and pass from the testis into the epididymis, where they mature and gain motility (the ability to move). Sperm, like ovum, contain only 23 chromosomes. When a sperm fertilises an ovum, they combine to have the same number of chromosomes as all the other cells in the human body (46).

The vas deferens is part of the spermatic cord and leads from the epididymis to meet the seminal vesicle at the ejaculatory duct. Mature sperm are transported along the vas deferens during ejaculation, a process controlled by the autonomic nervous system and consists of two phases: the emission phase and the expulsion phase. During the emission phase, muscular contractions move the sperm, along with a little fluid, from the epididymis and along the vas deferens. Sperm move up to the ejaculatory ducts and through the prostate gland into the prostatic urethra. Fluid is added to sperm from the seminal vesicles and the prostate to make semen. Most of the volume of the semen is produced by the prostate and seminal vesicles.

During the expulsion phase, the bladder neck contracts to prevent semen from entering the bladder, and the pelvic muscles contract rhythmically to propel the semen, which is discharged from the urethra through the urethral meatus.

23.3 Disorders of the female reproductive system

LEARNING OBJECTIVE 23.3 Identify common disorders of the female reproductive system and nursing management

Menstrual disorders

There is a wide spectrum of menstrual disorders or disturbances, which are generally not life-threatening, although women with heavy menstrual bleeding (HMB) can experience chronic anaemia and decreased quality of life. Common menstrual disorders include:

- HMB
- dysmenorrhoea (painful periods)
- premenstrual syndrome (PMS) — physical and emotional symptoms that may occur in the lead up to menstruation
- intermenstrual **postcoital** bleeding
- postmenopausal bleeding
- amenorrhoea (lack of periods)
- menstrual dysfunction in the **peri-menopause**, which can cause changes in cycle length and flow
- polycystic ovarian syndrome (PCOS)

Benign tumours of the female reproductive tract

Table 23.1 describes benign tumours and their management.

TABLE 23.1 Benign tumours of the female reproductive tract

Site	Type	Cause and presentation	Management
Vulva	Lipoma	Arises from fibrofatty and muscular tissues	Surgical excision if it causes discomfort or interferes with sexual intercourse
	Bartholin's cyst	Blockage of the duct by mucus Common Painful Can develop into an abscess	Marsupialisation of the cyst Stitching back of the cyst wall to allow drainage, followed by packing of the cavity Need to exclude infective causes
Vagina	Inclusion cysts	Trauma Imperfect repairs of the perineum	Surgical removal only if there is pain or discomfort
Cervix	Polyps	Small growths that arise from the • **Endocervical** mucosa • Surface of the cervix May be asymptomatic Cause intermenstrual and postcoital bleeding Recur	Removal by avulsion or resection
	Nabothian cysts	Mucus retention cysts Seen on the surface of the cervix	No treatment unless there are signs of cervicitis, for which cryotherapy may help
Uterus	Polyps	A focal overgrowth of endometrial glands and stroma Cause irregular bleeding Approximately 1% are malignant More common after the menopause	Hysteroscopic resection
	Fibroids (leiomyomas)	Tumours that arise from the smooth muscle of the myometrium Their size and position define the symptoms	None Myomectomy Hysteroscopic resection Uterine artery embolisation Hysterectomy
Ovary	Ovarian cysts	Many different types	Nil Ovarian cystectomy Removal of ovary

Fibroids

Fibroids are the most common benign tumours of the reproductive tract and arise from the smooth muscle of the uterus; their prevalence is hard to define as they can be asymptomatic. Their cause is unknown, but they are more common in African-Caribbean women, and their growth is stimulated by oestrogen. Fibroids shrink after menopause. Types of fibroid (figure 23.7) include:

- intramural fibroids, contained within the wall of the uterus
- submucosal fibroids, which lie inside the cavity of the uterus
- subserosal fibroids, which are found outside the wall of the uterus and can be **pedunculated**
- cervical fibroids positioned within the cervix.

FIGURE 23.7 Fibroids

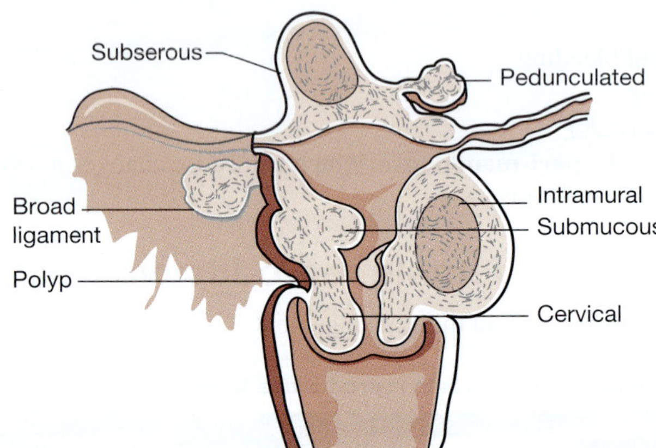

Source: Hamilton-Fairley (2008) *Lecture Notes: Obstetrics & Gynaecology*, with kind permission of Wiley Blackwell.

The signs and symptoms include:

- HMB or irregular bleeding
- pressure symptoms such as pain, swelling, pressure on the bowel or bladder (frequency of urination) and increased risk of thrombosis due to pressure on the venous return
- reproductive problems due to pressure on the ostia or tubes and intracavity problems
- pregnancy complications such as miscarriage, bleeding in pregnancy, degeneration of fibroids in pregnancy and pain.

If women are asymptomatic with fibroids and are then found on routine pelvic examination, no further assessment or treatment is needed. If women have symptoms suspicious of fibroids, a pelvic examination should be undertaken. An ultrasound, either vaginal or abdominal, will also give information about the fibroid's size and position. If there is any doubt or difficulty, a magnetic resonance imaging (MRI) scan can be used. In some cases, hysteroscopy or saline sonography can be used to assess the cavity.

Management of fibroids

Medical treatment, which is only really beneficial for women who have menstrual problems, includes:

- the combined oral contraceptive pill (COCP)
- tranexamic acid
- an intrauterine system (IUS) of contraception, but only if there are no submucosal fibroids
- GnRH analogues over a three-month course to induce temporary menopause, which can shrink the fibroids by up to 60 per cent, although they will grow again once treatment has been discontinued; GnRH analogues should not be used as a long-term treatment as they can cause bone density loss, but they can be useful before surgical intervention
- uterine artery **embolisation** (UAE), a procedure that aims to reduce the blood supply to the fibroids, causing them to shrink. The technique can be used on any fibroids except pedunculated ones. The procedure is carried out by an interventional radiologist and does not require a general anaesthetic. With a reduction in the size of the fibroids, there may be a reduction in the symptoms. Women should be advised that they are likely to have pain and bleeding after the procedure and vaginal discharge, which may persist for several months. Rarely they may have venous thromboembolism (VTE) (RANZCOG 2020).

The surgical treatment depends on the location, size and number of the fibroids. Myomectomy is the most common surgical treatment and can be carried out in different ways (table 23.2).

TABLE 23.2 Myomectomy

Procedure	Advantages	Disadvantages	Suitable for
Laparoscopic myomectomy	Quicker recovery Smaller incisions	A limited number of fibroids can be treated Not all gynaecologists offer this procedure	Women with fibroids no larger than 7 cm Subserosal or intramural fibroids only
Abdominal myomectomy	Removes more and larger fibroids	1% risk of needing a hysterectomy Length of time in hospital May need a second operation	Large uterus Multiple fibroids
Hysteroscopic myomectomy	Day case procedure No abdominal cuts	Not suitable for all fibroids Risk of perforation If fibroids are large, they may need a two-stage procedure Fluid overload	Submucosal only, with more than 50% in the uterine cavity
Hysterectomy	Cure	Length of stay Morbidity	All types

Ovarian cysts

The majority of cysts are fluid-filled, although some have solid elements within them; 90 per cent are likely to be benign. Ovarian cysts can arise from any cell type within the ovary:

- epithelium (mucinous cystadenomas, endometrioid tumours and Brenner tumours)
- germ cells (dermoid cysts, which may contain other materials such as hair, teeth and sebaceous matter)
- sex cord stroma (rarer granulosa cell tumours and theca cell tumours).

Some cysts may be functional, occurring during the menstrual cycle from corpus luteum cysts, and are generally asymptomatic. They arise during ovulation and resolve spontaneously.

Cysts may be asymptomatic and discovered on examination or ultrasound for a different presenting complaint. Some women may complain of:

- pain
- abdominal swelling
- pain on intercourse
- pressure symptoms such as a full feeling within the pelvis.

Progesterone-only contraception may also increase the risk of ovarian cysts. An acute onset of pain associated with nausea and vomiting may indicate torsion of the cyst, which will need immediate surgical intervention to prevent necrosis of the ovary. The assessment should include examination and ultrasonography. Some tumour markers can help distinguish whether there is a risk of malignancy:

- CA-125, although this is also raised with endometriosis, adenomyosis and fibroids
- alpha-fetoprotein (AFP), identified by a blood test
- human chorionic gonadotropin (hCG).

Management of ovarian cysts

There is no medical management available for ovarian cysts, but many do not need any intervention. Benign cysts less than 5 to 6 cm in size can be monitored with regular ultrasound scans. If women are prone to recurrent cysts, the COCP may be helpful to prevent them.

If there is any suspicion of malignancy for women experiencing symptoms or if the cysts are large (over eight centimetres), surgical removal is recommended. This may be achieved by laparoscopy and aspiration of the cyst, laparoscopic or open removal of the cyst, or oophorectomy (removal of the ovary). For postmenopausal women, the routine practice should be removing the ovary rather than just the cyst due to the risk of malignancy.

Cancers affecting the female reproductive tract

Cancer can occur in any part of the reproductive tract (table 23.3).

TABLE 23.3 Gynaecological cancers*

Type	Causes	Signs and symptoms	Diagnosis	Treatment
Vulval				
Accounts for less than 6% of gynaecological cancers Mainly squamous cell carcinomas More common in women >65 years On the increase in younger women	Has been linked to: • Human papilloma virus (HPV) • Smoking • A history of precancerous changes • Chronic skin conditions, e.g. lichen planus	Itching Ulceration Vulval pain Discharge Discolouration A mass	Vulval biopsy Check the vagina and cervix for coexisting disease EUA/MRI to check the extent of disease for staging	If early stage, wide local excision With wide spread, vulvectomy and possibly removal of the groin lymph nodes Radiotherapy if the margins are not clear Chemotherapy for inoperable or recurrent disease and metastases Complications of surgery include sexual dysfunction and wound breakdown
Cervix				
Rates have dropped in countries where there is a screening program The most common type is squamous cell (90%), adenocarcinomas making up the rest Most occur in the transformation zone as a result of dysplastic changes Cancers spread by direct invasion Spread in advanced cases is via lymph and blood	HPV types 16 and 18 Early sexual intercourse Multiple partners Non-use of barrier methods of contraception Smoking Immunosuppressants	None Vaginal discharge Postcoital bleeding Intermenstrual bleeding Back pain Late presentation — bladder and bowel dysfunction Fistula formation	Examination and colposcopy with biopsies EUA/MRI/CT Assess local spread: • Chest X-ray; • Sigmoidoscopy • Cystoscopy	Cervical screening HPV vaccination programs are available in the UK and Ireland Treatment depends on the stage If picked up in the precancerous stage (cervical screening), large loop excision Cone biopsy Trachelectomy (removal of the cervix) if fertility is an issue Early — radical hysterectomy Extensive — pelvic clearance Chemotherapy and radiotherapy, internal radiotherapy (brachytherapy) can be used with external beam radiotherapy

Endometrial				
[illegible] most common cancer and increasing in incidence Endometrioid adenocarcinoma is the most common type The majority are in postmenopausal women, with one-quarter being premenopausal	Oestrogen exposure No children and not breastfeeding Obesity Diabetes Tamoxifen Previous endometrial hyperplasia Unopposed oestrogen PCOS Family history	None Postmenopausal bleeding Vaginal bleeding Discharge Abnormal bleeding	Vaginal examination Ultrasound scan; a thin endometrium (under 4 mm) is normal in postmenopausal women If abnormal, hysteroscopy and biopsy is undertaken Further imaging for assessment of stage	Total abdominal hysterectomy, bilateral salpingo-oophorectomy and possibly removal of lymph nodes Radical hyster ectomy External or internal radiotherapy after surgery, depending on the stage or if the patient is not fit for operation Progesterone if the patient is not fit for operation and in palliative settings
Ovarian				
The fourth most common cause of cancer in women Are many different types: • Serous • Mucinous • Endometrioid • Clear cell cystade-nocarcinoma • Germ cell, and may be secondary	Related to ovulation The COCP and pregnancy have some protective effect BRAC1 and BRAC2 genetic mutations	Difficult to diagnose The patient may have no symptoms or may present with advanced disease Bloating Back and abdominal pain Tiredness Weight loss Urinary problems	Ultrasound MRI/CT Bloods for markers such as CA-125 (not always elevated and can also rise in other conditions, e.g. endometriosis) Risk malignancy index (RMI) is used in conjunction with physical examination and blood markers to determine a diagnosis (Yeoh 2015)	Total abdominal hysterectomy and bilateral salpingo-oophorectomy with lymph node removal and staging of the disease at the same time Alternatively, debulking surgery, chemotherapy and more surgery Chemotherapy

* CT = computed tomography; EUA = examination under anaesthesia; HPV = human papillomavirus.

Nursing management of female reproductive cancers

The diagnosis of cancer affects both the women and their families. Some treatments affect body image, sexuality and fertility, so referral to a psychosexual counsellor may be helpful. Treatment may also result in physical and functional changes that affect sexual function, such as vaginal problems after radiotherapy. All these changes will need to be discussed sensitively before and after treatment. Prior to surgery, fertility, plans for children, sexual activity and the nature of the surgery should be assessed and discussed (table 23.4).

TABLE 23.4 **Preoperative patient education**

Problem	Management
Loss of fertility	Preoperative counselling Fertility consultation (egg collection and storage)
Early menopause	Preoperative discussion Post-operative hormone replacement therapy, if indicated
Vaginal dryness	Dilators and lubrication
Changes in body image or sexuality and fertility	Specialist support
Unsure of the nature of the surgery	A full explanation of the operation: • What is removed • How the body will function post-operatively

Depending on the type of cancer and the treatment, women may need to be educated to expect or monitor for ascites (especially with ovarian cancer). Hormonal changes such as hot flushes may occur if the ovaries have been removed; an induced menopause may also result following chemotherapy or radiotherapy. If surgery involves lymph node removal, resultant lower limb oedema may occur. Women may experience anxiety and fatigue. Support is available from various agencies, including social services and national bodies available to all women, including the McGrath Foundation, Breast Cancer Network Australia and Cancer Council Australia. Women should also have access to a clinical nurse specialist who can guide them on what specialist support is available locally.

Prolapse

A prolapse is a protrusion of an organ from its normal position. In the female reproductive system, the urethra (urethrocele), bladder (cystocele), rectum (rectocele) or uterus may prolapse into the vagina. Uterine prolapse may be first degree (still within the vagina), second degree (where the cervix is at the introitus) or third degree (where the entire uterus has come out of the vagina).

A prolapse generally occurs due to a weakness of the pelvic floor muscles, which may be due to:

- damage from pregnancy and labour
- age-related changes
- lack of oestrogen after the menopause
- increased pressure in the abdomen due to heavy lifting, constipation or a pelvic mass.

Some women have no symptoms, whereas others may complain of feeling a mass or lump within the vagina. Women may experience pain, a dragging sensation, urinary problems or defecation problems. Discharge and bleeding may be present if there is a third-degree uterine prolapse.

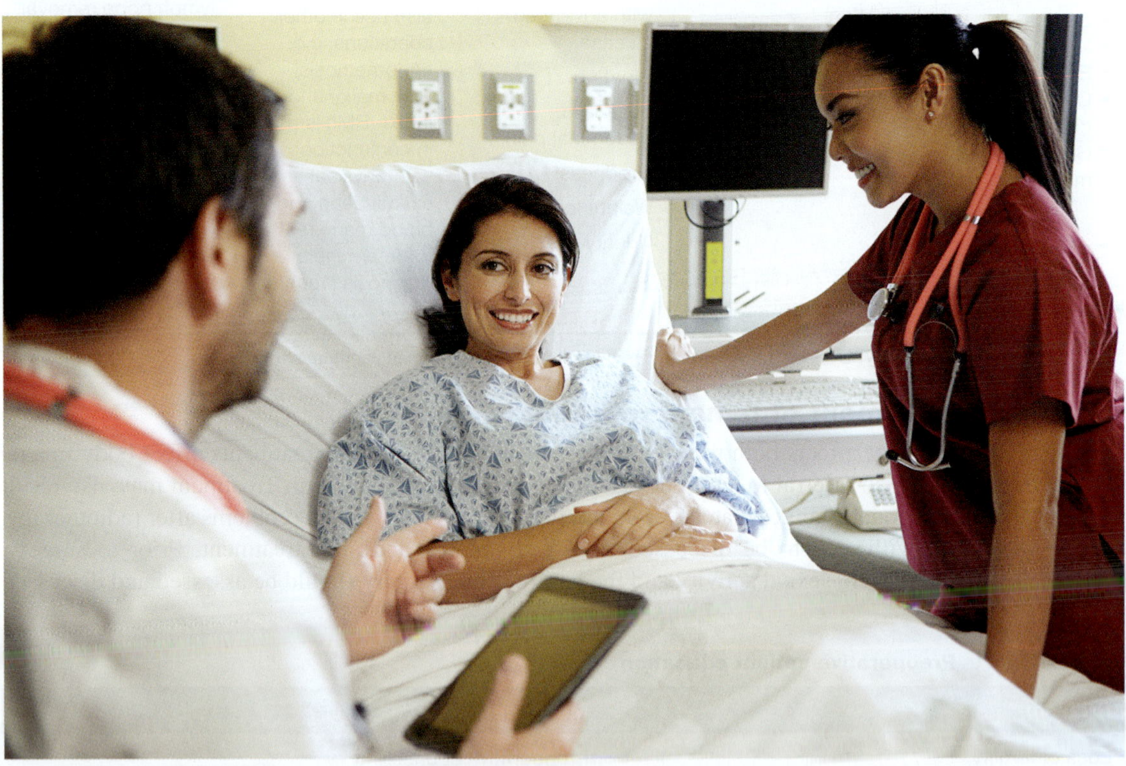

Management of prolapse

Women with mild symptoms should be taught to perform pelvic floor exercises to strengthen the pelvic floor muscles. In some cases, the insertion of a ring pessary may also help to support the pelvic floor. If the symptoms are severe and not helped by these measures, surgery may be performed to correct the anatomical problem (table 23.5).

TABLE 23.5 Surgery for prolapse

Surgery	Type of prolapse	Comments
Anterior repair	Urethrocele and cystocele	There may be: • urinary retention after surgery • painful intercourse
Vaginal hysterectomy	Uterine prolapse	Can be combined with anterior and posterior repairs
Sacrospinus fixation	Vault repair	Risk of post-operative cystocele and stress incontinence
Posterior repair	Rectocele	Painful intercourse post-operatively

Endometriosis

Endometriosis is a condition in which endometrial tissue is found outside the endometrial cavity but still responds to the influence of hormones. It can be found in the peritoneum over the uterosacral ligaments or in the ovaries, broad ligaments, fallopian tubes, pouch of Douglas, bowel and bladder. Less common sites include the diaphragm, lungs and brain. It is normally found in women of reproductive age, can be progressive and is linked with chronic pelvic pain, psychological problems and infertility. The symptoms will depend on the site of the endometriosis and may include:

- pelvic pain (which is not linked to the severity of the disease on laparoscopy)
- painful intercourse
- dysmenorrhoea
- infertility
- painful bowel movements
- painful micturition.

The exact aetiology of endometriosis is unknown. The endometrial deposits react to the influence of hormones and will bleed as if the tissue were in the uterine cavity. This bleeding can then cause inflammation, scarring and distortion of the pelvic anatomy. This may form as endometriomas, which are cysts on the ovary caused by endometriosis.

Management of endometriosis

Physical examination and ultrasound are used to assess and diagnose endometriosis, but the gold standard diagnostic tool is laparoscopy. Medical management will depend on the woman and her desired outcomes. Women who wish to avoid any hormonal treatment can be prescribed analgesia, which can be given during the menstrual period or when in pain (Dunselman et al. 2014). Hormonal treatment aims to suppress endometrial growth and proliferation. Treatment includes:

- COCPs taken continuously
- progesterone taken continuously to cause atrophy of the endometriosis
- an IUD for contraception
- GnRH analogues with add-back hormone replacement therapy (HRT) to reduce the side effects of menopause and stop bone density loss.

Endometriosis can be treated surgically. Approaches include laparoscopy combined with laser therapy or diathermy, which destroys the endometrial deposits. In addition to surgery, a combined approach with medical management is often used; any adhesions that have formed can be divided to try to restore the pelvic anatomy. Ablation of the deposits can help to improve fertility, but this may not relieve the symptoms, and repeated laparoscopy may be needed. The definitive surgery for women who do not wish to retain their fertility is a total abdominal hysterectomy and bilateral salpingo-oophorectomy. However, this may not cure long-standing pelvic pain. Continuous combined HRT may need to be prescribed to prevent the reactivation of any deposits.

Nurses need to provide patients with the following information:

- the impact the disease has on women's fertility
- an explanation of the condition
- the fact that many of the treatments are contraceptives
- information on coping strategies or adequate analgesia regimens that can be used to manage the chronic pelvic pain that is often associated with this condition.

Unplanned pregnancy loss

Unplanned pregnancy loss refers to either miscarriage or an ectopic pregnancy. Women who present with pain and or bleeding in pregnancy will need the following investigations:

- a urinary pregnancy test
- routine observations
- urinalysis
- a gentle bimanual and speculum examination to assess for pain and for whether the cervix is open
- blood samples for a full blood count, group and save, and levels of βhCG (which reflects pregnancy) and progesterone
- an ultrasound scan.

Risk factors for an ectopic pregnancy should be assessed, for example, previous ectopic pregnancies or a history of chlamydia infection or pelvic inflammatory disease (PID). Women should also be assessed for failed oral contraceptive pills or intrauterine contraceptive device, endometriosis and previous pelvic surgery.

Miscarriage

Miscarriage is defined as pregnancy loss before the 20th week of pregnancy and occurs in about one in four pregnancies. Miscarriage can be spontaneous, complete, incomplete, delayed or recurrent (which refers to more than three consecutive losses and occurs in one to two per cent of the population) (RANZCOG 2011).

Causes of miscarriage can be:

- foetal, for example, congenital malformations and genetic abnormalities (thought to be the most common cause and increasing with maternal age)
- maternal, for example, acute illness, infections, trauma, antiphospholipid (APL) syndrome, diabetes, hypothyroidism, abnormalities of the uterus, cervical incompetence, smoking, alcohol and drugs.

A molar pregnancy occurs when there is an overgrowth of the chorionic villi and is known as gestational trophoblastic disease. These are rare pregnancies and can be complete, partial or invasive; if left untreated, they can form choriocarcinomas.

Management of miscarriage

The management of miscarriage can be medical or expectant (NICE 2012). Expectant management involves monitoring to wait and see whether pregnancy tissue will be passed naturally without the need for surgical intervention. Medical management involves giving medication to expel the foetus or any remaining pregnancy tissue. The usual regimen is a combination of mifepristone, an antiprogesterone, followed 35–48 hours later by a prostaglandin.

If women fail to progress with conservative or medical management, or are unsuitable for such management, surgical intervention involving the evacuation of retained products of conception (ERPC) may be needed. Depending on the length of **gestation** and the amount of retained products visible on a scan, the cervix can be primed with a prostaglandin. ERPC may also be necessary when a molar pregnancy is suspected to ensure that the products can be sent for histology and when patients present with heavy bleeding and the condition is unstable.

Ectopic pregnancy

Ectopic pregnancies occur outside the uterus, predominantly in the fallopian tubes, but can also be ovarian, cervical or intra-abdominal (figure 23.8). They occur when the fertilised ovum does not implant in the correct place. This is generally due to tubal damage from infections and other conditions such as endometriosis, although the cause is sometimes unknown. The incidence of ectopic pregnancy is about 1–2 in 100 in Australia (Condous 2006).

Management of ectopic pregnancy

Ectopic pregnancies can be managed expectantly if the woman is stable and βhCG levels are decreasing, indicating a failing pregnancy. Medical management with methotrexate is the first-line treatment for women who can return for follow-up and meet criteria: no significant pain, unruptured ectopic pregnancy with no visible heartbeat, serum hCG level less than 1500 IU/litre, no intrauterine pregnancy. Methotrexate interferes with cell growth and will prevent the egg or ectopic pregnancy-related tissue from growing. Methotrexate is effective in about 90 per cent of cases. Surgery is the first-line treatment for ectopic pregnancy with significant pain, an adnexal mass of greater than 35 mm, foetal heartbeat visible on ultrasound or a serum hCG 5000 IU/litre or greater (NICE 2012).

FIGURE 23.8 Ectopic pregnancy

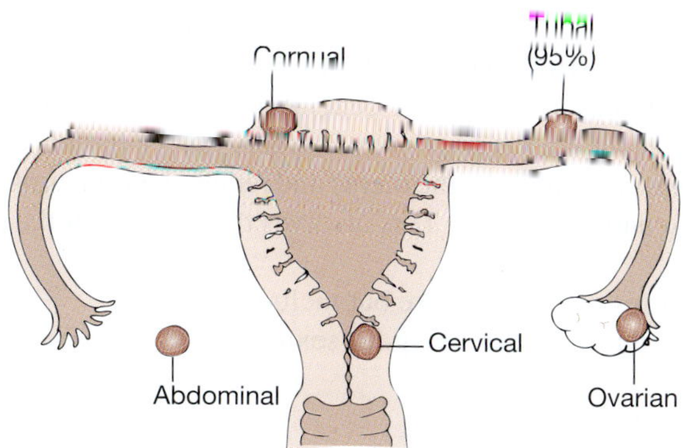

Source: Impey (2004) *Obstetrics & Gynaecology*, with kind permission of Wiley Blackwell.

The woman's clinical condition will determine whether she needs urgent surgical intervention as an ectopic pregnancy can still cause death. In haemodynamically unstable women, a laparotomy may be needed. An ectopic pregnancy is generally managed with laparoscopy and removal of the ectopic pregnancy by salpingostomy (opening the tube) or salpingectomy (removal of the tube).

Nurses need to support women with unplanned pregnancy loss by providing information on:

- bereavement counselling
- local or national support groups or charities
- future pregnancies
- the timing of future pregnancies
- the need for an early scan on the woman's next pregnancy
- determination of Rhesus (Rh) factor level and administration of anti-D if the woman is Rh-negative; this may be necessary after surgical instrumentation of the uterus or after 12 weeks gestation and acts to prevent Rh incompatibility in any subsequent pregnancies
- contraceptive advice (if necessary).

Termination of pregnancy

One-third of Australian women have an unintended pregnancy in their lifetime, and 30.4 per cent of these pregnancies end in a termination of pregnancy (TOP) or abortion. This is one in five Australian women. The rate of unintended pregnancy in socio-demographically disadvantaged women is disproportionately high (Mazza et al., 2020). For some, the only solution is a TOP. This is the removal of the contents of the uterus so it does not lead to the birth of a baby. The laws that govern TOP vary from country to country. In Australia, each state and territory have slightly different criteria for TOP, but it is legal up to 14 weeks gestation in all states and territories. Terminations are partially funded by Medicare and private insurers, which are both regulated by the federal government. Abortions and abortion advice is considered a health service. Termination over the gestational age of 14 weeks depends on the state or territory. While all states have slightly different laws concerning termination, doctors have the right to conscientious objection in performing this procedure. However, they are expected to advise the patient that they have a conscientious objection to the practice and should refer the patient to a suitable practitioner who does not object and ensures that the patients' health is not negatively impacted. The fine points of this are under discussion in some states.

Women will be referred to a range of clinics to discuss the TOP. Investigations include:

- the patient's history
- a full blood count
- vaginal swabs
- blood grouping for Rh factor
- ultrasound (if there is a doubt over the gestational age).

Medical management is undertaken for gestations up to nine weeks. The current regimen is oral mifepristone, which inhibits progesterone and prevents pregnancy progression and causes the placenta and embryo to detach from the endometrium. This is followed by vaginal misoprostol, a prostaglandin analogue, which works to induce contractions. There is a 95–97 per cent success rate for a complete TOP

(Mazza et al. 2020). Late medical TOP can be performed up to 24 weeks gestation. This is normally with mifepristone and then gemeprost up to two days later, causing the abortion; women need to deliver the foetus.

Surgical management can be performed in the first trimester between six and 14 weeks of gestation. The procedure involves vacuum aspiration under general or local anaesthetic. The cervix may be dilated preoperatively with prostaglandin, and at the time of surgery, an aspiration cannula is used to empty the uterus. Complications include perforation of the uterus and retained products of conception. After 15 weeks gestation, dilatation and evacuation are used. This involves the removal of the pregnancy with forceps via the cervix.

Complications from all forms of TOP are rare but include:

- infections, which can be reduced by screening for sexually transmitted infections
- haemorrhage
- failed TOP needing a repeat procedure
- uterine trauma such as perforation, which is more common with later gestations but lessened by using cervical preparations
- cervical lacerations, which the use of cervical preparations can lessen
- psychological problems — many women experience grief but also relief, and about 10 per cent will experience long-term problems.

Women should have access to counselling both before and after the procedure if needed and should be aware that there may be some bleeding and pain after the TOP. The Rh factor should also be checked prior to discharge and anti-D given if needed. Women should be offered advice regarding adequate contraception after the procedure.

Pelvic inflammatory disease

Pelvic inflammatory disease (PID) is an infection of the pelvic organs. This includes fallopian tubes, ovaries, cervix, endometrium and pelvic peritoneum. PID can be caused by several agents such as *Neisseria gonorrhoeae* and *Chlamydia trachomatis*, responsible for 80 per cent of all cases and dual infection is common. It may also be caused by *Escherichia coli* (part of the normal gut flora and found in faeces). This may be transmitted to the introitus of the vagina by wiping from anus to vagina after defaecating or by having anal sex.

PID may also be caused by insertion of IUDs, TOP, or surgery of the reproductive tract. In Australia, PID is not a notifiable disease. However, it is estimated that one million women experience PID per year, and as a result of the infection, more than 100 000 women become infertile. A large percentage of ectopic pregnancies are linked to PID.

PID is common in women 16–24 years of age who have had multiple partners and a history of STIs and can be associated with the recent fitting of an IUD (Fields & Moxham 2017). Symptoms may include:

- a lack of symptoms
- symptoms ranging from vague pain to peritonitis
- lower abdominal pain
- painful intercourse
- deep pain
- postcoital bleeding
- intermenstrual bleeding
- vaginal discharge.

On examination, women may present with:

- pyrexia
- guarding on bimanual examination
- cervical excitation (pain when the cervix is moved during examination)
- tenderness
- an adnexal mass if there is an abscess
- on speculum examination, discharge at the cervix (swabs and a midstream urine specimen will need to be obtained).

It is important to rule out the differential diagnoses of ectopic pregnancy, appendicitis, urinary tract infection, endometriosis and torsion of an ovarian cyst. This is done by ultrasound, blood tests (full blood count, C-reactive protein and erythrocyte sedimentation rate) and a pregnancy test.

Management of PID

Typical treatment is combination antibiotic therapy with at least two broad-spectrum antibiotics IV or orally, depending on the severity of symptoms. A GP can manage non-acute cases, but in acute cases, hospital admission will be needed. Abscesses that are present will need to be drained and if necessary, surgery to remove the uterus, ovaries and/or fallopian tubes (Field & Moxham 2017).

Nurses need to provide women with the following information.

- women may go on to develop chronic pelvic pain syndrome (possibly due to the formation of scar tissue)
- there is a risk of a second episode of PID
- women will have a sevenfold increased risk of ectopic pregnancy
- there is a risk of infertility, with 20 per cent of women having tubal damage after two episodes of PID
- PID is generally sexually transmitted; therefore:
  - the woman's partner needs to be contacted and treated
  - there should be no further sexual activity until both parties have completed the course of treatment
  - anxiety and relationship problems may arise if there has been infidelity.

23.4 Nursing care of women who have had gynaecological surgery

LEARNING OBJECTIVE 23.4 Identify the common types of female gynaecological surgery and the physical and psychological care required.

Surgery on the reproductive organs can be either diagnostic or therapeutic. The surgical approach can be vaginal, laparoscopic or via an open procedure, depending on the type of operation. With changes in care procedures and advances in technology over the last decade, many women no longer require surgery. The developments in laparoscopic surgical techniques and the increase in the number of procedures being performed in outpatients or day units means that nurses must spend a shorter time addressing the psychological care that is integral to women's health.

Preoperative nursing management for gynaecological surgery

In addition to carrying out standard preoperative checks and assessments, nurses should establish the date of the last menstrual period and check if there is any chance of pregnancy before any operation that may impact a woman's fertility prospects. Most units ensure that a urinary hCG test is carried out before a gynaecological operation.

Preoperative anxiety is normal, but in the case of gynaecological surgery, nurses must be aware that operations can be linked with fertility or infertility, loss of sexuality, loss of pregnancy and the onset of menopause. Women need additional support when undergoing operations, however minor they seem to the healthcare staff.

Post-operative nursing management following gynaecological surgery

Post-operative observations should be carried out to assess for signs of bleeding and infection. Bladder function should be monitored as there may be a risk of retention if catheterisation is not required. Wound sites should be regularly observed and vaginal bleeding assessed with each observation. Specific care related to gynaecological procedures is shown in table 23.6.

Hysterectomy

One of the more common gynaecological operations is a hysterectomy (figure 23.9). This can be carried out in many different ways: an open procedure, laparoscopically or per vagina. The approach used depends on the condition being treated. Hysterectomy via a laparotomy — a cut in the abdomen (either transverse or longitudinal) — can involve:

- a radical hysterectomy (usually indicated for cancer): complete removal of the uterus, cervix, upper vagina, parametrium, lymph nodes, ovaries and fallopian tubes
- a total hysterectomy: complete removal of the uterus and cervix
- a subtotal hysterectomy: removal of the uterus, leaving the cervix in situ.

TABLE 23.6 **Nursing care for specific gynaecological procedures**

Operation	Why	Where and anaesthetic	Specific care
ERPC	Removal of pregnancy tissue after miscarriage	Day surgery, sedation/ general anaesthetic Day surgery unit, general anaesthetic	Pregnancy loss Grief Check rhesus factor
Hysteroscopy	Diagnostic for bleeding Therapeutic resection of: • fibroids • polyps • removal of lost IUD	Day surgery, sedation Day surgery unit, general anaesthetic Inpatient procedure, general anaesthetic	Can bleed up for to 2 weeks, depending on the procedure
Laparoscopy	Diagnostic for pain Endometrial oblation Removal of cyst Ectopic pregnancy Sterilisation Removal of womb Fibroids	Day surgery unit, general anaesthetic Inpatient procedure, general anaesthetic	Pain under shoulder tip from carbon dioxide gas used in the procedure Dissolvable sutures or sutures that need to be removed after 5–7 days
Colposcopy	Large loop excision of the transformation zone Cone biopsy	Day surgery, sedation Day surgery unit, local or general anaesthetic	Risk of infection No sexual intercourse for up to 4 weeks No use of tampons for four weeks
Myomectomy	Removal of fibroids Can be: • laparoscopic • hysteroscopic • via open laparotomy	Day surgery, sedation Day surgery unit, general anaesthetic Inpatient procedure, general anaesthetic	As for laparotomy Wound care When to conceive will depend on the operation and whether the uterine cavity has been entered
Hysterectomy	Laparoscopic Open Vaginal	Day surgery unit, general anaesthetic Inpatient procedure, general anaesthetic	Psychological care Risk of early menopause If subtotal hysterectomy, stress need for future cervical screening See also figure 23.9
Bilateral salpingo-oophorectomy	Removal of both fallopian tubes and ovaries Laparotomy Laparoscopy	Day surgery unit, general anaesthetic Inpatient procedure, general anaesthetic	Same care as for hysterectomy Menopausal symptoms
Repairs	Anterior and posterior colporrhaphy	Day surgery unit, general anaesthetic Inpatient procedure, general anaesthetic	Care of the wound Avoidance of constipation and straining
Transvaginal tape	Mesh to support the urethra	Day surgery, sedation Day surgery unit, general anaesthetic Inpatient procedure, general anaesthetic	Avoidance of straining
TOP		Private clinic, day surgery, sedation/general anaesthetic	Check rhesus factor and if negative, give anti-D Contraception Psychological care

FIGURE 23.9 Post-operative nursing care following hysterectomy

Risk of bleeding

Monitor:

- the wound and dressings
- the wound drain, if used
- the vital signs
- vaginal loss.

If there has been a vaginal hysterectomy:

- monitor the loss using a vaginal pack.

Pain

- Provide regular analgesia

Risk of infection

- Temperature and pulse
- the wound
- Remove clips and sutures at 5–10 days, as directed
- Remove the pack at 24 hours if a vaginal hysterectomy has been carried out
- Monitor for vaginal discharge or wound haematomas

Urinary elimination

- A urinary catheter should be in place for 24–48 hours

Potential constipation

- Monitor the bowels
- Provide suppositories if the bowels have not opened by day 3. Offer a high fibre diet and adequate fluids.

Profound change in body image and sexual function

For women, the uterus is deeply tied to the concept and feeling of womanhood. It is symbolic of sexuality, femininity, fertility and motherhood. Whether the woman is pre or postmenopausal, this remains true. A hysterectomy may cause a profound change in a woman's perception of self (Erdogan et al. 2020).

- Allow the woman time to discuss her fears and concerns
- Warn of menopause if the ovaries have been removed
- Refer to a specialist counsellor

Discharge advice

- Seek medical help if signs of infection develop
- Access for ongoing psychological support if needed
- Carry out pelvic floor exercises
- Sexual activity can resume once it is comfortable to do so
- Housework and lifting should be limited for the first 6 weeks and gradually built up as is comfortable
- Driving can be resumed when the woman is comfortable enough to do an emergency stop
- Return to work at 6 weeks
- If the cervix has been removed and any smears were normal before surgery, no more cervical screening needs to be undertaken

A laparoscopic approach (figure 23.10) can be used for a laparoscopic hysterectomy or a laparoscopically assisted vaginal hysterectomy.

FIGURE 23.10 Laparoscopy

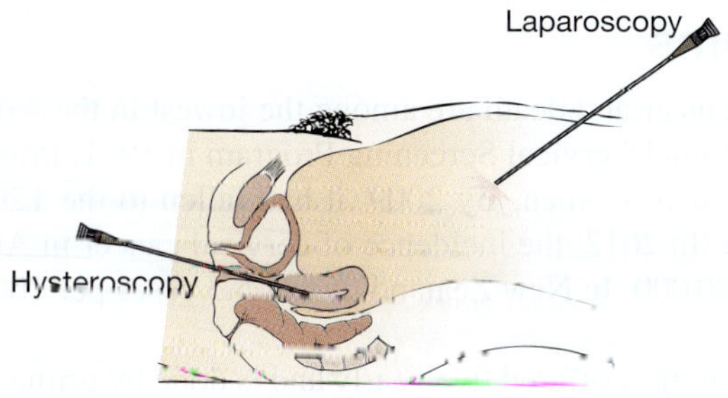

Source: Impey (2004) *Obstetrics & Gynaecology*, with kind permission of Wiley Blackwell.

23.5 Health promotion and contraception

LEARNING OBJECTIVE 23.5 Summarise the methods of contraception and identify screening programs available in women's health in Australia.

Sexually transmitted infections

Sexually transmitted infections (STIs) can be asymptomatic or cause symptoms in the form of discharge, itching, blisters and pain. Nurses should encourage women to reduce the risk of STIs by using barrier methods of contraception, possibly in addition to other methods of contraception, as infections can impact fertility and cause ectopic pregnancy and cervical cancer in later life.

Contraception

Contraception aims to prevent unplanned and unwanted pregnancies. Women's contraceptive needs change as they go through their reproductive life, and the use of contraception may also bring other health benefits, such as a reduction in menstrual loss with the COCP and IUDs.

Types of contraceptives include:

- male and female condoms
- male and female sterilisation
- female barrier methods (diaphragm/latex dome)
- the COCP
- the progestogen-only pill
- injections of progestogen
- implants, for example, a progestogen rod inserted subdermally into the arm
- intrauterine contraceptive devices (IUSs).

For more information on methods of contraception: www.familyplanningallianceaustralia.org.au.

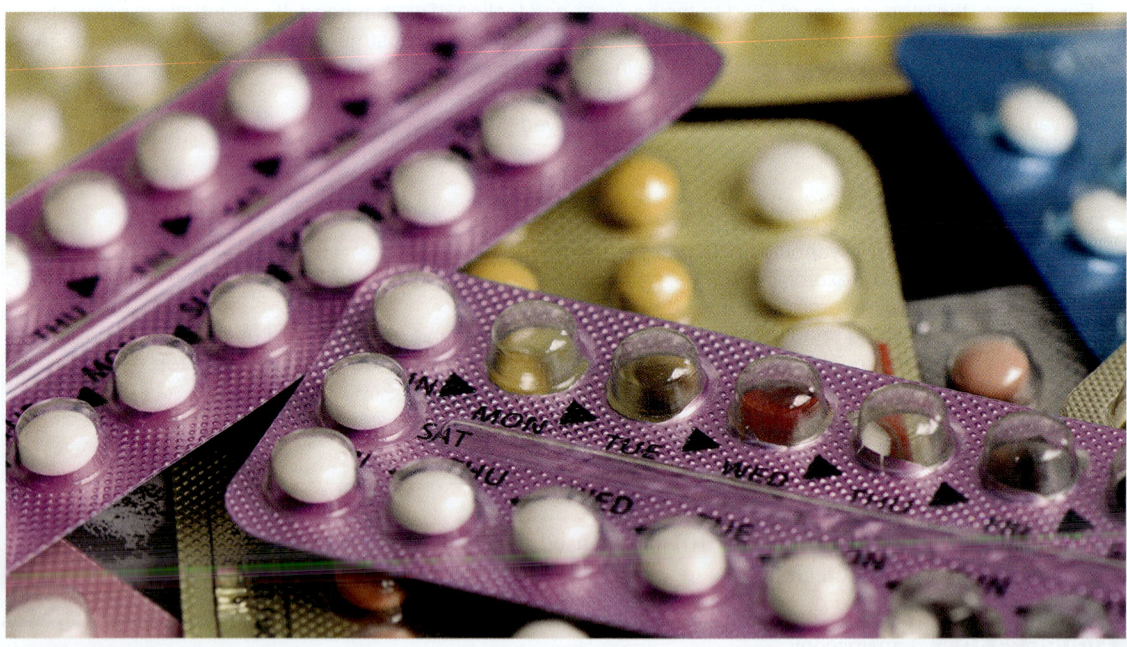

Screening programs

Australian rates of cervical cancer and death are among the lowest in the world. This is primarily related to the introduction of the National Cervical Screening Program in 1991. Prior to this, cervical cancer was the sixth most common cancer in women. By 2009, it had fallen to the 12th most common, a decrease of approximately 50 per cent. In 2012, the incidence of cervical cancer in Australia per 100 000 was 5.5, with a mortality of 1.6 per 100 000. In New Zealand, it was 5.3 cases per 100 000 with a mortality rate of 1.4 per 100 000.

In Australia, cervical screening is offered five yearly and is done by primary HPV screening with reflex liquid-based cytology for those women aged 25–74 years in whom oncogenic HPV is detected.

In New Zealand, cervical cytology remains the basis of the cervical screening approach, with HPV testing limited to assisting with clinical management in specific circumstances. It is expected that New Zealand will [illegible] to primary HPV screening soon (Bud & Hammond 2020).

Breast screening is a free service available every two years for females between the ages of 50–74 (Department of Health 2021). Breast screening involves having a low dose X-ray of the breasts called a mammogram. If the mammogram results cannot exclude a diagnosis of cancer, an ultrasound may also be performed. Between 1985–89 and 2011–15, the five year relative survival rates from breast cancer improved from 75 per cent to 94 per cent (Cancer Council 2020). Early detection gives women more treatment options to reduce illness and death and improve breast cancer survival rates. Unfortunately, the rate of accessing the free screening program is only approximately 55 per cent, a number that has remained stable since 2010 (AIHW 2020).

23.6 Disorders of the breast

LEARNING OBJECTIVE 23.6 Identify common breast disorders and discuss treatment options in breast cancer.

Breast problems are common (table 23.7). Women are concerned and worried that they may have breast cancer if they discover a breast lump; however, most lumps are benign. The incidence of breast cancer is increasing, with a lifetime risk of one in eight women developing this condition.

TABLE 23.7 **Common breast problems**

Condition	Signs and symptoms	Management
Mastalgia (breast pain)	Intermittent or cyclical in response to hormonal changes Can come from underlying structures such as ribs	A correctly fitting bra Analgesia Salt restriction Premenstrually, wearing a bra in bed Change hormonal contraception Evening primrose oil
Breast lumps (a variety of causes for non-cancerous lumps)	Fibroadenoma: • A firm oestrogen-sensitive nodule • Referred to as a breast mouse as it moves easily under the skin Cysts: • Can be large • Cause pain • More common in premenopausal women • Vary in number and size	No treatment unless >3 cm in size 20% will increase in size More common in younger women Ultrasound and possible aspiration
Nipple problems	Discharge Physiological Related to pregnancy Bloodstained discharge related to breast epithelial hyperplasia or ductal papilloma Galactorrhoea, caused by medications (dopamine agonists), pituitary tumours or hypothyroidism Pituitary adenoma: increased prolactin levels are associated with visual disturbances and menstrual problems	Reassurance Surgical excision Treatment is based on cause MRI of the pituitary and medication such as bromocriptine or cabergoline
Mastitis	Infection related: • Lactation • Smoking	Antibiotics Possible aspiration and culture

Breast cancer

As with gynaecological cancers, the incidence of breast cancer is increasing, and the condition has a profound psychological effect on women, their body image and their femininity. Risk factors include:

- age
- onset of menstruation before the age of 11 years
- menopause after 54 years of age
- first pregnancy when aged over 35
- a family history of breast cancer
- a high fat and alcohol intake
- obesity
- HRT
- possibly smoking.

The signs and symptoms include:

- any new lump
- pain (although this is present in only 10 per cent of women with cancer)
- newly occurring nipple retraction
- nipple eczema
- skin tethering or fixation
- ulceration.

Management of breast cancer

Clinical examination, ultrasound and biopsy (core biopsy or needle aspiration) are the standard methods of investigating breast lumps. If the results are positive for cancer, surgery is the treatment of choice. Several factors are taken into account when deciding what treatment is best:

- the stage and grade of the cancer (how big it is and how far it has spread)
- the patient's general health
- the menopausal status.

An MRI may give additional information about the extent of the disease. Women with cancer should be cared for by a multi-disciplinary team consisting of a specialist cancer surgeon, an oncologist (a radiotherapy and chemotherapy specialist), a radiologist, a pathologist, a radiographer, a reconstructive surgeon and a specialist nurse. Treatment options are outlined in table 23.8.

TABLE 23.8 Breast cancer treatment options

Treatment	Description	Nursing care
Lumpectomy	Removal of the lump only	See figure 22.11
Wide local excision	Excision around the cancer	See figure 22.11
Simple mastectomy	Removal of the breast	See figure 22.11
Modified radical mastectomy	Removal of the breast and chest wall muscles	See figure 22.11
Lymph node clearance	Removal of the lymph nodes, used with any of the above options	Post-operative lymphoedema
Radiotherapy	Used with local excision Takes place after surgery Can be a course of six weeks	Monitor for fatigue, sore throat, dry cough, nausea and anorexia
Chemotherapy	Can be given: • Before surgery • After surgery • After radiotherapy	Monitor for adverse effects of chemotherapy: • Bone marrow suppression • Nausea and vomiting • Alopecia • Gain or loss of weight • Fatigue • Stomatitis • Anxiety • Depression Discuss changes in diet if needed

Hormone therapy	Used if tumours are oestrogen receptor positive; an example is tamoxifen Aromatase inhibitors Trastuzumab for HER-2-positive breast cancer	Menopausal symptoms Risk of deep vein thrombosis Risk of fractures

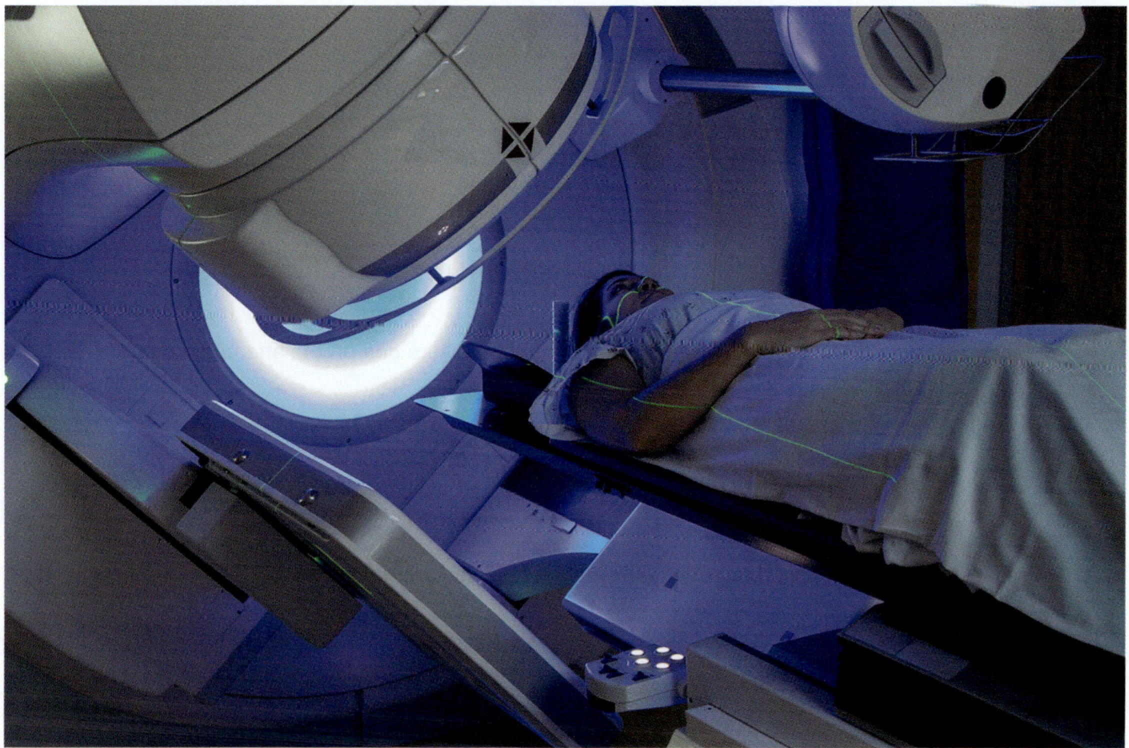

After surgery, breast cancers that are oestrogen and/or progestogen receptor positive are normally treated with antihormone medication such as tamoxifen or aromatase inhibitors to block the oestrogen receptors. Both of these medications have side effects similar to menopausal symptoms.

FIGURE 23.11 Post-operative care following breast surgery

Risk of bleeding

Observe the wound and dressings (the size of wound varies and depends on the surgical procedure that has been undertaken)

Monitor:

- the drain; if used, this may have been placed at the breast wound and/or in the axillary region
- the vital signs

Pain

- Provide regular analgesia
- Numbness, pins and needles in the axilla are common — reassure the patient

Risk of infection

Monitor:

- temperature and pulse
- the wound for haematoma or signs of infection
- remove clips and sutures after 5–10 days as directed
- wound drains, if present, are removed after post-operative day two

Profound change in body image and sexual function

- Allow the patient time to discuss fears and concerns
- Refer the patient to a specialist counsellor
- Provide advice on reconstruction or a prosthesis

Arm exercises following dissection of the axillary lymph nodes
- Women are at risk of developing problems with shoulder movement
- There is a need for specific arm exercises, usually taught by a physiotherapist; these can begin on day two post-operatively

Lymphoedema of the arm
Lymphoedema of the arm is a potential complication of axillary surgery and radiotherapy.
Educate patients on:
- the cause of lymphoedema
- the signs of lymphoedema
- preventing infection in the affected arm:
  - signs of infection
  - using gloves when gardening or doing household cleaning
  - avoiding the use of razors other than electric razors
  - cleaning any cuts and abrasions with antiseptic solutions
- moisturising the affected arm and hand
- carrying out arm and shoulder exercises
- elevating the affected arm, especially immediately post-operatively
- not carrying heavy objects with the affected arm
- not wearing heavy shoulder bags on the affected side
- avoiding injections, blood testing and the use of a blood pressure cuff on the affected arm

Discharge advice
- Seek medical help if signs of infection develop
- If needed, follow access for ongoing psychological support or support groups
- Attend outpatient follow-up appointments

After breast cancer, women need ongoing support and care and annual mammograms for at least 5 years. Follow-up includes:
- psychological care related to body image, fear of reoccurrence and fertility (as some treatments affect fertility)
- post-operative prosthetics following mastectomy; discussions with the patient may focus on reconstructive surgery
- monitoring of fatigue and strategies to avoid tiredness.

23.7 Disorders of the male reproductive system

LEARNING OBJECTIVE 23.7 Outline common testicular disorders and their management.

Testicular disorders

Men may present with pain, swelling, infection, inflammation and lumps in the testis, which may have various possible causes. Table 23.9 outlines the nursing care of common testicular disorders.

Testicular cancer

In Australia, testicular cancer affects 1.2 per cent of males. Testicular cancer accounts for one per cent of all cancers in men. It occurs most often in men aged 25–40, among whom it is the second most common cancer, excluding non-melanoma skin cancer. The rate of testicular cancer has increased by 50 per cent over the past 30 years. The increase is mostly in seminomas; the reasons for this are unknown (Cancer Council 2020). The two main types of testicular cancer are seminomas and non-seminoma cancers, including teratomas, embryonal carcinomas, choriocarcinomas and yolk sac tumours

Testicular cancer may present as:
- a lump in the testis, often painless
- an ache in the testis or abdomen
- breathlessness or backache if the cancer has spread.

Management of testicular cancer

Testicular cancer is diagnosed using ultrasound and markers in the blood, such as βhCG and AFP. If cancer is suspected, it is likely that the testicle will need to be removed (orchidectomy) (table 23.9). Other tests such as MRI or computed tomography scans and chest X-rays will be needed to look for signs of spread to the lymph nodes or other organs.

TABLE 23.9 Care of common testicular disorders

Patient problems	Nursing care
Pain and swelling due to infection and inflammation	Regular analgesia Supportive underwear Antibiotics Observation for worsening of the condition Discharge advice: • Ensure the scrotum is well supported • Avoid trauma or long periods of standing • Seek medical advice if pain or inflammation worsens after discharge from hospital
Post-operative care following orchidectomy, orchidopexy or hydrocele repair	Risk of bleeding: • Monitor vital signs, wound and wound drain if present • Observe for haematoma formation Pain: • Assess pain • Provide regular analgesia • Scrotal support or supportive underwear Psychological effects: • Testicular surgery (particularly orchidectomy) may cause fear and anxiety and a change in body image • Support should be offered along with information about local services • Men with a new diagnosis of testicular cancer should be given the details of the key worker, usually the clinical nurse specialist, who will take a lead role in coordinating their care. This promotes continuity of information and advice at different stages of the care pathway Discharge advice: • Check for signs of haematoma and infection and seek medical advice if necessary • Ensure the scrotum is well supported and avoid trauma and long periods of standing • Avoid sports and heavy lifting for four weeks or until comfortable • Avoid driving for two weeks (until able to perform an emergency stop safely)

Testicular cancer is primarily treated with orchidectomy (removal of the affected testis). Depending on the type of cancer and whether it has spread, chemotherapy and radiotherapy may also be used. Surgery may be required to remove tumours that have spread to other organs such as the lymph nodes and lungs. Men should be offered sperm storage as treatment may affect their future fertility. Testicular cancer has cure rates of over 97 per cent over five years (Cancer Council 2020).

Testicular pain and swelling

Testicular torsion is a serious and painful condition in which the spermatic cord twists, causing disruption to the testicular blood supply, leading to the death of the testicular tissue. It is a surgical emergency and has a peak presentation in males between the ages of 12–16 years. Quick surgical exploration is essential. If the testis is still viable, it may be untwisted and fixed to the scrotum (orchidopexy) to prevent recurrence. Otherwise, the testis must be removed (orchidectomy). The classical presentation of testicular torsion is acute pain often accompanied by nausea and vomiting, but it may also commonly present as generalised testicular pain at rest. Abdominal pain is also present in a significant number of presentations (Hyun 2018; Srinath 2013).

Other causes of testicular pain and swelling include inflammation and infection. This may affect the epididymis (epididymitis), the testis (orchitis) or both (epididymo-orchitis). The symptoms are similar to those of torsion, and a scan may be required to differentiate between the two. Unlike with torsion, the treatment involves analgesia, scrotal support and antibiotics. In severe cases, this will require admission for intravenous treatment.

A non-painful scrotal swelling may indicate a hydrocele, an accumulation of fluid between the layers of the tunica vaginalis. If this is painful or uncomfortable, the hydrocele can be drained or removed.

Penile disorders

The penis is made up of three columns of tissue. Two corpora cavernosa run along the dorsum (top) of the penile shaft, and below these two columns lies the corpus spongiosum. The corpus spongiosum surrounds the urethra along the ventral surface (underside) of the penis and forms the glans penis, which is the bulbous head of the penis. A fold of retractable skin covers the glans called the prepuce or foreskin, which is attached to the underside of the penis beneath the glans by a band of tissue called the frenulum.

A variety of disorders may affect the penis (table 23.10). Some are congenital, for example, hypospadias and epispadias, in which the urethral opening (meatus) is situated away from the tip of the glans and sometimes even on the shaft of the penis. Other disorders may result from trauma, infection, cancer or benign conditions that may develop later in life.

TABLE 23.10 Care of common penile disorders

Patient problems	Nursing care
Paraphimosis	Be aware of the risk of paraphimosis Replace the foreskin after retraction Observe for paraphimosis after instrumentation (e.g. catheterisation and cystoscopy) or examination
Post-operative care for circumcision	Carries risk of bleeding, so monitor the vital signs and wound Pain: • Regular analgesia • Anaesthetic gel if needed Oedema may require a supportive pad or underwear with the penis held in an upright position Discharge advice: • Counselling regarding sensitisation and later desensitisation of the glans • Most men can resume sexual intercourse after 4–6 weeks

Men may find it challenging to seek help for penile problems due to fear or embarrassment. Changes in body image due to the condition or its treatment may lead to depression, social isolation and sexual and relationship difficulties.

Phimosis and paraphimosis

Phimosis describes the condition in which the foreskin cannot be fully retracted over the glans. In paraphimosis, the foreskin becomes stuck behind the glans and cannot be pulled back. This may occur after the foreskin has been retracted for some time, for example, during catheterisation or other instrumentation, leading to the foreskin becoming swollen and oedematous. Care should always be taken to pull the foreskin forward following examination or catheterisation. This should be routinely documented when such procedures are performed.

Peyronie's disease

Peyronie's disease is a condition in which scar tissue or plaques form in the tunica albuginea (the fibrous layer of tissue that covers the corpora cavernosa). These plaques can cause pain, an abnormal bend in the penis, erectile dysfunction, indentations in the penis and penile shortening. If the penile bend is causing problems, either psychologically or with intercourse, an operation may correct it. In the Nesbit procedure, tissue is excised from the area opposite the plaque, and the area is sutured. This has the effect of 'shortening' the opposite side and thereby straightening the bend. Alternatively, tissue from, for example, the saphenous vein (the Lue procedure) may be grafted over the incised plaque area, thereby 'lengthening' the side with the defect. A penile prosthesis may be offered to patients with Peyronie's disease and ED.

Penile cancer

Penile cancer is rare and mostly affects men over the age of 60. Symptoms may include growths or sores on the penis that do not heal, bleeding from under the foreskin and a rash or colour change on the penis. The majority of penile cancers (90 per cent) are squamous cell cancers and tend to occur on the glans and foreskin. The likely outcome of treatment depends on how advanced the cancer is when diagnosed. Treatment may include radiotherapy, chemotherapy and surgery. The surgical options are shown in table 23.11.

TABLE 23.11 Surgery for penile cancer

Type of surgery	Description
Circumcision	Suitable if the cancer is only affecting the foreskin
Laser surgery or cryotherapy	Suitable for very early penile cancer Therapies use laser or liquid nitrogen to destroy the cancer cells
Simple excision	The tumour is removed with some surrounding skin. The wound edges can be simply sutured together
Wide local excision	The cancerous area is removed along with a border of healthy tissue. This may need a skin graft to cover the excised area
Glansectomy (removal of the glans)	Removal of the glans followed by a skin graft to reconstruct the head of the penis Sexual function may remain
Penectomy (removal of all or part of the penis)	Performed for extensive cancer A full penectomy is necessary if the cancer is deep or at the base of the penis It may be possible to perform reconstructive surgery
Removal of the lymph nodes	Lymph nodes in the groin may be removed if the surgeon suspects the cancer may have spread

Penile cancer and its treatment can affect sexual function, psychological well-being and quality of life and may also result in post-traumatic stress disorder (Novac et al. 2013). The nursing care for men undergoing penectomy is described in figure 23.12.

FIGURE 23.12 Post-operative nursing care following penectomy

- Risk of bleeding:
  - Observe the wound and dressings
  - Monitor vital signs
- Risk of oedema — maintain a supportive dressing with mild compression for 24 hours
- Pain — provide regular analgesia
- Risk of infection — monitor temperature
- Inability to pass urine — a urinary catheter should be in place for 48 hours
- Profound change in body image and sexual function:
  - Allow patients time to discuss their fears and concerns
  - Refer to a specialist counsellor
- Discharge advice:
  - Seek medical help if signs of infection develop
  - Provide access for ongoing psychological support

Erectile dysfunction

Erectile dysfunction (ED) is the inability (persistent or recurrent) to attain and or maintain a penile erection during sexual performance. In Australia, studies show a rate of 23.3 per cent ED in males 35–80 years of age. ED may be due to physical or psychological causes or a combination of the two. Some risk factors include advanced age, atherosclerosis, spinal cord disorders, obesity, medications, e.g. antihypertensives and alcohol or other substance abuse. Psychological causes may include partner-related stress, guilt and situational anxiety, self-image problems, history of sexual abuse, highly restricted sexual upbringing and psychiatric disorders such as depression and psychosis (Shoshony et al. 2017).

An erection occurs when physical or psychological stimuli cause arousal and stimulate the parasympathetic nervous system. Neurochemicals act on the smooth muscle walls of the penile blood vessels, causing vasodilation. The flow of blood into the penis increases and fills the corpora cavernosa. This engorgement causes compression of the small veins that drain the blood from the corpora, allowing the corpora to fill and become rigid. The sympathetic nervous system controls ejaculation, after which the penis loses rigidity (detumescence).

Men may have problems attaining or maintaining erections for several reasons. An erection is a complex event requiring hormones, nerves and blood vessels to work together. In addition, a low sex drive or psychological issues may lower the ability to become aroused or respond to stimuli. Psychological issues and the stress response may also interfere with parasympathetic nerve pathways.

Management of ED

Men often find it difficult to talk about sexual problems and often wait for months or years before discussing them with health professionals. Unfortunately, they often report that the response when they finally seek help is less than ideal. Nurses may be involved in the care and treatment of men with ED. As such, excellent communication and assessment skills and a non-judgemental attitude are essential. Given that ED is a common problem associated with many common diseases such as diabetes and cardiovascular disease, nurses must be aware of the need to ask about these issues and provide an environment where men feel supported and safe to discuss them.

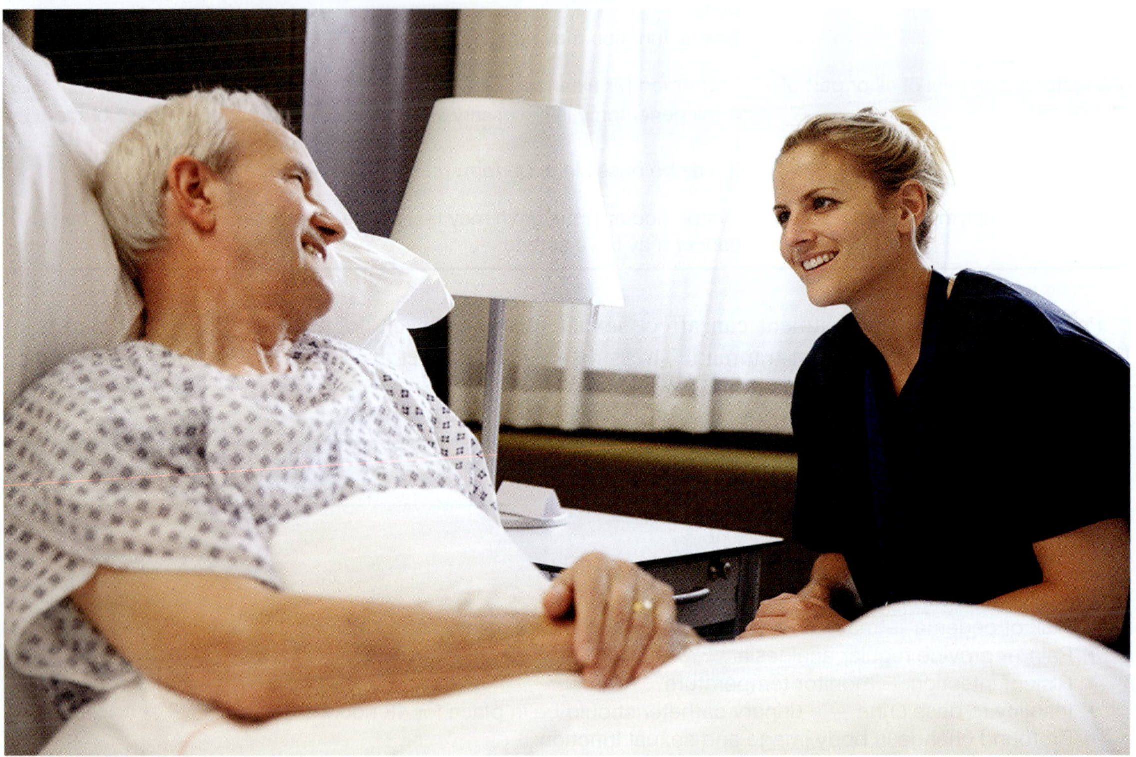

Management of ED includes lifestyle changes and some mechanical or pharmacological interventions to encourage erection (table 23.12). Men should be counselled that some causes of ED are irreversible and that management options may be required for the long term. The nursing care of men with ED is outlined in table 23.13.

TABLE 23.12 Managing ED

Treatment	Description
Lifestyle changes	Weight loss Smoking cessation Review of medication Stopping use of recreational drugs Relaxation Stress-relieving techniques
Oral medication	First-line treatment: • Phosphodiesterase type 5 inhibitors such as sildenafil (Viagra), tadalafil (Cialis) and vardenafil (Levitra) • Inhibition of phosphodiesterase type 5 increases nitrous oxide levels in the penile tissues, improves smooth muscle relaxation and facilitates erection This is contraindicated in men who take nitrate-based medications

Intracavernous injection	Alprostadil is a prostaglandin that is injected directly into the corpus cavernosum via a fine-bore needle This causes vascular smooth muscle relaxation, inflow of blood into the corpora cavernosa and erection The injection technique can be taught to the man or his partner There is a risk of priapism (prolonged erection)
Intraurethral medication	Alprostadil may be administered via the medicated urethral system for erection This contains higher doses of alprostadil, delivered as a pellet into the urethra with an applicator The alprostadil is absorbed via the urethra and corpus spongiosum
Vacuum constriction device	Vacuum constriction devices are mechanical devices consisting of a cylinder, a manual or battery-powered pump and a constriction ring The man is taught to put the penis inside the cylinder, forming a good seal The pump is operated, causing a vacuum inside the cylinder; negative pressure draws blood inside the penis to create an erection The constriction ring is applied at the base of the penis to maintain the erection once the cylinder has been removed
Psychosexual counselling	Techniques used may depend on the presenting factors Examples include behavioural techniques, cognitive techniques, psychotherapy and couple therapy An integrated approach combining medical and psychological therapies is the most effective treatment strategy
Penile prosthesis	A surgical procedure whereby implants are permanently inserted into the corpora cavernosum These may be semi-rigid silicone rods or inflatable sleeves that fill via a pump implanted in the scrotum This is only considered if the previous strategies fail It may also be useful in men with Peyronie's disease who have a severe curvature alongside ED

TABLE 23.13 **Nursing care for men with ED**

Area	Nursing care
General awareness and care	Be aware of the causes and risk factors for ED Encourage a sensitive and open discussion of sexual function Refer to specialist services if appropriate
Non-surgical treatments	Counsel regarding the availability and correct use of therapies
Penile prosthesis	Preoperative preparation to reduce risk of infection, as per local protocol Post-operative pain: • Elevate the penis with scrotal support or pad and pants • Provide regular analgesia Risk of bleeding and infection: • Give prophylactic antibiotics, as per local protocol • Monitor the vital signs • Observe the wound site for bleeding and breakdown Discharge advice: • Seek medical advice if signs of infection, haematoma or erosion (where the prosthesis breaks through the skin) develop • Resume sexual intercourse after 4–6 weeks

CASE STUDY 23.1

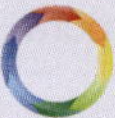

Nursing care of a patient with testicular torsion

A healthy 14-year-old boy presents to emergency with his mother complaining of pain in the left testicle of 4 hours duration, acute in onset. Pain persists when he is sitting still. He has nausea. He has not suffered any recent trauma in this area. The patient is pale and distressed.

Vital signs are:

- pain: 9/10 on movement and 6/10 when still
- temperature: 37.5°C
- heart rate: 86 beats per minute
- respiratory rate: 28 breaths per minute
- oxygen saturation: 100% on room air
- blood glucose level: 5.3 mmol/L.

Question

Using the information above, describe what action you would take as the nurse caring for this patient. Use the clinical reasoning cycle to guide you in this process.

Answer

- *Step: 1: Consider the patient.* 14-year-old boy with acute onset of unilateral testicular pain.
- *Step 2: Collect cues/information.* Collect cues/information: Include subjective and objective data here, including the patient's appearance and past medical history. Objective data will include measurable information such as vital signs.
- *Step 3: Process information.* Separate the relevant and irrelevant data — cluster the clues together to formulate an inference about the patient.

  Pain in a testicle is not normal. It is unilateral, involving one testicle only. Testicular torsion is most common in the 12 to 16 years age group. Testicular torsion occurs almost always unilaterally. Nausea is a common sign associated with testicular torsion.

  The patient has an elevated respiratory rate, but SpO_2 is 100%; therefore, it is likely that the increased respiratory rate is related to the pain, not to a respiratory cause.

  Temperature, SpO_2 and BGL are all within normal limits. Temp may be considered slightly elevated, but this would depend on the patient's usual baseline temp, so at this time, we will keep track of it in case it rises further.
- *Step 4: Identify problems/issues*. Patient and parent both concerned and anxious. The patient is in pain — likely testicular torsion. Immediate surgical intervention is needed, so the testicle does not become ischaemic.
- *Step 5: Establish goals*. The patient needs the doctor for immediate assessment and prep for potential surgery. Reassure both the patient and parent and give clear information and support.
- *Step 6: Take action*. The doctor is contacted to attend patient urgently for assessment. Administer analgesia if ordered; if not, may give nurse initiated analgesia.

  Fast patient in preparation for potential surgery, collect a urine sample, check weight, confirm last time that food and drink were ingested. Have consent form available if surgery is confirmed.

  Continue to communicate and reassure patient and parent.
- *Step 7: Evaluate outcomes*. Doctor confirms left-sided testicular torsion.

  Consent was obtained from the parent and the patient was prepped for theatre and understood that this was going to be beneficial.

  Testicular function was saved, and mother and son were relieved
- *Step 8: Reflect on the process and new learning.* Reflect on any aspects of care that could have been performed in a way to achieve an improved outcome.

CASE STUDY 23.2

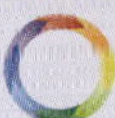

Nursing care of a patient undergoing a mastectomy

Mrs A, a 34-year-old female, was recently diagnosed with breast cancer of the left breast. She had a total left mastectomy with an axillary clearance 5 days ago. Prior to her surgery, she was a healthy, active female with no co-morbidities. She has a family history of breast cancer. When you go to introduce yourself to her and take her observations, you notice she appears very withdrawn and looks like she has been crying. She tells you the pain seems to be getting worse, and she is worried she is not getting better properly.

On examination, she has a dressing over the incision site on the left breast, which looks clean and dry and a smaller dressing at the axilla with a moderate amount of creamy exudate on the dressing. She also has a small dressing over the drain site, which also has pus coloured exudate.

Medications include paracetamol 1 gm 6-hourly and PRN (four hourly) Endone 5 mg, Clexane 40 mg mane subcutaneous, tamoxifen 20 mg daily.

Her observations are as:

- temperature: 37.9°C
- heart rate: 98 beats per minute
- blood pressure: 115/70 mmHg
- respiratory rate: 24 breaths per minute
- oxygen saturation: 99% on room air
- pain score: 7/10
- blood glucose level: 6.3 mmol/L
- redness and swelling noted at the axilla site with moderate creamy coloured exudate on dressing. Very tender and warm on palpation.

Question

Using the information above and charting on the approved colour coded/track and trigger chart used in your state or territory, describe what action you would take as the nurse caring for this patient. Use the clinical reasoning cycle to guide you through the process and devise a care plan for your patient.

Answer

- *Step 1: Consider the patient.* 34-year-old female five days post left mastectomy and axillary clearance.
- *Step 2: Collect cues.* Include subjective and objective data here, including the patient's appearance and past medical history. Objective data will include measurable information such as the vital signs.
- *Step 3: Process information*. Separate the relevant and irrelevant data — cluster the clues together to formulate an inference about the patient.

  Observations that are outside normal limits include temp 37.9 (this may indicate an infection) and HR 98 beats per minute. NB, while the temp and HR are still within the white zone of the chart, they are outside normal limits, and you note they have trended towards the danger zone.

  You know that you should not wait for these signs to trigger the need to call a doctor but should be proactive for the safety of the patient.

  Redness and swelling are not normal and are indicative of infection, as is the increased temperature. A hospital-acquired infection is likely to manifest approximately five days after contamination.

  Creamy exudate is also not normal and again indicates a possible infection. Increased pain is not normal.
- *Step 4: Identify problems/issues.* All signs at this time indicate this patient has a post-operative infection. She is also distressed by her pain and worried she is not healing properly.
- *Step 5: Establish goals*. This patient needs to be seen by a doctor for assessment and treatment initiated. We anticipate the need for antibiotic therapy to combat this infection. It is likely going to be ordered intravenously. We should be prepared for this as in order to commence IV therapy as soon as possible; it would be best if the doctor can insert an IV cannula stat.

  The patient needs pain relief and reassurance.
- *Step 6: Take action.* Ensure documentation up to date — document contemporaneous notes on the patient's condition. Speak reassuringly to the patient and explain you are going to call the doctor to come and assess her. Contact the surgical team and advise them of the patients' condition. Ask that they come and assess her. While awaiting the doctor, check her medication chart and give pain relief available at this time. Gather equipment for insertion of IV.
- *Step 7: Evaluate outcomes*. The patient is comforted and feels confident she will soon be back on the road to recovery. Pain relief is given with good effect.

  The doctor has taken a swab for culture and sensitivity and IV cannula inserted and IV broad-spectrum antibiotics commenced until results of swab are known. The care given was timely and appropriate.
- *Step 8: Reflect on the process and new learning*. Reflect on any aspects of care that could have been performed to achieve an improved outcome.

SUMMARY

The care of women and men with reproductive health issues is complex and multifaceted. This chapter has given an overview of the more common conditions that are seen in the hospital setting. The pathophysiology of these diseases is only one facet of any issue involving the reproductive system as this is always deeply entwined with social norms, roles, experiences and expectations. Humans are sexual beings, and reproductive illness can lead to guilt, social stigma and depression. A healthy reproductive system is integral to a person's sexuality and fertility and their deeply seated sense of manhood or womanhood. We must always acknowledge these factors and tailor our nursing care to be as holistic as possible.

KEY TERMS

embolisation A minimally invasive radiological procedure whereby a catheter is introduced to the blood vessel and embolysing agents are injected to block the vessel.

embryo A fertilised ova up to nine weeks post-fertilisation.

endocervical The inner part of the cervix lining the canal.

endometrium The inner layer of the uterine body made up of single-layer columnar epithelium, glands and stroma.

foetus By the end of the eighth week, all structures will be found in the full-term neonate. The embryo is now called a foetus.

gestation The time between conception and birth.

pedunculated To have a stalk or a stem.

peri-menopause Around menopause. This marks the time of natural transition through menopause marking the end of a woman's reproductive years. During this time, the ovaries gradually make less oestrogen until the time of menopause, when the ovaries cease releasing eggs.

postcoital Immediately following sexual intercourse.

REFERENCES

Australian Institute of Health and Welfare (AIHW). (2020) Breast cancer screening in Australia (fact sheet). www.aihw.gov.au/reports/cancer-screening/breastscreen-australia-monitoring-report-2020/contents/summary

Budd, A. & Hammond, I. (2020) 1. Cervical cancer in Australia. Cancer Council Australia cervical screening guidelines working party. https://Wiki.cancer.org/Australia/guidelines/cervicalcancerinAustralia

Cancer Council. (2020) Understanding testicular cancer. A guide for people with cancer their family and friends. https://www.cancer.org.au/assets/pdf/understanding-testicular-cancer-booklet

Condous, G. (2006) Ectopic pregnancy: risk factors and diagnosis. *Australian Family Physician.* 35(11): 854–857.

Department of Health. (2021) BreastScreen Australia Program. https://www.health.gov.au/initiatives-and-programs/breastscreen-australia-program/about-the-breastscreen-australia-program

Dunselman, G., Vermeulen, N., Becker, C., Calhaz-Jorge, C., D'Hooghe, T., De Bie, B., Heikinheimo, O., Horne, A., Kiesel, L., Nap, A., Prentice, A., Saridogan, E., Soriano, D. & Nelen, W. (2014) Eshre guideline management of women with endometriosis. *Human Reproduction.* (3): 400–412. doi: 10.1093/humrep/det457

Erdogan, E., Demir, S., Caliskan, B. & Bayrak, N. (2020) Effect of psychological care given to the women who underwent hysterectomy before and after the surgery on depressive symptoms, anxiety and the body image levels. *Journal of Obstetrics and Gynaecology.* 40(7): 981–987. doi: 10.1080/01443615.2019

Fields, L. & Moxham, L. (2017) 'Nursing care of people who have sexually transmitted disease'. In Lemone, Burke, Bauldoff, Gubrud, Levett-Jones, Hales, Berry, Carville, Dwyer, Knox, Moxham, Raymond & Reid-Searle (Eds.). *Medical-surgical nursing: Critical thinking for person-centered care*, 3rd ed. Pearson Australia.

Hogarth, K. (2017) 'The structure and function of the reproductive systems'. In Craft, J., Gordon, C., Huether, S., McLance, K., Brashers, V. & Rote, N. (Eds.). *Understanding pathophysiology*, 3rd ed. Chatswood, N.S.W: Elsevier.

Hyun, G. (2018) Testicular torsion. *Reviews in Urology.* 20(2): 104–106. www.ncbi.nlm.nih.gov/pmc/articles/PMC6168322

Mazza, D., Burton, G., Wilson, S., Boulton, E., Fairweather, J. & Black, K. (2020) Medical abortion. *Australian Journal of General Practice.* 49(6): 324–330. doi: 10.31128/AJGP-02-20-5223

National Institute for Health and Clinical Excellence (NICE). (2012) Ectopic pregnancy and miscarriage: Diagnosis and initial management in early pregnancy and miscarriage. Clinical Guideline 154. nice.org.uk/guidance.nice.org.uk/cg154

Novac, B., Ciobica, A., Dobrin, R., Ciobotaru, M. & Costache, C. (2013) Psychological/psychiatric trauma in patients with penile cancer and partial or total penectomy. *Archives of Biological Science.* 65(4): 1293–1298. doi: 10.2298/ABS1304293N

NSW Ministry of Health. (2019) *Summary of Abortion Law Reform Act 2019.* NSW Government. https://www.health.nsw.gov.au/women/pregnancyoptions/Factsheets/abortion-bill-summary.pdf

RANZCOG. (2011) *The investigation and treatment of couples with recurrent first trimester and second trimester miscarriage.* Green top guideline NO 17.

[illegible] *[illegible] for the treatment of uttering fibroids.* Statement provided for all health practitioners providing gynaecological [illegible]

[illegible] Katz, D. & Love, C. (2017) [illegible]ssment and treatment of erectile dysfunction by [illegible] *[illegible] Family Physician.* 46(9): [illegible]–704.

[illegible] scrotal pain. *Australian Family Physician.* 42(11): [illegible]–792.

[illegible] (2017) 'A person centred [illegible] the male and female reproductive systems'. In Lemone et al. (Eds.). *[illegible] Critical thinking for [illegible]* 3rd ed

United Nations. (1994) International Conference on [illegible] Development. Report of the [illegible] on Population and Development. Cairo, New York: United Nations.

Yeoh, M. (2015) Investigation and management of an ovarian mass. *Australian Family Physician.* 44(1-2): 48–52.

ACKNOWLEDGEMENTS

Figure 23.1: © Tortora, G.J. et. al., *Principles of Anatomy and Physiology*, 2nd Asia–Pacific Edition, figure 28.20, 2018. © John Wiley & Sons Inc. Reproduced with permission of John Wiley & Sons Inc.

Figure 23.2: © Tortora, G.J. et. al., *Principles of Anatomy and Physiology*, 2nd Asia–Pacific Edition, 2018. © John Wiley & Sons. Reproduced with permission of John Wiley & Sons inc.

Photo 23A: © Monkey Business Images / Shutterstock.com

Photo 23B: © areeya_ann / Shutterstock.com

Photo 23C: © Mark_Kostich / Shutterstock.com

Photo 23D: © Monkey Business Images / Shutterstock.com

CHAPTER 24

Principles of emergency and high dependency nursing

LEARNING OBJECTIVES

After studying this chapter, you should be able to:

24.1 identify key moments in the timeline of emergency nursing in Australia
24.2 explain the function of a high dependency unit
24.3 describe the principles of triage
24.4 describe the process of patient assessment in the emergency department (ED)
24.5 describe the assessment and stabilisation of emergency medical, surgical or trauma conditions
24.6 demonstrate an understanding of burns and their management
24.7 summarise the components of advanced life support
24.8 describe traumatic brain injury and use of the Glasgow Coma Scale
24.9 recognise behavioural disturbances and describe initial management in the ED
24.10 outline the care of patient and family who experience death in the ED.

Introduction

This chapter presents an overview of high dependency and emergency nursing. These are both areas designated as **critical care**. Critical care nursing is an umbrella term covering specialised areas where patients are too acutely unwell to be cared for in the ward environment. These areas include intensive care units (ICU), operating theatres (OT) and recovery units, coronary care units (CCU), neonatal intensive care units (NICU), emergency departments (ED), burns units, cardiothoracic units and **high dependency units (HDU)**. Key aspects of critical care relate to the severity of the patient's illness, the need for a higher ratio of nursing and medical staff available per patient and the specialised equipment and expertise required for the care of these patients.

24.1 Historical context of emergency nursing

LEARNING OBJECTIVE 24.1 Identify key moments in the timeline of emergency nursing in Australia.

Australia is a young country, as is the infrastructure of our health system. In the UK, EDs evolved from casualty departments in voluntary hospitals and workhouses from the 16th century. In Australia, we did not have 'poor houses' or workplaces to support the poor, nor did we have the social customs that obliged the wealthy to help those less fortunate. As our population grew, so did the dire consequences of poverty and illness. Australia's first charity was the Benevolent Society, which was established in 1813. In a short time, the services of this society were overwhelmed, and Australia's first hospital, The Rum Hospital, was built in 1816. In 1867, under the supervision of Lucy Osbourne, five nurses who had trained under Florence Nightingale arrived in Sydney. The Rum Hospital was renamed Sydney Hospital, and it was here that modern nursing in Australia was founded.

As with emergency medicine, emergency nursing is a relatively young specialist area of practice. Designated EDs were established in Australia in the early 1970s, and the evolution of emergency medicine and nursing has been congruent with developments in the UK, Canada, New Zealand and the USA. In 1967, the first full-time director of a 'casualty department' was appointed in Victoria, and in 1981, the Australasian Society of Emergency Medicine was established (National Museum of Australia 2021).

Emergency nursing in Australia has two national bodies. The Australian College of Emergency Nurses (ACEN), established in 2000, and the College of Emergency Nurses Australasia (CENA), established in 2002. Prior to establishing these national bodies, professional organisations were set up to support emergency nurses in this new specialty area. The Emergency Nurses Association was established in the UK in 1972, in Australia in 1983 and in New Zealand in 1990. Although there are two national organisations, each of the Australian states and territories have their own professional organisations for emergency nurses. Policies and guidelines for ED nurses are also state based. A number of educational institutions across the states offer postgraduate emergency nursing courses, as emergency nurses must have highly developed clinical skill sets and a highly evolved clinical reasoning ability. While it is estimated that nurses on a medical ward may engage in 50 clinical reasoning episodes per shift, emergency nurses face a clinical judgement or decision every 30 seconds (Levett-Jones & Hoffman 2013).

In Australia, the roles of individual EDs differ due to their geographical locations and available services. In urban areas, most metropolitan and regional hospitals have a designated ED. In rural and remote areas, designated treatment areas offer limited **resuscitation** services. To be designated an ED, facilities must have a specialist medical officer and nursing cover as well as onsite diagnostic services, OT and an ICU. In rural areas, nurses often assess and manage patients.

24.2 High dependency nursing

LEARNING OBJECTIVE 24.2 Explain the function of a high dependency unit.

A high dependency unit (HDU) is an area that is specially equipped and staffed to provide care that is intermediate between intensive care and general ward care. Patients may be admitted to a HDU as a step down from the ICU prior to transfer to the ward or be directly admitted from the ward as the need for care is escalated (CICE 2013).

Patients in HDU typically have single organ failure and are at risk of developing complications. Cardiac patients in facilities without a specified coronary care unit are often nursed in HDU until they are stable enough to go to the wards. Therefore, a HDU should have all the resources available to resuscitate and manage critically ill patients. The HDU should have equipment and suitably qualified staff available to manage short term emergencies, including ventilating a patient. Once a patient has been ventilated, they should be transferred to an ICU.

Single organ failure may include the following

- *Cardiovascular.* The nurse should have advanced skills in haemodynamic monitoring, including echocardiogram (ECG) interpretation and knowledge of common dysrhythmias, acute coronary syndromes, cardiogenic shock, heart failure and fluid and electrolyte disturbances.
- *Respiratory.* Skills needed include the ability to do a focused respiratory assessment, pulse oximetry, blood gas analysis, oxygen therapy, suctioning, intrapleural chest drain management, temporary and long-term tracheostomies and their care and non-invasive ventilation, e.g. CPAP and BiPAP.
- *Diabetic emergencies.* Such as diabetic ketoacidosis (DKA) may need a HDU in the early stages of resolution where the patient is acutely unstable and requires multiple lines, including IV insulin and fluids titrated to the patient's condition.
- *Renal.* Acute renal failure patients may need peritoneal dialysis. However, anyone needing haemodialysis will either have this in the ICU if they are acutely ill and have multisystem failure or will be cared for by a dialysis unit.
- *Gastrointestinal.* Disorders where the patient is acutely ill and requires close monitoring and fluid and electrolyte replacement therapy.
- *Other complications.* Acute liver dysfunction, acute neurological pathologies, haematological disorders and acute pain.

A HDU needs to provide routine monitoring of patients, including ECG, oximetry, invasive measurement of blood pressure, low-level inotropic support and non-invasive ventilation. The unit must be geographically part of the intensive care complex of a hospital and have 24-hour access to intensive care services, pharmacy, pathology, imaging services and operating theatres (CICE 2013).

The staffing in a HDU should include a nursing staff to patient ratio of 1:2. Nurses that have direct patient care must be registered nurses (RNs) and a majority should have post-registration qualifications. There must be a minimum of two RNs in the unit at all times that a patient is present. There must also be a medical director and at least one other specialist staff member who has an appropriate level of experience and is immediately available at all times (CICE 2013).

Generally, patients will be managed in a HDU for up to 72 hours, after which they should be reassessed in regard to whether they need to have their care escalated to ICU.

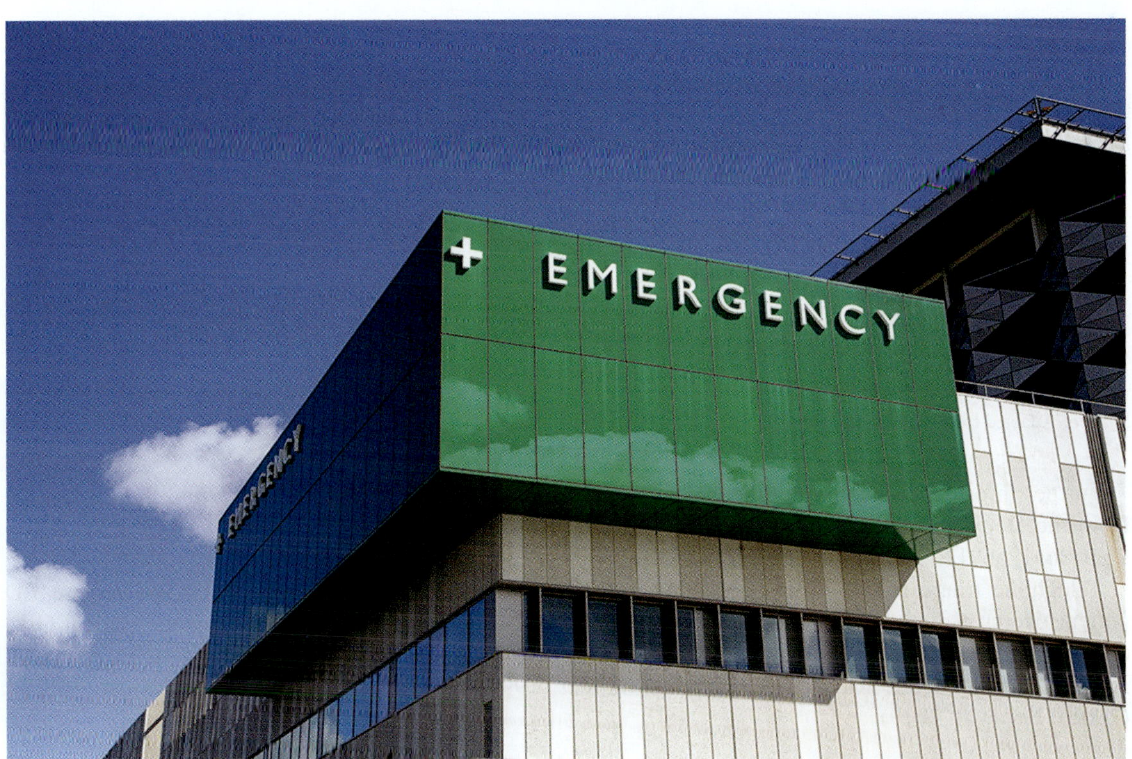

24.3 Triage principles

LEARNING OBJECTIVE 24.3 Describe the principles of triage.

The first step in the patients' journey through the ED is when they first present and are triaged to a category 1–5. The term comes from the French verb trier, meaning to pick or sort (Department of Health and Ageing 2009). **Triage** systems were first used in the Napoleonic wars and have been refined during subsequent wars treating the wounded behind the front lines. Triage has developed into a system of clinical risk management.

> The purpose of a triage system is to ensure that the level and quality of care that is delivered to the community is commensurate with clinical criteria, rather than administrative or organisational need. In this way, standardised triage systems aim to optimise the safety and the efficiency of hospital-based emergency services and to ensure equity of access to health services across the population (Department of Health and Ageing 2009).

Across the world, a number of triage systems exist. There is no universal standard, but most modern triage systems use a five-point **acuity** scale (Dippenaar 2019).

The years and countries in which each system was founded are:

- 1990 — Emergency Severity Index (ESI), USA
- 1993/4 — national triage scale (NTS), Australia. This formed a benchmark on which the Canadian and Manchester systems were based
- 1996 — Manchester Triage Scale (MTS), UK
- 1997 — Canadian Triage and Acuity Scale (CTAS), Canada
- 2001 — Australasian Triage Scale (ATS), Australasia. This is the scale currently used (Dippenaar 2019).

Table 24.1 outlines the triage categories and the times within which a patient must be seen to initiate assessment and treatment. Figure 24.1 outlines the recommended process of triage. Triage is the first point of contact a person has with the ED clinical staff. It should take no more than 2–5 minutes. Vital signs should only be measured to estimate urgency or if time permits. If a patient is identified as ATS category 1–2, they should immediately be moved to the appropriate treatment area. Nurse triage should only be undertaken by an experienced registered nurse in emergency care who has received specific training (Australian College of Emergency Medicine [ACEM] 2016).

TABLE 24.1 **The Australasian Triage Scale (ATS)**

Category	Name	Maximum target time (minutes) to first contact with the treating clinician
1	Resuscitation — immediately life-threatening	0
2	Emergency — imminently life-threatening	10 mins
3	Urgent — potentially life-threatening	30 mins
4	Semi urgent	60 mins
5	Non-urgent	120 mins

Source: Adapted from ACEM (2016).

Further information about the process of triage may be found in the *Emergency Triage Education Kit* from the Department of Health and Ageing (2009): www.acem.org.au/getmedia/c9ba86b7-c2ba-4701-9b4f-86a12ab91152/Triage-Education-Kit.aspx

Telephone triage has also developed in Australasia to reduce the burden on GPs and reduce ED patient overcrowding. Throughout Australasia, telephone triage systems can refer patients to local GPs, community services or EDs. In NZ, services include PlunketLine (1994) and Healthline (2005). In Australia, they include Kidsnet (1997), Healthdirect (1999), HealthConnect (2000) and Nurse on Call (2006) (Fry et al. 2019).

24.4 Patient assessment in the emergency department

LEARNING OBJECTIVE 24.4 Describe the process of patient assessment in the emergency department.

The management of patients presenting to the ED can be challenging due to the diverse and often complex surgical, medical and traumatic injuries as well as behavioural and social conditions. The emergency nurse is often the first healthcare professional to assess the patient presenting with an acute surgical condition; therefore, nursing assessment must be rapid, focused, accurate and continuous. The formulation of an accurate working diagnosis and timely appropriate management is essential to reduce overall morbidity and mortality. This requires good communication skills, a knowledge of anatomy, physiology and mechanisms of **trauma**, proficient assessment skills, critical thinking skills and common sense.

FIGURE 24.1 The recommended process of triage

1. Patient presents for triage — consider all safety aspects.
2. Quick evaluation. *Is the patient stable?* If NO, assign an appropriate ATS category in response to clinical assessment/data.
   - If patient is stable, continue assessment.
2. Assess the following — the most urgent clinical feature should be identified, and the triage allocation should be in response to this identified feature.
   - Chief complaint
   - General appearance
   - Airway
   - Breathing
   - Circulation
   - Disability
   - Environment/exposure
   - Limited history
   - Co-morbidities
3. Discriminate predictors of poor outcome from other data collected during the triage assessment.
4. Identify patients who are assessed as being at high risk of physiological instability.
5. Allocate an appropriate ATS category based on clinical assessment/data.
6. Allocate staff to patient. Give ISBAR handover to allocated staff members.
7. Proceed with care following ED model of care.

Source: Adapted from ACEM (2009).

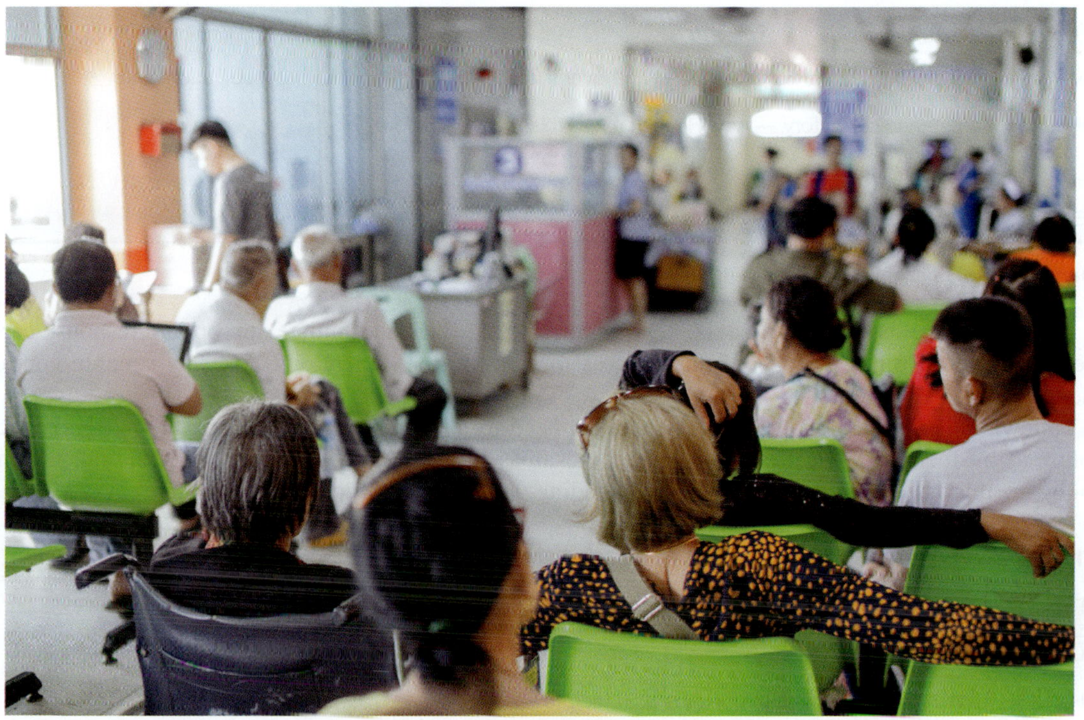

The principles of **advanced life support (ALS)** are used to assess all patients presenting to the ED. The primary and secondary assessment processes described here can be applied to any emergency admission and should be complete within 5 minutes. **Primary assessment** is conducted to identify potentially life-threatening situations and prioritise care. This should always begin with DRSABCDE (Danger, Response, Send for help, Airway, Breathing, Circulation, Disability, Exposure). Once this has been done, and the patient is judged to be stable, a more comprehensive (secondary) assessment can be attended. If at any time the patient deteriorates, always return to the DRSABCDE mnemonic pathway (table 24.2) (Munroe & Hutchinson 2019).

TABLE 24.2	Primary assessment
D	Check for danger
R	Check for patient responsiveness
S	Send for help
A	Airway (ensure cervical spine support for trauma patients) — check patient's colour; is the airway patent? Is the patient distressed?
B	Breathing — check rate, pattern, effort, sounds, chest movement, oxygen saturation
C	Circulation — check patient's colour, pulse rate, rhythm and strength, blood pressure, capillary refill time, blood loss, urine output
D	Disability — neurological assessment using AVPU (alert, responds to voice, pain, unresponsive), pupil reaction, blood sugar
E	Exposure — remove clothing to assess for any immediate threats to life or limb, rashes, wounds, scars and thrombosis

Source: Adapted from Munroe & Hutchinson (2019).

Secondary assessment includes a review of DRSABCDE and continues with the SAMPLE mnemonic (table 24.3) (Munroe & Hutchinson 2019) or other similar mnemonics.

TABLE 24.3	The SAMPLE mnemonic
S	Signs and symptoms of the chief complaint. Include pain history here — the PQRST mnemonic is useful here (see table 24.4).
A	Allergies
M	Medications, including prescribed and over the counter drugs and herbal medications, etc.
P	Past medical history — Ask 'Have you had this problem before?'
L	Last oral intake
E	Events leading up to the illness or injury

Source: Adapted from Munroe & Hutchinson (2019).

Throughout the assessment process, be alert for any red flags and initiate appropriate response early. Remember at all times throughout this process to reassure the patient and give any suitable comfort measures.

Following the primary and secondary survey, a head-to-toe assessment is done by the medical officer followed by focused clinical examination of the areas of concern. A detailed history is taken either following this assessment or concurrently, depending on the patient's condition.

TABLE 24.4	Pain assessment using PQRST mnemonic
P	What **provokes** the pain?
Q	What is the **quality** of the pain? E.g. sharp, dull, burning, etc.
R	What **region** is it in and does the pain radiate?

S	What is the **severity** of the pain? In the primary survey this is likely to be the only part of the pain assessment attended
T	How long has the patient had the pain? (**time**)

Source: Adapted from Munroe & Hutchinson (2019).

24.5 Assessment and stabilisation of emergency medical, surgical and trauma conditions

LEARNING OBJECTIVE 24.5 Describe the assessment and stabilisation of emergency medical, surgical and trauma conditions.

With any major trauma, surgical or medical emergency, the goal is to initiate appropriate treatment as soon as possible, requiring the patient to be transported from the ED to the specialty area best suited for that treatment. This may mean inter-hospital transfer or transfer from the ED to a specialised unit within the same hospital, whether this is the ICU, theatre or any other critical care unit. However, prior to this, the patient needs to be stabilised, and any life supporting measures must be initiated within the ED to enable the safe transfer of the patient.

Common surgical emergencies

Surgical emergencies are numerous and varied and commonly include conditions such as:

- neurological emergencies including skull fractures and head injuries
- cardiovascular emergencies such as abdominal or thoracic aortic aneurysms
- respiratory emergencies including traumatic chest injuries, for example, flail chest, haemothorax or rib/sternal fractures
- gastrointestinal emergencies including appendicitis, cholecystitis, abdominal trauma, pilonidal abscess, intestinal obstruction and perforated peptic ulcer
- genitourinary emergencies such as Bartholin's cyst/abscess and trauma to the bladder or genital area
- maxillofacial emergencies, for example, fractures and/or dislocation of the facial and mandibular bones
- musculoskeletal injuries, generally due to trauma and including fractures and/or dislocations of the upper and lower limbs, spine, pelvis and neck. Other musculoskeletal injuries include blast injuries and gunshot wounds.

Assessment for all patients presenting to the ED with abdominal pain includes:

- a DRSABCDE assessment
- urinalysis and culture and sensitivity
- blood tests (which may include a full blood count, urea and electrolytes and possibly liver function tests)
- an abdominal X-ray
- an ultrasound scan
- a computed tomography (CT) scan
- a magnetic resonance imaging scan.

Common medical emergencies

Medical emergencies are numerous and varied, as can be seen from the following list:

- neurological emergencies, including cerebrovascular accidents, meningitis, encephalitis, seizures and altered consciousness
- cardiovascular emergencies comprising chest pain, unstable angina, myocardial infarction, left ventricular failure, cardiogenic shock or anaphylaxis and deep venous thrombosis
- respiratory emergencies, such as acute exacerbation of asthma and heart failure, along with conditions such as pneumonia, pulmonary embolism and spontaneous pneumothorax
- gastrointestinal emergencies, for example, epigastric pain, peptic ulcer disease, pancreatitis, alcoholic liver disease, inflammatory bowel disease and gastroenteritis
- genitourinary emergencies including urinary tract infection, pyelonephritis, retention of urine, renal colic, sexually transmitted infections and priapism
- endocrine and metabolic emergencies such as hypoglycaemia, diabetic ketoacidosis, hypo- or hyperkalaemia/natraemia, thyrotoxic crisis and hypothyroidism

- clotting disorders such as haemophilia and sickle cell disease, which are the most common haematological emergencies
- skin emergencies, for example, burns, rashes, urticaria and leg ulcers
- ENT emergencies, including epistaxis, peritonsillar abscesses, tonsillitis and earache
- other medical emergencies, such as poisoning and drug/alcohol misuse.

Emergency trauma conditions

Worldwide, trauma causes nine per cent of all deaths and is the leading cause of death in the 15–44 year age group in developed countries. Neurotrauma is the most common cause of death in trauma. Thoracic trauma is responsible for 25 per cent of trauma deaths, and 10 per cent of deaths from trauma are due to abdominal injuries. These may be initially difficult to detect as the bleeding is likely to be internal, so the 'expose' aspect of the primary survey is vital. Noting bruising from seatbelt injury or other subtle signs may help swift diagnosis of internal bleeding (Cameron & O'Reilly 2020).

Australia has a large landmass with many sparsely populated areas — 38 per cent of the population live outside major cities. This has led to the development of a hub-and-spoke pattern of major trauma retrieval, facilitating the rapid transfer of trauma patients to designated trauma hospitals. One-third of major trauma patients are transferred to a second facility for optimum care (Warren et al. 2019).

The treatment of the seriously injured patient requires a rapid assessment and early intervention with life-saving therapy. Patients are assessed, and their treatment priorities established based on the cause and mechanism of their injuries, their vital signs and a primary assessment. The Advanced Trauma Life Support (ATLS) method was developed by the American College of Surgeons and provides a framework for the care of the trauma patient. In Australia, the Early Management of Severe Trauma (EMST) was introduced in 1988 and has become the national standard and is recognised as equivalent to ATLS. Similar courses exist for nurses. The hallmark of all programs is a systematic, concise approach to early care in the 'golden hour' after the injury has been sustained and is characterised by the need for rapid assessment and resuscitation, which are its fundamental principles. Handover from the retrieval/transport team follows the MIST protocol (mechanism of injury, injuries suspected, vital signs and treatment en route to hospital). The process is known as the 'initial assessment' and includes:

- preparation — the retrieval team will phone ahead and alert the hospital of their imminent arrival
- triage — patient will be triaged en route to the readied resuscitation area
- a primary survey (DRSABCDE)
- resuscitation
- adjuncts to the primary survey and resuscitation
- a secondary survey
- adjuncts to the secondary survey
- continued post-resuscitation monitoring and re-evaluation
- definitive care.

Minor trauma assessment and stabilisation

Minor trauma does not have a clear definition, but are patients whose injuries are not life-threatening. These patients can end up waiting for treatment, although their treatment time could be short with a clear diagnosis. Many EDs have recognised this and have set initiatives in place to expedite their movement through the ED. Specifically trained nurses are used in many EDs who can 'fast track' these patients' care. These nurses can undertake focused examination, order X-rays and routine blood work and provide analgesia. They may suture and dress wounds and provide other treatment measures. An increasing number of EDs are now utilising nurse practitioners in this role. Minor trauma/injuries may include sprains and abrasions, lacerations, bites, dislocations, minor non-displaced fractures and crush injuries, e.g. fingers in car doors (Jones & Rootham 2019).

24.6 Burns management

LEARNING OBJECTIVE 24.6 Demonstrate an understanding of burns and their management.

Burns are one of the most devastating injuries across all ages. Fortunately, in Australia and New Zealand, we have a lower rate of burn injuries than the US, and the incidence has been decreasing over the past 20 years; however, we still have a rate of one per cent per annum. Fifty-seven per cent of these occur in rural areas, which has significant implications in accessing prompt, vital treatment. As with all trauma cases,

Burns affect males more commonly than females at a rate of 1.6:1. Major burns have a relatively high mortality rate due to the systemic response that occurs and affects every organ in the body. These are initially caused by the release of inflammatory mediators with an immediate and profound effect on the circulation. Major burns are classified as 20 per cent total body surface area (TBSA) in adults and 10 per cent TBSA in children.

The severity and classification of the burn injury is based on assessing the extent and depth of the burn injury, the patient's age, any concomitant injuries, smoke inhalation and pre-existing health issues. There are many types of burn (table 24.5), and a key aspect of assessment is determining the victim's length of exposure to the source of the burn. This helps to accurately explain and assess the depth and extent of the burn. First aid should be attended by exposing the area to cool running water for 20 minutes. This is not only analgesic, but helps to stop the burning process and minimise further damage. Care must be taken to ensure the person does not become hypothermic during this process e.g. a child with extensive burns; however, this can be achieved by warming the environment or providing warm towels or a space blanket over the unburnt areas. The application of cool running water is still effective up to three hours post-injury (Holland & Quinn 2019; O'Reilly & Mitra 2020; NSW ACI 2018).

TABLE 24.5 Aetiology of burns

Types of burn	Mechanism of injury
Chemical	Direct contact with acid or alkaline chemicals. Alkaline substances cause more damage than acids
Contact	Direct contact with hot objects
Electrical	As electricity passes through the body, it meets resistance from the tissue. The smaller the area of contact, the more intense the heat and damage
Flame	Direct contact with open flame or fire
Flash	Exposure to the energy produced by explosive material
Friction	Rapid movement of a surface against the skin e.g. treadmill, motorbike accident etc.
Radiation	Exposure to solar energy, radiotherapy, laser or intense pulse light
Radiant heat	Heat radiating from heaters, open fireplaces etc
Reverse thermal	Frostbite This is caused by vasoconstriction of the peripheral blood vessels. Intra- and extracellular fluids freeze, forming crystals that damage the tissues
Scald	Direct contact with hot liquids
Thermal	Flame, flash, steam, liquid and contact burns

Source: NSW ACI (2018).

The depth of burns can be described as superficial partial thickness, deep partial thickness and full thickness, but it can take up to 48–72 hours to determine this accurately, owing to the formation of oedema and the compromised circulation.

The extent of a burn injury is determined using the Wallace Rule of Nines (figure 24.2) or the Lund and Browder table. Both the burned and unburned areas are calculated to ensure accuracy. The exception to using these charts is with electrical burns, where the percentage of body surface area is not used to describe the extent of the burn — in these cases, the injury is described anatomically.

Due to the loss of skin in burns, the emergency care of a burn injury focuses on preventing infection, **hypovolaemia** and maintaining a normal body temperature. Assessment includes the following steps:

- trauma survey — DRSABCDEF and assess the size and depth of the burn
- history:
  - time of injury
  - mechanism of burn
  - medical history
- reassure the patient and family:
  - what is happening now
  - what the plan is over the next 24–48 hours
  - what their level of understanding is.

FIGURE 24.2 Wallace Rule of Nines

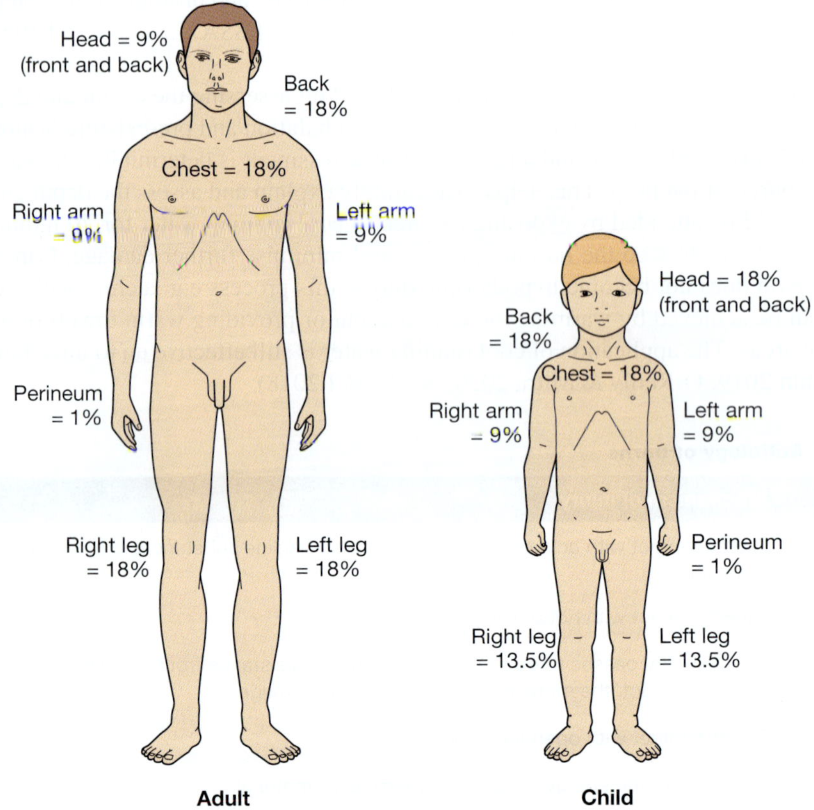

Source: Hettiarachty (2004) *ABC of Burns*, with kind permission of Wiley Blackwell.

If the burn injury is classified as major (affecting more than 20 per cent of the victim's TBSA), the following are the key points of care in stabilising the patient (Wraa 2010).

- All major burns patients should be given supplemental oxygen and placed on cardiac and oxygen saturation monitoring (O'Reilly & Mitra 2020).
- Stabilise and continually assess the airway. Burns of the face, neck and airways likely to cause oedema and result in upper airway obstruction. Be alert for inhalational damage and respiratory distress.
- Two large bore intravenous cannulae should be inserted and appropriate fluids given — administer all fluids through a fluid warmer.
- Take baseline blood samples.
- Insert a urinary catheter.
- Administer pain relief — short-acting narcotics.
- Dress the wound — wound should be cleaned with 0.1 per cent aqueous chlorhexidine or saline then covered with cling wrap or a clean, dry sheet. Any advice on burns can be obtained from the referral burns unit for your hospital (Holland & Quinn 2019).

24.7 Advanced life support

LEARNING OBJECTIVE 24.7 Summarise the components of advanced life support.

Advanced life support (ALS) is a generic term to describe resuscitation efforts that include a set of life-saving protocols and skills that extend basic life support to further support the circulation and provide an open airway and adequate ventilation (see figure 24.3). Emergency medical care for sustaining life may include defibrillation, airway management, drugs and medications.

ALS may commence in the pre-hospital setting before the patient arrives at the ED. Pre-hospital emergency care refers to any medical care or intervention that a seriously ill or injured person receives from trained personnel before being taken to hospital. ALS guidelines in Australia and New Zealand are produced by the Australian Resuscitation Council and New Zealand Resuscitation Council. The latest update to these guidelines was in 2016.

FIGURE 24.3 ALS guidelines*

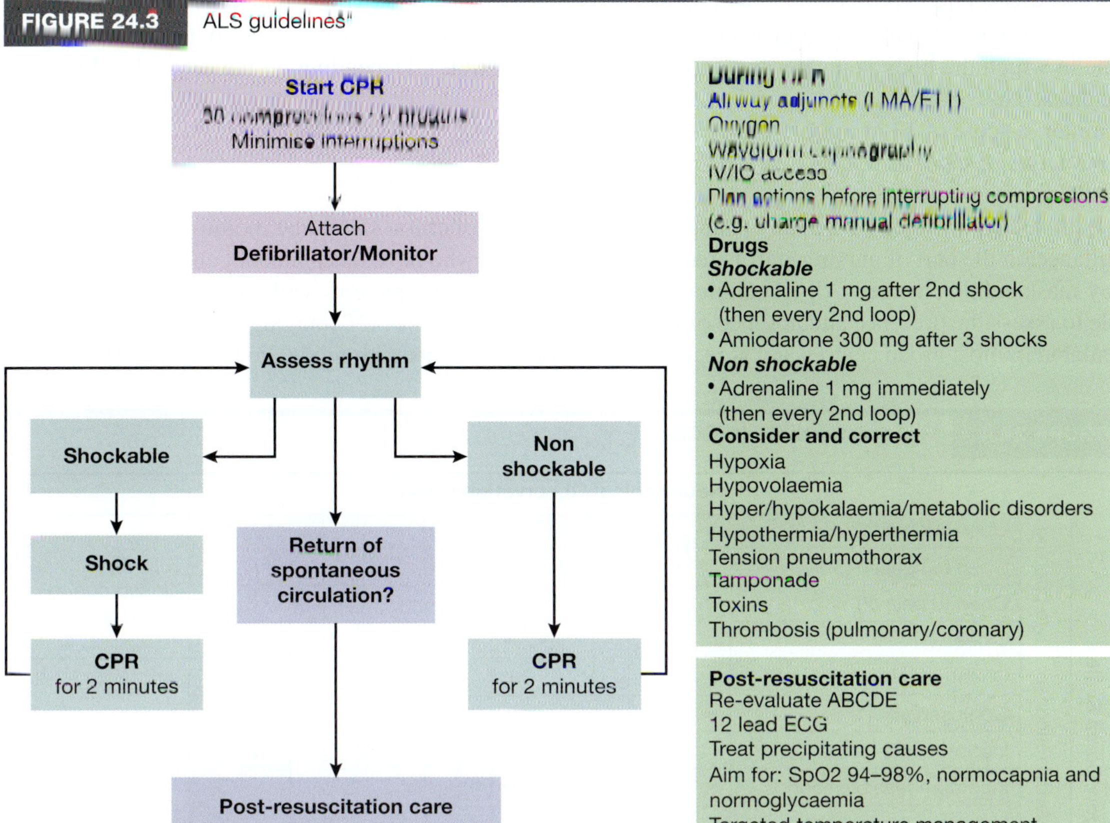

*CPR = cardiopulmonary resuscitation; PEA = pulseless electrical activity; VF = ventricular fibrillation; VT = ventricular tachycardia.
Source: Australian and New Zealand Committee on Resuscitation (ANZCOR) (2016).

24.8 Traumatic brain injury and the Glasgow Coma Scale

LEARNING OBJECTIVE 24.8 Describe traumatic brain injury and use of the Glasgow Coma Scale.

Neurotrauma is the leading cause of death in trauma cases causing between 30–50 per cent of all trauma deaths (O'Reilly & Cameron 2020). Traumatic brain injury is defined as 'an alteration in brain function or other evidence of brain pathology caused by an external force' (Sharpe & Cole 2019). Brain injuries are classified as mild, moderate or severe. The effects may range from mild, including **concussion**, to severe TBI, which can cause irreversible impairment or be fatal.

There were 22 710 hospitalisations for TBI in 2004–05 in Australia, and 14 000 are treated annually in New Zealand. The incidence of concussion is thought to be under-reported, with many people with mild TBI not presenting to hospital or seeking medical assistance. In New Zealand and Australia, the leading causes are falls and transport-related accidents, with 20 per cent acquired through sports. Alcohol is also a major contributing factor.

Concussion is a common presentation of mild brain injury. The pathophysiology of concussion is not well understood, but the current consensus is that it is a physiological disturbance rather than structural damage. Most concussion is associated with a loss of consciousness often followed by rapid recovery. If a person still has headaches or mild cognitive disturbance after 10–14 days, persistent vomiting, neck stiffness or drowsiness, this needs to be further investigated. Rugby league and Rugby Union have the highest concussion rates of any team sports in the world (Makdissie, Davis & McCrory 2015).

A primary and secondary survey should be conducted with particular attention to the Glasgow Coma Scale (GCS). The GCS (figure 24.4) provides an objective, standardised and easily interpreted tool for neurological assessment. The GCS allows healthcare professionals to assess how severely a person's brain has been damaged following a head injury. It scores people on:

- verbal responses (whether they can make any noise)
- physical reflexes (whether they can move)
- how easily they can open their eyes.

The highest possible score is 15, which means that the person knows where they are and can speak and move as instructed. The lowest possible score is 3, meaning that the body is in a deep coma (a sleep-like state in which the body is unconscious for a long period of time). Depending on the score, head injuries are classed as:

- minor: a score of 13 or more
- moderate: a score of 9–12
- severe: a score of 3–8.

With a GCS score of 13–15, any changes in the patient's condition should be monitored closely. Extra vigilance on the part of nursing staff is required with patients who have taken alcohol and/or drugs, which may mask subtle changes. All ED clinicians involved in assessing patients with head injuries should be able to assess the presence and absence of risk factors and the need for CT imaging. CT imaging is widely available in most urban centres and is recommended for all patients with moderate to severe TBI.

FIGURE 24.4 Glasgow Coma Scale (GCS)

Neurological Observation Chart																			
Glasgow Coma Scale	Eye opening	Open spontaneously (4)	•																(C) = Eyes closed due to swelling
		Open to speech (3)		•	•														
		Open to pain (2)				•	•												
		Closed (1)						•	•	•									
	Verbal response	Orientated (5)																	(T) = intubated
		Confused (4)	•	•	•														
		Inappropriate words (3)				•	•												
		Incomprehensible sounds (2)						•	•										
		No verbal response (1)								•									
	Motor response	Obeys commands (6)	•	•															Record best arm response
		Localises to pain (5)			•														
		Flexion withdrawal (4)				•	•												
		Abnormal flexion (3)						•											
		Extension to pain (2)							•										
		No movement (1)								•									
		Total (out of 15)	14	13	12	9	9	6	5	3									

Source: Woodward & Mestecky (2011) *Neuroscience nursing: Evidence Based Practice*, with kind permission of Wiley Blackwell.

Nursing assessment and examination should follow a set or systematic pattern regardless of how severe or trivial an injury may appear. The assessing clinician should establish the history, perform an examination and refer the patient for radiology as appropriate. More information on the assessment of TBI can be found in the chapter on conditions related to the neurological system.

Moderate and severe TBI are potentially life-threatening. Following the primary survey, the main considerations are to maintain the airway (patient is likely to be unconscious or semiconscious and unable to protect their own airway) and maintaining the cerebral perfusion pressure (CPP). Hypotension and hypoxia need to be addressed immediately. Systolic blood pressure should be maintained at 100 mmHg or above in patients aged 50–69 years and 110 systolic or greater if aged 15–49 years. If this is not done, the brain injury is likely to progress, which may be fatal (Sharpe & Cole 2019).

Most minor head injuries do not require treatment. Patients should be monitored for four hours, including GCS. If stable, they may be discharged home with instructions to represent if they have persistent vomiting, persistent drowsiness, confusion or disorientation, increased headache, localised weakness, blurred vision, seizure activity or neck stiffness (O'Reilly & Cameron 2020). If not stable, they should be admitted and continue to be monitored for 48 hours to check for any changes in their condition. After this time, they can be discharged with a head injury advice sheet to the care of a responsible adult.

24.9 Assessment and stabilisation of adverse behavioural presentations

LEARNING OBJECTIVE 24.9 Recognise behavioural disturbances and describe initial management in the ED

Behavioural disturbances and aggression in the ED are increasing problems confronting ED staff every day. The majority of attacks on healthcare workers, in general, occur in the ED. Patients may self-refer or be referred to the ED by concerned family members or other health professionals, such as GPs or community mental health teams, or may be transported by police or paramedics in an aroused and agitated state for assessment, management and the ruling out of an organic cause for their behaviour. It is the responsibility of the emergency nursing and medical staff to assess and manage these patients properly, without biases, and with the same thoroughness that every patient who presents to ED for treatment is afforded. The risk of violence, i.e. behaviour that involves either a threat of physical or psychological harm to oneself or others, is considered a critical predictor of urgency in mental health triage.

Patients with behavioural disturbance can challenge clinicians, the nursing and allied staff, and some can even be a challenge to the whole ED, including other patients and their relatives. These patients have a high morbidity and mortality rate and carry higher medicolegal risk from their behaviour, from injuries they may have obtained or the underlying organic illness that is causing their adverse behaviour. Emergency nurses and clinicians have a duty of care to these patients to provide assessment and treatment. The challenge is to carry out this duty of care while minimising the risks to the patient, staff and others in ED.

Patients presenting to the ED who are aggressive or hostile towards staff could be displaying behaviour that is symptomatic of a number of conditions, including:

- head injury
- substance abuse and intoxication
- underlying mental illness
- hypoxia
- hypoglycaemia
- infection — meningitis, encephalitis or sepsis
- hyperthermia or hypothermia
- seizures — post-ictally or status epilepticus
- vascular — stroke or subarachnoid haemorrhage.

The key in these cases initially is to de-escalate the behaviour to proceed to a safe primary survey and assessment. If de-escalation does not succeed, the patient may be sedated for the safety of themselves and others if other strategies have not been successful. The safety of the patient is paramount (MOH 2015).

24.10 Care of the critically ill and dying patient in the ED

LEARNING OBJECTIVE 24.10 Outline the care of patient and family who experience death in the ED.

Human life is precious and fragile. Despite the fact that we all know that we are not immortal few of us are prepared for death when it comes especially if it comes suddenly. As nurses we are in a unique position to provide strength and support for those who are dying and those who are losing a loved one. Our actions at this time are as important as any heroic measures performed during any resuscitation.

End of life in the ED

While the primary focus of the ED is the minimisation of mortality and morbidity, death is an ever-present reality. Fortunately, most patients are triaged, treated and discharged home or admitted to the hospital for further care. However, some are too critically ill and cannot be saved. Providing care for the person who is dying and supporting the family members is as important as any heroic life-saving activity. There are two main causes of death in the ED. The death of a person who has a chronic life-limiting illness is classified as an **'expected' death**. The other is the sudden death due to trauma or violence and is categorised as a 'sudden' or 'violent' death. Any death can be confronting for the practitioner, no matter how experienced. For families, it can be devastating. The care and compassion we give can have a major impact on the ability of the family to cope with what follows in their lives. Never underestimate the value of simple acts coming from a place of honest compassion, we are here to help those who are suffering, and the loved ones people leave behind may not have physical wounds, but they are suffering deeply and need comfort and support.

Approximately one-quarter of Australia's and New Zealand's populations were born overseas, so cultural competence is essential. For any situation, whether the death is expected or not, be aware of your own attitudes, values and beliefs about death and how these may impact the patient and their family. Ask clear questions about their culture and beliefs around death and dying, including any rituals that need to be observed. Nurses must show respect for others' beliefs — they are as valid as yours even if they are different. Communicate clearly as to what is happening to the patient and ensure access to interpreters.

Nursing care of an 'expected death'

Both Australia and New Zealand utilise advanced care plans as a means of ensuring that when patients come to hospital and are unable to communicate effectively that their wishes regarding their end of life treatment will be known and acted upon. The legislation differs from state to state and between Australia and New Zealand, but the basic process is the same (Ora, Robinson & Marshall 2019). The validity of any advanced care plan/directive may be strengthened by having a written document noting that the person was competent and not unduly influenced at the time of signing. It should relate to the current condition and should be appropriately worded so that the intention is clear. If the patient's wishes are known and acted upon, it can mean that aggressive and unwanted measures are avoided, the family are not subjected to making end of life decisions while in distress and potential conflicts between the healthcare team and family may be avoided (ACEM 2020). When care is not escalated it can be redirected to comfort and palliation. Nursing care should focus on sound, basic care provision, keeping the patient as comfortable as possible, offering oral fluids if they can tolerate any and always keeping the patient as pain-free as possible.

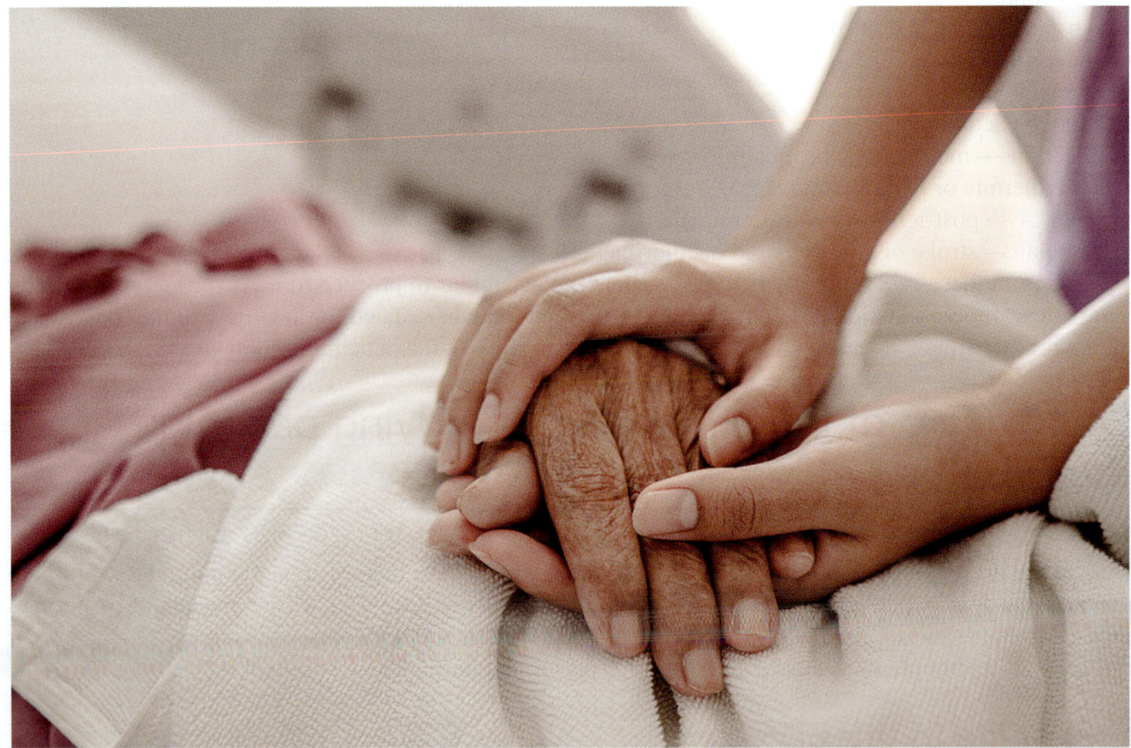

Sudden or unexpected death in the ED

This is always traumatic for family and loved ones. Understand that when people are confronted with the sudden death of a loved one, their responses will be different — no response is wrong unless it involves violence towards the staff. Each person is an individual, so each will behave differently, and different cultures have different ways of expressing loss. A lack of obvious emotion does not indicate a lack of internal grief; conversely, some people may be very vocal in their loss. All of the family and loved ones deserve non-judgemental support. Warmth, sympathy, genuineness, empathy, active listening and openness are skills needed by clinicians to support dying people and their families.

Family presence during resuscitation has been researched since the 1980s, and the Australian and New Zealans Committe on Resuscitation (ANZCOR) have provided guidelines concerning this. The evidence shows that with paediatric resuscitation, there are improved coping and more positive emotional outcomes. However, there have been reports of 'family presence stress' experienced by the staff. The family should be offered the opportunity to be present, preferably with an assigned support person (ANZCOR 2016; Ora, Robinson & Marshall 2019).

After death, nurses continue to care for the patient, which may include washing the patient, replacing dentures and dressing them in a clean gown or clothes. Assure the family that you will continue to care for their loved one with dignity and gentle care. Remember that the family may want to hold their loved one (especially a child) after death and ensure this is facilitated.

Death is confronting even to experienced clinicians, and sudden death even more so. Hospitals are expected to have provision for debriefing staff, which should be both formal and informal. Life and death are inextricably entwined in the cycle of life, and as nurses, we are privileged to participate in both.

Organ donation

Organ transplantation is an effective treatment for advanced organ failure. Australian organ transplantation survival rates are among the highest in the world (NHMRC 2016). In Australia, corneal transplant was first performed in 1941, kidneys in 1956, followed by liver and heart in 1968. In New Zealand, corneal grafting began in the 1940s, and the first kidney was transplanted in 1965. With the discovery of immune-suppressive agents in the 1960s, the modern era of transplantation began in Australia and New Zealand (Sgorbini et al. 2019). The clinical guidelines used in Australia and NZ were developed by the Transplant Society of Australia and New Zealand (TSANZ). 'Donation of organs is an act of altruism, solidarity and community reciprocity that provides significant benefits to those in medical need' (NHMRC 2016). The guidelines developed for transplantation of deceased donor organs in Australia and NZ articulate high ethical standards and align with the universal declaration of human rights. Deceased organ donation is only possible if a person dies in a hospital under defined circumstances. This is generally in an ED or ICU. Unless you are specifically trained to be a part of the team requesting and managing organ donation, the nurses' main role is support and care for the grieving family.

CASE STUDY 24.1

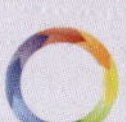

Head injury and minor TBI

An 18-year-old male presented to ED at 2300 hours via ambulance after being in an altercation outside a venue. He was ducking to avoid a punch and tripped on the curb, hitting the back of his head as he fell. He states an intake of approx. four drinks over 3 hours.

On arrival, he is conscious and orientated. He says he doesn't remember clearly what happened but doesn't think he lost consciousness. He has a headache pain score 4/10 and a laceration on the back of his head 3 cm in length — small blood loss; no longer bleeding.

Observations on arrival were:

- blood pressure: 120/80 mmHg
- respiratory rate: 16 breaths per minute
- heart rate: 86 beats per minute
- GCS: 15 — pupils 3 mm; both react to light
- triaged as category 3.

He is handed over to you for continuing care.

Question

Using the information above and the clinical reasoning cycle, describe what actions you will take as the nurse caring for this patient.

Answer

- *Step 1: Consider the patient.* An 18-year-old male with possible traumatic brain injury.
- *Step 2: Collect cues/information.* Include both subjective and objective data, include patient's appearance and past medical history.
  Medical history: asthma — well controlled with occasional PRN salbutamol. No other relevant history.
- *Step 3: Process information.* Patient has had blunt trauma to back of the head. This is classified as a TBI unless proven otherwise. This can be catastrophic. At present, his GCS and other observations are stable and within normal limits, but this is likely to change, and we need to maintain frequent monitoring of his vital signs and GCS to ensure any deterioration is quickly noted and addressed.

Considering his present condition, he is most likely to have concussion, but he will need a **CT scan (computed tomography scan)** to confirm no further damage due to the mechanism of injury and wound. The wound is minimal with no further bleeding but will need cleaning and dressing.

- *Step 4: Identify problems.* Potential for deterioration due to head trauma — open wound and pain.
- *Step 5: Establish goals*. Patient needs CT as soon as possible, as well as pain relief. He needs frequent (hourly) monitoring for potential deterioration and wound needs cleaning and dressing.
- *Step 6: Take action.* Patient was taken to CT and his wound was cleaned and dressed. Paracetamol was given for pain, and observations were attended hourly.
- *Step 7: Evaluate outcomes*. CT results: NAD (no abnormalities detected). No intracranial bleeds noted, no skull fracture detected. Observations remained within normal limits as per the track and trigger chart. Pain decreased to 2/10.
  Patient was monitored hourly for four hours and then discharged home with instructions to return if headache persists after 10 days, or if he has persistent vomiting, drowsiness, seizures or neck stiffness.
- *Step 8: Reflect on the process and new learning*. Reflect on any aspects of care that could have been performed in a way to achieve an improved outcome. This young man seems to have been lucky. He had a potentially critical incident, which could have caused severe brain injury. He was looked after following all policies and had timely appropriate care.

CASE STUDY 24.2

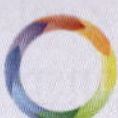

Nursing care of a child suffering from a burn

A three-year-old male child is brought into emergency, following accidentally spilling a hot cup of tea over their bare chest. The tea had just been made and was on the kitchen bench. The parents have come immediately to the ED following the incident.

The child is otherwise healthy and meeting their milestones of development.

Observations at triage were:

- redness over top half of chest — child is in obvious distress crying and screaming. Alert and responding to mother
- airway patent
- breathing: taking deep breaths between crying, colour other than chest pink and well perfused
- heart rate: strong pulse palpated; rate not counted at this time
- patient is triaged as category 2: this is due to the severity of the pain.

You are working in the paediatric section of your ED, and this patient is handed over to your care.

Question

Using the information above and your knowledge of burns what action would you take as the nurse caring for this patient?

Answer

- *Step 1: Consider the patient.* See presentation of patient to ED.
- *Step 2: Collect cues/information.* Include both objective and subjective data here. Objective data will include vital signs.
  In addition to the previously gathered information, you note the mother is very distressed. She is concerned about the pain her child is in and voices feelings of guilt at the accident.
- *Step 3: Process information*. A clear description of the cause of the burn has been given (scald), which is the most common type of burn in this age group. At this time, there is no reason to look further for a diagnosis. The mechanism of injury described correlates with the signs and symptoms noted in ED.
  ABCD no life-threatening abnormalities detected.
  Child has obvious pain that needs to be addressed. The level of pain will be the rationale for the category 2 triage. Nurse initiated medication is available, but the level of pain may need opioid analgesia that a doctor must prescribe.
  Using the 'rule of nines', you estimate the child has a burn covering 9 per cent TBSA. Fluid will be lost from the vascular spaces due to blister formation and inflammatory response. At this time, they will not need IV rehydration but should be encouraged with oral fluids.
  Child has not had any first aid measures, and cooling the area is paramount and should occur as soon as possible. After first aid the wound will need dressing to protect the area from infection.
  A set of vital signs should be taken, but until the pain is under control, this will only increase distress to the child at this time.
  Mother is distressed; this is a normal maternal response, but we must remember when treating a child, we need to include the families in our care planning as the health of the parent/carer is integral to the recovery of the child.

- *Step 4: Identify problems/issues*. Severe pain; potential for dehydration, infection and ongoing damage to the area; distressed parent.
- *Step 5: Establish goals*. Child needs pain relief as soon as possible. Burn must be cooled with running water to ease the pain and inhibit further dermal damage. Provide oral fluids and apply suitable dressing. A full set of observations should be attended as soon as possible to provide a baseline to measure the efficacy of the treatment against and to monitor for potential deterioration.
- *Step 6: Take action*. Give paracetamol dose to weight calculated (15 mg/kg) nurse initiated. Get stat order from Dr for analgesia to have available if paracetamol and cooling are ineffective in reducing pain. Get child under cool running water as soon as possible and protect from potential hypothermia by ensuring his body other than the area scalded is kept warm.
  When the child is calmer and in less pain, a set of vital signs must be attended. Child will be offered an ice block as a fluid intake, which should also help as a pain distraction. Dressing to be applied when the area has been cooled.
- *Step 7: Evaluate outcomes*. Patient was wrapped in a space blanket and towels, and mother and nurse helped keep child's chest under cool running water for 20 minutes. The cool water and paracetamol had a good effect on the level of pain. Child was able to use faces pain scale to show it had dropped to 3/10. Iceblock worked as a distraction from pain as well as ensuring fluid intake maintained. Dr quickly wrote up an order for stat IMI morphine if required (this was not needed).
  As the child's pain decreased, the mother began to relax and was reassured that it was not her fault and that accidents happen and that this is the most common burn in children. She also self-noted that she would make sure that anything potentially dangerous was kept away from the possible reach of a quickly growing child.
  A dressing was attended. Observations attended — all were within normal limits.
- *Step 8: Reflect on the process and new learning*. Reflect on any aspects of care that could have been performed in a way to achieve an improved outcome. This child had a common household accident. While care must be taken to prevent accidents as often as possible, children are unpredictable, and even with the best of intentions, scalds are relatively common. The mother was not judged in the care given but was supported. The child was triaged appropriately and was given care promptly, which meant that the burn did not continue to damage further tissue, the pain was quickly controlled, and both child and mother were happy. They were discharged home within three hours with a referral to the burns outpatient clinic.

SUMMARY

An ED is a dynamic, fast-paced environment. The skills required include teamwork, communication and sound clinical reasoning skills allied with genuine compassion. While HDU is generally a little less fast-paced, the patients are critically ill and require the same high level of skills. During a clinical placement, nursing students will experience or witness the emergency care of patients with a wide variety of acute and possibly life-threatening trauma injuries, acute medical/surgical and behavioural conditions. They will understand the role of the nurse in the emergency care team and observe or participate in the skills of triage, rapid assessment, resuscitation, care of the dying/dead patient and support of family and friends.

KEY TERMS

acuity The severity of a patient's illness.

advanced life support (ALS) A set of life saving skills and protocols that extend beyond basic life support. This includes fluid resuscitation, intubation and drug protocols as well as advanced diagnostic assessment to guide the process.

concussion A mild traumatic brain injury that causes a physiological alteration to brain function that is generally short term.

critical care An area whose primary purpose is to provide care for patients where the effectiveness of that care largely depends on time-sensitive and often rapid intervention (also known as acute care).

CT scan (computed tomography scan) A medical imaging technique that uses multiple X-ray measurements from different angles to show detailed images of internal organs.

expected death A death where the individual is diagnosed with a terminal illness or condition who is not expected to improve and where there are no further treatments available. This may be in the case of a long-term illness such as cancer or COPD.

high dependency unit (HDU) An area that provides high acuity care with a staff ratio of one nurse per two patients. It is an intermediate unit between ward and ICU. Once a patient needs to be ventilated, they will be transferred to ICU.

hypovolaemia Abnormal decrease in the volume of blood plasma.

primary assessment A rapid structured initial assessment using the ABCDE algorithm to identify and manage impending or actual life-threatening conditions.

resuscitation The procedure of restoring to life, e.g. cardiopulmonary resuscitation.

trauma An injury to tissue caused by an external agent.

triage The first step in the process 'to sort' the priority of care needed for patients that present to ED.

REFERENCES

Australasian College of Emergency Medicine (ACEM). (2016) Guidelines on the implementation of the Australasian Triage scale in Emergency Departments.

Australasian College of Emergency Medicine (ACEM). (2020) End of life and palliative care in the Emergency Department. Policy document P455.

Australian and New Zealand Committe on Resuscitation (ANZCOR). (2016) The Australian Resuscitation Council Guidelines [online]. https://resus.org/guidelines.

Cameron, P. & O'Reilly, G. (2020) 'Trauma'. In Cameron, P., Little, M., Mitra, B. & Deasy, C. (Eds.). *Textbook of adult emergency medicine*, 5th ed. Elsevier.

College for Intensive Care Medicine of Australia and New Zealand (CICE). (2013) Guidelines on standards for high dependency units for training in intensive care medicine.

Department of Health and Ageing. (2009) *Emergency triage education kit*. https://acem.org.au/getmedia/c9ba8667-c2ba-4701-9b4f-86a12ab91152/Triage-Education-Kit.aspx

Dippenaar, E. (2019) Triage systems around the world: A historical evolution. *International Paramedic Practice*. https://www.internationaljpp.com/features/article/triage-systems-around-the-world-a-historical-evolution

Fry, M., Shaban, R. & Considine, J. (2019) 'Emergency nursing in Australia and New Zealand'. In Curtis, K., Ramsden, C., Shaban, R., Fry, M. & Considine, J. (Eds.). *Emergency and trauma care for nurses and paramedics*, 3rd ed. Elsevier.

Holland, A. & Quinn, L. (2019) 'Burns trauma'. In Curtis, K., Ramsden, C., Shaban, R., Fry, M. & Considine, J. (Eds.). *Emergency and trauma care for nurses and paramedics*, 3rd ed. Elsevier.

Jones, K. & Rootham, E. (2019) 'Minor injury and management'. In Curtis, K., Ramsden, C., Shaban, R., Fry, M. & Considine, J. (Eds.). *Emergency and trauma care for nurses and paramedics*, 3rd ed. Elsevier.

Levett-Jones, T. & Hoffman, K. (2013) 'Clinical reasoning: What it is and why it matters'. In T. Levett-Jones (Ed.). *Clinical Reasoning, Learning to think like a nurse*. Pearson.

Makdissi, M., Davis, G. & McCrory, P. (2014) Updated guidelines for the management of sports related concussion in general practice. *Australian Family Physician*. 43(3): 94–99.

Ministry of Health, NSW. (2015) Management of patients with acute severe behavioural disturbance in emergency departments. Guideline document number GL2015_007.

Munroe, B. & Hutchinson, C. (2019) 'Patient assessment and essentials of care'. In Curtis, K., Ramsden, C., Shaban, R., Fry, M. & Considine, J. (Eds.). *Emergency and trauma care for nurses and paramedics*, 3rd ed. Elsevier.

National Museum of Australia. (2021) *Defining moments: First public hospital*. https://www.nma.gov.au/defining-moments/resources/first-public-hospital

NHMRC. (2016) Ethical guidelines for organ transplantation from deceased donors.

NSW Agency for Clinical Innovation. (2018)*Burn Patient Management: Summary of Evidence*, 4th ed. Chatswood: ACI.

Ora, L., Robinson, D. W. & Marshall, J. (2019) 'End of life'. In Curtis, K., Ramsden, C., Shaban, R., Fry, M. & Considine, J. (Eds.). *Emergency and trauma care for nurses and paramedics*, 3rd ed. Elsevier.

O'Reilly, G. & Cameron, P. (2020) 'Neurotrauma'. In Cameron, P., Little, M., Mitra, B. & Deasy, C. (Eds.). *Textbook of adult emergency medicine*, 5th ed. Elsevier.

O'Reilly, G. & Mitra, B. (2020) 'Burns'. In Cameron, P., Little, M., Mitra, B. & Deasy, C. (Eds.). *Textbook of adult emergency medicine*, 5th ed. Elsevier.

Sgorbini, M., McKay, L., Treloggen, J. & Alvaro, C. (2019) 'Organ and tissue donation'. In Curtis, K., Ramsden, C., Shaban, R., Fry, M. & Considine, J. (Eds.). *Emergency and trauma care for nurses and paramedics*, 3rd ed. Elsevier.

Sharpe, J. & Cole, T. (2019) 'Traumatic brain injury'. In Curtis, K., Ramsden, C., Shaban, R., Fry, M. & Considine, J. (Eds.). *Emergency and trauma care for nurses and paramedics*, 3rd ed. Elsevier.

Warren, K. -R., Morrey, C., Oppy, A., Pirpiris, M. & Balogh, Z. (2019) The overview of the Australian trauma system. *International Orthopaedic Trauma Association*. 2(S1): e018.

Woodward, S. & Mestecky, A. -M. (2011) *Neuroscience nursing: Evidence based practice*. Wiley Blackwell.

Wraa, C. (2010) 'Burns'. In Kunz Howard, P. & Steinmann R. A. (Eds.). *Sheehy's Emergency Nursing Principles and Practice*, 6th ed. (pp. 340–354). St Louis: Mosby.

ACKNOWLEDGEMENTS

Figure 24.3: © Advanced Life Support for Adults. © New Zealand Resuscitation Council. Reproduced with permission of New Zealand Resuscitation Council. https://www.nzrc.org.nz/assets/Uploads/Advanced-Life-Support-for-Adults-Jan-2016.pdf

Table 24.1: © Australian College for Emergency Medicine. Reproduced with permission from Australian College for Emergency Medicine. https://acem.org.au/Content-Sources/Advancing-Emergency-Medicine/Better-Outcomes-for-Patients/Triage

Photo 24A: © PomInPerth / Shutterstock.com

Photo 24B: © suvita style / Shutterstock.com

CHAPTER 25

Antipodean considerations

LEARNING OBJECTIVES

After studying this chapter, you should be able to:

25.1 describe the incidence and basic pathophysiology of snakebites
25.2 describe the incidence and basic pathophysiology of spider bites
25.3 describe the incidence and basic pathophysiology of a box jellyfish sting
25.4 identify the signs and symptoms of a patient presenting with a snakebite
25.5 identify the signs and symptoms of a patient presenting with a spider bite
25.6 identify the signs and symptoms of a patient presenting with a box jellyfish sting
25.7 understand the nursing assessment and management of a patient with a snakebite
25.8 understand the nursing assessment and management of a patient with a spider bite
25.9 understand the nursing assessment and management of a patient with a box jellyfish sting.

Introduction

Australia is well known for poisonous and venomous creatures, both in the ocean and on the land. It is home to some of the deadliest snakes and spiders in the world, including the world's most venomous, the Sydney funnel-web spider (*Atrax robustus*) and the inland or western taipan (*Oxyuranus microlepidotus*) (Queensland Health 2020). In addition, several marine creatures can cause severe illness or death, including the box jellyfish, stonefish and sharks. In Australia, venomous stings and bites resulted in almost 42 000 hospitalisations and 64 deaths during 2000–13 (Gardner 2017). Bees and wasps were responsible for just over one-third (33 per cent) of hospital admissions, spider bites were responsible for 30 per cent, and 15 per cent were due to snakebites (Gardner 2017). Despite there being many dangerous species in Australia, it is not possible to address them all. Therefore, this chapter will focus on the nursing care of some of the most common antipodean presentations in Australian hospitals, including snakebites, spider bites and box jellyfish stings.

25.1 The incidence and pathophysiology of snakebites

LEARNING OBJECTIVE 25.1 Describe the incidence and basic pathophysiology of snakebites.

There are over 30 different snakes species within Australia, with a variety of snakes within each category. Common snakes seen in Australia include brown snakes (see figure 25.1), tiger snakes, death adders, black snakes (see figure 25.2), the taipan and sea snakes. While the mortality rate from snakebites is one to three people yearly (Queensland Health 2020), this is largely due to improved education and first aid and **antivenom** availability in emergency departments across Australia. The number of people hospitalised due to snakebites between 2001 and 2013 was 6123. Some people can be bitten by a snake and not envenomated enough to cause systemic effects — this is known as a 'dry' bite (Naik 2017). In contrast, some people can be envenomated and receive a full dose of the snake's venom. If an envenomation is left untreated, it will likely result in severe morbidity or death (Ferraz et al. 2019).

FIGURE 25.1 An eastern brown snake

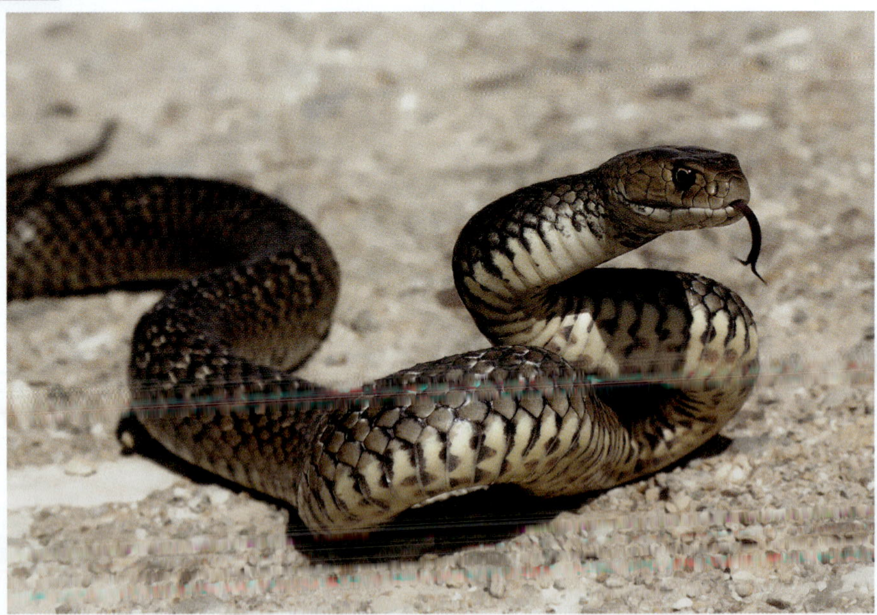

Snake **venom** is transported via the lymphatic system, not the vascular system. This is important when understanding the initial treatment and management of a snakebite. Once the venom is transported through the body via the lymphatic system, the venom's toxins lead to systemic effects within the body. These effects can be broadly categorised into three types: **neurotoxic**, **haemotoxic** and **myotoxic** effects (Ferraz et al. 2019).

Haemotoxic effects

Some snake venoms interfere with platelet function at various stages of the clotting cascade. This can lead to activation or inhibition of blood coagulation resulting in both blood clots and bleeding at the same time (de Queiroz et al. 2017). This can be difficult to manage and lead to a variety of complications, including haemorrhage.

FIGURE 25.2 A red-bellied black snake

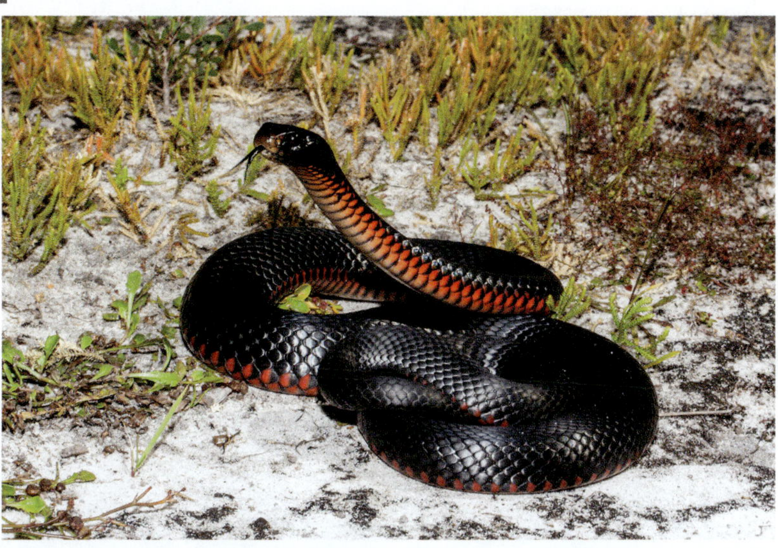

Neurotoxic effects

Snake venom neurotoxins primarily target the neuromuscular junction of skeletal muscles and can lead to severe pain and paralysis if left untreated (Ferraz et al. 2019; Isbister 2006). The paralysis is due to presynaptic or postsynaptic neurotoxins in the venom, depending on the type of snake. Presynaptic neurotoxins can occur due to bites from tiger snakes, copperhead snakes, taipans, rough-scaled snakes and occasionally, brown snakes (White 2018). This paralysis is referred to as '**descending paralysis**', which means that the paralysis starts at the top of the body and spreads downwards as the neurotoxins take hold. Nurses must be aware of this. One of the early clinical manifestations of a neurotoxic envenomation can be ptosis (drooping eyelids), which then progresses to paralysis of the respiratory muscles, leading to respiratory arrest and death if left untreated (de Queiroz et al. 2017; White 2018). This type of paralysis may take days to resolve and may not be reversed by antivenom, depending on the type of toxin (White 2018). The patient's breathing will need to be supported with mechanical ventilation until the paralysis has resolved (Silva et al. 2017).

Myotoxic effects

Some snakes have venom containing myotoxins. The myotoxins cause the skeletal muscles to break down, a condition known as rhabdomyolysis. This breakdown of skeletal muscle leads to the release of intracellular muscle components, including myoglobin, creatine kinase (CK) and electrolytes such as potassium into the bloodstream (Torres et al. 2015). This complication is referred to as rhabdomyolysis and can lead to acute kidney injury due to the exposure of the renal tubular epithelium to myoglobin (Nishimura et al. 2016; Torres et al. 2015).

25.2 The incidence and pathophysiology of spider bites

LEARNING OBJECTIVE 25.2 Describe the incidence and basic pathophysiology of spider bites.

Spider bites are a common problem in Australia, with many hospital presentations annually. Most spider bites do not require treatment and only result in minor effects. However, the funnel-web spider is the deadliest in the world. Its venom can kill a human within 15 minutes (Verhagen 2017). There are over 40 species of funnel-web, but the Sydney funnel-web (*Atrax robustus*) is the deadliest and is located in the highly populated east coast of Australia (Binstead & Nappe 2021). Several different toxins in funnel-web venom are referred to as atracotoxin (Binstead & Nappe 2021). This toxin causes severe effects on the nervous system inducing repetitive and spontaneous firing of action potentials in presynaptic autonomic and motor neurons (Binstead & Nappe 2021; Verhagen 2017). This leads to a surge in catecholamines, resulting in a number of symptoms including high blood pressure, tachycardia, numbness around the mouth and dyspnoea (Binstead & Nappe 2021; Murray et al. 2019; Verhagen 2017). Funnel-web spider bites can be deadly if left untreated.

Red-back spiders are endemic throughout Australia. They are responsible for the largest number of hospital presentations from spider bites in Australia, with 5000–10 000 bites occurring and 250 people receiving antivenom annually in Australia (Murray et al. 2019; Australian Museum 2020). It is the bite from the female red-back that can lead to serious illness. Some deaths have been reported, but in the majority of cases, the red-back spider is unlikely to cause significant envenomation (The Royal Children's Hospital Melbourne 2019; Australian Museum 2020). Despite the red-back spider being reclusive and not aggressive, some people may be bitten if they accidentally disturb the spider. Female red-back spiders are black with a characteristic red or orange stripe on the upper abdomen, as shown in figure 25.3 (Australian Museum 2020).

FIGURE 25.3 A female red-back spider

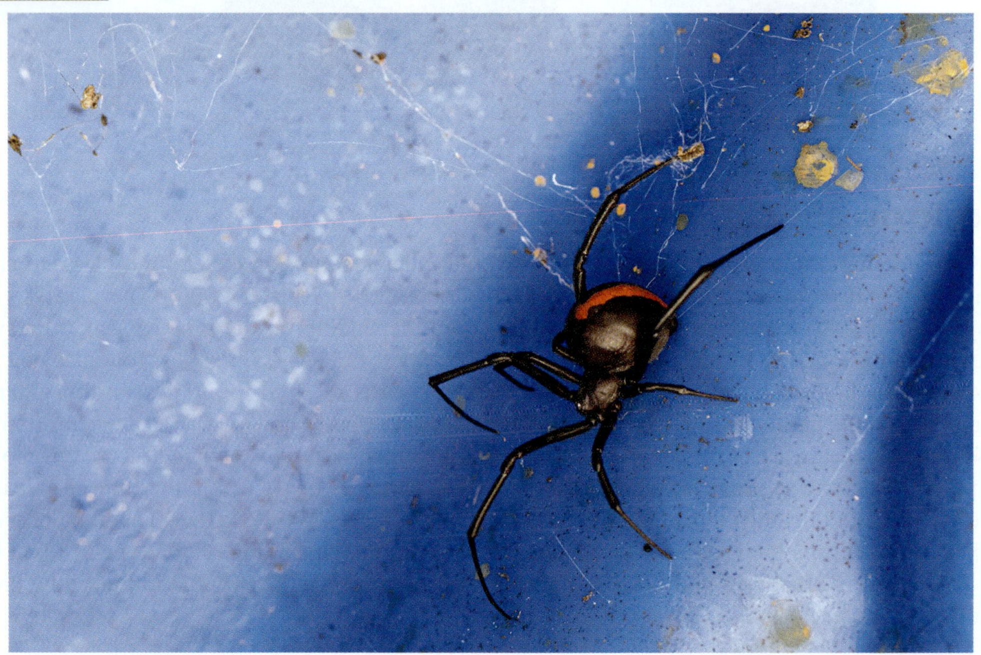

25.3 The incidence and pathophysiology of a box jellyfish sting

LEARNING OBJECTIVE 25.3 Describe the incidence and basic pathophysiology of a box jellyfish sting.

Box jellyfish are endemic in the tropical waters of the northern regions of Australia. They are distributed across tropical Australia from Dampier, WA south to Agnes Water, Queensland (Queensland Museum n.d.). The north Australian box jellyfish (*Chironex fleckeri*) is the deadliest. It is armed with millions of microscopic stinging cells (nematocysts) that discharge potent venom upon contact with skin. Their tentacles can stretch up to 10 feet in length (see figure 25.4). There were approximately 3707 hospitalisations due to jellyfish stings between 2001 and 2013 in Australia, and there have been at least 70 deaths recorded, the most recent in February 2021 (Rigby 2021). The specific components in the box jellyfish venom remain unknown; however, they affect sodium and calcium channels leading to abnormal membrane ion transport. The effects of this rapidly spread when the venom circulates systemically. Cardiac failure and death can occur within 5 minutes if significant envenomation has occurred (Cadogen 2020a; Murray et al. 2019).

FIGURE 25.4 Box jellyfish

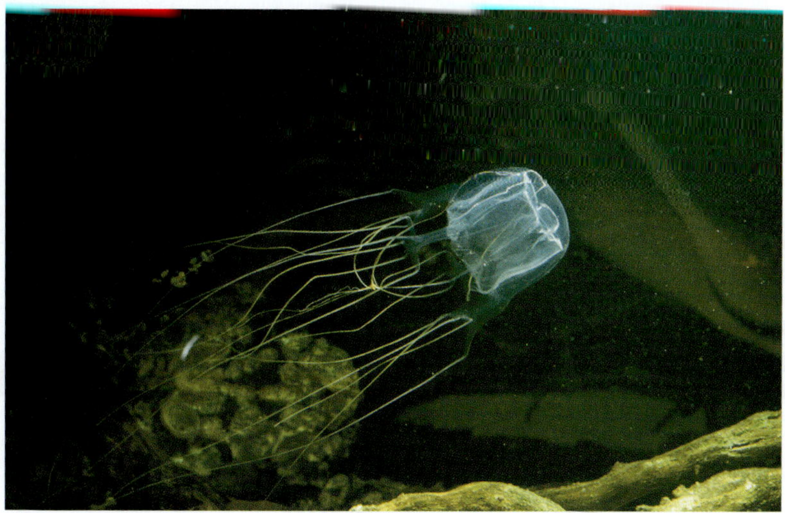

25.4 Signs and symptoms of snakebite

LEARNING OBJECTIVE 25.4 Identify the signs and symptoms of a patient presenting with a snakebite.

Snakebites can result in many signs and symptoms that depend on the extent of the bite and the type of toxin. 'Dry' bites can result in local effects such as erythema, pain and oedema. A snakebite's myotoxic effect can manifest by muscle weakness, pain and **myoglobinuria** from **rhabdomyolysis**. Myoglobinuria is characterised by tea-stained urine. The haemotoxic effect of snakebites can cause coagulopathies in patients, leading to bleeding at the puncture site and **haematuria** (blood in the urine). The neurotoxic effects are characterised by descending paralysis, starting with ptosis of the eyes, double vision, muscle weakness, followed by respiratory weakness and paralysis. A summary of the effects of Australian snakebites has been provided in table 25.1.

TABLE 25.1 **Complications of snake envenomation**

Effects of Australian snakebites			
Category	**Coagulopathy**	**Neurotoxicity**	**Myotoxicity**
Brown snake	Always present	Rare	Not present
Tiger snake	Always present	Not common	Not common
Death adders	Not present	Present	Not present
Black snakes	May have a mild anticoagulant effect	Not present	Present
Taipan	Always present	Present	Rare
Sea snakes	Not present	Not common	Present

Source: Adapted from Murray et al. (2019).

25.5 Signs and symptoms of a spider bite

LEARNING OBJECTIVE 25.5 Identify the signs and symptoms of a patient presenting with a spider bite.

Envenomation from a funnel-web spider is potentially lethal and needs to be differentiated from the red back spider. One characteristic difference between the two bites is the onset of pain. The pain following a funnel web spider bite is immediate, and the onset of the clinical syndrome associated with the bite will occur rapidly — within minutes. Fang marks are usually visible following a funnel-web spider bite. In contrast, the bite from a red-back spider is not immediately painful; however, pain at the bite site develops, increasing over minutes to hours. This pain then characteristically radiates from the bite site to regional areas, including the affected limb, before spreading systemically, including the chest or back. A classic triad of pain, sweating and piloerection (goosebumps) to the affected limb are characteristic of red-back spider envenomation (Cadogen 2020b; Murray et al. 2019).

Early symptoms of a funnel-web spider envenomation include severe local pain without erythema. Fang marks are usually present. Systemic envenomation from a funnel-web spider bite can lead to a rapid progression of symptoms, including facial paraesthesia, nausea, vomiting, profuse diaphoresis, drooling and shortness of breath (Binstead & Nappe 2021; Murray et al. 2019). The neurological effects of the venom can lead to patients becoming agitated, confused and ultimately comatose (Binstead & Nappe 2021). Hypertension and tachycardia can occur and lead to pulmonary and/or cerebral oedema. Pulmonary oedema or profound hypotension can lead to death (Binstead & Nappe 2021).

A summary of the signs and symptoms of spider bites has been provided in table 25.2.

TABLE 25.2 **Summary of the signs and symptoms of spider bites**

Red-back spider	Funnel-web spider
Pain onset 5–10 minutes	Pain onset: immediate
Localised erythema (mild)	No erythema
Headache	Headache
Irritability and agitation	Agitation
Lethargy	Profound diaphoresis (sweating) and excessive drooling
Nausea and vomiting	Nausea and vomiting
Myalgia and neck spasm may occur	Hypertension or hypotension Tachycardia or bradycardia
Triad of pain, sweating and piloerection (goosebumps to the affected limb)	Facial paraesthesia (paralysis)
Rarely: rhabdomyolysis, myocarditis	Acute pulmonary oedema, which can lead to death
Fang marks rarely visible	Fang marks usually visible

25.6 Signs and symptoms of a box jellyfish sting

LEARNING OBJECTIVE 25.6 Identify the signs and symptoms of a patient presenting with a box jellyfish sting.

The initial symptoms experienced include the sudden onset of severe pain, lasting up to 8 hours. Linear welts may also be present, occurring in a crosshatched pattern, as shown in figure 25.5. Some of the jellyfish tentacles may still be present. Systemic envenomation from the box jellyfish may cause collapse or sudden death, occurring within a few minutes of the sting. The cardiovascular effects of box jellyfish envenomation include hypertension, hypotension, tachycardia, impaired cardiac contraction and arrhythmias. Delayed allergic reactions occur in at least 50 per cent of patients and manifest as a pruritic rash (raised, itchy rash) at the original sting site, 7–14 days after the sting (Murray et al. 2019; White 2018).

FIGURE 25.5 Box jellyfish welts

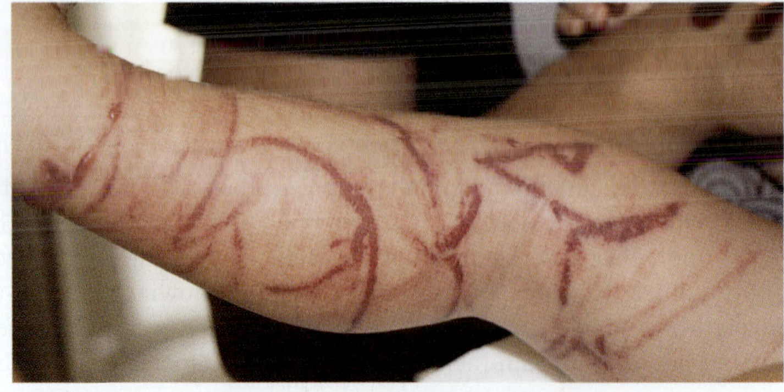

25.7 Nursing assessment and management of snakebite

LEARNING OBJECTIVE 25.7 Understand the nursing assessment and management of a patient with a snakebite

Nursing assessment of a patient presenting with a bite or sting should always commence with an A to E assessment to address any immediate life-threatening issues. Additional assessments are required depending on the type of bite or sting. The ABCDE approach below is not exhaustive but should include:

- assessing the patient for a response
- airway — check patency
- breathing — check respiratory rate, expansion, effort, percussion, breath sounds, SpO_2. Tidal volumes will decrease if the patient has been envenomated with a venom containing neurotoxins
- circulation— check pulse, blood pressure, capillary refill, urine output. Carry out an ECG or apply cardiac monitoring to monitor for cardiac arrhythmias due to the effects of envenomation
- disability — assess conscious level (AVPU, GCS) and pupils, check eyes for ptosis (drooping), measure blood glucose levels
- exposure — check temperature, assess the whole patient, look for evidence of haemorrhage, non-blanching rashes etc.

Snakebites are a medical emergency; therefore, the patient should be assessed as a matter of urgency. Some patients may present to the emergency department (ED) or local health facility with a snake bandage in place if they have received adequate first aid. A snake bandage is a compression bandage that stops the flow of lymphatic circulation, thereby halting the venom's effects. A snake bandage will need to be applied by the nurse if there isn't already one in place.

The doctor should order blood tests to monitor the patient for pathological signs of envenomation. The blood tests should include the following:

- coagulation studies (INR, aPTT, fibrinogen, d-dimer) to test for haemotoxic effects. An INR >2 usually indicates a coagulopathy
- full blood count (FBC)
- urea, electrolytes and creatinine (UEC) to assess kidney function and electrolyte imbalance such as hyperkalaemia, which would be present if the snake venom contained mycotoxins. Elevated creatinine or urea or oliguria/anuria indicates renal damage
- creatinine kinase (CK). There would be a rapid and profound rise in CK if rhabdomyolysis was present. A CK >1500 IU/l indicates muscle breakdown.

Snake venom detection kit

It is important to identify the type of snake to determine the correct antivenom to administer to a patient. Polyvalent antivenom, designed to neutralise the venom of most snakes encountered in Australia, is available. However, it carries an increased risk of anaphylaxis; therefore, it should only be used when it is not possible to identify the snake.

Advancements in technology have now made it possible to determine the type of snake using a snake venom detection kit. A swab of the bite site is necessary to test the venom. The nurse would need to cut away a section of the bandage covering the snakebite to take the swab. The results are usually available within 25 minutes. If it is impossible to access the bite site, then urine can be tested; however, systemic envenomation must be present to detect venom in urine (Silva et al. 2017; White 2018).

Snakebite management

If the patient presents with a severe degree of envenomation, the nurse must be prepared to resuscitate the patient. If **pressure bandage** and immobilisation have not been administered as first aid, they need to be applied in the ED to stop the venom from spreading (Murray et al. 2019). Please refer to figure 25.6 for guidance with the pressure immobilisation technique for snakebites. Administration of antivenom should be prioritised once the correct venom has been identified via the snake detection kit. Many types of monovalent (single venom) are available, including one for brown snakes, mulga snake, red-bellied black snakes and tiger snakes. If it is not possible to determine the type of snake, a polyvalent antivenom should be administered. The nurse must always have adrenaline ready in the case of anaphylaxis (White 2018).

FIGURE 25.6 Pressure immobilisation technique

One method of immobilisation for bites on a limb. There may be other PIT methods that are acceptable to use.

Step 1

Apply pressure bandage*

Lay patient down and stop them from moving

Apply firm pressure on bite

Apply a broad pressure bandage over the bite as firm as for a sprained ankle

(You should not be able to easily slide a finger between the bandage and the skin)

*Elasticised bandages 10–15cm wide are preferred, if unavailable, use clothing or other material, torn into strips if possible

Step 2

Apply second pressure bandage*

Apply a pressure bandage

Start at the fingers or toes of the bitten limb

Continue upward covering as much of the limb as possible

*No second bandage? – apply the initial bandage to fingers, or toes of the bitten limb, and work up the limb as far as possible

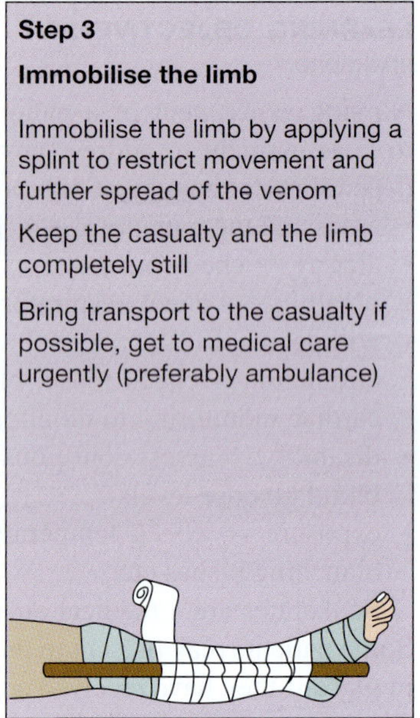

If the patient has been envenomated with a neurotoxin, they may need early intubation and mechanical ventilation in intensive care unit (ICU) to support their breathing due to the paralysis. If rhabdomyolysis is present, rigorous intravenous hydration is needed to increase urinary flow, reducing the renal tubular epithelium's exposure to myoglobin (Nishimura et al. 2016). This can reduce the likelihood of the patient developing acute kidney injury. The patient would need to have a catheter inserted to monitor urine output and check for myoglobinuria or haematuria.

Paediatric patients should receive the same dose of antivenom as an adult as it is not based on a patient's weight, rather the amount of venom.

25.8 Nursing assessment and management of a spider bite

LEARNING OBJECTIVE 25.8 Understand the nursing assessment and management of a patient with a spider bite.

Patients presenting with a spider bite must have a thorough history obtained. The nurse should obtain a description of the spider and the time of the bite. A pain assessment should also be conducted, although the bite from a red-back spider is not immediately painful; intense, localised pain develops 5–10 minutes after the bite. A patient's skin should also be assessed for fang marks and erythema at the bite site. This may be mild, with red-back spiders, and fang marks may not always be visible. Along with the localised skin assessment, the patient should be assessed for diaphoresis (sweating), as this is one of the classic symptoms of a red-back spider bite.

Blood tests are usually not needed to identify red-back spider bites, but there have been rare instances of myocarditis (inflammation of the myocardium) and rhabdomyolysis. If these are suspected, then a blood test to check for CK could identify rhabdomyolysis, and an ECG could identify myocarditis (The Royal Children's Hospital Melbourne 2019, Murray et al. 2010).

Paediatric considerations

Acute pain may present as inconsolable crying in an infant, and an appropriate pain assessment will need to be conducted on them as they are unable to voice their pain. The FLACC pain assessment tool can be used to assess infants and children unable to voice their pain. The acronym FLACC stands for face, legs, activity, cry and consolability, which the nurse will assess and give a total score out of 10. Please refer to figure 25.7 for the FLACC Scale.

FIGURE 25.7 The FLACC Scale

Face	0 No particular expression or smile	1 Occasional grimace or frown, withdrawn, disinterested	2 Frequent to constant frown, clenched jaw, quivering chin
Legs	0 Normal position or relaxed	1 Uneasy, restless, tense	2 Kicking, or legs drawn up
Activity	0 Lying quietly, normal position, moves easily	1 Squirming, shifting back and forth, tense	2 Arched, rigid, or jerking
Cry	0 No cry (awake or asleep)	1 Moans or whimpers, occasional complaints	2 Crying steadily, screams or sobs, frequent complaints
Consolability	0 Content, relaxed	1 Reassured by occasional touching, hugging or 'talking to'. Distractable	2 Difficult to console or comfort

Source: Merkel S, Voepel-Lewis T, Shayevitz JR, et al. (1997).

Older children can be assessed using the Wong-Baker faces rated scale as shown in figure 25.8.

FIGURE 25.8 The Wong-Baker FACES Pain Rating Scale

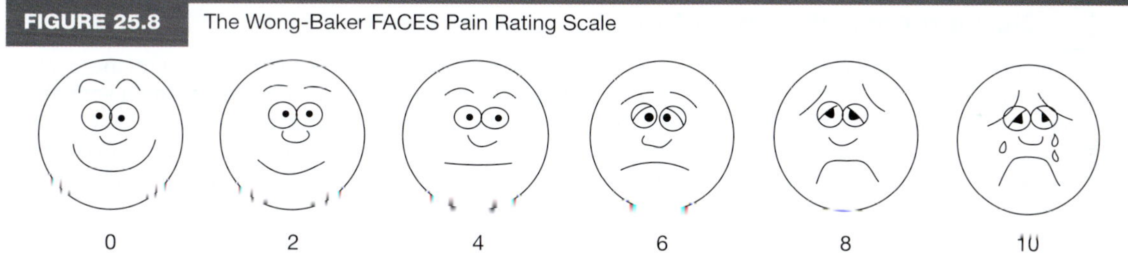

Source: Wong-Baker FACES Foundation (1983).

Spider bite management

Pre-hospital treatment of a funnel-web spider bite should include cleansing the area with soap and water and applying a pressure bandage and immobilisation to prevent the spread of the venom (Binstead & Nappe 2021). The patient should be transferred to the hospital immediately. Patients should be closely monitored and may need to be resuscitated if they develop respiratory failure, cardiac failure or a coma. If symptoms of systemic envenomation are present, then funnel-web spider antivenom should be administered. The initial dose is two vials, but a patient may need four vials if they have severe envenomation or are in cardiac arrest (Murray et al. 2019).

Pre-hospital treatment of a red back spider bite does not require a pressure bandage and immobilisation. An ice pack should be applied to the bite site to reduce pain and erythema if present. This can be supported with simple analgesia such as paracetamol (Murray et al. 2019; White 2018). If severe pain or systemic envenomation symptoms are present, red-back spider antivenom may be administered (Murray et al. 2019; White 2018).

25.9 Nursing assessment and management of a box jellyfish sting

LEARNING OBJECTIVE 25.9 Understand the nursing assessment and management of a patient with a box jellyfish sting.

In addition to an A to E assessment, a patient presenting with box jellyfish envenomation should have a 12 lead ECG and continuous cardiac monitoring (if available) to monitor for signs of cardiac arrhythmias, including tachycardia, sinus arrhythmia, bigeminy and bundle branch blocks (Murray et al. 2019). A chest X-ray may be ordered by the doctor, which could identify pulmonary oedema secondary to cardiac failure. While blood tests are not useful in detecting the presence of box jellyfish venom, they may be required in patients presenting with the symptoms of systemic envenomation to rule out any other causes of the symptoms and to identify any complications or damage to other organs within the body. Blood tests should include FBC, UEC, CK, troponin, magnesium, calcium and phosphate (Murray et al. 2019).

Box jellyfish management

The initial management of a patient with a box jellyfish sting depends on the extent of the envenomation. A patient may need immediate resuscitation if severe envenomation and systemic response have occurred. In a pre-hospital environment, the patient may run out of the water and suffer cardiac arrest on the beach. In this instance, CPR will need to be performed until paramedics arrive. Large volumes of undiluted vinegar should be applied to all visible sting sites as this deactivates the undischarged sting cells in the tentacles.

Once a patient is transferred to hospital, they need to be monitored for the severe effects of envenomation, including cardiac arrest, cardiac arrhythmias, hypotension or hypertension. If a patient presents with significant systemic effects from box jellyfish envenomation, such as hypotension, cardiac arrhythmia or cardiac arrest, box jellyfish antivenom should be administered. Morphine may be required for adequate pain relief (Murray et al. 2019).

CASE STUDY 25.1

Nursing care of a snakebite

Mr Peter Brown is a 29-year-old landscape gardener from Queensland who presented to the ED of the local University Hospital complaining of erythema (redness) and swelling in his right leg after feeling a scratch when working in a client's garden. Initial examination revealed a fully conscious patient with stable vital signs and. Local examination of the patient's right leg showed oedema, erythema (redness) and mild pain in the area. There were no obvious puncture sites, but the gardener believed that it could have been a snakebite.

Question

Using the information above, describe how you would provide nursing care for this patient in the ED. What action would you take as the nurse caring for this patient? Use the clinical reasoning cycle to guide you through the process and devise a care plan for your patient.

Answer

- *Step 1: Consider the patient*. Mr Peter Brown is a 29-year old landscape gardener who presented to his local ED with a swollen, painful leg.
- *Step 2: Collect cues/information*. Mr Brown was working in a client's garden when he felt a scratch on his leg. He now has swelling, redness and pain in his leg and believes it could be a snakebite. His observations are normal.
- *Step 3: Process information*. Mr Brown's description of a 'scratch' is a common description when a snake may have bitten people without visualising what type of snake it is. Mr Brown is experiencing some local effects of a snakebite, but there are no obvious systemic effects at this stage.
- *Step 4: Identify problems/issues*. Several nursing diagnoses are relevant for this patient. Despite there not being a nursing diagnosis that aligns with envenomation, the following were identified as priority nursing diagnoses for Mr Brown: poisoning, risk of shock and impaired skin integrity.
- *Step 5: Establish goals*. The goal of care for Mr Brown is to reduce the risk of envenomation and cardiac arrest within the next 2 hours.
- *Step 6: Take action*. A nurse must act rapidly to carry out an A to E assessment, determine the type of snake venom using a snake detection kit and apply pressure bandage and immobilisation as soon as possible to stop the spread of snake venom through his lymphatic system.

- *Step 7: Evaluate outcomes*. The medical team will review the results of the snake venom detection kit and determine whether the patient needs to have antivenom administered or whether the effects are localised only, in which case, this would be considered a 'dry' bite and no antivenom will be required.
- *Step 8: Reflect on the process and new learning*. Upon reflection of this case, the nurse must be aware of the differences between a 'dry' bite and systemic envenomation. Another key finding from this case is the patient presented to hospital without adequate first aid. The nurse should provide education around first aid for snakebites, especially because of Mr Brown's high-risk job as a landscape gardener in Queensland.

CASE STUDY 25.2

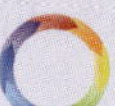

Nursing care of a patient with a box jellyfish sting

An 11-year-old Indigenous girl called Lilly is brought to a remote area health clinic screaming in agony with linear welts to her chest. Her family provides a brief history of Lilly swimming in the ocean when she started screaming and ran out of the water. Another family member witnessed what they thought was a plastic bag floating next to Lilly. They are worried that it could have been a box jellyfish.

On examination, Lilly has the following observations:

- respiratory rate: 36 breaths per minute
- heart rate: 146 beats per minute
- blood pressure 80/40 mmHg
- temperature: 36.5° Celsius
- oxygen saturation: 89% on room air.

Visible, linear welts are present on her abdomen and chest and right arm. She describes the pain as 'big mob' pain and is visibly uncomfortable and writhing around the bed.

Question

As the remote area nurse on shift, what action do you take, and what do you think has caused this reaction? Use the clinical reasoning cycle to support your answer.

Answer

- *Step 1: Consider the patient*. Lilly, an 11-year-old Indigenous girl, brought to the clinic in intense pain.
- *Step 2: Collect cues/information*. Include subjective and objective data here, including the patient's appearance (visible linear welts are present to her chest, abdomen and right arm) and past medical history. Objective data will include measurable information such as vital signs.
- *Step 3: Process information*. A family member witnessed what could have been a box jellyfish in the water. This aligns with the immediate, intense pain that Lilly is currently enduring. She has tachypnoea (a fast respiratory rate), tachycardia (fast heart rate), hypotension (low blood pressure) and low oxygen saturations. These all indicate that Lilly is suffering from the severe systemic effects of a box jellyfish sting.
- *Step 4: Identify problems/issues*. Ineffective tissue perfusion would be a priority nursing diagnosis due to the patient's fast heart rate and low blood pressure. She is also experiencing hypoxia and a fast respiratory rate, which could signify pulmonary oedema development.
- *Step 5: Establish goals*. For the patient's blood pressure to be within normal limits within the next 2 hours.
- *Step 6: Take action*. The remote area nurse should call for assistance from the doctor, either in person or via phone. An A to E assessment should also be conducted, and vinegar should be applied to the remaining stingers as a priority. The nurse should also be prepared to resuscitate the patient as they are critically unwell. Morphine will need to be administered for pain relief, and box jellyfish antivenom should be administered to Lilly.
- *Step 7: Evaluate outcomes*. Lilly was administered the box jellyfish antivenom and morphine and made a rapid improvement. She was evacuated to the nearest hospital over 700 kms away via CareFlight and monitored on the medical ward for a few days before she was discharged home. She made a full recovery.
- *Step 8: Reflect on the process and new learning*. Lilly suffered from a severe box jellyfish envenomation and was lucky to make it to the health centre and receive the antivenom.

SUMMARY

This chapter discussed the nursing assessment and care of patients presenting with antipodean specific considerations. The incidence, pathophysiology, nursing assessment and care of patients presenting with snakebites, spider bites and box jellyfish stings have been discussed. Although these presentations may not be as common as others throughout this text, nurses need to be aware of the seriousness of snake and spider bites and box jellyfish stings as they can lead to severe illness or death if left untreated. Nurses should always be prepared to resuscitate patients in either a pre-hospital or hospital environment.

KEY TERMS

antivenom A treatment that reverses the effects of venom from a number of different species including snakebites, spider bites and jellyfish.

box jellyfish The north Australian box jellyfish (*Chironex fleckeri*) is a box-shaped jellyfish and the deadliest in Australia.

descending paralysis A form of paralysis that gradually descends from the head down the body, ptosis (eye drooping) is one of the early symptoms.

haematuria Blood in the urine.

haemotoxic The haemotoxic effects of snake bites disrupt the clotting cascade leading to simultaneous bleeding and clotting.

myoglobinuria The presence of an excess amount of myoglobin in the urine. It is mostly caused by muscle breakdown, releasing a high amount of myoglobin in the blood. It can lead to acute kidney injury.

myotoxic The toxic effect on muscles leading to muscle breakdown that can result from some snake venom.

neurotoxic Neurological toxicity that produces an adverse effect on the structure or function of the central and/or peripheral nervous system, often resulting in a descending paralysis.

pressure bandage A compression bandage that exerts pressure to impede, for example, the flow of venom through the lymphatic system.

rhabdomyolysis A potentially life-threatening syndrome resulting from the breakdown of skeletal muscle fibres with leakage of muscle contents into the circulation.

venom A toxic substance that can be harmful to humans if it enters the human body.

REFERENCES

Australian Museum. (2020) *Redback spider*. NSW Government. https://australian.museum/learn/animals/spiders/redback-spider/#:~:text=Redback%20Spider%20Identification&text=Female%20Redback%20Spiders%20are%20black,the%20underside%20of%20the%20abdomen

Binstead, J. T. & Nappe, T. M. (2021) *Funnel web spider toxicity.* www.ncbi.nlm.nih.gov/books/NBK535394

Cadogen, M. (2020a) *Box jellyfish (Chironex fleckeri).* https://litfl.com/box-jellyfish-chironex-fleckeri

Cadogen, M. (2020b) *Red-back spider envenoming*. https://litfl.com/redback-spider-envenoming

de Queiroz, M. R., de Sousa, B. B., da Cunha Pereira, D. F., Mamede, C. C. N., Matias, M. S., de Morais, N. C. G., de Oliveira Costa, J. & de Oliveira, F. (2017) The role of platelets in hemostasis and the effects of snake venom toxins on platelet function. *Toxicon.* 133: 33–47. https://doi.org/https://doi.org/10.1016/j.toxicon.2017.04.013

Ferraz, C. R., Arrahman, A., Xie, C., Casewell, N. R., Lewis, R. J., Kool, J. & Cardoso, F. C. (2019). Multifunctional toxins in snake venoms and therapeutic implications: From pain to hemorrhage and necrosis [Review]. *Frontiers in Ecology and Evolution.* 7(218). https://doi.org/10.3389/fevo.2019.00218

Gardner, J. (2017) Venomous stings and bites lie close to home. https://pursuit.unimelb.edu.au/articles/venomous-stings-and-bites-lie-close-to-home

Isbister, G. K. (2006) Snake bite: a current approach to management. *Australian Prescriber* 29: 125–129. https://doi.org/10.18773/austprescr.2006.079

Murray, L., Little, M., Pascu, O. & Hogget, K. (2019) *Toxicology Handbook*, 3rd ed. Chatswood, NSW: Elsevier, Australia.

Naik, B. S. (2017). 'Dry bite'.In Venomous snakes: A review. *Toxicon.* 133: 63–67. https://doi.org/https://doi.org/10.1016/j.toxicon.2017.04.015

Nishimura, H., Enokida, H., Kawahira, S., Kagara, I., Hayami, H. & Nakagawa, M. (2016) Acute kidney injury and rhabdomyolysis after protobothrops flavoviridis bite: A retrospective survey of 86 patients in a tertiary care center. *The American Journal of Tropical Medicine and Hygiene.* 94(2): 474–479. https://doi.org/10.4269/ajtmh.15-0549

Queensland Health. (2020) *What are Queensland's most dangerous creatures? How to avoid and respond to attacks.* www.health.qld.gov.au/news-events/news/dangerous-creatures-animals-queensland-treatment-attack-prevention-spiders-snakes-sharks-bite-sting-poison

Queensland Museum. (n.d.) *Northern Australian box jellyfish*. Queensland Government. www.qm.qld.gov.au/Explore/Find+out+about/Animals+of+Queensland/Sea+Life/Corals+and+relatives+Cnidaria/Cubozoans/Northern+Australian+Box+Jellyfish

Rigby, M. (2021) *[illegible]*. Australian Broadcasting Corporation. www.abc.net.au/news/2021-03-

Royal Children's Hospital Melbourne. (2019) Spider bite — Redback spider. www.rch.org.au/clinicalguide/guideline_index/Spider_Bite_%E2%80%93_Redback_Spider

Silva, A., Hodgson, W. C. & Isbister, G. K. (2017) Antivenom for neuromuscular paralysis resulting from snake envenoming. *Toxins*. 9(4). 143. https://doi.org/10.3390/toxins9040143

Torres, P. A., Helmstetter, J. A., Kaye, A. M. & Kaye, A. D. (2015, Spring). Rhabdomyolysis: pathogenesis, diagnosis, and treatment. *The Ochsner Journal*. 15(1): 58–69. https://pubmed.ncbi.nlm.nih.gov/25829882

Verhagen, S. (2017) World's deadliest spider: the funnel-web. *Australian Geographic*. www.australiangeographic.com.au/topics/wildlife/2017/02/worlds-deadliest-spider-the-sydney-funnel-web

White, J. (2018) *Snakebite and spiderbite management guidelines: South Australia*. Department of Health. www.sahealth.sa.gov.au/wps/wcm/connect/85950800457e1fda87c5d7519b2d33fa/Snakebite-Spiderbite-Guidelines-SAHealth-2018.pdf?MOD=AJPERES&CACHEID=ROOTWORKSPACE-85950800457e1fda87c5d7519b2d33fa-niQBfJ6

ACKNOWLEDGEMENTS

Figure 25.1: © Kristian Bell / Shutterstock.com
Figure 25.2: © Ken Griffiths / Shutterstock.com
Figure 25.3: © whitejellybeans / Shutterstock.com
Figure 25.4: © Auscape / Getty Images
Figure 25.5: © DonyaHHI / Shutterstock.com
Figure 25.7: © Merkel, S,. Voepel-Lewis, T., Shayevitz, J. R., et al. (1997). The FLACC: A behavioural scale for scoring postoperative pain in young children. *Pediatric nursing,* 23: 293–297. © 2002, The Regents of the University of Michigan. Reproduced with permission. All Rights Reserved.
Figure 25.8: © The Wong-Baker FACES Pain Rating Scale. Retrieved from: https://wongbakerfaces.org.

INDEX